BMA

Obstetrics & Gynaecology

CRC Press
Taylor & Francis Group
6000 Broken Sound Parkway NW, Suite 300
Boca Raton, FL 33487-2742

© 2016 by Taylor & Francis Group, LLC
CRC Press is an imprint of Taylor & Francis Group, an Informa business

No claim to original U.S. Government works

Printed and bound in India by Replika Press Pvt. Ltd.

Printed on acid-free paper
Version Date: 20151006

International Standard Book Number-13: 978-1-4822-3382-7 (Pack - Book and Ebook)

Visit the Taylor & Francis Web site at
http://www.taylorandfrancis.com

and the CRC Press Web site at
http://www.crcpress.com

Obstetrics & Gynaecology

An Evidence-based Text for the **MRCOG**

THIRD EDITION

David M. Luesley
University of Birmingham, UK

Mark D. Kilby
University of Birmingham, UK

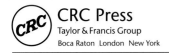
CRC Press
Taylor & Francis Group
Boca Raton London New York

CRC Press is an imprint of the
Taylor & Francis Group, an **informa** business

Contents

SECTION ONE   INTRODUCTORY/GENERAL   Section Editor: James Drife

SECTION TWO   ANTENATAL OBSTETRICS   Section Editor: Mark Kilby

SECTION THREE   FETAL CONDITIONS   Section Editor: Mark Kilby

SECTION FOUR   LATE PREGNANCY AND INTRAPARTUM EVENTS
Section Editor: Mark Kilby

SECTION FIVE   FIRST STAGE OF LABOUR
Section Editor: Mark Kilby

SECTION SIX   SECOND STAGE OF LABOUR
Section Editor: Mark Kilby

SECTION SEVEN   POSTPARTUM COMPLICATIONS
Section Editor: Mark Kilby

SECTION EIGHT   REPRODUCTIVE GYNAECOLOGY
Section Editor: Arri Coomarasamy

SECTION NINE   UROGYNAECOLOGY AND SEXUAL HEALTH AND WELLBEING

Section Editors: Linda Cardozo and Dudley Robinson

SECTION TEN   LOWER GENITAL TRACT

Section Editor: Simon Leeson

SECTION ELEVEN   GYNAECOLOGICAL ONCOLOGY

Section Editors: David Luesley and Simon Leeson

INDEX   **927**

Contributors

Adam H Balen DSc FRCOG
Professor of Reproductive Medicine and Surgery, Chair of The British Fertility Society, The Leeds Centre for Reproductive Medicine, Seacroft Hospital, Leeds

Smriti Bhatta MBBS MD MRCOG
Senior Clinical Fellow, Aberdeen Fertility Centre, University of Aberdeen, Aberdeen, Scotland

Siladitya Bhattacharya MBBS MRCOG MD
Professor of Reproductive Medicine & Head, Division of Applied Health Sciences, University of Aberdeen, Aberdeen, Scotland

Jenny Blackman
Post CCT Fellow, Royal Devon and Exeter Hospital, Exeter

Kate Bramham
Women's Health Academic Centre, St Thomas' Hospital, King's College London, London

Linda Cardozo OBE MD FRCOG
Professor of Urogynaecology, King's College Hospital, London

Susan V Carr FFSRH DRCOG MPhil
Associate Professor, Department of Obstetrics and Gynaecology, University of Melbourne, and Head of Psychosexual Service, Royal Womens Hospital, Melbourne and Chair Australian Society of Psychosocial Obstetrics and Gynaecology, Melbourne, Australia

Ying Cheong MD FRCOG
Associate Professor & Honorary Consultant in Obstetrics and Gynaecology, Subspecialist in Reproductive Medicine and Surgery, Faculty of Medicine University of Southampton, Southampton

Ben Chisnall
Foundation Year 1 Doctor at Oxford University Hospitals NHS Trust, Oxford

Duncan S Cochran MBBS(Lond) FCARCSI
Consultant Anaesthetist, Sandwell and West Birmingham NHS Trust, Birmingham

Arri Coomarasamy MBChB MD FRCOG
Professor of Gynaecology and Reproductive Medicine, College of Medical and Dental Sciences, University of Birmingham and Consultant in Gynaecology, Reproductive Medicine and Surgery, Birmingham Women's NHS Foundation Trust, Birmingham

Sarah M Creighton MD FRCOG
Consultant Gynaecologist, University College London Hospital, UCL Institute of Women's Health, London

Hilary OD Critchley BSc MBChB MD FRCOG FRANZCOG FFRSH FMedSci
Professor of Reproductive Medicine, Honorary Consultant Obstetrician and Gynaecologist, University of Edinburgh, Centre for Reproductive Biology, Edinburgh, Scotland

Margaret Cruickshank MB ChB MD FRCOG
Professor of Gynaecology, Department of Obstetrics and Gynaecology, Aberdeen Maternity Hospital, Aberdeen, Scotland

Andrew Currie BM DCH FRCPCH FRCP Ed
Consultant Neonatologist, Leicester Royal Infirmary, University Hospitals of Leicester NHS Trust, Leicester

Rebecca Deans MBBS MMED RANZCOG CREI
Lecturer and Gynaecologist, University of New South Wales, Royal Hospital for Women, and Sydney Children's Hospital, Sydney, Australia

Rima Dhillon
Specialist Trainee in Obstetrics and Gynaecology, University Hospital Coventry and Warwickshire, Coventry

Shuchi Dixit
Consultant Obstetrician and Gynaecologist, Derby Teaching Hospitals NHS Foundation Trust, Derby

Gabrielle Downey MD FRCOG
Consultant Obstetrician and Lead Colposcopist at City Hospital, Dudley Road, Birmingham

Timothy Draycott
Consultant Obstetrician, University of Bristol, Bristol

James Drife MD FRCOG FRCPEd FRCSEd FCOGSA FFSRH
Emeritus professor of Obstetrics and Gynaecology, University of Leeds, Leeds

Abey Eapen
Clinical Research Fellow, University of Birmingham/Birmingham Women's Hospital, Birmingham

Diana Fothergill BSc Med Sci Hons MB ChB FRCOG
Emeritus Consultant Obstetrician and Gynaecologist, The Jessop Wing, Sheffield Teaching Hospitals NHS Trust, Sheffield

Caroline Fox MBChB MD MRCOG
Subspecialty Trainee in Maternal and Fetal Medicine, Birmingham Women's Foundation NHS Trust, Birmingham

Fieke E M Froeling MD PhD MRCP
NIHR Academic Clinical Lecturer, Specialist Registrar in Medical Oncology, Division of Cancer, Department of Surgery and Cancer, Imperial College London, London

Islam Gamaleldin
Speciality Registrar Obstetrics and Gynaecology, Southmead Hospital, Bristol

Ilias Giarenis MRCOG
Subspecialty Trainee in Urogynaecology, King's College Hospital, London

Joanna Girling
Consultant Obstetrician and Gynaecologist, Lead Division 3 and Speciality Lead Reproductive Health & Childbirth NW London CRN, West Middlesex University Hospital, Isleworth

Mahalakshmi Gurumurthy MRCOG
Consultant Gyanecological Oncologist, Aberdeen Royal Infirmary, Aberdeen, Scotland

Lubna Haque MBBS MRCOG
Consultant Gynaecologist & Colposcopist, Luton & Dunstable University Hospital NHS Foundation Trust, Luton

Hoda Maaly Harb
Specialist Registrar in Obstetrics and Gynaecology, University of Birmingham, Birmingham

Alexander Heazell MBChB (Hons) PhD MRCOG
Senior Clinical Lecturer in Obstetrics, Maternal and Fetal Health Research Centre, University of Manchester and St Mary's Hosptial, Manchester

Mary Higgins
Consultant in Obstetrics, Gynaecology, Sub-specialist in Maternal Fetal Medicine, National Maternity Hospital / University College Dublin, Dublin

James Hounslow
Senior Registrar in Obstetrics and Gynaecology, Princess Anne Hospital, Southampton

Kulsum Jaffer BSc MBBS FRCOG FFSRH
Consultant in Sexual and Reproductive Health, Heart of Birmingham Teaching Primary Care Trust, St Patrick's Centre, Birmingham

Nina Johns BSc MBChB MRCOG
Consultant Obstetrician, Birmingham Women's Hospital, Birmingham

Tracey A Johnston MD FRCOG
Consultant in Maternal Fetal Medicine, Birmingham Women's NHS Foundation Trust, Birmingham

Davor Jurkovic
Department of Obstetrics and Gynaecology, University College Hospital, London

Lucy Kean DM FRCOG
Consultant Obstetrician Subspecialist in Maternal and Fetal Medicine, Nottingham University Hospitals, Nottingham

Louise Kenny MB ChB hons PhD MRCOG
Professor of Obstetrics and Gynaecology, University College Cork, Consultant Obstetrician and Gynaecologist, Cork University Maternity Hospital, Director, The Irish Centre for Fetal and Neonatal Translational Research (INFANT), Cork, Ireland

Mohammed Khairy MD MRCOG
Subspecialty Trainee in Reproductive Medicine and Surgery, Birmingham Women's Fertility Centre, Birmingham Women's Hosptial, Birmingham

Yakoub Khalaf MB BCh MSc MD FRCOG
Consultant Gynaecologist & Sub-Specialist in Reproductive Medicine and Surgery, Director of the Assisted Conception Unit & HFEA Person Responsible, Guy's and St Thomas' Hospital Foundation Trust, Guy's Hospital, London

Mark D Kilby DSc MB BS MD FRCOG FRCPI
Professor in Fetal Medicine, Centre for Women's and Children's Health, University of Birmingham, and Fetal Medicine Centre, Birmingham Women's Foundation Trust, Birmingham

Sailesh Kumar MB BS MMed O&G FRCS MRCOG FRANZCOG DPhil Oxon
Honorary Senior Lecturer and Consultant in Maternal and Fetal Medicine, Centre for Fetal Care, Imperial College London, Queen Charlotte's and Chelsea Hospital, London

William L Ledger MA DPhil Oxon MB ChB FRCOG
Head of School, Women's & Children's Health, UNSW Australia and Head of Reproductive Medicine Department, Royal Hospital for Women, Randwick, Australia

Simon Leeson FRCOG
Consultant Gynaecologist and Oncologist, Betsi Cadwaladr University Health Board, Wales

Will Lester
Consultant Haematologist, University Hospital Birmingham and Birmingham Women's Hospital, Birmingham

David M Levy FRCA
Consultant Obstetric Anaesthetist, Anaesthetics Directorate, Nottingham University Hospitals, Queens Medical Centre Campus, Nottingham

David M Luesley MA MD FRCOG
Emeritus Professor of Gynaecological Oncology, University of Birmingham, Birmingham

Sheila McLean LLB MLitt PhD LLD FRSE FRCGP FRCP(Edin) FRSA
Emeritus Professor of Law and Ethics in Medicine, University of Glasgow, Glasgow, Scotland

Fiona L Mackie MRes, MBChB
Clinical Research Fellow, University of Birmingham, and Birmingham Women's NHS Foundation Trust, Birmingham

Melanie C Mann FRCOG FFFP Dip GUM
Consultant in Sexual and Reproductive Health, Worcestershire Health and Care Trust, Alexandra Hospital, Redditch

Bill Martin
Consultant in Maternal and Fetal Medicine, Birmingham Women's Hospital, Birmingham

Pierre L Martin-Hirsch MRCOG
Consultant Gynaecological Oncologist, Central Lancashire Teaching Hospitals, Preston

Abi Merriel MRCOG
Clinical Research Fellow, University of Birmingham, Birmingham

Mostafa Metwally MD FRCOG
Consultant Gynaecologist and Subspecialist in Reproductive Medicine, The Jessop Wing and Royal Hallamshire Hospital, Sheffield

Michele P Mohajer BM BS FRCOG MD
Consultant in Maternal and Fetal Medicine, Royal Shrewsbury Hospital, Shrewsbury

R Katie Morris PhD MRCOG
Senior Clinical Lecturer in Fetal Medicine, Centre for Women's and Children's Health, University of Birmingham, and Fetal Medicine Centre, Birmingham Women's Foundation Trust, Birmingham

Rajeshwari Myagerimath
Consultant Obstetrician and Gynaecologist, Arrowe Park Hospital, Wirral University Teaching Hospital NHS Foundation Trust, Wirral

Catherine Nelson-Piercy MA FRCP
Consultant Obstetric Physician, Guy's and St Thomas' Foundation Trust and Imperial College Healthcare Trust, and Professor of Obstetric Medicine, King's College London, London

David Nunns MD MRCOG
Consultant Gynaecological Oncologist, Nottingham City Hospital, Nottingham

Sue Pavord MBChB FRCP FRCPath
Consultant Haematologist, Oxford University Hospitals NHS Foundation Trust, Oxford

Alexander M Pirie MB ChB(Edin) BSc(Hons) FRCP(Edin) FRCOG
Consultant in Obstetrics & Maternal Medicine, Honorary Senior Clinical Lecturer, Birmingham Women's Hospital, Birmingham

Richard Porter MA MSc FRCOG
Consultant Obstetrician and Gynaecologist, Royal United Hospital, Bath

Sam Pretlove MBChB PhD MRCOG
Consultant in Maternal & Fetal Medicine, Birmingham Women's Foundation Trust, Birmingham

Nirmala Rai
Cancer Sciences, University of Birmingham, Birmingham

Angie Rantell BSC HONS RN
Lead Nurse Urogynaecology / Nurse Cystoscopist, King's College Hospital, London

Nicholas Reed MRCP(UK), FRCR, FRCP&S (Glas)
Consultant Clinical Oncologist, Beatson Oncology Centre Gartnavel General Hospital, Glasgow, Scotland

Fiona M Reid MD MRCOG
Consultant Urogynaecologist, The Warrell Unit, St Mary's Hospital, Manchester

Alexandra Rice
Registrar in Obstetrics and Gynaecology, South East Scotland Deanery, Edinburgh, Scotland

Devender Roberts
Consultant in Maternal and Fetal Medicine, Liverpool Women's Hospital, Crown Street, Liverpool

Dudley Robinson MBBS MD MRCOG
Consultant Urogynaecologist and Honorary Senior Lecturer, Department of Obstetrics and Gynaecology, King's College Hospital, London

Lynne Robinson
Consultant Obstetrician and Gynaecologist, Birmingham Women's Foundation Trust, Birmingham

Stuart Rundle MRCOG
Speciality Trainee in Obstetrics and Gynaecology, Royal Devon and Exeter NHS Foundation Trust, Child and Women's Health, Exeter

Janice Rymer MD FRCOG FRANZCOG FHEA
Professor of Gynaecology, School of Medical Education, King's College London, London

Ghada Salman
Department of Obstetrics and Gynaecology, University College Hospital, London

Michael J Seckl BSc MBBS PhD FRCP
Professor of Molecular Oncology, Charing Cross Hospital Campus of Imperial College London, London

Tara Jayne Selman MRCOG PhD
Consultant in Fetal Medicine, Birmingham Women's NHS Foundation Trust, Birmingham

Andrew Shennan MB BS MD FRCOG
Professor of Obstetrics, Women's Health Academic Centre, St Thomas Hospital, Kings College London, London

Sushma Srikrishna FRCOG
Consultant Urogynaecologist, Department of Urogynaecology, King's College Hospital, London

Sudha Sundar
Senior Clinical Lecturer/Consultant in Gynaecological Oncology, Pan Birmingham Gynaecological Cancer Centre, City Hospital and School of Cancer Sciences, University of Birmingham, Birmingham

Jennifer A Tamblyn
Clinical Research Fellow Obstetrics & Gynaecology, Institute of Metabolism and Systems Research, College of Medical and Dental Sciences, University of Birmingham, Birmingham

Myles Taylor BA MRCOG PhD
Consultant Obstetrician & Gynaecologist, Subspecialist in Fetal & Maternal Medicine, Royal Devon and Exeter NHS Foundation Trust, Child and Women's Health, Exeter

Ganesh Thiagamoorthy MBBS MRCOG
Subspeciality Trainee in Urogynaecology, Department of Urogynaecology, King's College Hospital, London

Jane Thomas MBChB MSC MRCOG MFSRH
Editor Cochrane Gynaecology and Fertility Group, Gynaecologist, University College London Hospital, London

Peter J Thompson MB BS FRCOG
Consultant Obstetrician, Birmingham Women's Hospital, Birmingham

John Tidy BSc MD FRCOG
Professor of Gynaecological Oncology, Royal Hallamshire Hospital, Sheffield

Clare Tower MBCHB PHD MRCOG
Consultant in Obstetrics and Fetal Maternal Medicine, St Mary's Hospital, Manchester

Graham Tydeman BSc FRCOG
Consultant Obstetrician and Gynaecologist, NHS Fife, Scotland

Tina Sara Verghese
Clinical Research Fellow, University of Birmingham and Birmingham Women's NHS Foundation Trust, Birmingham

Christine P West MD FRCOG
Consultant Gynaecologist, Royal Infirmary of Edinburgh, Edinburgh, Scotland

Sarah Wharin
Leicester Royal Infirmary, University Hospitals Leicester NHS Trust, Leicester

Catherine White
Clinical Director, St Mary's Sexual Assault Referral Centre, St Mary's Hospital, Manchester

Denise Williams MSc FRCP
Consultant Clinical Geneticist, Birmingham Women's NHS Foundation Trust, Birmingham

Jenny Williamson FFSRH
Menopause Trainer and Chair of the West Midlands Menopause Society, University of Birmingham and Birmingham Women's NHS Foundation Trust, Birmingham

Nowmi Zaman
Specialty Trainee Year 3 in Obstetrics and Gynaecology, Birmingham Women's NHS Foundation Trust, Birmingham

Preface

It is often difficult to know when a new edition of an established textbook is required. It certainly feels as if the intervals get shorter and the demands of updating are greater with each new edition. However, there are constant revisions of our professional guidelines and new developments in the specialities of obstetrics and gynaecology are emerging.

Comparing the content of this, the third edition, with the first edition published in 2004 is both rewarding and somewhat frightening. The rapid pace at which new knowledge and new evidence becomes available seems likely to overwhelm our ability to organise and present it in a format that will fulfil the requirements of aspiring obstetricians and gynaecologists and continue to provide an easily accessible source of information for those practising as specialists.

The popularity of the previous two editions signifies that we are achieving these objectives and the tested template of aligning the text to the RCOG curriculum appears to meet the needs of most readers. The basic core knowledge upon which our discipline is built does not evolve as rapidly as other aspects of our specialism and an in-depth understanding of this core knowledge is an essential prerequisite to success in the MRCOG examination and a solid basis on which to build a career as a practising specialist. It is natural with the passage of time that contributors to our previous editions will have retired or moved on elsewhere and it is right to bring in new contributors who have enthusiasm and often bring a fresh perspective to their subject matter.

We remain of course immensely grateful for the grounding provided by our previous contributors. It is their previous efforts, and the skilful updating and rewriting of our new contributors, that have maintained the high quality of the presented material. Updating, adding and omitting provides a massive editorial challenge if the 'feel' of the text is to be preserved. We believe that we have done the best that we can and that this textbook will continue to be an invaluable companion to the higher training of obstetricians and gynaecologists and a useful repository of knowledge and evidence for those in established practice.

To reiterate the final paragraph of our last preface: *Textbooks do not make good doctors but good doctors must practise from a sound basis of knowledge.* We believe that this, the third edition, continues to satisfy the goals that were laid out in the first edition.

Acknowledgements

The editors are very grateful to the following, who kindly contributed to the previous edition: Harold Gee, Joanna C Gillham, Barry W Hancock, Richard Hayman, Susan J Houghton, Griff Jones, Henry C Kitchener, Ellen Knox, Murray Luckas, Ismaiel Mahfouz, Dimitrios Nikolaou, Michael Paterson, Charles Redman, Arasee Renganathan, Karina Reynolds, Jane Rufford, Anthony RB Smith, John AD Spencer, Elias Tzakas, Aarti Umranikar, and Linda Watkins.

List of abbreviations used

5-FU	5-fluorouracil
7-DHCO	7-dehydrocholesterol
AAA	arterio-arterial anastamatosis
ABC	airway, breathing, circulation
AC	abdominal circumference
ACE	angiotensin-converting enzyme
ACEI	angiotensin-converting enzyme inhibitor
AChE	acetylcholinesterase
ACHOIS	Australian Carbohydrate Intolerance Study in Pregnant Women
aCL	anticardiolipin
ACOG	American Congress of Obstetricians and Gynecologists
ACTH	adrenocorticotrophic hormone
ADPKD	autosomal dominant polycystic kidney disease
AEDF	absent end-diastolic flow
AED	anti-epileptic drug
AF	amniotic fluid
AFC	antral follicular count
AFE	amniotic fluid embolism
AFI	amniotic fluid index
AFLP	acute fatty liver of pregnancy
AFP	alpha-fetoprotein
AFS	American Fertility Society
AFV	amniotic fluid volume
AGA	appropriate for gestational age
AHA	American Heart Association
AIDS	acquired immunodeficiency syndrome
AIS	adenocarcinoma *in situ*
ALF	acute liver failure
ALO	*Actinomyces*-like organism
ALSO	advanced life support in obstetrics
ALT	alanine transaminase
AMH	anti-Müllerian hormone
ANA	antinuclear antibody
AP	antecedent pregnancy; anterior to posterior
APACHE	Acute Physiology and Chronic Health Evaluation
APH	antepartum haemorrhage
APL	antiphospholipid
APLS/APS	antiphospholipid syndrome
APSN	atypical placental site nodule
APTT	activated partial thromboplastin time
AR	androgen receptor
ARB	angiotensin II type 1 receptor blocker (angiotensin receptor antagonist)
ARC	antenatal result and choice
AREDV	absent or reversed end-diastolic flow
ARM	artificial rupture of membranes
ART	antiretroviral therapy; assisted reproduction technique

ASA	American Society of Anesthesiologists
ASCUS	atypical squamous cells of undetermined significance
ASD	atrial septal defect
ASRM	American Society of Reproductive Medicine
AST	aspartate aminotransferase (aspartate transaminase)
ATP	adenosine triphosphate
AUB	abnormal uterine bleeding
AUM	ambulatory urodynamic monitoring
AVA	arteriovenous vessel
AVM	arteriovenous malformation
AZT	zidovudine
β-hCG	beta-human chorionic gonadotrophin
β-IFN	beta-interferon
BASHH	British Association for Sexual Health and HIV
BCG	bacille Calmette Guérin
BCPT	Breast Cancer Prevention Trial
BCSH	British Committee for Standards in Haemotology
BEP	bleomycin, etoposide, cisplatin
BFLUTS	Bristol Female Lower Urinary Tract Symptoms
BG	blood glucose
BHIVA	British HIV Association
BMD	bone mineral density
BMI	body mass index
BMJ	British Medical Journal
BNF	British National Formulary
BP	blood pressure
BPD	biparietal diameter
bpm	beats per minute
BPP	biophysical profile
BPS	bladder pain syndrome
BSAC	British Society for Antimicrobial Chemotherapy
BSCC	British Society for Cervical Cytology
BSO	bilateral salpingo-oopherectomy
BV	bacterial vaginosis
bvm	bag–valve–mask
BW	birthweight
CAH	chronic active hepatitis; congenital adrenal hyperplasia
CAIS	complete androgen insensitivity syndrome
cAMP	cyclic adenyl monophosphate
CASA	computer-assisted sperm analysis
CBT	cognitive behavioural therapy
CC	clomifene citrate
CCC	clear-cell carcinoma

CCAML	congenital cystic adenomatous malformation of the lung
CCG	Clinical Commissioning Group
CCP	cyclic citrullinated peptide
CCSS	Childhood Cancer Survivor Study
CDSR	Cochrane Database of Systematic Reviews
CEA	carcinoembryonic antigen
CEE	conjugated equine oestrogen
CEFM	continuous electronic fetal monitoring
CEMACH	Confidential Enquiry into Maternal and Child Health
CEMD	Confidential Enquiry into Maternal Death
CEPOD	Confidential Enquiry into Perioperative Death
CESDI	Confidential Enquiry into Stillbirth and Death in Infancy
CEU	Clinical Effectiveness Unit
CF	cystic fibrosis
cffDNA	cell free fetal DNA
CFU	colony-forming units
CGH	comparative genomic hybridisation
CGIN	cervical glandular intraepithelial neoplasia
CHC	combined hormonal contraception
CHIVA	Children's HIV Association
CHM	complete hydatidiform mole
CI	confidence interval
CIGN	cervical intraepithelial glandular neoplasia
CIN	cervical intraepithelial neoplasia
CIS	carcinoma *in situ*
CKD	chronic kidney disease
CL	corpus luteum
CMA	Canadian Medical Association
CMACE	Centre for Maternal and Child Enquiries
CMV	cytomegalovirus
CNS	central nervous system
CNV	copy number variant
COC(P)	combined oral contraceptive (pill)
CODAC	cause of death and associated conditions
COH	controlled ovarian hyperstimulation
COMET	Comparative Obstetric Mobile Epidural Trial
COS	controlled ovarian stimulation
COX-2	cyclooxygenase-2
CP	cerebral palsy
CPD	cephalo-pelvic disproportion
CPM	confined placental mosaicism
CPR	cardiopulmonary resuscitation
CQC	Care Quality Commission
CRH	corticotrophin-releasing hormone
CRL	crown–rump length
CRP	C-reactive protein
CS	caesarean section
CSA	child sexual abuse
CSE	child sexual exploitation; combined spinal–epidural
CSF	cerebrospinal fluid
CSII	continuous subcutaneous insulin infusion
CSM	Committee on Safety of Medicines
CT	computed tomography
CTG	cardiotocography
CTOCS	collaborative trial of ovarian cancer screening
CTPA	computed tomography pulmonary angiogram
CVA	cerebrovascular accident
CVP	central venous pressure
CVS	chorionic villus sampling
CXR	chest X-ray
CYP	cytochrome p450
D&C	dilatation and curettage
D&E	dilatation and evacuation
DARE	Database of Reviews of Effectiveness
DAT	direct antiglobulin test
DC	dichorionic
DC/DA	dichorionic diamniotic
DES	diethylstilbestrol
DEXA	bone mineral density scan
DF	degrees of freedom
DFID	Department for International Development
DH	Department of Health
DHEA	dehydroepiandrosterone
DHT	dihydrotestosterone
DI	donor insemination
DIC	disseminated intravascular coagulopathy
DKA	diabetic ketoacidosis
DLE	diathermy loop excision
DM	diabetes mellitus
DMPA	depot medroxyprogesterone acetate
DMSO	dimethyl sulphoxide
DOB	date of birth
DS	donated sperm
DSD	disorders of sex development
dsDNA	double-stranded DNA
DV	ductus venosus
DVP	deepest vertical pool/pocket
DVT	deep venous thrombosis
DySIS	dynamic spectral imaging system
DXA	dual-energy X-ray absorptiometry
E2(V)	oestradiol (valerate)
E3	oestriol
E3G	oestrone-3-glucuronide
EAS	external anal sphincter
EBM	evidence-based medicine
EC	emergency contraception; endometrial carcinoma
ECG	electrocardiogram
ECL	echogenic cystic lesion

ECOG	Eastern Cooperative Oncology Group
ECV	external cephalic version
EDF	end-diastolic flow
EDTA	ethylenediaminetetraacetic acid
EE	ethinylestradiol
EEG	electroencephalogram
EFM	electronic fetal monitoring
EFW	estimated fetal weight
EGF	epidermal growth factor
eGFR	estimated glomerular filtration rate
EIA	enzyme immunoassay
EMA	etoposide, methotrexate, actinomycin D
EMG	electromyography
ENA	extractable nuclear antigen
ENG	etonogestrel
EPA	early pregnancy assessment
ER	extended-release; oestrogen receptor
ERCP	endoscopic retrograde cholangiopancreatography
ERCS	elective repeat caesarean section
ERP	enhanced recovery programme
ERPC	evacuation of products of conception
ERT	oestrogen replacement therapy
ESA	erythropoiesis-stimulating agent
eSET	elective single embryo transfer
ESG	European Society of Gynaecology
ESHRE	European Society of Human Reproduction and Embryology
ESMO	European Society of Medical Oncology
ESR	erythrocyte sedimentation rate
ESSIC	European Society for the Study of Bladder Pain Syndrome/Interstitial Cystitis
ET	embryo transfer
ETT	endotracheal tube; epithelial trophoblastic tumour
FA	fertility awareness
FAI	free androgen index
FAS	fetal alcohol syndrome
FBC	full blood count
FBS	fetal blood sampling
FDA	Food and Drug Administration (USA)
FDP	fibrin degradation product
FDV	first desire to void
FET	frozen embryo transfer
FEV	forced expiratory volume
FFLM	Faculty of Forensic and Legal Medicine
fFN	fetal fibronectin
FFP	fresh frozen plasma
FFPRHC	Faculty of Family Planning and Reproductive Healthcare
FGM	female genital mutilation
FGR	fetal growth restriction
FHR	fetal heart rate

FIGO	International Federation of Gynaecology and Obstetrics
FISH	fluorescence in-situ hybridisation
FL	femur length
FM	fetal movement
FMAIT	fetal maternal alloimmune thrombocytopenia
FME	forensic medical examiner, previously known as a police surgeon
FOCSS	familial ovarian cancer screening study
FRHM	familial recurrent hydatidiform mole
FSH	follicle stimulating hormone
FSRH	Faculty of Sexual and Reproductive Healthcare
FTA-Abs	fluorescent treponemal antibody absorption (test)
FTP	failure to progress
FVL	factor V Leiden
GA	general anaesthetic; gestational age
GABA-A	gamma-aminobutyric acid type A
GAG	glycosaminoglycan
GBS	group B *Streptococcus*
GCIG	Gynaecologic Cancer Intergroup
G-CSF	granulocyte colony-stimulating factor
GDF	growth differentiation factor
GDG	Guideline Development Group
GDM	gestational diabetes mellitus
GH	growth hormone
GHRH	growth hormone-releasing hormone
GI	glycaemic index
GIFT	gamete intrafallopian tube transfer
GMC	General Medical Council
GnRH	gonadotrophin-releasing hormone
GOG	Gynecologic Oncology Group
GP	general practitioner
GR	glucocorticoid receptor
GRADE	grading of recommendations, assessment, development and evaluation
GRIT	Growth Restriction Intervention Trial
GS	gestational sac
GT	gestational thrombocytopenia
GTD	gestational trophoblastic disease
GTN	gestational trophoblastic neoplasia; glyceryl trinitrate
GTT	gestational trophoblastic tumour
GUM	genito-urinary medicine
HAART	highly active antiretroviral therapy
HAPO	hyperglycaemia and adverse pregnancy outcomes
Hb	haemoglobin
HbSS	sickle cell anaemia
HBV	hepatitis B virus; honour-based violence
HC	head circumference; hybrid capture
hCG	human chorionic gonadotrophin
HCM	hypertrophic cardiomyopathy
HCV	hepatitis C virus

HDFN	haemolytic disease of the fetus and newborn	IDDM	insulin-dependent diabetes mellitus
HDL	high-density lipoprotein	IDU	injecting drug user
HDN	haemolytic disease of the newborn	IE	infective endocarditis
HDU	high dependency unit	Ig	immunoglobulin
HELLP	syndrome of haemolysis, increased liver enzymes and low platelets	IGF-1/2	insulin-like growth factor 1/2
		IGFBP	insulin-like growth factor binding protein
HERS	Heart and Oestrogen Progestogen Study	IgG	immunoglobulin G
HES	Hospital Episode Statistics	IgM	immunoglobulin M
HFEA	Human Fertilisation and Embryology Authority	IGT	impaired glucose tolerance
		IH	immune hydrops
HGSC	high-grade serous carcinoma	IHD	ischaemic heart disease
HGUS	high-grade undifferentiated sarcoma	IIQ	Incontinence Impact Questionnaire
HIE	hypoxic–ischaemic encephalopathy	ILCOR	International Liaison Committee on Resuscitation
HIV	human immunodeficiency virus		
HLA	human leukocyte antigen	IM	intramuscular
HMB	heavy menstrual bleeding	IMB	intermenstrual bleeding
hMG	human menopausal gonadotrophins	IMSI	intracytoplasmic morphological sperm injection
HNPCC	hereditary non-polyposis colorectal cancer		
		INI	integrase inhibitor
HP	hidradenoma papilliferum	IOL	induction of labour
hPL	human placental lactogen	IQ	intelligence quotient
HPLC	high-performance liquid chromatography	IQR	interquartile range
HPO	hypothalamic–pituitary–ovarian	ISD	intrinsic sphincter deficiency
HPV	human papilloma virus	ISSHP	International Society for the Study of Hypertension in Pregnancy
HQIP	Healthcare Quality Improvement Partnership		
		ISSVD	International Society for the Study of Vulvovaginal Diseases
HR	hazard ratio; high risk		
HRQoL	health-related quality of life	ISVA	independent sexual violence advisor
HRT	hormone replacement therapy	ITP	idiopathic/immune thrombocytopenic purpura
HS	harmonic scalpel; hidradenitis suppurativa		
		ITT	intention to treat
HSDD	hypoactive sexual desire disorder	IUCD	intrauterine contraceptive device
HSG	hysterosalpingography	IUD	intrauterine death; intrauterine device
HSIL	high-grade squamous intraepithelial lesions	IUFD	intrauterine fetal death
		IUGA	International Urogynaecology Association
HSV	herpes simplex virus		
HSV-1	herpes simplex type 1 virus	IUGR	intrauterine growth restriction
HSV-2	herpes simplex type 2 virus	IUI	intrauterine insemination
HTA	Health Technology Assessment Database; Human Tissue Authority	IUS	intrauterine system
		IUT	intrauterine transfusion
HUS	haemolytic uraemic syndrome	IV	intravenous
IADPSG	International Association of Diabetes and Pregnancy Study Group	IVD	instrumental vaginal delivery
		IVF	in-vitro fertilisation
IBD	inflammatory bowel disease	IVF-ET	IVF and embryo transfer
IBIS	International Breast Cancer Intervention Study	IVM	in-vitro maturation
		IVS	intravaginal slingplasty
IBS	irritable bowel syndrome	IVU or IVP	intravenous urogram
IC	interstitial cystitis	KHQ	King's Health Questionnaire
ICH	intracranial haemorrhage	LAC	lupus anticoagulant
ICIQ	International Consultation on Incontinence Questionnaire	LAM	lactational amenorrhoea method
		LARC	long-acting reversible contraception
ICP	intracranial pressure	LBC	liquid-based cytology
ICS	International Continence Society; intra-operative cell salvage	LDH	lactate dehydrogenase
		LDL	low-density lipoprotein
ICSI	intracytoplasmic sperm injection	LEEP	loop electrosurgical excision procedure
ICU	intensive care unit	LFT	liver function test

LGESS	low-grade endometrial stromal sarcoma
LGSC	low-grade serous carcinoma
LH	luteinising hormone
LHCGR	shared leutinizing hormone/hCG receptor
LLETZ	large loop excision of the transformation zone
LMP	last menstrual period
LMS	leiomyosarcoma
LMWH	low-molecular-weight heparin
LN	lymph node
LNG	levonorgestrel
LNG-IUS	levonorgestrel-releasing intrauterine system
LoC-IUT/SDI	letter of competence in intrauterine techniques/subdermal implants
LOD	laparoscopic ovarian drilling
LP	lichen planus
LS	lichen sclerosus
LSIL	low-grade squamous intraepithelial lesion
LUNA	laparoscopic uterine nerve ablation
LUTS	lower urinary tract symptom
LV	liquor volume
MA	monoamniotic
MAOI	monoamine oxidase inhibitor
MAP	mean arterial pressure; morbidly adherent placenta
MAR	mixed antibody reaction
MAS	McCune–Albright syndrome; meconium aspiration syndrome
MBRRACE-UK	Mothers and Babies: Reducing Risk through Audits and Confidential Enquiries across the UK
MC	monochorionic; mucinous carcinoma
MCA	Mental Capacity Act; middle cerebral artery
MCAD	medium-chain acyl-coenzyme A dehydrogenase deficiency
MC/DA	monochorionic diamniotic
MCH	mean corpuscular haemoglobin
MCHC	mean cell haemoglobin concentration
MCV	mean cell volume
MCP-1	monocyte chemotactic peptide-1
MDG	Millennium Development Goal
MDKD	multicystic dysplastic kidney disease
MDMA	3,4-methylenedioxymethamphetamine
MDR	multidrug-resistant
MDRD	modified diet in renal disease
MDT	multidisciplinary team
MEA	microwave endometrial ablation
MeSH	medical subject heading
MEWS	modified early warning system
MFPR	multi-fetal pregnancy reduction
MG	myasthenia gravis
MHRA	Medicines and Healthcare products Regulatory Agency
MI	myocardial infarction
MIG	metformin with insulin in gestational diabetes
MIN	multicentric intraepithelial neoplasia
MIS	Müllerian inhibiting substance
MLPA	multiplex ligation-dependent probe amplification
MLS	Maternal Lifestyles Study
MMF	mycophenolate mofetil
MMP	matrix metalloproteinase
MMR	maternal mortality rate
MMT	methadone maintenance treatment
MNC	modified natural cycle
MOET	managing obstetric emergencies and trauma
MoM	multiple of the normal median
MPA	medroxyprogesterone acetate
MPD	maximum pool/pocket depth
MRC	Medical Research Council
MRCS	maternal request caesarean section
MRg-FUS	magnetic resonance-guided focused ultrasound
MRI	magnetic resonance imaging
MRKH	Mayer–Rokitanksy–Kuster–Hauser syndrome
MRSA	methicillin-resistant *Staphylococcus aureus*
MS	multiple sclerosis
MSAFP	maternal serum alpha-fetoprotein
MSH	melanocyte-stimulating hormone
MSM	men who have sex with men
MSU	midstream urine
MSV	Mauriceau–Smellie–Veit
MTCT	mother-to-child transmission
MTX/FA	methotrexate with folinic acid
MUP	motor nerve unit potential
MVA	manual vacuum aspiration
MVP	maximum vertical pool/pocket
NAAT	nucleic acid amplification tests
NANC	non-adrenergic non-cholinergic
NAS	neonatal abstinence syndrome
NCCN	National Comprehensive Cancer Network
NCEPOD	National Confidential Enquiry into Patient Outcome and Death
NCSP	National Chlamydia Screening Programme
NET-EN	norethisterone enanthate
NFP	natural family planning
NGF	nerve growth factor
NHS	National Health Service
NHSCSP	National Health Service Cervical Screening Programme
NHSLA	NHS Litigation Authority
NICE	National Institute for Health and Care Excellence

NICHD	National Institute of Child Health and Human Development	PEPSE	post-exposure prophylaxis for HIV following sexual exposure
NICU	neonatal intensive care unit	PET	positron emission tomography; pre-eclampsia
NIDDM	non-insulin-dependent diabetes mellitus	PFMT	pelvic floor muscle training
NIH	National Institute of Health; non-immune hydrops	PFR	peak flow rate
		PG	prostaglandin
NIPT	non-invasive prenatal testing	PHM	partial hydatidiform mole
NMG	neonatal myasthenia gravis	PI	pulsatility index
NNT	number needed to treat	PICO	population, intervention, comparison, outcome
NNTB	number needed to treat to benefit		
NOMAC	nomegoestrol acetate	PID	pelvic inflammatory disease
NPEU	National Perinatal Epidemiology Unit	PIH	pregnancy-induced hypertension
NPSA	National Patient Safety Agency	PI/r	ritonavir-boosted protease inhibitor
NRTI	nucleoside reverse transcriptase inhibitor	PIVKA	prothrombin induced by vitamin K absence
NSAID	non-steroidal anti-inflammatory drug	PLCO	prostate, lung, colon and ovarian cancer
NSC	National Screening Committee	PlGF	placental growth factor
NST	non-stress test	PM	postmortem
NT	nuchal translucency	PMB	post-menopausal bleeding
NTD	neural tube defect	PMCS	perimortem caesarean section
NYHA	New York Heart Association	PMDD	premenstrual dysphoric disorder
OA	occiput anterior	PMR	perinatal mortality rate
OAA	Obstetric Anaesthetists' Association	PMS	premenstrual syndrome
OAB	overactive bladder	PND	perinatal death notification
OC	obstetric cholestasis	POEC	progesterone-only emergency contraception
OCP	oral contraceptive pill		
OCR	optical character recognition	POI	premature ovarian insufficiency; progestogen-only implant
OGTT	oral glucose tolerance test		
OHSS	ovarian hyperstimulation syndrome	POIC	progestogen-only injectable contraception
OI	ovulation induction		
OMR	optical mark reader	POP	progestogen-only pill
ONS	Office for National Statistics	POP-Q	Pelvic Organ Prolapse Quantification
OR	odds ratio	PORTEC	postoperative radiation therapy in endometrial carcinoma
OROS	oxybutynin preparation using an osmotic system		
		PORTO	prospective observational trial to optimise paediatric health in IUGR
OSAT	objective structured assessment of technical skill		
		PPH	postpartum haemorrhage
OWAM	organisation with a memory	PPI	proton pump inhibitor
PAIS	partial androgen insensitivity syndrome	PPIUS	Patient Perception of Intensity of Urgency Scale
PAMG-1	placental alpha macroglobulin-1		
PAPP-A	pregnancy-associated plasma protein-A	PPROM(T)	preterm premature rupture of membranes (close to term)
PARP	poly ADP ribose polymerase		
PBC	primary biliary cirrhosis	PPS	pentosan polysulphate
PCA	patient-controlled analgesia	PPT	postpartum thyroiditis
PCB	postcoital bleeding	PR	progesterone receptors
PCEA	patient-controlled epidural analgesia	PROM	pre-labour rupture of membranes
PCOS	polycystic ovary syndrome	PROMPT	Practical Obstetric Multiprofessional Training
PCR	polymerase chain reaction		
PDA	patent ductus arteriosus	PSN	placental site nodule
PDS	polydioxanone suture	PSN	presacral neurectomy
PE	pulmonary embolism	PSTT	placental site trophoblastic tumour
PECOT	population, exposure, comparison, outcome and time	PT	prothrombin time
		PTNS	posterior tibial nerve stimulation
PEEP	positive end-expiratory pressure	PTSD	post-traumatic stress disorder
PEFR	peak expiratory flow rate	PTU	propylthiouracil
PEP	post-exposure prophylaxis	PUFA	polyunsaturated fatty acids

PUL	pregnancy of unknown location	SGA	small for gestational age
PUVA	psoralens and ultraviolet A	SGOT	serum glutamic-oxaloacetic transaminase
QALY	quality-adjusted life years		
QF-PCR	quantitative fluorescence polymerase chain reaction	SGPT	serum glutamic pyruvic transaminase
		SHBG	sex hormone-binding globulin
QoL	quality of life	SIADH	syndrome of inappropriate anti-diuretic hormone
RA	rheumatoid arthritis		
RAADP	routine antenatal anti-D prophylaxis	SIDS	sudden infant death syndrome
RCA	root cause analysis	SIGN	Scottish Intercollegiate Guidelines Network
RCM	Royal College of Midwives		
RCOG	Royal College of Obstetricians and Gynaecologists	SIMS	single-incision mini sling
		SLE	systemic lupus erythematosus
RCPCH	Royal College of Paediatrics and Child Health	SMBE	simulation-based medical education
		SMD	standardised mean difference
RCR	Royal College of Radiologists	SMR	severe mental retardation
RCT	randomised controlled trial	SNRI	serotonin noradrenaline reuptake inhibitors
ReCoDe	Relevant Condition at Death		
REDF	reversed end-diastolic flow	SOA	Sexual Offences Act
REM	rapid eye movement	SOAP	subjective, objective, assessment, plan
RFM	reduced fetal movement	SPR	screen positive rate
rFSH	recombinant FSH	SPRM	selective progesterone modulator
Rh	Rhesus	SROM	spontaneous rupture of membranes
RI	resistance index	SRY	sex-determining region of the Y chromosome
RiCoF	ristocetin-induced cofactor activity		
RITA	radiofrequency interstitial thermal oblation	SSR	surgical sperm retrieval
		SSRI	selective serotonin reuptake inhibitor
RLU/PC	relative light unit/positive controls	STAN	ST analysis
RMI	risk of malignancy index	STD	sexually transmitted disease
ROBUST	RCOG operative birth simulation training	STI	sexually transmitted infection
		STIC	serous tubal intraepithelial carcinoma
RPOC	retained products of conception	STUMP	smooth muscle tumour of unknown malignant potential
RPR	rapid plasma reagin		
RR	relative risk	STV	short-term variability
RRSO	risk-reducing salpingo-oopherectomy	SUDEP	sudden unexpected death in epilepsy
RTA	road traffic accident	SVD	spontaneous vaginal delivery
RT-PCR	reverse transcriptase–polymerase chain reaction	SVT	supraventricular tachycardia
		T3	triiodothyronine
SADS	sudden adult death syndrome	T4	thyroxine
SANDS	Stillbirth and Neonatal Death Society	TA	transabdominal
SARC	sexual assault referral centre	TAH	total abdominal hysterectomy
SCBU	special care baby unit	TAMBA	Twins and Multiple Births Association
SCC	squamous cell carcinoma	TAP	transversus abdominis plane
SCCOHT	small-cell cancer of hypercalcaemic type	TAPS	twin anaemia polycythaemia sequence
SCCOPT	small-cell cancer of pulmonary type	TB	tuberculosis
SCD	sickle cell disease	TBA	thermal balloon ablation
SCD	sudden cardiac death	TBG	thyroid-binding globulin
SCI	spinal cord injury	TCA	tricyclic antidepressant
SCJ	squamo-columnar junction	TDF	testis-determining factor
SD	standard deviation	TED	thromboembolic deterrent/disease
SDP	single deepest pool/pocket	TENS	transcutaneous electrical nerve stimulation
SDV	strong desire to void		
sEMG	static and dynamic surface electromyography	TIA	transient ischaemic attack
		TIBC	total iron-binding capacity
sENG	endoglin	TLH	total laparoscopic hysterectomy
SERM	selective oestrogen receptor modulator	TM-ET	transmyometrial embryo transfer
SFH	symphisio-fundal height	TPHA	*Treponema pallidum* haemagglutination assay
sFLT	soluble fms-like tyrosine kinase-1		

TRAP	twin reversed arterial perfusion		UT	uterus
TRH	thyrotrophin-releasing hormone		UTI	urinary tract infection
TRUFFLE	Trial of Randomised Umbilical and Fetal Flow in Europe		UV	umbilical vein
			VACTERL	vertebral, anal, cardiac, trachea-oesophageal, renal, limb association
TSH	thyroid-stimulating hormone			
TTN	transient tachypnoea of the newborn		VaIN	vaginal intraepithelial neoplasia
TTP	thrombotic thrombocytopenic purpura		VAS	vibro-acoustic stimulation
TTTS	twin–twin transfusion syndrome		VBAC	vaginal birth after caesarean section
TV	*Trichomonas vaginalis*		VCU	videocystourethrogram
TVS	transvaginal ultrasound scanning		VDRL	Venereal Disease Research Laboratory
TVT	tension-free vaginal tape		VEGF	vascular endothelial growth factor
UA	umbilical artery		VIN	vulval intraepithelial neoplasia
UAE	uterine artery embolisation		VLP	virus-like particles
UDCA	ursodeoxycholic acid		VP	vasa praevia
UDI	urogenital distress inventory		VSD	ventricular septal defect
U&E	urea and electrolyte		VT	ventricular tachycardia
uE3	unconjugated oestriol		VTE	venous thromboembolism
UFH	unfractionated heparin		VVA	veno-venous anastomatoses
UGT	uridine 5'-diphosphate glucuronosyltransferase		vWD	von Willebrand's disease
			vWF	von Willebrand factor
UKGTN	UK Genetic Testing Network		VZIG	varicella zoster IgG
UKMEC	UK Medical Eligibility Criteria		VZV	varicella-zoster virus
UKOSS	UK Obstetric Surveillance System		WBC	white blood cell
UPA	ulipristal acetate		WHI	Women's Health Initiative
UPP	urethral pressure profilometry		WHO	World Health Organization
UPSI	unprotected sexual intercourse		WHOMEC	WHO Medical Eligibility Criteria
US(S)	ultrasound (scan)		WY	woman years
USI	urodynamic stress incontinence		ZIFT	zygote intrafallopian transfer

How to use this book

The following features are used throughout the book to highlight the key information and to clearly identify the evidence base.

MRCOG standards

An MRCOG standards box at the start of a chapter lists the relevant standards and/or theoretical and practical skills relating to the topic. Where there are no standards specified in the MRCOG curriculum, we have given a summary of best practice.

EBM

Evidence-based medicine boxes are included to provide a rapid summary of the evidence relating to the interventions and treatments discussed in each chapter. Where evidence is limited, this is also stated.

KEY POINTS

Key points boxes summarise the main points in a section or chapter.

Evidence scoring

It is one of the key principles of this book that doctors assess the quality and applicability of available evidence.

The evidence considered by the authors has been graded according to the structure below, in accordance with the system used in Guidelines published by the RCOG.

Classification of evidence levels

A   systematic review or meta-analysis

B   one or more well-designed randomised controlled trials

C   non-randomised controlled trials, cohort study, etc.

D   retrospective, uncontrolled

E   'expert opinion'

SECTION ONE
Introductory/General

Chapter 1 Evidence-based medicine and medical informatics

Jane Thomas

MRCOG standards: Epidemiology and statistics

- Demonstrate the skills needed to critically appraise scientific trials and literature
- Understand the production and application of clinical standards, guidelines and care pathways and protocols
- Understand the difference between audit and research
- Understand how to perform, interpret and use clinical audit cycles
- Understand how to plan a research project
- Demonstrate a full understanding of common usage of computing systems, including the principles of data collection, storage, retrieval, analysis and presentation

INTRODUCTION

This chapter outlines some key concepts of clinical epidemiology and statistics that will help you to understand the terms used within this book, in clinical research and in the MRCOG examination.

Traditionally, medical practice was based on pathophysiological mechanisms of disease and the experience of authoritative experts. The term 'evidence-based medicine' (EBM) was first coined by Gordon Guyatt around 1990 to describe the process of bringing critical appraisal of research evidence to the bedside and basing clinical decisions on clinical research evidence, clinical expertise and patients' values.[1] This title was intentionally provocative.[2] Developing in parallel with EBM there was recognition that randomised controlled trials are the best way of establishing the effectiveness of treatments, and recognition, that whilst a single study is useful, pooling the findings from all studies provides the best evidence.[3] *Effective Care in Pregnancy and Childbirth*[4] was the first attempt in medicine to look thoroughly for research evidence and

systematically summarise the effect of treatments in a clinical area. This led on to the setting up in 1993 of the Cochrane Collaboration, an international network to prepare, maintain and disseminate systematic reviews.

EBM has evolved, and there is now greater emphasis on evidence in the context of patients' values and preferences. Critical appraisal of a body of evidence takes time, and it is inefficient use of resources to search the literature for every treatment of every patient. Increasingly, therefore, processed research, such as systematic reviews, summary digests of reviews or evidence-based clinical guidelines, can offer the highest level evidence on which to base decisions.[2] Nevertheless, it remains important that clinicians can appreciate the principles of EBM so that they can distinguish what is trustworthy reliable evidence from what is not.[2] *Testing Treatments*[3] and the website 'Bad Science' provide an accessible introduction to the use and abuse of evidence.[5]

The practice of EBM comprises five steps:[6] these steps are also used by guideline developers to develop evidence-based clinical guidelines:

1. defining a clinical question,
2. finding the best evidence,
3. appraising the evidence for its validity (closeness to the truth), impact (size of effect) and applicability (usefulness in clinical practice),
4. integrating the findings of the critical appraisal with clinical expertise and patient values,
5. reviewing (auditing) clinical practice and the efficiency of the above steps.

STEP 1. SETTING THE CLINICAL QUESTION

Generating an answerable clinical question that is precise and specific is the basis of EBM. The development of a search strategy will flow from this. Focused clinical questions include four components, abbreviated as 'PICO':[6,7]

- **P** – the population: a description of the patients, such as their age, parity, clinical problem and the healthcare setting;

- **I** – the intervention(s) (or exposure): these are the main actions, such as treatment, diagnostic test or risk factor;
- **C** – the comparison group: for example, placebo or an alternative treatment;
- **O** – the outcome: for example, the change in health expected as a result of the intervention.

The type of study that will be sought is determined by the type of clinical question. For example, for a question about treatment, the highest level of evidence is based on randomised controlled trials (RCTs); for diagnostic test accuracy, studies that compare the 'new' test to a 'gold standard' test are needed; for questions about prognosis, studies that follow up groups of patients for a specified period of time (cohort studies) are needed. For a question about risk factors, cohort or 'case–control studies may be more appropriate. For cohort studies, the intervention may be an exposure (rather than a treatment intervention) and additional factors (length of follow-up or time) may be included. This is sometimes a population, exposure, comparison, outcome and time (PECOT) question.[7]

An example of a vague clinical question is: 'Should we use antibiotic prophylaxis at caesarean section?' This question could be focused in a number of ways.

- *Population:* are you interested in all caesarean sections, or a specific subgroup such as emergency or repeat caesarean section? The country in which you are practising, and the resources available, may also be important to specify.
- *Intervention:* antibiotic prophylaxis. Do you want to specify the antibiotic? Are you interested in the dose/duration of use?
- *Comparison:* is this compared with no antibiotics or with another intervention or another antibiotic – or to a different dose or treatment schedule?
- *Outcome:* what will be different as a result of giving the antibiotics? Will they reduce postoperative wound infection, or other outcomes such as endometritis or urinary tract infection (UTI), or other measures of febrile or infective morbidity such as length of hospital stay? What are the possible adverse effects or risks, for example allergy? What are the longer-term problems for mother or baby?

An example of a focused question is: 'For women having emergency caesarean section, does co-amoxiclav reduce the risk of postoperative endometritis compared with amoxicillin?' This is a question about treatment, so we would look for systematic reviews of randomised control trials.

STEP 2. FINDING THE BEST EVIDENCE

Where to search

There are numerous different library databases; different databases index different journals and they may be general or topic specific. MEDLINE is produced by the US National Library of Medicine and is widely available free of charge through PubMed. EMBASE has a greater European emphasis in terms of the journals it indexes and has a higher level of pharmacologic, content. Nursing and midwifery research may not be indexed by MEDLINE or EMBASE: to find such research, databases such as MIDIRS, BNI and CINAHL should be searched. Psychological literature is indexed on Psychinfo or Psychlit. The best resource for high-quality systematic reviews is the Cochrane Library:

- Cochrane Database of Systematic Reviews (CDSR)
- Database of Reviews of Effectiveness (DARE)
- Health Technology Assessment Database (HTA) (this includes UK and international HTA assessments).

DARE and HTA are also available on www.tripdatabase.com and www.crd.york.ac.uk. The latter also includes a new database, PROSPERO, an international prospective database of systematic reviews in health and social care. Systematic reviews are often also published in peer-reviewed journals and are indexed on library databases. The Cochrane Library has the Cochrane Central Register of Controlled Trials (CENTRAL). In addition, it can be useful to include a citation search of ISI Web of Science or SCOPUS, which will locate research papers that have referenced the papers you intend to include in your research.

There are two online databases specifically for guidelines:

1. AHRQ National Guidelines Clearing House, www.guideline.gov (2500 guidelines, free to search and with links to most guidelines)
2. The Guidelines International Network library, http://www.g-i-n.net/library/international-guidelines-library, with 6500 guidelines, is free to search but you need membership to access guidelines.

Summaries of guidelines are now often also published in journals. If included in the guidelines clearing house they can be found through PubMed, a search of Turning Research Into Practice (TRIP) www.tripdatabase.com or alternatively an internet search for the websites of guideline producers such as NICE SIGN or specialist societies.

- Scottish Intercollegiate Guidelines Network (SIGN) (http://www.sign.ac.uk/index.html)
- National Institute for Health and Care Excellence (NICE) (http://guidance.nice.org.uk/CG/Published)
- Royal College of Obstetricians and Gynaecologists (RCOG): http://www.rcog.org.uk
- Canadian Medical Association (CMA) (http://www.cma.ca/clinicalresources/practiceguidelines)

Developing a search strategy

Within general library databases, methodological indexing of study design has greatly improved. Specific strings of search terms that identify study designs, for example systematic reviews or RCTs, are available: these are designed to have high sensitivity. A good example of these is available in the Cochrane Handbook[8] – search filters. There are methodological filters, which aim to include all relevant papers, but this may result in relatively low precision. Making your search more precise may be at the expense of sensitivity, i.e. a higher proportion of citations retrieved by your search may be relevant, but it might not include all relevant citations on the topic if these have not been indexed in a way that the filters would pick up.

Developing a search strategy usually involves combining free text and controlled text terms. Using the components of your clinical question (population, intervention, comparison, outcome and study design), make a list of the synonyms, abbreviations and spelling variations (e.g. labor or labour) that might have been used by the authors to describe the concept. If you already know of relevant papers, scan them for more possible search terms. This list can be your 'free text' terms.

The next stage is to list useful controlled text terms or subject headings. In MEDLINE, these are known as MeSH (Medical Subject Headings). In most databases they will be found in the thesaurus or index. If you know of a relevant paper, check the subject headings under which it is indexed.

Having developed a focused four-part question (PICO), create a separate search strategy for each component. The next stage is to combine these searches. Combination is achieved by 'Boolean Logic' and works in a manner similar to combining numbers in algebra. Boolean Logic uses the terms 'and', 'or' and 'not' to create a set of results that should contain papers relevant to the clinical question. For example, combining cervical *and* cancer will retrieve all the papers that contain both terms. Combining cervical *or* cancer will retrieve all papers in which either one or both terms are found. To find papers relating to postoperative infection, it would be necessary to combine both the lists of controlled and free text terms for both words with *or*. Combining induction *not* labour will retrieve all papers that contain the word induction but do not also include the term labour. Care should be used when combining terms with *not*, as it will exclude any papers that discuss both the term of interest and the one to be excluded. All databases also have useful search commands and symbols, but these vary among databases.

If you are conducting a systematic review, either for publication or as the evidence base for a guideline, it is good practice to keep your search strategies and record:

- how many articles were found by the search,
- the number and source of any other records identified,
- any duplicate reports, which should be removed
- the number of records screened
- the number of full text records assessed,
- those included in a qualitative and quantitative assessment (a meta-analysis),
- exclusions – with the reason.

This information should be combined into a flow chart and published along with your review.[9]

STEP 3. APPRAISING THE EVIDENCE

The best evidence for guiding practice is an accurate, complete summation of current research knowledge such as systematic reviews.[3] In order to minimise bias, the methods of a systematic review should be explicit and well structured[9] and should include clearly defined PICO questions, an extensive search of the literature, appraising the quality of studies located by the search with explicit criteria, and analysing the research findings using appropriate methods. Data from each of the individual studies may be pooled and analysed using a technique known as meta-analysis. Clinical guidelines should be based on systematic reviews, so it is important that you are able to understand the principles of appraising clinical guidelines, systematic reviews and the primary studies on which they are based, so that you are able to judge the validity and applicability of the conclusions to your specific circumstances.

Improved reporting standards of primary and secondary research through statements such as PRISMA,[9] CONSORT 2010,[10] STARD[11] and STROBE[12] ensure the information necessary for critical appraisal is more likely to be available. In addition there are numerous guides to critical appraisal.[6,13]

Critical appraisal is the process of deciding if the research you have found can help you in answering your clinical question. The first filter is: 'Does this paper address my clinical question?' (i.e. is PICO the same or similar to that in your question?) If there are some slight differences, what are these?[6]

The second stage is to look at the study design (the methods section of a paper). The acceptable study design is determined by your clinical question. For questions about treatment interventions, RCTs or systematic reviews of RCTs provide the least biased estimate of effectiveness.[3,6,8] For diagnostic test accuracy, studies that compare the 'new' test to a 'gold standard' test are needed. For questions about prognosis, studies that follow up groups of patients for a specified period of time (cohort studies) are needed.

Bias

A systematic review summarises the results from a body of research, usually RCTs but also observational studies. Quality assessment is an essential part of the process of systematic review. If the 'constituent studies' are flawed, the conclusions of systematic reviews may also not be valid.[6,13] Bias is a systematic difference between groups that distorts the comparison so that the 'true' effect is either exaggerated or reduced. The quality of a study is the degree to which the study design, conduct and analysis have minimised bias. External validity examines the extent to which the results of a study are applicable to other clinical circumstances, i.e. its generalisability. Internal validity examines the extent to which systematic error (or bias) is minimised within the study. Such biases include:

- **selection bias** – the difference in the patient characteristics (such as prognosis) between comparison groups. In an RCT this is minimised by the method of randomisation (only non-predictable is acceptable) and by keeping allocation concealed to prevent subversion;

- **performance bias** – differences in the provision of care apart from the treatment under evaluation (achieved through blinding patients, assessors and analysts);
- **detection bias** – differences in the measurement or assessment of outcomes;
- **attrition bias** – the occurrence and handling of patient withdrawals or attrition;
- **reporting bias** – many outcomes may be measured but may not all be reported, reporting is varied dependent on findings, positive findings are more likely to be published and published sooner.

Different study types are prone to different biases; therefore, there are different validity checklists for different studies based on the conduct, design and analysis.[6,8] Appraising the quality of a study is dependent not only on what was done but on how the study was reported, and it is essential that the research is published so that the findings contribute to what is known.[5]

Understanding RCTs and systematic reviews of RCTs

For the MRCOG, it is important to understand the design of an RCT and of reviews of RCTs; therefore, the rest of this section focuses only on appraising RCTs. The RCT is the 'gold standard' method for evaluating the effectiveness of therapeutic interventions as it gives the least biased estimate of effect of treatment interventions.[3,5]

A confounder is a factor (such as disease severity) that may influence the choice of treatment and the outcome of care. Confounding is one reason for the tendency of non-randomised trials to overestimate treatment effects when compared with RCTs. With a well-conducted RCT, randomisation will create groups that are comparable with respect to any known or unknown potential confounding factors (providing the sample size is sufficiently large). The key questions to ask when appraising (assessing possible bias and quality) an RCT are outlined below, with an explanation of why these are important.[8] The first four questions relate to study validity, and the fifth to interpreting the results.

1. Was the assignment of treatment randomised?

The process of randomisation requires that those recruiting to a trial or participating in the trial cannot predict which group the subjects will be allocated to. The process of randomisation involves two stages:

(i) generation of an unpredictable allocation sequence (random number),
(ii) concealment of this sequence from those enrolling participants in the trials.

Failure to secure the concealment of the sequence may allow selective enrolment depending on prognostic factors.

A trial in which it is possible to predict the treatment allocation is more likely to be biased. The 'gold standard' for randomisation used in large multicentre trials is 'central computer' randomisation. The use of sealed envelopes (especially if they are not sequentially numbered) may be subverted (for example by holding the envelope up to the light); methods that could be predictable are date of birth, alternate days and hospital number.

2. Were the groups similar at the start of the trial?

The aim of randomisation is the creation of groups that are comparable with respect to any known or unknown potential confounding factors (providing the sample size is sufficiently large). Randomisation reduces bias in those selected for treatment and guarantees that treatment assignment is not based on patients' prognosis. RCTs will have eligibility criteria, but within these trials report the characteristics of the patients according to the treatment received in Table 1 of the results section. The characteristics (such as age, parity) of the two groups should not be different.

3. Were the groups treated equally?

Apart from the intervention being studied, the groups should be treated identically – differences in treatment between groups may occur if treatment allocation is known. This is called performance bias and can be minimised by standardisation of the care protocol and by 'blinding'. RCTs may blind patients, and those administering treatment, assessing outcomes and analysing the data. If they are aware of allocation, the treatment of both patient groups may differ or patients themselves may deviate from protocols because of awareness of allocation.

Detection (or measurement) bias applies to the measurement or assessment of the outcome. This should be standardised across all patients. Again, knowledge of treatment allocation may influence assessors. For an objective outcome (such as death), this may be less important, but, for outcomes that are subjective, interpretation may differ if the assessor has prior knowledge of allocation. This bias can be minimised by using objective outcomes and by ensuring that those assessing outcomes are unaware of treatment allocation. This approach is used in surgical RCTs: although the surgeon undertaking the treatment has to be aware of the treatment allocation, identical surgical dressings are used for all patients, and the assessment of recovery is done by another person who is not aware of treatment allocation.

4. Are all the patients accounted for at the conclusion?

The process of randomisation gives us comparable groups at the start of a trial, but results are valid only if we can account for all these patients at the end of the trial. Therefore, once randomised, a patient should be included in the analysis of that group even if he or she discontinues therapy, crosses over or never receives treatment. Loss of patients to follow-up or exclusion of patients from the analysis can lead to bias. Some losses may occur even in the best-quality studies, but this should not differ between groups, should be of similar types of patients and should not exceed the outcome event rate. Loss to follow-up of more than 20 per cent of recruits poses a serious threat to the validity of a study.

Intention to treat (ITT) analysis of RCTs ensures that comparisons of effects of care are made only between patients in the groups to which they were originally randomly allocated. ITT analysis includes all patients regardless of the treatment actually received or subsequent withdrawal or deviation from the protocol. Some treatments may result in large numbers of drop-outs, for example if side effects are unpleasant. Failure to account for these when examining interventions may cause false conclusions to be reached. These attritional issues are central to the generalisability of a treatment's final effect in clinical practice.

5. Are these findings important?

The analysis of RCTs is often a simple comparison of percentages. The difference in the event rate (outcome of interest) in the treatment group compared with that in the comparison group is:

Control event rate (%) – experimental event rate (%)
= absolute risk reduction or risk difference (%)

If an effect is seen in a trial, the final question is: 'Could this difference have arisen by chance?' In general, it is accepted that there is a 5 per cent chance of our concluding that there is a difference when in fact there is not – this is a 5 per cent chance of making a type 1 error, and hence we use a 95 per cent confidence interval (95% CI). Also by convention we accept an 80 per cent chance that we will detect a difference if one exists (this is the 'power' of a study). Increasing the number of patients in a study will reduce the chance of either error or increase the certainty of our estimates. The chance of these errors is also related to the size of difference we want to detect (we will need a larger study to detect a small difference between the two groups) and the frequency of the event (evaluating a very rare outcome such as occurs in 1:1000 people will need more people than an outcome that occurs in 1:100 or 1:10 people).

CIs can be calculated for this risk difference. The CI estimates the range of values likely to include the 'true' value. Usually, we use 95% CIs.

Finally, if you have a result that suggests a significant difference in outcome between two groups, you may want to consider what this means in practice. An alternative way of expressing this difference is the 'number needed to treat' (NNT). The NNT is simply 1 divided by the absolute risk reduction.

When communicating information about the benefits and risks of a treatment, a screening test is best done using natural frequencies rather than probabilities, so, for example, a 90% chance is expressed as 90 out of 100 patients or 9 out of 10 patients. It is preferable to keep the denominator constant and as small as possible.[14]

STEP 4. INTEGRATING THE EVIDENCE

In this section, we will consider how to apply evidence in clinical practice and when producing clinical guidelines. Clinical practice guidelines are defined by the Institute of Medicine as 'statements that include recommendations intended to optimise patient care, that are informed by a systematic review of evidence and an assessment of the benefits and harms of alternative care options'.[15]

Clinical decision-making can be complex. Guidelines have the potential to help clinicians and patients with complex choices, to improve the quality of care, and to help ensure the best use of limited resources.[16,17] To ensure that guidelines inform rather than misinform, it is important that they build on the best available research evidence, and make explicit and transparent value judgements that are incorporated in reaching these recommendations. A systematic review identified 40 appraisal tools for guidelines; the most well-known and validated tool is AGREE 11.[18,19]

In addition to your first filter, 'Does this paper address my clinical question?', the key features of guidelines that make an impact on their validity are:

- Guideline developers: did they include all relevant professional groups and patients?
- PICO format clinical questions, with outcomes important to patients specified
- Systematic review of the literature with explicit criteria for selecting the evidence
- A summary of the quality of the evidence – balance of risks and benefits for critical outcomes
- A clear process for moving from evidence to recommendations (e.g. using GRADE,[20] see below)
- External peer review and piloting
- Editorial independence and declaration of potential conflicts of interests of the group.

Formulating recommendations

The Grading of Recommendations Assessment, Development and Evaluation (GRADE) Working Group emphasised the link between the quality of a body of evidence and a recommendation.[20] Systematic reviews of RCTs provide high-quality evidence, but GRADE allows for factors that may reduce the assessment of quality and diminish our confidence in the findings such as:

1   RCTs within a systematic review are of poor quality so the risk of bias is increased;
2   inconsistency – heterogeneity in the findings of different studies not explained by clinical differences;
3   indirectness – any part of the PICO question may be slightly different to those in your question;

Table 1.1 A summary of the GRADE approach to grading the quality of evidence for each outcome[21]

Source of body of evidence	Initial rating of quality	Factors that may reduce the quality	Factors that may increase the quality	Final quality of a body of evidence*
RCTs or SR of RCTs	High	1. Risk of bias 2. Inconsistency 3. Indirectness 4. Imprecision	1. Large effect 2. Dose-response 3. All plausible residual confounding would reduce the demonstrated effect or would suggest a spurious effect if no effect was observed	High [⊕⊕⊕⊕ or A] Moderate [⊕⊕⊕◯ or B] Low [⊕⊕◯◯ or C)]
Observational studies	Low	5. Publication bias		Very low [⊕◯◯◯ or D]

*The final grade for quality of a body of evidence [Level of evidence] is given letters (A,B,C,D) rather than numbers (I–IV) as previously used by SIGN and RCOG. There are only two grades of recommendation: strong or weak.

4 imprecision – where studies are too underpowered to be certain of the effect size;

5 publication bias.

Observational studies start as low quality, but in some circumstances, such as when looking at evidence of adverse effects, risks or harm, our confidence may be increased where there is a large effect, or a dose–response, and/or where all plausible residual confounding would reduce the demonstrated effect or would suggest a spurious effect if no effect were observed. This is because such adverse effects should be rare events and RCTs are powered to look at benefits and are usually not large enough to provide accurate estimates for rare events.

High-quality evidence [Level I, Grade A] can be interpreted as 'further research is very unlikely to change confidence in the estimate of effect'. Moderate quality [Level II, Grade B] means that further research is likely to have an important impact on confidence in the estimate of effect and may change the estimate: this is often RCT-based evidence with limitations. Low quality [Level III, Grade C] means further research is very likely to have an important impact on confidence in the estimate of effect and is likely to change the estimate. Low-quality evidence mainly comes from observational studies. Most observational evidence will be low quality whether it comes from case–control studies, cohort studies or other forms of observation. The final category is very low [Level IV, Grade D], in which any estimate of effect is very uncertain. For each guideline question the overall quality of evidence is usually determined by the lowest quality of evidence for any of the outcomes (benefits or risks) selected. In addition, within GRADE 'expert opinion' is not considered a form of evidence but an interpretation of sometimes unsystematic evidence. RCTs may include a variety of different outcomes so the quality of evidence for each outcome in a systematic review may vary. Quality assessments for evidence on different outcomes can now be seen in Summary of Findings tables within Cochrane systematic reviews, in journals and in the evidence tables within guidelines.[8]

Within GRADE there are only two grades of recommendation: strong or weak. When there is less confidence in estimates of benefits and harms of an intervention, weaker recommendations are more likely to be made. Strong recommendations are made when it is very certain that benefits outweigh risks and costs or vice versa. A strong recommendation implies that virtually all informed patients would make the same choice. Weak recommendations are made when the benefits, risks and burdens appear to be finely balanced, or when there is appreciable uncertainty about the magnitude of benefits and risks: they imply that different values and preferences may play a crucial role in an individual's decision.

Implementation

One of the consistent findings of health services research is the gap between research evidence and practice.[23] It is a challenge for clinicians to keep up to date, but perhaps even harder is the challenge to alter established patterns of care. This can be a challenge not only for individuals, but also for the organisations they work in. If the change required is complex or involves change in the organisation and/or patients' attitudes, it is harder to achieve. There is no single strategy for getting research into practice that is sufficient on its own or significantly better than alternative strategies. Therefore a number of approaches are needed.

Research evidence is more likely to influence practice if it confirms our preconceptions.[22] In interpreting research evidence, we also need to be aware of our own biases; we are likely to be less questioning of research evidence that affirms our own beliefs or practice, while scrutinising more closely the evidence that challenges them.[23]

STEP 5. AUDIT

Research is concerned with discovering the right thing to do; audit is concerned with ensuring that the right thing is done. The purpose of clinical audit is to improve the quality of patient care and outcomes through systematic evaluation of care against explicit criteria (setting a standard of care and measuring practice against this standard) and the implementation of change (improvement where possible).[24] A review of the evidence has concluded that audit is an effective method of improving the quality of care.[25] The same review also describes the audit methods associated with successful audit projects. In the UK, the General Medical Council (GMC) requires that you demonstrate that you regularly participate in 'robust, systematic and relevant' quality improvement activity such as clinical audit or a review of clinical outcomes.

Audit may evaluate the outcome of care against an agreed standard, or the process of care, or the structure (organisation or provision) of services. For example, research evidence suggests that the outcome for patients with ovarian cancer is better if they are operated on by an appropriately subspecialty-trained gynaecological oncologist and managed within the framework of a multidisciplinary team. An audit of the referral and management of patients with ovarian cancer can provide an overview of service provision in this area.

Process measures are the 'interventions' in your PICO question: they are practices that have good-quality research evidence to show for their influence on outcomes. For example, the use of antenatal steroids has improved perinatal outcome; evaluation of this process of care would entail measuring the proportion of appropriate cases (women at risk of giving birth preterm) who received antenatal steroids.

An outcome measure (as used to develop the PICO questions above) is the physical or behavioural response to an intervention. Most interventions are carried out with the intention of improving health outcomes but they also carry the risk of adverse effects. The assessment of outcomes such as cancer survival rates, or live birth rates following IVF (in vitro fertilisation), is fundamental to measuring quality of care, but outcomes are not a direct measure of the quality of care provided. Good outcomes are more likely if the quality of care is good but are influenced by other factors such as disease stage, co-morbidity, level of education and deprivation; therefore, mechanisms to take these differences into account are required (e.g. case-mix adjustment for co-morbidity or standardised measures such as mortality ratios). Outcomes may be delayed, and not all patients who experience substandard care will have a poor outcome, but the purpose of healthcare is to improve health outcomes so outcome measures provide essential information.

When differences arise thought and care are needed to explore the possible reasons for them. It should not be assumed that poor outcomes equate to poor care;[26,27] differences in case mix and inconsistent coding can influence disease rates and adjustments. For example, the availability of hospices for palliative care will influence the number of patients receiving palliative care and the mortality rates within hospitals, and the frequency of coding for palliative care within a hospital will also have an impact. Ranking, as used in league tables, is a weak test and has not yet been shown to lead to improvements in healthcare: such tables create perverse incentives and encourage 'gaming', reducing access to care for patients with a poor prognosis and changing coding patterns. 'Critical

incident' or 'adverse event' reporting involves the identification of patients who have experienced an adverse event (e.g. to the NHS National Patient Safety Agency). Clinical activity, outcome indicators and adverse events are included in clinical dashboards such as the maternity dashboard.

Undertaking audit

Audit can be considered to have five principal steps (commonly referred to as the audit cycle):

(i)   select a topic,
(ii) identify an appropriate standard,
(iii) collect data to assess performance against the prespecified standard,
(iv) implement change to improve care, if necessary,
(v)   collect data for a second, or subsequent, time to determine whether care has improved.

It is essential to establish clear aims and objectives when choosing what to audit, so that the audit is focused towards addressing specific issues within the selected topic. A key consideration is: 'How will we use the results of this audit to change or improve practice?' Priority should be given to common health problems, areas associated with high rates of mortality, morbidity or disability, and those for which good-quality research evidence is available to inform practice (strong guideline recommendations), or aspects of care that use considerable resources. It is important to involve those who will be implementing change, those using the service and your local audit department at the planning stage. Good planning and resources are also necessary to ensure their success.

In audit, review criteria are generally used for assessing care. The criterion is the reference point against which current practice is measured. The first four steps above should be the starting point for developing criteria. Audit standards are often included in clinical guidelines. Review criteria should be explicit rather than implicit and need to lead to valid judgements about the quality of care, and relate to aspects of care that are important to patients or impact on clinical outcomes. The standard/target level of performance is defined as 'the percentage of events that should comply with the criterion' (e.g. the proportion of women delivered by caesarean section who received thromboprophylaxis, or the proportion of women with dysfunctional uterine bleeding who were offered endometrial ablation). 'Benchmarking' is defined as 'the process of defining a level of care set as a goal to be attained', such as used to define levels within clinical dashboards. There is insufficient evidence to determine whether it is necessary to set target levels of performance in audit.

Data collection

Data collection in criterion-based audit is generally undertaken to determine the proportion of cases in which care is in accordance with the criteria. In practice, the following points need to be considered. The methods of data collection, data handling and analysis described here for audit could also be used for a research project.

Consideration needs to be given to which data items are needed in order to answer the audit question. For example, if undertaking an audit on caesarean section (CS) rates, collecting information on the number of caesarean sections alone will not give sufficient information to measure the CS rate. Data on the number of other births that took place are also required, and in addition factors that may influence the likelihood of CS are needed, such as maternal age, parity, and previous CS. The availability of data-sets and the data items within sets is a key consideration. Many data-sets classify disease using ICD-10 codes and treatments using OPCS-4 co-morbidity (patients' other diagnostic or treatment) codes. Clarity about the codes to be used is needed; for example, if collecting data on rupture of membranes, you may need to specify whether this is spontaneous or artificial.

Data handlers should always be aware of their responsibilities to the Data Protection Act 1998. Data in obstetrics and gynaecology are likely to be personal, with identifiers such as name, date of birth (DOB) and address, confidential and sensitive. Consent is required for data sharing. Anonymisation (using a computer program) and restricting access (encryption and password protection) to data is good practice to protect integrity. It is an offence to collect personal data of an individual without consent. Personal information such as age, ethnicity and postcode may enable factors that influence healthcare to be taken into account when interpreting findings such as deprivation. There has been consensus that clinical audit is part of direct patient care (assessing care and improving quality) and therefore consent to the use of data for audit can be implied through consent to treatment, if patients are informed that their data may be used in this way. It is not generally acceptable to use patient identifiers such as names and addresses, but some form of pseudo-anonymised identifiers (NHS number, DOB, postcode) may be used. However, current plans by NHS England to link data-sets (general practice to Hospital Episode Statistics [HES] care data) using pseudo-anonymous data have been delayed because of concerns (presumed consent for data sharing, the sensitive nature of information and the risk of identification). Audit (measuring practice against an agreed standard) does not need Research Ethics Committee approval. Aggregate data for providers is published by the NHS but application and approval are required for individual data or linking data-sets.

Routinely collected data should be used where possible, if the data items required are available and the completeness and coverage are known to be satisfactory. Where the data source is clinical records, training data abstractors and the use of a standard pro forma can improve the accuracy and reliability of data collection. The use of multiple sources of data may also be helpful, but this can also be problematic as it will require linking of data from different sources with common unique identifiers.

Designing data collection tools and questionnaires

Questionnaires are often used as a tool for data collection. Questions may be open or closed. Generally, questionnaire design using open questions (e.g. 'What was the indication for caesarean section?' followed by space for free text response) is easier, but analysis of these data is difficult, as there will be a range of responses, and interpretation can be problematic. Open questions may be more difficult and time-consuming for respondents to answer and can lead to non-response, resulting in loss of data.

Questionnaires can be composed entirely of closed questions (i.e. with all possible answers predetermined). More time needs to be spent in developing this type of questionnaire, but the analysis is generally easier. The following is an example of this.[28]

'Which of the following statements most accurately describes the urgency of this caesarean section?

A   Immediate threat to the life of the fetus and the mother.
B   Maternal or fetal compromise that is not immediately life threatening.
C   No maternal or fetal compromise but needs early delivery.
D   Delivery timed to suit the woman and staff.'

Closed questions assume that all possible answers to the question are known but not the distribution of responses. Time and consideration need to be given to the options available for response because, if a desired response is not available, the question may just be missed out, it may put people off completing the rest of the questionnaire or they may tick an available but inaccurate category. The 'other' category can be used with the option 'please specify', which gives an opportunity for the respondent to write in a response. If this is used, however, thought must be given beforehand as to how these free text responses will be coded and analysed. In some situations, not having an 'other' category may lead to the question not being answered at all, which means data will be lost.

If questionnaires are developed for a specific project, they need to be piloted and refined to ensure their validity and reliability before use as a tool for data collection. Whilst those who developed the questionnaire understand the questions being asked, the aim of piloting is to check that those who have to fill in the questionnaire are able to understand and respond with ease. Questionnaires that are not user friendly are associated with lower response rates and the quality of data collected will be poor, hence the results will be of little value. Thought also needs to be given to how the data are going to be collected and by whom, as well as to the time and resources that will be involved.

Analysing the data

When data from an existing source are used, the formats and compatibility of software need to be checked. Data can be transferred using statistical transfer software but this can introduce errors and so data must be checked after transfer. Data that are collected on paper forms are usually entered on to electronic databases or spreadsheets such as Microsoft Access, Epi Info or Excel for cleaning and analysis. Data entry may be done by Optical Character Recognition (OCR) software, Optical Mark Readers (OMR) or manually. OCR is most accurate for questionnaire data using tick boxes but less accurate for free text responses. The method of data entry needs to be taken into account when designing the questionnaire or data collection sheet. For manual data entry, accuracy is improved if double data entry is used, but this can be a time-consuming exercise. If the facilities and resources are available, electronic collection of data can be considered. In this case, data are entered immediately at source into a computer and saved on to disks. Whilst this is quick and requires minimal storage space, it can be difficult to handle unexpected responses. As information is entered directly into a computer, it cannot be verified or double entered.

Consideration also needs to be given to the coding of responses on the database. For ease of analysis of closed questions, it is generally better to have numerical codes for responses. For example, yes/no responses can be coded to take the value 0 for no and 1 for yes. Missing data will also need to be coded, for example with the number 9. The code assigned for missing data should be distinguished from the code used when the response is 'not known' (if this was an option on the questionnaire). To minimise errors, it is advisable to incorporate consistency checks as data are being entered.

Simple statistics are often all that is required. Statistical methods are used to summarise data for presentation in the form of summary statistics (means, medians or percentages) and graphs. Statistical tests are used to find out the likelihood that the data obtained have arisen by chance, and how likely it is that a real difference exists between two groups. Before data collection has started, it is essential to know what data items will be collected, whether comparisons will be made, and the statistical methods that will be used to make these comparisons.[18]

Data items that have categorical responses (e.g. yes/no or A/B/C/D) can be expressed as percentages. Some data items are collected as continuous variables, for example mother's age, height and weight. Either these can be categorised into relevant categories and then expressed as percentages or, if they are normally distributed (bell-shaped curve), the mean and standard deviations may be reported. If they are not normally distributed, a median and range can be used. These summary statistics (percentages and means) are useful for describing the process, outcome or service provision that was measured.

Comparisons of percentages between different groups can be made using a x^2 test; t-tests can be used to compare means between two groups, assuming these are normally distributed. Non-parametric statistical methods can be used for data that are non-normally distributed. These comparisons are useful in order to determine if there are any real differences in the observed findings, for example when comparing audit results obtained at different time points or in different settings. In some situations, a sample size calculation may be necessary to ensure that the audit is large enough to detect a clinically significant difference between groups if one exists. In this situation, it is important to consult a statistician during the planning stages of the audit project. These simple statistics can be easily done on Microsoft Excel spreadsheets and Access databases. Other useful statistical software packages include Epi Info, SAS, SPSS, STATA and Minitab.

Implementation of findings

Data analysis and interpretation will lead to the identification of areas of clinical practice that need to change. Several methods may be needed to ensure this change takes place, but simple strategies such as feeding back findings are sometimes effective. Change does not always occur in audit, and consideration of the reasons for failure may take place after the second data collection. Resistance to change among local professionals or in the organisational environment or team should be considered. Patients themselves may have preferences for care that make change difficult.

ACKNOWLEDGEMENT

This chapter was written for the first edition of the book by Fiona M. Reid and Anthony R.B. Smith. It has been updated for both second and third editions by Fiona M. Reid.

GLOSSARY OF TERMS

Auditable standard An agreed standard against which practice can be assessed.

Case–control study The study reviews exposures or risk factors, comparing the exposure in people who have the outcome of interest, for example the disease or condition (i.e. the cases), with patients from the same population who do not have the outcome (i.e. controls).

Cohort study The study involves the identification of two groups (cohorts) of patients, one of which has received the exposure of interest and one of which has not. These groups are followed forward to see if they develop the outcome (i.e. the disease or condition) of interest.

Confounder A factor that may offer an alternative explanation for the observed association between an exposure and the outcome of interest.

Cross-sectional study The observation of a defined population at a single point in time or time interval. Exposure and outcome are determined simultaneously.

Denominator data Data describing the population within which a study group has been identified (e.g. in a hospital study of caesarean section the denominator data refer to every birth that occurred within the unit during the audited period, irrespective of the type of delivery that was undertaken).

HES Hospital Episode Statistics To receive payment for care delivered, every NHS hospital in England must submit information about activity including admissions, outpatient appointments and A&E attendances. Each HES episode contains a wide range of information, including:

- clinical information about diagnoses and operations (as ICD10 and OPCS-4 codes)
- information about the patient, such as age group, gender and ethnicity (demographics)
- administrative information, such as time waited, and dates and methods of admission and discharge
- geographical information such as where patients are treated and the area where they live.

It contains admitted patient care data from 1989 onwards, outpatient attendance data from 2003 onwards and A&E data from 2007 onwards. The HSCIC (Health and social care infromation centre) provides data, IT and information for the NHS. It publishes aggregated data and synthesised information. The NHS can access data for quality improvement activity. The primary purpose of HES is administrative, the quality of the data has been critised but it has been used in research and audit (eg by the RCOG). The sale of the information has raised concerns about confidentiality and data protection. Plans to merge it with GP datasets in care.data are currently stalled. If anonymised population data is invaluable for research and is available in Scotland and much of Scandinavia.

ICD10 = ICD-10 is the 10th revision of the International Statistical Classification of Diseases and Related Health Problems (ICD), a medical classification list by the World Health Organization (WHO). It contains codes for diseases, signs and symptoms, abnormal findings, complaints, social circumstances, and external causes of injury or diseases. ICD-10 was first mandated for use in the UK in 1995. The ICD-10 4th Edition was approved for NHS implementation on 1 April 2012 by the Information Standards Board for Health and Social Care.

Mean This is the summary statistic used when the data follow a normal distribution. It is the sum of all the values divided by the number of values. The standard deviation gives a measure of the spread of individual values about the mean.

Median If the data are arranged in an increasing order, the middle value is the median. The range is the difference between the largest and smallest values. The interquartile range (IQR) is the difference between the bottom quarter and top quarter of the data. This is the summary statistic used when the data are not normally distributed.

Meta-analysis An overview of a group of studies that uses quantitative methods to produce a summary of the results.

Number needed to treat This is the number of patients who need to be treated to prevent one outcome.

Odds ratio This describes the odds that a case (a person with the condition) has been exposed to a risk factor relative to the odds that a control (a person without the condition) has been exposed to the risk. The crude odds ratio describes the association without taking into consideration the possible effect of any confounders. Adjusted odds ratios describe the association having been adjusted for the effect of confounders.

OPCS-4 an alphanumeric nomenclature, with a 4 character code system similar to that found in ICD-10, but OPCS-4 classifies procedures and interventions, rather than diagnoses. It is used throughout the NHS in the UK to codify procedures and interventions performed during in-patient stays, day case surgery and some out-patient treatments. It is based on the earlier Office of Population Censuses and Surveys Classification of Surgical Operations and Procedures (4th revision), it retains the OPCS abbreviation from this now defunct publication.

Positive predictive value This describes the percentage of people who have a positive test who really have the condition. The predictive value is dependent upon the prevalence of the disease in the population being tested, i.e. if the disease is rare, the predictive value is low, due to the greater influence of false-positive tests.

Power The chance that we will detect a difference if one exists; by convention this is often set at an 80 per cent chance that we will detect a difference if one exists. Power is increased with an increased study size and reduced with a smaller study.

Randomised controlled trial A group of patients is randomised into an experimental group and a control group. These groups are followed up for the variables and outcomes of interest. This study is similar to a cohort study, but the exposure is randomly assigned. Randomisation should ensure that both groups are equivalent in all aspects except for the exposure of interest.

Risk difference The difference in risk of developing the outcome of interest between the exposed and control groups.

Risk ratio Risk is a proportion or percentage. The risk ratio is the ratio of risk of developing the outcome of interest in an exposed group compared with the risk of developing the same outcome in the control group. It is used in RCTs and cohort studies.

Sensitivity The ability of a test to detect those who have the disease, i.e. the proportion (percentage) of people with the condition who are detected as having it by the test.

Specificity The ability of the test to identify those without the disease, i.e. the proportion of people without the condition who are correctly reassured by a negative test.

Systematic review (SR) A literature review that aims to minimise bias and random errors by using a system that is documented in a materials and methods section, and which may or may not include meta-analysis.

Key References

1. Guyatt GH. Evidence-based medicine. *ACP J Club* March/April 1991;A-16.
2. Smith R, Rennie D. Evidence-based medicine–an oral history. *JAMA* 2014;311:365–7.
3. Evans I, Thornton H, Chalmers I, Glasziou P. *Testing Treatments, Evidence-based Medicines 2nd edn. Better Research for Better Healthcare,* London: Pinter & Martin, 2011. Available for free download from several sites including http://www.jameslindlibrary.org/.

4. Chalmers I, Enkin M, Keirse MJNC. *Effective Care in Pregnancy and Childbirth*. Oxford: Oxford University Press; 1989.

5. Goldacre B. *Bad Science* Published 2008 and *Bad Pharma* Published 2012, London: Fourth Estate. Available from: http://www.badscience.net/

6. Sackett DL, Straus S, Scott Richardson W, Rosenburg W, Haynes RB. *How to Practise and Teach Evidence-Based Medicine*, 2nd ed. London: Churchill Livingstone, 2000.

7. Jackson R. EPIQ (Effective Practice, Informatics and Quality Improvement). <http://www.fmhs.auckland.ac.nz/soph/depts/epi/epiq/ebp.aspx>.

8. Higgins JPT, Green S (editors). *Cochrane Handbook for Systematic Reviews of Interventions* Version 5.1.0 [updated March 2011]. The Cochrane Collaboration, 2011. Available free from www.cochrane-handbook.org.

9. Liberati A, Altman DG, Tetzlaff J, Mulrow C, Gøtzsche PC, *et al*. The PRISMA statement for reporting systematic reviews and meta-analyses of studies that evaluate health care interventions: explanation and elaboration. *PLoS Med* 2009;6(7):e1000100.

10. Schulz KF, Altman DG, Moher D, for the CONSORT Group. CONSORT 2010 Statement: updated guidelines for reporting parallel group randomised trials. *BMJ* 2010;340:698-702.

11. Bossuyt PM, Reitsma JB, Bruns DE, *et al*. The STARD initiative: Standards for Reporting of Diagnostic Accuracy. Toward complete and accurate reporting of studies of diagnostic accuracy. *BMJ* 2003;326:41–4.

12. von Elm E, Altman DG, Egger M, Pocock SJ, Gøtzsche PC, Vandenbroucke JP. STROBE Initiative. The Strengthening the Reporting of Observational Studies in Epidemiology (STROBE) statement: guidelines for reporting observational studies. *PLoS Med* 2007;4:e296.

13. Khan KS, Kuntz R, Kleijnen J, Antes G. *Systematic Reviews to Support Evidence-Based Medicine. How to Review and Apply Findings of Healthcare Research*. London: Royal Society of Medicine Press, 2003.

14. Gigerenzer G. What are natural frequencies? Doctors need to find better ways to communicate risk to patients. *BMJ* 2011;343:d6386 and Making sense of health statistics. *Bull World Health Organ* 2009;87:567 (uses example MRHA COCP risks). http://www.tedxzurich.com/speaker/gerd-gigerenzer/.

15. IOM (Institute of Medicine). *Clinical Practice Guidelines We Can Trust*. Washington DC: The National Academies Press, 2011.

16. Grimshaw J, Eccles M, Tetroe J. Implementing clinical guidelines: current evidence and future implications. *J Contin Educ Health Prof* 2004;24(Suppl 1):S31–7.

17. Grimshaw JM, Thomas RE, MacLennan G, Fraser C, Ramsay CR, *et al*. Effectiveness and efficiency of guideline dissemination and implementation strategies. *Health Technol Assess* 2004;8(6):iii–iiv, 1–72.

18. Brouwers M, Kho ME, Browman GP, *et al*. for the AGREE Next Steps Consortium. AGREE II: Advancing guideline development, reporting and evaluation in healthcare. *Can Med Assoc J* 2010;182:E839–42. http://www.agreetrust.org/.

19. Siering U, Eikermann M, Hausner E, Hoffmann-Eßer W, Neugebauer EA. Appraisal tools for clinical practice guidelines: a systematic review. *PLoS ONE* 2013;8(12):e82915.

20. Guyatt GH, Oxman AD, Vist G, *et al*. for the GRADE Working Group. GRADE: an emerging consensus on rating quality of evidence and strength of recommendations. *BMJ* 2008;336:924–6.

21. Woolf S, Schünemann HJ, Eccles M, Grimshaw J, Shekelle P. Developing clinical practice guidelines: types of evidence and outcomes; values and economics, synthesis, grading, and presentation and deriving recommendations. *Implementat Sci* 2012;7:61.

22. Kaptchuk EJ. Effect of interpretive bias on research evidence. *BMJ* 2003;326:1453–5.

23. Grol R, Grimshaw J. From best evidence to best practice: effective implementation of change in patients' care. *Lancet* 2003;362:1225–30.

24. Royal College of Obstetricians and Gynaecologists. *Understanding Audit*. Clinical Governance Advice No. 5. London: RCOG Press, 2003.

25. NHS, National Institute for Clinical Excellence, Commission for Health Improvement, Royal College of Nursing, University of Leicester. *Review of the Evidence. Principles for Best Practice in Clinical Audit*. London: NICE, 2002.

26. Lilford R, Mohammed MA, Spiegelhalter D, Thomson R. Use and misuse of process and outcome data in managing performance of acute medical care: avoiding institutional stigma. *Lancet* 2004;363:1147–54.

27. Spiegelhalter D. Have there been 13 000 needless deaths at 14 NHS trusts? *BMJ* 2013;347:f4893.

28. Thomas J, Paranjothy S, and Royal College of Obstetricians and Gynaecologists: Clinical Effectiveness Support Unit. *The National Sentinel Caesarean Section Audit Report*. London: RCOG Press, 2001.

Online resources: look for talks/websites by organisations (Cochrane, BMJ) and the authors Ben Goldacre, David Spiegelhalter, Gerd Gigerenzer, Amanda Burls and Hans Rosling.

Chapter 2 The general principles of surgery

Fiona M Reid

INTRODUCTION

'Choose well, cut well, get well.' Surgery has three phases. In the preoperative phase, the correct operation should be chosen for a patient, who should be in an optimal condition. A well-trained, competent surgeon should then perform the surgery in a safe environment. During the postoperative phase, the patient should be monitored, encouraged and advised. Each phase is equally important. These are the basic principles of surgery, and this chapter examines how they may be achieved.

THE PREOPERATIVE PHASE

There is always more than one treatment option and it is the role of a gynaecologist to counsel the patient about the appropriate options. The process of selecting the best procedure for a patient is inseparable from that of obtaining informed consent. A booklet of guidelines to obtaining consent is available from the General Medical Council or on the internet at www.gmc-uk.org.

When counselling patients about treatment options, effective communication is imperative. This may necessitate the use of written material or visual aids. It may require the use of interpreters for foreign or sign language. Preferably, interpreters should be independent professionals and not family members, who could have a vested interest in a particular treatment.

Patients should be informed of the advantages and disadvantages of each procedure, the success rates, failure rates, side effects and common complications. Risk should be quantified rather than being described subjectively with terms such as 'slight' or 'rare'.

Increasingly, the adequacy of consent is assessed legally by the concept of 'material risk'. A risk is material if:

In the circumstances of the case, a reasonable person in the patient's position, if warned of the risk, would be likely to attach significance to it or if the medical practitioner is, or should reasonably be, aware that the particular patient, if warned of the risk, would be likely to attach significance to it.[1]

In practice, this implies that even rare complications that are serious or that carry significance to an individual's social life or employment should be addressed.

Patients should have adequate time to reflect on the information they have been given prior to making a decision. It should not be assumed that a patient understands the general risks of surgery such as anaesthetic complications.

The General Medical Council's guidelines on informed consent state that ultimately it is the responsibility of the person performing the procedure to ensure informed consent has been obtained.

Optimising preoperative health

Although most gynaecological surgery is performed on relatively healthy women, it is imperative that all patients undergoing surgery are in their optimum condition. Smokers should be encouraged to stop at least 24 hours before surgery to reduce the level of carboxyhaemoglobin in the blood and minimise the cardiovascular effect of nicotine.[2] Screening for sexually transmitted infections or bacterial vaginosis prior to pelvic procedures should be considered.[3]

Basic preoperative screening involves a detailed history and a general examination. Routine screening blood tests have not been shown to influence cancellations or perioperative complications, and the majority of abnormal results could have been predicted from the history and examination.[4] A study by Golub *et al.*[5] in the USA demonstrated that avoiding batteries of routine preoperative tests could save US$397 per patient.

Ideally, preoperative investigations should be specific to each individual. Even routine sickle testing of at-risk adults has been challenged because patients with sickle cell disease would already have been detected as children due to chronic haemolytic anaemia. Also no sickling complications have been reported in sickle cell trait patients for the past 15 years.[6]

The morbidity and mortality of surgery and anaesthesia are increased in patients with coexisting disease (Box 2.1).[7]

Elective surgery should be delayed for 6 months after a myocardial infarct because 35 per cent will re-infarct before 3 months and this risk falls to 4 per cent after 6 months.[8] Of the deaths reported in the National Confidential Enquiries into Perioperative Deaths (CEPOD) Report 2001, 60 per cent of patients had ischaemic heart disease.[9] The history is as important as the investigations: a preoperative electrocardiogram

Box 2.1 Medical conditions most commonly associated with increased surgical morbidity

Ischaemic heart disease

Congestive cardiac failure

Arterial hypertension

Chronic respiratory disease

Diabetes mellitus

Cardiac arrhythmia

Anaemia

Box 2.2 The American Society of Anesthesiologists' (ASA) physical status classification system

ASA 1 Normal healthy patient

ASA 2 Patient with mild controlled systemic disease which does not affect normal activity

ASA 3 Patient with severe systemic disease which limits activity

ASA 4 Patient with severe systemic disease which is incapacitating and a constant threat to life

ASA 5 Moribund patient not expected to survive 24 hours with or without operation

Box 2.3 Patient-related risk factors of venous thromboembolism

Active cancer or cancer treatment

Age over 60 years

Critical care admission

Dehydration

Known thrombophilias

Obesity (BMI >30 kg/m^2)

One or more significant medical co-morbidities (e.g. heart disease; metabolic, endocrine or respiratory pathologies; acute infections; inflammatory conditions)

Use of HRT

Use of oestrogen-containing contraceptive therapy

Personal or first-degree relative with a history of VTE

Pregnancy or up to 6 weeks postpartum

Use of oral contraception or hormone replacement therapy (HRT)

Varicose veins with phlebitis

Table 2.1 Risk factors for venous thromboembolism (VTE)

Medical admissions	If mobility significantly reduced for ≥3 days **OR**
	If expected to have ongoing reduced mobility relative to normal state plus any VTE risk factor
Surgical admissions	If total anaesthetic + surgical time >90 minutes **or**
	If surgery involves pelvis or lower limb and total anaesthetic + surgical time >60 minutes **or**
	If acute surgical admission with inflammatory or intra-abdominal condition **or**
	If expected to have significant reduction in mobility **or**
	If any VTE risk factor present

(ECG) on patients with proven ischaemia will be normal in 20–50 per cent of cases.[10]

Protocols should be available on the ward for the management of common conditions such as diabetes mellitus.

It is the surgeon's responsibility to liaise with the anaesthetist and other specialties if patients have concurrent illness. At times it can be difficult to convey the complexity of a patient's condition, and the American Society of Anesthesiologists' (ASA) scoring system[11] can be a useful communication tool (Box 2.2).

Venous thrombosis embolism (VTE) is one of the most serious complications of surgery. An estimated 25,000 people in the UK die from preventable hospital-acquired VTE every year. The 2010 NICE guidance CG92[12] recommends that the risk of thromboembolism should be assessed in all hospital patients. All units should have clear protocols for thromboprophylaxis. Risk factors for thrombosis are shown in Box 2.3. A risk assessment is summarised in Table 2.1. Thromboprophylaxis should be prescribed after considering the balance of risk of bleeding and risk of VTE. Flow charts for specific clinical scenarios can be found on the NICE website for CG92 (www.NICE.org.uk). This includes continuing VTE prophylaxis for 28 days following major gynaecology procedures.

The Department of Health has recommended that all patients undergoing elective surgery should be screened preoperatively for meticillin-resistant *Staphylococcus aureus* (MRSA). All patients with positive skin screen for MRSA should undergo skin decolonisation therapy with a recommended skin wash. For procedures that require antibiotic prophylaxis patients with current or previous MRSA colonisation should receive teicoplanin or vancomycin intravenously.

Over the last 10 years enhanced recovery programmes (ERPs) which started in colorectal surgery have spread to gynaecology. A recent systematic review of 5099 patients in 38 trials found ERPs reduced the length of stay and reduced the risk of all complications within 30 days.[13]

There are four elements to the enhanced recovery programme:

1 Preoperative assessment, planning and preparation before admission;
2 Reducing the physical stress of the operation;
3 A structured approach to immediate postoperative management including pain relief;
4 Early mobilisation.

KEY POINTS

Consent

Selecting the best procedure is inseparable from gaining informed consent.

It is the operator's responsibility to ensure that informed consent has been obtained.

Effective communication is imperative: interpreters or visual aids may be necessary.

Patients should receive detailed information on benefits and risks.

Patients should have adequate time to reflect on this information.

Optimising preoperative health

Smoking should be stopped 24 hours before surgery.

Combined oral contraceptives should be stopped 1 month before major surgery.

Preoperative screening should be by history and examination; routine blood tests are rarely helpful.

Routine surgery should be delayed for 6 months after myocardial infarction.

If there is concurrent illness, liaison with the anaesthetist and other specialists is essential.

All units should have clear protocols for thromboprophylaxis.

All patients undergoing elective surgery should be screened for MRSA.

INTRAOPERATIVE CARE

A full knowledge of abdominal and pelvic anatomy is essential for gynaecological surgery. In cases in which the anatomy is distorted, the surgeon should attempt to restore normal anatomy and work from first principles. Tissue planes should be utilised and tissues should be handled gently. Many gynaecologists gain most of their early surgical experience in the obstetric theatre, where speed tends to be valued above all else. Technique should be valued above speed.

Adequate access is essential. A senior surgeon called to a difficult case often first improves access. This includes good bowel packing.

Asepsis is obviously important, but some aseptic practices are traditions and are not based on evidence. Preoperative shaving, for example, is aesthetic to the surgeon and allows for the painless removal of the dressing postoperatively, but it does not appear to alter wound infection rates.[14] The use of a single dose of prophylactic antibiotics to prevent wound infection or septicaemia is now widely accepted.[15] However, prolonged courses of antibiotics or use of unnecessary antibiotics should be avoided due to the risk of *Clostridium difficile* infection.

NICE has published guidance stating antimicrobial prophylaxis against infective endocarditis is not required in patients undergoing urological, gynaecological and obstetric procedures where infection is not already present.[16]

Box 2.4 Adults at risk of infective endocarditis

Acquired valvular heart disease

Valve replacement

Structural congenital heart disease including surgically corrected defects but excluding isolated atrial septal defects, fully repaired ventricular septal defects or fully repaired patent ductus arteriosus, and closed devices that are judged to be epithelialised

Hypertrophic cardiomyopathy

Previous infective endocarditis

If infection is present then patients at high risk of endocarditis should receive antibiotics to cover the organisms that cause infective endocarditis. Patients considered to be at risk of infective endocarditis are shown in Box 2.4.

Facemasks in general abdominal surgery and certainly in laparoscopic procedures do not appear to affect infection rates. However, eye protection or face shields to protect the surgeon's mucous membranes from the patient's bodily fluids are sensible. Without serum testing it is impossible to know if a patient has hepatitis or human immunodeficiency virus (HIV) and therefore all patients are a potential risk. All healthcare workers should be immunised against hepatitis B. Cotton gowns provide protection of one's nakedness only!

Drains may be used if clinically indicated and not as an alternative to good haemostasis. There is no robust evidence to support their use. A drain is probably advisable when a urinary tract injury has been repaired, in case of urinary leakage. Possible complications of drains include trauma during insertion, blockage, infection, erosion of adjacent tissue and retention of a foreign body.

TECHNICAL EQUIPMENT FOR SURGERY

Surgeons should have an understanding of the principles of the equipment they use.

Diathermy (electrocautery) involves the passage of electrical current through the patient's body. Electrocution does not occur because the frequency of current used in diathermy is much higher than that of mains electricity. Mains electricity is a low-frequency alternating current (50 Hz in the UK). Low-frequency currents cause depolarisation and neuromuscular stimulation. Diathermy utilises a very-high-frequency (400 kHz to 10 MHz) alternating current. It does not cause depolarisation but it does excite ions, and this causes heat, particularly when in a high-density form.

In monopolar diathermy, the active electrodes and the return electrode are some distance apart. In bipolar diathermy, the two electrodes are only millimetres apart.

Factors that influence the diathermy effect are current density, the resistance of the tissue, the waveform and the duration of activation.

At high current density, heat is produced. The size of the electrode influences current density. At the tip of an active electrode the current density is high, and therefore heat is generated. The return electrode's surface area is large, so the current density is low and no heating occurs.

The resistance of tissues is indirectly proportional to their water content: higher water content reduces resistance. Tissues with high resistance require a higher output (watts), from the diathermy generator, to generate heat.

Cutting is achieved by using a low-voltage but high-frequency current that is constantly flowing. The current is concentrated in a very small area and the high energy level causes so much ion excitation that the cells explode, releasing steam. If coagulation is required, an intermittent high-voltage current is used, with current flowing for only 6 per cent of the time. Thus a cutting current is inherently safer because of the lower voltage reducing the risk of inadvertent current discharge.

The safety of diathermy systems is continually improving. Initially, grounded generators were used, whereby current could return to ground via the path of least resistance. Since 1968, solid-state isolated generators have been used. These avoid burns at other sites such as drip stands because current will not flow unless current is returning to the generator. However, return electrode burns can still occur if the pad is not attached completely. Systems of contact quality monitoring have been available since the 1980s to prevent return electrode burns.

There are some specific hazards related to electrosurgery in laparoscopic procedures.

Direct coupling is the inadvertent flow of current from one instrument to another and may be secondary to insulation failure. Insulation failure can result from damaged equipment or the use of excessive voltage with coagulation current. Capacitance coupling can occur if a capacitor is created. Two conductors separated by an insulator form a capacitor, for example an insulated laparoscopic instrument passing through a metal port. The current stored in the capacitor can discharge into the patient, causing burns. The higher the current passing through the instrument, the greater will be the capacitance current. Plastic ports do not eliminate the risk of capacitance coupling because the patient's bowel or omentum can act as the second conductor. Capacitance coupling can be avoided with active electrode monitoring systems.

Other causes of diathermy burns are careless technique, not checking the dial setting before use, the use of spirit-based skin preparation near diathermy, or someone other than the surgeon activating the current flow.

Diathermy is the most commonly used energy source for tissue dissection and haemostasis, but others are used. These include ultrasonic energy (Harmonic Scalpel – HS) and laser (light amplification by stimulated emission of radiation). In the HS electrical energy is supplied to a piezoelectric ceramic element that expands and contracts rapidly (55,500 Hz). The ultrasonic energy mechanically breaks hydrogen bonds leading to protein denaturation and coagulation. The advantages of HS are lower temperatures, no current flow, no smoke or tissue charring, very little vapour and less lateral spread.

Two laser systems established themselves in gynaecological practice during the 1980s: carbon dioxide laser and the neodymium:yttrium–aluminium–garnet (Nd:YAG) laser. Both require specialised training.

KEY POINTS

Technique should be valued above speed.
Adequate access is essential.
Asepsis is important but some practices are not evidence based.
Single-dose antibiotic prophylaxis is now widely accepted.
All patients are a potential risk and all healthcare workers should be immunised against hepatitis B.
Drains should be used only when clinically indicated.
Surgeons should understand the principles of the equipment they use: this applies particularly to diathermy.

Minimal access surgery

Diseases that harm call for treatments that harm less.

William Osler (1849–1919)

The most common endoscopic techniques used in gynaecology are laparoscopy and hysteroscopy.

Laparoscopy

The possible benefits of laparoscopy are shown in Box 2.5. Many of these purported benefits have not undergone robust analysis. In a randomised trial of open versus laparoscopic colposuspension, in which the patients were blinded to the type of surgery, there was no significant difference in the length of hospital stay, but the laparoscopic group returned to normal activities significantly earlier than the open group.[17]

Many complications specific to laparoscopic surgery are related to the method of entry into the peritoneal cavity. The risk is as great for a diagnostic laparoscopy as it is for a

Box 2.5 Benefits of laparoscopy

Patients
Less pain[17]
Less blood loss[17,18]
Less scarring
Faster recovery[17]
Surgeon
Safer 'closed/no touch surgery'
Better display of anatomy
Healthcare providers
Reduced inpatient stay
Reduced social cost

major operative laparoscopic procedure. The risk of bowel injury is 0.4–3 per 1000 and of vascular injury 0.2–1 per 1000 laparoscopies.[19] Bowel adhesions to the anterior abdominal wall occur in 0.5 per cent of patients with no previous surgery, increasing to 20 per cent if they have had a previous pfannenstiel incision and to 50 per cent if they have had a midline incision.[20] To minimise this risk, safe entry techniques have been recommended (Box 2.6). Open laparoscopy has been advocated, particularly by general surgeons, because it appears to reduce the risk of vascular injury, but it does not reduce the risk of bowel injury. Microlaparoscopy at Palmers' point can also be used. Published recommendations on safe entry are formed from expert opinion,[19] [E] not clinical trials, because the number of subjects required to perform trials to investigate entry techniques is prohibitively large.

Hysteroscopy

This common procedure has specific safety issues. Distension media for hysteroscopy include carbon dioxide, 0.9% saline or glycine. Water is not used as a distension medium because it is hypo-osmolar and, once absorbed, causes haemolysis.

If intrauterine electrosurgery is to be performed using monopolar equipment, the solution must be non-conductive so that the electrical current is not dissipated. Solutions containing electrolytes can be used with recently developed bipolar electrosurgery equipment.

The complications of hysteroscopy include uterine perforation and fluid absorption. Uterine perforation can be associated with damage to the bowel or intraperitoneal haemorrhage. A high index of suspicion and early recourse to diagnostic laparoscopy are advisable.

Fluid may be absorbed at the time of hysteroscopy. If excessive, it can result in hyponatraemia and hypo-osmolality, clinically characterised by nausea, vomiting, seizures, coma and even death. The amount of fluid absorbed is dependent on the volume infused and the infusion pressure. Owing to the short duration of a diagnostic procedure, excessive fluid retention is unlikely to be a problem.

Large-volume fluid absorption is most likely when large vessels are opened at endometrial resection. The main precaution to avoid excessive absorption is accurate measurement of the fluid deficit throughout the procedure.

Fluid absorption increases significantly when the intrauterine pressure exceeds the mean arterial pressure (MAP). When gravity (the height of the bag) is used to drive the fluid, the lowest pressure (height) to distend the cavity should be used. It should not exceed the MAP. If the giving set contains a drip chamber, the height of the fluid is taken from the drip chamber, but, if this fills, the pressure is calculated from the fluid level in the bag.

KEY POINTS

Laparoscopy

Many of the purported benefits have not undergone robust analysis.

Many of the complications relate to the method of entry into the peritoneal cavity: safe entry techniques, formed from expert opinion, have been published [E].

Hysteroscopy

Non-conducting distension media must be used for intrauterine electrosurgery with monopolar equipment.

Uterine perforation may occur: a high index of suspicion is needed, with early recourse to laparoscopy.

Excessive fluid absorption may lead to seizures and even death. Accurate measurement of fluid deficit is needed throughout the procedure.

Local anaesthetic

Two common complications to consider when using local anaesthetic are systemic toxicity and delayed haemorrhage if it is combined with adrenaline. The duration of action and safe dosages are shown in Table 2.2.

Initial symptoms of toxicity are perioral paraesthesiae, tinnitus or visual disturbance. These may be followed by convulsions or cardiotoxicity, arrhythmia, complete heart block or cardiac arrest.

Sedation

A trained doctor should administer sedation. This doctor should be responsible only for administering the sedation and

Box 2.6 A safe entry technique for laparoscopy

The patient should be lying flat
Ensure the bladder is empty and check the abdomen for masses
Make the primary incision at the base of the umbilicus
Insert the Veress needle through the base of the umbilicus, sensing a double click
Insert 2–3 mL of saline through the Veress; it should run in freely
Aspirate back: nothing should be aspirated
Fill with CO_2 to a pressure of 25 mmHg
Repeat the saline test
Insert the primary trocar

Table 2.2 Properties of local anaesthetic agents

Agent	Duration of action (hours)	Maximum dosage	
		Plain solution	**With adrenaline**
Lidocaine	1–3	3	7
Bupivacaine	1–4	2	2
Prilocaine	1–3	4	8

cardiorespiratory monitoring. He or she should not perform the surgery.

The objective is to produce a level of sedation at which the patient is relaxed, calm and rational, and verbal communication is continuously possible. Sedation can result in unconsciousness or general anaesthesia. Facilities must be available to manage an anaesthetised patient.

All patients should be monitored with a pulse oximeter during sedation. Reversal agents should be avoided as their half-life may be shorter than the sedative, leading to delayed respiratory depression. Patients should be observed for at least 2 hours prior to discharge.

KEY POINTS

Local anaesthetic

Common complications of local anaesthetic are systemic toxicity and (if combined with adrenaline) delayed haemorrhage.

Sedation should be administered by a trained doctor who is not performing the surgery.

Facilities must be available to manage an anaesthetized patient.

Patients should be observed for at least 2 hours prior to discharge.

POSTOPERATIVE CARE

This can be divided into three phases:

1 immediate: theatre recovery;
2 early: until discharge from hospital;
3 late: home.

Theatre recovery

Airway, breathing and circulation (ABC) are the important parameters immediately after the operation. All staff should maintain life-support skills. Up-to-date resuscitation guidelines are available on the internet (www.resus.org.uk). Patients should be stable when they leave the recovery area. This includes the relief of pain.

Ward care

A doctor should review postoperative patients at least daily. A useful acronym for daily postoperative assessments is SOAP (subjective, objective, assessment, plan) (Box 2.7).

Modified early warning scores (MEWS) are now widely used in hospitals, and various different scoring systems have been used. A score of 5 or more on the one shown in Table 2.3 is associated with a statistically significant risk of admission to intensive care or death.[21] Many hospitals now link their early warning score to a 'track-and-trigger' system in which a high score will electronically trigger a call to a medical practitioner.

Adequate analgesia should be prescribed. Units can rationalise prescribing using guidelines, for example an analgesic ladder – paracetamol, non-steroidal anti-inflammatory drugs (NSAIDs), patient-controlled analgesia (PCA)/opioid and epidural.

Fluid balance is important. Most gynaecological patients will tolerate a 'standard fluid recipe' of 2500 mL/day. However, careless prescribing can lead to hyponatraemia or pulmonary oedema. Evidence-based practice of postoperative fluid management is sparse and equivocal but recent NICE guidance CG174 now provides useful algorithms for intravenous (IV) fluid therapy.[22] Patients requiring IV fluids for maintenance should receive 25–30 mL/kg per day of water. Daily requirements of sodium and potassium are 1 mmol/kg. However, the effects of stress hormones associated with surgery are poorly understood, and electrolytes should be checked every 24–48 hours if a patient remains on IV fluids, to guide fluid prescription.

Glucose 50–100 g/day should also be prescribed to limit starvation ketosis.

Box 2.7 Daily postoperative assessment

SOAP

Subjective: how does the patient feel?

Objective: blood pressure, temperature and fluid balance

Assessment: physical examination

Plan: plan of care for the next 24 hours

Table 2.3 MEWS

Score	3	2	1	0	1	2	3
Systolic BP (% below or above normal)	<45	30	15	Normal	15	30	>45
Heart rate		<40	41-50	50-100	101-110	111-129	>0 .130
Respiratory rate		<9		9-14	15-20	21-29	>30
Temperature (°C)		<35		35-38.4		>38.5	
AVPU				A	V	P	U

Oliguria is a urine output of less than 20 mL/h, in each of two consecutive hours. Oliguria due to hypovolaemia may result from:

- active haemorrhage;
- unreplaced blood loss;
- ileus: fluid loss into the gastrointestinal tract;
- loss of plasma into the abdomen;
- oedema.

If fluid balance is difficult, it may require central venous pressure monitoring and transfer to a high-dependency unit (HDU) or intensive care unit (ICU). The National CEPOD 2001 enquiry found that 16 per cent of patients were not admitted to ICU/HDU despite there being a demonstrable need.[9]

Fluids for volume expansion should be 500 mL bolus of crystalloid or blood. In the management of critically ill patients in intensive care, the TRICC study found that the group managed with a conservative transfusion strategy (Hb 7–9 g/dL) did significantly better than a group given a liberal transfusion management (Hb 10–12 g/dL) in terms of in-hospital mortality, adverse cardiac events, rate of organ dysfunction and overall transfusion rates[23] [D]. Further up-to-date guidance on all aspects of blood transfusion can be found at http://www.transfusionguidelines.org.uk.

DISCHARGE

Discharge should be planned. The patient should be aware of normal recovery rates, and be given advice about when to return to work, social activities and sexual intercourse. However, this information is usually based on traditional practice rather than evidence.

The general practitioner (GP) should be informed of the patient's treatment. An effective way to inform GPs is to give a brief discharge letter to the patient to take to the GP, followed by a formal letter. It may be necessary for social services, Macmillan nurses or district nurses to be involved in discharge procedures.

The need for follow-up visits is dependent on the surgery performed. The advantages and disadvantages are listed in Box 2.8.

DAY CASE SURGERY

There are special considerations to be accounted for in day case surgery, including patient selection and discharge arrangements.

Day surgery units should have clear protocols for patient selection to ensure patient safety and minimise cancellations (Box 2.9): patients should be generally fit and ambulant; they

Box 2.8 Follow-up clinics

| **Advantages** |
| Audit |
| Proactive detection of complications |
| Provide ongoing treatment |
| Completeness of treatment episode |
| **Disadvantages** |
| Delay in reviewing complication |
| Anxiety waiting for results |
| Time spent seeing well people |
| Cost to the health service |
| Cost to the patient in travel and time off work |

KEY POINTS

POSTOPERATIVE CARE

Immediate
All staff should maintain life support skills.

Early
A doctor should review patients at least daily.
Analgesia and fluid balance are important.

Discharge
Patients should be given full advice about recovery rates and activities.
The GP and, if necessary, other services should be promptly informed.
Not all procedures require routine follow-up.

Box 2.9 Common conditions that require further assessment

| Uncontrolled hypertension, BP >170/100 mmHg |
| Cardiac failure |
| MI/TIA/CVA in past 6 months |
| Severe asthma/respiratory disease |
| Diabetes – type 1 or poorly controlled type 2 (BG >11 mmol/L) |
| Renal or hepatic disease |
| Alcoholism or narcotic addiction |
| Advanced multiple sclerosis or myasthenia |
| Severe cervical spondylosis |
| Severe psychiatric disease |
| Drugs: MAOIs, digoxin, steroids, anticoagulants, GTN, diuretics and antiarrhythmics |

BP, blood pressure; MI, myocardial infarction; TIA, transient ischaemic attack; CVA, cerebrovascular accident; BG, blood glucose; MAOIs, monoamine oxidase inhibitors; GTN, glyceryl trinitrate.

should be able to climb one flight of stairs; they should not be grossly obese (BMI >35 kg/m²).[24]

Day surgery units should have written criteria for patients' discharge.[25,26] Patients should have stable vital signs, be oriented in time and place, and able to tolerate oral fluids; they should be able to dress and walk unaided; they must have a responsible and physically able adult to collect them and care for them overnight; they should have adequate analgesia and be aware of the action to take in the event of complications. A contact telephone number should be given for advice after discharge.

KEY POINTS

DAY CASE SURGERY
There should be:
- clear protocols for patient selection;
- written criteria for discharge.

RISK MANAGEMENT

Risk management is the process of examining procedures to prevent accidents and assessing incidents to prevent recurrence. Some of the most serious mistakes occur from the simplest system errors.

The introduction of simple protocols can avoid common mistakes such as retained swabs and ensure that the correct operation is performed on the correct patient.

The positive impact of a simple surgical checklist was demonstrated in a large multinational study. Data on clinical processes and outcomes were collected on 3733 patients undergoing non-cardiac surgery in 8 different countries. Following the introduction of a 19-item Surgical Safety Checklist, data were collected on 3955 patients. The death rate was 1.5% before the checklist was introduced and declined to 0.8% afterwards ($P = 0.003$). Inpatient complications occurred in 11% of patients at baseline and in 7% after introduction of the check list ($P < 0.001$)[27] [C].

Examining 'near misses' is as important as examining actual 'incidents'. Hospitals should have a reporting procedure that is accessible to all staff.

KEY POINTS

RISK MANAGEMENT
There should be reporting systems for incidents and 'near misses'.

CONCLUSIONS

Technicians can perform procedures, whilst surgeons should orchestrate care.

Surgeons have a responsibility to ensure they are adequately trained, have counselled the patient preoperatively and are performing the correct operation, and to provide postoperative care.

Audit is important to review practice and should be part of a surgeon's remit. Surgeons must be provided with the time and resources required to audit their practice. League tables of surgical care will be informative only when all aspects of care are included in the assessment. The National Confidential Enquiry into Perioperative Deaths is a national surgical audit that can be found at www.ncepod.org.uk.

ACKNOWLEDGEMENT

This chapter was written for the first edition of the book by Fiona M Reid and Anthony RB Smith. It has been updated for both second and third editions by Fiona M Reid.

Key References

1. Rogers vs Whitaker, *CRL* [1992]479.
2. Jones R. Smoking before surgery: the case for stopping. *BMJ* 1985;290:1763–4.
3. Department of Health. *National Strategy for Sexual Health and HIV*. London: Department of Health, 2001.
4. Johnson H, Knee-Iloi S, Butler T, *et al.* Are routine preoperative laboratory screening tests necessary to evaluate ambulatory surgical patients? *Surgery* 1988;104:639–45.
5. Golub R, Cantu R, Sorrento J, *et al.* Efficacy of preadmission testing in ambulatory surgical patients. *Am J Surg* 1992;163:565–71.
6. Wong E-M, Tillyer M, Saunders P. Pre-operative screening for sickle cell trait in adult day surgery; is it necessary? *Ambulatory Surg* 1996;4:41–5.
7. Campling A, Devlin H, Hoile R, Lunn J. *The Report of the National Confidential Enquiry into Perioperative Deaths, 1991/1992*. London: NCEPOD, 1993.
8. Portal R. Elective surgery after myocardial infarction. *BMJ* 1982;284:843–4.
9. National Confidential Enquiry into Perioperative Deaths. *Changing the way we operate: National Confidential Enquiry into Perioperative Deaths*. London: NCEPOD, 2001.
10. Jones R. Influence of coexisting disease. *In*: Kirk R, Mansfield A, Cochrane J (eds). *Clinical Surgery in General*. London: Churchill Livingstone, 1996, 67–83.
11. Robinson P, Hall G. Preoperative assessment. *In*: *How to Survive in Anaesthesia*. London: BMJ Publishing Group, 1997, 98.
12. NICE. *Venous Thromboembolism: Reducing the risk of venous thromboembolism (deep vein thrombosis and pulmonary embolism) in inpatients undergoing surgery*. NICE guideline CG92. London: NICE, 2010.
13. Nicholson A, Lowe MC, Parker J, Lewis SR, Alderson P, Smith AF. Systematic review and meta-analysis of

enhanced recovery programmes in surgical patients. *Br J Surg* 2014;101:172–88.

14. Leaper D. Surgical access, incisions and the management of wounds. *In*: Kirk R, Mansfield A, Cochrane J (eds). *Clinical Surgery in General*. London: Churchill Livingstone, 1996: 201–7.

15. Pollock A. Surgical prophylaxis – the emerging picture. *Lancet* 1988;i:225–30.

16. NICE. Prophylaxis against infective endocarditis. Available from www.nice.org.uk/CG64.

17. Carey M, Rosamilla G, Maher C, *et al*. Laparoscopic versus open colposuspension: a prospective multicentre randomised single blind trial. *Neuro Urodyn* 2000; 19:389–90.

18. Fatthy H, El Hao M, Samaha I, Abdallah K. Modified Burch colposuspension: laparoscopy versus laparotomy. *J Am Assoc Gynecol Laparoscopists* 2001;8(1):99–106.

19. *Preventing Entry-related Gynaecological Laparoscopic Injuries*. RCOG Green-top guideline No. 49. London: RCOG, 2008.

20. Audebert A, Gomel V. Role of microlaparoscopy in the diagnosis of peritoneal and visceral adhesions and the prevention of bowel injury associated with blind trocar insertion. *Fertil Steril* 2000;73:631–5.

21. Subbe CP, Kruger M, Gemmel L. Validation of a modified Early Warning Score in medical admissions. *Quarterly J Med* 2001;94:521–6.

22. NICE. *Intravenous Fluid Therapy in Adults in Hospital* (CG174). London: NICE, 2013.

23. Hebert PC, Wells G, Martin C, *et al*. A Canadian survey of transfusion practices in critically ill patients. Transfusion Requirements in Critical Care Investigators and the Canadian Critical Care Trials Group. *Crit Care Med* 1998;26:482–7.

24. Millar J, Rudkin G, Hitchcock M. *Practical Anaesthesia and Analgesia for Day Surgery*. Oxford: BIOS Scientific Publishers, 1997.

25. Korttila K. Recovery from outpatient anaesthesia. *Anaesthesia* 1995;50(Suppl):22–8.

26. Chung F. Discharge criteria – a new trend. *Can J Anaesth* 1995;42:1056–8.

27. Haynes A, Weiser G, Berry W, *et al*. A surgical checklist to reduce morbidity and mortality in a global population. *N Engl J Med* 2009;360: 491–9.

Chapter 3 Communication and counselling

Richard Porter

MRCOG standards

There are no specific standards in the MRCOG curriculum for this topic. Everything in this chapter is – or should be – self-evident. Communication is the foundation stone of our clinical practice.

INTRODUCTION

Humans communicate in myriad ways. Doctors do not always give the impression of being entirely alert to this. It is possible to be a proficient diagnostician or a highly competent surgeon, or both, and to be a poor communicator with patients. But I would argue that it is not possible to be a good doctor in the modern world without being a good communicator. After all, communication with patients is what principally distinguishes us from veterinary surgeons – with all due respect to veterinary surgeons.

This chapter does not presume to list the methods used in medical schools to improve patient–doctor communication. Medical school (undergraduate) curricula have developed teaching programmes that focus on this topic, and there is a body of academic research that underpins the strategies used by clinicians in eliciting and imparting information from and to patients as effectively as possible. Primary care training rightly regards the teaching of communication skills as one of the most important parts of the introduction of a trainee to general practice. However, in specialist training in obstetrics and gynaecology, one might be forgiven for thinking that there is a belief that the lessons have been adequately learned in medical school, so little formal teaching is given on the topic in many training schemes.

This is, however, being addressed. Examination for membership of the Royal College of Obstetricians and Gynaecologists includes Objective Structured Clinical Examination (OSCE) stations that incorporate contact with actors, who indeed give feedback on the standards of the doctors.

However, it is important to remember that doctors do not only communicate with patients and their relatives.

This chapter is an attempt to apply a sideways and personal look at the broader area of communication in clinical practice: communication between doctor and patient, between doctor and doctor, and between doctors and other professionals – in other words, the wider picture.

COMMUNICATION WITH PATIENTS (AND THEIR RELATIVES AND FRIENDS)

In obstetrics and gynaecology, good communication with patients generally requires:

- *Respect for the patient as an individual.* Even if she holds opinions and beliefs that may not be the same as ours.
- *Respect for women.* In cultures where this is not automatic, it is frequently observed that communication is at a lamentably low level, even when women interact with other women doctors. At its most extreme, women will simply avoid contact with medical services, with dire consequences for health outcomes, such as maternal and perinatal mortality. If an obstetrician/gynaecologist does not respect patients as women, it is difficult to understand why such a doctor remains in this specialty.
- *The ability of the doctor to understand the patient, and the patient to understand the doctor.* Language barriers are not a justification for substandard clinical care on either a medico-legal or a moral level.[1] We may require the use of interpreters, but we must remember that the problem may not just be with the words used. Even when a doctor and a patient ostensibly speak the same language, they may not be using the words in the same way, and this can be a cause of major and potentially dangerous misunderstanding.
- *The ability to listen.* This is not an open-ended commitment: some patients will want to tell us far more than we need, want or have time to hear. But achieving the right balance is essential, and sometimes very challenging.
- *Flexibility.* Any doctor who says that he or she takes a history in the same way under all circumstances is being

Verbal communication with patients

Assuming that you and the patient are speaking (literally) more or less the same language:

- *Do you introduce yourself?* The recent '*My name is …*' campaign is a simple but effective wake-up call for the medical profession. The campaign arose from the experience of a medically qualified patient who had been told of her terminal diagnosis by a doctor who did not introduce him- or herself. Was this perhaps shyness, or possibly difficulty handling the exchange of painful information? Who knows – but whatever else it was deeply wounding to the patient, and wholly avoidably insensitive.

- *Are you using a vocabulary that is appropriate to her?* I well remember watching a brilliant researcher explaining in detail to a totally bemused mother the physics of Doppler waveforms. This was in response to her anxious question – while being scanned at 34 weeks' gestation – 'Whassat doing then?' This was (to be honest) hilarious to watch – but a tragic illustration of the limitations of intelligence.

- *Are you going too fast?* How often do we see colleagues checking with patients, after imparting manageable (bite-sized?) chunks of information, whether or not they have understood? Not nearly often enough, I would predict. If we wait until the end of a long discussion, with masses of pieces of information, can we be surprised if the patient surrenders and says that she has understood – just to make us go away? In fact, I cherish the lesson I learnt from a patient who, after I had explained that she needed her urodynamics repeating (I assumed that she knew what I was talking about because she had had the test before), was asked by the sister when leaving the room, 'So, did you understand all that?', and said loudly (she was a bit deaf), 'Not a word dear'.

- *Are you 'talking down' to her?* In this new era of patients accessing information on the internet, few things are more likely to raise hackles than giving the impression that you assume that they are ignorant.

- *Are you giving her more information than she wants?* This is one of the most difficult areas in current practice (see Obtaining consent, p. 26). How much is enough, and how much too much? In oncology care, this is a particularly important issue, and is beyond the scope of this chapter. The problem is compounded by perceptions about a litigious environment. Yet we must recognise that we have a duty of care to our patients, and that may mean that we should make judgements about the appropriateness or otherwise of imparting every iota of information. (In this area the RCOG Consent Advice documents [available on-line from www.rcog.org.uk] are, on the one hand, particularly helpful templates and, on the other, arguably examples of potential information overload. Different patients will respond differently, and individualisation should be the nature of the interaction.)

- *Do you recognise the cultural sensitivities influencing her decisions?* In our multicultural society, we are becoming better at not trampling on the sensitivities of, for example, women who have religious reasons for not wanting to see men in a medical context, but it is still incumbent upon us to be alert to the possibility of unexpected beliefs and taboos.

- *Do you involve the patient in the decision-making?* Joseph-Williams et al. (2014) (*Power Imbalance Prevents Shared Decision Making*)[2] demonstrate how complex this dynamic is. We act as doctors in an environment that is considerably more complex than used to be the case. Gone – fortunately – are the days of unarguable 'top-down' distribution of medical decisions, but many doctors are unaware of the subtly coercive position we still occupy (even though that may be the polar opposite of what we might intend). This is of course not merely a moral and ethical challenge, it is also one underpinning an increasing amount of litigation in our specialty. Joseph-Williams et al. make the point that attitudinal issues are pre-eminent in this area.

Non-verbal communication with patients

A patient is more often than not in a state of some unease when meeting a doctor, and she will be responding to far more than what is said or not said. The nature of the space where the meeting takes place, the smells of the environment, the extraneous noises – all will influence both her perception of the event and the way in which she takes the information on board. A doctor cannot often immediately influence these factors, but can certainly add to or detract from the experience by means of non-verbal communication.

Much of this is a matter of common courtesy, but it is easy to let our standards slip on occasion – and patients notice it, you can be sure. Surely the guiding principle here is that you should act towards your patients exactly as you would wish to be acted towards yourself – and the use of the word 'act' is not accidental, for every contact with a patient is to a degree a theatrical event.

The following are some examples.

- *How do you greet the patient?* Do you stand up? Do you have your back to her when she comes in? Do you shake her hand? Do you invite her to sit? I suspect that we have all seen 'eminent' doctors greet a patient by continuing to talk to medical students. What sort of an impression does that give?

- *What is your facial expression?* A smile, a furrowed brow, a scowl, a deadpan expression – all will convey some message to the patient. Is the message the one you want to convey? The problem can, of course, get slightly out of hand: the phoney facial expression is just as unsettling as the unthinking one. Think of a politician delivering an unpalatable message with a sanctimonious look. None of us would like to be compared with politicians, I assume.

- *Do you look her in the eye when talking to her, or do you stare at the floor?* This again may reflect your cultural background, or even perhaps your innate modesty, but it may lead to unintended inferences by the patient. Would you propose marriage while looking at the floor? (Of course some might: I am reminded of the schoolmaster who did so by asking his intended if she wanted his surname on her gravestone. Tastes differ … .)

- *How do you sit during a consultation?* Are you leaning forward in an attentive pose, or slouching in the chair? Body language is powerful, and can be deeply unsettling for your patient.

- *When you stand (e.g. in a bedside consultation), how far away are you?* Are you too close for the patient's comfort, or are you so far that you give the impression that you regard the patient as another life form? Remember that differences in height – e.g. when you stand over a patient who is lying on a bed – can result in, to put it mildly, unintended distortions in communication.

- *Have you ensured that she is at her ease?* Is she embarrassed (more than is usual) by her state of undress? As ever, the question is: would you or your nearest and dearest want to be treated like this?

I have no doubt that every reader of this chapter can add other examples of good and bad practice that they have encountered in their professional lives. None of us succeeds at all times in making good communication with patients and their families and friends, but we should at least strive to stand back at times and analyse our performance, and to continue to improve.

Communication with a complaining or angry patient

I personally know of no more challenging area of communication, and this is clearly not an area where 'dry runs' are particularly easy to construct. However, for better or for worse, these situations are becoming more common as patients and their families become more vocal – and beyond doubt more critical (rightly or wrongly). Good communication can make the difference between a problem that is resolved there and then and one that lingers, often with complex ramifications. The principles of communication are essentially the same as above, but the application of the principles may prove exceedingly difficult. Staying calm may prove to be the most difficult part of the equation.

COMMUNICATION WITH OTHER STAFF

Although communication with patients is of paramount importance, the issue of communication with other professionals is also crucial. In hospital medicine, there is no such thing as a single-handed department, and dysfunction all too easily follows from poor inter-professional communication.

Any trainee who has worked in a department where rivalries pollute the atmosphere will know how destructive that can be. Many of these problems themselves arise from poor communication skills, but poor communication will surely follow from these rivalries.

The areas of importance are discussed below.

Doctor–doctor communication

Juniors need to communicate with other more senior doctors (and vice versa), and doctors of the same grade as themselves. Now that trainers are themselves being more commonly trained to train, and in the increasingly informal atmosphere in which we work in hospital practice, it should follow that this 'vertical downward' communication will be better handled. This is also assisted by the reduction in 'patronage' over the last few years, which makes for a far healthier training environment. However, that is beyond the scope of this chapter.

Yet, strangely perhaps, few if any trainees have been taught how to communicate 'upwards' with their trainers. Does this need to be taught? I would suggest that it does. Consider the 2 a.m. phone call to the consultant on call. Does the trainee have any idea what this feels like for the recipient of the call, roused from sleep? Possibly the best advice I received about this was the suggestion that the caller should be taught immediately to communicate the status of the call. Was it a call that (a) required the consultant's presence, (b) required the consultant's advice or (c) was merely to inform the consultant?

This is an example of learned communication that hugely enhances the transfer of information, almost certainly to the advantage of the patient.

The most formal type of doctor–doctor communication is case presentation. This is a skill and, like many others in postgraduate training, it is currently barely, if at all, taught. Yet without this skill there can be serious difficulties within the clinical team.

The simplest advice is, I believe, the best: present cases in three parts – the synopsis, the detail and the summary (or, in other words, tell them what you are going to say, tell them what you want to say and then remind them what you have just told them).

All trainees should practise these skills as often as possible, and should learn to teach them to the next generation.

Doctor–midwife/nurse communication

The other area of inter-professional communication – doctor–midwife/nurse communication – is just as important. Gone, thankfully, are the days of the presumed superiority of doctors. Instead we now respect the professional contributions of each other for what they are: interdependent and worthy of mutual respect. Nevertheless, all have to work to maintain the best possible level of communication at all times. Examples abound of departments where communication has failed – and the overall departmental dysfunction that ensues is massive, detrimental to patient care and wholly unnecessary. Like any relationship, this one will have ups and downs. The mark of maturity is when the system can tolerate these, and learn from them.

Written communication

The two areas are clinical records and letters to other professionals. The skills required are similar, but different in detail.

Clinical records

The quality of clinical records is of vital importance. Well-constructed clinical records communicate with other professionals and protect patients. They may also protect the writer from future medico-legal attack. Poor-quality clinical records, by contrast, confuse other professionals and endanger patients. Records should be (as far as possible for those of us whose handwriting is only marginally more decipherable than Egyptian hieroglyphs) legible. They must also be dated, timed and signed (identifiably), if referring to an inpatient. There should be no exceptions to this.

The thicker clinical records become, the less useful they are as modes of information transfer. Thought must therefore be given to what and how much you write. Write only what is necessary and sufficient. Historically, midwives have written more than is necessary, and doctors far less than is necessary. Fortunately, that gap has recently narrowed considerably. Nevertheless, all those involved in medico-legal practice express continuing concern about the quality of note keeping.

Letters

A generation ago, letters between doctors were more stylish, idiosyncratic and interesting. Unfortunately, they were also far less useful in transferring medical information. We live in an era in which letters are increasingly computer generated. Whether these letters are more effective in transferring information is yet to be determined, but I would suggest that the best letters are a compromise. If they are too short, they will be easily read, but they may omit relevant and necessary detail. If they are needlessly long, they risk losing the attention of the reader and remaining unread. Your letter should be relevant to the recipient. I remain astonished by some letters in clinical practice, written by highly intelligent clinicians, which seem not to recognise what the aim of the exercise is (it is communication, not intellectual gratification).

You must also remember that letters are crucially important medico-legal documents: you must ensure that what is typed is what you intended.

OBTAINING CONSENT

This is an area in which communication skills are sorely tested. How much information is required to enable a patient to give truly informed consent? For example, all surgery could lead to death, but is it necessary to include that in the discussion? As it stands, it is probably fair to say that today's practice will appear wrong within a short time. Even the test of 'How much would you like to know if it were you signing the consent form?' is probably an unreliable yardstick. The sensitive clinician will increasingly need to enter into the discussion with an open mind and good antennae, as well as (in UK practice) familiarity with the General Medical Council requirements in this field.[3] (See also the RCOG Consent Advice documents referred to above.)

COUNSELLING

As obstetricians and gynaecologists, we become involved in counselling in several types of difficult circumstances (e.g. malignant disease, prenatal screening dilemmas, preconception counselling). As stated above, counselling is the application of the full range of communication skills in a specific area of professional expertise. There is no added magic in the process.

CONCLUSIONS

This is an area where common sense rules. Integrity and respect for others are 'all' that is required. Always ask yourself if you, or your closest relatives, would want to be communicated with in this manner. Most of the time it really is that simple.

Key References

1. General Medical Council. *Good Medical Practice.* London: GMC, 2013. Available from: http://www.gmc-uk.org/guidance/good_medical_practice.asp.
2. Joseph-Williams N, Edwards A, Elwyn G. Power imbalance prevents shared decision making. *BMJ* 2014;348:g3178.
3. General Medical Council. *Consent: Patients and doctors making decisions together.* London: GMC, 2008. Available from: www.gmc-uk.org/static/documents/content/Consent_2008.pdf.

Chapter 4 The law, medicine and women's rights

Sheila McLean

INTRODUCTION

It is probably true to say that the relationship between law and medicine in the past has sometimes been characterised by confrontation, even hostility. Increasingly, however, doctors are turning to the law themselves as a way of obtaining guidance as to what is and what is not permissible in their practice. Thus, rather than law being seen simply as a mechanism for judging allegations of negligence, it has taken on the role of standard setter, particularly in some areas of medicine, such as obstetrics and gynaecology.

This change has arisen largely as a consequence of medicine's capacities in managing pregnancy. The ability to monitor fetal development in particular has radically altered the way in which physicians perceive their role in respect of the pregnant woman, and has in some cases led to legal action. It has been said that, in the past, women told their doctors about their pregnancies, but now doctors tell women. The ability to visualise the fetus in the womb means that it becomes endowed, however subconsciously, with the characteristics of a child much earlier in pregnancy than would previously have been the case. The temptation therefore is to treat the fetus as a separate and unique patient. As Harrison says:

The fetus has come a long way – from biblical 'seed' and mystical 'homunculus' to an individual with medical problems that can be diagnosed and treated. Although he cannot make an appointment and seldom even complains, this patient will at times need a physician.[1]

In some countries, this has led to a growing recognition of the alleged 'rights' of the fetus, which may on occasion conflict with the rights and interests of the pregnant woman. So common is this problem that it has been given a descriptive name of its own – maternal/fetal conflict – yet, as Hubbard says:

It makes no sense, biologically or socially, to pit fetal and maternal 'rights' against one another. Indeed, legal 'rights' do not offer a proper framework for assessing the situation of a pregnant woman and her fetus. As long as they are connected, nothing can happen to one that does not affect the other.[2]

However, one thing must be made clear at the outset. In law, the fetus has no rights, and therefore to talk about fetal rights is misleading. None the less, it is generally conceded that the embryo or fetus of the human species is worthy of some respect.[3] To say this, however, is quite different from asserting that it is a rights holder and worthy of equal consideration with the pregnant woman.

Most women will have no difficulty in behaving throughout their pregnancy in ways that maximise the potential health and safe delivery of their child. But not all women feel this way, or act this way, and this may be for reasons that appear to third parties unintelligible – even downright offensive or callous. However, the fact that women are free, autonomous actors means that their decisions – however unpalatable – must be given respect. This is not always easy for clinicians to accept, particularly when the woman's behaviour threatens the survival of an otherwise viable fetus. Indeed, a number of cases have reached courts in which doctors have asked that the choices of women should be overturned in the interests of fetal survival, as well as, sometimes, in the interests of saving the woman's life.

However, the basic legal position is clear. If a woman is otherwise legally competent, then her wishes must be respected, even if the result is her death or the death of an otherwise viable fetus. No matter how harsh this sounds, it is the law, and there are good reasons for the law to adopt this position. While recognising that this may be problematic for those caring for the pregnant woman, the fact of pregnancy does not reduce the rights of women to make autonomous, self-regarding decisions. The interests of the embryo or fetus are not completely ignored by the law, however. The general principle underpinning the law is to offer benefit to the embryo or fetus wherever possible (without, for example, breaching the rights of others). Once born alive, children are entitled to sue for damage they sustained prenatally (even pre-conception). This is based on the assumption that where a benefit should accrue, it is for the law to ensure that it does. But this is not to say that the law recognises the fetus as a rights holder before birth. Rather, it accepts that the injury arises at the moment the fetus becomes a child, and therefore is entitled to have rights attributed to it.

A BRIEF ANALYSIS OF CASE LAW

It is in the grey areas that problems have arisen, and an analysis of some of the leading cases will help to explore both the content of and the rationale for the law's attitude. Although the law is clear that the fetus has no rights, this does not mean that women's autonomous decisions about the management of their pregnancy and labour have always been respected. The first case to arise in the UK was that of *Re S.*[4] in 1992. In this case, a woman refused a caesarean section on religious grounds. Her doctors believed that both her life and the life of her fetus were at risk and sought court authority to proceed with the caesarean section, even in the face of her objections. A judge heard the case as a matter of urgency (the hearing took about 20 minutes) and authorised the carrying out of the operation.

Perhaps unsurprisingly, this judgment was widely criticised for a number of reasons. First, the speed of the hearing was felt to prevent the nuances of the case being properly considered. Sir Stephen Brown's judgment, which is extremely brief, merely comments that:

> *The consultant is emphatic. He says it is absolutely the case that the baby cannot be born alive if a caesarean operation is not carried out. He has described the medical condition. I am not going to go into it in detail because of the pressure of time.*[5]

Second, it is most unusual to interfere with people's religious commitments in this way and, given the passing of the Human Rights Act 1998, it is fairly certain that this judgment would not be compatible with the terms of the Act. Article 9 of the European Convention on Human Rights requires states to permit freedom of thought, conscience and religion, with the implication that this also includes the freedom to act on religious commitments. Manifestly, this right would be limited if, for example, X's freedom of religion threatened the life of Y. However, since the fetus – even at full term – is not a person for legal purposes, then this is not directly relevant. Equally, it is possible that Article 8 of the Convention – the right to respect for private and family life – could be called into play in such situations. This article of the Convention is generally described as being the one that most clearly supports autonomy.

Third, the woman was at no time represented at the hearing, which would also fall foul of Article 6 of the Convention on Human Rights: the right to a fair hearing. Finally, proceeding to surgery against the expressed wishes of a competent woman effectively means that she was the victim of an assault on her person (again in breach of the Convention, Article 5 – the right to liberty and security of the person) in the interests, in large part, of saving her fetus. Of course, the court was also concerned with the danger to the life of the woman, but, as courts have said on numerous occasions, a person is free to decline even life-saving treatment, no matter the reason for that choice, as long as they are competent.[6]

Subsequent cases, such as *St George's Healthcare NHS Trust v S, R v Collins and others, ex parte S,*[7] showed the lengths to which doctors and the law were prepared to go in forcing women to accept medical treatment deemed to be essential to save the fetus. S was diagnosed as suffering from severe pre-eclampsia, and was advised that an early delivery would be needed. She understood that both she and the fetus might die if surgery was not undertaken, but none the less refused it. On 26 April 1997 an order had been made which dispensed with her consent to the treatment. She had also been made subject to an order under the Mental Health Act 1983 to be admitted for 'assessment'. No treatment for her alleged depression was offered. S continued to record her extreme objections to the caesarean section. During her time in hospital, '… it was still believed by the psychiatrist who had played a significant part in the decision to admit her to hospital under s 2 that her capacity to consent was intact'.[8] It has already been indicated that a competent adult is free to refuse consent to life-saving treatment. As Lord Mustill said in the case of *Airedale NHS Trust v Bland*:[9]

> *If the patient is capable of making a decision on whether to permit treatment and decides not to permit it his choice must be obeyed, even if on any objective view it is contrary to his best interests. A doctor has no right to proceed in the face of objection, even if it is plain to all, including the patient, that adverse consequences and even death will or may ensue.*[10]

Given that the psychiatrist was willing to state that her competence was not in issue, the decision of the lower court to authorise the section flies in the face of the general rule of law, and was ultimately criticised by the Court of Appeal. However, one earlier case had suggested that the only situation in which the law might be different was where '… the choice may lead to the death of a viable fetus',[11] although the jurisprudential basis for this exception is unclear. As the court in *St George's NHS Trust v S* noted, it is not sufficient simply to ignore the interests of the fetus. But as was also said, in this case there was no conflict between the interests of the mother and the fetus, because '… the procedures to be adopted to preserve the mother and her unborn child did not involve a preference for one rather than the other'.[12]

In addition, the court hazarded a look into the future, noting that it may soon be the case that relatively minor medical intervention on an adult might save the life of an unborn fetus. In contemplating a refusal of consent in such a case, the court said:

> *The refusal would rightly be described as unreasonable, the benefit to another human life would be beyond value, and the motives of the doctor admirable. If, however, the adult were compelled to agree, or rendered helpless to resist, the principle of autonomy would be extinguished.*[13]

Finally, in the context of obstetrical intervention, it is worth restating the words of Butler-Sloss LJ in the case of *Re MB.*[14]

In this case she made an obiter explanation of the law as it currently stands:

> The fetus up to the moment of birth does not have any separate interests capable of being taken into account when a court has to consider an application for a declaration in respect of a caesarean section operation. The law does not have the jurisdiction to declare that such medical intervention is lawful to protect the interests of the unborn child even at the point of birth.[15]

Thus, even if we disapprove of the decisions of a pregnant woman, it is essential to ensure that her autonomy is respected where she is legally competent. Legal competence (or its absence) is now statutorily defined by the Adults with Incapacity (Scotland) Act 2000 and the Mental Capacity Act 2005. The issue of competence is, of course, central to the management of any disputes that arise between pregnant women and those caring for them. The Royal College of Obstetricians and Gynaecologists' Ethics Committee (https://www.rcog.org.uk) advises healthcare professionals as follows:

> If the patient's capacity is seriously in doubt, it should be assessed as a matter of priority by a medical practitioner experienced in such assessments (such as a consultant psychiatrist). If, following assessment, there remains a serious doubt about the patient's competence, legal advice should be sought.

One more recent case, widely reported in the media, further considers the question of the medical treatment of a non-competent pregnant woman. In August 2012, the Court of Protection considered the case of *Re AA*.[16] In this case, the woman, who was 39 weeks' pregnant, had been compulsorily detained under the Mental Health Act 1983. She reportedly suffered from psychotic episodes and delusional beliefs. Mr Justice Mostyn also held that she was lacking in legal capacity in terms of the Mental Capacity Act 2005. Following the judgment in *Re MB*, he authorised a caesarean section to proceed, a procedure that he believed to be in the interests of the woman herself, and of the fetus. Psychiatric evidence as to her mental health was clear and evidence from the obstetrician indicated that, should she proceed with a natural birth, there was a significant (perhaps as high as 1%) risk of a ruptured womb. Mr Justice Mostyn was constrained to reach a decision that was in her best interests which, in his view, was that the section should go ahead even though she lacked capacity to consent to it. Interestingly, in light of what has already been said, he was at pains to make it clear that – although the section would probably also be in the interests of the fetus – it was the best interests of the woman over which he had jurisdiction.

It would seem, therefore, taking each of these cases into account, that the law is now clear that a competent refusal by a pregnant woman of treatment designed to save the life or preserve the health of her fetus (and/or herself) must be respected. This conclusion doubtless will sit uncomfortably with those whose mission is to save life, particularly given the tendency to view the fetus as a separate entity from the woman. However, there are, as I have suggested, good reasons for the law to adopt this position, which – it should be noted – does not prevent those caring for pregnant women from using persuasion (not coercion) in advising women as to the clinically optimal path.

The principle of autonomy permeates our law and our ethics. It is a principle that can be freely exercised as part of our citizenship, subject only to the caveat that it may be restricted when its exercise threatens others. But as courts agreed in the case of *Paton v Trustees of BPAS*[17] – a case in which a man attempted to prevent his wife from terminating a pregnancy – and in *Re F (in utero)*[18] – a case in which an attempt was made to make a fetus a ward of court – the fetus does not have independent legal standing, and its interests cannot serve to outweigh the right of a woman to make autonomous decisions. This conclusion was further reinforced in the case of *Vo v France*.[19] In the case of *Re F*, Balcombe LJ made it clear that it was not for the courts to make decisions that would fly in the face of this conclusion. As he said:

> If the law is to be extended in this manner, so as to impose control over the mother of an unborn child, where such control may be necessary for the benefit of that child, then under our system of parliamentary democracy it is for Parliament to decide whether such controls can be imposed and, if so, subject to what limitations or conditions.[20]

That Parliament has declined to do this is a reflection of the interest which we all have in protecting autonomy, even when to do so is emotionally difficult. Just as it is not for judges to change the law, neither is it for doctors to do so.

But it is not just the protection of the abstract concept of autonomy that mandates the current legal response. In jurisdictions beyond those of the United Kingdom, decisions – often generated by doctors and handed down by courts – have served to demonstrate clearly the dangers of attributing rights to fetuses either during pregnancy or at the point of delivery. Medical recognition of the potential harm that can be caused by pregnant women to developing embryos and fetuses in the course of the pregnancy has in some countries resulted in the aggressive 'policing' of pregnancy – an egregious invasion of liberty. All too often, it appears that fetal interests have relatively easily been taken to trump women's rights. In the USA, for example, Kolder et al.[21] found that, of 21 applications for court orders by public hospitals, 86 per cent were successful. Interestingly – and arguably ominously – 81 per cent of the women affected were black, Hispanic or Asian, and 24 per cent did not have English as a first language. In addition, 46 per cent of heads of maternal medicine thought that women should be detained when they refused to follow medical advice and thereby endangered their fetuses.

In addition, as Sherman notes:

> Pregnant drug abusers have been jailed to keep them free of illegal substances that might harm fetuses. And laws have been expanded so that pregnant women who do ingest drugs harmful to the fetus can be charged with or investigated for child abuse.[22]

Whilst removing the availability of illicit substances might ultimately serve the long-term interests of the women (as well as benefiting the fetus), women in the USA have also been incarcerated because of their use of legal substances, such as alcohol. Moreover, those women addicted to illicit drugs are sometimes unable to gain access to programmes that might assist them in beating their addiction; locking them up or otherwise coercing them in the interests of their embryos/fetuses seems like a heavy-handed way of avoiding the need to address the fundamental problem head on.

In other cases, medical opinion that a natural delivery was too risky has been used to mandate coercion, but of course medical judgements can be wrong. In *Jefferson v Griffin Spaulding County Hosp. Auth.*,[23] for example, a court upheld an order for a forced caesarean section, although in fact the woman delivered naturally. Yet, at the time the order was sought, doctors had claimed that vaginal delivery carried a 99 per cent chance of fetal death and a 50 per cent chance of maternal death.

The consequences of coercion are perhaps most poignantly demonstrated by the US case of *In re AC*.[24] It was in fact on this case that the UK judge in *Re S*[25] depended for his authorisation of the forced intervention. Interestingly, he appeared to have failed to observe that *AC* had already been overturned on appeal.[26]

The facts of the case make tragic reading. Angela Carder was a young woman who had suffered from leukaemia as a child. Her condition had gone into remission; she married and became pregnant, but in the course of the pregnancy the leukaemia returned aggressively. It was clear that Angela Carder would die. At about 26½ weeks into the pregnancy, her doctors summoned a judge to the hospital and sought authority to carry out a caesarean section on Mrs Carder, despite her clear refusal to consent. When the case was first heard, the order was granted and the operation proceeded in the face of Mrs Carder's objections. Neither she nor the child survived, and indeed the section was listed as a contributing cause of death on the death certificate. In a trenchant criticism of this judgment, the distinguished American academic George Annas described what had happened as follows:

> They [the judges] treated a live woman as though she were already dead, forced her to undergo an abortion and then justified their brutal and unprincipled opinion on the basis that she was almost dead and her fetus's interests in life outweighed any interest that she might have in her own life and health.[27]

Why not intervene?

Despite the temptations to manage pregnancy and childbirth with substantial, if not primary, concern for the welfare of the developing embryo or fetus, it should be clear from consideration of these cases that unthinkingly adopting such a position is potentially dangerous. In respect of intervening in lifestyle choices during pregnancy, it seems clear that the women in the

cases discussed were treated differently from other competent adults solely on the basis of their biological capacities. The fact that we generally wish to protect the fetus does not give us a right to do so at the expense of the woman. Equally, since many of the harms likely to be caused will occur in the early stages of pregnancy – when the woman may not even know that she is pregnant – the logical conclusion of this would be that every fertile, sexually active woman would need to behave at all times as if she were pregnant, or run the risk of being accused of harming her fetus and perhaps even – in the USA at least – of being deprived of her liberty. Equally, as Draper says, 'it is one thing to show what a woman ought to do in relation to her unborn child and quite another thing to say that this obligation ought to be enforced'.[28]

Although some authors have suggested that the way forward is through a 'careful balancing of the offspring's welfare and the pregnant woman's interest in liberty and bodily integrity …',[29] such a balancing act is arguably at best inappropriate and at worst doomed to failure. The very act of 'balancing' automatically implies that there are relevant things to be balanced. It has already been agreed that the embryo or fetus of the human species is worthy of some respect, but this is not equivalent to saying that such respect is capable of being weighed in the scales against an existing person. Even in cases where a born person's life is threatened by the failure of another to undergo medical treatment in their aid, the law is unable to compel submission to treatment. This was clearly seen in one US case. In this case, the defendant refused to consent to a treatment that could have saved the life of the plaintiff. As the judge in that case said:

> Morally, this decision rests with the defendant, and in the view of the court, the refusal of the defendant is morally indefensible. For our law to compel the defendant to submit to an intrusion of his body would change every concept and principle upon which our society is founded. To do so would defeat the sanctity of the individual … .[30]

MATERNAL/FETAL CONFLICT

As has been said, the circumstances described above have come to be called maternal/fetal conflict. I have argued elsewhere[31] that this categorisation is inherently flawed, not least because it describes the pregnant woman as a 'mother' (which she is not yet) and assumes that conflict is possible. Arguably, conflict implies hostility and yet it is not obvious that a fetus can be hostile to the pregnant woman, nor that the pregnant woman's decisions are taken out of hostility for the fetus. None the less, this term has now become an accepted part of the language. Leaving aside these concerns, then, it is worth briefly analysing the implications of this purported conflict which is highly emotive because, as Lew says:

> Conflicts between a woman's needs and those of her fetus are vexing because they pit powerful cultural norms against one another; the ideal of autonomy and the ideal

of maternal self-sacrifice. Parents who make sacrifices for their children should be encouraged, even lauded, but the law should not require such sacrifices. Self-sacrifice is a gift. Forcing a pregnant woman to sacrifice her health for her fetus is simply slavery.[32]

Neither can it be presumed that it is always possible to measure the risk taken by the woman versus the risk to the fetus of non-intervention. A caesarean section carries risk (albeit that risk is lower given today's standards of medical treatment), but even if the risk is minimal, and the potential benefits to the fetus are considerable, we still do insult to the fundamental principles of law and ethics by compelling women to rescue their fetuses. No such ethical or legal principle is widely recognised and, as has been said, 'Even where there is a duty to rescue, the law never requires rescues which jeopardise life and limb'.[33]

CONCLUSION

The developing capacities of modern medicine have served both to enhance the care of pregnant women and to confront women and those caring for them with new dilemmas. During pregnancy, the widespread use of prenatal screening makes the actualisation of reproductive choice both more complex and more intangible. At the point of labour and birth, the clinical ability to rescue poses real tensions in cases where competent women wish to assert their own autonomy at the potential expense of both themselves and their fetuses. The consequences, as Gregg has said, are that:

Women's bodies increasingly have become medicalised as fertility testing, techniques of 'assisted conception', prenatal diagnosis, fetal monitoring, induced labour and caesarean sections have become normal, if not expected, interventions in women's procreative processes. Procreative technologies can enhance both the range of choices for women and the possibility of greater social control of women's choices.[34]

It is clear that, often encouraged by healthcare professionals, courts in particular have become increasingly intrusive into women's decision-making in the course of their pregnancy and at the point of birth. Medicine and the law make powerful allies in this venture, yet their collusion is a direct disavowal of the rights that we otherwise respect. The position in the UK now seems to have been clarified after a decade of highly dubious decisions, at least as far as forced caesarean sections are concerned, and the current legal position is endorsed by the Ethics Committee of the RCOG. It is to be hoped that, where the woman and physician share a relationship based on trust and the free exchange of relevant information, problematic cases will arise infrequently and, in the UK at least, this has proved to be the case. However, the impetus that triggered the call for courts to intervene in these decisions has not disappeared. The motivation of those caring for pregnant women is all too intelligible. However, no matter its source – religion,

professionalism or whatever – it does violence to other principles that have long been deemed essential to the proper functioning of society. All too often, the motivation for intervention is worthy, but it is no less a matter of concern for that. As Ikenotos has said:

To the extent that the state invokes the parens patriae *power to prevent harm to the fetus, the state subordinates the interests of the woman to those of the fetus. To the extent that the state regulates pregnant women to promote public health, safety, and morals – an exercise of the police power – it subordinates the interests of the woman to those of the rest of society. In either case, when the state regulates women as childbearers, it legislates the ideology of motherhood.*[35]

It is not necessary to adopt a particular woman-centred philosophy, such as feminism, to understand the damage done to respect for persons by treating pregnant women without regard for their views. To be sure, the commitment to respecting autonomy does not prevent healthcare professionals from making an attempt to inform women as to the risks they run both for themselves and for their fetuses if certain decisions are made, and to persuade them to think again. However, attempts to enforce the 'right' decision (clinically at least) by resort to the law mark a departure, which should be resisted, from the traditional relationship between doctor and patient. Such a relationship is ideally based on trust, not coercion, on respect, not condemnation. The ability to visualise and assess the development of an embryo or fetus, and to visualise and monitor in the womb, while often immensely helpful to pregnant women, is a technical, not an ethical, issue, and provides insufficient justification to invade the rights of a live, competent individual, however painful that conclusion may be.

KEY POINTS

- The law is no longer simply a mechanism for judging allegations of negligence, but has taken on the role of standard setter.

- Modern fetal imaging technology has increased the temptation to treat the fetus as a separate patient with unique 'rights'.

- Although the human fetus is worthy of respect, it does not, in law, have rights.

- Occasionally, a woman's decision or behaviour may threaten the survival of an otherwise viable fetus. The law says that if the woman is otherwise legally competent, her wishes must be respected.

- Children are entitled to sue for damage that they sustained prenatally, but this is still not the same as saying that the fetus has rights before birth.

- There have been cases of legally enforced obstetric intervention in the UK but the law has now been made clear: a competent refusal by a pregnant woman of treatment designed to save the life of her fetus (and/or herself) must be respected.

- In the USA, ominously, court-ordered treatment has mainly involved disadvantaged ethnic groups or women who did not have English as their first language.

- Pregnant women should not be treated differently from other competent adults.

- The concept of 'maternal/fetal conflict', in a legal context, is inherently flawed and is best avoided.

- The law and medicine make powerful allies. Attempts by the law to enforce the 'right' clinical decision are a departure from basic legal principles and should be resisted.

Key References

1. Harrison MR. Unborn: historical perspective of the fetus as patient. *Pharos* 1982;19:23–4.
2. Hubbard R. Legal and policy implications of recent advances in prenatal diagnosis and therapy. *Women's Rights Law Report* 1982;7:202–15.
3. See, for example, Review of the Guidance on the Research Use of Fetuses and Fetal Material (Polkinghorne Report) Cm 762/1989, para. 2.4. 'Central to our understanding is the acceptance of a special status for the living human fetus at every stage of its development which we wish to characterise as a profound respect based on its potential to develop into a fully-formed human being.'
4. Butterworth's Medico-Legal Reports No. 79, p. 69 (1992).
5. Butterworth's Medico-Legal Reports No. 9, p. 70 (1992).
6. See, for example, Re C (adult: refusal of medical treatment) 1994. All England Law Reports No. 1, p. 819: F v West Berkshire Health Authority (Mental Health Act Commission intervening) Butterworth's Medico-Legal Reports No. 4, p. 1 (1989).
7. Butterworth's Medico-Legal Reports No. 44, p. 160 (1998).
8. Butterworth's Medico-Legal Reports No. 44, p. 169 (1998).
9. Butterworth's Medico-Legal Reports No. 12, p. 64 (1993).
10. Butterworth's Medico-Legal Reports No. 12, p. 136 (1993).
11. Per Lord Donaldson in Re T (adult: refusal of medical treatment) Butterworth's Medico-Legal Reports No. 9, p. 46 (1992).
12. Butterworth's Medico-Legal Reports No. 9, p. 176 (1992).
13. *id.*
14. Butterworth's Medico-Legal Reports No. 38, p. 175 (1997).
15. Butterworth's Medico-Legal Reports No. 38, p. 186 (1997).
16. *In the Matter of Re AA*, 23 August 2012, transcript available at http://www.judiciary.gov.uk/Resources/JCO/Documents/Judgments/re-aa-approved-judgment.pdf (accessed on 30/12/2013).
17. All England Law Reports No. 2, p. 987 (1978).
18. All England Law Reports No. 2, p. 193 (1988).
19. *Vo v France* [2004] 2 FCR 577.
20. All England Law Reports No. 2, p. 200 (1988).
21. Kolder V, Gallagher J, Parsons MT. Court-ordered obstetrical interventions. *N Engl J Med* 1987;316:1192–6.
22. Sherman R. A pyrrhic victory, a court battle: forced caesarian. *Natl Law J* 1989; 16: 3.
23. 274 S.E. 2d 457 (Ga 1981).
24. 533 A.2d 611 (D.C. 1987).
25. 533 A.2d 611 (D.C. 1987). Note 4, supra.
26. In re A.C. 573 A.2d 1235 (D.C. 1990).
27. Annas G. She's going to die: the case of Angela C. Volume 18, No 1, Hastings Center Report, 1988, Volume 23, p. 25.
28. Draper H. Women, forced caesareans and antenatal responsibilities. Working Paper No. 1. Feminist Legal Research Unit, University of Liverpool, 1, 1992, p. 13.
29. Robertson J, Schulman J. Pregnancy and prenatal harm to offspring: the case of mothers with PKU. Volume 17, No. 4, Hastings Center Report, 1987, Volume 23, p. 32.
30. McFall v Shimp (1978) 127 Pitts Leg J 14.
31. McLean SAM. Moral status (who or what counts?). *In*: Bewley S, Ward RH (eds), *Ethics in Obstetrics and Gynaecology*. London: RCOG Press, 1994: 26–33.
32. Lew JB. Terminally ill and pregnant: state denial of a woman's right to refuse a caesarean section. *Buffalo Law Rev* 1990;38:619,621–2.
33. Lew JB. Terminally ill and pregnant: state denial of a woman's right to refuse a caesarean section. *Buffalo Law Rev* 1990; 38 note 30, supra, 641.
34. Gregg R. 'Choice' as a double-edged sword: information, guilt and mother-blaming in a high-tech age. *Women Health* 1993;20:53.
35. Ikenotos LC. Code of perfect pregnancy. *Ohio State Law J* 1992;53:1205,1284–5.

Chapter 5 Clinical risk

Sam Pretlove

INTRODUCTION

The vast majority of doctors subscribe to the basic principle of medicine, 'to do no harm', and very few clinicians ever want their patients to come to any harm. In contrast to this, however, when clinical risk and patient safety are discussed, clinicians can be suspicious, regarding the necessary processes as either meaningless tick-box exercises or something imposed by the financial or management team to reduce cost, rather than viewing clinical risk management as an opportunity to shape and improve healthcare and the systems around us. Rather than being a topic for a few medical managers, being able to understand and evaluate clinical risk enables us to give women and their babies the highest possible standard of care. The NHS Constitution[1] enshrines the principles that guide the NHS in all it does. Principle 3 states that 'the NHS aspires to the highest standards of excellence and professionalism' and principle 4 that 'the NHS aspires to put patients at the heart of everything it does'. These principles cannot be put into practice without understanding the risks in clinical practice and the steps that are required to make the minimisation of risks a reality. When whole hospitals (and other organisations) become aware of this, it changes the culture so everyone understands and practises in a way that maximises patient safety.

The specialty of obstetrics and gynaecology is well known for high levels of litigation.[2] Therefore having a good understanding of clinical risk is particularly important for obstetricians and gynaecologists, and is not separate from clinical work. For example, health professionals working in a large tertiary referral maternity unit may consider that, as they are dealing with a complicated case mix of women, postpartum haemorrhages are an inevitable complication of childbirth.[3] Obstetrics has particular challenges, as levels of risk can change very quickly. For example, a low-risk multiparous woman who has an abruption at 37 weeks' gestation immediately changes to a high-risk delivery.

This chapter aims to cover the basic principles of risk management and patient safety and to discuss how they relate to clinical governance and the NHS complaints procedure.

HISTORY OF RISK MANAGEMENT

The Confidential Enquiry into Maternal Deaths (CEMD) is the classic example of risk management where a multidisciplinary team of obstetricians, midwives and anaesthetists formed an independent group to determine the causes of the rare event of maternal death and then disseminated the findings. Although the CEMD started in 1952, risk management as we know it has gradually evolved from a combination of audit, large-scale incidents and insights from industry applied to healthcare from the 1990s onwards. One of the most helpful ways to understand risk management is to look at key documents and events that changed how clinical risk was approached. Some of these occurred in the NHS whilst other initiatives were transferred from lessons learnt in industry.

The North Sea Piper Alpha disaster

On 6 July 1988 Piper Alpha, an offshore oil platform, exploded, killing 167 men. Piper Alpha was located 120 miles north of Aberdeen, off the coast of Scotland. A routine safety valve check for Pump A took place but the crew were unable to complete this in the usual time frame. The crew sealed off the pipe, with permission, with a plan to complete the work the next day. The permission paperwork was stored near the pipe, as was the usual practice. Later that evening, Pump B failed and the team on duty checked the central log to confirm Pump A could be started. There was no central record of a problem with Pump A and so it was switched on. Without the safety valve working correctly, the pump could not cope with the pressure generated and gas came out of the pump and ignited. A series of events due to the design of the platform meant that gas continued to pour into the fire for 22 minutes after the initial explosion.

The Piper Alpha disaster was the largest man-made disaster at the time, with damages costing US$3.4 billion. The loss of life was so high that it ensured the practices on the platform were investigated and the disaster was not passed off as a 'freak accident'. The Cullen enquiry took place in 1990 and made 106 recommendations regarding practice in the offshore oil industry. Many of the lessons learned have been transferable to other industries and organisations. These included: the design of the platform, expansion to cope with a larger amount of gas than was originally intended, communication and handover practices, inadequate training of staff in safety procedures, minimal response to inspection findings and overlooking small safety issues to maintain productivity.

Bristol heart scandal

In the 1990s an anaesthetist recognised that an excessive number of children were dying during open heart surgery at Bristol Royal Infirmary. The 'switch' operation for transposition of the great arteries (where both great arteries are disconnected, switched round and re-plumbed in) was stopped in 1995 after 9 of 13 babies who had the operation before 1993 had died in the previous 18 months. The Kennedy report in 2002 identified many concerns about the care in Bristol. The report identified poor teamwork, with the cardiologists and the cardiac surgeons based on different sites. There were difficulties inherent in the building, with the operating theatre and intensive care on different floors. In addition, the lift between the two departments was available for general use at all times. Although the mortality data had been collected and discussed, clinicians were reluctant to draw adverse conclusions from it, and speaking out about how the department was run was not encouraged or accepted.

'Bristol' is important as it changed attitudes to clinical governance and how incidents should be reported in a no-blame culture. It changed how organisations respond to concerns raised about services and whistleblowing. Risk management as we know it today started to be implemented in the 1990s, as incident reporting became established in hospitals and clinical governance was introduced as a statutory duty for NHS chief executives.

The document, 'An organisation with a memory' (OWAM)[2], published in 2000, was the report of an expert group, chaired by the Chief Medical Officer, on learning from adverse events in the NHS. This released the figures for known reported harm in the NHS. Key concepts brought out by the report were the similarities seen between many of the adverse events and 'learning the lessons of experience'. It became clear that if an adverse incident causing patient harm occurred in Hospital A there was no systematic mechanism to make Hospital B aware of any issues surrounding the incident. In practice this meant that, until the same adverse incident occurred in Hospital B, the system in Hospital B would not be changed, despite some staff in the NHS having the knowledge to prevent the adverse event occurring. The report called for systematic incident reporting and active implementation of lessons learned in organisations.

WHAT IS RISK MANAGEMENT?

Risk management has been defined by the RCOG as follows: 'Methods for early identification of adverse events, using either staff reports or systematic screening of records. This should be followed by creation of a database to identify common patterns and develop a system of accountability to prevent future incidents.'[4] Risks are reduced by a process which includes risk identification, compiling a risk register, risk analysis and risk control.

Risk identification

Risks are identified by either internal or external sources. Internal sources reflect information gathered from events and situations in the organisation. External sources are risks that have often been identified nationally.

Systematic risk assessments should occur both in clinical areas (e.g. delivery suite, gynaecology theatres, gynaecology wards and outpatient departments) and in non-clinical areas (e.g. secretarial offices and canteen) to ensure areas are as safe as possible with minimal hazards. Staff should be encouraged to complete incident forms for specific triggers. A possible list of triggers is given in Table 5.1. An organisation needs to have a culture where the staff are able to report incidents and know they will be listened to, not blamed for the incident. Patient complaints and legal claims also provide insights into where problems may exist in systems in the hospital. Clinical audit can be a powerful tool for providing evidence of a clinical risk.

Patient safety indicators are inexpensive and readily available data-sets, such as return-to-theatre rates or number of cases of *Clostridium difficile* identified. Patient safety indicators can raise awareness in organisations of specific problems and how often they occur, without using large amounts of resources. Patient safety indicators do not distinguish between a true adverse event and medical error but can provide evidence of trends within an organisation.

Some risks are present in most hospitals, such as hospital-acquired infections, medication errors, thromboembolic disease and retained swabs. Other risks are specific to obstetrics and gynaecology and a suggested list of identified risks from the RCOG is shown in Tables 5.1 and 5.2[4].

External sources that can demonstrate risk include the RCOG guidelines. For example, the guideline on small-for-gestational-age (SGA) explains how often women with risk factors or proven SGA should be scanned.[5] This requires a significant resource involving sonographers, ultrasound machines and physical space. If the guideline cannot be implemented immediately, there is a risk of undetected SGA and the potential for an avoidable stillbirth to occur. NICE guidelines may also suggest changes to clinical care which require increased staff and resources. National confidential enquiries may highlight risks experienced in other organisations which need to be addressed. Alerts from the National

Table 5.1 Suggested trigger list for incident reporting in maternity

Maternal incident	Fetal/neonatal incident	Organisational incident
Maternal death	Stillbirth >500 g	Unavailability of health record
Undiagnosed breech	Neonatal death	Delay in responding to call for assistance
Shoulder dystocia	Apgar score <7 at 5 minutes	Unplanned home birth
Blood loss >1500 mL	Birth trauma	Faulty equipment
Return to theatre	Fetal laceration at caesarean section	Conflict over case management
Eclampsia	Cord pH <7.05 arterial or 7.01 venous	Potential service user complaint
Hysterectomy/laparotomy	Neonatal seizures	Medication error
Anaesthetic complications	Term baby admitted to the neonatal unit	Retained swab or instrument
Intensive care admission	Undiagnosed fetal anomaly	Hospital-acquired infection
Venous thromboembolism	European congenital anomalies and twins (Eurocat)	Violation of local protocol
Pulmonary embolism		
Third/fourth degree tears		
Unsuccessful Ventouse/forceps		
Uterine rupture		
Readmission of mother		

Table 5.2 Suggested trigger list for incident reporting in gynaecology

Clinical incident	Organisation incident
Damage to structures, e.g. bowel, bladder, vessel	Delay following call for assistance
Delayed or missed diagnosis, e.g. ectopic pregnancy	Faulty equipment
Anaesthetic complications	Conflict over case management
Venous thromboembolism	Potential service user complaint
Failed procedures, e.g. sterilisation, termination of pregnancy	Medication error
Unplanned intensive care admission	Retained swab or instrument
Omission of planned procedures (failure to insert intrauterine device after hysteroscopy)	Violation of local protocol
Unexpected blood loss >500mL	
Moderate/severe ovarian hyperstimulation (assisted conception)	
Procedure performed without consent (e.g. removal of ovaries at hysterectomy)	
Unplanned return to theatre	
Unplanned return to hospital within 30 days	

Patient Safety Agency (NPSA) can also identify areas where steps need to be taken to change practice. Information on risks can also be obtained from external visits such as those by the postgraduate dean or the Care Quality Commission (CQC). NHS England also describes 'never events' which are defined as 'serious, largely preventable patient safety incidents that should not occur if the available preventative measures have been implemented'. These include incidents such as: wrong site surgery, retained instrument post-operation and wrong route administration of chemotherapy.[6]

Risk register

Once the risks have been identified, the next step is to quantify the level of risk. This is most commonly done using risk registers.

Divisions and departments identify their own risks, which are then graded with the standard matrix demonstrated in Table 5.3. Risk registers are not restricted to clinical issues. Problems with buildings, such as breakdown of the heating system on delivery suite causing issues with cold babies, or staffing shortages, can also be entered into the risk register.

Risks are scored between zero and five in two ways. First, how serious the risk is, from negligible to an event that results in multiple fatalities. The second score reflects how likely the event is to occur, from impossible to certain. The two scores are then multiplied together to give the risk score so the risks can be ordered and placed in a risk register.[7]

The most serious risks are collated and entered into the trust risk register where they should be reviewed regularly.

Table 5.3 Method for producing a risk matrix

Consequences	Probability					
	Impossible 0	Rare 1	Unlikely 2	Moderate 3	Likely 4	Certain 5
Negligible – 0	0	0	0	0	0	0
Minor – 1	0	1	2	3	4	5
Serious – 2	0	2	4	6	8	10
Major – 3	0	3	6	9	12	15
Fatality – 4	0	4	8	12	16	20
Multiple Fatalities – 5	0	5	10	15	20	25

Discussions should focus on how reduction could be achieved in either the severity of the risk or the frequency of it occurring. The impact of a risk register depends on how often and how effectively the risks are reviewed and whether subsequently situations are changed to reduce the risk. Having a risk register that is not reviewed or discussed will not reduce the risks in an organisation.

Risk analysis

Risk analysis involves identifying what went wrong after an incident has occurred. The incident should be investigated using Reason's organisational accident model (Fig. 5.1).[8] This places importance on the latent failures in a system and the pre-existing working conditions rather than just the active mistakes made at the time of the incident. Instead of asking 'What went wrong?', a better question is 'Why didn't the barriers put in place to stop errors work?'. This is important in preventing the same incidents happening again and again.

This model has been adapted by the NPSA to use as the 'fishbone' for root cause analyses (Fig. 5.2).

Below is a fictitious example of a scenario that could be examined in a root cause analysis. Although this is not a real incident, it is based on events that can happen in maternity units:

A woman who is 37 weeks' pregnant with twins in her first pregnancy is admitted in labour at midnight with her cervix 4 cm dilated. Eight midwives were recorded on the rota to be on shift but three are sick. She is allocated a junior midwife who starts the cardiotocograph (CTG) but is unhappy with the trace of twin 2. She asks for the midwifery shift leader to review the CTG but the shift leader is looking after a woman who has pre-eclampsia and a previous caesarean section, and who is fully dilated and pushing. The shift leader advises calling the doctor as she cannot leave her woman. The junior midwife calls the doctor, an ST1 (specialist trainee year 1) who started his first Obs and Gynae job the week before. The doctor is unsure what to do and asks for the registrar to look at the CTG. The registrar is busy in theatre with a laparoscopic ectopic but says she will be finished soon. The junior midwife and the ST1 wait for the registrar to attend. When the registrar comes an hour later, she takes the woman to

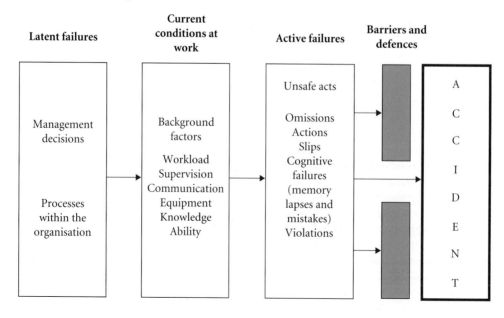

Fig. 5.1 Reason's organisational accident model

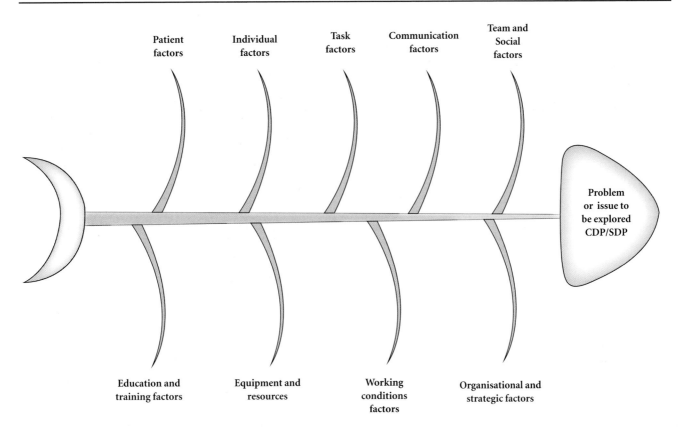

Fig. 5.2 The NPSA fishbone

theatre as a category 1 caesarean section and delivers the babies. Twin 2 suffers permanent hypoxic ischaemic brain damage.

The root cause analysis (RCA) is performed by staff who have undergone training in the process. Statements from those involved (the ST1, the registrar, the junior midwife and the shift leader) are collected and then the incident is presented. Instead of seeking to blame an individual for the events, the NPSA fishbone is used to systematically discuss where latent failures in the system occurred, the background to the incident and what, if any, part human error played. The staff are invited to attend and following the RCA are given individual feedback and support.

The incident is categorised according to whether or not suboptimal care was provided and, if there was suboptimal care, whether this had an impact on the outcome for the patient.

In the RCA, the team find there are ongoing problems with the midwifery rota system and that two of the midwives off sick that night were on long-term sick leave and should not have been on the rota. They also found that the gynaecology department struggled to get slots in the emergency theatre for women who appeared well and so the majority of emergency gynaecology was being performed out of hours, leaving the delivery suite exposed.

Rather than blaming the staff who were working that night, the RCA helped demonstrate the events that led to the situation where a woman's care was compromised. The staff had the opportunity to debrief with their supervisors and reflect on the events that had taken place in a structured and supported way.

Root cause analyses can be difficult and stressful for staff. Giving feedback in a helpful and constructive way can be time-consuming but is vital. If staff do not receive appropriate feedback they may disengage from the risk analysis process, reducing the quality of information gained and potentially reducing the impact of change identified through RCAs.

Risk control

Measures should then be put in place to reduce the risks. This can be by avoiding the risk, by substitution of an alternative lower risk or by implementing change to reduce the likelihood of the incident happening again. Ideally, this should be part of a coordinated approach to risk management, rather than individuals making small changes in different parts of the organisation without considering the impact in other areas.

An important clinical example of risk reduction is the World Health Organization (WHO) surgical safety checklist,[9] developed by Atul Gawande, an American endocrine surgeon:

Good checklists ... are precise. They are efficient, to the point, and easy to use even in the most difficult situations. They do not try to spell out everything – a checklist cannot fly a plane. Instead, they provide reminders of only the most critical and important steps – the ones that even the highly skilled professional using them could miss. Good checklists are, above all, practical. Atul Gawande.[11]

The checklist corresponds to the flow of work, with the sign-in check before anaesthesia is induced, the time-out check before the incision of the skin and the sign-out before the patient leaves the operating theatre. A large trial of its efficacy involved eight hospitals in eight different cities worldwide. This was not a randomised controlled trial but rather each site completed a baseline period followed by a second period where the checklist was introduced. Large numbers were recruited to the study ($n = 3733$ for the baseline period, and $n = 3955$ for second period). The trial demonstrated a significant reduction in death (from 1.5% to 0.8%, $P = 0.003$) during or after surgery. In addition the risk of any complication also dropped from 11.0% to 7.0%. Surgical site infection and unplanned return to theatre also dropped significantly. There was an increased adherence to appropriate antibiotic use from 56% to 83%.[10]

Inevitably there have been criticisms of the WHO surgical safety checklist, which have included concerns that it has less of an impact in high-income countries, that the success is dependent on the attitude of staff not the checklist itself, that implementation may result in unforeseen resource implications and that it can be difficult to administer in some settings (e.g. 'crash' caesarean section). Despite this the surgical checklist remains an important demonstration of how risk control can be effective clinically.

UNDERSTANDING THE COMPLAINTS PROCESS

Most complaints or issues can be resolved by talking directly to the complainant, acknowledging the situation and making a plan for the future. There are times when this does not resolve the complaint and a formal written complaint is made. Every NHS organisation has a complaints policy and process. Complaints can be made directly to the service provider but can also go to the Clinical Commissioning Group (CCG) or NHS England. If a complaint is made to a service provider and investigated, the same complaint cannot be taken to the CCG or NHS England. Usually complaints need to be made within 12 months of the incident to be valid.

If the matter cannot be resolved with the service provider, the complainant can refer to the Parliamentary and Health Service Ombudsman. Organisations are then obliged to put in place recommendations from the Ombudsman.

Complaints (and compliments) are an important source of patient feedback. Themes and recurring problems should be identified so that, where appropriate, changes can be made to the service provision to improve care. Complaints should be regularly audited to ensure that issues such as equality are considered. It could be presumed that not receiving complaints from some groups of the population means that they are happy with the service they receive. Alternatively, however, this may mean that some groups are unable to represent their problems and difficulties with the service, and remain unhappy and disengaged.

SUMMARY

Delivering high-quality care is a fundamental challenge for obstetricians and gynaecologists as we work in a high-risk specialty often delivering complex care. Understanding how to identify risks and develop systems that prevent or significantly reduce adverse events can enable us to give women and their babies the safe, effective and high-quality care they deserve.

Key References

1. The NHS Constitution. http://www.nhs.uk/choiceintheNHS/Rightsandpledges/NHSConstitution/Documents/2013/the-nhs-constitution-for-england-2013.pdf.

2. An organisation with a memory (OWAM). http://webarchive.nationalarchives.gov.uk/20130107105354/http://www.dh.gov.uk/prod_consum_dh/groups/dh_digitalassets/@dh/@en/documents/digitalasset/dh_4065086.pdf.

3. Vincent C. The measurement and monitoring of safety. The Health Foundation. http://www.health.org.uk/public/cms/75/76/313/4209/The%20measurement%20and%20monitoring%20of%20safety%20In%20brief.pdf?realName=jXdgR2.pdf.

4. Royal College of Obstetricians and Gynaecologists. *Improving patient safety: risk management for maternity and gynaecology.* RCOG Clinical Governance Advice No. 2. London: RCOG, 2009.

5. Royal College of Obstetricians and Gynaecologists. *Small for Gestational Age Fetus: Investigation and management.* RCOG Green-top guideline No. 31, 2013. London: RCOG. https://www.rcog.org.uk/en/guidelines-research-services/guidelines/gtg31/.

6. NHS England. Never events. Available at: http://www.england.nhs.uk/ourwork/patientsafety/never-events/.

7. Standards Association of Australia. Risk management AS/NZS 4360 Strathfield: Standards Association of Australia, 1999.

8. Reason JT. Understanding adverse events: human factors in. In: Vincent CA, ed. *Clinical Risk Management.* London: BMJ Publications, 1995: 31–54.

9. Editorial. WHO's patient-safety checklist for surgery. *Lancet* 2008;372:1.

10. Haynes AB, Weisser TG, Berry WR, Lipsitz SR, Breizat AH, Dellinger EP, *et al.* Safer Surgery Saves Lives Study Group. A surgical safety checklist to reduce morbidity and mortality in a global population. *N Engl J Med* 2009;360;491–9.

11. Gawande A. *The Checklist Manifesto.* New York: Picador, 2009.

Chapter 6 Rationale for advanced skills training

Timothy Draycott and Islam Gamaleldin

MRCOG standard

Competence in the management of shoulder dystocia, eclampsia and obstetric collapse is essential for completion of core training.

INTRODUCTION

Maternity care could and should be safer.[1] Adverse outcomes in maternity care are frequently avoidable and the cost of litigation for maternity care is rising for many health services across the world.[2–4] This is a tragedy for families for whom the injury was preventable, an enormous loss of resource to healthcare in general and possibly even a perverse incentive against best care.[5]

Poor care and avoidable harm are not confined to developing countries. In 2008, the UK-based King's Fund report, *Safe Births: Everybody's business*,[1] observed that, whilst the overwhelming majority of births in England are safe, some births are less safe than they could and should be. This observation may accurately describe obstetric care in the UK over the last century. There are similar problems with maternity care in France, Netherlands and the United States.[4]

Investigations of the root causes of maternal and perinatal mortality have consistently identified poor management of obstetric emergencies, including failure to recognise problems, failure to seek senior input, poor team working, poor communication and a need to improve these.[6–8]

Obstetric emergencies are rare, occurring rapidly and unpredictably. Their successful management requires a coordinated response by a multiprofessional team and although it is axiomatic that they should be managed by experienced staff – and indeed this is almost ubiquitously recommended – experience is difficult to acquire because of their rarity. This experience may be best gained in part through simulation.

This has led to repeated recommendations for obstetric emergency training, particularly simulation-based training, to prevent avoidable harm.

HARM AVOIDABLE WITH TRAINING

Poor team working, suboptimal communication and lack of effective training have been identified as possible contributors to preventable mortality and morbidity in maternity care.

Maternal mortality and morbidity

At least half of all maternal deaths are still considered avoidable. In the UK, the most recent Centre for Maternal and Child Enquiries (CMACE) report, *Saving Mothers' Lives*, published in 2011, identified substandard care in 70% of direct deaths and 55% of indirect deaths.[9] Absent and poor team working were repeatedly identified as significant contributors to substandard care.[10] Several other reports have demonstrated that accurate management of obstetric emergencies could have prevented significant maternal morbidities, including hysterectomy, multiple organ failure, shock, coma and admission to an intensive care unit.[11–14]

Women's experience of labour and birth has significant implications for breastfeeding, bonding, expectations for future birth and sexual function.[15,16] A unique challenge in obstetric emergencies is that mothers are most often awake with close relatives in attendance. A UK-based study demonstrated that over 25% of new mothers were not satisfied with communication by medical staff, which shows that training is needed to increase the overall satisfaction with care[17] and to decrease the risk of litigation.

Systematic reviews have demonstrated that debriefing after the emergency may not be helpful to parents,[18,19] and improved communication during the acute event is likely to be the most effective method of reducing the psychological morbidity. Therefore communication should be improved generally during the emergency, not just between other team members but also with the woman and her companions.

Perinatal mortality and morbidity

In 1917 the UK Medical Research Committee (MRC) reported that 52 per cent of infant deaths were avoidable, yet the 4th Confidential Enquiry into Stillbirth and Deaths in Infancy (CESDI) report, published 80 years later, in 1997, still identified that over 50% of intrapartum stillbirths were avoidable with better care.[20] Therefore although perinatal outcomes have improved significantly over the last century, the proportion of avoidable deaths has remained depressingly static.[20]

Litigation and complaints

This avoidable harm is extraordinarily expensive and the expense is rising.[2–4] Maternity claims represent the highest-value litigation claims reported to the NHS litigation authority (NHSLA). Substandard care and its sequelae cost the NHS £3.1 billion in the decade 2001–2010. Three (overlapping) categories accounted for 70% of the total value of claims: mistakes in fetal heart rate interpretation, mistakes in the management of labour and the development of cerebral palsy.[4]

Improved multiprofessional training appears to be one of the most promising strategies to improve perinatal outcomes across the world, localised for best fit, with a parallel evaluation of outcomes to ensure a positive effect.

SIMULATION TRAINING

The use of simulation in obstetrics is several centuries old. The earliest simulators were developed after 1600 and were known as 'phantoms'. They were used to teach midwives how to manage complicated deliveries.[21] This was followed by William Smellie, who developed a pelvis using human bones covered by leather, a fetus of wood and rubber, and a placenta also made of leather.[22] As early as 1760 a French midwife, Madame du Coudray, recognised that poor training of midwives around France could directly cause harm, and that training on a life-sized and anatomically correct mannequin phantom called 'The Machine' could potentially reduce these harms.[23]

More modern simulation models used for training in obstetrics range from very simple ones such as a bony pelvis with a baby, or trousers with red material to reproduce visual clues for postpartum haemorrhage,[24] through to complex, sophisticated simulators such as the SimMom, the NOELLE and the Practical Obstetric Multiprofessional Training (PROMPT) birth simulator. At one end of the spectrum, simple part-task trainers are less expensive and can be used alone to teach specific skills, for example instrumental deliveries or shoulder dystocia manoeuvres, or in combination with a simulated patient (hybrid simulation). At the other end of the spectrum, computer-based virtual reality simulator models can provide both kinaesthetic and visual feedback to learners. Both have their place depending on the skills that need to be practised and on available resources.

Both simple and advanced simulation models can be used to teach obstetric skills within structured training programmes. Such structured simulation-based training courses in obstetric emergencies were developed and implemented in 1990s. The 'Advanced Life Support in Obstetrics' (ALSO) course was introduced in 1991 in the United States,[25] followed by the 'Managing Obstetric Emergencies and Trauma' (MOET) course in 1998 to teach advanced skills to obstetricians and anaesthetists.[26] More recently, the PROMPT course was developed in the UK, as a training package for obstetricians, midwives and anaesthetists, allowing the implementation of local training in individual maternity units.[27]

Since 2003, a nascent evidence base for intrapartum skills training has emerged and we shall review the current evidence for effective training for obstetric emergencies.

EVIDENCE OF EFFECTIVENESS

Intrapartum care demands sensitivity, clinical skill and acumen from a multi-professional team of carers. Training should address all these elements, and this is likely to require a broad range of training techniques and tools. The King's Fund report[1] recognised that:

> Maternity units could easily provide their own simulation-based training .... Any such training should include clinical skills, communication, team working, and awareness of roles within the team.

A systematic review of obstetric emergencies training published in 2003 concluded that there was minimal evidence to support obstetric skills training.[28] Since 2003, however, several studies have been published evaluating the effectiveness of skills training for obstetric emergencies, not all of them positive.

Training is not magic, nor is it automatically effective, and the current literature is conflicting. There are a number of studies where training either did not improve clinical outcomes[29,30] or was associated with an increase in perinatal morbidity.[31]

We should demand the same robust research for training that we do for other obstetric interventions, to ensure that training passes the 'Ronseal' test. In 1975, Donald Kirkpatrick described the evaluation of training programmes using four interconnected levels[32] (Table 6.1). Ideally, training programmes should aim to show effectiveness on all levels including up to level four – change in clinical outcome.

We have reviewed the current evidence for obstetric emergency training using the Kirkpatrick levels as a framework and hierarchical evidence of effect.

Table 6.1 Kirkpatrick's levels of programme evaluation

Level	Description	Expansion
K1	Reaction	How participants felt about the training, e.g. self-perceived changes in confidence
K2	Learning	Formally evaluated changes in knowledge and/or skills following training, e.g. post-course questionnaires
K3	Behaviour	Demonstrable improvement in skill levels of participants, persisting through to the workplace of participants (i.e. actual clinical care)
K4	Outcomes	Changes in clinical outcomes following implementation of training, e.g. improvement in morbidity or mortality statistics

Eclampsia

Eclampsia is a rare and catastrophic obstetric emergency. Its incidence in the UK has been falling, whilst substandard care for eclampsia has increased, accounting for over 90% of pre-eclampsia and eclampsia deaths.[9] It appears that we have been getting better at preventing eclampsia after the publication of the Magpie trial,[33] but not getting better at managing eclampsia when it does happen, particularly now that it is even less common. This may be surprising given that one of the first reported obstetric drills was for the management of eclampsia,[34] and training has been recommended since at least 1996.[35] Moreover, a subsequent RCT[36] demonstrated marked improvement after training of maternity staff in interprofessional teams using realistic simulation. Following training there were significant increases in completion of basic tasks (including calling for help, stating the problem, calling for an anaesthetist, lowered head rest, recovery position and oxygen administration) (87% pre vs 100% post) and magnesium sulphate administration (61% pre vs 92% post) [K2].

There are data to inform best practice for women with eclampsia and these data have been used to produce a national guideline. There are also data that inform training for eclampsia, but clearly there has been a disconnection between the two. It is vital that we link these data to better understand the implementation of national guidance.

Shoulder dystocia

Training to manage shoulder dystocia is an excellent example of what can be achieved using simulation as both an implementation tool and a laboratory bench to understand and address the barriers preventing staff from providing best care.

There is wide variation in the reported incidence of shoulder dystocia[37] – from 0.58% to 3%.[38–43] Shoulder dystocia is rare, unpredictable and associated with significant perinatal morbidity (brachial plexus injury and hypoxic ischaemic encephalopathy) and mortality,[40] but it is probably the single most studied obstetric emergency, certainly in simulation research.

Practical shoulder dystocia training has been shown to improve knowledge,[44] confidence[45] and management of simulated shoulder dystocia.[46–49] Training has also been shown to improve patient-actors' perception of their care during simulated shoulder dystocia.[50]

Reports of the effect of training on perinatal outcomes, however, have been conflicting: an 8-year retrospective review of shoulder dystocia management before and after the introduction of annual shoulder dystocia training for all staff in one UK hospital demonstrated a significant reduction in neonatal injury at birth following shoulder dystocia: 9.3% pre-training, 2.3% post-training.[51] There are other reports of improvements after training,[52–54] but training has also been associated with no change in outcome[55] or even deterioration in neonatal outcome.[56]

The RCOG has recognised in their national guideline that:

Training associated with improvements in clinical management and neonatal outcome following shoulder dystocia was multiprofessional, with manoeuvres demonstrated and practised on a highfidelity mannequin.[51]

Teaching used the RCOG algorithm and staff were not taught mnemonics (e.g. HELPERR – [H: call for help, E: evaluate for episiotomy, L: legs, McRoberts maneuver, P: suprapubic pressure, E: enter: rotational maneuvers, R: remove the posterior arm, R: roll the patient to hands and knees.]) or eponyms (e.g. Rubin's and Wood's screws).[57]

Postpartum haemorrhage

Postpartum haemorrhage (PPH) contributes to 140,000 deaths worldwide annually.[58] Although PPH is more common in low-resource settings, it is still a significant problem for high-resource countries, complicating 4–6% of all deliveries,[59] and therefore both the Joint Commission on Accreditation of Healthcare and the UK CEMD have stressed the importance of simulation drills and regular training for all staff in reducing morbidity and mortality from PPH.[11,60]

Once again the data for training efficacy are conflicting. There are reports of no effect of simulation-based training for PPH in both Denmark[30] and the UK.[61] On the other hand, a group[62] who provided lectures and simulation-based training for all high- and mid-level providers involved in childbirth at a hospital in Tanzania demonstrated a decrease in PPH rates following training (33% pre vs 18% post), in parallel with an increase in the proportion of women with active management of the third stage (25.1% post vs 0.6% pre), including uterine massage, bimanual compression and oxytocin infusion [K4].

Once again there is a requirement to investigate the effect of simulation-based training and to define the active ingredients of effective training.

Cord prolapse

Cord prolapse is a rare obstetric emergency complicating 1% of deliveries,[63] but it is associated with a very high fetal mortality rate of 10%.[64] Because of the rarity of the condition, a randomised trial to determine the effectiveness of training would be impossible, and therefore there are only observational studies available. Recently, a retrospective cohort study demonstrated a statistically significant reduction in median diagnosis–delivery interval (25 minutes pre vs 14.5 minutes post) for women after cord prolapse following simulation-based training.[65] This improvement was associated with a consistent reduction in the rates of infants born with both low Apgar score and neonatal intensive care unit (NICU) admission [4]. Crucially, the simulation training programme was interprofessional, covered teamwork in principle and in action, and included 100% of maternity staff.

Maternal collapse

Maternal cardiac arrest is a rare complication occurring in approximately 1:30,000 pregnancies in the UK.[11] The national Confidential Enquiry reported in 2007[11] that resuscitation skills were unacceptably poor in a high number of maternal deaths. It was therefore recommended that all clinical staff should have regular training to improve basic, intermediate and advanced life support.

Simulation provides an opportunity to practise skills for this very rare problem, and improved care after cardiac arrest has been described after simulation training in a general hospital setting.[66] A small US study also found improved outcome in an obstetric setting.[67]

A retrospective cohort study evaluating the use of perimortem caesarean section (PMCS) in the Netherlands after the introduction of training showed that the utilisation rate of PMCS increased (12% pre vs 35% post).[68] The outcome, however, remained poor, possibly attributable to slow recognition, failure to initiate cardiopulmonary resuscitation (CPR), failure to display the uterus, poor communication, and delay in performing the procedure, as none was performed within 5 minutes of the arrest [K3]. Once again, it is not just individual decision-making and practical skills that make a difference to the clinical outcome of these rare situations, it is also the coordination and efficiency of the whole maternity team.

Instrumental delivery

The appropriate and safe use of forceps and vacuum instruments to assist vaginal birth should be one way to limit the ever-rising rate of caesarean section. This rise may be due to reduced senior supervision at night, leading most obstetric trainees to perform a caesarean section rather than attempt a difficult instrumental delivery. At the same time, UK obstetric trainees have identified that skills for operative birth, especially rotational operative births, are difficult to acquire and implement.[69] Simulation training may bridge the gap and help trainees build confidence and competence.

A high-fidelity model developed by Dupius et al. allows the trajectory of the application of forceps blades to be tracked using spatial sensors.[70] Following training, there was improvement in the abilities of junior doctors to perform instrumental deliveries.[70] Models have also been developed to train juniors in the appropriate traction. Both Moreau et al.[71] and Leslie et al.[72] found that correct forces and successful deliveries increased after simulating operative vaginal births [K3].

The RCOG has developed a new training course to meet the requirements for effective simulation-based training for operative vaginal birth: ROBUST (RCOG Operative Birth Simulation Training).

Communication and effect on patient perception

In obstetric care, complications commonly occur when the woman is conscious, and poor maternal experience is another significant complication of pregnancy and birth. UK-based research showed that over 25% of new mothers were not satisfied with communication by the medical staff, and there was a significant association between satisfaction with communication by medical staff and overall satisfaction with care.[73] Therefore training in communication with the women, their companions and among team members is crucial. This training can be delivered through simulation that can build confidence, which is then transmitted to the patient involved, creating a reciprocal feeling of safety and assurance that the situation is being managed appropriately and efficiently.

Communication with patient actors was improved after simulation training using the actors,[64,65] who reported improvement of safety perception with information about the cause of emergency, their baby's condition and the treatment plan [K3].

HOW SHOULD WE TRAIN?

It's not that practice makes perfect, but perfect practice leads to proficiency and perhaps perfection. Dr Andrew J Satin

Simulation-based training is a very promising intervention, but we should not overestimate the effect of simulation. A recent review of simulation-based medical education (SMBE) recognised that some but not all SMBE was associated with improvements in clinical outcome.[74]

There is an important need to test whether obstetric simulation training programmes are effective, sustainable and cost-effective. A review of the obstetric programmes associated with improvement in clinical outcome in 2009[75] highlighted the common features of clinically effective training:.

Multiprofessional training of all staff in an institution

Training should encourage active participation from all team members, including doctors, midwives, porters and healthcare assistants[76] and should take place in a non-threatening environment,[77,78] with everyone training in their professional role. Feedback should be given in a constructive way, stressing the positive attitudes of the participants, and possibly using a standardised checklist to be completed by peers, to reduce the authority gradient of facilitation by senior staff.

Training staff locally within their unit

Local (in-house) training can be less expensive than simulation centres; it helps units to recognise local safety issues and helps new staff members to familiarise themselves with their working environment.

In a previous study staff were able, after training, to identify and correct latent threats to patient safety in relation to emergency caesarean sections, peripartum hysterectomy and neonatal resuscitation.[79] Another study assessing local simulation demonstrated that the patient's bed could not pass through some labour ward rooms, resulting in unnecessary and potentially harmful delays. It appears to be the most effective way of improving outcome(s),[80] but it is not always feasible as small units will face problems in providing physical space and staff for training.

Realistic simulation

Environmental and training fidelity is important,[57] but high fidelity is not always synonymous with 'high technology'. There are a number of simulation-based courses that make use of simple, inexpensive tools to increase realism – e.g. trousers that 'bleed' red material and a perineum with prolapsed cord.[24]

Institutional-level incentives for training

Implementing and subsequently running a training programme is demanding and can be costly through staff release, space for training and funding of training equipment. However, institutions can justify, or offset, the cost of running training directly from reduced insurance premiums[4,63,75,81–83] and the insurers will recoup their investment downstream through better outcomes.

Interprofessional clinical training with integrated team work

Team training recognises that people make fewer errors when they work together. National bodies now recommend interprofessional training for the whole maternity team, comprising doctors, midwives and allied workers such as porters and healthcare assistants.[76]

Studies analysing the behaviour of teams in simulated emergencies have highlighted that good situational awareness is essential for good teamwork,[84,85] in particular three components of situational awareness for teams managing obstetric emergencies:

1 clinical situation awareness;
2 team awareness;
3 patient focus and involvement.[86]

In addition the most effective maternity teams in one study used 'closed-loop communication', where team members clearly direct a message to intended recipients (by touching, naming and establishing eye contact with them), who acknowledge the information on task allocation verbally and then confirm that it has been correctly acted upon.[87] Such clear and directed communication is associated with fewer errors and repetitions[88] and a shorter time interval to administer important drugs such as magnesium sulphate for eclampsia[89] and Syntometrine for PPH.[88,89]

Evidence-based training

Training should be based on, and implement, evidence-based practice.[11,60] Training can also be used to give local impact to national guidance[89–92] and develop implementation tools, e.g. CTG stickers, as mere availability of these guidelines is often not sufficient to change practice.

Evaluation of training

Ideally, training programmes should be formally evaluated, at least prior to distribution at scale. Moreover, it would be useful to understand implementation strategies and also the effect of the local context.

There is, however, minimal or no evidence that assessment of local practitioners is useful, or helpful.

Training in low-resource settings

The WHO Millennium Goals 4 and 5 aim to reduce infant mortality rates by two-thirds and maternal mortality rates by 75% by year 2015. Simulation will have a role in reaching these targets if it is not solely confined to the developed world. Training should be universal. Many candidates reading this book, particularly overseas candidates, will question the role of simulation training in obstetric emergencies. Even in busy units where emergencies such as eclampsia and shoulder dystocia are relatively more frequent, there is still an important role for simulation-based training. A recent WHO review of intrapartum training in low- and middle-income countries concluded that:

> Where in-service training can be provided at a low cost, it may be worthwhile to do so, given that some improvements in the care process can be expected. However, in general, such training may be associated with high cost and therefore for most settings it is difficult to justify the conduct of routine in-service neonatal and paediatric training courses primarily based on models developed in high-income countries.[93]

Care must be taken to avoid inappropriate 'square peg in a round hole' introduction of non-localised courses from high-income settings.

Once again the published data are conflicting: the introduction of training with the Essential Newborn Care course based in six countries (Argentina, Democratic Republic of Congo, Guatemala, India, Pakistan and Zambia) showed significant reduction in rate of stillbirths following training (23 per 1000 pre vs 15.9 per 1000 post),[94] whereas another study assessing the effect of training in improving outcomes done in a regional hospital in Tanzania showed that the introduction of ALSO training from the United States did not improve outcomes.[62]

Success of training programmes in low-resource settings depends on many factors such as appropriately skilled instructors, locally adapted training materials and time for training. More work is required to understand the specific requirements for, and local adaptation of training in, developing world settings.

CONCLUSION

Reducing avoidable harm is a priority for midwives, women and families across the world. Simulation-based training for obstetric emergencies appears to offer a direct route to improvement, but the effect of intrapartum training programmes has been inconsistent, if not conflicting.

Significant progress has been made at establishing an evidence base for training in obstetric emergencies since the publication of Black and Brocklehurst's paper in 2003.[28] However, those studies that demonstrate improvement in clinical outcomes are retrospective and only report neonatal outcome data, and there remains very little evidence for maternal outcomes. The next stage should be a well-designed RCT studying the effect of training on both maternal and neonatal outcomes across several hospitals while adjusting for baseline changes and temporal changes.

There is currently evidence of a positive impact of training on confidence, knowledge and skills, with emerging evidence of improvements for at least some perinatal outcomes. Therefore, based on the current available evidence, training for obstetric emergencies should be local, multiprofessional, mandatory for all staff and ideally supported by institutional incentives (most often insurance based) to train.

KEY POINTS

- Poor team working, suboptimal communication and lack of proper training can lead to preventable maternal and perinatal harm.
- Simulation-based training is one of the most promising strategies and can potentially reduce these avoidable complications by 50–70%.[6]
- Simulation-based training for maternity staff should be both effective and sustainable.
- Training programmes associated with improvements in perinatal outcome were all conducted 'in-house', trained 100% of staff, reported the introduction of system changes suggested by their staff after participating in the training, and trained all staff together, incorporating teamwork principles into clinical training scenarios.[76]
- Training in low-resource settings may be different and local adaptation of training courses is crucial for locally sustainable training programmes.

Key References

1. King's Fund. *Safe Births: Everybody's business. An independent inquiry into the safety of maternity services in England.* London: King's Fund, 2008.
2. Henary BY, Al-Yahia OA, Al-Gabanny SA, Al-Kharaz SM. Epidemiology of medico-legal litigations and related medical errors in Central and Northern Saudi Arabia. A retrospective prevalence study. *Saudi Med J* 2012;33:768–75.

3. Berkowitz RL. Of parachutes and patient care: a call to action. *Am J Obst Gynecol* 2011;205:7–9.

4. NHS Litigation Authority. *Ten Years of Maternity Claims: An analysis of NHS Litigation Authority data.* London: NHSLA, 2012.

5. Zwecker P, Azoulay L, Abenhaim HA. Effect of fear of litigation on obstetric care: a nationwide analysis on obstetric practice. *Am J Perinatol* 2011;28:277–84.6.

6. Lewis G (ed.) Saving mothers' lives: reviewing maternal deaths to make motherhood safer 2006–2008. *BJOG* 2011;118 (Suppl 1):1–205.

7. The Joint Commission. *Issue 30: Preventing infant death and injury during delivery.* Joint Commission, 1–2. /http://www.jointcommission.org/assets/1/18/SEA_30. PDFS; 2004. Accessed 06.12.12.

8. O'Mahony F, Settatree R, Platt C, Johanson R. Review of singleton fetal and neonatal deaths associated with cranial trauma and cephalic delivery during a national intrapartum-related confidential enquiry. *BJOG* 2005;112:619–26.

9. Draycott T, Lewis G, Stephens I. Executive Summary, Eighth Report of the Confidential Enquiries into Maternal Deaths in the UK. *BJOG* 2011;118(Suppl 1): e12–e21.

10. Confidential Enquiry into Stillbirths and Deaths in Infancy. *7th Annual report.* London: CESDI, 2000 106.

11. Lewis G (ed.). Confidential Enquiry into Maternal and Child Health (CEMACH). *Saving Mothers' Lives: Reviewing maternal deaths to make motherhood safer 2003–2005. The Seventh Report of the Confidential Enquiries into Maternal Deaths in the United Kingdom.* London: CEMACH, 2007.

12. Knight M, UKOSS. Antenatal pulmonary embolism: risk factors, management and outcomes. *BJOG* 2008;115:453–61.

13. Knight M, UKOSS. Peripartum hysterectomy in the UK: management and outcomes of the associated haemorrhage. *BJOG* 2007;114:1380–7.

14. Knight M, UKOSS. Eclampsia in the United Kingdom 2005. *BJOG* 2007;114:1072–8.

15. Goodman P, Mackey MC, Tavakoli AS. Factors related to childbirth satisfaction. *J Adv Nursing* 2004; 46:212–19.

16. Bahl R, Strachan B, Murphy DJ. Outcome of subsequent pregnancy three years after previous operative delivery in the second stage of labour: cohort study. *BMJ* 2004;328:311.

17. Kirke PN. Mothers' views of obstetric care. *Br J Obstet Gynaecol* 1980;87:1029–33.

18. Roberts N, Kitchiner NJ, Kenardy J *et al.* Multiple session early psychological interventions for the prevention of post-traumatic stress disorder. *Cochrane Database Syst Rev* 2009;8:CD006869.

19. Rowan C, Bick D, Bastos MH. Postnatal debriefing interventions to prevent maternal mental health problems after birth: exploring the gap between the evidence and UK policy and practice. *Worldviews Evid Based Nurs* 2007;4:97–105.

20. Maternal and Child Health Research Consortium, CESDI 4th Annual Report. *Care during Labour and Delivery.* London: CESDI, 1997: 35–44.

21. Buck GH. Development of simulators in medical education. *Gesnerus* 1991;48:7–28.

22. Wilson A. A new synthesis: William Smellie. *In: The Making of Man-Midwifery: Childbirth in England 1660–1770.* London: University College London Press, 1995.

23. Gelbert NR. *The King's Midwife: a history and mystery of Madame Du Coudray.* Vol. 1. Berkeley, CA: University of California Press, 1999.

24. Draycott T, Winter C, Crofts J, Barnfield S. *Practical Obstetric Multiprofessional Training (PROMPT) Trainer's Manual.* London: RCOG Press, 2008.

25. Beasley JW, Damos JR, Roberts RG, Nesbitt TS. The advanced life support in obstetrics course: a national program to enhance obstetric emergency skills and to support maternity care practice. *Arch Fam Med* 1994;3:1037–41.

26. Johanson R, Cox C, O'Donnell E *et al.* Managing obstetric emergencies and trauma (MOET): structured skills training using models and reality-based scenarios. *The Obstetrician & Gynaecologist* 1999;1:46–52.

27. Sibanda T, Crofts J, Barnfield S *et al.* PROMPT education and development: saving mothers' and babies' lives in resource-poor settings. *BJOG* 2009;116:868–9.

28. Black RS, Brocklehurst P. A systematic review of training in acute obstetric emergencies. *BJOG* 2003;110: 837–41.

29. Nielsen PE, Goldman MB, Mann S *et al.* Effects of teamwork training on adverse outcomes and process of care in labor and delivery: a randomized controlled trial. *Obstet Gynecol* 2007;109:48–55.

30. Markova V, Sorensen JL, Holm C *et al.* Evaluation of multiprofessional obstetric skills training for postpartum hemorrhage. *Acta Obstet Gynecol Scand* 2012;91:346–52.

31. MacKenzie IZ, Shah M, Lean K *et al.* Management of shoulder dystocia: trends in incidence and maternal and neonatal morbidity. *Obstet Gynecol* 2007;110:1059–68.

32. Kirkpatrick DL, Kirkpatrick JD. *Evaluating Training Programs*, Vol 3. San Francisco CA: Berrett-Koehler, 2009.

33. Altman D, Carroli G, Duley L, et al. Do women with pre-eclampsia and their babies, benefit from magnesium sulphate? The Magpie Trial: a randomised placebo-controlled trial. *Lancet* 2002;359:1877-90.

34. Draycott T, Broad G, Chidley K. The development of an eclampsia box and 'fire drill'. *Br J Midwifery* 2000;8:26–30.

35. Infancy. *Confidential Enquiries into Stillbirth and Deaths in Infancy, 5th Annual Report.* London: CESDI, 1996.

36. Ellis D, Crofts JF, Hunt LP *et al.* Hospital, simulation center, and teamwork training for eclampsia management: a randomized controlled trial. *Obstet Gynecol* 2008;111:723–31.

37. Gherman RB. Shoulder dystocia: an evidence-based evaluation of the obstetric nightmare. *Clin Obstet Gynecol* 2002;45:345–62.

38. McFarland M, Hod M, Piper JM *et al.* Are labor abnormalities more common in shoulder dystocia? *Am J Obstet Gynecol* 1995;173:1211–14.

39. Baskett TF, Allen AC. Perinatal implications of shoulder dystocia. *Obstet Gynecol* 1995;86:14–17.

40. Gherman RB, Ouzounian JG, Goodwin TM. Obstetric maneuvers for shoulder dystocia and associated fetal morbidity. *Am J Obstet Gynecol* 1998;178:1126–30.

41. McFarland MB, Langer O, Piper JM, Berkus MD. Perinatal outcome and the type and number of maneuvers in shoulder dystocia. *Int J Gynaecol Obstet* 1996;55:219–24.

42. Ouzounian JG, Gherman RB. Shoulder dystocia: are historic risk factors reliable predictors? *Am J Obstet Gynecol* 2005;192:1933–5; discussion 1935–8.

43. Smith RB, Lane C, Pearson JF. Shoulder dystocia: what happens at the next delivery? *Br J Obstet Gynaecol* 1994;101:713–15.

44. Crofts JF, Ellis D, Draycott TJ *et al.* Change in knowledge of midwives and obstetricians following obstetric emergency training: a randomised controlled trial of local hospital, simulation centre and teamwork training. *BJOG* 2007;114:1534–41.

45. Sorensen JL, Lokkegaard E, Johansen M *et al.* The implementation and evaluation of a mandatory multiprofessional obstetric skills training program. *Acta Obstet Gynecol Scand* 2009;88:1107–17.

46. Goffman D, Heo H, Pardanani S *et al.* Improving shoulder dystocia management among resident and attending physicians using simulations. *Am J Obstet Gynecol* 2008;199:294.e1–5.

47. Crofts JF, Bartlett C, Ellis D *et al.* Training for shoulder dystocia: a trial of simulation using low-fidelity and high-fidelity mannequins. *Obstet Gynecol* 2006;108:1477–85.

48. Crofts JF, Attilakos G, Read M *et al.* Shoulder dystocia training using a new birth training mannequin. *BJOG* 2005;112:997–9.

49. Deering S, Poggi S, Macedonia C *et al.* Improving resident competency in the management of shoulder dystocia with simulation training. *Obstet Gynecol* 2004;103:1224–8.

50. Crofts JF, Bartlett C, Ellis D *et al.* Patient-actor perception of care: a comparison of obstetric emergency training using mannequins and patient-actors. *Qual Saf Health Care* 2008;17:20–4.

51. Draycott TJ, Crofts JF, Ash JP *et al.* Improving neonatal outcome through practical shoulder dystocia training. *Obstet Gynecol* 2008;112:14–20.

52. Grobman, W., Miller D, Burke C *et al.* Outcomes associated with introduction of a shoulder dystocia protocol. *Am J Obstet Gynecol* 2011;205:513–7.

53. Inglis SR, Feier N, Chetivaar JB *et al.* Effects of shoulder dystocia training on the incidence of brachial plexus injury. *Am J Obstet Gynecol* 2011;204:322 e1–6.

54. Weiner C, Samuelson L, Collins L, Satterwhite C. 5-year experience with PROMPT (PRactical Obstetric Multiprofessional Training) reveals sustained and progressive improvements in obstetric outcomes at a US hospital. *Am J Obstet Gynecol* 2014;210 (Suppl 1):S40.

55. Walsh JM, Kandamany N, Ni Shuibhne N *et al.* Neonatal brachial plexus injury: comparison of incidence and antecedents between 2 decades. *Am J Obstet Gynecol* 2011;204:324 e1–6.

56. MacKenzie IZ, Shah M, Lean K *et al.* Management of shoulder dystocia: trends in incidence and maternal and neonatal morbidity. *Obstet Gynecol* 2007;110:1059–68.

57. Crofts J, Draycott TJ, Montague I *et al.* Shoulder Dystocia. RCOG Green top Guideline 42. London: RCOG, 2012.

58. AbouZahr C: Global burden of maternal death and disability. *Br Med Bull* 2003;67:1–11.

59. Deering SH, Chinn M, Hodor J *et al.* Use of a postpartum hemorrhage simulator for instruction and evaluation of residents. *J Grad Med Ed* 2009;1:260–3.

60. Joint Commission on Accreditation of Healthcare Organizations: Sentinel Event Alert Issue 302004, 2004. Available at: http://www.jointcommission.org/sentinel_event_alert_issue_30_preventing_infant_death_and_injury_during_delivery/.

61. Whittle R, Quenby S, Scholefield H. Does training in obstetric emergencies improve outcomes for women with postpartum haemorrhage? *BJOG* 2008;115:125.

62. Sorensen BL, Rasch V, Massawe S *et al.* Advanced Life Support in Obstetrics (ALSO) and postpartum hemorrhage: a prospective intervention study in Tanzania. *Acta Obstet Gynecol Scand* 2011;90:609–14.

63. Lin MG. Umbilical cord prolapse. *Obstet Gynecol Surv* 2006;61:269–77.

64. Murphy DJ, MacKenzie IZ. The mortality and morbidity associated with umbilical cord prolapse. *Br J Obstet Gynaecol* 1995;102:826–30.

65. Siassakos D, Hasafa Z, Sibanda T *et al.* Retrospective cohort study of diagnosis–delivery interval with umbilical cord prolapse: the effect of team training. *BJOG* 2009;116:1089–96.

66. Wayne DB, Didwania A, Feinglass J *et al.* Simulation-based education improves quality of care during cardiac arrest team responses at an academic teaching hospital: a case-control study. *Chest* 2008;133:56–61.

67. Fisher N. Eisen LA, Bavva JV *et al.* Improved performance of maternal-fetal medicine staff after maternal cardiac arrest simulation-based training. *Am J Obstet Gynecol* 2011; 205:239. e1–5.

68. Dijkman A, Huisman C, Smit M JV *et al.* Cardiac arrest in pregnancy: increasing use of perimortem caesarean section due to emergency skills training? *BJOG* 2010;117:282–7.

69. RCOG. *RCOG Trainees' Survey.* London: RCOG, 2009.

70. Dupuis O, Moreau R, Silveira R *et al.* A new obstetric forceps for the training of junior doctors: a comparison of the spatial dispersion of forceps blade trajectories between junior and senior obstetricians. *Am J Obstet Gynecol* 2006;194:1524–31.

71. Moreau R, Pham MT, Brun X *et al.* Assessment of forceps use in obstetrics during a simulated childbirth. *Int J Med Robot* 2008;4:373–80.

72. Leslie KK, Dipasquale-Lehnerz P, Smith M. Obstetric forceps training using visual feedback and the isometric strength testing unit. *Obstet Gynecol* 2005;105:377–82.

73. Kirke PN. Mothers' views of care in labour. *Br J Obstet Gynaecol* 1980; 87:1034–8.

74. McGaghie WC, Draycott TJ, Dunn WF *et al.* Evaluating the impact of simulation on translational patient outcomes. *Simul Healthc* 2011 (Suppl) S42–7.

75. Siassakos D, Crofts JF, Winter C *et al.* The active components of effective training in obstetric emergencies. *BJOG* 2009;116:1028–32.

76. Royal College of Obstetricians and Gynaecologists and Royal College of Midwives. *The Clinical Learning Environment and Recruitment: Report of a joint working party.* London: RCOG Press, 2008.

77. Lyndon A. Communication and teamwork in patient care: how much can we learn from aviation? *J Obstet Gynecol Neonatal Nurs* 2006;35:538–46.

78. Fraser DM, Symonds I, Cullen L. Multiprofessional or interprofessional education in obstetrics and gynaecology. *Obstet Gynaecol* 2005;7:271–5.

79. Siassakos D, Crofts J, Winter C, Draycott T; SaFE Study Group. Multiprofessional 'fire-drill' training in the labour ward. *The Obstetrician & Gynaecologist* 2009;11:55–60.

80. Hamman WR, Beaudin-Seiler BM, Beaubien JM *et al.* Using in situ simulation to identify and resolve latent environmental threats to patient safety: case study involving a labour and delivery ward. *J Patient Saf* 2009;5:184–7.

81. Draycott TJ, Crofts JF, Ash JP *et al.* Improving neonatal outcome through practical shoulder dystocia training. *Obstet Gynecol* 2008;112:14–20.

82. Kingdon C, Neilson J, Singleton V *et al.* Choice and birth method: mixed-method study of caesarean delivery for maternal request. *BJOG* 2009;116:886–95.

83. Phipps MG, Lindquist DG, McConaughey E *et al.* Outcomes from a labor and delivery team training program with simulation component. *Am J Obstet Gynecol* 2012;206:3–9.

84. Fletcher G, Flin R, McGeorge P *et al.* Anaesthetists' non-technical skills (ANTS): evaluation of a behavioural marker system. *Br J Anaesthesia* 2003;90:580–8.

85. Yule S, Flin R, Maran N *et al.* Surgeons' non-technical skills in the operating room: reliability testing of the (NOTSS) behaviour rating system. *World J Surg* 2008;32:548–56.

86. Bristowe K, Siassakos D, Hambly H *et al.* Teamwork for clinical emergencies: interprofessional focus group analysis and triangulation with simulation. *Qual Health Res* 2012;22:1383–94.

87. Siassakos D, Bristowe K, Draycott TJ *et al.* Clinical efficiency in a simulated emergency and relationship to team behaviours: a multisite cross-sectional study. *BJOG* 2011;118:596–607.

88. Siassakos D, Draycott T, Montague I, Harris M. Content analysis of team communication in an obstetric emergency scenario. *J Obstet Gynaecol* 2009;29:499–503.

89. Strachan B. How effective is training to help staff deal with obstetric emergencies. *J Health Services Res Policy* 2011;15(Suppl 1):37–9.

90. Crofts JF, Fox R, Ellis D *et al.* Observations from 450 shoulder dystocia simulations: lessons for skills training. *Obstet Gynecol* 2008;112:906–12.

91. Pratt S, Mann S, Salisbury M *et al.* John M. Eisenberg Patient Safety and Quality Awards. Impact of CRM-based team training on obstetric outcomes and clinicians', patient safety attitudes. *Jt Comm J Qual Patient Saf* 2007;33:720–5.

92. ACOG Committee Opinion No. 353. Medical emergency preparedness. *Obstet Gynecol* 2006;108:1597–9.

93. Kawaguchi A, Mori R. The in-service training for health professionals to improve care of the seriously ill newborn or child in low- and middle-income countries. In: *The WHO Reproductive Health Library* 2010. Geneva: World Health Organization.

94. Carlo WA, Goudar SS, Jehan I *et al.* Newborn-care training and perinatal mortality in developing countries. *N Engl J Med* 2010;362:614–23.

SECTION TWO

Antenatal Obstetrics

Chapter 7 Routine antenatal care: an overview

Nina Johns

MRCOG standards

- Candidates should be able to recognise and manage pre-existing and developing problems from pre-conceptual period through to delivery.
- Candidates should be able to evaluate the clinical risk for patients and make the decision whether for Midwifery led or Obstetrician led antenatal care and set out frequency of appointments.
- Demonstrate skill in listening and conveying complex information (e.g. concerning risk) and be able to deal with the diversity of maternal choices in antenatal and intrapartum care.
- Show understanding of the roles of other professionals (within a multidisciplinary team) and demonstrate skills in liaison and empathetic teamwork.

Practical skills

- Undertake pregnant and non-pregnant abdominal examination.
- Take an obstetric history and make the relevant referral as a result of domestic violence.
- Conduct a booking visit and arrange (and counsel for) appropriate investigations.
- Conduct follow-up prenatal visits.
- Have the skills to liaise with midwives and other health professionals to optimise care of the woman (a holistic approach).
- Show awareness of the need to identify and deal appropriately with domestic violence and have a working knowledge of child protection issues.
- Demonstrate an ability to explain the detection rates and limitations of maternal and fetal screening programme (sensitivity and specificity).

Theoretical skills

- A revision of the knowledge and high level of understanding of normal antenatal processes and progress.

- An understanding and judgement of the different models of antenatal care.
- Be fully conversant with the principles of prenatal diagnosis and screening (in its widest sense).
- Have good knowledge of the use of ultrasound in antenatal care.
- Demonstrate the use of appropriate protocols and guidelines and knowledge of National Guidance on Routine Antenatal Care (NICE, 2008).[1]

INTRODUCTION

Routine antenatal care describes the standard schedule of appointments, investigations and interventions offered to all pregnant women from healthcare services. It is perhaps important to emphasise here that in an ideal world all pregnant women and their partners would also have received pre-conceptual counselling and information, in either a primary care setting (low risk) or a secondary/tertiary care setting (complex-risk women, often with pre-existing medical problems). Pregnancy is a unique physiological state which may be associated with complications due to pre-existing medical conditions and gestation-specific conditions arising in otherwise healthy women. Antenatal care aims to identify risk factors for the development of complications in pregnancy and birth, prevent or treat these complications if they occur, and offer screening for specific pathologies in both the woman and the baby. The package of care also aims to provide the woman and her family with information to enable an improved experience of pregnancy, birth and early parenthood.

Evidence from observational studies has shown that women who receive antenatal care have lower maternal and perinatal mortality and better pregnancy outcomes. These studies appear to demonstrate that the number of antenatal appointments and the time of the initiation of care also affect pregnancy outcomes.[2] A systematic review by the WHO evaluated different models of antenatal care and found that a reduced number of antenatal visits could be as effective, in terms of preventing maternal and neonatal mortality and morbidity, as schemes with a higher number of visits. However, women were less satisfied with fewer antenatal visits.[3,4]

The aims of antenatal care are to:

- provide high-quality information that can be easily understood;
- provide an informed choice about the pathways of antenatal care;
- offer evidence-based treatment options for medical conditions pre-existing or arising in pregnancy;
- identify and screen for maternal and fetal complications;
- assess maternal and fetal wellbeing throughout pregnancy;
- provide advice and education on the normal symptoms of pregnancy.

Historically, the current model of antenatal care began in the UK following a review of maternal health by the RCOG in 1944 and came into practice with the creation of the NHS in 1948. The pattern of care – with monthly visits to an antenatal clinic until 32 weeks' gestation, fortnightly until 36 weeks and weekly until birth – has changed only marginally to the current recommended schedule of appointments.

More recently, the *Changing Childbirth* report (1993) and *Maternity Matters* (2007) recommended that the focus of maternity care should be woman centred, with an emphasis on providing choice, easy access and continuity of care.[5,6] These reports highlighted that care during pregnancy should enable women to make informed decisions and provide clear evidence-based information.

The management of antenatal care is subject to clear national and international guidance with NICE clinical guidelines[1] and WHO recommendations.[7] Local pathways of care and clinical decisions should therefore reflect this guidance and be based on the evidence available.

The recommended NICE clinical antenatal care pathway can be found within the guidance and website link: http://pathways.nice.org.uk/pathways/antenatal-care#content=view-index&path=view%3A/pathways/antenatal-care/routine-care-for-all-pregnant-women.xml (Fig. 7.1).

PRINCIPLES OF RISK ASSESSMENT AND SCREENING

The basic principles of routine antenatal care are those of risk assessment and population screening.

Antenatal risk assessments aim to identify the level and frequency of care that the woman needs due to medical, obstetric or social risk factors in her previous or current pregnancy. This risk assessment should initially occur at the booking visit, and is repeated in the second and third trimesters, to ensure that the woman is receiving the appropriate care and to identify any need for changes in care when risks have been identified.

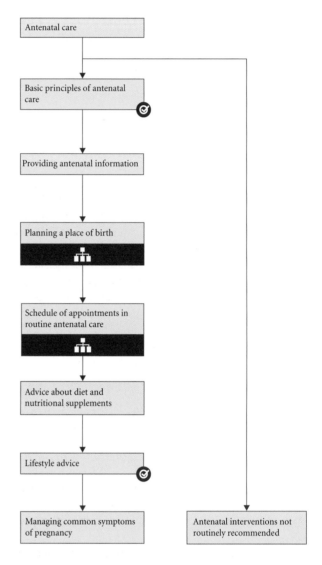

Fig. 7.1 NICE clinical antenatal care pathway

Potential risks in pregnancy include: significant pre-existing medical conditions, such as diabetes or hypertension; substantial obstetric factors, such as previous history of fetal growth restriction; or important social issues, such as domestic violence. The recognition of risk factors is empirical to the success of appropriate antenatal care and planning of multidisciplinary support and surveillance for the planning, birth and postnatal period.

Each part of antenatal care should also fulfil the criteria for effective screening programmes. These are that:

1 the condition being screened for is an important health problem;
2 the screening test (further diagnostic test and treatment) is safe and acceptable;
3 the natural history of the condition is understood;
4 early detection and treatment have benefit over later detection and treatment;
5 the screening test is valid and reliable;

6   treatments or interventions should be effective;

7   there are adequate facilities for confirming the test results and resources for treatment;

8   the objectives of screening justify the costs.

Maternal screening

Antenatal screening for pre-existing maternal conditions forms an essential part of the initial and on-going risk assessment and planning for care in pregnancy.

At the booking appointment women should be offered screening blood tests for anaemia, haematological conditions by electrophoresis (such as sickle cell diseases and thalassaemias), blood group and rhesus status testing, and red cell antibody screen. Screening for anaemia and red cell antibodies should also be repeated at 28 weeks' gestation.[1]

It is likely that women with haematological diseases such as sickle cell and thalassaemias will be aware of their diagnosis prior to pregnancy and may have received preconception counselling (see Chapter 12). However, women may be unaware that they are carriers and, if identified as a carrier of a clinically significant haemoglobinopathy, then the father of the baby should be offered counselling and appropriate screening as soon as possible.[1]

Anaemia in pregnancy is reviewed in detail in Chapter 21. Once identified by screening, it is recommended that routine antenatal anti-D prophylaxis is offered to all non-sensitised pregnant women who are rhesus D negative at 28 weeks.[1]

Women with clinically significant atypical red cell alloantibodies should be offered referral to a specialist centre for further investigation and advice on subsequent antenatal management.[1]

Screening for maternal infections enables potential intervention to reduce the risk to both mother and baby, and enables planning for appropriate specialist antenatal, intrapartum and postnatal care. Routine antenatal serological screening for hepatitis B, HIV, syphilis and rubella immunity are currently recommended.[1]

Serological screening for hepatitis B virus should be offered to pregnant women at booking and has been part of the routine screening programme in the UK since 2000. Identification of active or carrier status will enable referral to secondary obstetric care and facilitate effective postnatal intervention to be offered to decrease the risk of mother-to-child transmission. Mother-to-child transmission is approximately 95% preventable through administration of vaccine and immunoglobulin to the baby at birth.[1]

Routine screening for HIV infection in early pregnancy allows the identification of women with asymptomatic infection, referral to appropriate specialist services and treatment with antiretroviral therapy, and planning for labour and birth and treatment of the baby. In the UK, the mother-to-child transmission of HIV has dropped from 25.6% in 1993 to 0.57% in 2007–2011. In addition to this reduction in transmission the number of vaginal births has increased from 15% to 40%. (BHIVA paper 2014).[8]

Syphilis is a rare condition in the UK (but prevalence is increasing worldwide). The routine screening for syphilis should be offered to all pregnant women at booking as treatment is beneficial to the mother, and mother-to-child transmission of syphilis in pregnancy is associated with neonatal death and severe growth restriction, and is a cause of fetal hydrops fetalis. Congenital syphilis, which may cause long-term disability, is associated with stillbirth and preterm birth. In pregnant women with early untreated syphilis, 70–100% of infants will be infected and one-third will be stillborn.[1] Parenteral penicillin effectively prevents mother-to-child transmission of syphilis and is not associated with any difference in adverse pregnancy outcomes.

The national recommendation to screen for rubella susceptibility in antenatal care aims to identify women at risk of contracting rubella infection and to enable vaccination in the postnatal period for the protection of future pregnancies.[1]

In addition to serological screening women should be offered routine screening for asymptomatic bacteriuria via midstream urine culture at the booking appointment.[1] Studies in the UK have shown that asymptomatic bacteriuria occurs in 2–5% of pregnant women and is associated with increased rates of maternal pyelonephritis and preterm birth. However, evidence from RCTs shows that antibiotic treatment is of benefit only to reduce the risk of pyelonephritis.[1]

In addition to screening for those maternal conditions that are present prior to pregnancy, antenatal care also includes screening for those maternal medical conditions that develop without symptoms in pregnancy.

Screening for gestational diabetes should be targeted at women with risk factors such as: body mass index (BMI) >30 kg/m²; previous macrosomic baby weighing 4.5 kg or above; previous gestational diabetes; family history of diabetes (first-degree relative with diabetes); or family origin with a high prevalence of diabetes. Women with any one of these risk factors should be offered testing for gestational diabetes using an oral glucose tolerance at 26 weeks' gestation, or earlier at 16 weeks' gestation if there is a previous history of gestational diabetes.[1]

At every antenatal appointment and contact with a healthcare professional, blood pressure measurement and urinalysis for protein should be carried out to screen for pre-eclampsia.[1] Additional risk factors for development of pre-eclampsia, such as age 40 years or older, first pregnancy, pregnancy interval of more than 10 years, family history of pre-eclampsia, previous history of pre-eclampsia, BMI 30 kg/m² or above, pre-existing vascular disease such as hypertension, pre-existing renal disease or multiple pregnancy, should be identified at the booking visit. At present, there is no predictive diagnostic test for pre-eclampsia or proven intervention; however, more frequent blood pressure measurements should be considered for pregnant women who have any of the above risk factors. In addition, all pregnant women should be made aware of the need to seek immediate advice if they experience symptoms of pre-eclampsia, such as severe headache, problems with vision, vomiting, or swelling of face, hands or feet.[1]

Fetal screening

Screening for fetal anomalies is discussed in detail in Chapters 29 and 30.

At the first contact in a pregnancy, women should be given information about the purpose and implications of fetal screening. Information given to women should include the screening pathway for both biochemical and ultrasound screening, the decisions that need to be made at each point along the pathway, the fact that screening does not provide a definitive diagnosis, and a full explanation of the risk score obtained following combined first trimester testing. Giving accurate information will enable women and families to make an informed choice as to whether to accept the offers of screening and the implications and limitations of the results provided.

The purpose of screening for fetal anomalies and identifying fetal anomalies is to enable women to make reproductive choices (which may include termination of pregnancy), assist parents to prepare (for any treatment/disability/palliative care/termination of pregnancy), facilitate birth in a specialist centre if required, and allow intrauterine therapy if available.

The current antenatal and newborn screening opportunities are summarised in Fig. 7.2.

ANTENATAL INFORMATION

Routine antenatal appointments/visits also provide multiple opportunities for sharing information with women and their families. The majority of such visits in the UK are provided by midwives. However, worldwide other models of delivery exist. National guidance recommends that the information given is evidence based, easy to understand and accessible to women in different languages, and with additional sensory or learning requirements.[1] Some antenatal information is gestation specific and can be found in the relevant sections of this chapter. The following includes antenatal information that may be discussed at any time in the pregnancy.

Nutrition

Evidence from systematic review, RCTs and cohort studies has shown that antenatal advice on dietary intake can improve

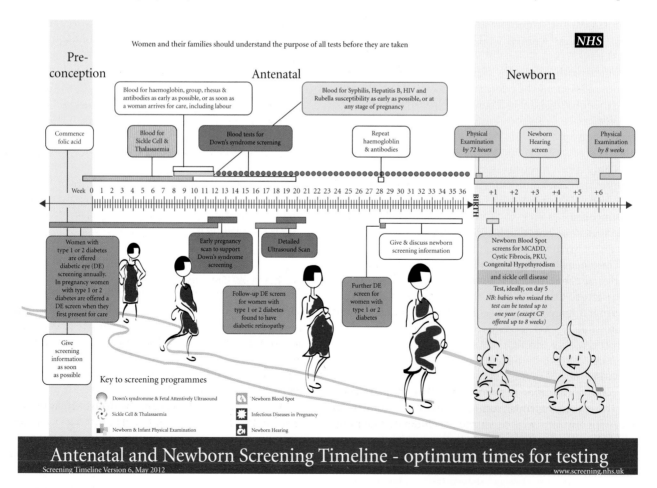

Fig. 7.2 The current antenatal and newborn screening opportunities summary: http://cpd.screening.nhs.uk/timeline

women's knowledge and healthy eating, but does not appear to affect pregnancy outcomes.[1] More recent reviews have confirmed that lower weight gain in pregnancy may be associated with less weight retention afterwards and that diet and exercise interventions may reduce the amount of weight gained in pregnancy.[9]

Smoking

Smoking in pregnancy is associated with increased risk of miscarriage, preterm premature rupture of membranes, preterm birth, small for gestational age (SGA), low birthweight, placental abruption, perinatal mortality and sudden infant death.

Systematic reviews show a reduction in smoking rates associated with structured cessation programmes, rewards and social support, and this was associated with lower rates of low birthweights and preterm birth.[1]

Alcohol

RCOG guidance and patient information recommend that women should be informed that high intake of alcohol during the first trimester increases the risk of miscarriage and chronic use may lead to fetal alcohol spectrum disorder.[10] It further recommends that women should avoid alcohol in pregnancy, but if they do drink alcohol they should limit intake to national recommendations (1–2 units, not more than twice a week) and avoid binge drinking. However a recent cohort study showed that women who drank regularly before pregnancy (more than weekly) continued to consume alcohol in the antenatal period, despite national guidelines recommending abstinence.[11]

Working

National guidance recommends that most pregnant women can be reassured that it is safe to continue working during pregnancy and there is some evidence that employment is beneficial.[1] However, identification of potential occupational hazards (e.g. ionising radiation) for pregnancy need to be explored. There is some evidence that employment that involves heavy lifting or shift work may be associated with a small increased risk of preterm birth; however, the studies are small and systematic review showed no difference.[12]

Exercise

Systematic review of evidence confirms that, in the absence of any obstetric or medical complications, most women can begin or maintain a regular exercise regimen during pregnancy without complications. It is recommended that pregnant women should avoid exercise that involves the risk of abdominal trauma, falls or excessive joint stress, and also scuba diving (increased incidence of fetal anomaly and risk of fetal decompression disease).[1]

Travel

RCOG guidance on travel in pregnancy concentrates on air travel and the scientific impact paper concludes that there is no clear evidence that air travel increases the risk of pregnancy complications such as preterm labour, rupture of membranes or abruption. However, flights of more than 4 hours' duration are associated with a small increased risk of venous thrombosis, and the paper states that graduated elastic compression stockings for all women, and low-molecular-weight heparin (LMWH) for those with significant risk factors, are likely to be of benefit, but that low-dose aspirin should not be used for thromboprophylaxis.[13] The guidance suggests avoidance of air travel from 37 weeks' gestation in a singleton pregnancy and from 32 weeks' gestation if there are significant risk factors for preterm birth.

Who provides antenatal care?

Midwives and GPs should provide care for women with an uncomplicated pregnancy. Care should be provided by small groups or teams of carers (usually midwives) and with continuity of care throughout the antenatal period. Systematic review of evidence shows that the routine involvement of obstetricians in the care of women with an uncomplicated pregnancy at scheduled times does not appear to improve perinatal outcomes compared with involving obstetricians when complications arise.[1] A system of clear referral paths should be established so that, if additional care is required, women can be seen and treated by the appropriate specialist teams. Obstetricians and specialist teams should be involved if pre-existing medical conditions are present, or when maternal or fetal complications arise.

National guidance recommends that antenatal appointments should take place in a location that women can easily access and that maternity records should be standardised, containing an agreed minimum data-set and held by the woman.[1]

Schedule for appointments

The NICE recommendation for schedule of antenatal appointments can be found within the guidance and website link: http://pathways.nice.org.uk/pathways/antenatal-care#path=view%3A/pathways/antenatal-care/schedule-of-appointments-in-routine-antenatal-care.xml&content=view-index (Fig. 7.3).

Women in their first pregnancy, with no complications arising, should receive ten appointments and those in subsequent pregnancies require seven appointments.[1] An individualised schedule of appointments may need to include additional visits if complications arise within the pregnancy or other

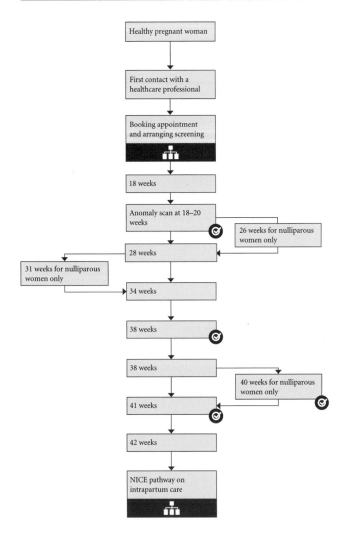

Fig. 7.3 NICE recommendation for schedule of antenatal appointments

risk factors are identified. Wherever possible, appointments should incorporate routine tests and investigations to minimise inconvenience to women.[1]

First contact with healthcare professional

At their initial appointment with a healthcare professional, women should receive information regarding food hygiene and lifestyle advice, including smoking cessation, and the implications of recreational drug use and alcohol consumption in pregnancy. Women should also be advised to take folic acid supplementation and, if at increased risk (previous neural tube anomaly, maternal epilepsy or diabetes), offered a prescription for high-dose folic acid (5 mg). Information on the risks and benefits of antenatal screening tests and advice on who is likely to provide care and schedule of next appointments should also be given.

Booking visit

This antenatal appointment should occur ideally between 10 and 12 weeks' gestation and should include:

- Gestational age assessment with ultrasound scan offered between 11+0 weeks and 13+6 weeks, to determine gestational age, detect multiple pregnancies and offer nuchal translucency (NT) measurement for screening;
- Assessment of maternal and obstetric risk factors to identify women who may require additional antenatal care;
- Ask about any past or present severe mental illness or psychiatric treatment;
- Ask about the woman's occupation, to identify potential risks;
- Plan lead care professional (midwife or obstetrician);
- Plan pattern of care for pregnancy;
- Discussion on antenatal screening;
- Offer blood tests to check blood group and rhesus D status, and screening for anaemia, haemoglobinopathies, red-cell alloantibodies, hepatitis B virus, HIV, rubella susceptibility and syphilis;
- Measure height and weight and calculate BMI;
- Measure blood pressure and test urine for proteinuria;
- Offer screening for asymptomatic bacteriuria;
- Information on how the baby develops during pregnancy, nutrition, diet (including vitamin D supplements if necessary) and exercise;
- Monitor smoking status and offer smoking cessation advice and information on the specific risks of smoking during pregnancy (such as low birthweight and preterm birth);
- Information on pregnancy care pathway including parent education and infant feeding;
- Information on options for place of birth and different modes of birth.

First trimester

If the booking appointment occurs prior to 11 weeks' gestation, offer an additional appointment for ultrasound examination between 11+0 and 13+6 weeks to determine gestational age, detect multiple pregnancies and offer NT measurement for screening with the combined serum screening for Down's syndrome.

If ultrasound measurement of NT is not possible at ultrasound, or a woman presents after 13+6 weeks, then serum screening test (triple or quadruple test) between 15+0 and 20+0 weeks can be offered.

Second trimester

Routine antenatal appointment at 16 weeks' gestation for all women should include:

- Review, discuss and record the results of screening tests;
- Measure blood pressure and test urine for proteinuria;

- Investigate a haemoglobin level below 11 g/100 mL and consider iron supplements;
- Information on the routine anomaly scan.

An ultrasound scan should be offered to all women and, if accepted, be performed between 18+0 weeks and 20+6 weeks to detect structural anomalies. If structural differences are identified, appropriate information should be given and potential referral to a fetal medicine specialist considered. If ultrasound examination identifies a low-lying placenta, an additional scan at 32 weeks should be offered.

Routine appointment at 24–25 weeks' gestation is recommended only for women in their first pregnancy. This appointment should include:

- Measure blood pressure and test urine for proteinuria;
- Measure and plot symphysis–fundal height.

Third trimester

Routine antenatal appointment at 28 weeks' gestation for all women should include:

- Measure blood pressure and test urine for proteinuria;
- Offer blood tests to check for anaemia and atypical red-cell alloantibodies;
- Investigate a haemoglobin level below 10.5 g/100 mL and consider iron supplements;
- Offer anti-D prophylaxis to women who are rhesus D negative;
- Measure and plot symphysis–fundal height.

Routine appointment at 31 weeks' gestation is recommended only for women in their first pregnancy. This appointment should include:

- Review, discuss and record the results of blood tests undertaken at 28 weeks;
- Measure blood pressure and test urine for proteinuria;
- Measure and plot symphysis–fundal height.

Routine antenatal appointment at 34 weeks' gestation for all women should include:

- Review, discuss and record the results of blood tests undertaken at 28 weeks;
- Measure blood pressure and test urine for proteinuria;
- Measure and plot symphysis–fundal height;
- Give information on preparation for labour and birth, including the birth plan, recognising active labour and coping with pain.

Routine antenatal appointment at 36 weeks' gestation for all women should include:

- Measure blood pressure and test urine for proteinuria;
- Measure and plot symphysis–fundal height;
- Check the presentation of the baby (refer if breech presentation suspected);

- Give information on infant feeding, care of the new baby, vitamin K prophylaxis, newborn screening tests, and postnatal self-care.

Routine antenatal appointment at 38 weeks' gestation for all women should include:

- Measure blood pressure and test urine for proteinuria;
- Measure and plot symphysis–fundal height;
- Give information on options for management of prolonged pregnancy.

Routine antenatal appointment at 40 weeks' gestation is recommended only for women in their first pregnancy. This appointment should include:

- Measure blood pressure and test urine for proteinuria;
- Measure and plot symphysis–fundal height;
- Further discussion of management of prolonged pregnancy and offer membrane sweep.

Routine antenatal appointment at 41 weeks' gestation for all women should include:

- Measure blood pressure and test urine for proteinuria;
- Measure and plot symphysis–fundal height;
- Further discussion of management of prolonged pregnancy and offer membrane sweep and date for admission for induction of labour.

This plan of care relates to uncomplicated singleton pregnancies. In multiple pregnancy, NICE guidelines outline a regimen of care.

MANAGEMENT OF COMMON SYMPTOMS IN PREGNANCY

Multiple symptoms occur in a healthy uncomplicated pregnancy; most can be managed with conservative treatments and maternal reassurance. However, further investigation may be required to exclude unusual or insidious presentations of other pathologies.

Nausea and vomiting

It is estimated that nausea is experienced in 80–85% of all pregnancies and associated with vomiting in approximately 50%. The condition of hyperemesis gravidarum can be diagnosed if these symptoms lead to fluid, electrolyte or nutritional imbalance requiring hospital treatment.

For the majority of women symptoms of nausea and vomiting in pregnancy resolve spontaneously within 16 to 20 weeks of gestation and are not usually associated with a poor pregnancy outcome. Systematic review of evidence and RCT data show that dietary ginger, wrist acupressure and prescribed antihistamines appear to be effective in reducing symptoms.[1]

Heartburn

Symptoms of heartburn are caused by gastro-oesophageal acid reflux due to relaxation of the distal oesophageal sphincter and reduced gastric motility in pregnancy, and are not associated with any adverse outcomes in pregnancy, but generally worsen with gestation. Symptoms of heartburn should be differentiated from presenting epigastric pain in pre-eclampsia by checking maternal blood pressure and urinalysis.

Current guidance recommends that women should be offered information regarding lifestyle and diet modification (timing of meals, portion size and posture). If symptoms remain, RCT data show that antacids are safe and effective at relieving heartburn.[1]

Constipation

Symptoms of constipation are due to reduced gastric motility and transit in pregnancy, and appear to improve with gestation. Systematic review of RCT data show that dietary changes with wheat or bran fibre supplements improve symptoms and, though laxative treatment is effective, it is associated with increased abdominal pain and diarrhoea.[1]

Haemorrhoids

Observational studies estimate the incidence of haemorrhoids in the third trimester as 8%. There is currently no evidence for the safety or effectiveness of topical treatments in pregnancy. Women should be offered information concerning dietary changes (to increase fibre content) and advised that, if symptoms remain, standard haemorrhoid creams may be considered.[1]

Varicose veins

Varicose veins are caused by the pooling of blood in the surface veins, commonly in the legs, due to inefficient valves and relative pelvic obstruction. RCT evidence shows that compression stockings do not prevent varicose veins occurring, but appear to improve leg symptoms for women in pregnancy.[1]

Backache

Back pain affects 30–60% of pregnant women and worsen with gestation. A number of RCTs have investigated interventions such as shaped pillows, exercises in water, massage, back care classes and acupuncture with small numbers, but have failed to identify clear effectiveness or safety. Current guidance recommends that exercising in water, massage therapy and group or individual back care classes might help to ease backache during pregnancy.[1]

Symphysis pubis dysfunction

Pelvis girdle pain is estimated to affect at least 20% of pregnant women.[12] Systematic review of the limited evidence available shows that normal activity, exercises to improve posture

and acupuncture may improve symptoms. Pharmacological pain-relief options have not been investigated for effectiveness, but guidance highlights that medications prescribed must be appropriate for pregnancy.[1,14]

SUMMARY

Routine antenatal care describes the standard schedule of appointments, investigations and interventions offered to all pregnant women from healthcare services. Women who receive antenatal care have lower maternal and perinatal mortality and better pregnancy outcomes. Antenatal care aims to identify risk factors for the development of complications in pregnancy and birth, prevent or treat these complications if they occur, and offer screening for specific pathologies in both the woman and the baby. The package of care also aims to provide the woman and her family with information to enable an improved experience of pregnancy, birth and early parenthood.

KEY POINTS

The aims of antenatal care are to:
- Provide high-quality information that can be easily understood;
- Provide an informed choice about the pathways of antenatal care;
- Offered evidence-based treatment options for medical conditions pre-existing or arising in pregnancy;
- Identify and screen for maternal and fetal complications;
- Assess maternal and fetal wellbeing throughout pregnancy;
- Provide advice and education on the normal symptoms of pregnancy.

The recommended NICE clinical antenatal care pathway can be found within the guidance and website link: http://pathways.nice.org.uk/pathways/antenatal-care#content=view-index&path=view%3A/pathways/antenatal-care/routine-care-for-all-pregnant-women.xml.

Key References

1. National Collaborating Centre for Women's and Children's Health. *Antenatal Care: Routine care for the healthy pregnant woman.* NICE Clinical guideline Number 62. CG062. London: NICE, 2008 Mar.
2. Carroli G, Villar J, Piaggio G, Khan-Neelofur D, Gülmezoglu M, Mugford M, Lumbiganon P, Farnot U, Bersgjø P; WHO Antenatal Care Trial Research Group. WHO systematic review of randomised controlled trials of routine antenatal care. *Lancet* 2001;357:1565–70.
3. Villar J, Carroli G, Khan-Neelofur D, Piaggio G, Gülmezoglu M. Patterns of routine antenatal care for low-risk pregnancy. *Cochrane Database Syst Rev*

2001;4:CD000934. Review. Update in: *Cochrane Database Syst Rev* 2010;10:CD000934.

4. Dowswell T, Carroli G, Duley L *et al.* Alternative versus standard packages of antenatal care for low-risk pregnancy. *Cochrane Database Syst Rev* 2010;10:CD000934.

5. Department of Health (1993). *Changing Childbirth.* Report of the Expert Maternity Group. London: HMSO.

6. Department of Health. *Maternity Matters: Choice, access and continuity of care in a safe service.* London: Department of Health, 2007. Available from: http://www.dh.gov. uk/en/Publicationsandstatistics/Publications/ PublicationsPolicyAndGuidance/DH_073312.

7. Banta D (2003). What is the efficacy/effectiveness of antenatal care and the financial and organizational implications? Copenhagen: WHO Regional Office for Europe Health Evidence Network (HEN) report. December 2013. Available from: http://www.euro.who. int/Document/E82996.pdf.

8. British HIV Association guidelines for the management of HIV infection in pregnant women 2012 (2014 interim review). *HIV Medicine* 2014;15:1–77. http://www.bhiva. org/documents/Guidelines/Pregnancy/2012/BHIVA-Pregnancy-guidelines-update-2014.pdf.

9. NICE Antenatal Care: Evidence Update May 2013. A summary of selected new evidence relevant to NICE clinical guideline 62 'Antenatal Care' (2008) Evidence Update 41.

10. RCOG. Alcohol consumption and the outcomes of pregnancy. Statement No. 5. London: RCOG: 2006.

11. Anderson A, Hure A, Forder P, Powers J, Kay-Lambkin F, Loxton D. Predictors of antenatal alcohol use among Australian women: a prospective cohort study. *BJOG* 2013;120:1366–74.

12. Royal College of Physicians. *Physical and Shift Work in Pregnancy. Occupational aspects of management. A national guideline.* London: RCP, 2009.

13. RCOG. Air travel and pregnancy. Scientific Impact Paper No. 1. London: RCOG, May 2013. Available from: www. rcog.org.uk/womens-health/clinical-guidance/ air-travel-and-pregnancy.

14. Vleeming A, Albert HB, Ostgaard HC, Sturesson B, Stuge B. European guidelines for the diagnosis and treatment of pelvic girdle pain. *Eur Spine J* 2008;17:794–819.

Chapter 8 Chronic hypertension

Kate Bramham and Andrew Shennan

MRCOG standards

We would suggest the following:

Theoretical knowledge
Definition of chronic hypertension.
Describe the aetiology of chronic hypertension.
Relationship between chronic hypertension and pregnancy pathology.

Practical
Be able to recognise and diagnose secondary causes of hypertension.
Know how to manage moderate hypertension in pregnancy.

INTRODUCTION

Pre-existing or chronic hypertension is one of the most common conditions in women of child-bearing age, and is becoming more prevalent[1] due to trends of increasing maternal age[2] and obesity.[3] Chronic hypertension is estimated to affect 1–5% of pregnant women,[4] and is frequently diagnosed for the first time during antenatal care. Underlying pathology for secondary hypertension is identified in a small proportion of women, and should be sought in all women who are newly diagnosed during pregnancy. Similarly hypertension recognised postnatally should be monitored, and if persistent investigated appropriately.

Women with chronic hypertension have worse pregnancy outcomes than normotensive women, with both maternal and neonatal complications being reported. Pre-pregnancy counselling, increased antenatal surveillance and postpartum review are therefore recommended.

DEFINITION

Chronic hypertension is defined as:

- The presence of hypertension before 20 weeks' gestation (in the absence of a hydatiform mole)
- OR persistent hypertension beyond 6 weeks postpartum.

NICE guidelines also include threshold values of >140 mmHg systolic or 90 mmHg diastolic blood pressure;[5] however, there is a linear relationship between blood pressure at first antenatal visit and frequency of adverse obstetric events.[6]

AETIOLOGY

The cause of primary hypertension is considered to be multifactorial, with both genetic and environmental contributions. Secondary hypertension is identified only in less than 5% of the general population but has been shown to be present in 14% of women of child-bearing age.[1] Renal disease is the most common cause of secondary hypertension in pregnancy. Chronic kidney disease affects up to 3% of women age 20–39 years[7] and pregnancy may be the first time it is identified.

HISTORY AND EXAMINATION

The majority of women will be asymptomatic; however, a careful history for end-organ damage and potential underlying aetiology should be taken. Questioning about late enuresis and recurrent urinary tract infections in childhood may suggest reflux nephropathy, and a detailed family history may confirm a genetic basis for primary hypertension, or identify familial renal disease. Paroxysmal or severe hypertension associated with headache and sweating or palpitations may be indicative of a phaeochromocytoma.

Examination should include fundoscopy to identify hypertensive retinopathy (mild vessel tortuosity, silver wiring and arteriovenous nipping), and assessment for radiofemoral delay (coarctation of the aorta). Other findings may include enlarged kidneys (polycystic kidneys), a renal bruit (renal artery stenosis) and clinical features of endocrine disease (e.g. hyperthyroidism – tachycardia, goitre, proptosis).

INVESTIGATIONS

Any woman of child-bearing age identified as having hypertension should have confirmation with 24-hour ambulatory monitoring,[8] and be investigated for end-organ damage including an echocardiogram to assess for left ventricular hypertrophy and assessment of renal function and proteinuria. Referral for investigation for secondary causes should be made to an appropriate specialist depending on local expertise and interest (e.g. nephrology, clinical pharmacology, cardiology, endocrinology).

Investigations and causes for secondary hypertension are given in Table 8.1.

Chronic kidney disease

The most common causes of renal disease in women of child-bearing age are reflux nephropathy, lupus nephritis,

IgA nephropathy and autosomal dominant polycystic kidney disease (ADPKD), although hypertensive nephropathy and obesity-related focal segmental glomerulosclerosis are becoming increasingly common. Women with reflux nephropathy and ADPKD may have affected family members but both conditions can also occur spontaneously. The modified diet in renal disease formula (MDRD), which provides an estimate of glomerular filtration rate (eGFR), is not valid in pregnancy as it underestimates the GFR by approximately 20%.[9]

Endocrine disorders

Many endocrine disorders are associated with hypertension, the most common being hyperthyroidism in women of child-bearing age. A careful clinical history and examination may identify features of other conditions including primary hyperparathyroidism, phaeochromocytoma, carcinoid and acromegaly.

Table 8.1 Causes and investigations of secondary hypertension (adapted from[20])

Cause of hypertension	Features	Investigations
Primary		
Essential hypertension	Family history of hypertension, raised BMI, >35 years, black ethnicity, maternal low birthweight, pre-eclampsia or hypertension Secondary causes must be excluded to make a diagnosis	Confirmation with 24-hour ambulatory monitoring
Secondary		
Renal		
Chronic kidney disease	Family history of renal disease Clinical features of autoimmune disease (e.g. rash, arthritis, mouth ulcers) History of recurrent UTIs in childhood or primary enuresis (reflux nephropathy); micturition difficulties including incomplete bladder emptying; renal calculi; epidodes of haematuria (IgA nephropathy)	Creatinine Urinalysis Ultrasound of renal tract Immunoglobulins DMSA (^{99m}Tc-dimercaptosuccinic acid)to confirm scarring if clinically indicated Antinuclear antibodies/complement C3 and C4: if positive, extractable nuclear antigen/ antiphospholipid screen
Renal artery stenosis (usually fibromuscular dysplasia)	Possible audible renal bruit	Renal artery Doppler
Renin-producing tumours		Plasma aldosterone:renin ratio
Drug induced or drug related	History of taking oral contraceptives, glucocorticoids, liquorice (mimics primary aldosteronism), cocaine or other illicit drugs, or history of taking nephrotoxic agents including non-prescribed over-the-counter medications, e.g.NSAIDs, calcineurin inhibitors	
Endocrine		

ANTENATAL OBSTETRICS

(continued)

Table 8.1 Causes and investigations of secondary hypertension (adapted from[20]) (*continued*)

Cause of hypertension	Features	Investigations
Primary aldosteronism (Conn's syndrome) and other mineralocorticoid excess states	Myalgia, weakness and headaches, hypokalaemia	Plasma aldosterone:renin ratio Serum potassium (low)
Cushing's syndrome and other glucocorticoid excess states including chronic steroid therapy	History of steroid use or rapid weight gain, polyuria/polydipsia, skin changes including acne, skin thinning, telangiectasia	24-hour urine cortisol
Phaeochromocytoma	History of episodic headache, tachycardia and sweating	Plasma metanephrines 24-hour urine catecholamines
Thyroid or parathyroid disease	Clinical features of hyper- or hypothyroidism, or hyperparathyroidism (hypercalcaemia)	Thyroid function tests Parathyroid hormone, vitamin D and calcium
Acromegaly	Carpal tunnel syndrome, sweating, enlarged feet, hands, jaw, tongue, muscle weakness	IGF-1 Growth hormone suppression test
Carcinoid tumours	Diarrhoea, flushing, wheezing, weight loss	Chromogranin-A 24-hour urine 5-hydroxyindoleacetic acid
Neurological disorders		
Sleep apnoea	History of snoring and episodic apnoea and high BMI	Overnight oximetry
Increased intracranial pressure	Symptoms/signs of intracerebral tumours	Cerebral imaging
Spinal cord injury	Quadriplegia, paraplegia, Guillain–Barré syndrome	
Coarctation of the aorta	Radio-radial or radio-femoral pulse delay, differential blood pressure in arms	Echocardiogram CT/MR angiography Chest X-ray (rib notching)

TREATMENT

First-line treatment for non-pregnant women of African or Caribbean origin is a calcium channel blocker such as nifedipine, whereas angiotensin-converting enzyme inhibitors (ACEIs) or angiotensin receptor blockers (ARBs) are the drugs of choice for other ethnicities.[8] Modification of treatment may be required prior to, or at, conception. Medications which are considered safe in pregnancy are shown in Table 8.2. Currently there is no evidence that any agent is preferable during pregnancy and treatment should be chosen according to tolerability and dosing regimen. Single-agent dose should be maximised before a second agent is introduced.

ACEIs/ARBs

Women taking ACEIs or ARBs should be informed that these medications are contraindicated in pregnancy and should be stopped before or at conception. If they are being used to reduce proteinuria, for renal or cardiac protection it is suggested that they are continued until a positive pregnancy test, provided that conception can be reliably identified. For women using these agents as antihypertensives alone, an alternative agent should be offered which is safe in pregnancy, e.g. amlodipine, nifedipine, labetolol.

ACEIs/ARBs are associated with a fetopathy when taken in the second trimester, and some reports suggest teratogenicity,[10,11] although others suggest that these congenital abnormalities are associated with hypertension itself, rather than the ACEIs or ARBs.[12]

Beta blockers

Some beta blockers have been associated with intrauterine growth restriction and therefore are usually avoided in pregnancy.[13] Labetolol is a combined alpha and beta blocker which has a good safety profile in pregnancy and breastfeeding, but may require three times daily dosing to achieve an adequate response. Women should be questioned about a history of asthma before prescribing, as it may exacerbate bronchoconstriction.

Table 8.2 Safety data for commonly used antihypertensives in pregnancy (adapted from NICE[5])

Drug	Route	Safety data maternal	Safety data fetal/neonatal
Centrally acting			
Methyl-dopa	Oral	Fatigue, headache, transaminitis (rare)	Mild hypotension in babies in first 2 days of life No obvious association with congenital abnormalities
Beta blocker			
Labetolol	Oral/IV	Exacerbation of maternal asthma	No obvious association with congenital abnormalities Rare mild hypotension in first 24 hours in neonate
Very rare hypoglycaemia			
Atenolol	Oral	Exacerbation of maternal asthma	No obvious association with congenital abnormalities Low birthweight/placental weight Decreased fetal heart rate
Alpha blocker			
Prazocin	Oral		No obvious association with congenital abnormalities
Calcium channel blockers			
Nifedipine	Oral	Headache Ankle oedema	No obvious association with congenital abnormalities
Amlodipine	Oral	Headache Ankle oedema	No reports
Verapamil	Oral/IV	Headache Ankle oedema	No obvious association with congenital abnormalities
Diuretics			
Chlorothiazide	Oral	Possible electrolyte imbalance Hypovolaemia	Possible association with congenital abnormalities Possible neonatal thrombocytopenia Possible neonatal hypoglycaemia/hypovolaemia Possible electrolyte imbalance
Bendroflumethiazide	Oral	Possible electrolyte imbalance Hypovolaemia	No obvious adverse fetal effects
Furosemide	Oral/IV	Possible electrolyte imbalance Hypovolaemia	No obvious adverse fetal effects
Vasodilators			
Hydralazine	Oral/IV		No obvious association with congenital abnormalities
Diazoxide	IV	May inhibit uterine contractions Profound hypotension possible	Neonatal hypoglycaemia

α-Methyl-dopa

Methyl-dopa has an excellent safety profile, and has been used for decades. However, side effects are common and include tiredness, headache and depression, and occasionally hepatitis. It is no longer recommended during breastfeeding in order to avoid exacerbation of postnatal depression.[5]

Vasodilators

Hydralazine crosses the placenta but has been shown to be safe in pregnancy. It can also be given intravenously for management of severe hypertension.

Diuretics

Very occasionally diuretics may be required for symptomatic relief of oedema in women with renal disease; however, their use for the treatment of hypertension is not recommended, as they reduce plasma volume. Chlorothiazide has recently been shown to be associated with increased risk of congenital abnormalities, and ideally should be switched before conception.[5]

PRE-PREGNANCY ASSESSMENT AND COUNSELLING

Pre-pregnancy counselling is essential for all women with chronic hypertension in order to optimise their hypertensive control, to plan switching of teratogenic medication to alternative agents, and to inform women about potential complications in the pregnancy. In addition, exacerbating factors can be addressed with lifestyle adaptation such as weight loss, reduced alcohol intake, a low-salt diet and exercise.[8] Smoking cessation should be recommended for all women who continue to smoke.

MANAGEMENT OF HYPERTENSION IN PREGNANCY

If hypertension is diagnosed for the first time in pregnancy, secondary causes should be sought. The majority of investigations described in Table 8.1 are safe in pregnancy, but should be discussed with a specialist. Women should have increased frequency of antenatal contacts, but this should be tailored to individual requirements.

Target blood pressure in pregnancy for women with chronic hypertension is unknown, but NICE guidelines recommend that treatment is given to keep blood pressure lower than 150/100 mmHg, and lower than 140/90 mmHg if there is evidence of end-organ damage (e.g. left ventricular hypertrophy) or renal disease. Studies of blood pressure control in women with chronic or gestational hypertension have reported that individuals with 'tighter' control were less likely to develop severe hypertension or be admitted to hospital, and their babies were less likely to be born preterm.[14,15] There is an association between low birthweight and low diastolic blood pressure, therefore treatment should be reduced if diastolic blood pressure is persistently <80 mmHg.[5,16]

Hypertension may improve in early pregnancy due to gestational physiological changes and some women may be able to stop their medication for several weeks. However, vigilance should be maintained, as the normal physiological rise in blood pressure with later gestation may require dose titration or the introduction of additional agents. In addition to antihypertensive therapy, lifestyle measures including a low-salt diet and weight loss, if necessary, should also be discussed.

MATERNAL COMPLICATIONS

The incidence of superimposed pre-eclampsia in women with chronic hypertension is approximately 1 in 5,[17] and is higher in women with secondary hypertension.[1] All women should be advised to take aspirin 75 mg in order to reduce the risk of pre-eclampsia.[5] It is recommended that aspirin should be offered from 12 weeks onwards, as this is the earliest gestational age for which evidence supporting benefit is available.[18] Women with chronic hypertension may have undetectable renal damage which is revealed only by pregnancy, therefore a quantitative assessment of proteinuria should be performed at booking, for comparison in later pregnancy.

Evidence for uterine artery Doppler velocimetry in women with chronic hypertension is of poor quality and currently is insufficient to recommend any changes in antenatal care based on Doppler findings.[5]

Superimposed pre-eclampsia may be difficult to distinguish from physiological changes but the following features are suggestive of the condition:[19]

- A rapid rise in hypertension;
- New onset or doubling of proteinuria;
- Other laboratory parameters, e.g. low platelets, raised liver enzymes or creatinine.

Timing of delivery

Preterm delivery is more common in women with chronic hypertension compared with the general population.[1] Frequently this is iatrogenic for maternal and/or fetal indications. Timing of delivery should be guided by the severity of hypertension, the presence of proteinuria and fetal compromise. NICE guidelines suggest that delivery for women with chronic hypertension should be managed the same as for women with gestational hypertension, or if proteinuria is present as for pre-eclampsia.[5] Additional recommendations are given below:

- Do not offer birth to women with chronic hypertension whose blood pressure is lower than 160/110 mmHg with or without antihypertensive treatment, before 37 weeks.
- For women with chronic hypertension whose blood pressure is lower than 160/110 mmHg after 37 weeks

with or without antihypertensive treatment, timing of birth, and maternal and fetal indications for birth, should be agreed between the woman and the senior obstetrician.

- Offer birth to women with refractory severe chronic hypertension, after a course of corticosteroids (if required) has been completed.

Neonatal complications

Neonatal complications are also more commonly reported for women with chronic hypertension than for normotensive women, including higher rates of perinatal mortality, fetal growth restriction and admission to neonatal special care.[1]

POSTPARTUM MANAGEMENT

Peak postpartum blood pressure usually occurs at 3–5 days. It is recommended that women with chronic hypertension should have blood pressure measured at the following times postpartum, and treatment titrated to keep blood pressure lower than 140/90 mmHg:[5]

- Daily for the first 2 days postpartum;
- At least once between day 3 and day 5 postpartum;
- As clinically indicated if antihypertensive treatment is changed after delivery.

Women with previously diagnosed chronic hypertension can be discharged when their blood pressure is stable and <140/90 mmHg or <150/100 mmHg with treatment.[20] Medications that are safe for breastfeeding are listed in Table 8.3. Usually women can continue taking their antenatal antihypertensive agent. Enalapril is a good alternative for women with proteinuria associated with renal disease. It is the only ACEI/ARB that has been investigated for excretion into breast milk and is found in only small amounts.[21]

Hypertension may also be diagnosed postpartum, if blood pressure remains persistently elevated after 6 weeks. Community care should be alerted to the presence of unresolved hypertension and instructed to monitor and investigate appropriately.

All women with chronic hypertension should be offered a medical review at the postnatal review (6–8 weeks after delivery) for future pre-pregnancy counselling.[5] Assessment of future cardiovascular risk should also be made including serum lipids, family history and smoking history. Each 2-mmHg rise in systolic blood pressure is associated with a 7% increased risk of mortality from ischaemic heart disease and a 10% increased risk of mortality from stroke.[8] Women should be advised that statin and fibrate treatment should be stopped before or at conception.[22]

It is recommended that oestrogen-containing contraceptives be avoided in women with hypertension, due to their potential to exacerbate sodium retention[23] and hypertension.[24]

Table 8.3 Drugs safety in breastfeeding (adapted from Bramham et al.[20])

Drug	Dose	Comments
NICE recommendation and widely used in UK		
Alpha and/or beta blockers		
Labetalol	100–600 mg 2–3 times daily	Only small quantities detected in breast milk
Atenolol	25–100 mg once daily	Second-line use for women who require once-daily formulation
Calcium channel antagonists		
Nifedipine SR	10–20 mg twice daily	Amount in breast milk too small to be harmful; manufacturer suggests avoid but widely used without reports of neonatal side effects
Amlodipine	5–10 mg once daily	Second-line use for women who require once-daily formulation. Amount in breast milk too small to be harmful. Manufacturer suggests avoid but used in clinical practice without report of harm
Nifedipine MR	30–60 mg once daily	
Angiotensin-converting enzyme inhibitor (ACEI)		
Enalapril	5–20 mg twice daily	Can be used in breastfeeding when previously on ACEI; other first-choice agents cannot be used or cardiac/renal protection needed. Excreted into breast milk in low concentrations but amount probably too small to be harmful

(continued)

Table 8.3 Drugs safety in breastfeeding (adapted from *Bramham et al.*[20]) (*continued*)

Drug	Dose	Comments
NICE recommendation and widely used in UK		
Contraindicated		
Other ACEIs and ARBs	Not recommended	Minimal data on use during lactation. Manufacturers suggest avoid
Diuretics	Not recommended	Excessive thirst in breastfeeding women; large doses may suppress lactation

CONCLUSION

Women with chronic hypertension in pregnancy have increased maternal and neonatal morbidity, and require pre-pregnancy counselling and heightened antenatal surveillance. Hypertension identified for the first time in pregnancy should be investigated for secondary causes and evidence of end-organ damage. All women should be offered low-dose aspirin, and lifestyle modifications advised to reduce risk of complications.

Key References

1. Bateman BT, Bansil P, Hernandez-Diaz S, Mhyre JM, Callaghan WM, Kuklina EV. Prevalence, trends, and outcomes of chronic hypertension: a nationwide sample of delivery admissions. *Am J Obstet Gynecol*. 2012;206:134.e131–8.
2. Mathews TJ, Hamilton BE. Delayed child-bearing: more women are having their first child later in life. *National Center for Health Statistics Data Brief*. Bethesda, MA: CDC, 2009:21.
3. Kelly T, Yang W, Chen CS, Reynolds K, He J. Global burden of obesity in 2005 and projections to 2030. *Int J Obesity* 2008;32:1431–7.
4. Livingston JC, Sibai BM. Chronic hypertension in pregnancy. *Obstet Gynecol Clin North Am* 2001;28:447–63.
5. National Institute for Clinical Excellence. *Hypertension in Pregnancy: The management of hypertensive disorders during pregnancy* Clinical Guideline 107. London: NICE, 2010 wwwniceorguk/CG107.2010.
6. Cnossen JS, Vollebregt KC, de Vrieze N, et al. Accuracy of mean arterial pressure and blood pressure measurements in predicting pre-eclampsia: systematic review and meta-analysis. *BMJ* 2008;336:1117–20.
7. Coresh J, Selvin E, Stevens LA *et al.* Prevalence of chronic kidney disease in the United States. *JAMA*. 2007;298:2038–2047.
8. NICE. *Clinical Management of Primary Hypertension in Adults*. Clinical Guideline 127. London: NICE, 2011 www.nice.org.uk/CG127. 2011.
9. Smith MC, Moran P, Ward MK, Davison JM. Assessment of glomerular filtration rate during pregnancy using the MDRD formula. *BJOG* 2008;115:109–12.
10. Cooper WO, Hernandez-Diaz S, Arbogast PG *et al.* Major congenital malformations after first-trimester exposure to ACE inhibitors. *N Engl J Med* 2006;354:2443–51.
11. Bullo M, Tschumi S, Bucher BS, Bianchetti MG, Simonetti GD. Pregnancy outcome following exposure to angiotensin-converting enzyme inhibitors or angiotensin receptor antagonists: a systematic review. *Hypertension* 2012;60:444–50.
12. Li DK, Yang C, Andrade S, Tavares V, Ferber JR. Maternal exposure to angiotensin converting enzyme inhibitors in the first trimester and risk of malformations in offspring: a retrospective cohort study. *BMJ* 2011;343:5931.
13. Butters L, Kennedy S, Rubin PC. Atenolol in essential hypertension during pregnancy. *BMJ* 1990;301:587–9.
14. El Guindy AA, Nabhan AF. A randomized trial of tight vs. less tight control of mild essential and gestational hypertension in pregnancy. *J Perinat Med* 2008;36:413–18.
15. Magee LA, von Dadelszen P, Chan S *et al.* The Control of Hypertension In Pregnancy Study pilot trial. *BJOG*. 2007;114:770. e713–20.
16. von Dadelszen P, Ornstein MP, Bull SB, Logan AG, Koren G, Magee LA. Fall in mean arterial pressure and fetal growth restriction in pregnancy hypertension: a meta-analysis. *Lancet* 2000;355:87–92.
17. Chappell LC, Enye S, Seed P, Briley AL, Poston L, Shennan AH. Adverse perinatal outcomes and risk factors for preeclampsia in women with chronic hypertension: a prospective study. *Hypertension* 2008;51:1002–9.
18. Duley L, Henderson-Smart DJ, Meher S, King JF. Antiplatelet agents for preventing pre-eclampsia and its complications. *Cochrane Database Syst Rev* 2007;2:CD004659.
19. Brown MA, Lindheimer MD, de Swiet M, Van Assche A, Moutquin JM. The classification and diagnosis of the hypertensive disorders of pregnancy: statement from the International Society for the Study of Hypertension in Pregnancy (ISSHP). *Hypertens Pregnancy* 2001;20:IX–XIV.

20. Bramham K, Nelson-Piercy C, Brown MJ, Chappell LC. Postpartum management of hypertension. *BMJ* 2013;346:894.

21. Redman CW, Kelly JG, Cooper WD. The excretion of enalapril and enalaprilat in human breast milk. *Eur J Clin Pharmacol* 1990;38:99.

22. Pechère-Bertschi A, Maillard M, Stalder H, Bischof P, Fathi M, Brunner HR, Burnier M. Renal hemodynamic and tubular responses to salt in women using oral contraceptives. *Kidney Int* 2003;64:1374–80.

23. Williamson PM, Buddle ML, Brown MA, Whitworth JA. Ambulatory blood pressure monitoring (ABPM) in the normal menstrual cycle and in women using oral contraceptives: Comparison with conventional blood pressure measurement. *Am J Hypertens* 1996; 9:953–8.

24. Briggs GG, Freeman RK, Yaffe SJ (eds). *Drugs in Pregnancy and Lactation: A reference guide to fetal and neonatal risk,* 9th edn. 2011, Philadelphia, PA: Lippincott Williams & Wilkins.

Chapter 9 Diabetes mellitus

Clare L Tower

INTRODUCTION

Diabetes mellitus (DM) is a collection of metabolic disorders with hyperglycaemia as the common feature and is predominantly classified outside pregnancy into two major subtypes, type 1 and type 2. Type 1 is typically due to a deficiency of insulin and tends to present in a younger age group, whereas type 2 is considered to be a disease of insulin resistance presenting in an older age group. Persistent hyperglycaemia in both disorders causes organ damage affecting the eyes, kidneys, nerves and cardiovascular system. Pre-existing diabetes (type 1 or type 2) is associated with a higher risk of a poor obstetric outcome. In 1990, the St Vincent Declaration set a series of targets to improve the outcome of pregnant women with diabetes, with the aim that the risks should approximate those of the non-diabetic populations. Unfortunately, the 2007 CEMACH (Confidential Enquiry into Maternal and Child Health) report on diabetes in pregnancy found that current care falls well short of this target.[1]

PREVALENCE

Diabetes is the commonest medical condition encountered during pregnancy in the UK (and probably around the world), with up to 5% of pregnancies being complicated by either pre-existing or gestational diabetes. Overall, for adults in the UK with diabetes, 90% have type 2 diabetes and 10% type 1. However, in pregnant women, with diabetes this pattern is reversed, with 5%% having type 2 diabetes, 7.5% having type 1 Diabetes, and the majority, 87.5% having Gestational diabetes.[2] Overall, 0.27% of births are affected by type 1 diabetes, and 0.1% are affected by type 2.[2]

EPIDEMIOLOGY

Type 2 diabetes is typically associated with advancing age, obesity and particular ethnic groups including those of African, black Caribbean, south Asian, Middle Eastern and Chinese origin. As such, the incidence of type 2 diabetes is increasing in the population as a whole, and also therefore in pregnant women. Type 1 diabetes is usually diagnosed before the age of 30 years and is also increasing in incidence at a rate of 4% per year, being commoner in Scandinavian countries (Finland has the highest incidence). In contrast to type 2 diabetes, type 1 is not thought to be associated with lifestyle factors, but is an autoimmune disorder. The reason for the increasing incidence is unclear.

CAUSES

Physiological changes in pregnancy

Pregnant women have considerably altered carbohydrate metabolism. There is hyperplasia of the pancreatic islet cells which leads to a doubling in insulin production between the first and the third trimesters. Although there is an initial increase in insulin sensitivity during the first trimester, the release of insulin-resistant hormones (human placental lactogen, glucagons, progesterone and corticotrophin-releasing hormone) from the placenta results in progressive glucose intolerance (insulin resistance) with advancing gestation. In addition to the increased glucose uptake of the fetus, there is increased peripheral uptake, increased glycogenesis and reduced hepatic gluconeogenesis. The renal tubular threshold for glucose falls, such that glycosuria is common. Overall, fasting glucose levels fall by 10–20% and postprandial levels are higher.

Pathogenesis of type 1 diabetes

Type 1 DM (juvenile onset) is an autoimmune disease that usually presents in childhood or young adulthood. Autoimmune destruction of the pancreatic islet cells results in insulin deficiency and causes symptoms of thirst, polyuria, blurred vision, weight loss and, if untreated, progression to life-threatening diabetic ketoacidosis. There is a genetic component and it is associated with human leukocyte antigen (HLA)-DR3 and HLA-DR4. It is not associated with obesity. The baby of an affected mother has a 2% risk of developing diabetes, whilst the child of an affected father faces an 8% risk. If both parents have type 1 diabetes, there is a 30% risk to their offspring.

Pathogenesis of type 2 diabetes

Type 2 disease (maturity onset) is a disease of peripheral insulin resistance rather than deficiency. Although it more commonly occurs over the age of 40 years, it often occurs at a younger age (25 years and upwards) in those of south Asian and African Caribbean origin. The incidence increases with age and body-weight and there is a stronger genetic component than in type 1. Hyperglycaemia is commonly present for a prolonged period prior to diagnosis and, although these patients sometimes require insulin treatment, they do not become ketotic if it is withdrawn. The prevalence of type 2 diabetes is expected to rise with increasing maternal obesity, age and social deprivation.[1] The risks of affected offspring are higher than in type 1 diabetes. Offspring of an affected mother or father have a 15% risk, and if both parents are affected the risk is 75%.

Women with type 1 or type 2 diabetes are at risk of vascular complications (both macro- and microvascular), resulting in a reduced life expectancy. The CEMACH report confirmed that all women with pre-existing diabetes (type 1 and type 2) have uniformly poorer outcomes than women without diabetes.[3]

MANAGEMENT

Pre-conception

Optimising pre-conception care in women with diabetes has been shown to improve outcome. Despite this, the CEMACH report found that only 35% of pregnant women with diabetes received adequate pre-conceptional counselling and care.[3] Studies have shown lower rates of congenital abnormalities and pregnancy complications in women who received multidisciplinary preconception care[4,5] [C].

Type 1 (Box 9.1)

The risk of major congenital malformations, in particular cardiac and neural tube defects, increases with poor control of blood glucose during the first 8 weeks of pregnancy. Levels of glycated haemoglobin, HbA1c, are used to reflect long-term glycaemic control, and in general, all congenital malformations are associated with poor control in the first trimester. If significantly raised, to greater than 69–80 mmol/mol (8.5–9.5%), malformation rates of around 20% have been reported, and these risks fall if levels of HbA1c can be reduced.[1,6] Therefore, women should be advised that optimising diabetic control pre-pregnancy will improve outcome of pregnancy. Good glycaemic control will also reduce the risks of miscarriage, stillbirth and neonatal death. The NICE guidelines 2015 recommend that information about planning pregnancy and the importance of good control of blood glucose be explained at each contact with health professionals from adolescence and that this information be given in a supportive environment with other family members encouraged to attend.[2] Smoking and diet should also be discussed and women with a body mass index of greater than 27kg/m[2] be supported to lose weight. Risks of pregnancy should also be outlined, and the need for frequent and regular attendance at clinics during the antenatal period. Targets for self monitoring of blood glucose should be agreed with the woman, and these should consider individual risks of hypoglycaemia. These targets should be the same ranges as recommended for all people with type 1 diabetes. Monthly testing of HBA1c should be offered to women planning pregnancy and women advised to aim for an HbA1c of less than 48 mmol/mol (6.5% [C]) as long as this does not cause difficulties with hypoglycaemia.[2] Women with an HbA1c greater than 86 mmol/mol (10%) should be strongly advised to avoid pregnancy until better control is achieved.[2] The 2010 SIGN guidelines state that pre-pregnancy glycaemic control should be as close to the non-diabetic range as possible.[5] Goals should be set with the woman, involving other members of the multidisciplinary team. More rigorous control will increase the risks of hypoglycaemia, so this should be discussed, and women and

Box 9.1 Pre-conceptual counselling

Multidisciplinary management
Optimise glycaemic control – aim HbA1c 43 mmol/mol or less
Discuss hypoglycaemia
Review diet and weight loss
Discuss complications of pregnancy
Prescribe folic acid 5 mg
Review renal function and blood pressure
Retinal assessment
Review other medications, e.g. ACE inhibitors, statins
Smoking cessation

ANTENATAL OBSTETRICS

their families should be aware of the treatments for this (see below). Women planning pregnancy should also be offered ketone testing strips and a meter and be advised to self-monitor for ketonaemia if they become unwell or hyperglycaemic.[2] The opportunity should also be taken to counsel about diet, weight control and smoking cessation. Women should be prescribed 5 mg of folic acid to be taken pre-conception and for the first 12 weeks of pregnancy [D–E]. The risks of other complications of pregnancy, including pre-eclampsia, birth trauma, fetal macrosomia and the increased risk of caesarean section, should also be discussed.

Other aspects of the women's diabetes should also be reviewed, such as blood pressure, renal function and retinal assessment. Retinal assessment should be offered preconception unless this has been performed within the last 6 months. The use of any medications that are contraindicated in pregnancy should be assessed, and changed if a suitable alternative exists. Typical drugs falling into this category are statins, angiotensin II-converting enzyme (ACE) inhibitors and angiotensin receptor blockers (ARBs). ACE inhbitors, ARBs and statins should be discontinued prior to pregnancy, or as soon as pregnancy is confirmed and antihypertensive agents suitable for use in pregnancy be used. Renal function should be checked and women with creatinine levels greater than 120 μmol/L, a urinary albumin:creatinine ratio >30mg/mmol or a glomerular filtration rate of less than 45ml/min/1.73m^2 should be referred to a renal physician prior to stopping contraception use.

Women who have significant retinopathy or nephropathy should be advised that pregnancy may accelerate these pathological processes. Some women, with severe end-organ damage, such as diabetic nephropathy with glomerular filtration rate of <30%, severe cardiac damage or neuropathy, face significant maternal risk in pregnancy and may be better advised to avoid pregnancy.[7] Due to the close association with other autoimmune disorders, some advocate screening for thyroid dysfunction.[7]

Type 2

It is estimated that there may be around half a million individuals in the UK with undiagnosed diabetes, usually type 2. Therefore, type 2 diabetes is often unrecognised prior to pregnancy and may be misdiagnosed as gestational diabetes during pregnancy. However, recent data suggest that women with type 2 diabetes have a similar increase in risk of congenital abnormality to those with type 1, at around double that of women without diabetes.[6] Therefore, the pre-conception advice is the same as that for type 1 diabetes. This group of women is more likely to be overweight and should be helped to reduce their weight if their body mass index is greater than 27 kg/m^2. Women taking oral hypoglycaemic agents should have their medication reviewed. Metformin is safe to take in pregnancy so can be continued, but current advice is that other oral hypoglycaemics should be changed. Some women may achieve better control by converting to insulin, and this should be discussed with the woman.

Box 9.2 Complications of pregnancy associated with diabetes

Fetal risks
Miscarriage
Congenital anomaly
Stillbirth
Prematurity
Macrosomia
Shoulder dystocia and birth injury
Respiratory distress
Neonatal hypoglycaemia and poor feeding
Risk of diabetes
Maternal risks
Hypoglycaemia
Diabetic ketoacidosis
Operative delivery
Worsening of retinal disease
Worsening of pre-existing renal impairment
Pre-eclampsia

Antenatal care

The risks and complications of pregnancy in a woman with diabetes are summarised in Box 9.2. The aim of antenatal care is to target and reduce these risks. There is no doubt that pregnant women with diabetes are best managed in a multidisciplinary clinic involving diabetologists, obstetricians, dieticians, specialist midwives and nurses. Unfortunately, the CEMACH survey found that a third of maternity units in England, Northern Ireland and Wales did not provide such specialist services.[1] Women should be booked for care early in pregnancy, preferably before 10 weeks. An early ultrasound scan (7-9 weeks) will enable viability and dating to be confirmed. At this early appointment, a full clinical history and medication review should be conducted. If retinal or renal assessment has not occurred during the preceding 3 months, these should be arranged. NICE guidelines 2015 recommend digital imaging retinal assessment using tropicamide mydriasis both following booking and again at 28 weeks.[2] If there is any retinopathy present at booking, repeat assessment is recommended at 16-20 weeks. If the woman has a raised creatinine > 120mmol/l or proteinuria greater than 2g/day or a urinary albumin:creatinine ratio of >30mg/mmol then referral to a renal physician should be considered. Women with proteinuria >5g/day should be offered thromboprophylaxis. Due to the risk of pre-eclampsia, all women with diabetes should be offered 75 mg aspirin from the first trimester.[8] The usual nutritional assessments offered to all pregnant women, including iron and vitamin D, should also be discussed.[9]

In common with all women, women with diabetes should be offered screening for Down's syndrome. The recommended first-trimester test which reaches the current required criteria of a detection rate of 75% and a false-positive rate of less than

3% is the combined test, consisting of nuchal translucency (NT), human β-chorionic gonadotrophin (β-hCG) and pregnancy-associated plasma protein A (PAPP-A). If women present too late, or the NT is unobtainable or not available, they should be offered the triple (β-hCG, unconjugated oestriol [uE$_3$], α-fetoprotein [AFP]) or quadruple test (triple + inhibin A) in the second trimester. The NT measurement is unaffected by diabetes. However, diabetes is associated with lower levels of AFP and uE$_3$ in the second trimester, hence risk adjustments need to be made. Recent data have also suggested that first trimester PAPP-A and β-hCG may be reduced, although the data are conflicting. Current practice is to reduce PAPP-A measurements in women with preexisting diabetes. Maternal weight and poor diabetic control are two factors that may also reduce the levels of these markers, thus explaining the differences between these studies.

Management of diabetic complications

The longer the duration of the diabetes, the higher the chance of a patient having pre-existing vasculopathy, renal dysfunction, neuropathy and diabetic retinopathy. The presence of these complications increases the risks of pre-eclampsia and fetal growth restriction. Pregnancy is associated with progression of pre-existing retinopathy, and this is more likely with increased severity of the pre-existing disease, duration of diabetes, poor glycaemic control and rapid improvements in control [C]. However, NICE considers that the benefits of improved glycaemic control overall outweigh the risks of progression of diabetic retinopathy[2] [E]. The presence of hypertension also worsens progression of retinopathy, thus it has been suggested that, in women with these complications, blood pressure should be kept at 120–130/70–80 mmHg. Beta blockers should be avoided as antihypertensives due to their possible adverse effects of glucose metabolism. There is evidence that some diabetic retinopathy may regress after delivery, but women with retinopathy should undergo further retinal assessment by 6 months postpartum.

Diabetic nephropathy is considered as a continuous spectrum from microalbuminuria, proteinuria and impaired renal function to end-stage renal disease in which there is increasing serum urea and creatinine. Overall, with the exception of women with pre-existing renal failure, nephropathy does not deteriorate with pregnancy. However, there is an increased risk of growth restriction, pre-eclampsia and preterm birth. Thus increased surveillance is required in these women.

Congenital anomalies

The CEMACH enquiry found the prevalence of confirmed major anomalies to be 41.8/1000 total births in pregnant women with diabetes.[3] The commonest are cardiac abnormalities in which there is a 3 to 5-fold relative increased risk. Although caudal regression (sacral agenesis) is the most well-known associated abnormality (200-fold increased risk), the prevalence is low. Diabetes conveys a 2 to 10-fold increased risk

of neural tube defects. Thus, all women with diabetes should have a detailed fetal anatomy scan at 20 weeks, which should include the four-chamber cardiac view, 3 vessel view and the outflow tracts. NICE and SIGN currently do not recommend specialist fetal echocardiography for women with diabetes.[2,5]

MEDICATIONS

Good glycaemic control is the key to improving the outcome of pregnancy in women with diabetes. This can be achieved using a combination of diet, insulin and oral hypoglycaemic agents.

Oral hypoglycaemic agents

The oral hypoglycaemic agents used in patients with type 2 diabetes are given in Box 9.3. With the exception of metformin and glibenclamide, there are few available data regarding the safety of most of these drugs in pregnancy, or whether they cross the placenta. Metformin is increasingly used in women with polycystic ovarian syndrome as it reduces the risk of first-trimester miscarriage and reduces the risk of developing gestational diabetes. Metformin is known to cross the placenta; use in early pregnancy does not increase the risk of congenital malformations.[10] Glibenclamide may cross the placenta in small amounts and some small observational studies suggest that it may reduce morbidity and mortality in developing countries in which insulin use is impractical and expensive. Of the other sulfonylureas, chlorpropamide and tolbutamide, although probably not associated with congenital malformations, may be associated with prolonged neonatal hypoglycaemia and seizures. There are very

Box 9.3 Oral hypoglycemic agents

Sulfonylureas
Chlorpropamide
Glibenclamide
Gliclazide
Glimepiride
Glipizide
Gliquidone
Tolbutamide
Biguanides
Metformin
α-Glucosidase inhibitors
Acarbose
Thiazolidinediones
Pioglitazone
Rosiglitazone
Drugs stimulating insulin release
Nateglinide
Repaglinide

few data relating to the newer classes of drugs, and it is largely unknown whether drugs such as nateglinide are able to cross the placenta.

Current recommended practice is for women who conceive on oral hypoglycaemic agents to be switched to insulin therapy as soon as they are pregnant. However, there is growing interest in the use of metformin and glibenclamide in the management of type 2 diabetes or gestational diabetes. These drugs are cheaper, easier and more convenient, have less risk of hypoglycaemia and may have beneficial effects on long-term prognosis. An RCT of glibenclamide compared with insulin for the treatment of gestational diabetes found no significant differences in the major outcomes of macrosomia, blood glucose, neonatal hypoglycaemia or admissions to neonatal intensive care.[11] An RCT comparing metformin with insulin in gestational diabetes (MIG trial) has recently confirmed the safety and benefit of metformin treatment in women with gestational diabetes after 20 weeks' gestation.[12] Current NICE recommendations are that metformin may be considered as an alternative to insulin therapy in pregnant women with type 2 diabetes.[2] Individual risks and benefits should be considered and the patient should be involved in the decision. However, this remains the exception rather than the rule in current practice, with most women with pre-existing diabetes managed on insulin therapy.

Insulin

Insulin is the current recommended treatment for the majority of pregnant women with diabetes. Initially, insulin available for human use was cow or pig insulin. However, the majority of insulins in current use are recombinant insulins or their analogues. These analogues have a modified amino acid structure to improve absorption profile such that risks of hypoglycaemia are less and more stable blood glucose levels are achieved. There are four main types of insulin available for use, categorised by duration of action (summarised in Table 9.1). The newer long-acting insulin analogues may be associated with fewer hypoglycaemic episodes as they provide steady background levels without peaks. Some insulin preparations are described as biphasic as they contain a combination of two types of insulin, for example Mixtard 30, which contains a short-acting insulin, together with intermediate insulin, given twice a day. Commonly, type 2 diabetics may be able to achieve good control following conversion from oral agents with these preparations. Insulin regimens vary with the individual, but will typically consist of a long-acting basal insulin, given once or twice a day, with additional boluses given via a pen to cover meal times. This is known as the multiple daily injection (MDI) regimen. The short acting insulins, aspart and lispro, have been associated with less hypoglycaamia, and better glycameic control overall, therefore use of these preparations should be considered in pregnancy.[2]

Continuous subcutaneous insulin infusion (CSII) pumps were initially introduced in the 1970s, are growing in popularity. Regular and short-acting insulin can be delivered via a pump and the benefits include less risks of hyper- and hypoglycaemia and better compliance. Therefore, they are particularly useful in patients with unstable diabetes and troublesome hypoglycaemia. The pumps consist of a cannula that is inserted into the subcutaneous abdominal tissue (site changed every 3 days) through which a continuous basal level of fast-acting insulin is administered. Additional boluses are also given through the pump for meal times. Outside pregnancy, pumps are associated with better quality of life and better control of blood glucose. In general, studies have shown CSII is associated with improved HbA1c and lower hypoglycaemia rates, although to date minimal maternal and fetal benefits have been reported in studies of pregnancy.[7] NICE (2015) rcommends that CSII pumps be offered to pregnant women if their MDI regimen does not achieve adequate control without problematic hypoglycaemia.[2]

GLYCAEMIC CONTROL

Although good glycaemic control during pregnancy is likely to reduce the risks of macrosomia, stillbirth, neonatal hypoglycaemia and respiratory distress syndrome,[5] the evidence for the timing and frequency of testing, or target blood glucose ranges, is of poor quality and at times conflicting. Although some data have suggested that obtaining good glycaemic

Table 9.1 Types of insulin

Type	Examples	Onset	Peak	Duration
Rapid acting	Lispro (Humalog) Aspart (NovoRapid) Glulisine (Apidra)	15 min	30–90 min	5 hours
Short acting	Regular	30 min	2–4 hours	4–8 hours
Intermediate acting	NPH (isophane), lente	2–6 hours	4–14 hours	14–20 hours
Long acting	Ultralente	6–14 hours	Small (or none) 10–16 hours	20–24 hours
	Glargine Detemir	1–2 hours	None	24 hours

control, as indicated by a satisfactory HbA1c level, does not reduce the risk of macrosomia,[13] other observational studies have demonstrated that postprandial blood glucose measurements in the third trimester correlated with macrosomia [B]. The risks of respiratory distress and preterm labour also increase with worsening glycaemic control [C]. Women with diabetes also have an increased risk of stillbirth. The recent CEMACH report found that women whose babies had congenital malformations, or suffered a stillbirth or neonatal death, had worse glycaemic control (as monitored by higher HbA1c levels) throughout pregnancy[3] [D]. Two small RCTs of preprandial and postprandial blood glucose monitoring have found improved outcomes in women in the postprandial group [B]. The HAPO study[5] found that there was no threshold level of blood glucose which complications were increased and that there was a continuous linear association between blood glucose levels and complications such as macrosomia. With these reservations in mind, the NICE guidelines 2015 recommended that individualized targets for blood glucose measurements should be set with the woman, taking into account the risk of hypoglycaemia. Suggested targets for capillary plasma glucose are:

- Fasting less than 5.3mmol/l and
- 1 hour post meal less than 7.8mmol/l or 2 hours post meal less than 6.4mmol/l

Women taking insulin or glibenclamide should be advised to keep blood glucose greater than 4mmol/l.

Box 9.4 Glycaemic control - recommended levels[2]

Pre-conception

HbA1c <48 mmol/mol

Avoid pregnancy if HbA1c >86 mmol/mol

Aim for same capillary plasma blood glucose as recommended for all people with type 1 diabetes

Throughout pregnancy:

Fasting blood glucose <5.3 mmol/L

1 hour Postprandial blood glucose <7.8 mmol/L or

2 hour postprandial blood glucose <6.4mmol/L

Women on insulin or glibenclamide should aim to keep capilliary plasma glucose level greater than 4mmol/L

Use of HbA1c not routinely recommended for monitoring

Monitoring

All women should test daily

Type 1 diabetes or those on multiple daily insulin doses:

Fasting levels

Pre meal and 1 hour after every meal

Bedtime

Those on diet, oral treatment or single insulin doses:

Fasting and 1 hour post meal

Women taking insulin should also test before bedtime

Women with type 1 diabetes should be offered ketone testing strips for use if they become hyperglycaemic or feel unwell.

Medical review on a regular basis (1-2 weekly)

Women with type 1 diabetes or those on an MDI regimen should be advised to test their fasting, pre-meal and 1 hour post meal and bedtime capillary blood glucose every day during pregnancy. Women receiving diet, oral hypoglycaemics or single daily dose insulin should also test a daily fasting glucose and 1 hour after meals.[2] SIGN guidelines suggest fasting levels of 4–6 mmol/L, <8 mmol/L 1 hour postprandially, <7 mmol/L 2 hours postprandially and >6 mmol/L before bed.[5] The physiological adaptations of pregnancy result in increasing insulin requirements with gestation, and obtaining good control necessitates frequent review by a diabetic team at 1- to 2-weekly intervals.

HbA1c represents blood glucose levels in the preceding 4–12 weeks, and does not reflect subtle changes in blood glucose, in particular postprandial levels. Furthermore, it falls in response to the physiological changes in pregnancy, and the timescale may not be appropriate in pregnant women. Although American guidelines recommend monitoring HbA1c in type 1 diabetes,[7] UK NICE guidelines (2015) and SIGN guidelines (2010) do not recommend it is used routinely to monitor blood glucose control in the the second and third trimesters. It is recommended at booking in order to determine the overall risk to the pregnancy from poor pre-existing control and can be considered for women with pre-existing diabetes to aid assessment of ongoing risk.[2] This is because risks increase when HbA1C is greater than 48nmol/l or 6.5%.

There is growing interest in the use of continuous blood glucose monitoring, using a subcutaneous sensor to measure interstitial blood glucose as frequently as every 10 seconds, with the aim of maintaining blood glucose within a physiological range, and avoiding the inevitable peaks and troughs that occur with intermittent monitoring. Although there is evidence for the benefit of such monitoring outside pregnancy, there are limited studies to support the use in pregnant women, although it offers a promising technology for the future.[15] NICE guidelines currently do not recommend routine use of this technology, but it can be considered in women with problematic hypoglycaemia, unstable blood glucose levels or in order to gain information about blood glucose variability.[2]

Hypoglycaemia

Tighter glycaemic control in pregnancy is associated with an increase in the risk of hypoglycaemia. This is compounded by the fact that pregnant women also have an altered hormonal response to hypoglycaemia and reduced awareness, often worsened by pregnancy-related nausea and vomiting. Studies have shown that the highest risk time for hypoglycaemic episodes is between 8 and 16 weeks.[7] The recent CEMACH report found that women with type 1 diabetes are much more likely to suffer recurrent hypoglycaemia (61%) than those with type 2 (21%).[3] It is therefore vital that pregnant women who are taking insulin, and their families, are fully educated about the symptoms and treatment of hypoglycaemia. Women taking insulin should be advised to have a fast-acting form of glucose with them at all times and glucagon should also be provided to all pregnant women with type 1 diabetes, and the woman and her family should be educated in how to use it.[2] NICE defines hypoglycaemia as a blood glucose of <3.5mmol/L, and this level of blood glucose should be treated even if the patient is asymptomatic. If the patient is conscious, this should be by consuming 10–15 g of glucose (approximates to 4 teaspoons of sugar or half a can of juice or 3 glucose tablets). Alternatives include a glucose gel (2 tubes of HypoStop/Glucogel) which can be rubbed on the inside of the cheek. This should be followed by a slower-releasing carbohydrate such as bread or a sandwich. If unconscious, a family member can administer glucagon (0.5–1 mg) intramuscularly. This has a rapid onset and lasts approximately 90 minutes. For these reasons, it is recommended that patients carry information identifying them as having diabetes. Patients in hospital can be given 150 mL of 10% dextrose intravenously. Once a patient is conscious, they should be given oral therapy as above. If after 10 minutes the blood glucose remains less than 5 mmol/L, the treatment should be repeated. Insulin doses with the next meal should not be withheld but may require modification.

Diabetic ketoacidosis

Diabetic ketoacidosis (DKA) occurs when there is insufficient insulin to metabolise blood glucose. This can be caused by failure to appreciate the increasing insulin requirements in pregnancy, missed insulin doses or pump failure, concurrent illness such as infection, steroid therapy and stress, and is more common in pregnancy.[16] It is defined as a plasma glucose over 12 mmol/L, an arterial pH of less than 7.3, with ketonuria or ketonaemia, and is associated with poor maternal and fetal outcome. CTG abnormalities are typical in the third trimester and resolve with treatment of the hyperglycaemia. Management should involve the diabetic teams and treatment of the precipitating cause, and will usually require intravenous insulin via a sliding scale. Volume replacement with careful monitoring and replacement of potassium are also needed. It is recommended that this therapy is administered within a level 2 critical care unit, where both medical and obstetric care is available. A continuous CTG may be necessary, but should be given careful consideration. CTG abnormalities are to be expected in a woman with DKA, and it would be unsafe to perform an emergency caesarean until the woman is stable from metabolic and haemodynamic perspectives. Severe hyperglycaemia requiring intensive treatment is defined as persistent pre-meal blood glucose values of greater than 12 mmol/L on 2 consecutive occasions, or a random level of more than 15 mmol/L. Involvement of diabetologists is recommended as it is important to ensure that the hyperglycaemia is at variance to the patients' usual level of control. Because of the dangers of DKA, NICE guidelines 2015 recommend that all pregnant women with type 1 diabetes should be given testing strips and a meter for blood ketones and instructed in their use. They should be advised to test if they become hyperglycaemic or feel unwell.[2] Similarly, a pregnant woman present with hyperglycaemia or feeling unwell should be tested for ketonaemia. Women with type 2 or gestational diabetes should be advised to seek medical advice urgently if they have hyperglycaemia or feel unwell.

Administration of corticosteroids

Corticosteroids, given to reduce neonatal morbidity and mortality associated with prematurity, almost always have an adverse effect on glucose tolerance, resulting in an increased insulin requirement in diabetic women. This can be managed by increasing subcutaneous doses, or by the use of intravenous insulin via a sliding scale.[2] The peaks in blood glucose usually occur between 9 and 15 hours after the first dose and 8–15 hours after the second dose. Diabetes should not be considered a contraindication to the use of antenatal steroids, but close monitoring and additional insulin will probably be needed, often requiring a sliding scale.

FETAL MONITORING

The aim of fetal monitoring is to detect the two extremes of fetal weight and to reduce the risk of stillbirth. Women, usually those with long-standing type 1 disease involving end-organ damage, are at risk of pre-eclampsia and fetal growth restriction. The CEMACH report found that the stillbirth rate after 24 weeks was 26.8 per 1000 live births and stillbirths, compared with the national background rate of 5.7 per 1000.[3] The stillbirth rate varied with gestation, with 17.2% occurring at 24–27 weeks, 13.8% at 28–31, 41.4% at 32–36 weeks and 27.6% at 31–41 weeks [D]. More commonly, however, the risk is of fetal overgrowth and macrosomia.

RCOG guidelines list women with diabetes and vascular disease as having a major risk factor for the development of growth restriction.[17] The odds ratio for a birthweight less than the 10th centile is 6 but with a wide 95% CI of 1.5–23.3 [D].[18] This study also found a 3.5-fold (95% CI 1.28–9.53) increase in risk of pre-eclampsia. Although uterine artery Doppler at 20–22 weeks' gestation can be used to aid prediction of growth restriction, the negative likelihood ratio is not good enough to negate the risk or alter the management of regular growth scans starting from 26–28 weeks gestation. Therefore, the RCOG do not recommend uterine artery Doppler for these women.[17]

Fetal macrosomia, defined by either a birthweight greater than 4 kg or a birthweight centile greater than 90, is associated with increased rates of caesarean section, and birth injury such as shoulder dystocia, fractures and brachial plexus injury. Most macrosomic infants are uniformly or symmetrically large (70%), although asymmetrically large infants in whom the thoracic and abdominal circumference is greater than the head circumference are at greatest risk of shoulder dystocia.

Monitoring strategies aimed at reducing these risks consist of regular ultrasound scans and CTGs, but there is no good evidence for the use of any of these in the care of women with diabetes. CTG interpretation can be challenging as diabetes may reduce the variability and increase the baseline fetal heart rate. There may also be fewer movements and thus fewer accelerations. Therefore, patterns of change may be a better indicator of deterioration in fetal wellbeing.

NICE guidelines recommend regular ultrasound scans for growth, liquor volume and umbilical artery Doppler in women with diabetes at 4-weekly intervals, guided by findings and control of blood glucose betweeen 28 and 36 weeks.[2] Ultrasound estimation of fetal weight to detect macrosomia is subject to inaccuracy, with sensitivities and positive predictive values 36–76% and 51–85% respectively, and there is evidence that this increases caesarean section rate without clinical benefit.[5] The negative predictive value is better at 80–96%, hence there is probably a role for ultrasound in the exclusion of macrosomia. Overall, growth velocity and, in particular, crossing centiles are of use in identifying the development of macrosomia and growth restriction. Routine monitoring before 38 weeks of biophysical profile or CTG is not recommended unless there is a particular risk of growth restriction.[2]

MODE AND TIMING OF DELIVERY

The CEMACH enquiry found high rates of induction of labour and caesarean section in women with diabetes with induction rates of 39% (background 21%), and a caesarean section rate of 67%3 [D]. There is evidence to suggest that induction of labour at 38 weeks may reduce the risk of shoulder dystocia in macrosomic infants of women with diabetes. An RCT compared induction with expectant management in women requiring insulin (most had gestational diabetes) and found that expectant management did not reduce caesarean section rates and increased the rates of large babies and shoulder dystocia[19] [B]. A further case–control trial from Israel compared induction at 38–39 weeks with expectant management in type 1 diabetes. The rate of shoulder dystocia was lower in the induction group[20] [C]. Interestingly, there are also retrospective data suggesting that induction is associated with a reduction in caesarean section rates in women with diabetes [D]. Current NICE (2015) guidelines advise that timing and mode of delivery should be discussed with women with diabetes, and that women with any pre-existing diabetes without compliations be offered an elective birth between 37+0 and 38+6 weeks gestation.[2] SIGN (2010) guidance is that women with diabetes and a normally grown baby should be offered delivery (induction or caesarean section if indicated)

Table 9.2 Example sliding scale for use during labour in pregnant women taking insulin

Hourly blood glucose (mmol/L)	Insulin rate (units per hour = mL per hour)	Other action
3.0 or less	0	Repeat glucose test, **give glucose*** If <3.1, check all lines and infusion pumps, call consultant
3.1–3.9	0.5	Repeat glucose test, **give glucose if <4.0 and symptomatic*** If hypo confirmed, check all lines and infusion pumps
4.0–6.9	1	
7.0–7.9	2	
8.0–8.9	3	
9.0–10.9	4	Call consultant
11.0–16	6	Stop dextrose, start 0.9% saline, call consultant
>16	8	Stop dextrose, start 0.9% saline, call consultant

*Treat hypoglycaemia with three glucose tablets, 60 ml lucozade or 150 ml of intravenous 10% dextrose.
- Serious clinical incidents including death have occurred with sliding-scale insulin regimens. Please follow protocol precisely.
- Setting up the insulin sliding scale should always be done in consultation with the consultant physician. Some patients required higher or lower insulin infusion rates especially if they are receiving high doses of insulin (>60 units/day).
- The insulin infusion rate should be reduced immediately after delivery – the consultant physician will advise.
- The aim is to keep blood glucose concentration between **4–7 mmol/L**.
- If blood glucose levels do not fall into the 4-7 mmol/L range after 3 hours of IV insulin contact the consultant physician, the diabetes specialist midwife or the on-call medical team.
- Set up the following infusions that can be given through the same Venflon using a Y-connector
  - IVAC Drip - 10% dextrose 500 ml at - 83 ml/h
  - Infusion syringe pump - 50 units Actrapid insulin in 50 ml 0.9% saline.
- It is very important that the lines and pumps are checked hourly, AND if there is unexplained hyper- or hypoglycaemia – failure of either IVAC pump or line can cause unexplained dangerous hyper- or hypoglycaemia.
- The rate of the insulin pump is adjusted based on hourly blood glucose measurements.

Taken from St Mary's Hospital guidelines, Central Manchester University Hospitals NHS Foundation Trust, Dr Martin Rutter and Dr Mike Maresh.

after 38 completed weeks, and certainly by 40 weeks. Women with pre-existing diabetes and any complications may need to be offered delivery before 37 weeks. Women with an ultrasound diagnosis of macrosomia should be informed of the risks and benefits of induction of labour, vaginal birth and caesarean section.[2] One retrospective case–control study suggested that caesarean section was safer with estimated fetal weights greater than 4.25 kg; thus some advocate this fetal weight as a cut-off, but this is poor quality data [D]. Diabetes is not a contraindication for attempting a vaginal birth after Caesarean section.

INTRAPARTUM CARE

Good control of maternal blood glucose during labour is important as maternal hyperglycaemia is associated with neonatal hypoglycaemia. Some infants produce high levels of insulin antenatally in response to high levels of glucose crossing the placenta. After delivery, there is withdrawal of the maternal glucose but a persistent high level of neonatal insulin production, resulting in neonatal hypoglycaemia. More recently, data have suggested that short-term control of maternal blood glucose, i.e. during labour, may impact on neonatal hypoglycaemia. A maternal blood glucose of greater than 7.1 mmol/L is associated with neonatal hypoglycaemia [C]. Furthermore, maternal hyperglycaemia is also associated with 'perinatal asphyxia' and 'fetal distress' [C]. Thus, current guidance is that maternal blood glucose should be kept between 4 and 7 mmol/L during labour and delivery.[2,5] However, there are no studies investigating the best method of achieving this. Blood glucose should be tested hourly and women not maintaining their blood glucose within this range should be commenced on an intravenous insulin and dextrose infusion via a sliding scale. Sliding scales should be developed together with local diabetologists, but an example is given in Table 9.2. This may be considered at the onset of labour for women with type 1 diabetes, particularly if their oral intake is reduced. It will also be required for women delivered by elective caesarean section. However, some women, particularly those with a CSII pump, may manage the required level of control without the use of a sliding scale. Care should be taken with the use of sliding scales, and the intravenous infusions regularly checked (preferably hourly), as severe clinical incidents and death have occurred when infusions have become blocked or run too fast.

Induction of labour in women with diabetes is conducted in the same way as women without diabetes (Syntocinon infusions should be administered in saline), and NICE guidelines state that diabetes alone is not a contraindication to allowing a vaginal birth after a caesarean section.[2]

There are very few studies of the use of analgesia during labour and delivery. Thus NICE guidelines state that analgesia for women with diabetes should be managed in the usual way.[2] Diabetes may be associated with delayed gastric emptying, thus increasing risks for women requiring a general anaesthetic.

General anaesthesia also increases risks of hypoglycaemia and reduces awareness, thus these women should have blood glucose monitoring every 30 minutes until fully conscious. Since women with other co-morbidities such as autonomic neuropathy or obesity face additional risks, these women should be offered anaesthetic review during the third trimester.

POSTPARTUM CARE

With delivery of the placenta, insulin requirements dramatically decrease, thus all women will require a reduction in insulin dose. Consultant diabetologist involvement is very important at this time, and especially when the patient is converted back to pre-pregnancy insulin regimens. Advice varies regarding the subcutaneous insulin dose following delivery for women with pre-existing diabetes. Some suggest changing insulin regimens to the pre-pregnancy dosing, others suggest halving of insulin doses, and this should be carefully planned by the diabetic team. Careful capillary blood glucose monitoring is recommended to aid insulin dose adjustment for the first 2–3 days following delivery, aiming for values of 5–9 mmol/L. Hypoglycaemia is a major risk for women with type 1 diabetes at this time, especially in overweight or obese women who experience a large increase in their insulin requirements during pregnancy. Women who have undergone caesarean section will require continuation of the sliding scale until normal eating has been resumed. Women with type 2 diabetes can change from insulin back to their oral hypoglycaemic agents.

Breastfeeding

Glycaemic control is better in women who exclusively breastfeed than in those who bottlefeed [D], so overall breastfeeding should be supported.[5] Small cohort studies have demonstrated that breastfeeding increases the frequency of hypoglycaemia in type 1 diabetics [C]. Thus women should be advised to have a snack before or during breastfeeding and be advised of this risk. Oral hypoglycaemic agents cross into breast milk in small quantities. NICE currently recommends that women with pre-existing type 2 diabetes can safely take metformin and glibenclamide while breastfeeding.[2]

Contraception and follow-up

Women with pre-existing diabetes should be referred back to their routine diabetic care team. Contraception should be discussed, and the need for planning of future pregnancies should be emphasised. The CEMACH report found that women with a poor obstetric outcome were less likely to receive such advice.[3] UK Medical Eligibility Criteria (UKMEC) for contraceptive use should be followed and, for all hormonal methods, benefits usually outweigh risks for diabetic women in the absence of co-morbidity such as vascular disease or obesity.[21]

KEY POINTS

- Women with diabetes have poorer pregnancy outcomes than women without diabetes.
- Good glycaemic control pre-conception and in the first 8 weeks reduces the risk of congenital abnormalities.
- Pregnant women with diabetes should be managed in a joint obstetric/diabetic clinic involving the input of obstetricians, diabetologists, dieticians, specialist nurses and midwives.
- Insulin requirements usually increase during pregnancy.
- Fasting blood glucose should be less than 5.3 mmol/L.
- Postprandial levels at one hour should be less than 7.8 mmol/L.
- Tight glycaemic control results in a higher incidence of hypoglycaemia, hence education of the woman and her family about these risks is paramount.
- Diabetic ketoacidosis is associated with poor maternal and fetal outcome.
- Women with diabetes should be offered 4 weekly ultrasound monitoring of fetal growth and wellbeing, although there is no good evidence that these monitoring strategies reduce the risks of stillbirth and macrosomia.
- Women with pre-existing diabetes and no complications should be offered delivery after between 37+0 and 38+6 weeks.
- Women with macrosomia should have the risks and benefits of different modes of delivery discussed with them.
- Maternal blood glucose should be kept between 4 and 7 mmol/L during labour and delivery to reduce the risks of neonatal hypoglycaemia. This may require an insulin/dextrose infusion.
- Insulin requirements fall rapidly postnatally.
- Breastfeeding is associated with better glycaemic control and a risk of hypoglycaemia.
- All women should receive postnatal advice regarding contraception and planning of their next pregnancy.

CONCLUSIONS

Pregnancy represents a high-risk time for women with pre-existing diabetes. Management in a multidisciplinary team environment is imperative, with good glycaemic control being key to improving outcomes.

Key References

1. CEMACH. *Diabetes in Pregnancy: are we providing the best care? Findings of a National Enquiry: England, Wales and Northern Ireland.* London: CEMACH, 2007.
2. *Diabetes in Pregnancy. Management of diabetes and its complications from preconception to the postnatal period.* NICE guideline. London: National collaborating Centre for Women's and Children's health 2015.
3. CEMACH. *Pregnancy in Women with Type 1 and Type 2 Diabetes in 2002–3.* London: CEMACH, 2005.
4. Metzger BE, Lowe LP, Dyer AR *et al.* Hyperglycemia and Adverse Pregnancy Outcome (HAPO) Study: associations with neonatal anthropometrics. *Diabetes* 2009;58:453–9.
5. SIGN. *Management of Diabetes. A national clinical guideline.* Edinburgh: SIGN, 2010.
6. Macintosh MC, Fleming KM, Bailey JA *et al.* Perinatal mortality and congenital anomalies in babies of women with type 1 or type 2 diabetes in England, Wales and Northern Ireland: population based study. *BMJ* 2006;333:177.
7. Ringholm L, Mathiesen ER, Kelstrup L, Damm P. Managing type 1 diabetes mellitus in pregnancy – from planning to breastfeeding. *Nat Rev Endocrinol* 2012;8:659–67.
8. NICE. *Hypertension in Pregnancy. The management of hypertensive disorders during pregnancy.* NICE Clinical Guideline 107. London: NICE, 2010.
9. NICE. *Antenatal Care.* NICE Clinical Guideline 62. London: NICE, 2008.
10. Gilbert C, Valois M, Koren G. Pregnancy outcome after first-trimester exposure to metformin: a meta-analysis. *Fertil Steril* 2006;86:658–63.
11. Langer O, Conway DL, Berkus MD *et al.* A comparison of glyburide and insulin in women with gestational diabetes mellitus. *N Engl J Med.* 2000 Oct 19;343(16):1134–8.
12. Rowan JA, Hague WM, Gao W *et al.* Metformin versus insulin for the treatment of gestational diabetes. *N Engl J Med* 2008;358:2003–15.
13. Evers IM, de Valk HW, Mol BW *et al.* Macrosomia despite good glycaemic control in Type I diabetic pregnancy; results of a nationwide study in The Netherlands. *Diabetologia* 2002;45:1484–9.
14. Prutsky GJ, Domecq JP, Wang Z *et al.* Glucose targets in pregnant women with diabetes: a systematic review and meta-analysis. *J Clin Endocrinol Metab* 2013;98:4319–24.
15. Sung JF, Taslimi MM, Faig JC. Continuous glucose monitoring in pregnancy: new frontiers in clinical applications and research. *J Diabetes Sci Technol* 2012;6:1478–85.
16. de Veciana M. Diabetes ketoacidosis in pregnancy. *Semin Perinatol* 2013;37:267–73.
17. RCOG. *The Investigation and Management of the Small for Gestational Age Fetus.* Green-top Guideline No.31, London: RCOG, 2013.
18. Howarth C, Gazis A, James D. Associations of Type 1 diabetes mellitus, maternal vascular disease and complications of pregnancy. *Diabet Med* 2007;24:1229–34.
19. Kjos SL, Henry OA, Montoro M *et al.* Insulin-requiring diabetes in pregnancy: a randomized trial of active induction of labor and expectant management. *Am J Obstet Gynecol* 1993;169:611–15.
20. Lurie S, Insler V, Hagay ZJ. Induction of labor at 38 to 39 weeks of gestation reduces the incidence of shoulder dystocia in gestational diabetic patients class A2. *Am J Perinatol* 1996;13:293–6.
21. FSRH. UK Medical eligibility criteria for contraceptive use – summary sheets. London: Faculty of Sexual and Reproductive Healthcare of the RCOG, 2010.

Chapter 10 Cardiac disease

Catherine Nelson-Piercy

MRCOG standards

Relevant standards
To understand and demonstrate appropriate knowledge skills and attitudes in relation to pregnant women with heart disease.

Theoretical skills
Understand the epidemiology, aetiology, pathophysiology, clinical characteristics, prognostic features and management of women with heart disease.

Practical skills
Be able to manage under direct supervision pregnant women with congenital, rheumatic or ischaemic heart disease, and those with:

* an artificial heart valve,
* arrhythmia,
* peripartum cardiomyopathy.

INTRODUCTION

Cardiac disease in pregnancy is rare in the UK, but common in developing countries. This chapter covers the most important conditions relevant to pregnancy, including arrhythmias, pulmonary hypertension, aortic dissection, myocardial infarction, mitral stenosis and mechanical heart valves. Peripartum cardiomyopathy is included as it is specific to the pregnant or postpartum state.

PHYSIOLOGICAL CHANGES IN PREGNANCY

Cardiac output increases by 40 per cent, reaching a maximum by the mid-second trimester. There is peripheral vasodilatation, an increase in heart rate, and a fall in systemic and pulmonary vascular resistance. Labour and delivery are associated with further increases in cardiac output. Palpitations, extrasystoles, sinus tachycardia and ejection systolic murmurs are common in pregnancy but rarely represent underlying pathology. The ECG changes associated with normal pregnancy include atrial and ventricular extrasystoles, a 'left shift' in the QRS axis, a small Q wave and inverted T wave in lead III, and ST segment depression and T wave inversion in the inferior and lateral leads.

INCIDENCE

Although cardiac disease in pregnancy is rare (<1 per cent) in the UK, cardiac disease is the most common cause of maternal death.[1] Ischaemic heart disease is becoming more common in pregnancy, and deaths in pregnancy and the puerperium from myocardial infarction and ischaemic heart disease are increasing.[1]

Congenital heart disease is encountered more frequently as those who have received corrective surgery as children reach child-bearing age. Rheumatic heart disease is less common in the UK, but is encountered increasingly in migrant women from developing countries.

AETIOLOGY

The aetiology of heart disease may be divided into congenital and acquired causes. The most common congenital heart diseases encountered in pregnancy are ventricular and atrial septal defects (VSD, ASD), patent ductus arteriosus (PDA) and aortic coarctation. These are mostly diagnosed before pregnancy and septal defects and PDA are usually either haemodynamically insignificant or corrected. Acquired causes of cardiac disease include ischaemic heart disease, rheumatic heart disease, cardiomyopathies, and aneurysms and dissection of the aorta or its branches.

GENERAL PRINCIPLES

In pregnant women with heart disease, it is important to remember that the outcome and safety of pregnancy

Table 10.1 New York Heart Association (NYHA) functional classification

NYHA	Symptoms
I	No symptoms and no limitation in ordinary physical activity
II	Mild symptoms and slight limitation during ordinary activity
III	Marked limitation in activity due to symptoms, even during less than ordinary activity. Only comfortable at rest
IV	Severe limitations. Experiences symptoms even at rest

are related to the presence and severity of pulmonary hypertension, the presence of cyanosis, the haemodynamic significance of the lesion and the functional class [D]. The functional class is determined by the level of activity that leads to dyspnoea (Table 10.1). In addition, women with previous cardiac events including transient ischaemic attacks, arrhythmia, pulmonary oedema or heart failure, and those with left-sided lesions (e.g. aortic or mitral stenosis) or myocardial dysfunction, are at risk in pregnancy.[3] Women with congenital heart disease are at increased risk of having a baby with congenital heart disease, and should therefore be offered detailed fetal scanning for cardiac anomalies. During pregnancy, women with heart disease require multidisciplinary team care,[2] with regular antenatal visits and judicious monitoring to avoid or treat expediently any anaemia, infection or hypertension. There should be early involvement of obstetric anaesthetists and a carefully documented plan for delivery.[2]

PULMONARY HYPERTENSION

The most common forms of pulmonary hypertension encountered in women of child-bearing age are idiopathic pulmonary arterial hypertension, Eisenmenger's syndrome (when pulmonary hypertension develops secondary to a large left-to-right shunt such as a VSD, and the shunt is reversed to become right to left, with consequent cyanosis), secondary to chronic pulmonary thromboembolic disease, secondary to connective tissue disorders particularly scleroderma and sickle cell disease, and secondary to cardiac lesions causing raised pulmonary capillary wedge pressure such as mitral stenosis. Pulmonary hypertension from any cause is dangerous and maternal mortality is 25 to 40 per cent [D],[4,5] although this may be decreasing.[6] The danger relates to fixed pulmonary vascular resistance and an inability to increase pulmonary blood flow, with refractory hypoxaemia. Most pregnancy-associated deaths can be attributed to thromboembolism, hypovolaemia or pre-eclampsia.

Management

Women with pulmonary hypertension should be advised to avoid pregnancy or, in the event of unplanned pregnancy, to have a therapeutic termination [D].[5,7] If such advice is declined, multidisciplinary care in a pulmonary hypertension centre is recommended [D].[4] Vasodilatation therapies such as sildenafil, nebulised or intravenous prostacyclin should be continued or instituted in pregnancy as indicated. Endothelin antagonists (e.g. Bosentan) are usually avoided as they are teratogenic in rats, although it is not known whether there are similar risks in humans.

EBM

- Most published evidence relating to pulmonary hypertension comes from retrospective cohorts and case series.
- All the literature supports a high risk of maternal death sufficient to make this condition one of the absolute contraindications to pregnancy.
- There is no evidence that monitoring the pulmonary artery pressure prepartum or intrapartum improves outcome.

AORTIC DISSECTION

Aortic dissection is a common cause of cardiac death in pregnancy,[1] and pregnancy increases the risk of aortic dissection. Most cases occur in late pregnancy at or near term or in the early puerperium. Certain conditions predispose to aortic dissection. These include bicuspid aortic valve, aortic coarctation, Turner's syndrome, Ehlers–Danlos syndrome (vascular type IV) and Marfan's syndrome.[8]

Marfan's syndrome is an autosomal dominant condition with typical skeletal and other features including tall stature, a high arched palate, scoliosis and lens dislocation. Progressive aortic root dilatation and an aortic root dimension >4 cm are associated with increased risk [D].[9] Conversely, in women with minimal cardiac involvement and an aortic root <4 cm, pregnancy outcome is good [C]. Overall, pregnancy is associated with a 5-fold increased risk of aortic complications in women with Marfan's syndrome.[10]

Management

Acute aortic dissection should be suspected if a woman in late pregnancy presents with severe chest or interscapular pain, particularly if associated with systolic hypertension, different blood pressures in each arm or an early diastolic murmur, especially if she has predisposing risk factors. Urgent imaging with CT, MRI or echocardiography is essential, as well as rapid and effective control of blood pressure. Women with aortic roots >4.5 cm should be advised to delay pregnancy. Management in women with Marfan's syndrome or dilated aortic roots from other causes should include serial echocardiograms and beta-blockers. Vaginal delivery is appropriate for those with stable aortic root measurements <4.5 cm, but elective caesarean section with epidural is usually recommended if there is an enlarged (>4.5 cm) or dilating aortic root [D].[9]

EBM

- Most published evidence relating to Marfan's syndrome comes from retrospective cohorts and case series.
- The literature supports a higher risk of aortic rupture and maternal death if the aortic root is >4 cm.

MITRAL STENOSIS

Mitral stenosis is increasingly encountered in migrant women, who may or may not have had the diagnosis made prior to pregnancy.[11] A history of previous mitral valvotomy does not preclude restenosis. Mitral stenosis is the most common rheumatic heart disease and is important in pregnancy because women may deteriorate secondary to tachycardia, arrhythmias or the increased cardiac output. The commonest complication is pulmonary oedema secondary to increased left atrial pressure and precipitated by increased heart rate or increased volume (such as occurs during the third stage of labour) [C].[11] The risk is increased with severe mitral stenosis, moderate or severe symptoms prior to pregnancy, and in those diagnosed late in pregnancy [C].[12]

Management

Women with severe mitral stenosis should be advised to delay pregnancy until after balloon, open or closed mitral valvotomy or mitral valve replacement. Beta-blockers decrease heart rate and the risk of pulmonary oedema [D],[11] but if medical therapy fails or for those with severe mitral stenosis, balloon mitral valvotomy may be safely and successfully used in pregnancy [D].[11]

Women with mitral stenosis should avoid the supine and lithotomy positions as much as possible for labour and delivery. Fluid overload must be avoided [E]. Pulmonary oedema should be treated in the usual way with oxygen and diuretics.

EBM

- Most published evidence relating to mitral stenosis comes from retrospective cohorts and case series.
- The literature supports a higher risk of pulmonary oedema in severe mitral stenosis.
- Beta-blockers, diuretics and balloon valvotomy are safe in pregnancy.

MECHANICAL HEART VALVES

Women with mechanical heart valves require lifelong anticoagulation, and this is the reason they have such high-risk pregnancies. Pregnancy itself increases the risk of thrombosis. Warfarin is associated with warfarin embryopathy[13] and increased risks of miscarriage, stillbirth and fetal intracerebral haemorrhage.[14] Heparin, even in full anticoagulant doses, is associated with increased risks of valve thrombosis and embolic events [C].[13,14]

Management

The safest option for some mothers is to continue warfarin throughout pregnancy [C].[13,14] Other management strategies include replacing the warfarin with high-dose low-molecular-weight heparin (LMWH), either from 6 to 12 weeks' gestation to avoid warfarin embryopathy or throughout pregnancy.[15] Since the risk of thrombosis is less with the newer bileaflet valves (e.g. Carbomedics), and valves in the aortic position, it may be that high doses of LMWH throughout pregnancy are appropriate in women with these valves [E]. If LMWH is used, doses should be adjusted according to anti-factor Xa levels and low-dose aspirin is usually also given.[15] Both strategies carry risk; with warfarin the risk is predominantly fetal and with LMWH the risk is of maternal valve thrombosis or stroke. Whichever management option is chosen, warfarin should be discontinued and substituted with LMWH for 10 days prior to delivery to allow clearance of warfarin from the fetal circulation. For delivery itself, heparin therapy is interrupted, but restarted postpartum. Warfarin is recommended 5–7 days postpartum [E]. In the event of bleeding or the need for urgent delivery in a fully anticoagulated patient, warfarin may be reversed with prothrombinase complex and vitamin K, and heparin with protamine sulphate. If heparin is used, this should be in full anticoagulant doses, adjusted according to regular monitoring.

EBM

- Most published evidence relating to mechanical heart valves comes from retrospective cohorts and case series of women.
- The literature supports a lower risk of thromboembolic events if warfarin is continued throughout pregnancy, and a lower risk of fetal loss, fetal haemorrhage and anomalies if LMWH is used.

ISCHAEMIC HEART DISEASE/ MYOCARDIAL INFARCTION

Ischaemic heart disease in pregnancy is becoming more common as maternal age and obesity increase.[1,16] The risk of myocardial infarction (MI) is increased in women over 35 years old, multigravid women, those who smoke, and women with diabetes, obesity, hypertension and hypercholesterolaemia [C].[16] Acute coronary syndromes may be diagnosed as in the non-pregnant patient with raised troponin levels, which are not altered by pregnancy, and ECG changes. Infarction most commonly occurs in the postpartum period. The maternal death rate is about 10 per cent.[16] In pregnancy, other underlying aetiologies for MI, such as coronary artery thrombosis or dissection, are more common than outside pregnancy and should be considered [C].[1]

Management

Management of acute MI is as for the non-pregnant woman [D]. Coronary angiography should not be withheld in pregnant patients. Percutaneous coronary intervention may provide a better alternative to thrombolysis in pregnancy as it is associated with less bleeding risk and also allows management of spontaneous dissections with coronary artery stents. However, stent implantation may be associated with an increased risk of coronary dissection in a vulnerable vessel [D]. For secondary prevention in women with known ischaemic heart disease, both aspirin and beta-blockers are safe in pregnancy [A]. Statins should be discontinued prior to and for the duration of pregnancy [E].

ENDOCARDITIS PROPHYLAXIS

The current UK recommendations from NICE (2008) are that antibiotic prophylaxis against infective endocarditis (IE) is not required for childbirth. The British Society for Antimicrobial Chemotherapy (BSAC 2006) and the American Heart Association (AHA) have recommended cover only for patients deemed to be at high risk of developing IE (such as women with previous IE) and for those who have the poorest outcome if they develop IE (such as those with cyanotic congenital heart disease) (see below under Published guidelines). If antibiotic prophylaxis is used, it should be with amoxicillin 2 g IV plus gentamicin 120 mg IV at the onset of labour or ruptured membranes or prior to caesarean section, followed by amoxicillin 500 mg orally (or intramuscular [IM]/IV depending on the patient's condition) 6 hours later. For women who are penicillin allergic, vancomycin 1 g IV or teicoplanin 400 mg IV may be used instead of amoxicillin.[17]

HYPERTROPHIC CARDIOMYOPATHY

Most cases of hypertrophic cardiomyopathy (HCM) are familial, inherited as autosomal dominant. Women may be asymptomatic, especially if diagnosed because of family screening, or may experience syncope or 'angina-like' chest pain. The danger relates to left ventricular outflow tract obstruction which may be precipitated by hypotension or hypovolaemia. Provided that these are avoided, pregnancy is usually well tolerated. Risk factors for sudden cardiac death (SCD) are non-sustained ventricular tachycardia (VT), failure of the systolic blood pressure to rise during exercise and a family history of SCD. Beta-blockers should be continued in pregnancy or initiated for symptomatic women [D].[18]

PERIPARTUM CARDIOMYOPATHY

This pregnancy-specific condition is defined as heart failure secondary to left ventricular (LV) systolic dysfunction towards the end of pregnancy or in the months following delivery, where no other cause of heart failure is found. It is a diagnosis of exclusion. The left ventricle may not be dilated but the ejection fraction is always reduced below 45% [C].[18] Risk factors include multiple pregnancy, hypertension, multiparity, increased age and African–Caribbean race [D].[2]

Diagnosis should be suspected in puerperal women or those in late pregnancy with breathlessness and signs of heart failure. It is confirmed with echocardiography showing LV dysfunction and often dilatation of all four chambers of the heart. Treatment is as for other causes of heart failure, with oxygen, diuretics, vasodilators, ACE inhibitors if postpartum and inotropes if required. Prognosis and recurrence depend on the normalisation of LV size and function within 6 months of delivery [C].[2,18]

ARRYTHMIAS

A sinus tachycardia requires investigation for possible underlying pathology such as blood loss, infection, heart failure, thyrotoxicosis or pulmonary embolus, but no treatment is required if such causes are excluded. The most common arrhythmia encountered in pregnancy is supraventricular tachycardia (SVT). An SVT that does not respond to vagal manoeuvres may be safely terminated in pregnancy with adenosine [D] or intravenous verapamil or beta blockers.

KEY POINTS

- Heart disease is the commonest cause of maternal mortality in the UK.
- Eisenmenger's syndrome, other causes of pulmonary hypertension, severe mitral stenosis, Marfan's syndrome with marked or increasing aortic root dilatation and severe cardiomyopathy are contraindications to pregnancy.
- The safest option for some women with mechanical heart valves is to continue warfarin in pregnancy, notwithstanding the associated fetal risks.
- Antibiotic prophylaxis against endocarditis is no longer recommended peripartum in women with heart disease.

ANTENATAL OBSTETRICS

Published Guidelines

ESG; Association for European Paediatric Cardiology (AEPC); German Society for Gender Medicine (DGesGM), Regitz-Zagrosek V, Blomstrom Lundqvist C, Borghi C, Cifkova R, Ferreira R, Foidart JM, Gibbs JS, Gohlke-Baerwolf C, Gorenek B, Iung B, Kirby M, Maas AH, Morais J, Nihoyannopoulos P, Pieper PG, Presbitero P, Roos-Hesselink JW, Schaufelberger M, Seeland U, Torracca L; ESC Committee for Practice Guidelines. *Eur Heart J* 2011;32:3147-97.

European Society of Gynecology (ESC) Guidelines on the management of cardiovascular diseases during pregnancy: the Task Force on the Management of Cardiovascular Diseases during Pregnancy of the European Society of Cardiology (ESC).

NICE Clinical Guideline. Prophylaxis against infective endocarditis. March 2008. http://www.nice.org.uk/nicemedia/pdf/CG64NICEguidance.pdf

Key References

1. Nelson-Piercy C. Cardiac disease. *In* Lewis G (ed). CMACE. Saving Mothers' Lives: reviewing maternal deaths to make motherhood safer: 2006-2008. The Eighth Report of the Confidential Enquiries into Maternal Deaths in the UK. *BJOG* 2011;118,suppl(1):109-15.

2. Steer P, Gatzoulis M, Baker P (eds) *Cardiac Disease in Pregnancy*. London: RCOG Press, 2006.

3. Siu SC, Sermer M, Colman JM et al. Prospective multicenter study of pregnancy outcomes in women with heart disease. *Circulation* 2001;104:515–21.

4. Yentis SM, Steer PJ, Plaat F. Eisenmenger's syndrome in pregnancy: maternal and fetal mortality in the 1990s. *Br J Obstet Gynaecol* 1998;105:921–2.

5. Bédard E, Dimopoulos K, Gatzoulis MA. Has there been any progress made on pregnancy outcomes among women with pulmonary arterial hypertension? *Eur Heart J* 2009;30:256–65.

6. Kiely DG, Condliffe R, Wilson VJ, Gandhi SV, Elliot CA. *Obstet Med* 2013;6:144–54.

7. Thorne SA, Nelson-Piercy C, MacGregor A. Risks of contraception and pregnancy in heart disease. *Heart* 2006;92:1520–25.

8. Immer FF, Bansi AG, Immer-Bansi AS et al. Aortic dissection in pregnancy: analysis of risk factors and outcome. *Ann Thorac Surg* 2003;76:309–14.

9. Lipscomb KJ, Clayton Smith J, Clarke B et al. Outcome of pregnancy in women with Marfan's syndrome. *Br J Obstet Gynaecol* 1997;104:201–6.

10. Pacini L, Digne F, Boumendil A et al. Maternal complication of pregnancy in Marfan syndrome. *Int J Cardiol* 2009;136:156–61.

11. Tsiaras S, Poppas A. Mitral valve disease in pregnancy: outcomes and management. *Obstet Med* 2009;2:6–10.

12. Silversides CK, Colman JM, Sermer M, Siu SC. Cardiac risk in pregnant women with rheumatic mitral stenosis. *Am J Cardiol* 2003;91:1382–5.

13. Chan WS, Anand S, Ginsberg JS. Anticoagulation of pregnant women with mechanical heart valves. *Arch Intern Med* 2000;160:191–6.

14. Sadler L, McCowan L, White H et al. Pregnancy outcomes and cardiac complications in women with mechanical, bioprosthetic and homograft valves. *Br J Obstet Gynaecol* 2000;107:245–53.

15. Oran B, Lee-Parritz A, Ansell J. Low molecular weight heparin for the prophylaxis of thromboembolism in women with prosthetic mechanical heart valves during pregnancy. *Thromb Haemostat* 2004;92:747–51.

16. Ladner HE, Danielsen B, Gilbert WM. Acute myocardial infarction in pregnancy and the puerperium: a population-based study. *Obstet Gynecol* 2005; 105:480–4.

17. Dajani AS, Taubert KA, Wilson W et al. Prevention of bacterial endocarditis. Recommendations by the American Heart Association. *JAMA* 1997;277:1794–801.

18. Adamson D, Dhanjal MK, Nelson-Piercy C (eds). *Oxford Specialist Handbooks in Cardiology. Heart Disease in Pregnancy*. Oxford: Oxford University Press, 2011.

19. Pearson GD, Veille JC, Rahimtoola S et al. Peripartum cardiomyopathy. National Heart, Lung and Blood Institute and Office of Rare Diseases (NIH). Workshop Recommendations and Review. *JAMA* 2000;283:1183–8.

Chapter 11 Thyroid disease

Andrew Shennan and Joanna Girling

INTRODUCTION: PHYSIOLOGY OF THYROID FUNCTION

Maternal physiology

Thyroid disease occurs in more than 1 per cent of the population and is the most common pre-existing endocrine disorder in pregnant women. A fundamental understanding of thyroid function in pregnancy is essential.

Thyroid-stimulating hormone (TSH) is released from the anterior pituitary in 1 to 2-hourly cycles. It increases both the synthesis and release of thyroxine (T_4) and triiodothyronine (T_3) by the thyroid gland. The T_3 and T_4 are mostly protein bound – to thyroid-binding globulin (TBG), albumin and transthyretin. Although the concentration of TBG is low, the binding affinity is high, and TBG binds more than 75 per cent of thyroid hormones. The unbound thyroid hormones have biological activity; only 0.04 per cent of T_4 and 0.05 per cent of T_3 are free; the bound thyroid hormones do not have biological activity.

Iodide is essential for the synthesis of thyroid hormones, and the thyroid gland actively traps iodine, which is then bound to a tyrosine molecule on a thyroglobulin molecule. Each molecule carries three or, more commonly, four molecules of iodine, making T_3 or T_4 respectively. Most circulating T_3 is produced by peripheral deiodination of T_4, by deiodinase enzyme, and is three times more potent than T_4. Although the production of T_3 is lower than that of T_4, more T_3 is available as a free, inactive compound.

In pregnancy, there is altered TBG production as a result of increased oestrogen synthesis. Levels of TBG increase in the first 2 weeks of pregnancy, and triple to reach a plateau by 20 weeks, due to glycosylation that is oestrogen driven. The half-life extends from 15 minutes to 3 days in this time. The increase in TBG leads to an increase in the serum concentrations of total T_4 and T_3, but there are no major changes in the amount of free circulating (unbound) thyroid hormones, although these must be interpreted within pregnancy-specific reference ranges.

There is relative iodine deficiency in pregnancy as a result of loss through increased glomerular filtration and increased maternal production of T_4 and T_3. This results in increased uptake by the thyroid gland, which can result in enlargement and the appearance of a goitre. Fetal thyroid activity also depletes the maternal iodide pool from the second trimester, probably via diffusion along a concentration gradient.

As human chorionic gonadotrophin (hCG) and TSH share a common alpha subunit and have similar beta subunits, TSH receptors are prone to stimulation by hCG. In conditions such as molar pregnancy, hyperemesis gravidarum and multiple pregnancy, increased thyroid activity has been noted, associated with high levels of hCG. Even in normal pregnancy, a fall in TSH levels is associated with peak hCG concentrations, and there is a correlation between levels of T_4 and hCG. In pregnancy, there is also placental conversion of T_4 to T_3. Low levels of T_4 will increase this activity, producing more active thyroid hormone. Deiodination also occurs in trophoblasts, preventing excess thyroid hormone exposure to the baby and perhaps explaining the fall in T_4 found in the mother in later pregnancy.[1]

Fetal thyroid function

During the first trimester, the fetus requires maternal T_4 for normal fetal brain development. It is likely that T_4 crosses the placenta in small amounts before 12 weeks' gestation to facilitate this (otherwise, T_3, T_4 and TSH do not cross the placenta). From 10 weeks' gestation, the fetal thyroid gland produces both T_4 and T_3. From this point onwards, the fetal thyroid axis is independent of the mother, and requires only transplacental iodine; there is little relationship between maternal and fetal thyroid hormone levels. Fetal levels reach those of the adult by 36 weeks' gestation. Although fetal TSH concentrations are greater than maternal TSH levels, T_3 is lower in the fetus, probably as a result of little peripheral conversion and a good placental barrier. Both thyrotrophin-releasing hormone (TRH) and iodine freely cross the placenta. (TRH has unsuccessfully been investigated as a method of stimulating thyroid function to enhance fetal lung maturity.)

Congenital hyperthyroidism can occur when TSH receptor-stimulating antibodies cross the placenta (see below). Very rarely, mutations of the TSH receptor result in either congenital hyperthyroidism or hypothyroidism.

Thyroid function tests in pregnancy

In pregnancy, it is important to measure free T_4 and T_3 and to base management decisions principally on these levels [C]; TSH is often suppressed, especially in the first trimester, and then can only be detected with new, ultrasensitive assays.

Pregnancy-specific reference ranges should be used: as T_4 levels fall slightly during pregnancy, the lower limit of normal for free T_4 is below that of non-pregnant women. As there is more conversion of T_4 to T_3, low levels of T_4 are not necessarily indicative of hypothyroidism.[2]

Thyroid hormones are involved in the metabolism of alpha-fetoprotein (AFP), and there has been some concern that AFP measurements may be unreliable. However, in women suspected of having thyroid disease, the available evidence suggests AFP measurements can still be used if required for the quadruple Down's serum screening test [D].

AETIOLOGY AND MANAGEMENT OF THYROID DISEASE

Iodine

Women in areas of iodine deficiency may have goitres and reduced reproductive success.[3] In iodine deficiency, the maternal thyroid gland has a greater affinity for iodine than

the placenta and the fetuses are thus prone to cretinism – the leading preventable cause of learning disability worldwide.

The fetal cochlea, cerebral neocortex and basal ganglia are particularly sensitive to iodine deficiency.[4] Iodine administration prior to conception and up to the second trimester will improve neurological outcome by allowing normal thyroid hormone production by the fetus, therefore protecting the fetal brain. Iodination of water, salt or flour, or even annual injections for reproductive-age women, can easily achieve this.

The introduction of iodine supplementation in certain areas of the developing world has also reduced both the miscarriage and the stillbirth rates. However, high levels of iodine intake can cause fetal hyperthyroidism. Therefore, some cough medicines and eye drops containing iodine should be avoided, as should radiological procedures utilising iodinated contrast dyes. Similarly, amiodarone, which is rich in iodine, should be avoided in pregnancy unless absolutely necessary for life-threatening arrhythmias. In these cases, neonatal assessment must be made regarding thyroid function. Radioactive iodine, which destroys the fetal thyroid, must never be used, even in early pregnancy, as damage can occur before there is active fetal tissue.

Hyperemesis gravidarum

In women with hyperemesis, T_4 levels may be elevated with suppression of TSH. These changes probably result from high levels of hCG, particularly if there are higher levels of subtypes of hCG which have a greater affinity for the thyroid gland TSH receptor: these stimulate the TSH receptors[5] and occur in approximately 40 per cent of hyperemesis cases (particularly in those with more severe disease). This usually resolves by 20 weeks' gestation. The clinical signs of thyrotoxicosis are generally absent and, as the condition improves, T_4 levels only remain elevated if true hyperthyroidism ensues.

Antithyroid medication should not be used in hyperemesis as the thyroid abnormality is biochemical and self-limiting and is not related to an overactive thyroid [D]. When used, this type of medication is generally ineffective or required in unusually high doses.

Hyperthyroidism

Hyperthyroidism occurs in approximately 1 in 500 pregnancies and is usually diagnosed and treated prior to the pregnancy, since untreated thyrotoxicosis is associated with reduced fertility. It is usually due to Graves' disease (autoimmune thyrotoxicosis). Less than 5 per cent of cases result from a toxic nodule, thyroiditis or a carcinoma. If pregnant women present with hyperthyroidism, hyperemesis or a molar pregnancy must be considered.

Graves' disease is associated with a hyperplastic goitre and often with exophthalmos. Disease activity and severity are correlated to immunoglobulin G (IgG) thyrotrophin (TSH) receptor-stimulating antibody titres. The immunosuppressive effect of pregnancy means that the disease typically remits in the last two trimesters,[6] and doses of antithyroid medication should be reduced accordingly, to minimise the likelihood of either maternal or fetal side effects; in approximately one-third of women treatment may be discontinued. Postnatally the TSH-receptor-stimulating antibody titre usually returns to its pre-pregnancy value, and so treatment needs to be restarted or the dose increased for most women.

Typical symptoms and signs of hyperthyroidism are difficult to separate from those of normal pregnancy, but poor weight gain in the presence of a good appetite or a tachycardia >100 beats per minute that is unresponsive to a Valsalva manoeuvre may indicate the disease. Onycholysis does reflect disease activity, unlike the eye signs and pretibial myxo-edema, which may persist after Graves' disease has resolved. Unfortunately, many other symptoms, such as fatigue, warm peripheries, amenorrhoea, hair thinning and heat intolerance, are common in pregnancy and are not useful.

It is essential to maintain euthyroidism in pregnancy, as uncontrolled disease is associated with maternal and fetal complications, including thyroid storm, heart failure and maternal hypertension. Observational studies have reported increased rates of premature labour, growth restriction and stillbirth. Treatment is similar to that for non-pregnant women, although radioactive iodine must not be given [D]. Surgery may be considered if medical treatment fails or there is a clinical suspicion of cancer or compressive symptoms due to a goitre. With well-controlled disease, normal pregnancy outcomes can be expected.

Medical treatment involves blocking thyroid hormone synthesis. Propylthiouracil (PTU) and carbimazole both reduce the titre of TSH-receptor antibodies, directly influencing the aetiology of Graves' disease. PTU was previously the preferred therapy, as it not only inhibits T_4 synthesis by blocking the incorporation of iodine into tyrosine, but also inhibits the peripheral conversion of T_4 to T_3. However, both drugs probably cross the placenta in the same proportion and there is no need to change from carbimazole to PTU [D]. Both drugs are equally beneficial and the dose of either can be titrated against maternal wellbeing and biochemical status [D].[7] Neither PTU nor carbimazole is thought to be teratogenic, and indeed studies have shown that pregnancies conceived with pharmacologically achieved biochemical control have a better outcome than those that are not controlled; the relationship previously found between aplasia cutis of the scalp and these drugs is unlikely to exist. Antithyroid drugs can cause agranulocytosis and so a sore throat should prompt a full blood count.

It is recommended that thyroid function tests be performed every 4–6 weeks during pregnancy. When Graves' disease is unstable, beta blockers can be used to control the symptoms of tachycardia or tremor, and propranolol is the recommended therapy [D].

As both PTU and carbimazole cross the placenta, both may make the fetus hypothyroid.[8] The minimal dose required in the mother should therefore be used, and it is usual to aim for free T_4 levels at the upper limit of normal [E]. Even if the

fetus does become hypothyroid, neurodevelopmental status is preserved, although careful control can still lead to neonatal hypothyroidism and even neonatal goitre. The goitres are generally small, clinically unimportant and tend to resolve within 2 weeks. No long-term fetal side effects of antithyroid drugs have been demonstrated, although the studies performed have been small and retrospective.

Both drugs are expressed in breast milk, but have little effect on thyroid function.

Fetal and neonatal hyperthyroidism

When maternal TSH-receptor-stimulating antibodies cross the placenta, they can cause fetal thyrotoxicosis, although, as many women are taking antithyroid medication which also crosses the placenta, this is relatively uncommon. Women who had their Graves' disease treated by radioactive iodine or surgery may still have TSH-receptor antibodies, but will no longer be taking antithyroid medication (and in fact are likely to be taking thyroxine), and they have a greater likelihood of developing fetal hyperthyroidism. The fetal thyroid is capable of responding to these antibodies after 20 weeks' gestation, and potential effects should be monitored in the second half of pregnancy. Assessment should include maternal perception of fetal movements, standard growth assessments (symphyseal–fundal height) and measurement of the fetal heart rate, which, if sustained above 160 beats/min, may be indicative of fetal thyrotoxicosis.

An ultrasound scan can be used to exclude a fetal goitre or clinically undetected fetal growth restriction. In suspected cases, the diagnosis can be made clinically or cordocentesis for free T_4 and TSH determination can be performed and is preferable to amniocentesis [D].

Fetal hyperthyroidism is associated with premature delivery. Fetal cardiac failure can result, leading to hydrops fetalis and death; fetal goitre can cause polyhydramnios or an obstructed delivery. The condition is also associated with craniosynostosis and intellectual impairment. The fetus can be effectively treated in one of two ways, either by maternal administration of antithyroid agents, which cross the placenta, or by delivery. The fetal heart rate can be used to titrate the dose of antithyroid drugs. The mother can be treated with T_4 to offset any hypothyroid effects, as T_4 will not cross the placenta [C]. As thyroid TSH receptor stimulating antibodies have a long half-life (3 weeks), which exceeds that of placentally transferred antithyroid medication, they can also cause neonatal hyperthyroidism. The symptoms may therefore present in the baby only after a week and tend to be non-specific, such as poor weight gain, feeding and sleeping.

A goitre may also cause problems with breathing and feeding. Untreated fetal/neonatal hyperthyroidism is responsible for substantial mortality.

TSH-receptor-stimulating antibody titres should be measured in women with active Graves' disease, as well as those whose disease was cured by surgery or radioactive iodine. As long as antibody levels are low, involvement of the fetus is unlikely. If antibody levels are high, fetal/neonatal thyroid function should be checked, both in cord samples and in peripheral samples taken approximately a week after delivery.

Hypothyroidism

Hypothyroidism occurs in nearly 1 per cent of pregnant women and is usually due to autoimmune Hashimoto's thyroiditis or idiopathic myxoedema; the condition can also occur following treatment of hyperthyroidism. Direct pituitary causes are rare.

In pregnancies complicated by hypothyroidism, babies are normally grown and do not seem to have an increased risk of congenital anomalies. Large studies have not yet confirmed this apparent lack of adverse events. Aberrant thyroid function has been implicated in the aetiology of recurrent miscarriage, but the evidence for this is weak, and the current RCOG guidelines suggest against routine testing of thyroid function in the investigation of recurrent miscarriage.

There is a reduced intelligence quotient (IQ) in babies of women with profound hypothyroidism that is not adequately treated, or that goes unrecognised. The insult is likely to occur in the first trimester, and therefore pre-conceptual optimisation of T_4 therapy is important [D];[9,10] ideally contraception should be used until euthyroidism is achieved. Referral to a physician or obstetrician interested in the field would seem prudent.

As hypothyroidism is associated with subfertility, it is rare to make a new diagnosis in pregnancy. The classic symptoms of hypothyroidism, such as tiredness, constipation, anaemia, weight gain, carpal tunnel syndrome and hair changes, are common in pregnancy and cannot be relied upon to discriminate onset or worsening of the disease. Treatment is with thyroxine, which is safe in pregnancy and lactation [C]. Thyroxine dose is titrated against biochemical results.

As long as the patient is clinically euthyroid, thyroid function tests should be performed every few months, such as at booking and at 28 weeks. More frequent measurements are made if the clinical or biochemical condition is deranged [E]. Most pregnant women do not need any increase in therapy [C].[11] Some authors have advocated a routine increase in the first trimester, but, as there have been some reports of adverse events with thyroxine therapy, such as miscarriage, it would seem prudent to titrate therapy to biochemistry.[12] A low free T_4 level indicates a need for increased therapy, rather than a raised TSH [D].[13] Beyond the end of the first trimester, placental pharmacokinetics prevent transfer of maternal T_4, whether endogenous or exogenous, to the fetus, and therefore at this stage treatment is aimed only at normalising the biochemical picture and minimising maternal symptoms; it does not have a direct action on the fetus.

Fetal hypothyroidism

Although in Hashimoto's hypothyroidism autoantibodies cross the placenta, these do not affect fetal thyroid development. However, very rarely, TSH-receptor-blocking antibodies can cause a transient hypothyroidism in either a fetus or a baby.

Postpartum thyroiditis

Postpartum thyroiditis (PPT) can occur up to a year following delivery and can manifest as hyper- or hypothyroidism. The incidence varies widely and, when diagnosed biochemically, has been reported to be as low as 2 per cent in New York and as high as 17 per cent in Wales. Most women will not have clinically apparent disease, and may present with depression or be diagnosed as having Hashimoto's hypothyroidism as they tend to present to general practitioners, who may be unaware of PPT. Women on long-term T_4 treatment following an onset soon after pregnancy should have this diagnosis considered.

The condition is thought to be autoimmune and presents postpartum following a return to normal immunity after delivery. Ninety per cent of women will have thyroid antiperoxidase antibodies (compared with 10 per cent of the normal population). Histology from thyroid biopsies suggests a chronic thyroiditis with lymphocytic infiltration but not fibrosis (which is a typical feature of Hashimoto's thyroiditis).

The disease may present initially between 1 and 3 months postpartum with thyrotoxicosis and later with hypothyroidism. Radioactive iodine or technetium uptake tests can help distinguish between postpartum thyroiditis (low uptake) and Graves' disease (high uptake), but lactation should not continue during testing [D]. If symptomatic with hyperthyoidism, beta blockers can be used; antithyroid drugs are inappropriate, as T_4 production is not increased [D]. Hyperthyroidism is due to destruction of thyroid follicles and the release of pre-formed hormones. The destruction of thyroid follicles ultimately leads to the hypothyroid phase, which is more likely to be associated with symptoms such as tiredness and cold intolerance, and even a goitre. At this stage, the differential diagnosis includes Hashimoto's thyroiditis and Sheehan's syndrome. A course of T_4 may be necessary. If the symptoms of hypothyroidism are due to Hashimoto's thyroiditis, withdrawing treatment will result in relapse, but cessation of T_4 is probably the only way to avoid unnecessary long-term treatment.

The period of hypothyroid state is variable, and permanent hypothyroidism can result (approximately 5 per cent of antibody-positive postpartum thyroiditis sufferers). The condition will recur in 70 per cent of future pregnancies and women with postpartum thyroiditis should be followed up to ensure that permanent hypothyroidism does not occur [E]. This would usually involve annual TSH and T_4 measurement.

THYROID CANCER IN PREGNANCY

Thyroid cancer is two to three times more common in women than men, and 50 per cent of cases occur within the reproductive age group. Pregnancy itself does not appear to influence the survival rates of women diagnosed with thyroid cancer. It is recommended that pregnancy should be delayed after treatment with radioactive iodine, probably for a period of a year

[D], in view of the higher incidence of congenital anomalies that follow this treatment.

If a pregnant woman presents with a thyroid nodule, thyroid function tests and an ultrasound are indicated. Thyrotoxicosis occurring with cystic nodules is unlikely to be malignant, but other nodules should be investigated with a fine-needle aspirate. Cellular cytology from a fine-needle aspirate may suggest an underlying malignancy, and serial ultrasound should be performed. Removal of nodules that are increasing in size should be considered. A thyroidectomy can be performed, usually in the second trimester of pregnancy. If radioactive iodine is required, this should not be administered during pregnancy or breastfeeding [D].

Thyroid globulin concentration cannot be used to detect a relapse of thyroid cancer in pregnancy, as it is already elevated. Women on suppressive doses of T_4 may continue this therapy, with the usual aim of reducing TSH to undetectable levels.

KEY POINTS

- Management decisions should be based on free T_4 and T_3 measurements in pregnancy; T_4 is found at the lower limits of normal in pregnancy and trimester-specific reference ranges should be used for all assessments of thyroid function in pregnancy.
- Management of hypothyroidism should be optimised prior to conception, and pregnant women may need to alter their dose of thyroxine from early pregnancy.
- Forty per cent of women with hyperemesis gravidarum have elevated T_4 (and suppressed TSH); they do not require antithyroid treatment. This will usually resolve by 20 weeks' gestation.
- Graves' disease is the most common cause of hyperthyroidism, and euthyroidism should be maintained in pregnancy with antithyroid drugs. Thyroid status should be checked every 4–6 weeks. Treatment can be reduced in the third trimester to prevent fetal hyperthyroidism, then restored postnatally.
- Women with hypothyroidism should be euthyroid prior to conception to avoid intellectual impairment in the baby. The fetus requires maternal thyroxine in early pregnancy.

Key References

1. Koopdonk-Kool JM, de Vijlder JJM, Veenboer GHM *et al.* Type II and type III deiodinase activity in human placenta as a function of gestational age. *J Clin Endocrinol Metab* 1996;81:2154–8.
2. Cotzias C, Wong SJ, Taylor E, Seed P, Girling J. A study to establish gestation-specific reference intervals for thyroid function tests in normal singleton pregnancy. *Eur J Obstet Gynecol Reprod Biol* 2008;137:61–6.
3. Dillon JC, Milliez J. Reproductive failure in women living in iodine deficient areas of West Africa. *Br J Obstet Gynaecol* 2000;107:631–6.
4. Cao XY, Jiang XM, Dou ZH *et al.* Timing of vulnerability of the brain to iodine deficiency in endemic cretinism. *N Engl J Med* 1994;331:1739–44.
5. Kimura M, Amino N, Tamaki H. Gestational thyrotoxicosis and hyperemesis gravidarum: possible role of hCG with higher stimulating activity. *Clin Endocrinol* 1993;38:345–50.
6. Kung AWC, Jones BM. A change from stimulatory to blocking antibody activity in Graves' disease during pregnancy. *J Clin Endocrinol Metab* 1998;83:514–18.
7. Wing DA, Miller LK, Cunnings PP *et al.* A comparison of propylthiouracil versus methimazole in the treatment of hyperthyroidism in pregnancy. *Am J Obstet Gynecol* 1994;170:90–95.
8. Momotani N, Noh JY, Ishikawa N, Ito K. Effects of propylthiouracil and methimazole on fetal thyroid status in mothers with Graves' hyperthyroidism. *J Clin Endocrinol Metab* 1997;82:3633–6.
9. Haddow JE, Palomaki GE, Allan WC *et al.* Maternal thyroid deficiency during pregnancy and subsequent neuropsychological development of the child. *N Engl J Med* 1999;341:549–55.
10. Pop VJ, Kuijpens JL, van Baar AI *et al.* Low maternal free thyroxine concentrations during early pregnancy are associated with impaired psychomotor development in infancy. *Clin Endocrinol* 1999;50:149–55.
11. Girling JC, de Swiet M. Thyroxine dosage during pregnancy in women with primary hypothyroidism. *Br J Obstet Gynaecol* 1992;99:368–70.
12. Anselmo J, Cao D, Karrison T *et al.* Fetal loss associated with excess thyroid hormone exposure. *JAMA* 2004;292:691–5.
13. Hypothyroidism in the pregnant woman. *Drug Ther Bull* 2006; 44:53–6.

Chapter 12 Haematological conditions

Sarah Wharin and Sue Pavord

INTRODUCTION

Over the last two decades there has been increasing recognition of the impact of haematological conditions on pregnancy, delivery and the puerperium. However in many areas there is a lack of evidence to guide practice. Established standards for haematological conditions relate mainly to haemoglobinopathies. For the other topics, we have suggested points for guidance and identified key areas of knowledge and technique.

NORMAL HAEMATOLOGICAL CHANGES IN PREGNANCY

Red cells

During pregnancy, blood volume increases by around 1500 mL. Plasma volume expands by 25–80%, approximately twice the simultaneous expansion in the red cell mass. This results in a net reduction in haemoglobin (Hb) concentration, despite the 10–15% rise in Hb mass. There is a small physiological rise in the mean cell volume (MCV) due to increased red cell production and a higher proportion of larger immature erythrocytes.

Increased leukocyte production in pregnancy is manifest by a 'left shift', with increased band forms and the occasional presence of more immature neutrophil precursors. This is most marked in the third trimester and peaks at delivery. Lymphocytes are slightly reduced in number and monocytes increase, whilst the eosinophil and basophil counts remain the same.

Platelets

The platelet count usually remains constant but around 6% of women develop a gestational thrombocytopenia in the second half of pregnancy, related to increased peripheral clearance of platelets and a shorter platelet lifespan. The investigation and management of thrombocytopenia in pregnancy are covered later in the chapter.

Haemostasis

Pregnancy confers a hypercoagulable state which persists for up to 12 weeks postpartum. This is secondary to physiological changes in all elements of the haemostatic system, preparing the body for delivery. The haemostatic system is a fine balance between mechanisms to form a platelet-fibrin plug, mechanisms to control and localise its formation, and mechanisms to break it down. The main changes in the coagulation factors, natural anticoagulants and fibrinolytic system are outlined below in the Key Points.

KEY POINTS: NORMAL CHANGES TO HAEMATOLOGICAL PARAMETERS IN PREGNANCY

Red cells: ↑ plasma volume > ↑ red cell mass = ↓Hb ↓haematocrit ↑MCV

White cells: ↑ white cell count: ↑ neutrophils, ↑ monocytes ↓ lymphocytes

Platelets: ↓ platelet count in around 6% of women

Routine coagulation tests: ↓PT, ↓APTT

Coagulation factors: ↑ factors VII, VIII, fX, fibrinogen and von Willebrand's factor. Possible rise in fII and fV

Anticoagulants: ↓ protein S, activated protein C resistance ↑ fibrin but ↓ fibrinolytic activity ↑ D-dimers

Whilst these normal physiological changes provide some protection against haemorrhage at delivery, they can have a detrimental effect for some women if they result in venous thromboembolism. The risk is particularly high around the time of delivery and persists for a number of weeks after.

HAEMOGLOBINOPATHIES

Background

The haemoglobinopathies are inherited disorders of Hb synthesis and are largely classified into those that display a qualitative defect in the globin chains, namely sickle cell disease, or those with reduced synthesis of globin chains, thalassaemia.

Epidemiology

Haemoglobinopathies are most common in people whose family origins are in Africa, the Caribbean, the Middle East and Mediterranean areas, and hence are becoming more prevalent in the UK as the world's population becomes more mobile. It is estimated that sickle cell diseases affect one in every 200 births in the UK and 240,000 people are carriers. Beta-thalassaemia affects more than 700 people in the UK and the carrier rate is around 214,000.[1]

Normal Hb structure

Haemoglobin A (HbA) consists of 2 alpha chains and 2 beta chains ($\alpha_2\beta_2$). In the adult, HbA makes up 95% of red cell haemoglobin. Up to 3% is HbA2 ($\alpha_2\delta_2$), and a small amount of fetal Hb ($\alpha_2\gamma_2$) persists into adulthood. HbA is the predominant haemoglobin by 3 months of age and reaches adult levels by 9 months of age. Alpha-chains are coded for by a total of four genes, i.e. two from each parent. These are found on chromosome 16. The beta-chain is encoded for by two genes, one from each parent, found on chromosome 11.

Thalassaemia pathophysiology and clinical features

Thalassaemia is a quantitative defect in Hb production and includes alpha-thalassaemia and beta-thalassaemia. Some mutations cause complete absence of globin chain synthesis, denoted α^0 or β^0, whilst others produce chains at a reduced rate, α^+ or β^+.

Alpha-thalassaemia

If four affected alpha genes are inherited, no alpha chain is produced and Hb Barts, with four gamma chains, accumulates in red blood cells. The extremely high affinity for oxygen makes it incompatible with life, and death from hydrops fetalis occurs shortly before or after delivery. Conversely inheritance of only one abnormal gene is not associated with morbidity and the blood count may be completely normal. Two affected genes gives rise to alpha-thalassaemia trait, with hypochromic, microcytic anaemia. Three affected genes (two from one parent, one from the other) lead to an accumulation of beta- globin chains known as HbH bodies. This results in chronic haemolysis, anaemia and splenomegaly. Patients are usually transfusion dependent and susceptible to haemolytic crises, often triggered by infection.

Beta-thalassaemia

One abnormal beta gene gives rise to an asymptomatic carrier state: β-thalassaemia trait. Two defective genes results in clinical disease, with varying phenotype depending on the underlying mutations. This ranges from mild anaemia requiring only occasional blood transfusion (β-thalassaemia intermedia) to transfusion dependence (β-thalassaemia major) and the consequent iron accumulation in the heart, liver and endocrine system. Iron chelation therapy is necessary to prevent death from cardiac failure.

Management of pregnant women with thalassaemia

Physiological haemodilution of pregnancy exacerbates the anaemia of thalassaemia but women with thalassaemia trait usually remain asymptomatic. A serum ferritin is required to exclude coexisting iron deficiency, which should be treated with iron supplements. Iron should not be given to women with HbH disease who are at risk of iron overload, particularly if receiving blood transfusion. The chronic haemolysis renders them folate depleted and folate supplements should be routine. Pregnancy is uncommon in transfusion-dependent thalassaemia major and there are few data to guide management. However, with advances in iron chelation, fertility and life expectancy have improved over recent years and successful pregnancy outcomes are possible if women are adequately transfused and chelated prior to conception.[2] Complications predominantly relate to iron overload, particularly cardiomyopathy, and transfusion-related issues. Risks to the fetus include an increased incidence of intrauterine growth restriction (IUGR) and early and late pregnancy loss.[3,4]

Prior to pregnancy in women with β-thalassaemia major, iron chelation therapy should be optimised, to minimise organ dysfunction. Assessment of hepatic and cardiac function should be performed, the latter with T2-weighted magnetic resonance imaging (MRI). Iron chelation is potentially teratogenic and should be discontinued.

Blood count, serum ferritin and liver function tests should be monitored regularly throughout pregnancy, as well as serial growth scans. Transfusion regimens may need

---

KEY POINTS: MANAGEMENT OF THALASSAEMIA IN PREGNANCY

- Partner testing and prenatal diagnosis
- Echocardiogram to assess ventricular function
- Monitor full blood count (FBC) and ferritin. Transfuse as required
- Serial growth scans
- Give extended phenotype blood due to the risk of alloimmunisation
- Monitor liver function tests (LFTs).

altering to minimise large fluid shifts and iron chelation therapy may be necessary at delivery to reduce the toxic effect of free iron on the fetus.

Sickle cell disease pathophysiology and clinical features

Sickle cell disease (SCD) is caused by the production of defective beta chains due to a single amino acid shift in the beta-globin gene from glutamine to valine. Sickle cell anaemia (HbSS) is the most common of the sickling disorders. However SCD is also caused by a combination of sickle haemoglobin in the heterozygous state with a thalassaemia or another haemoglobin variant. Significant sickling syndromes occur with HbSC, HbSβ-Thal, HbSD$_{Punjab}$, HbSLepore, HbSE and HbSO$_{Arab}$. The prevalence of SCD varies geographically and is classically associated with areas where malaria is endemic. Highly prevalent areas include West and Central Africa, Asia, the Caribbean and northern Greece.

When Haemoglobin Sickle [HbS] is in a deoxygenated state, it forms large polymers with other Hb tetramers. This leads to 'sickling' of the red cells which are more rigid and less 'deformable' in the circulation. The consequences of this are vaso-occlusion and a state of chronic haemolysis. Patients encounter 'crises' which can be vaso-occlusive (painful), aplastic (characteristically triggered by parvovirus B19 infection), acute chest syndrome and splenic sequestration (predominantly in children). Situations in which sickling increases include hypoxia, hypothermia and acidosis. The clinical manifestations of SCD are vast and are largely the consequence of vaso-occlusive disease. Heterozygous HbS carriers are usually asymptomatic.

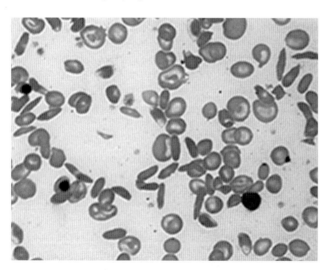

Fig. 12.1 Blood film of a patient with HbSS during a sickle crisis. Note the presence of numerous sickle cells, polychromasia and nucleated red cells

KEY POINTS: SICKLE CELL DISEASE

Chronic complications

- Haemolytic anaemia
- Hyposplenism and increased risk of infection
- Bone disease
- Renal disease
- Retinopathy
- Neurological
- Thromboembolic disease
- Pulmonary hypertension
- Hepatobiliary disease

Acute crises

- Painful (vaso-occlusive)
- Chest syndrome
- Splenic sequestration (infants)
- Aplastic crisis

Prenatal diagnosis and counselling

Any woman who has a haemoglobinopathy or is a known carrier should ideally undergo prenatal counselling in a specialist centre. Possible risks of pregnancy to the mother and the fetus should be outlined and the option of pre-implantation genetic diagnosis discussed.

Screening

Due to the increasing incidence of haemoglobinopathies in the UK population and the resulting morbidity, a screening programme was initiated in 2005 and updated in 2011.[5] The aim of the programme is to detect women who are carriers of a thalassaemia or Hb variant and thereby assess their risk of having an affected child. Mother and partner testing should be completed before 12 weeks' gestation, to allow the parents enough time to make a decision regarding prenatal diagnosis. Antenatal screening is offered to all women; the exact method varies depending on whether the area has a high or low prevalence of haemoglobinopathies. In high-prevalence areas, FBC and haemoglobin analysis via high pressure liquid chromatography (HPLC) are performed on all women in conjunction with a family origin questionnaire. In low-prevalence areas, FBC is performed initially, with a family origin questionnaire and HPLC undertaken if the fetus is deemed to be at risk. β-thalassaemia is suspected if red cell indices are hypochromic (mean corpuscular Hb [MCH]<27) and microcytic (MCV <75 fL) in conjunction with a raised HbA$_2$. Alpha-thalassaemia trait results in similar red cell indices but a normal HbA$_2$. A family origin questionnaire will identify if the woman is from a high-risk population group for alpha-thalassaemia. Haemoglobin variants, such as HbS, HbE or HbD Lepore, will be detected by HPLC. Any abnormal results should prompt partner testing to assess potential risk to the fetus. If the child is at risk, prenatal testing should be offered; the usual method of choice is chorionic villous sampling in the first trimester.

Sickle cell disease in pregnancy

There are 150–250 deliveries each year in women with sickle cell disease.[6] SCD in pregnancy has consequences for both the mother and the fetus; maternal morbidity and mortality are significantly higher than those for healthy women. Painful episodes may become more common, particularly in the third trimester, and the risk of infections and thromboembolic disease is amplified. A recent nationwide surveillance study of pregnant women with SCD in the UK over a 12-month period found that 52% suffered a painful crisis, with 25% requiring admission to hospital (Fig. 12.1).[6]

Anaemia is exacerbated by physiological changes and increased maternal demands, and cardiac complications are increased by pulmonary hypertension and iron overload. Specific obstetric complications include an increased risk of pre-eclampsia and antepartum haemorrhage, and the rate of miscarriage, intrauterine growth restriction and neonatal death is substantially increased.[7] These complications are less apparent in HbSC disease.[8]

Management in pregnancy

Health should be optimised before pregnancy and iron overload aggressively treated with chelation prior to conception. An up-to-date echocardiogram should be performed to look for evidence of pulmonary hypertension. Vaccinations must be up to date. Hydroxycarbamide should be discontinued at least 3 months prior to conception and ACE inhibitors or ARBs should be stopped.

Routine antenatal care
During pregnancy, women should be cared for by a specialist obstetric haematology team, where available. The increased incidence of infections, painful crises and acute chest syndrome should be discussed, highlighting the need to avoid triggering factors such as cold, exertion and dehydration, and to seek medical attention early if pain is not relieved by simple analgesia or vomiting occurs, increasing the risk of dehydration and subsequent crisis. Three litres of oral fluid is needed daily, due to the reduced ability of the kidneys to concentrate urine.

Full blood count, renal and liver function tests, and serum ferritin should be performed at booking, with urine dipstick for blood and protein. These should be repeated regularly throughout the course of the pregnancy. Blood group and antibody screen are important to exclude alloimmune antibodies caused by blood transfusion. Continued folic acid 5 mg daily and phenoxymethylpenicillin prophylaxis should be ensured.

Sickle cell disease is a risk factor for pre-eclampsia and women should receive aspirin prophylaxis.[9] A large study of 18,000 deliveries to SCD mothers in the USA showed that these women had a six-fold increased risk of venous thromboembolic disease.[10] It is therefore recommended that these women receive graded compression stockings and thromboprophylaxis during hospital admissions and the postpartum period.[11]

> **KEY POINTS: SICKLE CELL DISEASE IN PREGNANCY**
>
> - Pre-conception counselling
> - Partner testing and prenatal diagnosis
> - Folic acid, phenoxymethylpenicillin for all women
> - Avoidance of triggers
> - Treat infections early
> - Consider aspirin and LMWH
> - Monitor FBC, ferritin, urea & electrolytes (U&Es), urine dip
> - 4-weekly growth scans after 20/40

Women should be offered a viability scan at 7–9 weeks, routine first-trimester scan at 11–14 weeks and a detailed anomaly scan at 20 weeks. Thereafter, 4-weekly growth scans should be performed.[11]

Blood transfusions
There is little evidence to support prophylactic blood transfusions, with no apparent improvement in morbidity in mother or fetus.[12] If blood is transfused it should be matched according to an extended phenotype, and should be cytomegalovirus (CMV) negative and sickle negative.

Management of acute painful crisis (Box 12.1)
Women need to be admitted and assessed immediately and managed by obstetric and haematology teams. They should be offered adequate analgesia, working up the analgesia ladder. NSAIDs can be given between weeks 12 and 28. Pethidine should be avoided due to the risk of seizure but other strong opioids such as morphine may be given. Particular attention needs to be paid to treatment of infection, prevention of dehydration with intravenous fluids and early detection of acute chest syndrome. Supplemental oxygen should be given to treat

Box 12.1 Management of an acute crisis

- Early and frequent analgesia
- Maintain good hydration and oxygenation
- Treat any underlying infection
- Monitor Hb; top-up transfusion may be required
- Early recognition of chest syndrome
- Thromboprophylaxis during inpatient stay

hypoxia and close liaison with critical care teams should be maintained. Top-up transfusions and possibly exchange transfusion may be required. Consideration should be given to early delivery at 38–40 weeks. Mode of delivery should be decided by obstetric factors. Women need to be closely monitored with pulse oximetry and kept well hydrated. Thromboprophylaxis is essential postnatally.

PLATELET DISORDERS IN PREGNANCY

Platelets are formed from megakaryocytes, which are large multinucleate cells found in the bone marrow. Their differentiation and proliferation is under the control of

Box 12.2 Causes of thrombocytopenia in pregnancy

- Gestational thrombocytopenia
- Isoimmune (idiopathic) thrombocytopenic purpura (ITP)
- Pre-eclampsia
- Haemolysis, increased liver enzymes and low platelets (HELLP) syndrome
- Disseminated intravascular coagulation
- Thrombotic thrombocytopenic purpura
- Haemolytic uraemic syndrome
- Antiphospholipid syndrome (APLS)

Box 12.3 Investigation of thrombocytopenia in pregnancy

- Full history and examination
- Blood film
- Prothrombin time (PT), activated partial thromboplastin time (APTT), fibrinogen
- Liver function tests
- Reticulocyte count
- Haptoglobin, lactate dehydrogenase (LDH)
- Consider systemic lupus erythematosus (SLE) serology
- Consider APLS screen
- Hepatitis/HIV serology

thrombopoietin. Each megakaryocyte can generate 2000–3000 platelets. Thrombocytopenia in pregnancy is relatively common and there are a number of possible causes. Platelet function disorders are less common but do occur so will be covered briefly.

Thrombocytopenia in pregnancy

Thrombocytopenia affects 6–10% of all pregnant women and after anaemia is the most frequent haematological disorder in pregnancy. There are many possible causes, some specific to pregnancy and others that can also occur in the non-pregnant population (Boxes 12.2 and 12.3).

Gestational thrombocytopenia

Gestational thrombocytopenia (GT) is the most common cause of thrombocytopenia and accounts for 75% of the cases.[13] The fall in platelet count is secondary to haemodilution and increased platelet activation and clearance. Inevitably, as the platelet count falls in pregnancy, some will fall into the thrombocytopenic range. In these patients, the platelet count outside pregnancy is normal and it usually resolves 1–2 months postnatally. The platelet count usually remains above 70×10^9/L and it is diagnosed after other causes of thrombocytopenia have been considered. It is often not possible to distinguish between GT and mild ITP and the platelet count should be monitored 4 weekly throughout pregnancy. Affected women do not suffer with bleeding symptoms, there is no associated morbidity in the fetus and the risk of neonatal thrombocytopenia is not increased.

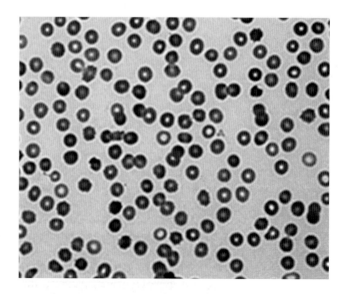

Fig. 12.2 ITP; note normal red cell morphology

Immune thrombocytopenia

Immune thrombocytopenia (ITP, Fig. 12.2) affects 1 in 1000–10,000 pregnancies.[14] It occurs as a first presentation in a third of cases and as a relapse in women with pre-existing disease in the other two-thirds. Unlike GT, the platelet count can fall significantly and these women may suffer associated symptoms of mucosal bleeding. It may present at any point in pregnancy and, unlike gestational thrombocytopenia, may present in the first trimester. Investigations may be necessary to exclude alternative diagnoses or associated conditions.

The aim of management in ITP in pregnancy is to control bleeding symptoms and to allow for a safe delivery. Bleeding symptoms rarely occur with a platelet count $>20 \times 10^9$/L and therefore asymptomatic women with platelet counts above this threshold are unlikely to require treatment in the first two trimesters. Treatment should be initiated if bleeding or excessive bruising occurs or the platelet count falls $<20 \times 10^9$/L. Around the time of delivery, the platelet count needs to be raised to a threshold to ensure minimal haemorrhagic complications. There should be close collaboration of the obstetricians, the haematologist and the obstetric anaesthetist. A platelet count of $>50 \times 10^9$/L is acceptable for a vaginal delivery or caesarean section; however, whilst there is no evidence base, it is recommended that the platelet count should be $>75 \times 10^9$/L for spinal anaesthesia.[15]

First-line treatment of ITP in pregnancy is corticosteroids, which achieve good response in 70–80% of women. Side effects include increased risk of gestational diabetes, pregnancy-induced hypertension and postpartum psychiatric disorders. Steroids are not teratogenic but may be associated with premature rupture of membranes and placental abruption. To avoid unnecessary adverse effects, the minimal therapeutic dose possible should be used, with dose escalation if response is poor. An appropriate starting dose of prednisolone is 20 mg daily.[15]

For refractory cases, or where a rapid increase in platelet count is required, intravenous immunoglobulin (IVIg) can be given (1 g/kg). Women often report headaches and more serious complications, such as aseptic meningitis and renal impairment, have been known. Although vigorous viral safety measures are ensured, women should be counselled about the use of blood products. The rise in platelets lasts around 6 weeks but this can become shorter as pregnancy advances. The cost is high and shortage of supply not infrequent.

There is some experience of using anti-D but higher doses are needed than for prevention of rhesus D (RhD) alloimmunisation and there is concern about theoretical risk of fetal haemolysis. It does not appear to add any advantages over IVIg except perhaps the lower volume. Azathioprine appears to be safe in pregnancy (teratology information service) and can be helpful for persistent or refractory disease; however, full effect takes 3 months, limiting its value if started late in gestation. Platelet transfusions are reserved for emergency bleeding or for delivery of women with platelet counts $<50 \times 10^9$/L. The response is brief due to clearance by the circulating antibody.

Transplacental transfer of maternal antiplatelet antibodies may cause thrombocytopenia in the infant. The incidence is around 25%;[16] however, severe thrombocytopenia is uncommon. Approximately 15% of neonates will have platelet counts of <100, <10% have platelet counts $<50 \times 10^9$/L and the incidence of neonatal intracranial haemorrhage or other haemorrhagic complications is <1%. There are no reliable factors that predict the risk to the baby other than the occurrence in an older sibling,[17] where the ability for transplacental passage of the antibody has clearly been demonstrated. Other alarm bells are a history of splenectomy and severe and/or refractory ITP.

Cordocentesis is not recommended as the risks outweigh the benefits, given that the random platelets transfused will be rapidly destroyed by antibody (in contrast to fetal alloimmune thrombocytopenia, where compatible platelets can be used). The mode of delivery should be determined by obstetric indications. However to minimise trauma, fetal scalp electrodes, blood sampling and use of Ventouse or rotational forceps should be avoided. Lift-out forceps can be used.

A cord platelet count should be taken and intramuscular vitamin K withheld until the count is known, or given orally. A count $<70 \times 10^9$/L necessitates a repeat sample at day 5, when the nadir is reached due to splenic development. Babies with a platelet count of $<30 \times 10^9$/L require platelet transfusion and intracranial ultrasound performed.

KEY POINTS: MANAGEMENT OF ITP IN PREGNANCY

Should be managed in collaboration with obstetrician, haematologist and anaesthetist.

Desired platelet counts

First and second trimester: Treatment only required if platelet count is $<20 \times 10^9$/L or patient is symptomatic.
36 weeks onwards: Treatment required if platelets $<50 \times 10^9$/L.
Vaginal delivery: Platelet count $>50 \times 10^9$/L.
Caesarean section: Platelet count $>50 \times 10^9$/L.
Spinal anaesthesia: Platelet count $>75 \times 10^9$/L.

Maternal treatment strategies

First-line treatment: Corticosteroids.
Second-line treatment: Intravenous immunoglobulin.
Emergency/rapid response required: Platelet transfusion + IVIg + IV methylprednisolone.

Management of fetus

Routine cordocentesis not recommended.
Avoid fetal scalp sampling.
Avoid Ventouse and rotational forceps.
Check FBC from cord sample.
Intracranial Doppler in the neonate if platelet count $<30 \times 10^9$/L.

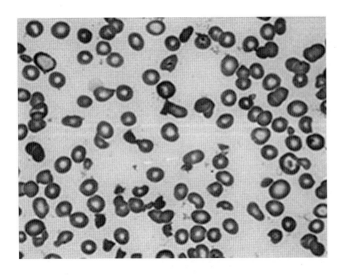

Fig. 12.3 TTP; schistocytes (red cell fragments), polychromasia and spherocytes

Pre-eclampsia and HELLP

Consumptive thrombocytopenia occurs in around 30% of women with pre-eclampsia and may precede other signs and symptoms. HELLP is the combination of thrombocytopenia with microangiopathic haemolytic anaemia and elevated liver enzymes. These disorders are discussed in detail in other chapters.

Thrombotic thrombocytopenic purpura

Thrombotic thrombocytopenic purpura (TTP, Fig. 12.3) is a relatively rare but important cause of thrombocytopenia in pregnancy as it carries a high mortality and morbidity rate which can be avoided if treatment is started early. It is defined by the combination of microangiopathic haemolytic anaemia and thrombocytopenia, usually accompanied by neurological symptoms and sometimes fever. Renal impairment can also occur. In the acute setting, TTP can be difficult to distinguish from severe pre-eclampsia and HELLP and, like these disorders, the main therapeutic manoeuvre is to deliver the baby.

TTP is caused by reduced levels of ADAMTS-13 (a disintegrin and metalloproteinase with a thrombospondin type 1 motif, member 13), a metalloprotease required for the cleavage of ultra-large von Willebrand's factor (vWF) multimers. This leads to the formation of platelet aggregates in the microvasculature, leading to tissue ischaemia and sometimes infarction. This process particularly affects the lung, renal and cerebral vasculature. Most cases are acquired, with an autoimmune antibody to ADAMTS-13; however, some cases are familial and may present for the first time in pregnancy.

The mortality rate of untreated TTP is 80% which reduces to around 10% with plasma exchange, with intracerebral and cardiac events being the main cause of death. A high index of suspicion is crucial to ensure rapid diagnosis and treatment. If

KEY POINTS: TTP IN PREGNANCY	
Clinical:	Typical 'pentad' of fever, renal impairment, neurological symptoms, thrombocytopenia and microangiopathic haemolytic anaemia.
	May be difficult to distinguish from pre-eclampsia and HELLP.
	Obstetric emergency: up to 90% mortality rate if left untreated.
Investigations:	FBC and film: schistocytes (fragments), polychromasia, thrombocytopenia.
	U&Es, LFT ($\uparrow$ bilirubin), LDH ($\uparrow$), reticulocytes ($\uparrow$), haptoglobin ($\downarrow$).
	Clotting (will be normal in TTP).
	The Direct Antiglobulin Test (DAT) (will be negative in TTP).
	ADAMTS-13 level and ADAMTS-13 antibody (ADAMTS-13 level may be low in HELLP but with no antibody detected).
Management Immediate:	Contact haematologist.
	Start infusion of solvent-treated FFP.
	If in third trimester, consider delivery of baby.
	Arrange for urgent plasma exchange.
	Start IV methylprednisolone (3 days, then switch to oral corticosteroids).
Continuing:	Start folic acid 5 mg once daily.
	Start aspirin and LMWH when platelets are >50.
	Continue plasma exchange until platelet count is normal.
	If fetus not delivered immediately, serial growth scans with uterine artery Doppler.
Future:	Warn about risk of recurrence in future pregnancies.
	Avoid oral contraceptive pill.

any doubt remains regarding the diagnosis, an ADAMTS level should be taken and plasma exchange initiated until the diagnosis can be definitively confirmed or refuted. If there is likely to be a delay in starting plasma exchange, solvent-treated fresh frozen plasma (FFP) should be infused, to provide the missing protease.

Plasma exchange needs to continue daily, in addition to corticosteroids. Folic acid supplements are necessary to support erythropoiesis and thromboprophylaxis with LMWH and aspirin should be started as soon as the platelet count is >50 × 10⁹/L. Serial growth scans with uterine artery Doppler will be required to monitor placental function and the fetus should be delivered as early as possible. Recovery after delivery

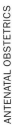

of the baby is not necessarily prompt and repeated plasma exchanges are necessary until the platelet count normalises. Women should be counselled about the risk of recurrence in further pregnancies and should be advised to avoid the oral contraceptive pill.

Platelet function disorders

Congenital platelet function disorders reflect the inability of platelets to aggregate under normal conditions, or the defective release of platelet granule constituents. Pre-conception counselling is necessary to explain the risks of inheritance where these are known and the management for pregnancy. The clinical picture in these disorders is very variable and ranges from asymptomatic mild mucosal-type bleeding to a severe bleeding phenotype. The description of the individual disorders is beyond the scope of this chapter; however patients should be managed in close liaison with a haematologist. Desmopressin (trade name DDAVP) is usually the agent of choice and, as these are heritable conditions, care should be taken in the delivery of the baby.

Alloimmune conditions in pregnancy

Blood group antigens are found on the red cell surface. The ABO and Rh groups of antigens are the most clinically significant in clinical transfusion practice. There are numerous other red cell antigens and these can become more significant in multiply transfused patients and during pregnancy. Platelets also have antigens on their cell surface and both red cell and platelet antigens are inherited in a mendelian fashion. Fetal red cells and platelets therefore express both maternal and paternal antigens. As maternal circulation is in contact with fetal cells, maternal antibodies can be formed against the paternally derived antigens, if they are not present on maternal cells. Red cell alloimmunisation can result in fetal or neonatal haemolytic disease. Alloimmunisation against fetal platelet antigens can cause fetal or neonatal alloimmune thrombocytopenia.

Red cell alloimmunisation and haemolytic disease of the fetus and newborn (HDFN)

Maternal antibodies to paternally derived fetal red cell antigens may cross the placenta and coat fetal red cells, leading to their destruction. If this process exceeds the rate at which erythropoiesis occurs in the fetus, anaemia ensues. This can lead to heart failure, oedema and, in the most severe cases, hydrops fetalis and fetal death. Severe haemolysis can occur in neonates, with a risk of kernicterus as the immature liver is unable to process the unconjugated bilirubin.

The most significant antibodies are anti-D, anti-C and anti-K, of which anti-D is the most common and will be the

Box 12.4 Antenatal 'sensitising' events with risk of isoimmunisation

- Miscarriage or threatened miscarriage >12 weeks' gestation
- Medical or surgical termination of pregnancy at any gestation
- Ectopic pregnancy
- Hydatidiform mole
- Prenatal diagnostic procedures: chorionic villous sampling (CVS) or amniocentesis
- Abdominal trauma
- External cephalic version
- Antepartum haemorrhage
- Stillbirth
- Traumatic delivery including caesarean section
- Manual removal of placenta

focus of this text. The D antigen is one of the Rh group of antigens, formally known as rhesus antigens. Most RhD-negative women have a complete absence of the RhD antigen whilst a small minority have a qualitative or quantitative deficiency of the D antigen, known as partial D or weak D respectively. In the UK, 10% of deliveries are RhD-positive babies born to RhD-negative women. In one in six RhD-negative women, isoimmunisation will occur after delivery of an RhD-positive baby.

Isoimmunisation is precipitated by fetomaternal haemorrhage (FMH). Most commonly this is at delivery and, in the majority of cases, HDFN does not affect the first pregnancy but is a risk for subsequent pregnancies. However, as little as 0.25 mL of fetal blood can be sufficient to cause isoimmunisation and, in order to prevent this, anti-D should be given to the mother after all potentially sensitising events (Box 12.4).

Anti-D is a virally inactivated, plasma-derived product from US donors. A dose of 500 units of anti-D will neutralise an FMH of up to 4 mL. For women with sensitising events before 20 weeks' gestation 250 IU is sufficient. For events after 20 weeks' gestation 500 IU should be administered immediately, within 72 hours,[18] with further doses depending on estimation of the size of the FMH.

Estimation of fetomaternal haemorrhage
Estimation of FMH should be undertaken:

- in an RhD-negative woman following delivery of an RhD-positive baby;
- following any sensitising events after 20 weeks' gestation.

estimation for FMH is not required when:

- events occur before 20 weeks' gestation;
- the fetus is known to be RhD negative;
- the mother is RhD positive;
- the mother is known to have immune anti-D.

Two main methods exist for estimating FMH.

Kleihauer (acid elution method). Fetal haemoglobin (HbF) is more resistant than adult haemoglobin (HbA) to acid and alkali conditions. Dried maternal blood is fixed and exposed to acid; the HbA is denatured and eluted leaving 'red cell ghosts'. The HbF remains and can be stained, allowing estimation of the fetal red cell volume. This method detects the presence of fetal cells but does not distinguish between RhD-positive and RhD-negative cells.

Flow cytometry method. This test is performed after Kleihauer, to confirm the volume of FMH and determine whether the fetal cells are RhD positive or negative. A fluoro-chrome is conjugated to an IgG antibody which recognises the RhD antigen. If flow cytometry is negative when a Kleihauer test is positive, it suggests that the fetus is RhD negative. Unfortunately this test is not readily available in all centres.

If the FMH is estimated to be <2 mL by Kleihauer test, 500 IU anti-D is sufficient and no further action is required. If the FMH is >2 mL, the volume should be confirmed by flow cytometry. If the FMH is >4 mL, a further dose should be calculated on the basis that 125 IU anti-D will neutralise 1 mL of FMH. Follow-up testing should be performed after 72 hours to confirm that the fetal cells have been cleared.

Postnatal anti-D

The guideline published by the British Committee for Standards in Haematology (BCSH)[19] states that every RhD-negative woman should receive at least 500 IU of anti-D within 72 hours of delivery of an RhD-positive baby. However 1% of women will have an FMH of >4 mL and therefore it is important to be able to accurately estimate the FMH volume and a maternal blood sample for FMH estimation should be sent within 2 hours.[18] Some centres give a single anti-D 1500 IU dose postnatally, which is adequate to neutralise a 15 mL bleed; however, some FMH are >15 mL.

A fetal cord blood sample should also be sent to confirm the infant's blood group and Rh status. If the pregnancy is non-viable and fetal blood sampling is not possible, anti-D should be given to an Rh-negative non-sensitised mother within 72 hours of the diagnosis of fetal death, regardless of the timing of delivery.[19] If the Kleihauer test estimates an FMH of >2 mL, this should be confirmed by flow cytometry and additional anti-D should be administered if required. Follow-up testing should be performed 72 hours after the dose.

If intraoperative cell salvage (ICS) is used during caesarean section, a dose of at least 1500 IU of anti-D should be given. This is to allow for the fact that, during ICS, fetal cells can be re-infused into the maternal circulation and a dose of up to 20 mL has been reported. Estimation of FMH should then occur 35–40 minutes after re-infusion of red cells to establish whether any further anti-D is required.[19]

Sensitising events prior to 20 weeks' gestation

Prior to 12 weeks' gestation anti-D is required after surgical evacuation of the uterus, termination and ectopic pregnancy. Spontaneous miscarriage does not require anti-D prophylaxis if there is no instrumentation of the uterus and if there is only mild painless bleeding. However, a recent update of the BCSH guidelines state that anti-D should also be given before 12 weeks if there is prolonged heavy bleeding or bleeding accompanied by abdominal pain.[19] Anti-D is required following a spontaneous miscarriage after 12 weeks' gestation.

KEY POINTS: MANAGEMENT OF SENSITISING EVENTS IN RHD-NEGATIVE WOMEN

- <20 weeks' gestation: administer 250 IU anti-D within 72 hours.
- >20 weeks' gestation: administer 500 IU anti-D and perform estimation of FMH.
- If FMH >4 mL, administer 125 IU for each additional 1 mL.
- Re-check FMH estimation after 72 hours to ensure neutralisation of fetal red cells.

Sensitising event after 20 weeks' gestation

Prophylaxis should be given for any sensitising event after 20 weeks' gestation at a dose of 500 IU. FMH should then be estimated. For recurrent intrauterine bleeding after 20 weeks' gestation, women should receive anti-D at least 6 weekly. An FMH sample should be tested 2 weekly and, if positive, extra anti-D should be given.[19]

Routine antenatal anti-D prophylaxis (RAADP)

In addition to overt clinical events, it became clear that isoimmunisation can result from occult, low-volume FMH occurring in normal pregnancy. RAADP has been shown to significantly reduce rates of sensitisation[20] and NICE now recommend RAADP for all RhD-negative women.

Anti-D prophylaxis can either be given as a single dose of 1500 IU at 28 weeks or as two separate doses of 500 IU at 28 and 34 weeks' gestation with no evidence of difference in efficacy.[18] RAADP should still be offered if prophylactic anti-D was administered earlier in pregnancy after a sensitising event and, conversely, prophylactic anti-D still needs to be administered after sensitising events even if RAADP has been given previously.

It is important to note that passive anti-D can be detected up to 8 weeks post-prophylaxis and laboratory tests are unable to distinguish between passive and immune anti-D. Therefore if anti-D has been given early in pregnancy, anti-D antibodies may be detected at the 28-week routine screen. Passive anti-D is usually <1 IU/mL. If there is doubt, the woman should be treated as non-immune and RAADP should continue.

Management of alloimmunisation

Despite efforts with prophylaxis, isoimmunisation may still occur. This is usually because guidelines for RAADP have not been followed, women fail to attend in a timely manner after sensitising events, 'silent' FMH occurs before 28 weeks' gestation or a woman has been exposed to Rh antigens during transfusion. If immune anti-D is detected, close monitoring in a fetomaternal medicine unit is needed. Investigations should be undertaken to try to determine the cause of the immune anti-D and to assess the risk of haemolytic disease of the newborn (HDFN)in the current pregnancy. This involves a full history of previous pregnancies, transfusion history and testing of the partner to determine heterozygosity or homozygosity for the RhD antigen. The level of the anti-D antibody at booking can give valuable information regarding the risk of HDFN. If it <4 IU/mL, HDFN is unlikely; if >15 IU/mL, there is a high risk of hydrops. The antibody level should be monitored closely throughout pregnancy: 4 weekly to 28 weeks' gestation then 2 weekly thereafter.

The Rh status of the fetus should be determined if the father is heterozygous or if he is not available for testing. This is achieved by testing for free fetal DNA in maternal blood. This can be done from the first trimester but testing is more sensitive and therefore usually performed after 16 weeks' gestation.

Fetal anaemia can be predicted by measuring fetal blood flow velocity in the middle cerebral artery (MCA) by Doppler. It is a non-invasive yet accurate and sensitive test which detects fetal anaemia in the early stages. If there is evidence of anaemia, fetal blood sampling is undertaken and an intrauterine transfusion (IUT) programme initiated. IUT is particularly hazardous prior to 20 weeks' gestation and carries a mortality rate of around 10%. After 20 weeks' gestation the risk of fetal loss, membrane rupture, fetal bleeding or bradycardia is around 2–4%. Blood used for IUT should be cross-matched against the maternal blood and should be CMV negative, irradiated and less than 5 days old. The transfused blood should have a haematocrit of >75–80% to reduce the volume of transfusion and should be given at a rate of <5 mL/min. The mother is usually sedated for the procedure. Transfusions may need to be repeated every 2–3 weeks until 34–36 weeks' gestation, at which point delivery should be arranged. Close communication should be maintained with the neonatology team.

After delivery, the infant should have cord blood sent for grouping, direct coombs' test (DCT) and bilirubin level. Phototherapy may be required and, in severe cases, exchange transfusion may be necessary. Exchange transfusions can be very hazardous for the baby and should be avoided if possible. IVIg may reduce the need for exchange transfusion.[21] The baby may need repeated transfusions over the first 4–6 months of life as maternal antibodies circulate for 4–6 months and normal erythropoiesis may be suppressed by the newborn and intrauterine transfusions. Parents should be carefully counselled about the risk of recurrence in subsequent pregnancies.

KEY POINTS: MANAGEMENT OF ANTI-D DURING PREGNANCY

- Management by fetal–maternal medicine unit.
- Quantify anti-D level at booking.
- Establish RhD status of father with full genotype.
- If father is heterozygous for RhD, establish RhD status of the fetus by testing free fetal DNA in the maternal blood after 16 weeks' gestation.
- If the fetus is RhD positive, monitor anti-D levels at 4-weekly intervals until 28 weeks' gestation then 2 weekly thereafter.
- Perform MCA Doppler ultrasound at 20 weeks' gestation.
- If evidence of anaemia arrange fetal blood sampling and IUT programme.

Other clinically significant red cell antigens causing haemolytic disease of fetus and newborn (HDFN)

Anti-C antibodies and anti-K antibodies can also cause significant HDFN, with the latter suppressing erythropoiesis as well as causing increased haemolysis. If detected at booking, a similar approach should be taken as with detection of anti-D antibodies. The father should be typed and, if heterozygous or not available, the fetal red cells should be typed from a maternal blood sample. Presence of fetal anaemia should be monitored with MCA Doppler ultrasound from 20 weeks' gestation and an IUT programme initiated if necessary. Other antibodies at high titre of more than 1:32 dilution may result in neonatal anaemia.

Fetal maternal alloimmune thrombocytopenia

Fetal maternal alloimmune thrombocytopenia (FMAIT) is the most common cause of severe fetal and neonatal thrombocytopenia and of intracranial haemorrhage in term neonates. It results from the formation of maternal antibodies against the fetal platelet alloantigens that are paternally derived. Transplacental passage of the maternal IgG antibody can cause thrombocytopenia in the fetus or neonate. It is thought to affect 1:1000 pregnancies. The most common platelet antigens implicated in FMAIT are HPA-1a, which accounts for 80% of cases, and HPA-5b, which accounts for 15% of cases. Two per cent of mothers are homozygous for HPA-1b and therefore lack the HPA-1a antigen. Only 10% of these will form anti-HPA-1a antibodies. Unlike HDFN, approximately 50% of cases of FMAIT occur in the first pregnancy.

The most severe complication of FMAIT is intracranial bleeding which may occur *in utero* or after birth. This complicates 10% of cases and often results in death or long-term neurological damage. In most other cases, there is a finding of severe thrombocytopenia in an otherwise well baby with

Table 12.1 Clinical and laboratory diagnosis of FMAIT

FMAIT diagnosis	
When to suspect FMAIT in the fetus	**When to suspect FMAIT in the newborn**
Previous history of neonatal thrombocytopenia	Incidental finding of neonatal thrombocytopenia
Fetal intracranial haemorrhage, hydrocephalus or ventriculomegaly	If there are signs or symptoms of bruising, bleeding or unexplained intracerebral haemorrhage
Family history of FMAIT	Platelets $<50 \times 10^9$/L with otherwise normal counts and absence of other causes of neonatal thrombocytopenia – sepsis, DIC, maternal ITP
Unexplained late fetal loss	
Samples required for diagnosis	
Maternal	6 mL EDTA blood for analysis of platelet antigens + 6 mL clotted blood for antibody detection
Paternal	6 mL EDTA blood for platelet antigen analysis
Neonate	1 mL EDTA for analysis of platelet antigens

- DIC, disseminated intravascular coagulation; EDTA, Ethylenediaminetetraacetic acid .

purpura or bruising. The platelet nadir is usually around day 3–4. The condition is self-limiting and usually resolves within 2–8 weeks. The presence of anti HPA-1a antibodies results in a more severe clinical picture than HPA-5b antibodies.

Investigation and management of FMAIT

Diagnosis (Table 12.1) requires the demonstration of maternal platelet antibodies that react against platelet-specific antigens present in the father and neonate but not in the mother. Samples therefore need to be sent from both parents and the neonate to the transfusion laboratory.

In a term healthy infant platelet transfusions should be given to maintain the platelet count $> 30 \times 10^9$/L. The platelets should be kept higher at 50×10^9/L in the presence of bleeding

Table 12.2 Risk of FMAIT in subsequent pregnancies

Risk to fetus	History of older sibling
Standard	Neonatal thrombocytopenia with no ICH
High	ICH occurring in third trimester
Very high	ICH occurring before 28 weeks' gestation

or in preterm infants. HPA-1a- and -5b- negative platelets will be compatible with 90–95% of cases of FMAIT and should be used in preference to random platelets, which would be destroyed by maternal antibody in the neonate. Platelets should also be irradiated and CMV negative.

Information must be given to the parents about FMAIT, in particular the risk of recurrence in future pregnancies and the antenatal management options. It should be suggested that female relatives of the mother are also tested. Paternal testing for the HPA antigen should be performed to see if the father is homozygous or heterozygous for the causative HPA antigen.

Management of subsequent pregnancies

The rate of recurrence in subsequent pregnancies is 75–90% and, with each subsequent affected pregnancy, the thrombocytopenia usually occurs earlier in gestation and unfortunately tends to be more severe. The risk of intracranial haemorrhage (ICH) following a previous pregnancy of FMAIT with ICH is estimated to be around 70%. Women should be managed in a hospital with a dedicated fetomaternal medicine unit and in collaboration with a haematologist.

Fetal blood sampling (FBS) and intrauterine platelet transfusions used to be the mainstay of treatment but, given the associated morbidity and fetal mortality, focus has diverted to maternal treatment early in gestation, to control antibody production. There is much debate regarding the agents given, the exact timing of treatment and whether or not FBS should be performed. Practice varies between centres but, as there is good correlation between the severity of FMAIT in siblings, most stratify risk according to the history of the older sibling, as shown in Table 12.2.[22]

Treatment comprises IVIg with or without steroids. Berkowitz *et al.* randomised high-risk women to receive IVIg alone or combined with prednisolone 1 mg/kg per day and found a satisfactory increase in platelet count, by 20 weeks, in 89% on combined therapy compared with 35% with IVIg alone (P=<0.05).[23] No differences were seen in responses of standard-risk women. A management model that avoids fetal blood sampling has been proposed by Pachecho *et al.*[22] (Fig. 12.4).

Intrapartum management

There is debate regarding the optimal route of delivery, however, vaginal delivery is considered safe if the fetal platelet count is $>100 \times 10^9$/L. In cases where the fetal platelet count is $<50 \times 10^9$/L, the options are to perform a caesarean section or allow normal vaginal delivery within 5 days of an intrauterine platelet transfusion. If the fetus is to be delivered vaginally, trauma should be minimised with avoidance of Ventouse, rotational forceps, scalp monitoring and fetal blood sampling.

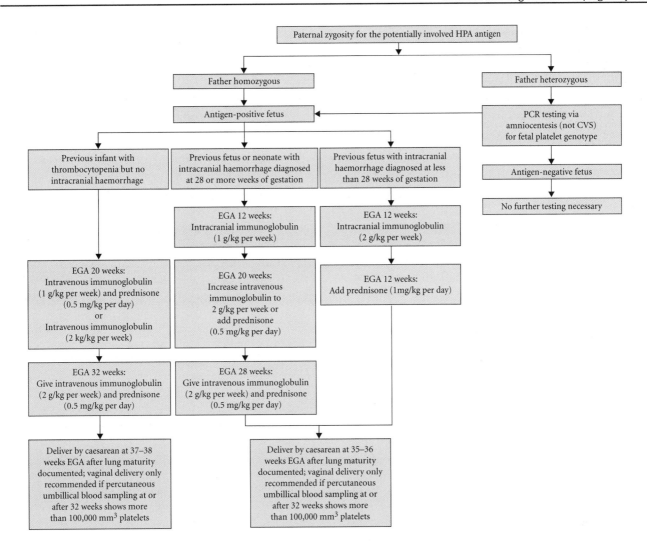

Fig. 12.4 Algorithm for antenatal management of FMAIT.[22]

INHERITED BLEEDING DISORDERS IN PREGNANCY

Managing women with bleeding disorders in pregnancy is challenging. Attention must be given to prevention of bleeding complications in the mother as well as considering the risk of inheritance and bleeding for the baby. Conditions that are considered here are disorders of primary haemostasis including von Willebrand's disease and platelet function disorders, and inherited coagulation defects, including haemophilia A and B and the rare coagulopathies.

Von Willebrand's disease

Von Willebrand's disease (vWD) is the most common inherited bleeding disorder, with an incidence of around 1% of the population. VWF is a large multimeric glycoprotein required for platelet adhesion. It also acts as a carrier for factor VIII, maintaining its stability in the circulation. There are three main types of vWD: type 1 is due to a quantitative reduction in vWF levels and accounts for around 80% of cases of vWD; type 2 is due to a functional deficiency in vWF and is subdivided by the particular defect. These types have autosomal dominant inheritance but clinical penetrance is variable and the severity of bleeding problems is not consistent in family members. Type 3 vWD is characterised by complete absence of vWF, due to autosomal recessive homozygosity or compound heterozygosity.

KEY POINTS: VON WILLEBRAND'S DISEASE

Type 1: Quantitative deficiency of vWF
Type 2: Qualitative deficiency of vWF
Type 3: Complete absence of vWF
Laboratory diagnosis: APTT may be normal.
                            Test for vWF:Ag, factor VIII, vWF:RCo, vWF:CBA.

Symptoms consist of mucosal bleeding and bleeding after surgery or trauma associated with failure of primary plug formation. Most affected individuals will be diagnosed in childhood, but in some women, childbirth may present the first significant haemostatic challenge.

Laboratory tests show reduced vWF antigen (vWF:Ag), with or without accompanying low factor VIII levels and reduced functional ability of vWF with ristocetin (vWF:RCo) and collagen-binding activity (vWF:CBA). In type 1 disease, both the vWF level and function are reduced in parallel. In type 2 disease the vWF:RCo is disproportionately reduced.

Management of von Willebrand's disease in pregnancy

Patients should be managed in conjunction with a haemophilia centre. VWF and fVIII levels rise from 6 weeks' gestation and often reach three times their baseline level by delivery. For most patients with type 1 disease, this rise is significant, enough to bring their vWF levels into the normal range, so that no special precautions are required for delivery.

Pre-pregnancy care

Management should begin with pre-pregnancy counselling of the couple, outlining the inheritance patterns and potential risks to the mother and fetus. Individual bleeding risk and response to treatment should be assessed. Women should be warned about the potential need for plasma products during delivery and consented appropriately. Antenatal diagnosis is not usually offered owing to the mild bleeding phenotype in these disorders, except where both parents have the condition and the baby is at risk of type 3 vWD.[24] Women should be vaccinated against hepatitis A and B if this has not already been done.

Antenatal care

Given the physiological rise in vWF in pregnancy, many women with type 1 disease will achieve levels of above 50 IU/dL, which is the lower limit of normal. vWF levels, including vWF:Ag, factor VIII and ristocetin cofactor activity (RiCof) should be performed at booking, at 28 weeks' gestation and prior to any invasive procedures. If the levels have risen adequately, no further testing is required. However, if levels are below 50 IU/dL, testing should be repeated at 34 weeks.

Treatment options for vWD in pregnancy

Treatment options include DDAVP or plasma concentrates. DDAVP is a synthetic vasopressin (antidiuretic hormone) analogue and stimulates the release of vWF multimers from endothelial cells. It can be given intravenously or subcutaneously. A trial of DDAVP should be done before pregnancy to assess its utility in each individual case. It is particularly useful in patients with type 1 vWD, but may also be beneficial in some patients with type 2 disease, although the release of abnormal vWF means that the functional deficit may not be

overcome. It should not be used in type 2B, which is associated with increased platelet binding, as it may exacerbate the thrombocytopenia. It is of no use in type 3 vWD. It is also contraindicated in patients with arterial disease or pre-eclampsia as there are reports of myocardial and cerebral infarction. Due to the antidiuretic effect, DDAVP will cause fluid retention and women should be advised to restrict their fluid intake to only quenching thirst, for 24 hours.

In cases where DDAVP is contraindicated, or does not produce significant improvement in vWF levels or where the response is unknown, factor concentrates will be required. There are a number of virally inactivated plasma-derived vWF/FVIII concentrates available. Treatment should be given 1 hour preoperatively or at the onset of established labour.[24]

KEY POINTS: MANAGEMENT OF PREGNANCY IN WOMEN WITH vWD

Pre-pregnancy:	Pre-conceptual counselling with inheritance risk.
	Discuss prenatal diagnosis in severe cases.
	Assess maternal bleeding risk and treatment options.
	Perform DDAVP trial in type 1 and type 2 disease.
	Consent for use of plasma products.
	Ensure immunity against hepatitis A and B.
Antenatal:	Check vWF levels at booking, 28 weeks and 34 weeks if low.
	Cover procedures with DDVAP or factor concentrates if vWF or vWF:RCo <50 IU/dL.
	Form an intrapartum care plan.
Intrapartum:	Maintain levels >50 IU/dL.
	Avoid fetal scalp monitoring, Ventouse, rotational forceps.
Postnatal:	Risk of delayed PPH so monitor bleeding symptoms and Hb in all cases and vWF levels in severe cases.
	Tranexamic acid 1 g three times daily for 2 weeks.
Neonate:	Minimise trauma at birth.
	Avoid intramuscular vitamin K.
	Test cord blood for vWF:Ag and vWF:RCo.
	Consider cranial ultrasound scan in affected infants.

Intrapartum management

Particular risks for the mother in the intrapartum period include postpartum haemorrhage (PPH) and perineal haematoma. The consensus expert opinion is that both vWF:Ag and vWF:RCo should be above 50 IU/dL for safe vaginal delivery or caesarean section.[25] Due to the risk of intracranial bleeding in the fetus, traumatic delivery should be avoided as far as possible. Prolonged labour, fetal scalp monitoring and vacuum extraction or rotational forceps should be avoided.

Postpartum management

Factor VIII and vWF levels can fall rapidly postpartum, occurring between 24 hours and 2 weeks. Women with vWD are therefore at risk of delayed postpartum haemorrhage and this occurs in 20–25% of cases. The average time of presentation of PPH in women with vWD is 10–20 days. The risk of PPH can be reduced by active management of the third stage of labour and by minimising perineal trauma. Women should be warned of the risk of delayed bleeding and advised to seek help early. Hb should be monitored and oral tranexamic acid given for 2 weeks. Those with type 2 and type 3 disease will need close observation with measurement of vWF levels. Women with type 3 disease or those who have a caesarean section should continue to receive treatment for 7 days after delivery.

Diagnosis of vWD in the neonate

A cord blood sample should be tested for vWF:RCo and oral vitamin K should be given in place of intramuscular vitamin K while the result is awaited.

Haemophilia

Haemophilia is the clinical syndrome produced by the deficiency of either factor VIII (haemophilia A), or factor IX (haemophilia B or Christmas disease). The genes for both factor VIII and IX are found on the X chromosome and the disorders are X-linked recessive. Therefore males are clinically affected and females are carriers. Females may have reduced factor levels due to a skew in the X-chromosome inactivation (unbalanced lyonisation). The incidence of haemophilia A is 1:5000 male births and 1:30,000 for haemophilia B.

Haemophilias can be classified according to the residual activity of the coagulation factor in question, which is also predictive of their bleeding symptoms:

Mild: >5%

Moderate: 1–5%

Severe: <1%

Patients with mild haemophilia are likely to bleed in response to trauma or other haemostatic challenges but spontaneous bleeding is rare. In contrast, boys with severe

---

KEY POINTS: HAEMOPHILIA

Genetics: X-linked recessive, males are affected, females are carriers.

Clinical: Classified as mild, moderate or severe. Muscle and joint bleeds, bleeding after trauma.

Haemophilia A: Deficiency in factor VIII.

Haemophilia B: Deficiency in factor IX.

---

haemophilia suffer with spontaneous major bleeding events affecting joints and muscles, resulting in chronic joint arthropathy, if attention is not given to effective prophylaxis.

Haemophilia in pregnancy

Pregnancy should be managed in a comprehensive care centre by a team of obstetricians, haematologists and anaesthetists who are experienced in managing patients with haemophilia and where there is 24-hour access to suitable laboratory facilities. Good communication between these teams and the neonatologist is paramount. There should be a written intrapartum care plan accessible to all staff involved with the patient's care.

Levels of factor VIII rise steadily in pregnancy from 6 weeks, therefore most women with low factor VIII will have achieved normal levels by delivery. Factor IX levels remain unchanged and women with low levels are likely to need treatment around the time of delivery.

Pre-pregnancy management

The risk of inheritance should be discussed with the parents prior to conception. Female carriers of the haemophilia gene have a 50% chance of having an affected male and a 50% chance of having a daughter who is a carrier. Sons born to affected males are not affected but daughters are obligate carriers. The severity of the bleeding pattern tends to follow in family lines and therefore it can be predicted whether the child will be mildly, moderately or severely affected. The role of prenatal diagnosis should be discussed. Fetal sex can be determined by maternal blood sampling, testing circulating fetal DNA for Y-chromosome-specific sequences.[26] This can be done from 7 weeks' gestation and will obviate the need for further investigations in female fetuses.

If prenatal diagnosis is not wanted, fetal sex should be determined at the anomaly scan as this information is vital for the intrapartum care plan. For male fetuses some centres also perform third-trimester amniocentesis to determine the presence of haemophilia.[24]

Antenatal management

The mother should have her factor VIII levels checked at booking then again at 28 weeks' gestation. If levels are still low, they should be re-checked at 34 weeks' gestation. Factor IX levels do not change and therefore need to be checked only at booking. Factor levels should also be checked before invasive procedures such as amniocentesis or CVS or if there is spontaneous abortion or termination of the pregnancy.

Treatment options

DDAVP will usually give a significant rise in factor VIII levels, unless baseline levels are <15 IU/dL, in which case factor VIII concentrates may be required. DDAVP does not affect factor IX levels and women with low factor IX levels will need treatment with factor IX concentrates. Recombinant factor concentrates are the treatment of choice.

Intrapartum management

Expert consensus opinion is that factor levels should be >50 IU/dL for vaginal delivery and caesarean section. The level should be brought to >100 U/dL pre-delivery and maintained at >50 U/dL for 3–5 days post-partum. If the fetus is considered to be at risk, fetal trauma should be minimised by avoiding fetal blood sampling, fetal scalp electrodes, Ventouse delivery and the use of mid-cavity and rotational forceps.[27]

The use of spinal anaesthesia is controversial in women with bleeding disorders due to the risk of spinal haematoma; however, if the factor level is >50 U/dL, it is not contraindicated.

KEY POINTS: MANAGEMENT OF HAEMOPHILIA CARRIERS IN PREGNANCY

Pre-pregnancy:	Pre-conception counselling.
	Bleeding risk in mother and fetus.
	Offer pre-implantation or antenatal genetic diagnosis.
	Check baseline factor levels and consent for products.
	Ensure hepatitis immunity.
Antenatal:	Determine fetal sex at anomaly scan or by Y-chromosome testing after 10 weeks.
	Check factor VIII/factor IX levels at booking.
	Factor factor VIII levels rise in pregnancy therefore repeat at 28 weeks' gestation and 34 weeks' gestation.
	Factor levels need to be >50 U/dL for procedures.
	DDAVP can be used to increase factor VIII levels.
	Recombinant factor concentrates will be required for factor IX deficiency or with very low factor VIII levels.
Intrapartum:	Maintain levels >50 U/dL for vaginal delivery, caesarean section and spinal anaesthesia.
	Avoid fetal scalp monitoring, prolonged labour, Ventouse or forceps delivery.
Postpartum:	Maintain factor levels for 3-5 days.
	Consider the use of tranexamic acid.
Neonate:	Cord blood at delivery for factor levels.
	Avoid intramuscular vitamin K until results known.
	Cranial ultrasound (USS) for moderate or severe haemophilia.

It is equally important for factor levels to be sufficient when removing a spinal catheter, therefore levels should be rechecked prior to removal.

Postnatal management

The risk of PPH can be reduced by active management of the third stage of labour. One study of female haemophilia carriers found the rate of primary and secondary PPH to be 19% and 2% respectively.[28] Factor levels should be maintained for 3 days postpartum and for 5 days in women who have had a caesarean section. Tranexamic acid may be useful to reduce bleeding symptoms. Care must be taken to maintain levels <100 U/dL as there is an increased thrombotic risk with levels above this threshold.

Diagnosis of haemophilia in the neonate

Cord blood should be sent immediately after birth to test for factor VIII or factor IX levels. Oral vitamin K should be given in place of intramuscular vitamin K where the child is known to be affected or if the results are awaited. Cranial ultrasound should be undertaken in all infants with moderate or severe haemophilia prior to discharge.[27]

THROMBOEMBOLIC DISEASE AND PREGNANCY

Venous thromboembolic disease in pregnancy

Despite the risk of venous thromboembolism (VTE) being significantly increased by pregnancy and particularly the postpartum period, the absolute risk remains low, at around 1:1000. However pulmonary embolism is one of the leading causes of maternal mortality and deaths occur where management has been tardy or sub-standard (MMBRACE). Detection of VTE in pregnancy is particularly problematic and, whilst a high index of suspicion must be maintained, it is important not to undertake unnecessary investigations.

Deep vein thrombosis (DVT)

The three elements of Virchow's triad are alterations in blood flow (stasis), alterations in blood coagulability and damage to the vascular endothelium. Venous stasis occurs in pregnancy with a reduction of up to 50% in venous flow by 29 weeks' gestation. Hypercoagulability results from a rise in procoagulant factors, a fall in anticoagulant factors and a reduction in fibrinolytic activity. Vascular endothelial damage occurs at the time of delivery, contributing to the higher risk of VTE in the puerperium.

Almost 90% of DVTs occurring in advanced pregnancy develop in the left leg, with 70% involving the iliofemoral veins. These carry a significantly higher risk of embolisation to the pulmonary circulation than distal DVTs. The signs and symptoms of DVT are outlined in Table 12.3.

Diagnosis can be particularly difficult in pregnancy as the methods that would be relied upon in non-pregnant women are often inadequate. Clinical probability scores have not been adequately validated, although the LEFt rule shows promise. This combines three variables: symptoms in the left leg (L), calf circumference difference of 2 cm or more (E for oedema) and first-trimester presentation (Ft). Two studies with a combined total of 135 patients found that no one with a negative LEFt rule had DVT and propose its usefulness as a negative predictive test when used in conjunction with other tools, such as D-dimers and/or ultrasound.[29,30]

The value of negative D-dimers in excluding VTE in non-pregnant patients with a low clinical probability score has been well demonstrated. However, they rise progressively in pregnancy and by delivery are elevated to approximately three times normal. They are therefore less likely to be helpful in excluding VTE in pregnant patients. Thus professional bodies differ in their recommendations, but a pragmatic approach would be to consider their use for women presenting in the first and possibly second trimesters.

Compression duplex ultrasonography of the lower limb is both sensitive and specific for DVT. However, the calf veins may be difficult to visualise and, if it is negative but a high index of suspicion remains, anticoagulation should be continued and the scan repeated in a week (Green top, Grade C). If the repeat scan is negative, a DVT can be excluded and anticoagulation stopped.

Iliac vein thrombosis may not be detected by ultrasound scan and if there is entire leg swelling or unexplained back pain, magnetic resonance venography or contrast venography should be considered.

Pulmonary embolism

Signs and symptoms of PE are outlined in Table 12.3. The high frequency of non-specific chest pain and breathlessness in pregnancy leads to many women being scanned for PE, with a positive detection rate of only around 2%. Therefore non-invasive tests should be used wherever possible (Box 12.5).

A chest X-ray should be performed initially to exclude other pathology such as infection. This will be normal in about 50% of cases but changes associated with a PE may be seen, including atelectasis, effusion, focal opacities or pulmonary

Table 12.3 Signs and symptoms of venous thromboembolism

Symptoms and signs of venous thromboembolism	
DVT	Leg pain and swelling, (usually unilateral)
	Erythema
	Tenderness over the affected area
Pelvic vein thrombosis	Lower abdominal pain
	Back pain
PE	Shortness of breath,
	Chest pain, usually pleuritic
	Haemoptysis
Submassive/ massive PE	Collapse
	Cyanosis
	Pain and breathlessness
Non-specific features	Low-grade temperature
	Leukocytosis

- PE, pulmonary embolism.

Box 12.5 Non-invasive tests that may be helpful in the diagnosis of suspect PE

ECG: can show classic S1,Q3,T3 appearance or signs of right heart strain such as P pulmonale, right bundle-branch block or right axis deviation.

Pulse oximeter: although patients are rarely hypoxic.

D-dimers: may be helpful in first and second trimesters.

Leg ultrasound: should be done if there are signs and symptoms of DVT, as PE can be assumed without confirmation if DVT is detected.

Bilateral leg ultrasound: may be considered in women without signs and symptoms of DVT, as a positive result would obviate the need for lung scanning.

Table 12.4 Diagnostic imaging in suspected pulmonary embolism

	Advantages	Disadvantages
CTPA	Lower dose of radiation to fetus	Higher dose of radiation to the breast tissue with a 13.6% increased lifetime risk of developing breast cancer
	Better sensitivity and specificity to $\dot{V}/\dot{Q}$ scan	
	Can detect other pathology e.g. aortic dissection	May miss small peripheral PEs
	Readily available	
$\dot{V}/\dot{Q}$ scan	Lower dose of radiation to the breast tissue	$10 \times$ higher dose of radiation to the fetus
	The ventilation scan can often be omitted, further lowering the radiation dose	Scan may be delayed because of the availability of isotope
	High negative predictive value	

oedema. If any of these abnormalities are seen and/or there is a high clinical suspicion of PE, definitive imaging should be arranged. If the chest X-ray is normal, a bilateral Doppler ultrasound scan of the legs may be considered, which may indirectly confirm the presence of a PE without the need for further radiation exposure.

More definitive imaging requires computed tomography pulmonary angiogram (CTPA) or Ventilation–Perfusion ($\dot{V}/\dot{Q}$) scan. There are small radiation risks associated with both, which need to be discussed with the patient (Table 12.4); however, ultimately the choice of scan usually depends on availability and local protocols.

Initial treatment of acute VTE in pregnancy

Prior to starting anticoagulation, samples should be sent for full blood count, urea and electrolytes, liver function tests and coagulation screen. Thrombophilia testing is not recommended in the acute setting (see below for discussion of thrombophilia testing in pregnancy).

If there is likely to be a significant delay before investigations are complete or the index of suspicion is high, anticoagulation should be started until the diagnosis is confirmed or refuted. The anticoagulant of choice is LMWH.[31,32] Meta-analyses have shown that, in comparison with unfractionated heparin (UFH), LMWH is equally efficacious and has a reduced risk of haemorrhagic complications[33] and lower overall mortality. The risk of heparin-induced thrombocytopenia and osteoporosis is also significantly less. Vitamin K antagonists should not be used in pregnancy, as they are teratogenic in the first trimester and associated with haemorrhagic complications and central nervous system (CNS) anomalies at all stages of pregnancy.

The LMWHs commonly used in the UK include enoxaparin, dalteparin or tinzaparin. Due to altered pharmacokinetics in pregnancy, both enoxaparin and dalteparin are usually given as a twice-daily dose to begin with, with some centres reducing to a once-daily intermediate dose after 2–4 weeks, if symptoms and signs are resolving. Tinzaparin is given once daily. LMWH therapy does not require monitoring with anti-factor Xa levels, except for extremes of weight, renal disease or if VTE has occurred while on LMWH, when they may be helpful to guide dosing. Although the test is limited by lack of standardisation and wide inter-laboratory variation, in-house experience allows reasonable interpretation of the assay result and the activity level is considered therapeutic at 0.5–1.2 U/mL 3 hours after injection. Unfractionated heparin may be preferred if the acute thrombotic event occurs near term, as the half-life is short and it can be continued for longer before delivery. It is also more easily monitored, readily reversed and not a concern in renal impairment.

Duration of anticoagulation will be determined by the circumstances of the VTE but should continue throughout pregnancy and until at least 6 weeks postpartum.[32] A total of at least 3 months' therapy should be given and in the absence of any other provoking factors this should be extended to 6 months.

Heparin-induced thrombocytopenia is very rare in pregnant women on LMWH and routine platelet monitoring is not recommended. However, the risk is higher with UFH and, if patients are being treated with UFH or have received UFH prior to LMWH, the platelet count should be monitored every 3–4 days until 2 weeks.

Women should be advised to wear a class II graduated compression stocking on the affected leg for at least 2 years after the acute event. This reduces pain and swelling and lowers the risk of post-thrombotic syndrome. Knee-length stockings have been shown to be just as effective as thigh length and are easier to manage. Contrary to previous advice, once anticoagulation has been started, women should be encouraged to mobilise while wearing their compression hosiery.

Massive PE in pregnancy

There are a number of case reports regarding the successful use of thrombolytic therapy for acute massive PE in pregnancy. RCTs outside pregnancy show that, if restricted to massive PE, there is a lower rate of recurrent PE or death, compared with using heparin alone. However, maternal haemorrhage and/or fetal loss may occur in approximately 1–3%. As data are minimal, thrombolysis should be reserved for those women with life-threatening PE.[31]

Inferior vena caval filters

Inferior vena caval filters are rarely required but can be helpful if the thrombotic event has occurred within a week of delivery, or if PE has developed despite anticoagulation or where anticoagulation is contraindicated. Potential complications include migration, infection and an increased risk of DVT. Occasionally temporary filters cannot be retrieved and long-term anticoagulation is necessary to reduce the DVT risk.

Management at the time of delivery

The delivery should be planned by induction of labour or elective caesarean section. This minimises the risk of delivery while fully anticoagulated and allows the option of spinal anaesthesia.

An intraoperative care plan should be generated and coordination between obstetricians and anaesthetists is essential. The dose of LMWH should be reduced to once daily the day before procedure. If a spontaneous presentation occurs, the woman should be advised not to inject herself with LMWH once there are any signs of labour. To avoid the risk of spinal haematoma, neuraxial anaesthesia is contraindicated within 24 hours of a therapeutic dose of LMWH and LMWH should not be given within 4 hours of catheter removal. The risk of wound haematoma and postpartum haemorrhage is increased and women should be monitored for 1–2 days after delivery.

Postnatally, the patient should be given the choice of continuing on LMWH or switching to an oral anticoagulant. Neither warfarin nor LMWH is contraindicated in breastfeeding. The new oral anticoagulants should be avoided in pregnancy and breastfeeding. The ongoing risk of thrombosis and requirement for anticoagulation should be discussed postnatally, taking into account the circumstances surrounding the acute event, family history and ongoing risk factors. A thrombophilia screen should be performed if deemed appropriate.

Thrombophilia and antiphospholipid syndrome in pregnancy

The presence of a heritable or acquired thrombophilia increases the relative risk of VTE in pregnancy. A systematic review studied the increased risk associated with all the thrombophilias; homozygosity for factor V Leiden (FVL) was the most prothrombotic, with a 34-fold increase in the relative risk of thrombosis. Tests for inherited thrombophilia include measurement of protein C, protein S and antithrombin levels, and genotyping for FVL and prothrombin G20210A mutations. Antiphospholipid syndrome is an acquired thrombophilia and requires testing for anticardiolipin antibodies and lupus anticoagulant.

Thrombophilia testing

A thrombophilia screen should not be performed during an acute event as it may give misleading results. It may, however, have a role after a period of anticoagulation to determine management in a future pregnancy, although this is largely based on the clinical circumstances surrounding the initial thrombotic event and the presence of transient provoking factors. It is important to note that the protein S levels may not return to normal baseline for a number of weeks and therefore testing should be delayed until at least 12 weeks postpartum. The limitations of thrombophilia testing should be understood, as negative results do not guarantee the absence of an inherited factor and positive results may be given too much importance. Guidelines from the BCSH state that thrombophilia testing need not be performed in women who suffer an unprovoked VTE as in future pregnancies they will qualify for thromboprophylaxis on clinical grounds alone.[34] Conversely, if there was a clear provoking factor at the time of VTE, for example a lower-limb plaster cast, antenatal thromboprophylaxis is unlikely to be required in a future pregnancy. The difficulty lies with those patients in whom there was a weak provoking factor and it is in these cases that a thrombophilia screen may be most valuable in determining future risk.

Antiphospholipid syndrome

Antiphospholipid syndrome (APLS) is an autoimmune disorder that is characterised by vascular thrombi and/or pregnancy morbidity in the presence of persistent antiphospholipid (aPL) antibodies, specifically anticardiolipin antibodies (aCL), β_2-glycoprotein 1 antibodies or a lupus anticoagulant (LAC). It may be a primary disease or occur in association with other autoimmune disease as secondary APLS. It is not completely understood why the presence of anticardiolipin antibodies

results in a prothrombotic syndrome but it is thought that antibodies against a particular domain of β_2-glycoprotein 1 play a major role. β_2-glycoprotein is an apolipoprotein that has a role in the regulation of haemostasis as well as many other physiological functions. It has been shown that the presence of LAC is most predictive of thrombosis.[35] Conversely, the sole presence of ACL antibodies does not appear to be associated with an increased thrombotic risk but is associated with increased pregnancy morbidity.[36]

Obstetric complications include early miscarriage, late pregnancy loss, premature delivery and early onset pre-eclampsia. Thrombosis may occur in the placental bed, inflammatory cell infiltrate results from activation of complement and aPL may cause direct damage to the trophoblasts, affecting invasive ability.[37]

Epidemiology

Antiphospholipid antibodies are found in 3–5% of healthy individuals and in up to 30% of individuals with SLE. Among patients suffering recurrent pregnancy loss, 10–20% have detectable aPL antibodies and up to 90% will have further fetal loss if left untreated.

Diagnosis requires the presence of one clinical criterion and one laboratory criterion; it therefore follows that testing should be performed in the clinical situations described (Box 12.6).

Box 12.6 Diagnostic criteria for antiphospholipid syndrome (Sapporo's criteria)

Clinical criteria

- Vascular thrombosis: one or more episodes of arterial, venous or small-vessel thrombosis.

- Pregnancy morbidity:

  (a) One or more unexplained deaths of a morphologically normal fetus at or beyond week 10 of gestation.

  (b) One or more preterm births of a morphologically normal neonate before week 34 of gestation because of (i) eclampsia or severe pre-eclampsia or (ii) recognised features of placental insufficiency.

  (c) Three or more unexplained consecutive spontaneous miscarriages before week10 of gestation, with maternal anatomical or hormonal abnormalities and paternal and maternal chromosomal causes excluded.

Laboratory criteria

- The LAC present in plasma, on two or more occasions at least 12 weeks apart.

- The aCL antibody of IgG and/or IgM isotype in serum or plasma, on two or more occasions, at least 12 weeks apart.

- Anti-β_2-glycoprotein 1 antibody of IgG and/or IgM isotype in serum or plasma, present on two or more occasions at least 12 weeks apart.

Management of APLS and pregnancy

APLS associated with VTE

These women should be managed as other women who have previously suffered an unprovoked VTE. They may well be on long-term oral anticoagulation and should be advised to stop this and start taking LMWH as soon as they have confirmation of pregnancy. This should be at a high or an intermediate dose. If the previous thrombotic event was associated with a clear provoking factor then prophylactic LMWH may be sufficient. Each case should be considered individually to assess current risk factors for thromboembolic disease. Aspirin 75 mg daily should also be given from 12 weeks' gestation. The patient should be regularly reviewed to assess ongoing thrombotic risk and should be offered serial growth scans with uterine artery Doppler to ensure adequate placental function.

APLS associated with pregnancy morbidity

A Cochrane review of 13 studies found that aspirin and unfractionated heparin are superior to aspirin alone in preventing miscarriage.[38] Smaller studies have shown the benefit of LMWH and aspirin and there is now vast experience of using LMWH, which remains the agent of choice[39] due to its ease of use and more favourable safety profile. There is less evidence to confirm its benefit in reducing late-pregnancy morbidity, pre-eclampsia, preterm birth and IUGR associated with APLS but aspirin is proven to improve outcomes in these conditions.

Thromboprophylaxis

Whilst VTE remains one of the leading causes of maternal death, the fact is that many of these cases could have been avoided. Several CEMACH/national audit reports have highlighted the need to identify those women who are at risk and ensure that adequate thromboprophylactic measures are taken. In 2008, a case–control study undertaken by the UK Obstetric Surveillance System (UKOSS) revealed that, of 143 cases of pulmonary embolism, only 9 should have received thromboprophylaxis on risk assessment criteria of the time, and only 3 of these had actually done so. Also six women had a PE whilst on thromboprophylaxis, three of whom were on an inadequate dose. The risk is greatest postnatally with studies showing as high as a 60-fold increase compared with the non-pregnant population.[40] Whilst risk increases as pregnancy advances, many studies have shown that the incidence of VTE in the first trimester is also significantly increased compared with the non-pregnant state, with one American study revealing 44% of DVTs occurring in the first trimester.[41]

Reducing risk of VTE

All women should undergo a VTE risk assessment early on in pregnancy which should be reassessed if the woman is admitted to hospital or if her clinical situation changes in any way.

The 2009 Green-top guideline, which is due to be updated shortly, defines the approach to risk assessment and thromboprophylaxis in pregnant women. Education of midwives and pregnant women pays a significant part in reducing the occurrence and early identification of VTE in pregnancy.

General antithrombotic advice should be given to all women – the importance of maintaining good hydration and mobility and, in times of unavoidable immobility, for example travel situations or illness, to regularly perform feet and ankle

Table 12.5 Adapted from Robertson *et al.* Risk of VTE with associated thrombophilias[44]

Thrombophilic defect	Adjusted OR for risk of VTE
AT deficiency	4.7
Protein C deficiency	4.8
Protein S deficiency	3.2
FVL heterozygous	8.3
Prothrombin G20210A heterozygous	6.8
FVL homozygous	34.4
Prothrombin G20210A homozygous	26.4

- OR, odds ratio.

Table 12.6 Additional risk factors for VTE in pregnancy and the puerperium

Pre-existing	New onset or transient	Specific to postpartum
Age >35 years	Ovarian hyperstimulation syndrome	Caesarean section (especially emergency)
Obesity (BMI >30 kg/m²)	Hyperemesis	Prolonged labour
Parity >3	Dehydration	Mid-cavity instrumental delivery
Gross varicose veins	Severe infection	Postpartum haemorrhage
Sickle cell disease	Long-distance travel	Immobility after delivery
Smoking	Immobility	
Paraplegia	Pre-eclampsia	
Inflammatory bowel disease	Hospital admission/surgical procedure	
Medical disorders: pre-existing diabetes		
Family history in first-degree relative especially in presence of thrombophilia		

exercises. The signs and symptoms of a DVT or PE should be outlined to all women to increase the chance of early diagnosis and treatment.

Assessing individual risk (Table 12.5)

Early identification of those women at risk of VTE can allow counselling and commencement of thromboprophylaxis. The single greatest risk factor for VTE in pregnancy is a previous thrombotic event. One retrospective study of 1104 pregnant women with previous VTE found an incidence of recurrent VTE of 5.8%. This was increased if the first event was unprovoked, or related to pregnancy or hormonal therapy. The rate of recurrence in the puerperium was 15% if the first VTE was pregnancy related.[42] Conversely, there was no increased risk of recurrence if the previous event was provoked by a transient risk factor. For women with a weak provoking factor, the risk of recurrence is less clear and a thrombophilia screen may be helpful in guiding the use of thromboprophylaxis.

Up to 50% of women who suffer a VTE in pregnancy will have an underlying thrombophilia; however, some thrombophilias confer a greater risk than others; homozygotes for FVL or prothrombin gene mutation, compound heterozygotes and women with antithrombin deficiency have the highest risks and intermediate to high doses of LMWH are required throughout pregnancy and for at least 6 weeks postnatally.[43]

A number of other factors have been shown to significantly increase the risk of VTE in pregnancy and are listed in Table 12.6. In reality the individual risk is an interplay of many factors: the more factors present, the higher the risk of VTE. Some risk factors carry more weight than others and it is therefore difficult to validate a scoring system that is appropriately weighted. For simplicity and applicability, RCOG suggest adding the number of risk factors with the recognition that coexistent risk factors have an additive effect.

A large Norwegian case–control study of over 600,000 pregnancies showed that the overall incidence of VTE was 1:1000 and antenatal risk factors associated with increased risk were assisted reproduction, gestational diabetes, age older than 35 years and multiple pregnancies. Postnatal risk factors were caesarean section, pre-eclampsia, assisted reproduction, placental abruption and placenta previa.[45] The UKOSS 2008 study also showed that the strongest risk factors for VTE were multiparity and obesity.[46] A recently published UK cohort study of >300,000 deliveries[47] suggested that the risk factors traditionally associated with increased VTE risk in pregnancy and postnatally were associated only with moderately increased risk. However, during the antepartum period, varicose veins, inflammatory bowel disease, urinary tract infection and pre-existing diabetes were associated with a significant increased risk for VTE. Postpartum the strongest risk factor was stillbirth; however, medical co-morbidities, including varicose veins, inflammatory bowel disease (IBD) and cardiac disease, a BMI of 30 kg/m² or higher, obstetric haemorrhage, preterm delivery, and caesarean section were

Table 12.7 Prophylactic dosing schedules for LMWH in pregnancy

Dose	Enoxaparin	Dalteparin	Tinzaparin
Standard prophylactic			
<50 kg	20 mg OD	2500 units OD	3500 units OD
50–90 kg	40 mg OD	5000 units OD	4500 units OD
91–130 kg	60 mg OD or 40 mg BD	7500 units OD or 5000 units BD	7000 units OD
131–170 kg	80 mg OD or 40 mg BD	10,000 units OD or 5000 units BD	
High prophylactic			
	40 mg BD	5000 units BD	4500 units BD
Treatment/therapeutic			
	1 mg/kg BD	100 units/ kg BD	175 units/ kg OD

- BD, twice daily; OD, once daily.

also all associated with increased risk. The same group also confirmed the significant risk associated with hospital admission, increased by 17.5 times.[48]

Management

All women should undergo risk assessment for VTE in early pregnancy or pre-pregnancy. The history and circumstances of any previous events should be assessed, along with family history and any known thrombophilic defects. Risk assessment should be repeated if the situation changes to take account of additional transient risk factors. A thrombophilia screen may help to determine risk in cases where there is a personal history of VTE with a weak provoking factor, or if there is no personal history but a strong family history of unprovoked VTE.

Pharmacological

LMWHs are the agent of choice due to ease of use and a large body of experience supporting their safety and efficacy. Dalteparin, enoxaparin or tinzaparin is the LMWH used in the UK. The dose should take account of the patient's early pregnancy weight; patients <50 kg will require a reduced dose whilst those >90 kg will require a higher dose (Table 12.7).

Duration, dose and timing of LMWH will depend on the risk group. The RCOG have divided women with a previous history of VTE into three risk groups:

– Very high risk: recurrent VTE, or VTE associated with a high-risk thrombophilia. These women should receive an intermediate to high dose of LMWH.

– High risk: previous unprovoked or hormone-related VTE or a previous VTE with other risk factors or a family history suggesting thrombophilia. These women should be considered for standard-dose LMWH antenatally and for 6 weeks postpartum.

– Intermediate risk: previous VTE was provoked by a major risk factor which is no longer present. These women may not need LMWH but should be reassessed regularly through pregnancy and LMWH should be given if any additional risk factor arises. They should receive LMWH for 6 weeks postpartum.

For those without a previous history of VTE but with a thrombophilia, or a family history, thromboprophylaxis is likely to be required postnatally and should be considered antenatally if other risk factors are present. For women with multiple risk factors as outlined above, thromboprophylaxis should be given postnatally for 6 weeks and should be considered antenatally. Table 12.8 shows indications for postpartum thromboprophylaxis.

Table 12.8 Indications for postpartum thromboprophylaxis

Indication	Usual duration of LMWH (weeks)
Received antenatal prophylaxis	6
Previous VTE	6
Class III obesity	1
Emergency caesarian section	1
Elective caesarian section with one or more additional risk factors	1
Presence of some thrombophilias without personal history of VTE	1

Aspirin

The role of aspirin in preventing VTE in pregnancy has not been validated and there are no recommendations for its use or otherwise for thromboprophylaxis in pregnant women. Outside pregnancy it has been shown to reduce the risk of recurrent VTE by 40% compared with placebo, with no increase in major bleeding.[49]

Graduated elastic compression stockings

If correctly applied, anti-embolic stockings may reduce the occurrence of VTE. They are advised for women with previous VTE, those undertaking long journeys and hospitalised women in whom LMWH is contraindicated. They are also recommended in addition to LMWH for women post-caesarean section with multiple additional risk factors.

Management of labour

Women should be advised to withhold any further doses of LMWH as soon as there are signs of labour or if they have any vaginal bleeding. Regional anaesthesia should not be used for

12 hours after a prophylactic dose of LMWH. Women should be encouraged to stay hydrated and to remain as mobile as possible.

Key References

1. Streetly A, Latinovic R and Henthorn J. Positive screening and carrier results for the England-wide universal newborn sickle cell screening programme by ethnicity and area for 2005-07. *Journal of Clinical Pathology* 2010;63:626–629.

2. Aessopos A, Karabatsos F, Farmakis D *et al.* Pregnancy in patients with well-treated β-thalassemia: outcome for mothers and newborn infants. *Am J Obstet Gynecol* 1999;180(2 Pt 1):360–5.

3. Nassar AH, Naja M, Cesaretti C, Eprassi B, Cappellini MD, Taher A. Pregnancy outcome in patients with β-thalassemia intermedia at two tertiary care centers, in Beirut and Milan. *Haematologica* 2008;93:1586–7

4. Nassar AH, Usta IM, Rechdan JB, Koussa S, Inati A, Taher AT. Pregnancy in patients with β-thalassemia intermedia: outcome of mothers and newborns. *Am J Hematol* 2006; 81:499–502.

5. NHS Screening Programmes. *NHS Sickle and Thalassaemia Screening Programme.* Standards for the linked antenatal and newborn screening programme, 2ed. London: UK National Screening Committee, 2011.

6. UKOSS: UK Obstetric Surveillance Team. Annual Report. 2012.

7. Villers MS, Jamison MG, De Castro LM, James AH. Morbidity associated with sickle cell disease in pregnancy. *Am J Obstet Gynecol* 2008;199:125.e1–5.

8. Serjeant GR, Hambleton I, Thame M. Fecundity and pregnancy outcome in a cohort with sickle cell–haemoglobin C disease followed from birth. *BJOG* 2005;112:1308–14.

9. NICE. *Hypertension in Pregnancy. The management of hypertensive disorders during pregnancy.* NICE clinical guideline 107. London: NICE, 2010.

10. James AH, Jamison MG, Brancazio LR, Myers ER. Venous thromboembolism during pregnancy and the postpartum period: incidence, risk factors, and mortality. *Am J Obstet Gynecol* 2006;194:1311–15.

11. RCOG. *Management of Sickle Cell Disease in Pregnancy.* Green-top Guideline No. 61, 2011.

12. Okusanya BO, Oladapo OT. Blood transfusion policies for sickle cell disease in pregnancy. Cochrane Database Published online: 2013.

13. McCrae KR. Thrombocytopenia in pregnancy. In: Michelson AD, ed. *Platelets.* New York: Elsevier, 2006, 925–33.

14. Gill KK, Kelton JG. Management of idiopathic thrombocytopenic purpura in pregnancy. *Semin Hematol* 2000;37:275–89.

15. Provan D, Stasi R, Newland AC *et al.* International consensus report on the investigation and management of primary immune thrombocytopenia. *Blood* 2010;115.168–86.

16. Webert KE, Mittal R, Sigouin C, Heddle NM and Kelton JG. A retrospective 11-year analysis of obstetric patients with idiopathic thrombocytopenic purpura. *Blood* 2003;102:4306–11.

17. Christiaens GC, Niewenhuis HK, Bussel JB. Comparison of platelet counts in first and second newborns of mothers with immune thrombocytopenic purpura. *Obstetrics and Gynaecology* 1997;90:546–52.

18. RCOG. *The Use of Anti-D Immunoglobulin for Rhesus D Prophylaxis*. Green-top Guideline No. 22, 2011.

19. Qureshi H, Massey E, Kirwan D *et al*. BCSH guideline for the use of anti-D immunoglobulin for the prevention of haemolytic disease of the fetus and newborn. *Transfusion Medicine* 2014;24:8–20.

20. MacKenzie IZ, Bowell P, Gregory H, Pratt G, Guest C, Entwistle CC. Routine antenatal Rhesus D immunoglobulin prophylaxis: the results of a prospective 10 year study. *Br J Obstet Gynaecol* 1999;106:492–7.

21. Alcock GS, Liley H. Immunoglobulin infusion for isoimmune haemolytic jaundice in neonates. Cochrane Database of Systematic Reviews 2002; CD003313.

22. Pacheco LD, Berkowitz RL, Moise KJ Jr *et al*. Fetal and neonatal alloimmune thrombocytopenia: a management algorithm based on risk stratification. *Obstet Gynecol* 2011;118:1157.

23. Berkowitz RL, Kolb EA, McFarland JG. *et al*. Parallel randomized trials of risk-based therapy for fetal alloimmune thrombocytopenia. *Obstet Gynecol* 2006;107:91.

24. Lee CA, Chi C, Pavord SR. *et al*. The obstetric and gynaecological management of women with inherited bleeding disorders – review with guidelines produced by a taskforce of UK Haemophilia Centre Doctors Organization. *Haemophilia* 2006;12:301–336.

25. Pasi KJ, Collins PW, Keeling DM. *et al*. Management of von Willebrand disease: a guideline from the UK Haemophilia Centre Doctors' Organization. *Haemophilia* 2004;10:218–31.

26. Bustamante-Aragones A, Rodriguez de Alba M, Gonzalez-Gonzalez C *et al*. Foetal sex determination in maternal blood from seventh week of gestation and its role in diagnosing haemophilia in the foetuses of female carriers. *Haemophilia* 2008; 14:593–8.

27. Chalmers E, Williams M, Brennand J, Liesner R, Collins P, Richards M. Guideline on the management of haemophilia in the fetus and neonate. *British Journal of Haematology* 2011;154:208–15.

28. Chi C, Lee CA, Shiltagh N, Khan A, Pollard D, Kadir RA. Pregnancy in carriers of haemophilia. *Haemophilia* 2008;14:56–64.

29. Chan WS, Lee A, Spencer FA. *et al*. Predicting deep venous thrombosis in pregnancy: out in 'LEFt' field?. *Ann Intern Med* 2009;151: 85–92.

30. Righini M, Jobic C, Boehlen F. *et al*. and the EDVIGE study group. Predicting deep venous thrombosis in pregnancy: external validation of the LEFt clinical prediction rule. *Haematologica* 2013;98:545–8.

31. Bates SM, Greer IA, Middeldorp S, Veenstra DL, Prabulos AM, Vandvik PO. VTE, thrombophilia, antithrombotic therapy, and pregnancy VTE, Thrombophilia, Antithrombotic Therapy, and Pregnancy: antithrombotic therapy and prevention of thrombosis, 9th ed: American College of Chest Physicians Evidence-Based Clinical Practice Guidelines. *Chest* 2012;141:e691S-e736S.

32. RCOG. *The Acute Management of Thrombosis and Embolism During Pregnancy and the Puerperium*. Green-top Guigeline No. 37b, 2007. London, RCOG.

33. Greer IA, Nelson-Piercy C. Low-molecular-weight heparins for thromboprophylaxis and treatment of venous thromboembolism in pregnancy: a systematic review of safety and efficacy. *Blood* 2005;106:401–7.

34. Baglin T, Gray E, Greaves M *et al*. Clinical guidelines for testing for heritable thrombophilia. *British Journal of Haematology* 2010;149:209–20.

35. Galli M, Luciani D, Bertolini G, Barbui T. Lupus anticoagulants are stronger risk factors for thrombosis than anticardiolipin antibodies in the antiphospholipid syndrome: a systematic review of the literature. *Blood* 2003;101:1827–32.

36. Pengo V, Biasiolo A, Pegoraro C, Cucchini U, Noventa F and Iliceto S. Antibody profiles for the diagnosis of antiphospholipid syndrome. *Thromb Haemost* 2005;93:1147–52.

37. D'Ippolito S, Di Simone N, Di Nicuolo F, Castellani R, Caruso A. Antiphospholipid antibodies: effects on trophoblast and endothelial cells. *Am J Reprod Immunol* 2007;58:150–8.

38. Empson M, Lassere M, Craig, Scott J. Prevention of recurrent miscarriage for women with antiphospholipid antibody or lupus anticoagulant. The Cochrane Library, 2005.

39. Keeling D, Mackie I, Moore GW, Greer IA, Greaves M and BCSH. Guidelines on the investigation and management of antiphospholipid syndrome. *British Journal of Haematology* 2012;157:47–58.

40. Pomp ER, Lenselink AM, Rosendaal FR, Doggen CJ. Pregnancy, the postpartum period and prothrombotic defects: risk of venous thrombosis in the MEGA study. *J Thromb Haemost* 2008;6:632–7.

41. James AH, Tapson VF, Goldhaber SZ. Thrombosis during pregnancy and the postpartum period. *American Journal of Obstetrics and gynaecology* 2005;193:216–19.

42. De Stefano V, Martinelli I, Rossie E *et al*. The risk of recurrent venous thromboembolism in pregnancy and puerperium without antithrombotic prophylaxis. *British Journal of Haematology* 2006;135:386–91.

43. RCOG. *Reducing the Risk of Thrombosis and Embolism During Pregnancy and the Puerperium*. Green-top Guideline No. 37a, 2009. London, RCOG.

44. Robertson L, Wu O, Langhorne P *et al*. Thrombosis: risk and economic assessment of thrombophilia screening (TREATS) study. Thrombophilia in pregnancy: a systematic review. *Br J Haematol* 2005;132:171–96.

45. Jacobsen AF, Skjeldestad FE, Sandset PM. Incidence and risk patterns of venous thromboembolism in pregnancy and puerperium – a register-based case-control study. *Am J Obstet Gynecol* 2008;198:233.

46. Knight M on behalf of UKOSS. Antenatal pulmonary embolism: risk factors, management and outcomes. *BJOG* 2008;115:453–61.

47. Sultan AA, Tata LJ, West J *et al.* Risk factors for first venous thromboembolism around pregnancy: a population-based cohort study from the United Kingdom. *Blood* 2013;121:19.

48. Sultan AA, West J, Tata LJ, Fleming KM, Nelson-Piercy C, Grainge MJ. Risk of first venous thromboembolism in pregnant women in hospital: population based cohort study from England. *BMJ* 2013;347:f6099.

49. Becattini C, Agnelli G, Schenone A *et al.* for the WARFASA Investigators. Aspirin for preventing the recurrence of venous thromboembolism. *N Engl J Med* 2012;366:1959–67.

Chapter 13 Renal disease

Catherine Nelson-Piercy

MRCOG standards

Relevant standards

To understand and demonstrate appropriate knowledge, skills and attitudes in relation to pregnant women with kidney disease.

Theoretical skills

Understand the epidemiology, aetiology, pathophysiology, clinical characteristics, prognostic features and management of women with kidney disease.

Practical skills

Be able to manage independently:
- urinary tract infection,
- pyelonephritis.

Be able to manage under direct supervision pregnant women with:
- chronic kidney disease,
- a renal transplant,
- acute kidney injury.

INTRODUCTION

Urinary tract infection (UTI) is a common cause of maternal morbidity and a potential cause of perinatal morbidity and mortality via preterm delivery. Renal disease is an important predisposing factor for pre-eclampsia and fetal growth restriction (FGR). The combination of hypertension and proteinuria at booking (provided that this is in the first or early second trimester) suggests pre-existing renal disease and should prompt further investigation. A serum creatinine is mandatory in such cases to exclude pre-existing chronic kidney disease (CKD).

The number of women with renal transplants considering pregnancy is increasing and success rates are high, but case selection is required. Acute kidney injury in pregnancy is most commonly due to obstetric conditions, particularly haemorrhage and pre-eclampsia.

PHYSIOLOGICAL CHANGES IN PREGNANCY

There is dilatation of the ureters and renal calyces in pregnancy. This must be remembered when interpreting ultrasound scans of the renal and urinary tract systems in pregnancy. Both renal plasma flow and glomerular filtration increase dramatically in pregnancy.[1] This results in an increased urinary protein excretion and increased creatinine clearance.[1] Thus, in the second trimester, the upper limit of normal for serum creatinine falls to around 65 μmol/L with a mean of 54 μmol/L,[1] and throughout pregnancy the upper limit of normal for proteinuria is taken as 300 mg/24 hours or a protein:creatinine ratio less than 30 mg/mmol.

URINARY TRACT INFECTION

Incidence

Urinary tract infection is more common in pregnancy because of the physiological dilatation of the upper renal tract. The incidence of asymptomatic bacteriuria in pregnancy ranges from 4 to 7 per cent, and up to 40 per cent of the women affected will develop symptomatic UTI in pregnancy. Cystitis complicates about 1 per cent of pregnancies, and 1–2 per cent of pregnant women develop pyelonephritis. Women who have a history of previous UTIs are at increased risk of a UTI in pregnancy, as are those with diabetes, receiving steroids or immunosuppression, or with polycystic kidneys, reflux nephropathy, congenital abnormalities of the renal tract (e.g. duplex kidney or ureter), neuropathic bladder (e.g. spina bifida or multiple sclerosis) or urinary tract calculi.

Presentation

A midstream urine (MSU) specimen performed as part of routine antenatal screening may reveal asymptomatic bacteriuria. Additional MSUs are indicated in pregnancy in those women at increased risk as described above, and those with symptoms of UTIs. Typical clinical features are urinary frequency, dysuria, suprapubic pain, haematuria, proteinuria and nitrites on urinalysis. Fever, loin and/or abdominal pain, vomiting and rigors suggest pyelonephritis.

Diagnosis

Much dipstick proteinuria in pregnancy is erroneously attributed to UTIs. Indeed, a diagnosis of pre-eclampsia may not be considered if it is assumed that proteinuria is due to UTI (see Chapter 26). Dipsticks for nitrites and leukocyte esterase may be used to help exclude UTIs, but their positive predictive value is low and therefore any positive dipstick should be followed up with an MSU. A clinical diagnosis should always be confirmed with culture of an MSU sample. Bacteriuria is considered significant if there are more than 100,000 organisms per millilitre of urine. Urine culture resulting in a non-significant or mixed growth should be repeated on a fresh MSU specimen.

Management

All bacteriuria in pregnancy requires treatment to prevent pyelonephritis and preterm delivery (Cochrane guideline A) (Box 13.1). Treatment for 3 days is sufficient for asymptomatic bacteriuria [E].[2] Regular urine cultures should be taken following treatment to ensure eradication of the organism. About 15 per cent of women will have recurrent bacteriuria during the pregnancy and will require a second course of antibiotics. The choice of antibiotic depends on the sensitivities of the causative organism, but, in suspected pyelonephritis, treatment should begin before the results of culture are available. Penicillins (amoxicillin) and cephalosporins are safe and appropriate antibiotics in pregnancy. Augmentin (co-amoxiclav) increases the risk of necrotising enterocolitis in the neonate. Cefadroxil 500 mg twice daily is effective against the majority of urinary pathogens. Nitrofurantoin should be avoided in the third trimester as it may cause haemolytic anaemia in the neonate and trimethoprim should be avoided in the first trimester because of its antifolate action. For acute cystitis, a 7-day course of antibiotics is recommended and antibiotics should be continued for 10–14 days for pyelonephritis [E].[2]

In pyelonephritis with vomiting or pyrexia, antibiotics should be given intravenously until the pyrexia settles; intravenous fluids may also be required. Renal function should be checked. Ultrasound examination of the renal tract is indicated in those with pyelonephritis or two or more proven UTIs. This is to exclude hydronephrosis, congenital abnormalities and renal calculi. Continuous prophylactic antibiotics are usually recommended only for those with two or more confirmed (with a positive culture) UTIs and either one of the above risk factors or in those with renal transplants.

Box 13.1 Suggested treatment regimens for urinary tract infection (UTI) in pregnancy

Oral antibiotics

Amoxicillin 500 mg three times daily

Cefadroxil 500 mg twice daily

Cephalexin 250 mg three times daily

Nitrofurantoin 100 mg three times daily (not third trimester)

Trimethoprim 200 mg twice daily (not first trimester)

Intravenous antibiotics for pyelonephritis

Cefuroxime 750 mg to 1.5 g three times daily

Amoxicillin 1 g three times daily

Gentamicin 5–7 mg/kg daily as one dose and then further doses as determined by serum gentamicin concentrations (for organisms resistant to, or women allergic to, penicillins and cephalosporins)

Duration of treatment

Asymptomatic bacteriuria: 3 days

Acute cystitis: 7 days

Pyelonephritis: 10–14 days

Prophylaxis of UTI

Cephalexin 250 mg once daily

Amoxicillin 250 mg once daily

CHRONIC KIDNEY DISEASE

Aetiology

In women of child-bearing age, the most common causes of CKD are reflux nephropathy, diabetes, SLE, other forms of glomerulonephritis and adult polycystic kidney disease. Conventionally, CKD is classified as CKD 1–5 depending on the degree of renal impairment[1] (Table 13.1). However, it must be remembered that the eGFR is not validated for use in pregnancy, so the serum creatinine level should be used. However, the serum creatinine is also dependent on the muscle mass, so a figure that represents moderate impairment in an 85-kg woman may represent severe impairment for a 50-kg

Table 13.1 Stages of chronic kidney disease

Stage	GFR (mL/min per 1.73 m^2)
1	>90
2	60–89
3	30–59
4	15–29
5	<15 or dialysis

ANTENATAL OBSTETRICS

woman. It has been estimated that around 1 in 750 pregnancies is complicated by CKD stages 3–5.

Presentation

If renal disease is not diagnosed pre-pregnancy, it is usually first recognised because of hypertension and proteinuria and/or haematuria in early pregnancy, prompting blood tests for urea and creatinine. However, a common caveat is to attribute hypertension and proteinuria to underlying renal disease rather than to the much more common pre-eclampsia, which may rarely present before 20 weeks' gestation. If there is no record of blood pressure or urinalysis in the first trimester to allow the hypertension and proteinuria to be designated 'new onset', a differentiation between pre-eclampsia and renal disease is more difficult.

Effect of pregnancy on renal impairment

In general, those with mild impairment (creatinine <125 µmol/L; CKD 1–2) tolerate pregnancy well and do not usually suffer deterioration in renal function as a result of the pregnancy. The serum creatinine will follow a trend similar to that in normal pregnancy, i.e. it will fall to a nadir in the second trimester and then rise again but remain below non-pregnant levels in the third trimester. Conversely, those with severe impairment of renal function (creatinine >180 µmol/L; CKD 3b–5) are at increased risk of permanent loss of function during and after the pregnancy (50 per cent will have a permanent decline in function) and even end-stage renal failure (35 per cent within 1 year) [C].[1]

Effect of CKD on pregnancy outcome

All women with renal impairment are at increased risk of pre-eclampsia, FGR, and spontaneous and iatrogenic preterm delivery [C].[1,3] Again, outcome depends on the level of impairment and the level of any pre-existing hypertension [C].[3–6] Those with severe renal impairment (creatinine >250 µmol/L) and hypertension have a less than 50 per cent chance of successful pregnancy, often developing severe, early-onset pre-eclampsia with marked FGR. Even in the absence of pre-eclampsia or uteroplacental dysfunction, one may be faced with the need to deliver a woman with rapidly worsening renal function (or to institute dialysis), resulting in a pre-viable or extremely preterm infant. For these reasons, it is usual to counsel women with severe renal impairment against pregnancy [C].[3–5] Women with severe renal impairment may also develop polyhydramnios and the risk of cord prolapse. This is probably the result of fetal polyuria in response to the high osmotic load from increased maternal urea. Those with nephrotic syndrome and heavy proteinuria also develop worsening hypoalbuminaemia in pregnancy, with the associated risks of pulmonary oedema and venous thrombosis.

Management

This should begin with pre-pregnancy counselling and should involve multidisciplinary care by clinicians with expertise in the management of these high-risk pregnancies.[3]

It is important to document baseline (pre-pregnancy and early pregnancy) values for creatinine, albumin and protein excretion. Some increase in proteinuria is inevitable in pregnancy and does not necessarily indicate superimposed pre-eclampsia or worsening renal disease. Deterioration in renal function at any stage in pregnancy should prompt a search for reversible causes such as UTI, obstruction or dehydration.

Tight control of any hypertension is important to minimise the risk of deterioration in renal function. Blood pressure should be maintained below 140/90 mmHg.[3] The choice of antihypertensive agents is no different in women with renal disease [E]. Many renal patients, especially those with significant proteinuria, are treated with ACEIs or ARBs. These should be discontinued prior to or in early pregnancy as they are teratogenic [C].[7] Diuretics are also usually discontinued and their use restricted to severe hypoalbuminaemia with fluid overload and incipient pulmonary oedema [D].

Not only are women with renal disease at high risk of pre-eclampsia, but it is also often difficult to diagnose in the presence of pre-existing hypertension and proteinuria. Admission should be considered with worsening hypertension, increasing serum creatinine, and large increases in proteinuria. Useful additional features to support a diagnosis of pre-eclampsia include FGR, thrombocytopenia and abnormal liver function. The use of prophylactic low-dose (75 mg/day) aspirin is appropriate to decrease the risk of pre-eclampsia in all those with CKD [A].[8] Serial scans for fetal growth and liquor volume, and serial haematology and biochemistry are essential in the monitoring of these pregnancies [D].[3,9]

If CKD is discovered for the first time in pregnancy, and the hypertension and proteinuria are not readily attributable to pre-eclampsia, investigation should include blood glucose (for diabetes), serum calcium, antinuclear antibodies (for SLE),[9] immunoglobulins (for IgA) and a renal tract ultrasound (e.g. for polycystic kidneys, reflux nephropathy with scarring or to demonstrate small kidneys suggestive of chronic renal failure) [D].

EBM

- The risks of obstetric complications such as pre-eclampsia, FGR and iatrogenic preterm delivery increase with increasing baseline serum creatinine.
- The chances of successful pregnancy decrease with increasing baseline serum creatinine.
- The risks of temporary and permanent deterioration in renal function increase with increased baseline serum creatinine.
- Women with severe renal impairment (creatinine >250 µmol/L; CKD 4-5) are usually advised against pregnancy.

Postpartum, continued close monitoring is necessary to ensure the renal function returns to pre-pregnancy levels. ACEIs may be safely used in breastfeeding women. Those with newly suspected underlying renal disease should be referred to a nephrologist.

RENAL TRANSPLANTS

The rates of successful pregnancy outcome in women with well-functioning renal transplants are similar to those of the general population. However, a recent UK-wide study of 105 renal transplant recipients found that 24% developed pre-eclampsia and the same percentage had an SGA baby; over 50% delivered before 37 weeks' gestation. Women are usually advised to delay pregnancy for a year after transplantation to allow graft function to stabilise and immunosuppression to reach maintenance levels [E]. The risks of adverse outcome in pregnancy relate to the pre-pregnancy level of function of the allograft and the presence of hypertension (C).[10,11]

In addition, these women are immunosuppressed and therefore more prone to infection. There are substantial data regarding the safety of immunosuppressive drugs in pregnancy. Prednisolone [C], azathioprine [C], ciclosporin[10] [C] and tacrolimus [C] are all considered safe. Recent data suggest that tacrolimus is not transferred to breast milk in significant quantities and women should be encouraged to breastfeed[12] [E]. Mycophenolate mofetil (MMF) is teratogenic in humans.[10] Women can usually be switched from MMF to azathioprine prior to pregnancy.

DIALYSIS

Because women with end-stage renal failure have markedly reduced fertility, pregnancy on dialysis is unusual. The chances of a successful pregnancy outcome are sufficiently low, and the attendant risks sufficiently high, to counsel women on dialysis against pregnancy [E].[3] Anaemia and haemorrhage are common, and the risks of miscarriage, fetal death, pre-eclampsia, preterm labour, preterm rupture of the membranes, polyhydramnios and placental abruption are increased [C].[13] Pregnancy outcome in CKD has improved with modern dialysis techniques and livebirth rates are up to 80 per cent,[14] but pregnancy is not advised in women on dialysis. Women who decide to continue with pregnancy require increasing frequency of dialysis in order to maintain the pre-dialysis urea, 15–20 mmol/L [C].[3,11] The incidence of poor obstetric outcome is similar with both haemodialysis and peritoneal dialysis.

ACUTE KIDNEY INJURY IN PREGNANCY

Acute kidney injury (AKI) is rare in pregnancy, the most common causes being pre-eclampsia and related syndromes, haemorrhage, infections, drugs, particularly NSAIDs, and obstruction due to a gravid uterus or ureteric damage or stones. Mild degrees of renal impairment are more common, and again are usually related to pre-eclampsia or blood loss. AKI most commonly complicates the early postpartum period. It is characterised by oliguria, a rising urea and creatinine, a metabolic acidosis and hyperkalaemia. In the obstetric situation, there may be an associated coagulopathy. An isolated rise in urea (without concomitant rise in creatinine) is often observed following antenatal corticosteroid administration. A rare cause of AKI that is most commonly encountered postpartum is haemolytic uraemic syndrome (HUS). The hallmark of this condition is a microangiopathic haemolytic anaemia (diagnosed with a blood film) associated with renal failure and thrombocytopenia.

Pre-eclampsia and renal failure

Oliguria is an almost universal finding in pre-eclampsia and is exacerbated by Syntocinon and caesarean section. It does not alone indicate AKI, but should prompt measurement of serum urea and creatinine. AKI is more common in acute fatty liver of pregnancy[15] (see Chapter 15), HELLP syndrome (7 per cent) [C][16] and eclampsia (6 per cent) than in 'straightforward' pre-eclampsia. HELLP syndrome is the most common cause (50 per cent) of AKI in the context of pre-eclampsia.

The management of AKI depends on the cause: blood volume replacement for haemorrhage, delivery for pre-eclampsia, cessation of nephrotoxic drugs. Postpartum management is largely conservative and supportive. Accurate assessment of fluid balance with the use of a central venous pressure (CVP) line is important. Provided that blood loss and volume depletion have been excluded as causes (CVP high or normal), fluids are given only to replace insensible losses and the previous hour's urine output. Iatrogenic fluid overload must be avoided in pre-eclampsia because these women are often hypoalbuminaemic and particularly susceptible to pulmonary oedema. Overzealous fluid administration is far more dangerous than oliguria. Dialysis may rarely become necessary, but a need for long-term renal replacement therapy is extremely unusual.

KEY POINTS

- UTIs are common in pregnancy, and bacteriuria requires treatment to prevent pyelonephritis and preterm labour.
- The risks of complications, such as pre-eclampsia and FGR, and deterioration in renal function are high, and the chances of successful pregnancy lower in women with severe renal impairment (CKD 4-5).
- Women with well-functioning renal allografts generally have successful pregnancies, but should be advised to delay pregnancy until a year after transplantation.
- Women on dialysis should be advised to delay pregnancy until they have received a renal transplant.
- Acute kidney injury is rare, but may complicate haemorrhage and pre-eclampsia.

Published Guidelines

NICE. *Hypertension in Pregnancy.* NICE Clinical Guideline 107. London: NICE, 2010. Available from: www.nice.org.

Vazquez JC, Abalos E. Treatments for symptomatic urinary tract infections during pregnancy. Cochrane Database of Systematic Reviews 2011: CD002256. DOI: 10.1002/14651858.CD002256.pub2.

Key References

1. Williams D, Davison J. Chronic kidney disease in pregnancy. *BMJ* 2008;336:211–15.
2. Cattell WR. Urinary tract infection in women. *J R Coll Phys Lond* 1997;31:130–33.
3. Davison J, Nelson-Piercy C, Kehoe S, Baker P (eds). *Renal Disease in Pregnancy.* Report of RCOG Study Group. London: RCOG, 2008.
4. Palma-Reis I, Vais A, Nelson-Piercy C, Banerjee A. Renal disease and hypertension in pregnancy. *Clin Med* 2013;13:57–62.
5. Jones DC, Hayslett JP. Outcome of pregnancy in women with moderate or severe renal insufficiency. *N Engl J Med* 1996;335:226–32.
6. Jungers P, Chauveau D. Pregnancy in renal disease. *Kidney Int* 1997;52:871–85.
7. Cooper WO, Hernandez-Diaz S, Arbogast PG *et al.* Major congenital malformations after first-trimester exposure to ACE inhibitors. *N Engl J Med* 2006;354: 2443–51.
8. Duley L, Henderson-Smart DJ, Knight M, King JF. Antiplatelet agents for preventing pre-eclampsia and its complications Cochrane Database of Systematic Reviews 2007;2:CD004659.
9. Bramham K, Soh MC, Nelson-Piercy C. Pregnancy and renal outcomes in lupus nephritis: an update and guide to management. *Lupus* 2012;21:1271–83.
10. Armenti VT, Constantinescu S, Moritz MJ, Davison JM. Pregnancy after transplantation. *Transplant Rev* 2008; 22:223–40.
11. Bramham K, Nelson-Piercy C, Gao H *et al.* Pregnancy in renal transplant recipients: A UK National Cohort Study. *Clin J Am Soc Nephrol* 2013;8:290–8.
12. Bramham K, Chusney G, Lee J, Lightstone L, Nelson-Piercy C. Breastfeeding and tacrolimus. Serial monitoring in breast- and bottle-fed infants. *Clin J Am Soc Nephrol* 2013;8:563–7.
13. Hou SH. Pregnancy in women with chronic renal insufficiency and end stage renal disease. *Am J Kidney Dis* 1999; 33: 235–52.
14. Yang L Y, Thia EWH, Tan LK. Obstetric outcomes in women with end-stage renal disease on chronic dialysis: a review *Obstetric Medicine* 2010;3:48–53.
15. Knight M, Nelson-Piercy C, Kurinczuk JJ *et al.* A prospective national study of acute fatty liver of pregnancy in the UK. *Gut* 2008;57: 951–6.
16. Drakeley AJ, Le Roux PA, Anthony J, Penny J. Acute renal failure complicating severe preeclampsia requiring admission to an obstetric intensive care unit. *Am J Obstet Gynecol* 2002;186: 253–6.

Chapter 14 Autoimmune conditions

Catherine Nelson-Piercy

INTRODUCTION

This chapter covers the autoimmune connective tissue diseases, including rheumatoid arthritis (RA), systemic lupus erythematosus (SLE) and antiphospholipid syndrome (APS), Sjögren's syndrome and scleroderma. Autoimmune thrombocytopenia is discussed in Chapter 12; myasthenia gravis in Chapter 17; and autoimmune thyroid disease in Chapter 11.

Changes in the immune system in pregnancy result in relatively suppressed cell-mediated immunity and enhanced humoral immunity. These changes revert postpartum when there is a sudden reduction of oestrogen, progesterone and cortisol levels. The postpartum period is therefore a time of theoretical susceptibility to autoimmune disorders. This means that some autoimmune conditions such as RA often improve in pregnancy and may flare, worsen or present anew in the postpartum period. In pregnancy, many of the issues for women with connective tissue disease relate to the safety of the drugs used to control their disease and to the degree of any systemic involvement of their disease.

RHEUMATOID ARTHRITIS

This is a chronic, inflammatory, symmetrical arthritis causing joint pain, stiffness and deformity. Systemic features include rheumatoid nodules, pulmonary granulomas, vasculitis, Sjögren's syndrome (see below) and scleritis. Haematological abnormalities include a normocytic anaemia and raised erythrocyte sedimentation rate (ESR). Rheumatoid arthritis is usually associated with positive rheumatoid factor and anti-cyclic citrullinated peptide (anti-CCP). Thirty per cent of cases are antinuclear antibody (ANA) positive. Up to 20–30 per cent are Ro/La positive (see below) and 5–10 per cent are antiphospholipid (aPL) antibody positive (see below), although APS is rare. Pregnancy is associated with a decrease in T-cell immunity that is reversed postpartum.[1] This may explain why 48–66 per cent of women with RA experience improvement in their symptoms during pregnancy and why those who improve usually flare postpartum.[2]

Rheumatoid arthritis has no adverse effect upon pregnancy outcome. Limitation of hip abduction is rarely severe enough to preclude vaginal delivery, and atlantoaxial subluxation is a rare complication of general anaesthesia for caesarean section. Severe joint deformity and disability may rarely necessitate the need for help with care of the infant.

Management

Assessment of disease activity is usually clinical. The ESR is raised in normal pregnancy and does not therefore provide a reliable marker of disease activity. As arthritis often improves in pregnancy, some reduction in analgesia may be possible.

DRUGS FOR AUTOIMMUNE CONDITIONS

Paracetamol is safe in pregnancy and may be instituted or continued in maximal doses if required. The commonly used drugs for connective tissue disease are summarised in Table 14.1.[3]

NSAIDs, such as ibuprofen and diclofenac, are often used in women with RA and SLE. They are normally avoided in pregnancy because they are detrimental to the fetal kidney, causing oligohydramnios, and they may cause premature closure of the ductus arteriosus, leading to pulmonary hypertension and fetal haemorrhage, in large doses. Neither aspirin nor the other NSAIDs are teratogenic, so it is not necessary to discontinue these drugs prior to conception [C]. However, there is an association between NSAIDs and infertility due to luteinized unruptured follicle syndrome.[4] They should therefore be withdrawn if there is a history of infertility [D]. Occasionally, they are used in pregnancy when alternatives, such as paracetamol, codeine and corticosteroids, are inadequate or inappropriate. In such cases, they should be discontinued by 32 weeks' gestation, as at later gestations the effects on the fetal renal function and the ductus are irreversible.[3] The selective cyclooxygenase-2 (COX-2) inhibitors are also contraindicated in pregnancy.

Corticosteroids are the first-line anti-inflammatory drugs in pregnancy.[3] They are used for many connective tissue diseases, not only for the arthritis manifestations, but also to treat vasculitis, skin involvement, renal lupus and thrombocytopenia. There is no evidence to support the premise that steroids will prevent flare, either antenatal or postnatal, but they remain the mainstay of management for these disorders in pregnancy. They must never be withheld because of erroneous fears concerning their effects on the fetus. Many women are understandably reluctant to use any drugs, but particularly steroids, in pregnancy and therefore, if they are used, this must be with adequate counselling regarding their safety in pregnancy to ensure concordance with therapy [E].

Table 14.1 Safety in pregnancy of drugs used for autoimmune conditions

Safe to continue or start in pregnancy	Discontinue or avoid in pregnancy
Paracetamol	NSAIDs
Hydroxychloroquine	Cyclophosphamide
Sulfasalazine	Gold
Corticosteroids	Penicillamine
Azathioprine	Methotrexate
	Chlorambucil
	Leflunamide
	Mycophenolate mofetil

Any possible small risk of teratogenesis (there are some data suggesting a small increased risk of oral clefting with first trimester exposure[5]) is dwarfed by the beneficial effects to the fetus of controlling the maternal disease process [C]. Caution is needed because the use of steroids in pregnancy is associated with an increased risk of infections and gestational diabetes. Large doses of steroids are associated with an increased risk of preterm rupture of the membranes.

Azathioprine is also safe in pregnancy. The fetal liver lacks the enzyme that converts azathioprine to its active metabolites. Azathioprine is used as a 'steroid-sparing' agent and there are reassuring data regarding a lack of adverse effects on babies born to mothers receiving this drug for renal transplants, inflammatory bowel disease[6] and connective tissue diseases [C].[3] A study has shown that there are no detectable levels of the metabolites of azathioprine in the blood of neonates who were fully breastfed by women receiving azathioprine [D].[7]

Antimalarials such as hydroxychloroquine are safe in pregnancy [C].[3] Discontinuation of this drug is associated with a risk of SLE flare.

Sulfasalazine is safe in pregnancy and breastfeeding. It is a dihydrofolate reductase inhibitor and therefore associated with an increased risk of neural tube, oral cleft and cardiovascular defects. Folate supplementation (5 mg/day) is advised [B].

Gold and D-penicillamine used in RA are usually avoided in pregnancy, although the risk of abnormalities is probably low. Cytotoxic drugs, such as cyclophosphamide, methotrexate and chlorambucil, are all highly teratogenic and must be discontinued prior to pregnancy.[3] Mycophenolate mofetil, used in lupus nephritis, is teratogenic and women should be changed to azathioprine prior to pregnancy.[8]

The anti-tumour necrosis factor (TNF) biologic agents (etanercept, adalimumab and infliximab) are used increasingly in inflammatory arthritis. Available data suggest that these agents are safe in pregnancy but that they should ideally be discontinued by about 28-30 weeks' gestation depending on the individual drug [D].[8,9] It is important that live vaccines are avoided in the child for 6 months after birth.[9]

SYSTEMIC LUPUS ERYTHEMATOSUS

SLE is a relapsing and remitting multisystem connective tissue disorder that predominantly affects women of childbearing age. The diagnostic criteria are shown in Table 14.2. It most commonly affects the joints (symmetrical non-erosive peripheral arthritis and arthralgia), the skin (malar rash, photosensitivity, discoid lupus, alopecia, vasculitis, Raynaud's phenomenon) and the kidneys (glomerulonephritis). There may be anaemia, lymphopenia, thrombocytopenia, hypocomplementaemia and a raised ESR. The C-reactive protein (CRP) is not raised.

SLE is associated with ANA and anti-double-stranded DNA (dsDNA) antibodies. There may be antibodies to extractable nuclear antigens (ENAs) including Ro and La, or aPL antibodies with or without APS.

ANTENATAL OBSTETRICS

Table 14.2 American College of Rheumatology criteria for SLE

Malar rash	Renal disorder
Discoid rash	Neurological disorder
Photosensitivity	Haematological disorder
Oral ulcers	Immunological disorder
Arthritis	Antinuclear antibody
Serositis (e.g. pleurisy, pericarditis)	

- For a diagnosis of SLE, four of these criteria are required simultaneously or serially.

Effect of pregnancy on SLE

Pregnancy is associated with an increased risk of SLE flare, which may occur at any stage of the pregnancy or postpartum. Neither the severity nor the type (e.g. renal or skin) of flare is altered by pregnancy. Flares may be harder to diagnose in pregnancy because many features, such as fatigue, erythema, anaemia and hair loss, are common to both.[10]

Pregnancy does not alter the antibody profile but increases the ESR and may exacerbate thrombocytopenia.

Effect of SLE on pregnancy outcome

In women who have quiescent SLE, have no renal involvement and are Ro/La and aPL negative, there is no adverse effect of their disease on pregnancy.[10] Active disease at conception, renal involvement and APS increase the risks of miscarriage, pre-eclampsia, FGR, preterm delivery and stillbirth.

Management

This should begin with pre-pregnancy counselling enabling an accurate risk assessment for individual women. Women should be advised to conceive during periods of disease remission. Once pregnancy is confirmed (or pre-pregnancy if there is a delay in conception), NSAIDs are discontinued. Hydroxychloroquine is continued because it is safe, withdrawal may precipitate flare and it has a very long half-life such that the fetus remains exposed for up to 3 months after the mother discontinues the drug.[10] Prednisolone and azathioprine are also continued. During pregnancy, SLE flares are treated with new or increased doses of steroids [C].[10,11]

Not only are women with renal lupus at increased risk of pre-eclampsia, but also pre-eclampsia may be harder to diagnose in such women, who already have hypertension and proteinuria. Low platelets, renal impairment, oedema, worsening hypertension and proteinuria may be attributable to either. Pointers to a renal lupus flare include red cells or red cell casts in the urine, hypocomplementaemia (falling levels of C3 and C4) and a rising anti-DNA titre. Pointers to a diagnosis of pre-eclampsia include raised transaminases and absence of other features of SLE flare. Those at high risk of pre-eclampsia and

FGR should be offered serial growth scans and tests of fetal wellbeing as indicated. Regular visits to a joint obstetric/rheumatology clinic are important to screen for pre-eclampsia and SLE flare.

NEONATAL LUPUS SYNDROMES

These are caused by anti-Ro or anti-La antibodies and manifest as cutaneous neonatal lupus, affecting 5 per cent of babies of Ro-positive women, and congenital heart block, affecting 2 per cent of babies of Ro-positive women. If the first child is affected, the risk to the second child is 10-fold higher, and once two children are affected the risk rises to about 50 per cent. Neonatal cutaneous lupus develops in the first 2 weeks of life and is a geographical skin lesion of the face or scalp. It may be precipitated by exposure to ultraviolet light and usually regresses spontaneously without scarring within 6 months. Congenital heart block develops *in utero* at 18–30 weeks' gestation. There is no treatment, and one in five affected babies dies *in utero* or as a neonate. About half of those surviving require pacemakers in early infancy and the rest by their teens.[10] Ro-positive women should be offered fetal cardiology screening [C]. Retrospective data suggest hydroxychloroquine may reduce the risk of congenital heart block.

ANTIPHOSPHOLIPID SYNDROME

This describes the association of aPLs (either aCL antibodies or lupus anticoagulant) with the clinical features shown in Table 14.3.[12]

Additional clinical features include thrombocytopenia, livedo reticularis, epilepsy, migraine, heart valve disease and

Table 14.3 Classification criteria for antiphospholipid syndrome

Clinical criteria	
Thrombosis	Venous
	Arterial
	Small vessel
Pregnancy morbidity	Three or more consecutive miscarriages (<10 weeks)
	One or more fetal death (>10 weeks)
	One or more premature birth (<35 weeks) due to severe pre-eclampsia or placental insufficiency
Laboratory criteria	
Anticardiolipin antibody	IgG or IgM
	Medium/high titre
	Two or more occasions >12 weeks apart
Lupus anticoagulant	Two or more occasions >12 weeks apart

pulmonary hypertension. APS may be primary or found in association with SLE, RA or other connective tissue disease. Therefore women with primary APS, even if based on a positive lupus anticoagulant, do not have 'lupus' unless there are features of SLE (see Table 14.1).

The pathogenesis of APS involves a co-factor, beta-2 glycoprotein. Antiphospholipid antibodies reduce hCG release and inhibit trophoblast invasion in vitro – a potential explanation for the association with miscarriage. However, the 'typical APS' fetal loss occurs in the second trimester and is associated with severe FGR, oligohydramnios and early onset pre-eclampsia.[13]

The common feature is defective or abnormal placentation, possibly related to thrombosis.

Pregnancy in women with APS is associated with an increased risk of thrombosis. This is particularly so for women with previous thrombosis. APS is an acquired thrombophilia and may therefore affect unusual sites such as the axillary or retinal veins. What makes APS particularly dangerous is the fact that thrombosis may also affect arterial and small vessels, causing, for example, stroke or renal disease. In general, those women who have had a previous venous thrombosis are at risk of recurrent venous thromboses, and those with previous arterial thrombosis at risk of recurrent arterial events. Pregnancy also increases the risk of, or may exacerbate, pre-existing thrombocytopenia.

The effect of APS on pregnancy is to increase the risk of early and late miscarriage, stillbirth, placental abruption, FGR and pre-eclampsia.[13]

Management

APS should be managed in pregnancy by multidisciplinary teams with expertise in caring for these high-risk pregnancies. Those women with a previous history of arterial or venous thrombosis will usually be on long-term treatment with warfarin or other oral anticoagulants. This should be converted to aspirin and high prophylactic or treatment doses of LMWH as soon as pregnancy is confirmed and at least before 6 weeks' gestation to avoid warfarin embropathy (see Chapter 27). LMWH is continued in high prophylactic doses throughout pregnancy and postpartum for 6 weeks or until warfarin is recommended.

For women without a previous history of thrombosis, there is agreement that low-dose aspirin (75 mg/day) is beneficial, although supportive evidence is mostly from retrospective, non-randomised studies. Indeed, randomised studies do not support a beneficial effect of aspirin, but this is because such studies have included very-low-risk groups of women, some without any previous history of adverse pregnancy outcome. Low-dose aspirin is safe and all centres with an interest in APS use aspirin sometimes from pre-conception [D].[13] The role of LMWH in addition to aspirin is more controversial.[14] Two prospective studies of women with aPLs and recurrent miscarriage demonstrated significantly increased livebirth rates in

groups allocated to aspirin and LMWH versus those receiving aspirin alone, and current RCOG guidelines advocate the use of LMWH in addition to aspirin for women with recurrent miscarriage and aPLs (see Published guidelines at the end of this chapter). However, both these studies had an unusually low livebirth rate in the aspirin-alone groups. Two more recent randomised studies failed to show any increased benefit of LMWH over and above aspirin alone in women with APS and recurrent pregnancy loss.[14] That said, in women who have suffered late fetal losses or neonatal deaths attributable to APS, the risk of adverse pregnancy outcomes is higher and it is common to recommend LMWH in these situations [D].[13,15]

EBM

- Evidence supports the use of high prophylactic doses of LMWH throughout pregnancy in women with APS who have had previous thromboses.
- Evidence from retrospective and cohort studies supports a role for low-dose aspirin for fetal indications.
- There is growing evidence that the use of LMWH in addition to aspirin for recurrent miscarriage provides no additional benefit.

A suggested management plan is given in Table 14.4. The risk of pre-eclampsia, abruption, FGR and preterm delivery is less for women with APS diagnosed as a result of recurrent early miscarriage compared with those women with APS diagnosed as a result of later pregnancy adverse outcome.[13,15] Past obstetric history is the best predictor of risk, although success rates for women diagnosed and treated for APS are about 70–80 per cent.[13-15] All women require careful and regular monitoring for pre-eclampsia, and serial growth scans and tests of fetal wellbeing as appropriate [D].[13] Liaison with obstetric anaesthetists is vital prior to delivery in women receiving LMWH for any indication. In those who have had previous thromboses, discontinuation of LMWH peripartum should be minimal, but, for those receiving LMWH for purely fetal indications, it may simplify the management of analgesia and anaesthesia for labour and delivery if the LMWH is discontinued prior to delivery.

Table 14.4 Management recommendations for APS pregnancies

aPL antibodies; no thrombosis or pregnancy loss	Aspirin 75 mg or nothing
Previous thrombosis	LMWH and aspirin
Previous recurrent (>3) miscarriages (<10 weeks)	Aspirin +/- LMWH (? stop LMWH at 13-20 weeks)
Fetal loss or severe pre-eclampsia/FGR/NND	Aspirin + LMWH

- NND, neonatal death.

SJÖGREN'S SYNDROME

This typically causes dry eyes and a dry mouth. The dry eyes may be confirmed objectively with Schirmer's tear test. Similar to APS, Sjögren's syndrome may be primary or associated with SLE, RA or other connective tissue disease. This syndrome is typically associated with positivity for Ro and La antibodies, and therefore the risk of neonatal lupus and congenital heart block (see above). Primary Sjögren's syndrome is associated with the finding of positive rheumatoid factor and positive ANA, and hypergammaglobulinaemia.

SCLERODERMA

Scleroderma may occur as a localised cutaneous form, as systemic sclerosis, or as part of the CREST syndrome (calcinosis, Raynaud's phenomenon, (o)esophageal involvement, sclerodactyly and telangiectasia). Skin involvement produces characteristic facies with a beaked nose and limited mouth opening, limiting facial expression. Systemic fibrosis involves the oesophagus, the lungs, the heart and the kidneys. There is no effective definitive treatment for scleroderma, although symptoms may be controlled with calcium antagonists, prostacyclin and specific treatments for renal involvement (ACEIs) and pulmonary hypertension (sildenafil, bosentan).

Adverse effects on pregnancy relate to the degree of any renal, lung or cardiac involvement. Women with early diffuse disease are at increased risk in pregnancy and therefore women should be advised to postpone pregnancy until the disease has stabilised.[16] Those with severe pulmonary fibrosis or pulmonary hypertension should be advised against pregnancy [E]. Those with renal involvement and hypertension are at increased risk of pre-eclampsia and FGR. Oesophageal symptoms often increase in pregnancy, but those of Raynaud's phenomenon may improve secondary to vasodilatation.

Management

Pre-pregnancy counselling is vital to inform women accurately about the potential risks of pregnancy. Formal lung function and echocardiography to assess the extent of systemic involvement are recommended. During pregnancy, regular multidisciplinary assessment is required, with screens of blood pressure, urinalysis, renal function and maternal symptoms. Scleroderma renal crises are extremely dangerous and ACEIs should not be stopped in pregnancy or withheld [E]. Raynaud's phenomenon may be ameliorated with heated gloves and calcium antagonists. High-dose corticosteroids, such as used to induce fetal lung maturation, should be avoided because they may precipitate a renal crisis. Assessment by an obstetric anaesthetist prior to delivery is essential. In women with scleroderma, there are often problems with blood pressure measurement, venous access, capillary oxygen saturation monitoring and difficult airways.

KEY POINTS

- RA commonly improves in pregnancy and deteriorates postpartum.
- SLE is more likely to flare in pregnancy.
- Adverse pregnancy outcome in SLE is related to the presence of APS, renal involvement, disease activity and the presence of anti-Ro and -La antibodies.
- Ro and La antibodies are associated with Sjögren's syndrome and may cause congenital heart block and neonatal lupus.
- APS may cause arterial, venous or capillary thrombosis, miscarriage, late fetal loss, early onset pre-eclampsia and severe FGR.
- APS is treated in pregnancy with low-dose aspirin and LMWH.
- Steroids are safe to treat connective tissue disease in pregnancy and are used in preference to NSAIDs.

Published Guidelines

RCOG guidelines for recurrent miscarriage/APS. Guideline No. 17. London: RCOG. Recurrent Miscarriage, Investigation and Treatment of Couples (Green-top Guideline No. 17) https://www.rcog.org.uk/en/guidelines-research-services/guidelines/gtg17/

Key References

1. Nelson JL, Ostensen M. Pregnancy and rheumatoid arthritis. *Rheum Dis Clin North Am* 1997;23:195–212.
2. de Man YA, Dolhain RJ, van de Geijn FE, Willemsen SP, Hazes JM. Disease activity of rheumatoid arthritis during pregnancy: results from a nationwide prospective study. *Arthritis Rheum* 2008;59:1241–8.
3. Ostensen M, Khamashta M, Lockshin M *et al*. Anti-inflammatory and immunosuppressive drugs and reproduction. *Arthritis Res Ther* 2006;8:209–38.
4. Mendonca LLF, Khamastha MA, Nelson-Piercy C *et al*. Non-steroidal anti-inflammatory drugs as a possible cause for reversible infertility. *Rheumatology* 2000; 39:880–25.
5. Carmichael SL, Shaw GM, Ma C *et al*. National Birth Defects Prevention Study. Maternal corticosteroid use and orofacial clefts. *Am J Obstet Gynecol* 2007;197: 585.e1–7.
6. Akbari M, Shah S, Velayos FS, Mahadevan U, Cheifetz AS. Systematic review and meta-analysis on the effects of thiopurines on birth outcomes from female and male patients with inflammatory bowel disease. *Inflamm Bowel Dis* 2013;19(1):15-22.
7. Sau A, Clarke S, Bass J *et al*. Azathioprine and breastfeeding: is it safe? *BJOG* 2007;114:498–501.

8. Østensen M, Förger F. How safe are anti-rheumatic drugs during pregnancy? *Curr Opin Pharmacol* 2013; 13:470-5.

9. Hyrich KL, Verstappen SM. Biologic therapies and pregnancy: the story so far. *Rheumatology* (Oxford). 2014;53:1377-85.

10. McKillop L, Germain S, Nelson-Piercy C. SLE in pregnancy. *BMJ* 2007;335:933–6.

11. Ateka O, Nelson-Piercy C. Connective tissue disease in pregnancy. *Clin Medicine* 2013;13:580-4.

12. Miyakis S, Lockshin MD, Atsumi T *et al.* International consensus statement on an update of the classification criteria for definite antiphospholipid syndrome (APS). *J Thromb Haemost* 2006;8:295–306.

13. Soh M-C, Nelson-Piercy C. The antiphospholipid syndrome in pregnancy. *Expert Review of Obstetrics & Gynaecology* 2010;5:741-61.

14. Laskin CA, Spitzer KA, Clark CA *et al.* Low molecular weight heparin and aspirin for recurrent pregnancy loss: results from the randomized controlled HepASA trial. *J Rheumatol* 2009;36:279–87.

15. Bramham K, Hunt BJ, Germain S *et al.* Pregnancy outcome in women with antiphospholipid syndrome: Management in a tertiary referral centre. *Lupus* 2010;19:58–64.

16. Steen VD. Pregnancy in women with systemic sclerosis. *Obstet Gynecol* 1999; 94:15–20.

Chapter 15 Liver and gastrointestinal disease

Catherine Nelson-Piercy

MRCOG standards

Theoretical skills

Understand the epidemiology, aetiology, pathophysiology, clinical characteristics, prognostic features and management of women with liver and gastrointestinal disease.

Practical skills

Be able to manage independently:

- irritable bowel syndrome,
- reflux oesophagitis,
- hyperemesis,
- obstetric cholestasis.

Be able to manage under direct supervision pregnant women with:

- Crohn's disease and ulcerative colitis,
- acute fatty liver of pregnancy,
- hepatitis.

INTRODUCTION

Liver disease in pregnancy is encountered relatively rarely, but gastrointestinal problems, including nausea, vomiting, oesophageal reflux and constipation, are almost universal. Liver disease can be dangerous for both the mother and the fetus. This chapter considers the liver conditions specific to pregnancy – obstetric cholestasis and acute fatty liver of pregnancy – and those that pre-date or coincide with pregnancy – viral hepatitis and chronic liver disease. HELLP syndrome is discussed in Chapter 26. Gastrointestinal diseases usually pre-date the pregnancy; inflammatory bowel disease (IBD) and irritable bowel syndrome are the most common. Gastrointestinal problems exacerbated or brought on by pregnancy, such as gastro-oesophageal reflux and hyperemesis, are also discussed.

PHYSIOLOGICAL CHANGES IN PREGNANCY

Pregnancy causes decreased lower oesophageal pressure, decreased gastric peristalsis and delayed gastric emptying. Gastrointestinal motility is reduced, with increased small-bowel and large-bowel transit times. There is a 20–40 per cent fall in serum albumin concentration, partly due to dilution resulting from the increase in total blood volume. Total serum protein concentration also decreases. The alkaline phosphatase concentration more than doubles due to production by the placenta, which increases with gestation. Levels of alanine transaminase (ALT), serum glutamic–pyruvic transaminase (SGPT), aspartate transaminase (AST) and serum glutamic–oxaloacetic transaminase (SGOT) fall, and there is a fall in the upper limit of the normal ranges for these enzymes (Table 15.1).[1] Thus a mildly abnormal level for transaminases that may be significant in the diagnosis of obstetric cholestasis

Table 15.1 Normal ranges for liver enzymes in non-pregnant and pregnant women

Liver enzyme	Non-pregnant	First trimester	Second trimester	Third trimester
AST (IU/L)	7–40	10–28	10–29	11–30
ALT (IU/L)	0–40	6–32	6–32	6–32
Bilirubin (μmol/L)	0–17	4–16	3–13	3–14
γ-Glutamyl transferase (γ GT) (IU/L)	11–50	5–37	5–43	3–41
Alkaline phosphatase (IU/L)	30–130	32–100	43–135	133–418

or in the assessment of pre-eclampsia may be overlooked unless pregnancy-specific ranges are used. The concentrations of other liver enzymes are not substantially altered and there is no significant change in bilirubin concentration during normal pregnancy.

NAUSEA, VOMITING AND HYPEREMESIS

Nausea and vomiting are common symptoms in early pregnancy, affecting over half of pregnant women. The onset of symptoms is usually early in the first trimester at around 5–6 weeks' gestation. Hyperemesis is less common, but causes much morbidity and repeated hospital admissions and can be dangerous if inadequately or inappropriately treated. Nausea and vomiting in pregnancy become hyperemesis if the woman is unable to maintain adequate hydration and nutrition, because of either severity or duration of symptoms. This is associated with marked weight loss, muscle wasting, ketonuria, dehydration and electrolyte disturbance, including hypokalaemia and a metabolic hypochloraemic alkalosis. A common associated symptom is ptyalism – the inability to swallow saliva. The risks associated with hyperemesis include FGR, maternal hyponat- raemia leading to central pontine myelinolysis, and thiamine deficiency leading to Wernicke's encephalopathy.[2] Markers of severity include weight loss >10 per cent, abnormal thyroid function tests with raised free T_4 and suppressed TSH, and abnormal liver function tests with raised transaminases.

Management

Other possible causes of nausea and vomiting should be considered, especially UTI (which often coincides with hyperemesis), hypercalcaemia, Addison's disease and thyrotoxicosis (weight loss, heat intolerance and tachycardia precede the pregnancy), and cholecystitis. An ultrasound scan of the uterus is important to exclude multiple pregnancy and hydatidiform mole, both of which increase the risk of hyperemesis. The most important component of management (Table 15.2) is to ensure adequate rehydration. This should be with 0.9% saline with added potassium chloride sufficient to correct tachycardia, hypotension and ketonuria, and return electrolyte levels to normal. Dextrose-containing fluids are avoided except in women with diabetes. High concentrations of dextrose in particular may precipitate Wernicke's encephalopathy. This is prevented by routine administration of oral or intravenous thiamine. Antiemetics may be liberally and safely used in pregnancy [A, C].[2–4] Women with severe hyperemesis may require regular parenteral doses of more than one antiemetic to control their symptoms. Even for women with nausea and vomiting in pregnancy that do not require hospital admissions

Table 15.2 Protocol for the management of hyperemesis

Investigations	U&Es, FBC, LFTs, TFTs
MSU	US scan of the uterus
Fluid therapy	0.9% saline 1 L + 20–40 mmol KCl 8-hourly
Vitamin therapy	Thiamine orally 25–50 mg t.d.s. *or* thiamine intravenously 100 mg in 100 mL 0.9% saline weekly
Antiemetic therapy	Possible regimens include: • Cyclizine 50 mg p.o./i.m./i.v. t.d.s. • Promethazine 25 mg p.o. nocte • Stemetil 5 mg p.o. t.d.s; 12.5 mg i.m./i.v. t.d.s. • Metoclopramide 10 mg p.o./i.m./i.v. t.d.s. • Domperidone 10 mg p.o. q.d.s.; 30–60 mg p.r. t.d.s. • Chlorpromazine 10–25 mg p.o.; 25 mg i.m. t.d.s. • Ondansetron 4–8mg p.o./i.v.

• i.m., intramuscularly; i.v., intravenously; p.o., orally; p.r., as required; q.d.s., four times daily; t.d.s., three times daily; US, ultrasound.

but interfere with work and home life, antiemetics may be appropriate. For women with severe hyperemesis who do not improve despite conventional treatment with IV fluids and electrolytes and regular antiemetics, a trial of ondansetron or corticosteroids may be considered [B].[2,5,6] Iron supplements may induce nausea and vomiting, and should be withheld until symptoms resolve.

EBM

• There are substantial data from systematic reviews[3] and cohort studies[2] to support the safety of conventional antiemetics in pregnancy, including the first trimester.
• Several RCTs[5] support a beneficial effect of corticosteroids for severe disease.

GASTRO-OESOPHAGEAL REFLUX

About two-thirds of women experience heartburn in pregnancy, commonly in the third trimester. This is partly because of increased reflux due to the decreased lower oesophageal pressure, decreased gastric peristalsis and delayed gastric emptying, and partly due to the enlarging uterus. Reflux of acid or alkaline gastric contents into the oesophagus causes inflammation of the oesophageal mucosa, leading to pain, waterbrash and dyspepsia.

Management

Postural changes, such as sleeping in a semi-recumbent position, may help, especially in late pregnancy. Avoiding food or fluid intake immediately before retiring may also prevent symptoms. Antacids are safe in pregnancy and may be used liberally. Liquid preparations are more effective and should be given to prevent and treat symptoms. Aluminium-containing antacids may cause constipation, and magnesium-containing antacids may cause diarrhoea. Metoclopramide increases lower oesophageal pressure and speeds gastric emptying, and may help relieve reflux. Sucralfate and histamine H_2-receptor blockers (e.g. ranitidine) are both safe throughout pregnancy. Proton-pump inhibitors (PPIs) such as omeprazole are more powerful suppressors of gastric acid secretion, and are also safe.[4] It should be reserved for reflux oesophagitis when H_2-receptor blockers have failed.

PEPTIC ULCER

Peptic ulceration is rare in pregnancy. Presentation is usually with epigastric pain rather than with complications such as haemorrhage or perforation. Prostaglandins induced by pregnancy have a protective effect on the gastric mucosa, thus explaining the reduced incidence compared with non-pregnant women. Gastrointestinal endoscopy (including the sedation used for the procedure) is safe in pregnancy and should be used to investigate all but minor haematemesis.

Management

Antacids, sucralfate and H_2-receptor blockers and PPIs are all safe in pregnancy. *Helicobacter pylori* has a causal role in peptic ulceration, but eradication therapy is usually deferred until after delivery. Misoprostol, a prostaglandin analogue, protects the gastric mucosa but is contraindicated during pregnancy because of the risk of miscarriage.

CONSTIPATION

This is another common symptom of normal pregnancy, probably due to reduced colonic motility. Poor dietary intake associated with nausea and vomiting, dehydration, opiate analgesia and iron supplements exacerbates constipation. Management includes advice regarding increased fluid intake and dietary fibre. Temporary cessation of oral iron supplements may help, and laxatives should be used only if the

---

> ## EBM Gastro-oesophageal reflux, dyspepsia, constipation
>
> - There are substantial data from systematic reviews[3] to support the safety of antacids, anti-emetics, sucralfate, H_2-receptor blockers and PPIs in pregnancy.
> - Misoprostol should be avoided.
> - Osmotic and stimulant laxatives are safe to use in pregnancy.

above measures fail. Osmotic laxatives, such as lactulose and magnesium hydrochloride, are safe. Stimulant laxatives, such as glycerol suppositories, and senna (Senokot®) tablets are also safe in pregnancy.

INFLAMMATORY BOWEL DISEASE

Both Crohn's disease and ulcerative colitis tend to present in young adulthood. Ulcerative colitis is more common in women and is encountered more commonly in pregnancy. The course of IBD is not usually affected by pregnancy. The risk of flare in pregnancy is reduced if the colitis is quiescent at the time of conception. Most exacerbations occur early in pregnancy and cause abdominal pain, diarrhoea, and passage of rectal mucus and blood. Women with Crohn's disease may experience postpartum flare. Pregnancy outcome is usually good in women with IBD, although active disease at the time of conception is associated with an increased risk of miscarriage, and active disease later in pregnancy may adversely affect pregnancy outcome, with an increased rate of pre-term delivery.[7,8] Prior surgery, including ileostomy, procto-colectomy and pouch surgery, does not preclude successful pregnancy.

Management

Women with IBD should be encouraged to conceive during periods of disease remission. Management is not substantially affected by pregnancy. Oral or rectal sulfasalazine (Salazopyrin), mesalazine (Asacol) and other 5-aminosalicylic acid drugs may be safely used throughout pregnancy and breastfeeding, although, as sulfasalazine is a dihydrofolate reductase inhibitor, 5 mg daily folic acid should be used pre-conception and in pregnancy to reduce the increased risk of neural tube defects, cardiovascular defects, oral clefts and folate deficiency. Oral and rectal preparations of corticosteroids may be required for acute treatment or maintenance and are safe in pregnancy. Azathioprine may be needed to maintain remission and this should be continued in pregnancy (see Chapter 14).[8] Biologic therapies such as the anti-TNF agents (infliximab and adalimumab) are used increasingly in IBD. Available data suggest that these agents are safe in pregnancy but should ideally be discontinued by 30 weeks' gestation [D].[9,10]

Clinicians must remain alert to the possible dangerous surgical complications of IBD, including intestinal obstruction, haemorrhage, perforation or toxic megacolon. Caesarean section may be indicated in the presence of severe perianal Crohn's disease with a deformed, inelastic or scarred rectum and perineum. Active perianal Crohn's may prevent healing of an episiotomy.

EBM Inflammatory bowel disease

- Evidence from systematic review[7] supports an association between conception during periods of active disease and adverse pregnancy outcome.
- Sulfasalazine and related drugs are safe in pregnancy, but folic acid 5 mg/day should be given concomitantly.
- Corticosteroids and azathioprine may safely be used for maintenance or acute management of disease flares.[7,8]

ACUTE AND CHRONIC VIRAL HEPATITIS

The course of most viral hepatitis is not altered by pregnancy. Pregnant women may contract acute hepatitis in the same way and with the same clinical features as non-pregnant women. Thus fever, malaise, anorexia, jaundice and possible recent exposure should alert the clinician to the diagnosis. The implications of acute hepatitis infection in pregnancy are discussed in Chapter 24. As with acute hepatitis B infections, neonates born to women with chronic hepatitis B virus (HBV) should be given hepatitis B immune globulin and HBV vaccine within 24 hours of birth. Immunisation is 85–95 per cent effective at preventing both HBV infection and the chronic carrier state. There is a significant risk (60–80 per cent) of hepatitis C infection progressing to chronic infection, and about 20 per cent of those with chronic infection develop slowly progressive cirrhosis over a period of 10–30 years. Detection of hepatitis C virus (HCV) antibody implies persistent infection rather than immunity. The risk of progressive liver disease with hepatitis C is lower in women and in those aged <40 years who do not abuse alcohol. Women with hepatitis C are at increased risk of obstetric cholestasis (see below).[11]

CHRONIC LIVER DISEASE

Severe hepatic impairment is associated with infertility. Liver disease may decompensate during pregnancy, and pregnancy should be discouraged in women with severe impairment of hepatic function. Those with portal hypertension and oesophageal varices are at risk from variceal bleeding, especially in the second and third trimesters.

OBSTETRIC CHOLESTASIS

This is a liver disease specific to pregnancy, characterised by pruritus affecting the whole body but particularly the palms and soles, and abnormal liver function tests. It is more common in women from South America, the Indian subcontinent and Scandinavia. The prevalence in the UK is about 0.7 per cent.[12] The aetiology is unknown, but relates to a genetic predisposition (one-third of patients have a positive family history) to the cholestatic effect of oestrogens.

Obstetric cholestasis most commonly presents in the third trimester at around 30–32 weeks' gestation.[12] Women with pruritus but without a rash, other than excoriations, should have liver function tests. These must be interpreted with reference to the normal ranges for pregnancy[1] since often in obstetric cholestasis the hepatic transaminases are only mildly elevated. The most usual abnormality is raised ALT or AST, although a small proportion of women have only a raised gamma GT or raised bile acids.[13] Although raised bile acids are not necessary to confirm the diagnosis, they are useful, especially in those women with typical clinical features but normal standard liver function tests.[13] There may be associated dark urine, pale stools, steatorrhoea and malaise. Obstetric cholestasis is a diagnosis of exclusion, and the differential diagnosis includes extrahepatic obstruction with gallstones, acute or chronic viral hepatitis, primary biliary cirrhosis (PBC) and chronic active hepatitis (CAH). Investigations should therefore include a liver ultrasound, serology for hepatitis A, B and C, and liver autoantibodies (anti-mitochondrial antibodies to exclude PBC and anti-smooth muscle antibodies to exclude CAH).

The risks with obstetric cholestasis include postpartum haemorrhage (related to vitamin K deficiency secondary to malabsorption of fat), preterm labour, meconium-stained liqor, fetal distress (CTG abnormalities) in labour and, rarely, intrauterine death (IUD).[14,15] The cause of the adverse effects on the fetus is unknown. The risk of IUD increases towards

EBM Obstetric cholestasis

- Evidence from prospective studies,[12,13] supports the need for a high index of clinical suspicion, and therefore serial measurement of liver function tests, in women with onset of pruritus affecting predominantly the palms and soles in the third trimester.
- The evidence also highlights significant increased risks of adverse perinatal outcomes in women with severe cholestasis.

ANTENATAL OBSTETRICS

and beyond term but does not correlate with either symptoms or transaminases. There is a correlation with bile acid levels.[14,15]

Management

This should involve counselling the woman regarding the above risks. Liver function tests and clotting times should be monitored regularly. Current guidelines suggest that there is insufficient evidence to support the common practice of expediting delivery at 37–38 weeks unless the bile acids exceed 40 µmol/l. Vitamin K should be given to the mother (10 mg orally daily) if the clotting is deranged to reduce the risk of postpartum haemorrhage. No specific method of fetal surveillance can be recommended to predict fetal complications in mothers with obstetric cholestasis. Although such monitoring may serve to reassure the mother and her carers, delivery is rarely indicated earlier than 37 weeks on the basis of such monitoring. Management strategies that involve elective early (by 38 weeks) delivery and fetal surveillance have shown a decreased risk of IUD compared with earlier studies, but also result in increased rates of caesarean section, prematurity and admissions to neonatal intensive care units.[12]

Control of symptoms may be achieved with a combination of antihistamines and emollients or, if these are insufficient, ursodeoxycholic acid (UDCA). This drug usually leads to rapid reduction in liver function tests and pruritus, but there is as yet no evidence for a reduction in fetal risk. A pilot RCT showed that UDCA significantly reduced pruritus and that early term delivery did not increase the caesarean section rate. A larger trial is planned.[16]

Following delivery, liver function tests return to normal and there is no permanent detrimental effect on maternal liver function. Symptoms may recur with menstruation (cyclical itching) or with oestrogen-containing oral contraceptives, which should therefore be avoided. Recurrence of obstetric cholestasis in subsequent pregnancies exceeds 90 per cent.

KEY POINTS

Obstetric cholestasis

- Liver function tests should be requested in any pregnant woman with pruritus without obvious rash.
- Liver function tests should be repeated serially if the itching involves the palms and soles.
- Other causes of pruritus and abnormal liver function tests, including viral hepatitis and gallstones causing extrahepatic obstruction, should be excluded.
- Severe cholestasis is associated with a significantly increased risk of preterm delivery and stillbirth.
- Fetal risks increase with increasing bile acid levels.
- UDCA improves symptoms and liver function tests

ACUTE FATTY LIVER OF PREGNANCY

This is another pregnancy-specific liver disease. It is rare and a recent UK-wide study found a prevalence of 5 per 100 000.[14]

Acute fatty liver of pregnancy (AFLP) is closely related to, and shares many features and probably pathophysiology with, pre-eclampsia. It usually presents in the third trimester with abdominal pain, nausea, vomiting, anorexia and sometimes jaundice. It is associated with markedly deranged liver function tests, renal impairment, a markedly elevated uric acid, a raised white cell count, hypoglycaemia and coagulopathy.[14]

Clinical features of pre-eclampsia may be mild or absent. It is more common in twin pregnancies. It may come to light only after delivery when coagulation is checked because of excessive bleeding. It is also associated with diabetes insipidus and may present with polyuria and polydypsia. Perinatal and maternal mortality and morbidity rates are increased (10 and 1.8 per cent, respectively).[14]

Management

This should involve a high-dependency or intensive care unit and a multidisciplinary team. Delivery should be expedited following adequate correction of any hypoglycaemia or coagulopathy with 50 per cent dextrose, intravenous vitamin K and fresh frozen plasma. Management after delivery is conservative, although early referral to a liver unit should be considered if liver function does not improve or if there are any features of hepatic encephalopathy.

Published Guidelines/Online Resources

Germain S, Nelson-Piercy C. Liver and gastrointestinal disease. Maternal Medicine Module. *RCOG Strat-OG* 2nd edn. London: RCOG, 2007.

RCOG. *Obstetric Cholestasis*. Green-top Guideline No. 43 London: RCOG, 2011. Available from: files/ GT43ObstetricCholestasis2006.pdf.

van der Woude CJ, Kolacek S, Dotan I, *et al.*; European Crohn's Colitis Organisation (ECCO). European evidenced-based consensus on reproduction in inflammatory bowel disease. *J Crohns Colitis* 2010:493–510.

Key References

1. Girling JC, Dow E, Smith JH. Liver function tests in pre-eclampsia: importance of comparison with a reference range derived for normal pregnancy. *Br J Obstet Gynaecol* 1997;104:246–50.
2. Jarvis S, Nelson-Piercy C. Nausea and vomiting in pregnancy *BMJ* 2011;342:d3606
3. Mazzotta P, Magee LA. A risk–benefit assessment of pharmacological and non-pharmacological treatments for nausea and vomiting of pregnancy. *Drugs* 2000;59:781–800.

4. Kametas N, Nelson-Piercy C. Hyperemesis gravidarum, gastrointestinal and liver disease in pregnancy. *Obstetrics Gynaecol Reprod Med* 2008;18:69–75.

5. Nelson-Piercy C, Fayers P, de Swiet M. Randomised, placebo-controlled trial of corticosteroids for hyperemesis gravidarum. *Br J Obstet Gynaecol* 2001;108:1–7.

6. Moran P, Taylor R. Management of hyperemesis gravidarum: the importance of weight loss as a criterion for steroid therapy. *QJM* 2002; 95:153–8.

7. Vermeire S, Carbonnel F, Coulie PG *et al.* Management of inflammatory bowel disease in pregnancy. *J Crohns Colitis* 2012;6:811–23.

8. Alstead EA, Nelson-Piercy C. Inflammatory bowel disease in pregnancy. *Gut* 2002;52:159–61.

9. Vinet E, Pineau C, Gordon C *et al.* Biologic therapy and pregnancy outcome in women with rheumatic diseases. *Arthritis Rheum* 2009;61:587–92.

10. Hyrich KL, Verstappen SM. Biologic therapies and pregnancy: the story so far. *Rheumatology* (Oxford). 2014;53:1377-85.

11. Locatelli A, Roncaglia N, Arreghini A *et al.* Hepatitis C virus infection is associated with a higher incidence of cholestasis of pregnancy. *Br J Obstet Gynaecol* 1999;106:498–500.

12. Kenyon AP, Nelson-Piercy C, Girling J *et al.* Obstetric cholestasis, outcome with active management: a series of 70 cases. *Br J Obstet Gynaecol* 2002;109:282–8.

13. Kenyon AP, Nelson-Piercy C, Girling J *et al.* Pruritus may precede abnormal liver function tests in pregnant women with obstetric cholestasis: a longitudinal analysis. *Br J Obstet Gynaecol* 2001;108:1190–2.

14. Glantz A, Marschall HU, Mattson LA. Intrahepatic cholestasis of pregnancy: relationship between bile acid levels and fetal complication rates. *Hepatology* 2004;40:467–74.

15. Geenes V, Chappell LC, Seed PT, Steer PJ, Knight M, Williamson C. Association of severe intrahepatic cholestasis of pregnancy with adverse pregnancy outcomes: A prospective population-based case-control study. *Hepatology* 2014;59:1482-91.

16. Chappell LC, Gurung V, Seed PT, Chambers J, Williamson C, Thornton JG; PITCH Study Consortium. Ursodeoxycholic acid versus placebo, and early term delivery versus expectant management, in women with intrahepatic cholestasis of pregnancy: semifactorial randomised clinical trial. *BMJ* 2012;344:e3799.

17. Knight M, Nelson-Piercy C, Kurinczuk JJ *et al.* A prospective national study of acute fatty liver of pregnancy in the UK. *Gut* 2008;**57**:951–6.

Chapter 16 Respiratory conditions

Louise Kenny

INTRODUCTION: PULMONARY DISEASE IN PREGNANCY

The physiological changes occurring within the respiratory system are summarised in Tables 16.1 and 16.2. Symptomatically, pregnant women may complain of new-onset rhinitis, which may result from oestrogen-induced oedema, hyperaemia and hypersecretion of the upper airways. Although mostly harmless, this contributes to the greater difficulties encountered during intubation of pregnant women. Much more common is the complaint of shortness of breath or 'air hunger'. This dyspnoea is experienced by approximately half of all pregnant women by 20 weeks' gestation and by three-quarters by 30 weeks. It rarely occurs at rest and does not significantly impair normal activities. The postulated mechanism is high

Table 16.1 Normal arterial blood gas values and the effect of pregnancy

	Pre-pregnancy	By term
PaO_2	11–13 kPa (83–98 mmHg)	13 kPa (98 mmHg)
$PaCO_2$	4.8–6.0 kPa (36–45 mmHg)	3.7–4.2 kPa (28–32 mmHg)
HCO_3^-	24–30 mmol/L	18–21 mmol/L
pH	7.35–7.45	7.4–7.45

Table 16.2 The effect of pregnancy on lung function

Lung function	Change by term	Actual volume change
Total lung capacity	4% decrease	200–400 mL
Functional residual	10–20% decrease	300–500 mL capacity
Expiratory reserve	15–20% decrease	100–300 mL volume
Tidal volume	30–50% increase	200 mL
Minute (or expired volume in 1 min) ventilation	30–50% increase	3 L/min
Residual volume	20–25% decrease	200–300 mL
Respiratory rate	No change	
Vital capacity	No change	
Peak flow	No change	
Metabolic rate	15% increase	
Oxygen consumption (V_{O2})	20–33% increase	

progesterone levels acting via the hypothalamus to increase respiratory drive.

Anatomically, the lower chest wall circumference increases by 5–7 cm, the diaphragm is elevated 4–5 cm by term and the costal angle widens. These changes occur due to pressure from the expanding uterus and the relaxation of thoracic ligaments. Diaphragmatic excursion is not reduced; however, the accessory muscles contribute proportionally more than the diaphragm to the increase in tidal volume found in pregnancy.

The metabolic rate becomes elevated in pregnancy, as demonstrated by a rise in resting oxygen uptake and carbon dioxide output. This extra oxygen turnover is of course necessary for the fetoplacental unit and the extra demands made by maternal physiology. Minute ventilation (or volume expired in a minute) and alveolar ventilation are both increased to meet this demand by an increase in tidal volume rather than by a change in respiratory rate, which remains constant. This state of relative hyperventilation causes a fall in $PaCO_2$, which results in a chronic respiratory alkalosis. Blood pH is kept within the normal range by a reactionary increase in renal bicarbonate excretion.

Airway function is maintained and peak expiratory flow rate (PEFR) and forced expiratory volume in 1 second (FEV_1) measurements are not affected by pregnancy.

Investigating pulmonary disease in pregnancy

The physiological changes occurring in pregnancy must also be considered when interpreting the results of investigations. The effect on arterial blood gas analysis is clear from Table 16.1. The chest X-ray must also be interpreted with caution. The cardiothoracic ratio is elevated, vascular markings may become more prominent, and small pleural effusions are even possible in normal pregnancy. Peak flow and spirometry tests can be interpreted in the usual manner.

Concern is often raised about the safety of various radiological examinations during pregnancy. For a fuller description of risks to the fetus, see Chapter 23. The maximum safe exposure for the fetus is often considered to be 5 cGy, although this is gestation dependent [D]. Chest X-ray, venography, pulmonary angiography and ventilation–perfusion (V/Q) scanning all expose the fetus to significantly lower levels than this, and the potential benefits of all these investigations are usually thought to outweigh the risks. However, exposure should be minimised where possible. For example:

- lateral chest X-rays are often unnecessary and carry a greater exposure risk than an anteroposterior (AP) erect chest film; they can mostly be avoided;
- a mobile chest X-ray carries greater exposure than a departmental film, so the patient should be moved where possible;
- the 'ventilation' component of V/Q scanning can be omitted in women with no previous history of chest disease;
- pulmonary angiography carries less fetal risk if a brachial route is used in preference to the femoral.

Shielding of the fetus should be used where the situation allows. CT scanning utilises much higher energy levels, and safer alternatives are usually available. However, if the indication is strong enough, even CT has its place. Spiral and non-contiguous axial imaging are techniques that may reduce exposure without compromising diagnostic accuracy. MRI involves no irradiation and is also considered safe.

ASTHMA

The incidence of asthma appears to be increasing globally. There is some geographical variation, with reported prevalence in pregnancy ranging from 4 per cent to 12 per cent. Consequently, asthma is the respiratory illness most likely to be encountered during pregnancy and up to 6 per cent of women are hospitalised on at least one occasions for asthma during pregnancy.

The effect of pregnancy on asthma

The true effect of pregnancy on asthma severity has been addressed by a number of prospective case-controlled studies which suggest that asthma will deteriorate, stay the same and improve in equal measure.[1] The potential benefits of pregnancy-induced immune system alterations and progesterone-mediated bronchodilatation may be opposed by the reluctance of patients and physicians to treat asthma appropriately for fear of harming the fetus through drug exposure. Women with severe asthma seem more likely to deteriorate, whilst those showing improvement during pregnancy are more likely to suffer postpartum relapse.[2] Approximately 1 in 10 women with asthma will suffer an acute attack in labour [C].

The effect of asthma on pregnancy

The precise effect that the asthma has on the pregnancy is unclear. Almost every conceivable obstetric complication has been found to be more common in pregnant women with asthma by one case–control study or another. However, the pattern of antenatal complications varies greatly among studies and this lack of consistency has cast doubt over the findings. Poor controls, varied case mixes and different treatment regimens make resolution of the data very difficult.

Several studies have reported an association with asthma and an elevated risk of hypertension in pregnancy. Recent evidence suggests that this risk is confined to women with pre-existing severe asthma and points to a mechanistic common pathway of mast cell–airway smooth muscle cell interactions.[3] Moderate-to-severe asthma and poorly controlled asthma with frequent exacerbations are associated with other adverse outcomes including intrauterine growth restriction and preterm rupture of membranes/labour so increased surveillance is justified [E].

Management of asthma in pregnancy

In the recent Eighth Report of the CEMD in the UK, there were five indirect deaths due to asthma (mortality of 0.22 per 100,000 maternities), a similar number to those in the two previous reports.[4] None of the five women who died had received specialist care in pregnancy even though three of them had many hospital admissions or a history of asthma that was particularly difficult to treat. This highlights the need for specialist input in pregnant women with severe asthma.

Asthma will usually have been diagnosed prior to pregnancy and treatment already instituted. However, this is not always the case, and the initial presenting signs and symptoms of asthma are the same as those of asthma that is inadequately treated:

- chest tightness and wheeziness;
- cough;
- breathlessness, especially in the early hours of the morning.

The management of asthma in pregnancy is essentially the same as in the non-pregnant patient and should be in line with current guidelines from British Thoracic Society/SIGN.[5]

Prevention is the key, and known triggers of exacerbations should be eliminated or avoided in the home and at work (Table 16.3).

Pharmacological treatment of asthma

This follows a step-by-step approach, more clearly outlined in the current guidelines from British Thoracic Society/SIGN. In general, the medicines used to treat asthma are safe in pregnancy. A large UK population-based case–control study found no increased risk of major congenital malformations in children of women receiving asthma treatment in the year before or during pregnancy. The risk of harm to the

Table 16.3 Triggers and provocative stimuli for exacerbations of asthma

Allergens	Pollen (seasonal)
	Dust mites, animal danders, moulds (non-seasonal)
Occupational	Industrial chemicals, metal salts, wood and vegetable dust
Infection	Viral and/or bacterial
Environmental pollution	Tobacco smoke, ozone
Pharmacological	Aspirin and NSAIDs, beta blockers
Emotional stress	
Exercise and cold air	

> ### EBM
>
> Counsel women with asthma regarding the importance and safety of continuing their asthma medications during pregnancy to ensure good asthma control [B]

fetus from severe or chronically under-treated asthma outweighs any small risk from the medications used to control asthma.

No significant association has been demonstrated between major congenital malformations or adverse perinatal outcome and exposure to short-acting or long-acting β_2 agonists, and these can be used with confidence in pregnancy.

A meta-analysis of four studies of inhaled corticosteroid use in pregnancy showed no increase in the rate of major malformations, preterm delivery, low birthweight or pregnancy-induced hypertension, and therefore inhaled steroids should be used as normal during pregnancy.

No significant association has been demonstrated between major congenital malformations or adverse perinatal outcome and exposure to methylxanthines.

Neonatal irritability and apnoea have been reported with theophylline; however, this uncommon side effect should not prohibit use of the drug if indication exists. For women requiring theophylline to maintain asthma control, measurement of theophylline levels is recommended. As protein binding decreases in pregnancy, resulting in increased free drug levels, a lower therapeutic range is probably appropriate.

No significant association has been demonstrated between major congenital malformations or adverse perinatal outcome and exposure to chromones, and these should therefore be used as normal during pregnancy.

Prednisolone is the oral steroid of choice for pregnancy, as 88 per cent of it is metabolised by the placenta, limiting fetal exposure. The teratogenic risk and possible harmful fetal effects of maternal steroid treatment remain an area of controversy. Initial worries about an association with isolated cleft lip have been allayed by a recent case–control study which did not support the original animal experimental work [B].[6] However, a subsequent meta-analysis has once again confused the debate with a statistically significant three-fold increase in oral clefting risk for steroid use in the first trimester [A].[6] Newer anxieties have arisen about associations with intrauterine growth restriction, neuronal development, long-term hypertension and preterm labour.

These associations are therefore not definite and, even if real, the benefit to the mother and the fetus of steroids for treating a life-threatening disease justifies the use of steroids in pregnancy.

Data regarding the safety of leukotriene receptor antagonists in pregnancy are limited but so far reassuring. Leukotriene antagonists may therefore be continued in women who have demonstrated significant improvement in asthma control with these agents prior to pregnancy not achievable with other medications.

There are as yet no clinical data on the use of immunomodulation therapies such as omalizumab for moderate-to-severe allergic asthma in pregnancy. There are some reassuring animal studies on teratogenicity (classed as FDA category B). A registry of pregnancy exposures is being undertaken.

Specific guidelines also exist for the management of acute asthma attacks and these should also be adhered to in pregnancy.[7] The severity of acute exacerbations is divided into three groups.

1 **Uncontrolled asthma in adults**. Speech must be normal, with a pulse of <110 beats/min and respiratory rate of <25/min. Peak flow should be >50 per cent of predicted or personal best. Treatment involves nebulised salbutamol or terbutaline. Failure to respond should prompt referral to hospital. Otherwise, normal treatment can be stepped up and a course of oral steroids may be prescribed.

2 **Acute severe attack**. These patients will not be able to complete sentences, will have a pulse >110 beats/min, a respiratory rate of >25/min and a peak flow of <50 per cent predicted or personal best. Acute treatment involves oxygen, nebulisers and oral prednisolone. Those not responding well should be transferred to hospital with an aminophylline infusion.

3 **Life-threatening asthma**. This most serious of asthma exacerbations is characterised by a 'silent chest', cyanosis, bradycardia or a peak flow of <33 per cent of predicted or personal best. Immediate hospital treatment is necessary with oxygen, nebulisers, intravenous aminophylline, oral steroids or intravenous hydrocortisone.

It is useful for all clinicians to remember these guidelines. However, there should be a low threshold for the involvement of appropriate physicians in cases of deteriorating asthma in pregnancy. Possible precipitating factors should be addressed with all acute exacerbations. For example, antibiotics are often prescribed for presumed chest infection.

Managing pregnancy in asthmatic patients

- Patients with well-controlled mild or moderate asthma will have a normal outcome with standard antenatal care [B]. For those with poorly controlled or severe asthma, care should be multidisciplinary, preferably through a high-risk antenatal clinic with general medical input [E].
- Baseline investigations, such as peak flow measurements, should be obtained at booking [E].
- Medical treatment should be optimised by following the above protocol, with repeated reassurance about the use of these drugs in pregnancy. A recent study has demonstrated that physicians are still reluctant to prescribe oral steroids during pregnancy.[2]
- In view of the uncertainty over the true impact of severe asthma on pregnancy outcome, the maternity team should remain vigilant for signs of preterm labour and follow fetal growth and wellbeing with ultrasound [E].

- Induction of labour and caesarean section will mostly be reserved for obstetric indications, although delivery may need to be expedited in the most severe cases [D].
- No form of analgesia is contraindicated, although regional anaesthesia is preferable rather than general for major operative procedures.
- Women taking prednisolone should be screened for glucose intolerance and measures taken to control this if it is found. Those taking prednisolone at the onset of labour should be given supplementary doses of 100 mg hydrocortisone 6–8 hourly until oral intake is resumed [B].
- Prostaglandin E_2 may safely be used for labour inductions [E].
- Prostaglandin $F_2\alpha$ (carboprost/hemabate®) used to treat postpartum haemorrhage due to uterine atony may cause bronchospasm and should be avoided if possible [E].
- Although ergometrine may cause bronchospasm, particularly in association with general anaesthesia, this is not a problem encountered when syntometrine (Syntocinon/ ergometrine) is used for postpartum haemorrhage prophylaxis [E].
- The risk of postnatal deterioration should be discussed with the woman.
- Breastfeeding is not contraindicated with any of the medications used.

CYSTIC FIBROSIS

The reporting of pregnancies in women with cystic fibrosis (CF) began in the 1960s and the initial outcomes seemed unfavourable. However, with improvements in the care of both individuals with CF and high-risk pregnancies in general, the outlook is more favourable. Although men with CF are usually infertile, this is not the case for women. Menarche is delayed by an average of 2 years and the incidence of anovulatory cycles and secondary amenorrhoea is indeed higher. Cervical mucus may be more tenacious. However, fertility is the general rule rather than the exception. Average life expectancy for those with CF continues to lengthen. According to the 2011 Annual Data Report from the Cystic Fibrosis Patient Registry, the median predicted age of survival is approaching 40 years. Consequently many women are now choosing to start a family and employing specialist assistance where subfertility exists.

The North American Cystic Fibrosis Foundation Patient Registry has reported approximately 140 pregnancies per annum since 1991, equating to 3–4 per cent of women aged over 17 becoming pregnant each year. Thus, pregnancy in women with CF is increasingly common and most adult CF centres and many paediatric centres will have had to care for a woman with CF and her pregnancy.

The spectrum of disease phenotype and severity is highly varied and only loosely correlated to genotype. Individual counselling, preferably prior to conception, is vital and it must be clearly understood that outcome predictors are imprecise.

Outcomes

Outcomes needing consideration are both the effect of the pregnancy on the CF and, conversely, the effect of the CF on the pregnancy.

A recent case–control study of women with CF compared 22 pregnant women with matched non-pregnant women and an average follow-up of 4.5 years. Nutritional outcomes, changes in lung function and exacerbation rates were compared. Pregnancy was not associated with immediate or medium-term adverse effects for CF patients.[9] This is broadly in line with two large previously reported case series from Toronto (n=92 pregnancies in 54 women)[10] and the UK (n=22 pregnancies in 20 women).[11]

A number of different markers of disease severity have been proposed as predictors of maternal and fetal outcome (Box 16.1) but the evidence base to support each of these markers is weak and in the recent case–control study the only significant predictors of decline were higher lung function at the beginning of the study and pancreatic insufficiency.

Effect of pregnancy on cystic fibrosis

No women in these three studies died during or within 6 weeks of pregnancy. However, only 79 per cent of the Canadian women were still alive 10 years after the delivery, the earliest death occurring 3 years after the birth. Only three-quarters were still alive 4 years after delivery in the UK study, the earliest death occurring only 6 months postpartum. These mortality rates are, however, no different from those for non-pregnant individuals with CF.

Death is a very crude measure of the effect of pregnancy on CF. Decline in lung function has also been examined. Edenborough found a 13 per cent loss in %FEV$_1$ during pregnancy, although this was mostly regained in the following year, and a net loss of 5 per cent in FEV$_1$ overall at 1 year following delivery. Gilljam's prediction of 3 per cent is similar; neither deterioration is significantly greater than that expected for the

Box 16.1 Predictors of maternal and fetal outcome in pregnancies complicated by cystic fibrosis

Absolute pre-pregnancy pulmonary function
Stability of pre-pregnancy pulmonary function
Colonisation with *Burkholderia cepacia*
Presence of pulmonary hypertension
Degree of pancreatic insufficiency
Glucose intolerance/diabetes (pre-dating pregnancy or gestational)
BMI
Maternal weight gain during pregnancy
Presence of liver disease and portal hypertension

normal CF population [B]. However, caution must be exercised in women with poor pre-pregnancy lung function (<50 per cent predicted %FEV$_1$). There is evidence suggesting that they do suffer a permanent pregnancy-associated decline in lung function,[10] although this, too, is disputed.[8]

The anatomical and physiological changes in cardiorespiratory function during pregnancy might be thought to impair mucus clearance, increase atelectasis and predispose to pulmonary infections. However, serious medical events would appear to be no more common in pregnancy than would be expected from the pre-pregnancy lung function tests.

Effect of cystic fibrosis on pregnancy

Studies have not shown an increase in miscarriage or anomaly risk over the general obstetric population,[8–12] although CF was diagnosed in two of the Canadian offspring. In one case, the diagnosis of maternal CF was not made until after the child was born, and, in the second, prenatal screening had indicated that there was only a very low risk that the child would be affected (see below). The mean gestation at delivery was >37 weeks in both studies, although one in three babies was born preterm in the UK study. The prematurity rate was no higher than for the general population in the Canadian group (8 per cent). Intrauterine growth restriction was not encountered more frequently than would normally be expected. Only one neonate died, sepsis being the cause following delivery at 31 weeks' gestation.

The average maternal weight gain of 10–12 kg during pregnancy demands an extra 300 kcal/day. Pancreatic insufficiency is very common in CF, and enzyme supplements are usually needed to aid digestion. Increasing nutritional intake during pregnancy may be very difficult, especially with confounding factors such as nausea, hyperemesis and indigestion. It is hardly surprising that average maternal weight gain is reduced by approximately half. Furthermore, a compromised pancreas may fail to fulfil its added endocrine responsibilities: gestational diabetes occurred in 8 per cent of those women in the Canadian group who did not have pre-existing diabetes.

Caesarean section is normally employed only for obstetric reasons in women with mild-to-moderate CF. However, one in three women was delivered by preterm section in the UK group, the most common indication being deteriorating lung function. Instrumental delivery rates do not appear to be increased.

The more recent retrospective reviews do suggest a generally good outcome for mother and baby. Problems such as prematurity and maternal death within 5 years of delivery are mostly confined to cases with poor pre-pregnancy lung function, pancreatic insufficiency (especially glucose intolerance) and lung colonisation with *Burkholderia cepacia*. A %FEV$_1$ of <50 per cent is often considered a relative contraindication to pregnancy. Good outcomes with prolonged maternal survival afterwards are nevertheless possible, even with values below this. The presence of pulmonary hypertension causes grave concern. Serious consideration should be given to termination of the pregnancy to prevent right-sided heart failure.

Management of cystic fibrosis during pregnancy

A recent and comprehensive guideline has been commissioned by the European Cystic Fibrosis Society, based on review of the literature and experience of paediatricians, adult and transplant physicians, nurses, physiotherapists, dieticians, pharmacists and psychologists experienced in CF, and anaesthetists and obstetricians with experience of CF in pregnancy.[13] This makes broad-based multidisciplinary recommendations for the management of pregnancy in CF, which should be undertaken in specialist centres.

- Ideally, a full discussion should take place prior to conception. Treatment can be optimised and the risks discussed. Patients with poor lung function or pulmonary hypertension may be advised to avoid pregnancy altogether.
- The average age of survival for women with CF in the UK is approximately 28 years. The effect on a child of losing a parent should be considered before conception.
- The issue of prenatal screening should be raised, although this must be done diplomatically, as the condition being screened for is, after all, present in the mother. As CF is an autosomal recessive condition, the offspring will either be all obligate carriers, if the partner is free of mutations, or one in two will be affected if he is a carrier himself. Approximately 1 in 25 individuals is a CF carrier in the UK. ΔF508 is the most common CF mutation in the UK, accounting for 80 per cent of the total. A 'rare' mutation screen may test for as many as 30 different mutations; however, this will still only detect approximately 90 per cent of all mutations. Hence, even when the partner of the woman with CF has a 'negative' mutation screen, there is still a 1 in 250 chance that he is a carrier (1/25 x 1/10) and therefore a 1 in 500 chance that the baby will have cystic fibrosis (1/250 x 1/2).
- Vigilance must be maintained for the complications of CF: haemoptysis, pneumothorax, atelectasis, respiratory failure and cor pulmonale.
- There should be no hesitation in performing chest X-rays where these are deemed necessary.
- Chest physiotherapy and bronchial drainage should continue.
- Serial lung function tests, e.g. spirometry and arterial blood gases, should be performed at regular intervals throughout pregnancy.
- Careful surveillance for signs of chest infection becomes even more important due to the complications of pneumonia in pregnancy (see below). *Pseudomonas aeruginosa* is the most common cause of chest infection in CF. Penicillins, cephalosporins and aminoglycosides are the most commonly used antibiotics (intravenously, orally or inhaled). All are considered safe in pregnancy, even gentamicin (the risk of fetal ototoxicity can be minimised

by ensuring maternal serum levels do not exceed recommended levels). The risks to the mother and fetus of withholding appropriate antibiotics are greater. Some antibiotic-dosing schedules will need to be adjusted due to the larger volume distribution and enhanced renal elimination found in pregnancy.

- Cardiovascular status should be observed during pregnancy, preferably by echocardiography.
- Pancreatic enzymes should be continued and insulin levels adjusted appropriately.
- Termination of pregnancy should be considered by women with very unfavourable features.
- Advice from dieticians will be essential to maintain caloric intake. Rarely, enteral (and even parenteral) feeding is necessary.
- Regular fetal monitoring with growth scans is advisable, especially in more severe cases of lung disease or poor maternal weight gain.
- Ideally, induction of labour and caesarean section are performed only for obstetric reasons. However, deterioration in lung function may prompt intervention. General anaesthesia should be avoided where possible.
- Facial oxygen may be required in labour, and exhaustion should be prevented by instrumental delivery if necessary. Prolonged Valsalva manoeuvres may predispose to pneumothoraces.

EBM

Retrospective studies suggest that pregnancy accelerates the loss of respiratory function only in 'severe' cases of cystic fibrosis.

TUBERCULOSIS

Infection with *Mycobacterium tuberculosis* most commonly presents in African and Indian ethnic groups, new immigrant populations, refugees and asylum seekers. HIV positivity is another well-recognised risk factor and this is one reason cited for the increasing incidence of tuberculosis (TB) since the 1980s. As deaths from TB appear to be increasing a prospective national study of TB in pregnancy was undertaken by UKOSS from February 2005 to August 2006.[14] Over this period, there were 52 confirmed cases, representing an incidence rate of 4.6 per 100,000 maternities with a 95% CI of 3.4–8.0. From these figures the estimated total number of cases of TB in the 2006–8 triennium was 266 (95% CI 184–374). In this same period, the Confidential Enquiry reported that two pregnant women died from TB, giving an estimated case fatality rate of TB in pregnancy in 2006–8 of 1:133 known cases (95% CI 1:92 to 1:187).

Treatment can be safe and effective in pregnancy and the outcome is normally good. Failure to diagnose the condition

EBM

There is no good evidence to suggest that pregnancy is an independent risk factor for infection with *Mycobacterium tuberculosis* or that the course and outcome of TB are altered by pregnancy.

and patient non-compliance with medication regimens put the mother and newborn at increased risk.

Primary infection is usually asymptomatic, although fever, cough, conjunctivitis and erythema nodosum may all occur. A cellular immune response can be detected 3–8 weeks later by a positive tuberculin test.

Any further clinical manifestations are known as 'post-primary tuberculosis' and include pulmonary disease (apical lung cavitation, pneumonia, pleural effusion), miliary TB (widespread disseminated TB), pericarditis, peritonitis, meningitis, bone and genitourinary TB. These may occur months or years after the primary infection following a period of 'latency'.

Public health policies towards TB prevention and detection have differed on each side of the Atlantic. In the USA, tuberculin testing (the Mantoux test) is used to screen high-risk groups during pregnancy. A positive result combined with specific risk factors may prompt a screening chest X-ray and sputum testing for mycobacteria. Based on the results of these, the patient is either treated for active TB or given prophylaxis with isoniazid, on the assumption that latent infection is present and could reactivate at any time. In the UK, widespread vaccination of schoolchildren with bacille Calmette–Guérin (BCG – said to prevent 70 per cent of infections) reduces the value of routine tuberculin testing, which will be positive in those who have been vaccinated. There is no screening programme for TB in pregnancy in the UK and clinicians must remain hypervigilant for signs and symptoms suggestive of the disease.

Pulmonary manifestations are the most common presenting features of TB, and a chest X-ray may show upper-lobe densities and cavitation, fibrosis, pleural effusion, empyema or calcifications. Sputum is examined for acid-fast bacilli using a Ziehl–Neelsen stain and subsequently cultured for antibiotic sensitivity testing. Bronchoscopic washings must be obtained if there is no sputum. Extrapulmonary TB is diagnosed using tissue biopsies in a similar way. Although the Mantoux test is considered safe in pregnancy, it is unable to distinguish active disease from previous disease and BCG vaccination.

Active TB infections are treated with a combination of antibiotics, determined by the results of the culture sensitivities. Although regimens vary, treatment usually includes therapy with rifampicin, isoniazid, pyrazinamide and sometimes ethambutol. Less well-known drugs may be necessary in cases of multi-drug resistance including amikacin, kanamycin and ethionamide.

The relationship between pregnancy and TB

It is generally agreed that pregnancy has no impact on the course of TB and that TB, if diagnosed and treated expeditiously, has no significant impact on the pregnancy [D]. Delayed or inadequate therapy would appear to be detrimental to both maternal and fetal outcomes; however, increasing the risks of prematurity and intrauterine growth restriction [D].

Presentation and diagnosis are unaffected by pregnancy, although misguided reluctance in performing chest X-rays may lead to further diagnostic delay.

Vertical transmission (congenital TB) is extremely rare and usually occurs only where maternal disease has gone untreated. Fewer than 300 cases have been reported, although placental infection is somewhat more common. Lateral transmission from the mother or other close contacts, occurring after delivery, is a much more likely cause of infant infection. Therefore strict criteria exist for the diagnosis of congenital TB. One of the following is necessary:

- lesions in the first week of life;
- a primary hepatic complex or caseating granuloma;
- histological evidence of placental or endometrial involvement;
- absence of TB in other carers of the child.

Congenital TB usually presents with fever, lymphadenopathy, hepatosplenomegaly and respiratory distress. It is fatal in one in five cases. In only half of all cases has the diagnosis of maternal TB already been made.

Treatment of TB during pregnancy

TB is most likely to be diagnosed by physicians, even during pregnancy, and the specialist advice of a respiratory consultant is essential along with close involvement by microbiologists [E].

Isoniazid, rifampicin and ethambutol are used initially. The ethambutol can be stopped when sensitivities show that the other two drugs are adequate. These are then continued for 9 months in total. The most significant toxic side effect of isoniazid in animal and human studies is demyelination (causing a peripheral neuropathy). This can be prevented by supplementation with pyridoxine (vitamin B_6). Hepatotoxicity may be more common in pregnancy, and liver function tests should be performed monthly [D]. Most studies do not show a significant elevation in the anomaly rate above the background 2–3 per cent in users of rifampicin in pregnancy [B]. Liver enzyme induction, with theoretical vitamin K deficiency, should prompt maternal oral vitamin K supplements in the third trimester to prevent haemorrhagic disease of the newborn. The theoretical risks of fetal ocular toxicity with ethambutol have not been borne out in practice. Although pyrizinamide is usually avoided in pregnancy, there are no data to suggest a harmful effect and it should be used if needed as a second-line agent. Streptomycin, a previous favourite in TB treatment, has well-recognised fetal ototoxicity. Safer alternatives are available.

Non-compliance with drug regimens outside pregnancy is a major problem. There is no reason to think that it is any less so during pregnancy. Supervision, encouragement and incentive schemes may be necessary to encourage proper use of the prescribed medications.

All the anti-tuberculous drugs mentioned in this section are compatible with breastfeeding [D].

There is often concern over the infectious nature of TB in a maternity setting. Provided that the prescribed drugs have been taken properly, an active TB sufferer will become non-infectious within 2 weeks of commencing treatment. If the mother is still sputum positive, specialist infection control nursing will be necessary. The newborn should be immunised with BCG and also given prophylactic antibiotics (usually isoniazid). Separation of the infant from its mother is not necessary unless she is non-compliant or another carer or family member is highly infectious.

It would seem prudent to send the placenta for microbiological investigation. Evidence of acid-fast bacilli should increase surveillance of the newborn.

PNEUMONIA

Pneumonia in otherwise healthy individuals is no more common in pregnancy than in an age-matched population as a whole, and the maternal outcome, in the main, is no better or worse. The incidence of pneumonia in pregnancy would appear to be on the rise, but this may be accounted for by an increase in the number of pregnancies in women with coexisting problems such as HIV and CF. Four women died in the 2006–2008 CEMD, most of whom had underlying social factors such as severe deprivation. Generally prompt diagnosis and treatment avoid poor maternal outcomes. In addition, fetal outcome may be affected, and prompt recognition and treatment of pneumonia in pregnancy are essential if this is to be avoided. The main risk would appear to be preterm labour, although growth restriction has also been reported (Box 16.2).

Box 16.2 Risk factors for pneumonia

History of recent upper respiratory tract infection
Chronic respiratory disease (e.g. asthma, cystic fibrosis)
Smoking
Immunocompromise (HIV, substance abuse, alcoholism, recurrent courses of antenatal steroids)
Anaemia
Farm workers (*Coxiella burnetii*)
General anaesthesia (aspiration pneumonitis)
HIV

Diagnosis of pneumonia in pregnancy

The symptoms and signs of pneumonia are not altered by pregnancy, but may be confused with physiological changes common to pregnancy. Reluctance to perform a chest X-ray may further delay the diagnosis. Obstetricians have a responsibility in educating other physicians that the fetal radiation exposure with appropriate shielding is minimal and that this examination is safe. This message is even more important if risk factors for pneumonia are present.

Sputum should be sent for microbiological examination and culture. Blood can be taken for serological testing for *Mycoplasma* and viral antibodies.

Treatment of pneumonia in pregnancy

Common organisms
Frequently, no infectious agent is found and the pneumonia is treated empirically. The most common bacteria causing community-acquired pneumonia are *Streptococcus pneumoniae* and *Haemophilus influenzae*, often occurring after a viral infection. Atypical pneumonias caused by *Mycoplasma* and, less commonly, *Legionella* must also be considered. Penicillins, macrolides and cephalosporins are the treatments of choice and none is contraindicated in pregnancy. Higher doses of amoxicillin should be used to counteract the increased renal clearance found in pregnancy. Erythromycin or clarithromycin should be added if there is suspicion of an atypical pneumonia, and cephalosporins used for penicillin-allergic individuals or hospital-acquired infections. Pneumonias requiring hospitalisation are usually treated with a third-generation cephalosporin (e.g. ceftriaxone) with erythromycin.

Common viral causes of pneumonia include the three subtypes of influenza myxovirus. Although amantadine and ribavirin antiviral agents have been used in pregnancy with no obvious harmful effects, their use is not recommended. The generally good outcome of viral pneumonia in pregnancy would support this.

Less common causes of pneumonia in pregnancy
More unusual pneumonias occur when there are underlying risk factors. *Klebsiella* is said to be typical of alcoholics, often associated with abscess formation. *Coxiella burnetii* is found in the aerosols produced by farm animals. Q fever, the pneumonia caused by this organism, is said to cause miscarriage, intrauterine death and stillbirth. *Staphylococcus aureus* is significantly more likely after influenza infections and may have a sudden and rapid course. Pneumonia following aspiration of stomach contents is rare, but carries a significant mortality, with anaerobic and Gram-negative organisms being the most common infectious agents.

S. pneumoniae and *Pseudomonas aeruginosa* are common causes of pneumonia in HIV-positive individuals. *Pneumocystis jirovecii* is an acquired immune deficiency syndrome (AIDS)-defining illness that carries a high mortality rate, whether or not it occurs in pregnancy. The theoretical risks of using Septrin (trimethoprim–sulfamethoxazole) in pregnancy include folate antagonism, and kernicterus or haemolysis in the newborn. The latter is extremely uncommon, and folate supplementation minimises the risks associated with trimethoprim. Pentamidine can be used as an alternative in pregnancy. Other unusual organisms to be considered in HIV-positive women, or those with other causes of significant immunocompromise, include atypical mycobacteria and cryptococci.

The true incidence of pneumonia in adult chickenpox infections is unclear, but mortality from varicella pneumonitis has been quoted as 11 per cent. Whether the depressed cell-mediated immunity of pregnancy truly influences the incidence and mortality of varicella pneumonia in pregnancy is unclear, although many reports suggest that it worsens outcome, with mortality quoted as being as high as 1 in 3. Varicella-zoster virus infections in pregnancy are discussed further in Chapter 24.

Key References

1. Murphy VE, Gibson PG. Asthma in pregnancy. *Clin Chest Med* 2011;32:93–110, ix.
2. Cydulka RK, Emerman CL, Schreiber D, Molander KH, Woodruff PG, Camargo CA. Acute asthma among pregnant women presenting to the emergency department. *Am J Respir Crit Care Med* 1999;160:887–92.
3. Siddiqui S, Goodman N, McKenna S, Goldie M, Waugh J, Brightling CE. Pre-eclampsia is associated with airway hyperresponsiveness. *BJOG* 2008;115:520–2.
4. CMACE. Saving mothers' lives: reviewing maternal deaths to make motherhood safer: 2006–08. The Eighth Report on Confidential Enquiries into Maternal Deaths in the United Kingdom. BJOG 2011; 118(Suppl 1):1–203.
5. British Thoracic Society/SIGN. British Guideline on the Management of Asthma (2008). *Thorax* 2008;63 (Suppl 4):1–21.
6. Czeizel AE, Rockenbauer M. Population-based case-control study of teratogenic potential of corticosteroids. *Teratology* 1997;56:335–40.
7. Park-Wyllie L, Mazzotta P, Pastuszak A *et al.* Birth defects after maternal exposure to corticosteroids: prospective cohort study and meta-analysis of epidemiological studies. *Teratology* 2000;62:385–92.
8. British Thoracic Society. The British guidelines on asthma management. *Thorax* 1997; 52(Suppl.):S1–21.
9. Hadeh A, Ferrin M, Hadjiliadis D, Ahluwalia M, Hoag JB, Cystic fibrosis and pregnancy in the modern era: a case-control study. *J Cystic Fibrosis* 2014;13:69–73.
10. Gilljam MD, Antoniou M, Shin J, Dupuis A, Corey M, Tullis E. Pregnancy in cystic fibrosis. Fetal and maternal outcome. *Chest* 2000;118:85–91.
11. Edenborough FP, Stableforth DE, Webb AK, Mackenzie WE, Smith DL. Outcome of pregnancy in women with cystic fibrosis. *Thorax* 1995;50:170–4.
12. Edenborough FP, Mackenzie WE, Conway SP *et al.* The effect of pregnancy on maternal cystic fibrosis vs nulliparous severity matched controls. *Thorax* 1996;51 (Suppl. 3):A50.
13. Edenborough FP, Borgo G, Knoop C *et al.* European Cystic Fibrosis Society. Guidelines for the management of pregnancy in women with cystic fibrosis. *J Cyst Fibros* 2008; 7 (Suppl 1):S2–32.
14. Knight M, Kurinczuk JJ, Spark P, Brocklehurst P. *UKOSS Annual Report 2007*. Oxford: National Perinatal Epidemiology Unit, 2007.

Chapter 17 Neurological conditions

Louise Kenny

INTRODUCTION

The focus of this section is mostly on pre-existing medical conditions and how they interact with pregnancy. Neurological disease is fortunately rare. The details of each and every neurological condition are well beyond the bounds of this textbook, and also of the MRCOG. Candidates sitting this examination are not expected to be obstetric physicians. However, competence is demanded in the management of several neurological conditions commonly encountered in the antenatal clinic. Epilepsy is common in women of reproductive age and the use of anticonvulsant drugs in pregnancy represents a model example of how benefits of treatment to the fetus and mother must be weighed against the risks. Multiple sclerosis demonstrates clearly how pregnancy can alter the clinical course of a disease. Myasthenia gravis illustrates how maternal conditions can continue to cause harm, even after delivery, and the 'triplet repeat diseases' highlight the need for specialised pre-pregnancy counselling and prenatal diagnostic services.

Strictly speaking, stroke need not be included here as it tends to feature more as a problem arising during pregnancy. However, in other respects it fits well with this discussion and it is important to recognise those women presenting with risk factors for stroke at booking, when the possibility of prevention exists.

EPILEPSY

Approximately 6 in every 1000 pregnancies are complicated by a past or current history of epilepsy, making it the most common pre-existing neurological condition complicating antenatal care. However, on occasion epilepsy can present for the first time during pregnancy and every obstetrician must have a working differential for the causes of seizure during pregnancy (Box 17.1). Familial, cryptogenic and trauma-related epilepsies account for the vast majority of cases with an established diagnosis at the onset of pregnancy. A minority of cases are caused by brain tumours, congenital abnormalities and vascular problems, and these may require even more specialised care during the pregnancy. Seizure frequency may increase, decrease or stay the same in pregnancy (37 per cent, 13 per cent and 50 per cent, respectively),[1] with labour being a particularly high-risk time for convulsions. A recent prospective study in the UK demonstrated no major differences in obstetric outcomes (excluding fetal abnormalities); however, an Icelandic retrospective study found a caesarean section rate almost double that of the control population.[2] A proportion of emergency caesarean sections were performed for seizures occurring during labour.

Box 17.1 A differential diagnosis of seizures during pregnancy and the postpartum period

Idiopathic epilepsy

Epilepsy secondary to a specific cause

    Previous trauma

    Antiphospholipid syndrome

    Intracranial mass lesions

    Gestational epilepsy (seizures secondary to pregnancy)

Intracranial infection

    Meningitis

    Encephalitis

    Brain abscess/subdural empyema

    Cerebral malaria

Vascular disease

    Cerebral infarction

    Subarachnoid and cerebral haemorrhage

    Hypertensive encephalopathy

    Eclampsia

    Cerebral vein thrombosis

    Thrombotic thrombocytopenic purpura

Metabolic

    Hyponatraemia/hypoglycaemia/hypocalcaemia

    Liver and renal failure

    Anoxia

    Alcohol withdrawal

Drug toxicity

    Local anaesthetics, e.g. lidocaine

    Tricyclic antidepressants

    Amphetamines

    Lithium

Pseudoepilepsy (factitious)

Therapeutic aspects

Antiepileptic drugs (AEDs) may affect the fetus and newborn in a number of ways (Box 17.2).

The evidence is confusing and often contradictory. There are no RCTs and studies are mostly retrospective with ascertainment bias. This makes patient counselling very difficult. However, a number of points are generally accepted.

- The incidence of congenital anomalies is increased significantly among the offspring of epileptic mothers [B].
- AEDs are responsible for most or all of this increase [B].
- The benefits of seizure control during pregnancy outweigh the risks [E].
- Polytherapy with more than one AED carries greater risks to the fetus than monotherapy [B].

Box 17.2 Effects of antiepileptic drugs on the fetus and newborn

Teratogenicity

    Major and minor congenital malformations

    Characteristic dysmorphic syndrome

Neonatal withdrawal effects

Vitamin K deficiency with haemorrhagic disease of the newborn

Developmental delay or behavioural difficulties

- Although certain AEDs are more strongly linked to particular congenital abnormalities, there is significant overlap, and the first-line agents can all cause the fetal anticonvulsant syndrome [B].

Other points are more controversial. No evidence grade is given for these points in view of this uncertainty.

- Women with a history of seizures who are not taking AEDs have a higher risk of congenital anomalies in their offspring than those with no history.
- Women with regular and severe seizure activity during pregnancy carry a higher congenital abnormality risk.
- Lower doses of AEDs carry a lower risk.
- The use of high-dose folic acid reduces the congenital anomaly risk.
- AED levels should be checked during each trimester as altered pharmacokinetics may disrupt seizure control.

Congenital abnormalities

The reported incidence of congenital abnormalities among the offspring of epileptic women varies among studies, mainly due to variations in case ascertainment and definition. Major abnormalities (which are less likely to go unreported) are found in 5–10 per cent of women who have taken AEDs [C].[2–4] The incidence of anomalies may actually be determined by a number of different factors:

- an inherent added risk associated with epilepsy, independent of AEDs;
- genetically inherited tendencies;
- the number and severity of seizures during pregnancy;
- the use of AEDs during pregnancy.

Until recently, it was generally agreed that, whether treated or not, women with a history of seizures had a higher fetal anomaly rate than those without such a history. A recent prospective study from Newcastle has supported this assertion, finding *major* abnormality rates among treated epileptics, untreated epileptics and controls to be 4.6 per cent, 8 per cent and 2.4 per cent respectively.[3] However, equivalent figures from the USA published in 2001 have suggested differently (5.7 per cent, 0 per cent and 1.8 per cent, respectively),[4] as did a study from Milan, which found severe structural anomalies in 5.3 per cent of AED-exposed pregnancies and none in the 25 pregnancies with a history of seizure but no treatment.[5]

There is similar disagreement over the impact that first- and second-trimester seizure activity has on congenital anomaly rates. These studies found no evidence of increased congenital anomaly rates in the offspring of women with higher-level seizure activity.

The medications themselves undoubtedly carry the greatest risk [B]. Non-epileptic women using these drugs for other reasons demonstrate similar anomaly rates.[4] The 'fetal hydantoin syndrome' described by Hanson and Smith in 1975 has been renamed the 'fetal anticonvulsant syndrome' after the realisation that AEDs other than phenytoin (carbamazepine, valproate, phenobarbital, benzodiazepines) could also cause a similar array of abnormalities (Table 17.1).

The incidence of this syndrome in AED-exposed pregnancies is two to three times higher than in controls [B]. Behavioural problems, learning difficulties, speech and gross motor delay, and features of autism were found in more than 50 per cent of children diagnosed with this syndrome when studied retrospectively [D].[6]

Despite this generic effect seen with most anticonvulsants, certain drugs are more closely associated with particular groups of anomalies. Valproate and, to a lesser extent, carbamazepine are thought to increase the risk of neural tube defects to between 1 and 2 per cent [B]. Doses >1000 mg/day of valproate seem more likely to be associated with this outcome [C]. Valproate may likewise increase the incidence of genitourinary anomalies and, along with phenytoin, cardiac abnormalities. Prospective studies have estimated a risk as high as one in five of developmental delay with phenytoin and carbamazepine therapy, although this is disputed.

The various studies do agree on one point: polytherapy carries greater risk than treatment with one drug alone [B].[4,5] Holmes and colleagues, for example, found the incidence of major malformations to be 5.7 per cent in the offspring of women using monotherapy but 8.6 per cent in those using two or more AEDs.[4]

The question is often asked: which anticonvulsant carries least risk of fetal harm? A recent systematic review[7] highlighted that women presenting already pregnant on AEDs should probably remain on their current regimen, as any teratogenic harm is likely to have occurred already. If a pregnancy is being planned, some have the opinion that valproate should be avoided, as it would appear to carry the greatest teratogenic risk and more recent reports suggest that it may also cause developmental delay. Newer drugs such as lamotrigine, gabapentin and tiagabine so far have a good record in animal studies, but experience in human pregnancies is still too limited to assess their safety confidently [E].

Other important drug effects

For reasons that are not entirely clear, carbamazepine, phenytoin, phenobarbital (and even valproate) cause vitamin K deficiency, perhaps by inducing liver enzymes responsible for its oxidative degradation. Vitamin K is required for the carboxylation of factors II (prothrombin), VII, IX and X, and deficiency in the neonate may cause haemorrhagic disease of the newborn, with catastrophic intracranial and gastrointestinal bleeding occurring in a few. Owing to the extremely low levels of vitamin K in a healthy neonate, deficiency must be measured indirectly by studying 'prothrombin induced by vitamin K absence' (PIVKA) levels. Use of these anticonvulsants has been shown to increase PIVKA levels [B]. This increase can be prevented by maternal therapy with vitamin K supplements in the third trimester [B]. Indeed, some have even postulated that vitamin K deficiency may contribute to some of the structural abnormalities found in the fetal anticonvulsant syndrome, raising the possibility that vitamin K supplements earlier in pregnancy might be warranted.

Neonatal withdrawal effects have been noted with maternal use of phenobarbital, carbamazepine and valproate, and range from poor feeding to jitteriness and convulsions. Such effects are uncommon now that phenobarbital is used less frequently.

Phenytoin and carbamazepine *may* also cause an increase in childhood cancers such as neuroblastoma, although the rarity of these makes statistical certainty difficult [C].

Drug pharmacokinetics

A number of factors during pregnancy serve to reduce effective serum concentrations of various AEDs:

- the increased volume distribution of pregnancy;
- the increased renal clearance;
- induction of hepatic enzyme metabolism by pregnancy and high folate levels;
- vomiting and delayed malabsorption.

The reduction in serum protein concentration during pregnancy means that a greater proportion of the drug is found in the free (active) state. This is especially true for those AEDs exhibiting strong protein-binding characteristics (Table 17.2).

Serum levels of AEDs include both the free and the protein-bound components. Keeping the total level in the low 'normal' range is therefore advised during pregnancy to limit the chances of maternal toxic side effects and fetal complications [E]. In reality, even free levels do not correlate

Table 17.1 The fetal anticonvulsant syndrome(s)

Major abnormalities	Minor abnormalities
Microcephaly	Hypertelorism
Cleft lip and palate	Distal digital and nail hypoplasia
Neural tube defects	Flat nasal bridge
Congenital heart defects	Low-set abnormal ears
Intrauterine growth restriction	Epicanthic folds
Developmental delay	Long philtrum

ANTENATAL OBSTETRICS

Table 17.2 Protein binding of anti-epileptic drugs

50% protein bound	50% protein bound
Clonazepam	Carbamazepine
Gabapentin	Phenytoin
Valproate	Lamotrigine
	Phenobarbital
	Vigabatrin

Table 17.3 Enzyme-inducing ability of antiepileptic drugs

Enzyme-inducing AEDs	Non-enzyme-inducing AEDs
Phenobarbital	Valproate
Phenytoin	Lamotrigine
Carbamazepine	Gabapentin
	Ethosuximide
	Clonazepam

well with seizure control [D] and some authorities disagree with routine testing of serum levels.

However, testing should be performed in a number of special cases [E]:

- suspected non-compliance (60 per cent of pregnancies in a recent survey);
- increasing seizure activity;
- concerns over toxic side effects;
- polypharmacy with drug interactions.

The enzyme-inducing AEDs may enhance their own metabolism and that of other agents (Table 17.3). Valproate may inhibit the enzyme epoxide hydrolase, which metabolises phenytoin and carbamazepine.

Managing epilepsy and pregnancy

There are no RCTs pertinent to the management of epilepsy in pregnancy. Guidelines such as the ones given below are based on evidence of grades C, D and E.[8,9] Retrospective studies highlight how poorly such guidelines are adhered to.

Pre-pregnancy counselling

As with diabetes, there is much to be gained by planning pregnancy carefully following detailed counselling from a joint team including obstetricians and neurologists [D].

- The diagnosis should be reviewed by a neurologist – this is dubious in a proportion of women using AEDs.
- Consideration should be given to stopping AEDs in those who have been seizure free for more than 2 years. The risk of relapse is 20–50 per cent, being higher for some forms of epilepsy (e.g. juvenile myoclonic epilepsy) than others (e.g. absence or tonic–clonic seizures) [C]. Serious health and social consequences may result from a recurrence of seizures (e.g. driving prohibition). If withdrawal is to be attempted, it should occur in small increments over a prolonged period, supervised by a specialist. The patient should not drive during this period.
- Where possible, treatment regimens should be simplified to a single AED and the lowest effective dose used to minimise the risk of congenital abnormalities [E].
- The risks to the mother and the fetus of non-compliance with prescribed medications, especially status epilepticus, must be discussed along with the AED-associated fetal risks [E].

- Folic acid 5 mg should be taken each day periconceptually. This is most important for women taking valproate and carbamazepine, although it is still unclear whether this reduces the risk of neural tube defects in this group [E].
- The risk to the offspring of epilepsy should also be discussed. Few cases of epilepsy exhibit autosomal dominant inheritance. However, having one parent with idiopathic epilepsy confers a 4 per cent risk of epilepsy in the offspring, increasing to 10 per cent when a parent and a sibling are affected, and to 15 per cent when both parents have epilepsy [C].

Antenatal management

- Care should be carried out by an obstetrician with a special interest in epilepsy, jointly with a neurologist [E].
- All pregnancies occurring in women on anticonvulsant drugs should be notified to the UK Register of Anti-epileptic Drugs in Pregnancy [E].
- Screening for fetal anomalies should be offered to all women with epilepsy, with particular attention paid to those anomalies more commonly found in this group. A fetal cardiac scan may be warranted at 22 weeks' gestation [E].
- Drug level monitoring may not need to be carried out as a routine but many clinicians like a 'starting' value and there are other situations that may prompt testing (see above) [E].
- Oral vitamin K supplements should be taken from 36 weeks onwards (10 mg per day) to prevent haemorrhagic disease of the newborn [C].
- If steroids are to be given for the usual obstetric indications, women using enzyme-inducing AEDs should be given 48 mg in total (two lots of 24 mg dexamethasone 24 hours apart) [E].

Intrapartum care

- Induction of labour and caesarean section are indicated for the usual obstetric indications. Vaginal delivery should otherwise be the aim [E].
- Labour carries a higher risk of seizure due to sleep disruption, reduced intake and absorption of AEDs, and hyperventilation, which may alter free levels of AEDs. Every effort must be made to administer anticonvulsants as usual. Intravenous phenytoin can be used if necessary, although it may cause arrhythmias.

ANTENATAL OBSTETRICS

- Seizures during labour are best controlled with IV benzodiazepines (e.g. clonazepam or diazepam). Rectal diazepam can be used in the absence of intravenous access. Provided that the fetal heart rate tracing remains reactive, this is not usually considered an indication for emergency caesarean section. However, status epilepticus or recurrent seizures in labour may warrant abdominal delivery for fetal reasons [E].

Postpartum care

- The serum levels of AEDs may rise in the postpartum period and monitoring may be necessary to prevent maternal toxic side effects. However, sleep deprivation may lower the normal threshold for seizure activity. If doses have been raised during pregnancy, a reduction in the immediate postpartum period may be necessary [E].
- All anticonvulsants reach breast milk. Neonatal side effects are rare, but sedation and withdrawal effects must be watched for, in particular where phenobarbital and benzodiazepines have been used. Breastfeeding is to be encouraged [C].
- A single 1 mg intramuscular vitamin K neonatal supplement is advised in order to prevent haemorrhagic disease of the newborn [C].
- Contraceptive advice should be given before discharge home. The enzyme inducers will reduce the contraceptive efficacy of the combined pill, minipill and Depo-Provera injections. A combined oral contraceptive pill containing 50 mg of oestrogen should be used, preferably with a shorter pill-free interval (5–6 days instead of 7). 'Tricycling' will further reduce the chances of ovulation. Depo-Provera should be given every 10 weeks instead of every 12. The Mirena intrauterine system is ideal, as the locally administered progestogen will not be affected by induced liver enzymes [C].
- Special advice should be given to new mothers who also have epilepsy [C].

    - Ask for extra help if you are not getting enough sleep.
    - Ensure that someone else is present when you bath your baby.
    - Surround yourself with cushions and pillows when you are holding your baby.
    - Feed and change your baby on the floor while leaning against a wall to prevent you falling on to the baby in the event of a seizure.

Unfortunately, a recent UK prospective study[3] has shown how poorly such recommendations are being followed. Less than 50 per cent of pregnancies were planned and only 1 in 10 epileptic women took folic acid appropriately. Most did not have pre-pregnancy counselling and 1 in 5 was using AEDs despite a fit-free interval of more than 2 years prior to the pregnancy. Sixty per cent were looked after solely by general practitioners, and vitamin K was given to only a third of those who should have received supplements in the third trimester.

Sudden unexpected death in epilepsy

Sudden unexpected death in epilepsy (SUDEP) is an uncommon and non-traumatic death that occurs suddenly and unexpectedly in a patient with epilepsy who was otherwise previously healthy. Deaths from SUDEP are usually not witnessed and may or may not occur during a seizure. It is without any obvious clinical or pathological explanations. SUDEPs account for 10% of all epilepsy-related deaths; 85% of these fatalities occur between the ages of 20 and 50 years. The incidence of SUDEP stands at approximately 1 in 1000 people with epilepsy per year, which is at least 10 times the sudden death rate found in the general population.

The latest Confidential Enquiry *Saving Mothers' Lives* investigated 14 deaths of women with epilepsy in the 2006–8 triennium – the highest number from any neurological disease and three times the number of deaths from asthma. The actual cause of death in 11 of the 14 women with epilepsy was categorised as SUDEP. The other three deaths were seizure-related deaths, one from status epilepticus, one from a fall and one death while bathing.

It is not clear whether pregnancy is an independent risk factor for SUDEP; it will, however, be an indirect risk factor since SUDEP is known to be more common in patients who do not take prescribed anticonvulsants and many women are reluctant to take anticonvulsants when pregnant or breastfeeding for fear of harming their babies.

MULTIPLE SCLEROSIS

Multiple sclerosis (MS) is a multifocal autoimmune disease of the CNS. Infiltrating lymphocytes and macrophages bring about inflammation, demyelination and axonal damage while further activating inherent CNS immune cells such as astrocytes and microglia. Optic nerve, brain and spinal cord may all be affected and this may manifest as almost any neurological deficit, symptom or sign. Most cases are characterised by a 'relapsing and remitting' natural history, with slow gradual decline. Less commonly, the MS follows a more rapidly progressive pattern. Diagnoses of MS are either 'probable' or 'definite', depending on whether the clinical features (probable) have been supported by the results of specialised investigations (oligoclonal abnormalities in cerebrospinal fluid, white matter lesions on MRI or prolonged latency of evoked potentials on neurophysiological testing). An inheritable genetic element to the disease does exist, but very rarely is a true mendelian pattern of autosomal dominance seen. Overall, the risk of the offspring developing MS with one affected parent appears to be approximately 4 per cent. The rate can, however, be as high as 30 per cent if both parents are affected [D]. Viral infection is likely to be a more important aetiological factor and indeed relapses are more common following non-specific viral illness [D].

Effect of pregnancy on MS

Various studies, both prospective and retrospective, suggest that pregnancy does not accelerate the course of MS, but relapses are more common in the puerperium. Pregnancy may have a protective effect.

The key part that the immune system plays in MS disease activity is highlighted by the effects of pregnancy on this condition. Pregnancy is characterised by a shift from type 1 (pro-inflammatory) to type 2 (anti-inflammatory) T-cell activity. Although various studies have reached slightly different conclusions, the combined evidence suggests that pregnancy itself is associated with a reduction in the number of relapses [C][10] and that this may even reduce the overall progression of the disease in the long term [D].[11] Also, the incidence of MS may be lower in multiparous women than in women who have never been pregnant [D].[11] As with rheumatoid arthritis, however, relapses in the puerperium are more common [C],[10] although this is not influenced by breastfeeding and one recent study has even reported a possible protective effect.[10] It is important to be aware of potential bias in such studies; women with more active disease are less likely to become pregnant for many reasons. However, the most recent reports have tried to avoid such bias and the above effects remain. Confavreux and colleagues[10] found a relapse rate of 0.2 per woman per year during the third trimester, compared with 0.7 in the year before pregnancy. In the first 3 months postpartum this rate increased to 1.2. The overall progression in disability scores was not altered by pregnancy over a 3-year time period. The effect of pregnancy on the course of the chronic progressive variant of MS is less clear.

Management of MS during pregnancy

Multiple sclerosis sufferers experience a wide variety of neurological symptoms and treatment should be tailored to the individual. Non-pharmacological therapy may be sufficient in some cases, but expert help should be requested from a neurologist.

A recent expert consensus report made several recommendations regarding pharmacological treatment of MS in pregnancy.[12]

Immunomodulator therapy such as beta-interferon (B-IFN) or glatiramer acetate (a synthetic amino acid polymer) has not been shown to be harmful to the fetus and can be safely continued until pregnancy is confirmed. In case of very active disease, continuation of immunomodulator therapy throughout the entire pregnancy may also be considered on a case-by-case basis, as there is a lack of evidence of toxicity from studies and pharmacovigilance registries.

There is a paucity of data in pregnancy for newer agents such as natalizumab and fingolimod. Natalizumab is a humanised monoclonal antibody against the cell adhesion molecule 4-integrin. Given the current absence of sufficient safety data in pregnancy the current recommendation is to discontinue this drug 3 months before conception.

Fingolimod is a sphingosine 1-phosphate receptor modulator, which sequesters lymphocytes in lymph nodes, preventing them from contributing to an autoimmune reaction. This drug should be discontinued at least 2 months before conception due to a presumed teratogenic risk shown in animals.

Urinary urgency may be treated with tricyclic antidepressants such as imipramine and this is safe to continue. Spasticity and paroxysmal pain may be treated with baclofen (probably safe in pregnancy) and anticonvulsant drugs (see Epilepsy). Mood alterations are also common in MS. Depression and hopelessness are just as typical as the frequently mentioned 'euphoria'. Treatment with tricyclic antidepressants is not contraindicated in pregnancy. Prophylaxis for MS remains an area of controversy.

Induction of labour and caesarean section are mostly reserved for obstetric indications [E], although serious disability may make vaginal delivery impractical and an exacerbation of urinary symptoms and limb spasm may warrant earlier planned delivery. The use of epidural anaesthesia is not contraindicated and does not cause an increased rate of disease progression [C].

Breastfeeding is not advised while using b-IFN, although harmful effects have not been noted.

MYASTHENIA GRAVIS

This relatively rare neurological condition deserves mention as it is more common in women of child-bearing years and illustrates well how maternal disease can interact with pregnancy in ways not yet covered in this chapter.

Myasthenia gravis (MG) is caused by autoimmune disruption at the nicotinic neuromuscular junction. It may present with double vision, difficulty swallowing, ptosis and respiratory muscle failure. Anti-acetylcholine receptor autoantibodies can be found in 85–90 per cent of patients, and thymic abnormalities (hyperplasia or thymoma) in somewhat fewer. However, these autoantibodies can also be found in women who do not have the disease, and the diagnosis instead is usually made by administration of edrophonium chloride (a short-acting anticholinesterase), which transiently improves symptoms, notably muscle strength, in those with MG (the Tensilon test). Longer-acting acetylcholinesterase inhibitors are the mainstay of treatment (neostigmine and pyridostigmine), but immunosuppressive therapy with corticosteroids, azathioprine, ciclosporin and methotrexate is a second-line option. Plasmapharesis and IV immunoglobulin infusions are used for serious exacerbations. Undertreatment and overtreatment both carry their own risks. 'Myasthenic crises' can be precipitated by infection, aminoglycosides, magnesium sulphate, local anaesthetics, beta blockers, beta-receptor agonists, narcotics and neuromuscular blockers (Table 17.4).

Table 17.4 Emergencies in myasthenia gravis

Myasthenic crisis	Cholinergic crisis
Nasal regurgitation	Abdominal 'colicky' pain
Dysphagia	Diarrhoea
Respiratory impairment	Excess salivation and sweating
	Severe weakness (depolarising block)
	Bradycardia

Interaction between myasthenia and pregnancy

The effect of pregnancy on MG is unpredictable and varies considerably among women and even between pregnancies in the same woman.

A recent retrospective review found deterioration in 19 per cent, improvement in 22 per cent and no change in 59 per cent.[13] Myasthenic symptoms worsened postpartum in approximately a third of the women in this study [D]. The severity of the pre-pregnancy disease did not predict well what would occur during the confinement, although women who have previously undergone thymectomy have been noted in other studies to be less likely to have an exacerbation [D].

The risk of maternal mortality is highest during the first year after diagnosis of MG, with the risk being minimal 7 years after diagnosis. Thus, women with MG should delay pregnancy for at least 2 years after disease onset. Despite these considerations, pregnancy has not been shown to adversely affect MG in the long term.

A recent study of 163 pregnant women with MG reported no statistically significant increase in preterm delivery, low birthweight of SGA infants and caesarean delivery, suggesting that MG does not adversely affect pregnancy outcome.

Anticholinesterases are considered safe in pregnancy, although neonatal intestinal tube muscular hypertrophy has been reported following a pregnancy exposed to very high doses. Although there have been concerns regarding the teratogenicity and fetal effects of corticosteroids and azathioprine, their use is not contraindicated [E] and most clinicians will continue to use them through pregnancy if an indication exists. Experience with ciclosporin in pregnancy is growing, although there remains an added possible risk of intrauterine growth restriction. Methotrexate should be avoided before and during pregnancy due to its teratogenic effects. The theoretical reduction in serum hormone levels brought about by plasmapharesis has not caused preterm labour in practice. Miscarriage rates and preterm delivery rates are not significantly different from those of a control population [C].

Due to the change in volume distribution of pregnancy, the dose of anticholinesterase inhibitors needed to control symptoms usually increases in pregnancy. Increasing the dosage frequency has been found to be more effective in some cases. Persistent vomiting in the first trimester will necessitate intravenous administration of anticholinesterases. Prolonged labour (associated with delayed gastric emptying and malabsorption) may also be an indication for parenteral drug delivery.

Transplacental passage of the IgG autoantibodies may cause two distinct fetal/neonatal problems:

1 Women with anticholinergic receptor antibodies occasionally deliver infants with arthrogryposis multiplex congenita, a serious congenital syndrome characterised by multiple joint contractures and pulmonary hypoplasia. Although the aetiology of this syndrome is diverse, severely reduced movement *in utero* is thought to be the basic mechanism. Animal experiments have shown that sera from women with anticholinergic receptor antibodies can cause a similar range of anomalies in vivo.

2 Neonatal myasthenia gravis (NMG) is a more common manifestation of these antibodies, affecting 10–50 per cent of newborns delivered to women with MG. The onset is usually within 24 hours and most cases are mild, presenting with generalized hypotonia, poor sucking, difficulty in feeding and weak cry. Less commonly, ventilation is required, sometimes for a number of weeks. The newborn is usually treated with anticholinesterases but exchange transfusions, plasma exchange and intravenous immunoglobulins have been used in more resistant cases. The correlation between maternal disease severity, or antibody titres, and the incidence and severity of NMG is not a strong one. However, seronegative mothers may be less likely to have an affected baby, and affected babies themselves are usually seropositive.

Clearly, the pregnancy should be managed in conjunction with a neurologist. Anaesthetic and paediatric colleagues should be informed [E]. Regular fetal surveillance is warranted and polyhydramnios should be excluded. Preterm delivery is necessary only in severe crises and a vaginal delivery should be aimed for [E]. Problems may occur in second stage due to skeletal muscle fatigue and there should be a low threshold for instrumental delivery. Advice should be taken before any medications are prescribed, as various drugs may precipitate a myasthenic crisis. Magnesium interferes with neuromuscular transmission by inhibiting release of (ACh). Magnesium competitively blocks calcium entry at the motor nerve terminal. Therefore, magnesium sulphate for the treatment of hypertension or eclampsia should be used with extreme caution. The neonate should be carefully observed for signs of NMG and caution should be exercised with breastfeeding when high doses of anticholinesterases have been used. Drug doses may need to be reduced slowly to pre-pregnancy levels.

ANTENATAL OBSTETRICS

INTRACRANIAL VASCULAR EVENTS: 'STROKE'

'Stroke' is a generic term used to describe a cerebrovascular accident, the causes of which are many and varied. Assigning a diagnosis to 'stroke' is vital for appropriate treatment and prevention of further events.

Stroke can be further classified as shown in Table 17.5.

Across all age groups, hypertension, diabetes and cigarette smoking are the most common 'causes' of stroke, working through a common atherosclerotic pathway.

Retrospective studies [D] consistently show that the incidence of stroke is increased during pregnancy, and that this increase is mostly confined to the postpartum period. The aetiology of pregnancy-associated stroke is very different from that of stroke in general.

Various studies have estimated a stroke risk of between 5 and 10 per 100,000 deliveries, although a Canadian retrospective review gave a six-fold higher risk than this.[14] Most do not find a significant increase in strokes antenatally compared with a female population of the same age distribution, but the increase in the postpartum period is striking. A US study published in 1996 found a relative risk for stroke in pregnancy of 2.4 overall (95 per cent CI 1.6–3.6); however, when subdivided into antepartum and postpartum periods, the relative risk in the first 6 weeks after delivery was found to be 9 for ischaemic stroke (infarcts) and 28 for haemorrhagic [D].[15] Evidence from other studies supports these findings.

In women under 40 years of age, infarcts are more common than haemorrhagic strokes. However, this predominance of infarcts is less marked in the pregnancy-associated group.

Causes of pregnancy-associated strokes

Below are the causes of pregnancy-associated strokes found in two recent studies.[14,15]
Infarcts

- Pre-eclampsia/eclampsia
- Primary CNS vasculopathy
- Carotid artery dissection
- Cardiac embolic events
- Coagulopathies (e.g. thrombophilias, APS)
- TTP
- Post-herpetic vasculitis.

Haemorrhagic

- Pre-eclampsia/eclampsia
- Disseminated intravascular coagulation

Table 17.5 Stroke classification

Ischaemic	Arterial
	Venous
Haemorrhagic	Subarachnoid
	Intracerebral

- Arteriovenous malformations
- Ruptured aneurysms
- Cocaine abuse
- Primary CNS vasculopathy
- Sarcoid vasculitis.

In a significant number of cases no underlying cause is found. The wide aetiology of stroke in pregnancy presents a diagnostic challenge. The subsequent treatment will depend very much on the diagnosis. Investigations undertaken to determine a cause may include:

- MRI/CT scanning
- cerebral angiography
- echocardiogram
- thrombophilia screen
- antiphospholipid testing.

Clearly, treatment and management of the pregnancy will depend on the diagnosis; anticoagulation, for example, may be necessary after a cerebral venous thrombosis. Haemorrhagic strokes caused by bleeding aneurysms or arteriovenous malformations (AVMs) carry a significant risk of re-bleeding if left untreated in pregnancy [D].[16] Ideally, such abnormalities would be diagnosed and treated before conception, but some will present for the first time in pregnancy. AVMs, in particular, may enlarge as pregnancy progresses, perhaps in response to hormonal changes. Outside pregnancy they are a much less common cause of subarachnoid haemorrhage than aneurysms. In the two studies cited above, AVMs were found to be the cause of subarachnoid haemorrhage in more cases than a bleeding aneurysm (8 vs 3) [D]. A few will present with recurrent headaches and neurological deficit, but without haemorrhage. Treatment in these cases is the same as in the pre-pregnant state, with surgery (excision of AVM, clipping of aneurysm) or obliteration with neuroradiological techniques. However, some consideration must be given to fetal radiation exposure. Subarachnoid haemorrhage may present with headache, vomiting, reduced consciousness, neck stiffness and focal neurology. In view of the high risk of re-bleeding, most advocate early treatment rather than an initial delay. Nimodipine is used to reduce vasospasm, and hypertension must be controlled. Neurosurgery is normally tolerated well by the pregnancy, although decision-making can be complicated by reduced maternal conscious level. Vaginal delivery is encouraged if there is confidence that the source of the bleeding has been treated adequately, although this can be difficult sometimes with AVMs. A longer passive second stage is usually encouraged to reduce the need for the Valsalva manoeuvre, with early recourse to instrumental delivery [E]. If the aneurysm or AVM has not been treated, or this treatment has occurred recently, an elective caesarean section is advocated, as labour is considered by many to be a high-risk time for a first bleed or a re-bleed [E]. Of note, however, is that only one death has occurred from subarachnoid haemorrhage during labour in the last 6 years in the UK, leading some to believe that this risk has been previously overstated. Poor maternal clinical state (coma, brain-stem death) is of course another indication for caesarean section. Epidurals can be used provided there is no evidence of raised intracranial pressure. Special anaesthetic techniques are used to limit the hypertensive responses found with intubation, which carry the risk of precipitating a re-bleed [E].

Investigation and treatment of the pregnant patient with stroke obviously require significant input from neurologists and neurosurgeons. However, all those in maternity care have an important part to play in stroke prevention. For example, women with APS and thrombophilias can be treated, once recognised, with prophylactic anticoagulation [D]. Optimal management of hypertension in pre-eclampsia and eclampsia will also help to reduce the associated stroke risk [D].

MIGRAINE AND HEADACHE

Tension headaches are more common in pregnancy, and migraines may present for the first time. Clinically they must be differentiated from much less common but far more serious causes of headache (see below). Making a diagnosis may involve special investigations and the help of a neurologist or radiologist. Treatment will depend on the cause.

A classic migraine attack in a woman with a history of migraines does not normally warrant review by a neurologist. Visual disturbance, aphasia and paraesthesia or numbness usually last no more than an hour or so, and are followed by a throbbing unilateral headache with associated nausea, vomiting and photophobia. However, as many as 1 in 10 women with migraine in pregnancy has no previous history [D]. In view of the considerable symptom overlap with other diagnoses, a specialised opinion may be warranted. This applies also to women with migraine who suffer a presumed attack with atypical or prolonged neurological deficits. Hemiplegic migraine, for example, may last for many hours and should raise the possibility of an alternative diagnosis.

Causes of headache in pregnancy

- Tension headache
- Migraine
- Pre-eclampsia
- Benign intracranial hypertension
- Cerebral vein thrombosis
- Meningitis
- Subarachnoid haemorrhage (see below)
- Intracranial mass
- Inadvertent dural puncture (spinal headache).

Between 60 and 70 per cent of women with migraine will improve, or be symptom free, during pregnancy [C]. Those women who have cycle-related migraines are most likely to note an improvement. No more than 10 per cent seem to deteriorate in pregnancy. Every effort should be made to avoid precipitating factors, such as chocolate and cheese. Non-drug therapies such as relaxation techniques, sleep, massage and ice packs can be tried. Acute attacks in pregnancy are normally treated with paracetamol (rectal may be better than oral administration) and/or codeine-based drugs along with an antiemetic such as metoclopramide. Occasional use of NSAIDs is permitted, but should be avoided after 32–34 weeks [C]. Stronger opiates are sometimes needed. Ergotamine derivatives should be avoided, although studies have failed to show obvious harm. Sumatriptan, a serotonin antagonist, is in common use outside pregnancy. Data from the 16-Year Sumatriptan Pregnancy Registry of unintended pregnancy exposures have demonstrated no clear problems.[17]

Prophylaxis against migraine attacks in pregnancy is best provided by low-dose aspirin or amitriptyline (commencing with low doses such as 10 mg per day). Propranolol and atenolol have been used, with the awareness of the associated potential for intrauterine growth restriction. The safety of pizotifen and methysergide in pregnancy is still in question.

PARAPLEGIA

Pregnancy in a woman with a spinal cord injury (SCI) can present challenges to the patient and her obstetrician. Some problems that occur in able-bodied women are more likely to occur in women with SCI such as UTI, anaemia and venous thrombosis. Other problems are specific to women with SCI and include neurogenic bladder, spasticity, decubitus ulcers and autonomic hyperreflexia.

Antenatal management

- Antenatal management should take into account the level of SCI and the degree of paralysis. A formal assessment of renal, urological or pulmonary status may be appropriate.
- Women with spinal cord lesions at T6 or above are at risk of autonomic hyperreflexia and should be cared for in a setting where invasive monitoring and physicians experienced with autonomic hyperreflexia are available.
- Pre-eclampsia, intrauterine growth restriction and stillbirth are NOT more common in this population and antenatal testing for fetal wellbeing is not indicated in the absence of other obstetric indications.
- Preterm labour may be slightly more common in this population. In addition, although the majority of patients with SCI are able to perceive labour, the subjective experience may be different to that of able-bodied women and may delay presentation. However, serial cervical assessment (using ultrasound) and home uterine contraction monitoring have not proven useful in detecting women at increased risk of preterm labour in this population.

Intrapartum care

- Previous recommendations against performing inductions of labour have been made because of concern over autonomic hyperreflexia. Most studies available do not provide enough detail to suggest that induced labour is more difficult to manage than spontaneous labour with regard to autonomic hyperreflexia and it is therefore reasonable to restrict inductions to obstetric indications.

- The mode of delivery in women with SCI is primarily determined by standard obstetric indications. However, spasticity and contractures can impair the ability to achieve a vaginal delivery. If the patient has limited abduction and rotation preventing use of the lithotomy position, she should be assessed for suitability of positioning on her side with flexion of the upper leg at the hip.
- A unique indication for caesarean section in women with SCI is intractable autonomic hyperreflexia unresponsive to pharmacological or anaesthetic manipulation. The surgery will continue to incite the process but can be life saving if the time to delivery seems remote.
- Attendant staff need to be aware of the risk of pressure ulcers and traumatic injuries in women with SCI; frequent changes in position are advised.
- Frequent bladder emptying or catheterisation will prevent overdistension in patients with a neurogenic bladder.
- The level and completeness of the spinal cord lesion determines the patient's perception of labour and the anaesthetic requirements:
  - Pain from the first stage of labour is transmitted by sympathetic fibres that enter the spinal cord at T10–12 and L1.
  - The second stage of labour involves pain from pressure and distension of perineal tissues. These signals travel along the pudendal nerve and enter the spinal cord at S2–4. Therefore patients with lesions above T10 may not perceive labour at all but those with lesions above T5–6 may benefit from anaesthesia to prevent autonomic hyperreflexia.
- SCI is not a contraindication to regional anaesthesia.

Postnatal care

- Once again, attendant staff need to be aware of the risk of pressure sores and traumatic injuries in the postnatal period.
- Care should be taken to avoid urinary retention, no matter what the mode of delivery, in order to prevent a deterioration in bladder function and to minimise the risk of urinary infection and autonomic hyperreflexia.
- Breastfeeding should be encouraged; no deficiency in the let-down reflex has been observed, even in patients with high cervical lesions.

PRENATAL DIAGNOSIS OF NEUROLOGICAL DISEASES

Although most severe neurological disorders limit life expectancy, many milder problems do not, and women suffering from these conditions may wish to become pregnant, or may present at the booking clinic. Alternatively, a healthy woman with a previously affected child may come under your care. Such individuals may or may not be interested in recurrence risks in their offspring. Good-quality information is needed so that an informed choice can be made. The first step is to seek out the true diagnosis. The term 'cerebral palsy', for example, does not give any indication of aetiology. Although cerebral palsy usually occurs as a result of various environmental factors, genetic factors are responsible for a few cases, raising the recurrence risk. 'Muscular dystrophy' is all too often assumed to be Duchenne's muscular dystrophy (an X-linked recessive condition); in fact, there are many different kinds of muscular dystrophy with different inheritance patterns. A careful family history is vital, but help is likely to be needed from neurologists, paediatricians and clinical geneticists.

Once the maternal diagnosis has been established, empirical recurrence risks can often be quoted. In a few cases genetic testing offers the possibility of more precise prenatal prediction. This entire process can take many weeks, and plans should be made before the woman actually becomes pregnant, if possible.

The *triplet repeat diseases* highlight best some of the complexities of prenatal testing. Huntington's disease, myotonic dystrophy, Friedreich's ataxia and fragile X all share a similar genetic abnormality. A three-basepair sequence (the 'triplet') which is repeated a variable number of times in the healthy gene becomes 'expanded', so that many more copies of the triplet are present and gene function becomes disrupted. To a degree, the disease severity may be related to the size of the expansion. Expanded sequences have a tendency to expand further, causing so-called 'anticipation', i.e. the condition becomes more severe in successive generations. Myotonic dystrophy provides the clearest example.

Myotonic dystrophy is the most common muscular dystrophy affecting pregnant women and occurs as a result of the disruption of a gene coding for a protein kinase on chromosome 19. The gene is disrupted by the expansion of a CTG triplet repeat; 5–35 CTG repeats is considered normal. More than 40 is abnormal, and mildly affected individuals will show a degree of expansion beyond this size. Severely affected individuals often have many thousands of repeats. Clinical features include muscle weakness, myotonia of hands and tongue, swallowing and speech disability, cataracts and cardiac arrhythmias, testicular atrophy and peripheral insulin resistance. Learning disability occurs in those affected severely from a young age.

Myotonic dystrophy is an autosomal dominant condition, affected individuals having one normal and one abnormal allele. Their offspring have a 50 per cent risk of inheriting the mutated allele. Quite how severely affected the child will be is difficult to predict with any degree of accuracy. A woman with moderate-to-severe disease herself is likely to have a significantly expanded mutation already. If this is inherited by the fetus, further expansion is likely and the neonate will be born with severe congenital myotonic dystrophy. Such a pregnancy may be characterised by polyhydramnios and poor fetal movements. Preterm delivery is more common, and severe hypotonia and respiratory difficulties are evident at birth. Talipes and facial diplegia may be present and survival beyond the neonatal period is followed by significant developmental delay in most cases. A woman with minimal or absent disease (and therefore a shorter expansion) has a risk of approximately 1 in 10 that her child will be severely affected. However, if such a woman has delivered a severely affected newborn in a previous pregnancy, the risk of another badly affected child is higher (approximately 40–80 per cent). This reflects the greater likelihood that she has an inherently unstable mutation.

Inheritance and further expansion of the mutated allele can be detected by molecular testing carried out on placental biopsy material, although precise analysis of expansion size and prediction of outcome can still be difficult.

Key References

1. Tomson T, Lindbom U, Ekqvist B, Sundqvist A. Epilepsy and pregnancy: a prospective study of seizure control in relation to free and total plasma concentrations of carbamazepine and phenytoin. *Epilepsia* 1994;35: 122–30.

2. Olafsson E, Hallgrimsson JT, Hauser WA, Ludvigsson P, Gugmundsson G. Pregnancies of women with epilepsy: a population-based study in Iceland. *Epilepsia* 1998; 39:887–92.

3. Fairgrieve SD, Jackson M, Jonas P *et al.* Population-based, prospective study of the care of women with epilepsy in pregnancy. *BMJ* 2000;321:674–5.

4. Holmes LB, Harvey EA, Coull BA *et al.* The teratogenicity of anticonvulsant drugs. *N Engl J Med* 2001;344: 1132–8.

5. Canger R, Battino D, Canevini MP *et al.* Malformations in offspring of women with epilepsy: a prospective study. *Epilepsia* 1999;40:1231–6.

6. Moore SJ, Turnpenny P, Quinn A *et al.* A clinical study of 57 children with fetal anticonvulsant syndromes. *J Med Genet* 2000;37:489–97.

7. Harden CL, Meador KJ, Pennell PB *et al.*; American Academy of Neurology; American Epilepsy Society. Practice parameter update: management issues for women with epilepsy: focus on pregnancy (an evidence-based review): teratogenesis and perinatal outcomes: report of the Quality Standards Subcommittee and Therapeutics and Technology Assessment Subcommittee of the American Academy of Neurology and American Epilepsy Society. *Neurology* 2009;73:133-41.

8. Brodie MJ, French J. Management of epilepsy in adolescents and adults. *Lancet* 2000;356:323–9.

9. Scottish Obstetric Guidelines and Audit Project; *The Management of Pregnancy in Women with Epilepsy*. A Clinical Practice Guideline for Professionals Involved in Maternity Care. Aberdeen, SOGAP, 1997.

10. Confavreux C, Hutchinson M, Marie Hours M, Cortinovis-Tourniaire P, Moreau T and the Pregnancy in Multiple Sclerosis Group. Rate of pregnancy-related relapse in multiple sclerosis. *N Engl J Med* 1998;339:285–91.

11. Rumarker B, Andersen O. Pregnancy is associated with a lower risk of onset and a better prognosis in multiple sclerosis. *Brain* 1995;118:253–61.

12. E. Bodiguel, C. Bensa, D. Brassat, D *et al.* Multiple sclerosis and pregnancy. *Revue Neurologique* 2014;170:247–65.

13. Wen JC, Liu TC, Chen YH, Chen SF, Lin HC, Tsai WC. No increased risk of adverse pregnancy outcomes for women with myasthenia gravis: a nationwide-based study. *Eur J Neurol* 2009;16:889-94.

14. Jaigobin C, Silver FL. Stroke and pregnancy. *Stroke* 2000;31:2948–51.

15. Kittner SJ, Stern BJ, Feeser BR *et al.* Pregnancy and the risk of stroke. *N Engl J Med* 1996;335:768–74.

16. Stoodley MA, Macdonald RL, Weir BK. Pregnancy and intracranial aneurysms. *Neurosurg Clin North Am* 1998;9:549–56.

17. Ephross SA, Sinclair SM. Final results from the 16-year sumatriptan, naratriptan, and treximet pregnancy registry. *Headache* 2014;54:1158-72.

Chapter 18 Dermatological conditions

Louise Kenny

INTRODUCTION

Although this section of the book deals with pre-existing diseases and their interaction with pregnancy, the dermatological conditions of most interest to the obstetrician are the 'dermatoses of pregnancy', i.e. the skin conditions peculiar to pregnancy. These are thus discussed alongside pre-existing conditions.

The skin may be the sole organ affected by a particular condition or it may be just one of many involved in a multisystem disease. Skin disorders occurring as part of multisystem disease (connective tissue disease, infections and malignancies) are considered in the appropriate chapters. It is worth remembering, however, that the skin manifestation of these disorders may be the initial presentation of these conditions.

PHYSIOLOGICAL SKIN CHANGES IN PREGNANCY

Physiological cutaneous skin changes during pregnancy are common and rarely cause major concern. Hyperpigmentation may occur of the nipples and areolae, axillae, linea alba (which becomes the linea nigra), face (melasma or cloasma), and pre-existing pigmented moles and freckles. Oestrogen is probably responsible for cutaneous vascular changes such as an increase in spider naevi, palmar erythema, and even the occurrence of head and neck haemangiomas. Oedema is almost universal, and venous varicosities of the legs, vulva and rectum often become more prominent or appear for the first time. Striae gravidarum are pinkish-purple linear markings on the lower abdomen and breast, which later fade to white and usually persist after pregnancy is over as depressed, irregular bands. Some women maintain that hair growth and condition improve in pregnancy. Postpartum alopecia, however, is a recognised phenomenon that is usually mild and transient.[1] Sebum secretion increases (see below), but apocrine activity may decline.

PRE-EXISTING CONDITIONS

Women with pre-existing skin problems are likely to present with a diagnosis already established. As with all pre-existing maternal conditions, one must consider the effect that both the disease and its therapies will have on the pregnancy, the labour, the fetus and the neonate. Conversely, the pregnancy may influence the course and nature of the condition itself.

The effect of pregnancy on atopic dermatitis (atopic eczema) and psoriasis is unpredictable.[2] The former often improves in pregnancy but may deteriorate postnatally, due to physical factors such as breastfeeding, environmental agents such as detergents or even immune factors. A generalised pustular psoriasis may occur in pregnancy (see below) and is more common in women with previous psoriasis. Sebum secretion increases in pregnancy and may be responsible for the common deterioration of acne during pregnancy. Apocrine gland activity, on the other hand, declines in pregnancy, meaning that the rare conditions affecting these glands (hidradenitis suppurativa and Fox–Fordyce disease) are likely to improve. The pregnancy-associated suppression of cell-mediated immunity is thought to cause the often marked increase in human papillomavirus warty lesions (condylomata acuminata). In rare cases, these may obstruct the vagina. Only then are they an indication for caesarean section.

Impact of pre-existing skin diseases on the pregnancy itself is usually minimal in the absence of any multisystem involvement (clearly, connective tissue disorders and infections with skin involvement are quite different).

Conditions affecting the abdominal wall may interfere with abdominal delivery and delay wound healing. Vulval problems may similarly affect vaginal delivery and the healing of tears and episiotomies. A rare condition called X-linked ichthyosis is associated with steroid sulphatase deficiency, and this in turn is said to delay the onset of labour, increasing the need for induction for prolonged pregnancy.

Certain skin conditions have a genetic component and the offspring may be at risk of the condition themselves. A few examples are cited in Box 18.1.

One of the most important factors to consider is the potential impact that dermatological drugs and therapies may have on a pregnancy.[3] A number of such treatments are confirmed teratogens and are absolutely contraindicated in pregnancy (Box 18.2). The retinoids are used to treat severe acne and psoriasis. Isotretinoin is especially harmful, causing CNS, craniofacial and cardiovascular abnormalities in as many as 50 per cent of exposed pregnancies.

Other drug treatments should be used only with careful consideration in pregnancy, including ciclosporin, hydroxyurea, penicillamine, psoralens and ultraviolet A (PUVA) and rifampicin.

A number of these medications may linger in body tissues for many months after treatment has ended. Great care must

Box 18.1 Examples of inheritable skin disorders

Autosomal dominant
Ichthyosis hystrix and vulgaris
Palmoplantar hyperkeratosis (tylosis)
Epidermolysis bullosa simplex
Ectodermal dysplasia (some forms)
X-linked recessive
X-linked icthyosis
Hypohidrotic ectodermal dysplasia
Multifactorial
Atopic eczema (the risk of some allergic problems may reach 50% in the offspring of a couple with one affected person; the risks are higher where both parents are eczema sufferers)
Psoriasis (the children of two psoriatic parents have a risk of approximately 50% of being affected themselves)

Box 18.2 Dermatological treatments to be avoided during pregnancy

Acitretin and tazarotene (retinoids used in psoriasis)
Isotretinoin (retinoid used to treat severe acne)
Griseofulvin (antifungal treatment)
Methotrexate (antimetabolite used to treat psoriasis)
Podophyllin (used for genital warts)
Tetracycline (used for skin infections/acne)
Thalidomide (leprosy treatment)

be taken that women undergoing such therapies are made aware of the vital role of reliable contraception, which may need to be continued long after the treatment has stopped. The *British National Formulary* advises the following periods of time during which conception should be avoided after the drugs have been stopped [E]:

- acitretin – 2 years;
- methotrexate – 6 months;
- griseofulvin – 1 month.

It should be noted that these drugs may also carry potential harm through an effect on the male gametes. Men who have used griseofulvin, for example, are advised against fathering offspring within 6 months of treatment ending.

Emollients, dithranol, coal tar and topical corticosteroids are safe in pregnancy, as is chlorpheniramine.

DERMATOSES PRECIPITATED BY PREGNANCY

This section covers two groups of conditions:

1 skin conditions in which pregnancy is just one of a number of precipitating factors;
2 skin conditions unique to pregnancy.

Acne, erythema multiforme, erythema nodosum and generalised pustular psoriasis form the first group. Pre-existing **acne** may deteriorate during pregnancy, but may also present anew. **Erythema multiforme** and **erythema nodosum** are both caused by a multitude of other aetiological factors, which must be excluded before it is possible to attribute the onset to pregnancy alone. **Generalised pustular psoriasis** describes a superficial sterile eruption occurring on the background of widespread erythema, which is associated with fever, systemic upset and hypocalcaemia (with tetany) in the more severe cases. It carries significant perinatal mortality and is more common in those with a history of plaque psoriasis. A clinically identical condition called **impetigo herpetiformis** was previously thought to be a pregnancy-specific dermatosis, but the two are now considered the same condition. Pregnancy appears to be one of a number of triggers for generalised pustular psoriasis.

ANTENATAL OBSTETRICS

Table 18.1 Pregnancy-specific dermatoses

Name	Incidence	Onset	Resolution	Clinical features	Histology	Immunofluorescence	Fetal effects	Recurrence	Management	Associated conditions
Polymorphic eruption of pregnancy (pruritic urticarial papules and plaques of pregnancy, toxaemic rash of pregnancy, toxic erythema of pregnancy)	1 in 250	27–40 weeks (usually late third trimester)	Usually within 2 weeks of delivery	Red urticarial papules and plaques. Rarely, vesicles and target lesions. Begins abdominally within striae. Umbilical sparing May spread to thighs and occasionally limbs	Epidermal/dermal oedema Perivascular infiltration Patchy parakeratosis	Negative	None	Uncommon	Calamine lotion 1% hydrocortisone aqueous cream Antihistamines Systemic steroids	None
Pemphigoid gestationis (herpes gestationis)	1 in 3000–60,000	Second/third trimester (occasionally postpartum)	Few weeks postpartum to 1 year	Erythematous urticarial plaques. Vesicles and bullae form at the centre or periphery of plaques. Often begins periumbilically. Spreads to trunk and extremities	Perivascular inflammation Subepidermal blister	Positive	Possible increased risk of IUGR and preterm labour	Common	Moderate/strong topical steroids Systemic steroids Antihistamines	Graves' disease and other autoimmune conditions
Prurigo of pregnancy	1 in 300	25–30 weeks	Several months	No urticated lesions Multiple excoriated papules Abdomen and limbs	See polymorphic eruption of pregnancy	Negative	None	Recorded	Aqueous cream Topical steroids Antihistamines	Atopy
Pruritic folliculitis of pregnancy	Uncertain	Second/third trimester	Within 2 weeks of delivery	Masses of itchy red follicular papules	Non-specific folliculitis	Negative	None	Uncertain	Topical 10% benzoyl peroxide Mild topical steroids Antihistamines	None

This leaves four reasonably well-defined dermatoses found only in pregnancy (Table 18.1).

A diagnosis can usually be made on clinical grounds alone; however, pemphigoid gestationis can be confused with polymorphic eruption of pregnancy if there are no vesicles present. The two conditions are easily distinguished by immunofluorescence studies of skin biopsies. Pemphigoid gestationis is characterised by C3 deposition along the epidermal/dermal junction. IgG deposition is usually another feature, the target protein being a 180-kDa component of hemidesmosomes. Immunofluorescence studies are negative in polymorphic eruption of pregnancy. Clinical distinction is appropriate as pemphigoid gestationis has been linked to increased rates of stillbirth, IUGR and preterm labour [D].

Although this may represent biased reporting of poor outcomes, extra surveillance would seem warranted in these pregnancies [E].

Key References

1. Schiff BL, Kern AB. A study of postpartum alopecia. *Arch Dermatol* 1963;87:609.
2. Winton GB. Skin diseases aggravated by pregnancy. *J Am Acad Dermatol* 1989;20:1–13.
3. Perlman SE, Rudy SJ, Carissa P, Townsend-Akpan C. Caring for women with childbearing potential taking teratogenic dermatologic drugs. *J Reprod Med* 2001;46(Suppl 2):153–61.

Chapter 19 Drug and alcohol misuse

Louise Kenny

INTRODUCTION

The incidence of substance misuse in the UK varies widely by geographical location. Three per cent of under-35s in the UK are said to have a drug problem, although London, Glasgow, Liverpool and Manchester have traditionally been considered the 'hotspots'. However, a recent cross-sectional audit of health records in a London specialist perinatal addictions outreach service reported that a total of 167 pregnant substance-using women were referred between 2002 and 2005. Compared with 1989–1991, there were significantly more pregnant women presenting at an older age, later gestation, with increased polysubstance use and a higher percentage of women from black or minority ethnic communities. Clearly the problem is increasing, and maternity services must have local guidelines and action plans in place to manage it. Alcohol is a particular concern. Recent data from a global cohort study of low-risk first-time mothers found that 34 per cent of women reported binge alcohol consumption in the 3 months before pregnancy, and 23 per cent of these participants reported binge alcohol consumption during the first 15 weeks of pregnancy.[1]

There is a tendency to focus attention on the medical aspects of substance abuse in pregnancy. Although these drugs may involve actual harm to the pregnancy, the associated social and health problems are as important, if not more so. Throughout this chapter it will become clear that separating the two is very difficult, and the contributions made first by the drugs themselves and second by the socio-economic environment are almost impossible to disentangle. Separating the two is of greater theoretical than practical importance. Substance-exposed pregnancies are 'high risk', and tailored antenatal care must be provided that tackles all the problems, both social and medical.

Substances of abuse are rarely used in isolation. 'Polysubstance' misuse is the norm, and heavy alcohol consumption and tobacco smoking compound the harm done by classified drugs. The following discussion therefore does not tackle each drug independently, but aims to explore their individual contributions to each problem encountered in the pregnancy. Many studies demonstrating harmful effects of substance abuse in pregnancy are retrospective and little or no effort is made to control for confounding factors. Clearly, there are no randomised studies. Better study design is often associated with negative results or a diminution in the harm reported. There is little doubt, however, that drug use during pregnancy *is linked* to poorer outcomes.

PHARMACOLOGY

It is valuable to revise the basic pharmacological actions of abused substances, as these actions help to explain both the short-term and the long-term effects on the pregnancy outcome.

Cocaine

Cocaine is a CNS stimulant. It prevents the re-uptake of neurotransmitters (adrenaline, noradrenaline, dopamine) at nerve terminals, causing an exaggerated response to these chemical messengers. Increased motor activity, tremors, convulsions, tachycardia, generalised vasoconstriction, hypertension and hyperpyrexia may result. The sense of euphoria occurs as a result of dopamine accumulation within the mesolimbic system. Chronic cocaine use brings about dopamine depletion. Use of cocaine with alcohol results in a more powerful vasoconstrictor called cocaethylene.

Opiates

Opiates (heroin, methadone, morphine, buprenorphine) mimic the actions of the endogenous opioid peptides widely distributed throughout the CNS, which bind to mu, delta or kappa opioid receptors. These compounds have a wide diversity of physical functions but are intimately linked with pain perception and mood control. The 'reward circuitry' of the mesolimbic dopaminergic system is influenced by endogenous and exogenous opioids and is responsible for both the pleasurable effects and the psychological dependence found with opiate abuse.

Amphetamines

Amphetamines similarly enhance the dopaminergic neurotransmitter system. Ecstasy (3, 4-methylenedioxymethamphetamine – MDMA) is a derivative of metamphetamine. It causes accumulation of synaptic serotonin and dopamine, but direct axonal damage and serotonin depletion can occur with prolonged use.

Alcohol and marijuana

Alcohol and marijuana have fundamental non-specific actions on the neural membrane, in common with the sedative–hypnotic–anaesthetic group of drugs. They differ somewhat in their actions due to differing lipid solubilities, routes of intake, metabolic pathways and different ratios of stimulant and depressant effects. Marijuana, unlike alcohol, has hallucinogenic properties.

Benzodiazepines

The actions of benzodiazepines (diazepam, temazepam) are mediated through the neuroinhibitory gamma-aminobutyric acid type A (GABA-A) receptor. GABA and benzodiazepines have anxiolytic, sedative and hypnotic effects, and also affect cognition. They bring about muscle relaxation and act as anticonvulsants. GABA has trophic effects and this may be important in neurodevelopment. Excessive benzodiazepine use leads to receptor down-regulation and tolerance.

MATERNAL EFFECTS

The effects of substance abuse on the mother may be acute or chronic and may be specific to the drug used or part of a general pattern of illness found among substance abusers. It is vital for obstetricians to have an understanding of these problems, as they may present in the antenatal clinic or as emergencies on the labour suite. Furthermore, they may be confused with complications of pregnancy.

Acute maternal effects

Drug abuse is associated with a wide range of health problems, which may present acutely to various different healthcare professionals.

Overdose
Excess alcohol intake causes ataxia, confusion, stupor and eventually coma.

Opiates in excess depress respiratory drive and may also cause coma.

Cocaine, amphetamines and ecstasy cause tachycardia, hypertension and hyperthermia, and predispose to cardiac arrhythmias, myocardial infarction, seizures and stroke. The potential for diagnostic confusion with fulminating pre-eclampsia and eclampsia is clear. Acute presentations also include aggression, paranoia and psychosis, particularly with the CNS stimulants such as amphetamines, ecstasy and cannabis.

Withdrawal
Withdrawal from the physically addictive substances may also present acutely. Alcohol withdrawal may result in blackouts, tremor, hallucinations, delirium and seizures. Opiate withdrawal is characterised by sweating, coryza and lacrimation. Pyrexia, nausea and vomiting, diarrhoea and abdominal pain, tachycardia and hypertension are also common.

Infections
Drug abuse is often associated with poor diet, poor hygiene and generalised immunosuppression. Pneumonia and TB may present acutely. Sexual disinhibition and prostitution increase the risk of sexually transmitted infections (STIs),

including HIV. Intravenous substance use predisposes to endocarditis, hepatitis and septicaemia (which may be fungal). Local infections such as cellulitis and osteomyelitis are not uncommon.

Other acute presentations

Hypoglycaemia, acute or chronic hepatic failure and Wernicke's encephalopathy may result from excessive alcohol consumption. Aspiration pneumonitis, subdural haematomas and rhabdomyolysis with acute renal failure are further examples of acute complications of substance abuse. All types of trauma, including road traffic accidents (RTAs) and grevious bodily harm, are more common among drug users.

Chronic maternal effects

The effects of HIV infection and chronic hepatitis (whether alcoholic or infectious) are well known. Nutritional deficiencies may cause peripheral neuropathy (vitamin B_1 and vitamin B_{12}), pellagra (niacin), cerebellar degeneration and Wernicke–Korsakoff syndrome (vitamin B_1). Poor venous access is common in IV substance users and this may cause difficulty during emergency situations (drug induced or pregnancy related). Femoral nerve neuropathy may result from frequent trauma during injection into the femoral vein. Obstructive and restrictive pulmonary lesions may occur, as can pulmonary hypertension.

OBSTETRIC PROBLEMS

Substance abuse has been associated with a number of obstetric complications, including:

- miscarriage
- preterm rupture of membranes
- preterm labour
- placenta praevia
- abruption
- pre-eclampsia
- breech presentation
- chorioamnionitis
- IUGR and IUD.

Although plausible biological explanations exist for why substances of abuse might cause these problems, the exact contribution from the drugs themselves is very difficult to isolate from the confounding factors such as smoking, poor nutrition and general health, lack of antenatal care and low socio-economic status.

Miscarriage

Studies examining rates of miscarriage in substance-exposed pregnancies are often retrospective and poorly controlled.

Confirmation by tissue diagnosis is often missing. Opiates, cocaine and CNS stimulants have all been implicated, but good-quality evidence is mostly lacking.

Most attention has been paid to the effect of alcohol on miscarriage rates, and large quantities have been shown to have abortive properties in animal experiments. There is general agreement that alcoholics have a higher rate of miscarriage, although it is almost impossible to separate the effect of the alcohol from the confounding effects of ill-health, poor nutrition and low socio-economic status. Alcohol consumption is closely related to smoking and caffeine use (coffee drinking), both of which have stronger causative relationships with miscarriage. North American studies have linked 'heavy drinking' (more than two drinks per day) with an increase in miscarriage rate, giving relative risk values of between 2 and 3. This association is not, on the whole, confirmed in European and Australian studies, where greater effort has been made to control for confounding factors.[2] Most agree, however, that more than six drinks a day for several days per week is associated with higher miscarriage risk [C].

There is no good evidence to suggest that the other substances discussed in this chapter cause miscarriage.

Teratogenicity

The only confirmed teratogen among this group of substances is alcohol. The **fetal alcohol syndrome** (FAS) describes a clearly defined group of problems caused by *in utero* alcohol exposure:

- prenatal or postnatal growth restriction/microcephaly;
- nervous system dysfunction (learning disability, intellectual impairment, ataxia, attention defects);
- characteristic facial appearance (mid-face hypoplasia, narrow palpebral fissures, underdeveloped philtrum, ptosis, rotated low-set ears).

Fetal alcohol spectrum is the term used to describe other alcohol-induced abnormalities that do not qualify for the 'full' diagnosis of FAS.

The relationship between alcohol consumption during early pregnancy and the incidence of FAS is not a simple one. Despite having the highest rates of worldwide alcohol consumption, France has a significantly lower rate of reported FAS than North America, where less alcohol is consumed. A number of reasons have been cited to explain this discrepancy, including a difference in drinking patterns between the two countries and a greater readiness to label newborns with the diagnosis of FAS in the USA. 'Heavy drinking' is defined as more than two drinks per day, or more than 45 per month. This group of women have an approximate incidence of FAS of 4 per cent. Alcoholics, or those drinking more than 18 units per day, carry a risk of one in three of their offspring having FAS. These figures are altered by socio-economic status, general health, smoking and possibly ethnicity, which all act as confounding factors. There is no clear threshold below which alcohol consumption is considered entirely safe; however, the incidence of alcohol-related birth defects and FAS increases sharply after 3 units per day [C].[3] 'Binge drinking' of more than 5 units in one session may be more harmful than taking the same quantity in 'divided doses', although there is no good evidence for this at present. Clearly this practice should be discouraged during pregnancy [E].

The relationship between benzodiazepine use in the first trimester and congenital anomalies, most notably cleft lip and palate, has been examined many times. A meta-analysis by Dolovich et al.[4] included the 23 most technically robust studies. The cohort studies could not significantly link benzodiazepine use with any fetal abnormalities. The case–control studies, however, gave a three-fold increase in risk for all major anomalies and an odds ratio of 1.79 (1.13–2.82) for oral clefting. They suggest detailed scanning for those pregnancies exposed in the first trimester.

There are good scientific reasons why ecstasy and cocaine might act as teratogens, although the better-controlled studies and meta-analyses have not confirmed the effects found in laboratory animals exposed to high concentrations of these drugs in utero. Neurotransmitters can be found in the fetal brain from very early gestation, and it is likely that they are involved in neuronal migration and establishment of synaptic circuitry. It is simple to imagine how these processes could be disturbed by exposure to such drugs and bring about the microcephaly said to be characteristic of cocaine-exposed neonates.

After maturation of the muscularis layer of fetal cerebral vessels, acute vasoconstriction may lead to infarction followed by the subsequent development of cavitary lesions (e.g. porencephalic cysts). Vascular disruption secondary to cocaine use has also been postulated as a cause for the increase in gut, genitourinary and limb defects reported by some authors. Controlled studies have failed to support these findings.

A recent prospective follow-up study[5] of 136 babies exposed to ecstasy in utero has reported a significant increase in the anomaly rate (15.4 per cent); however, almost half the women used other illegal substances or alcohol and most of the abnormalities were 'minor', raising the possibility of ascertainment bias. To reach statistical significance, the background congenital anomaly rate was quoted as 2–3 per cent; in fact, if minor abnormalities are included, it may be closer to 10 per cent.

Although congenital anomalies will undoubtedly complicate a proportion of pregnancies exposed to marijuana and opiates, no consistent pattern of abnormalities has been found. Most studies show no increase in anomaly risk or are uncontrolled and retrospective.

Preterm labour and abruption

The obstetric effects of cocaine have perhaps drawn the most attention. Its vasoconstrictive properties are thought to cause abnormal implantation, hypertensive episodes and abruption. Down-regulation of beta-adrenoreceptors in the myometrium may lead to increased uterine irritability and predispose

to preterm labour. Amphetamines and ecstasy may have similar effects, although there are far fewer data. Studies of cocaine use in pregnancy have confirmed the increased risk of preterm labour and abruption; however, these are often lost when confounders (alcohol use and smoking) have been accounted for.[6]

Opiate withdrawal is also thought to cause uterine excitability and result in preterm rupture of membranes and preterm labour [E]. However, smoking is more common amongst opiate abusers, and minimal antenatal care is the norm. Failure to consider the effect of these confounding factors means the effect of opiates itself is often overestimated.

The effect of prenatal alcohol exposure on the length of gestation remains unclear.

In utero growth and development

Intrauterine growth restriction and stillbirth more commonly occur in pregnancies exposed to high alcohol levels, opiates and cocaine. The vasoconstrictive properties of cocaine and ecstasy may cause placental insufficiency and predispose to abruption, uterine irritability and preterm labour. The high metabolic demands of a fetus alternately exposed to opiate 'highs' and withdrawals might also be responsible for IUGR and even stillbirth [E].

Fetal growth restriction is one of the three defining criteria for FAS. Although there are many reasons why growth might be restricted in pregnancies exposed to high levels of alcohol, it is generally held that alcohol itself has a growth-retarding action.

The OR of producing infants below the tenth centile of weight for gestational age compared with non-drinkers for women consuming less than 1 unit per day is 1.1 (95% CI 1.00–1.13), 1–2 units per day 1.62 (1.26–2.09) and 3–5 units per day 1.96 (1.16–3.31).[7] Among women who continue to drink more than 2 units per day throughout the third trimester, 45% had an infant with a birthweight below the tenth centile for gestational age, whereas in those who successfully reduced or discontinued their alcohol consumption during the last 3 months of pregnancy there was no excess of low birthweight with only 8% falling below the tenth centile. Although low birthweight, is a consistent finding in opiate-exposed pregnancies, a *causative* link between opiate use and IUGR has been difficult to prove due to the action of the following confounding factors:

- 'polydrug' use;
- tobacco smoking and alcohol consumption;
- chaotic and reduced attendance for antenatal care;
- high rates of HIV and other STIs;
- low socio-economic status;
- poor nutrition.

Substituting methadone for heroin has a beneficial effect on prenatal growth, but this may have more to do with increased levels of antenatal care than the action of the heroin itself (see below).

The vasoconstrictive properties of cocaine suggest it should cause prenatal growth restriction. The Maternal Lifestyles Study (MLS)[7] demonstrated a 450 g reduction in birthweight in cocaine-exposed pregnancies even after the effects of alcohol and tobacco were controlled for [C]. This growth limitation is thought to occur mostly in the third trimester.

NEONATAL EFFECTS

In the newborn period, substance-exposed infants are more likely to suffer low Apgar scores, infectious complications and CNS disturbance, and opiates may also cause neonatal respiratory depression. Prematurity, low birthweight and IUGR contribute as much to the neonatal problems as do the short-term actions of the drugs themselves.

Finnegan was the first to describe the **neonatal abstinence syndrome** (NAS). This results from the acute withdrawal of transplacental opioid which occurs at the delivery of a baby born to an opiate-abusing mother. The onset of the syndrome is normally within 24 hours of birth if the opiate used was short acting (e.g. heroin). It consists of:

- irritability, hypertonicity, tremor, exaggerated startle response and occasionally seizures;
- sweating and sneezing;
- abnormal sleep behaviour, high-pitched cry, poor feeding with weak suck and uncoordinated swallowing.

Methadone maintenance does not prevent NAS, but may delay its presentation until the second day of life due to its longer half-life.

Alcohol, cocaine and amphetamines have a less marked effect on neonatal behaviour, if any effect at all. Rare events such as neonatal hypertension, arrhythmias and necrotising enterocolitis are said to be more common in the offspring of cocaine users, although the confounding effects of prematurity are difficult to separate. Abnormal electroencephalogram (EEG) and brain-stem auditory-evoked responses have been demonstrated in these neonates, and the use of neonatal behavioural assessment scales has shown dampened arousal, poor orientation and reduced state control.

Amphetamine-exposed newborns occasionally demonstrate hyperactivity, poor feeding and disrupted sleep patterns. The neonatal effects of marijuana are debated. Greater irritability, tremors and startle responses have been reported, but a well-controlled Jamaican study[9] has suggested that once again the postnatal environment is more important than drug exposure itself. In fact, neonatal scores were found to be higher in the offspring of heavy marijuana users. In rural Jamaican society, these women tend to be wealthier and more highly educated. Benzodiazepines may cause neonatal respiratory depression, reduced tone and poor feeding.

CHILD DEVELOPMENT

Tests of child development are complex and beyond the scope of this chapter. They examine many aspects of behaviour, including language and motor skills, attention and play, cognition and problem-solving, and arousal and affective expression. They themselves are open to interpretation and bias.

Mothers willing to participate in longitudinal studies may be more highly motivated, and superior parenting skills in cooperative families may make the effects of the substance abuse appear less significant. Children, as they grow up, may find that society's low expectations of their substance-abusing mothers are reflected on to themselves.

Alcohol

Impaired development of the CNS is a key criterion of FAS. Although children with FAS have an average IQ of less than 70, the consequences of alcohol consumption that does not result in the full syndrome are less clear. The literature is confusing and does not offer clear guidance, perhaps because of the aetiological difficulties discussed above.

Opiates

Opiate use in pregnancy is indeed associated with poor developmental outcomes for the offspring; however, it seems that confounding factors are most likely to be responsible, rather than the drug itself. Results of child development tests have been found to be lower at 1 and 2 years of age by some researchers. However, a clear harmful effect of opioids themselves on child development is not strongly suggested by the literature.

Cocaine

Head circumference is inversely related to cocaine exposure during pregnancy. Along with the reported association with serious fetal/neonatal intracranial pathology, it is unsurprising that cocaine itself is thought to be directly damaging to neurodevelopment, with or without confounding social factors. Indeed, neurophysiological testing of such children suggests reduced numbers of oligodendrocytes and impaired myelination.

Closer examination of the data on neurodevelopmental outcome has challenged this view, and the two sides of the debate are difficult to reconcile. The meta-analysis performed by Frank and colleagues[10] selected 36 prospective and blinded studies in which polydrug use was uncommon. After controlling for confounding factors, there was no significant overall association between prenatal cocaine exposure and cognition, language and motor skills, behaviour, attention, affect or neurophysiology, up to 6 years of age [C].

This controversy is likely to continue. For practical purposes, cocaine use in pregnancy should be considered a marker of 'high risk'. Independent of any direct actions of the drug, pregnancy and neurodevelopmental outcomes are nevertheless poor and will improve only with better access to healthcare and social support.

SCREENING FOR SUBSTANCE ABUSE IN PREGNANCY

Pregnant women who use drugs may avoid antenatal care for fear of inciting closer scrutiny of their lifestyles, which may often include other criminal activities. They may fear that their child, or children, will be removed from them. Because of this, they may present needing help only at the time of a social, domestic or medical crisis. All those caring for pregnant women should be vigilant for substance abuse and take the opportunity to institute specialised antenatal care whenever presentation occurs. Enquiry about illicit substance use should be routinely made of all pregnant women in a matter-of-fact way. Be prepared to ask more than once. Covert urine testing may confirm substance abuse, but be careful when disclosing this information source, as it may be seen as underhand and untrustworthy and may damage the fragile relationship between the woman and the healthcare services.

Screening for heavy alcohol consumption can be quickly carried out in all pregnant women using the TACE questionnaire. Only four questions are asked:

Tolerance: *how many drinks does it take to make you feel high?* More than two suggests a degree of tolerance and scores 2 points.
Annoyance: *has anyone annoyed you by criticising your drinking?* Answering 'yes' scores 1 point.
Cutting down: *have you ever thought you needed to cut down your drinking?* Answering 'yes' scores 1 point.
Eye opener: *have you ever had a drink first thing in the morning to steady your nerves or to get rid of a hangover?* Answering yes scores 1 point.

A score of 2 or more points is considered a positive screen and carries a 70 per cent sensitivity for detection of heavy drinkers. Further questioning and assessment are needed of those who screen positive.

MANAGEMENT OF PREGNANCY COMPLICATED BY SUBSTANCE ABUSE

A multidisciplinary team approach is necessary to create a confidential, reassuring and non-judgemental environment in which the pregnancy outcome and childbirth experience can be optimised. This team will include social workers, specialist drug services, drug-liaison midwives, GPs, obstetricians and paediatricians.

'Harm minimisation' recognises the futility of simply telling users to stop using. It aims initially to promote a change in the nature of the drug taking, stabilise lifestyles and reduce criminal behaviour. Stopping drug abuse altogether is a much longer-term aim. Exchanging needles or moving to non-IV modes of delivery would be examples of harm reduction. Reducing alcohol and tobacco consumption and establishing methadone maintenance are particularly important aims in pregnancy.

Antenatal care

Significant improvements in pregnancy outcome are achieved by regular antenatal care, which should be tailored to the individual. Points to consider include:

- carefully targeted history taking;
- counselling about the possible effects of the drug abuse on the pregnancy;
- possible urine testing for illicit substances;
- discussion and delineation of achievable aims to reduce harm;
- ultrasound scanning to accurately date the pregnancy;
- screening for hepatitis B and C, HIV and possibly bacterial vaginosis;
- detailed anomaly scanning;
- serial growth scanning and fetal assessments as necessary;
- reflection on the need for a child protection case conference;
- communication with anaesthetic and paediatric services: cocaine and opiate abusers may pose particular problems for obstetric anaesthetists, and admission to a special care baby unit (SCBU) is very likely, even if only for observation.

Focused history taking from the pregnant drug abuser

- Type of drug(s) used, when, how often, how much and mode of administration.
- Does her partner use drugs?
- Has the woman particular fears or concerns of her own?
- Are there specific psychological or health problems leading to, or a consequence of, the drug abuse?
- What are the social/financial circumstances?
- Is she in any legal trouble?
- Does she drink alcohol or smoke tobacco?
- Does she practise safe sex?
- Does she share needles?

Women using street narcotics should be offered **methadone maintenance treatment** (MMT). Methadone has a longer half-life than heroin and blood levels remain more stable. Users are provided with a regular but limited supply, which offers the opportunity to remove themselves from the criminal high-risk behaviours often necessary to fund a street habit and which carry such risk to the pregnancy. Having to attend regularly to obtain prescriptions allows close antenatal surveillance and healthcare. The fetus avoids opiate 'highs' and withdrawals and other possible harmful contaminants of street drugs. Compliance with these regimens can reduce neonatal mortality and increase birthweight, although the benefits are lost if MMT is supplemented with street 'top-ups', which many abusers need for the 'highs' not provided by methadone. Negotiating the dose with the user is a difficult task. Low doses (60 mg/day) are associated with higher rates of non-compliance. Twice-daily dosing regimens may minimise the trough levels and reduce relapses.

Women established on MMT may consider gradual withdrawal (e.g. a reduction in dose of 2–2.5 mg every 7–10 days). Anecdotal evidence recommends that this should occur in the second trimester, as leaving it until later risks preterm labour [E]. The greater risk of withdrawal during pregnancy is a subsequent relapse of illegal narcotic use. This is considered to carry the greatest risk of fetal harm, and withdrawal during pregnancy should be attempted only in highly motivated women with a stable, supportive and drug-free environment to which they can return.

Unfortunately, there is no such 'replacement' regimen for cocaine users. Harm reduction must involve a reduction in cocaine use. Without an incentive, it may be very difficult to gain the trust and cooperation of pregnant users who fear reprisals for their substance abuse.

Pregnancy is a relative indication for inpatient alcohol detoxification. Most programmes choose to treat the pregnant, alcohol-dependent woman with short-acting barbiturates or benzodiazepines. Chlordiazepoxide and other benzodiazepines, such as diazepam and barbiturates, are valuable for symptomatic treatment during medical withdrawal from alcohol. They are also potentially teratogenic. Some clinicians, therefore, recommend avoiding their use if at all possible. The risks versus the possible benefits of their use need to be assessed.

Disulfiram (Antabuse) is contraindicated during pregnancy. Its use has been associated with club foot, VACTERL association (the non-random co-occurrence of birth defects vertebral anomalies, anal atresia, cardiac defects, tracheoesophageal fistula and/or oesophageal atresia, renal and radial anomalies and limb defects) and phocomelia of the lower extremities. The woman who conceives while taking this drug should receive counselling before deciding to continue the pregnancy.

EBM

Using methadone during pregnancy (as opposed to no opiates at all) is associated with an approximate doubling of neonatal mortality. Use of both methadone and heroin carries a six-fold increase in neonatal mortality risk.

Intrapartum care

Labour may be the first time a pregnant substance abuser presents to medical services. It should be managed as normal, with a few additional points to bear in mind.

- Recommend continuous CTG monitoring in view of the increased risk of placental insufficiency and fetal compromise.
- Be aware that opiates may influence the CTG and interpretation may be more difficult.
- Avoid, as far as possible, fetal blood sampling, scalp electrodes and episiotomies to reduce the vertical transmission risk of hepatitis and HIV.
- Elective caesarean section before membrane rupture reduces HIV vertical transmission and possibly that of hepatitis C[10] (although this needs confirmation).
- Give normal maintenance doses of methadone to prevent withdrawal. These will not provide analgesia, which should be offered in addition. Epidural analgesia may prove most effective if opioid receptors are already saturated by the illegal opiate.
- Those women who have undergone supervised withdrawal from opiates during the pregnancy should avoid systemic opiates in labour. Nitrous oxide and epidural analgesia are preferable.
- Naloxone should not be given to opiate-dependent mothers or their offspring – severe withdrawal effects may occur.
- In cocaine users, ephedrine may be less effective at reversing hypotension secondary to regional analgesia. Phenylephrine is a useful alternative.

Postnatal care

Above all, the new mother should be supported in her first few days, as any new parent should be. Indeed, she is likely to have minimal help when she leaves hospital. Ongoing assistance from the specialist midwife is vital.

- If the baby seems well it should be transferred to the postnatal ward with the mother. NAS usually presents in the first 2 days and the baby must be closely observed for signs of this. Methadone withdrawal may take a little longer, but will usually have begun by 4 days (the minimum time period that women are advised to stay in hospital). If the infant is demonstrating withdrawal symptoms, it will need special care facilities.
- Breastfeeding is encouraged in most women, even those on methadone. Infant weaning should occur gradually; fortunately the quantities of opiates reaching breast milk are small. HIV-positive women, those using large amounts of benzodiazepines and cocaine users are exceptions to this general rule. These women should be advised to bottlefeed. Hepatitis C is not a contraindication to breastfeeding.[11]

- Babies born to hepatitis-B-positive mothers should be immunised.
- Drug misuse by a parent does not necessarily equate with child neglect or abuse, and automatic child abuse registration will only discourage women from seeking antenatal care. Social services should be informed of the delivery and decisions made about the levels of support needed to ensure child safety.
- Appropriate contraceptive advice must be provided before discharge.

KEY POINTS

- There is an increasing body of evidence suggesting harm to the fetus from heavy alcohol consumption in pregnancy.
- Binge drinking in early pregnancy may be particularly harmful.
- There is considerable doubt as to whether infrequent low-level alcohol consumption conveys any long-term harm.
- Alcohol is the only clear teratogen, although benzodiazepines may predispose to oral clefting.
- Moreover, the effects of alcohol and other drugs on short-term and long-term child development are still in question. Potent cellular actions and devastating complications such as intracerebral haemorrhage are well recognised, but have a less striking impact on the results of larger population studies.
- Regardless of the direct harm caused by drug or alcohol abuse during pregnancy, such behaviour is a powerful marker of poor obstetric outcome and should prompt close antenatal surveillance by specialised healthcare workers.
- The aim of antenatal care should be to minimise harm by setting realistic goals.
- All units should have a dedicated team with defined guidelines to optimise outcomes for mother and baby.

Key references

1. McCarthy FP, O'Keeffe LM, Khashan AS *et al.* Association between maternal alcohol consumption in early pregnancy and pregnancy outcomes. *Obstet gynecol* 2013;122:830–7.
2. Abel EL. Maternal alcohol consumption and spontaneous abortion. *Alcohol* 1997;32:211–19.
3. Allebeck P, Olsen J. Alcohol and fetal damage. *Alcoholism: Clinical & Experimental Research* 1998;22:3295–325 (Suppl 7).
4. Dolovich LR, Addis A, Vaillancourt JM, Power JD, Koren G, Einarson TR. Benzodiazepine use in pregnancy and major malformations or oral cleft: meta-analysis of cohort and case-control studies. *BMJ* 1998;317:839–43.
5. McElhatton PR, Bateman DN, Evans C, Pughe KR, Thomas SHL. Congenital anomalies after pre-natal ecstasy exposure. *Lancet* 1999;354:1441–2.
6. Sprauve ME, Lindsay MK, Herbert S, Graves W. Adverse perinatal outcome in parturients who use crack cocaine. *Obstet Gynecol* 1997;89:674–8.
7. Mills JL, Graubard BI, Harley EE, Rhoads Gc, Berendes HW. Maternal alcohol consumption and birth weight. *J Am Med Assoc* 1984;252:1875-97.
8. Bada HS, Verter J, Bauer CR *et al.* MLS: Intra-uterine growth of infants exposed to cocaine/opiates in utero. *Paediatr Res* 1996;39:256.
9. Dreher MC, Nugent K, Hudgins R. Prenatal marijuana exposure and neonatal outcomes in Jamaica: an ethnographic study. *Pediatrics* 1994;93:254–60.
10. Frank DA, Augustyn M, Knight WG, Pell T, Zuckerman B. Growth, development and behaviour in early childhood following prenatal cocaine exposure. A systematic review. *J Am Med Assoc* 2001;285:1613–26.
11. Gibb DM, Goodall RL, Dunn DT *et al.* Mother-to-child transmission of hepatitis C virus: evidence for preventable peripartum transmission. *Lancet* 2000;356:904–7.

Chapter 20 Smoking

Andrew Shennan

INTRODUCTION

Smoking-related morbidity and mortality affect millions of individuals throughout the world. Each year, almost a quarter of all deaths in men can be attributed to a smoking-related cause and, although far fewer female deaths are related to smoking, the gap is rapidly closing. More women are becoming smokers in industrialised countries. The cause of this morbidity and mortality is largely related to the effects on cardiovascular disease although smoking is also a cause of cancer, particularly of the lung.

In the western world, almost a quarter of young women smoke and this affects their risks of developing gynaecological cancers such as cancer of the cervix. In recent years there is some evidence that this may be declining, particularly in countries where smoking has been banned in public places. Other risks, such as that of thromboembolic disease, are increased. Effects on the menopause and miscarriage, as well as low birthweight, have been reported. However, in spite of educational programmes to point out these obvious detrimental effects to fetal wellbeing, it has proved very difficult to introduce preventative strategies. Smoking remains a major preventable cause of low birthweight, preterm delivery and perinatal mortality; this section will review the relationship between smoking and pregnancy outcome, and management strategies to reduce adverse events.

INCIDENCE IN PREGNANCY

In the developed world approximately 20–30 per cent of pregnant women will report smoking; the figure of 27 per cent in the UK has been stable for some years although legislation banning smoking may now be influencing this and analysis of the impact is eagerly awaited. As with the non-pregnant population, there is a strong association with socio-economic background so that those from lower groups have considerably higher smoking rates. Generally actual smoking rates are about 3 per cent higher than reported rates, as evidenced by cotinine levels.[1]

It has been reported that women who continue to smoke in spite of knowledge of the detrimental effects are more likely to have problems at work and, in general, are less well supported on a psychosocial basis. Women without partners, and who already have children, are less likely to stop.

AETIOLOGY AND CLINICAL EFFECTS

Prematurity

There is good epidemiological evidence that smoking is related to the risk of premature delivery, including early preterm birth. There is also an established relationship with perinatal death [C]. The association is strong and often dose related which, therefore, adds considerable evidence that the effect is causative and not related to other associated factors [C].

Women who smoke have approximately double the risk of premature delivery. This is principally due to spontaneous preterm delivery but it can also increase the risk of the need for iatrogenic delivery through association with placental abruption and placenta praevia [C]. Smoking is also a risk factor for preterm premature rupture of the fetal membranes.[2]

Lower mean birthweight has been associated with a high mean systolic blood pressure in later life in the children of mothers who smoke. Smoking may therefore be contributing to the possible *in utero* programming effects with which reduce fetal growth potential is now thought to be associated.

Intrauterine growth restriction

It is established that low birthweight for gestation is more common in women who smoke.[3] On average, babies will be approximately 200 g lighter as a result of smoking. There is a dose relationship to this effect and it is established that women who smoke more than ten a day will have lower birthweight than those who smoke less than this number, the effects being greater in male fetuses [C]. Even passive smoking can reduce birthweight.[4]

IQ

Cognitive performance is reduced in the children of mothers who smoke during pregnancy, even after adjustment for other confounding variables.[5] Longer-term effects on the children may include influence on respiratory illness, over and above that which may be caused by the children living in a family where smoking continues [C].

Smoking and pre-eclampsia

There are many studies now that demonstrate an association between a reduced risk of pre-eclampsia and smoking [C].[6] However, it is clear that any possible benefit in this reduction is completely superseded by the harmful effects of smoking [D]. Indeed, women who smoke and show the clinical signs of pre-eclampsia have much more severe disease. In these women there are increased rates of perinatal mortality, abruption and IUGR.

Infertility, ectopics and miscarriage

There is now evidence that both ovarian function and implantation may be affected by smoking, thus reducing the fertility of these women. There is also an increased incidence of ectopic pregnancy that is apparent from recent meta-analyses. The risk of miscarriage is also increased.

MANAGEMENT: SMOKING CESSATION IN PREGNANCY

A minority of women will stop smoking when they become pregnant. These individuals frequently smoke less and have better support from home, including a partner who gives up or is a non-smoker. Programmes that encourage smoking cessation have been associated with some improved outcome, in terms of less low birthweight and premature delivery [C]. However, these programmes are highly intensive before they are successful and standard advice from midwives and other clinicians to stop smoking has had little impact on overall quitting rates during pregnancy [C]. Approximately 7 per cent of pregnant women who undergo focused counselling will give up smoking. However, a small number of individuals do stop on brief advice and, as this is inexpensive, it is worthwhile [E].

Specialist staff are known to be more effective than others, with more than a doubling of cessation rates [B].[7] Unfortunately few women are willing to, or have the opportunity to, use these counselling services. Self-help material has some benefit in approximately 4 per cent of smokers. The effectiveness and safety of nicotine replacement have enabled improved cessation rates, and at 2 years there may be less unimpaired development of the baby.[8]

There is good evidence that stopping smoking will reduce the adverse effects of smoking in pregnancy, and result in an improvement in birthweight and early birth [B].[9] In 72 trials, in spite of a modest reduction in the number of women who quit (6 per cent), there was a 10–15 per cent reduction in important obstetrics outcomes such as birthweight and preterm birth.[10] Of note, those countries that have evaluated smoking bans following legislation have noted benefit in the post-ban period. For example, in Ireland there was a reduction in SGA.[11]

KEY POINTS

- A quarter of pregnant women in the developed world smoke in pregnancy.
- Smoking in pregnancy is associated with prematurity, low birthweight and perinatal death, and is the single most preventable cause of these adverse events.
- In childhood, smoking in pregnancy is known to increase the risk of sudden infant death syndrome (SIDS).
- Most adverse events are dose related and reversed if pregnant women stop smoking.
- The children of mothers who smoke have lower IQs.

EBM

Specialist staff trained in counselling women about smoking are more likely to succeed in cessation programmes.

Key references

1. Tapen DM, Forward RP, Wilde CJ. Smoking at the end of pregnancy measured by cord blood cotanine assay. *NZ Medical Journal* 1995;108:108–9.
2. Harger JH, Hissing AW, Tamala RE. Risk factors for preterm premature rupture of membranes; a multicentre case control study. *AMJOG* 1990;163:130–7.

3. Harrod CS, Reynolds RM, Chasan-Taber L *et al.* Quantity and timing of maternal pre-natal smoking on neonatal body composition: the Healthy Start Study. *Pediatr* 2014;165:707-12.

4. Ruben DH, Krazeldondikoff PA, Leventhal JM, Weel B, Bergnet A. Effect of passive smoking on low birthweight. *Lancet* 1986; Aug 23;2(8504):415-7.

5. Sexton M, Fox NL, Hebble RL. Pre-natal exposure to tobacco and effects on cognitive functioning at age 3. *International Journal of Epidemiology* 1990;19:72–7.

6. Cnattingius S, Mills JL, Ewan J, Erikson *et al.* The paradoxical effect of smoking in pre-eclamptic pregnancies. Smoking reduced the incidence with increases of rates of perinatal mortality and abruption *AMJOG* 1997;177:156–61.

7. West R. Helping patients in hospital to quit smoking. Dedicated counselling services are effective – others are not. *BMJ* 2002;324:64.

8. Cooper S, Taggar J, Lewis S *et al.*; for the Smoking, Nicotine and Pregnancy (SNAP) Trial Team. Effect of nicotine patches in pregnancy on infant and maternal outcomes at 2 years: follow-up from the randomised, double-blind, placebo-controlled SNAP trial. *Lancet Respir Med* 2014;2:728-37.

9. Sexton M, Hebble JR. A clinical trial of change in maternal smoking and its effect on birthweight. *JAMA* 1984;251:911–15.

10. Lumley J, Chamberlain C, Dowswell T, Oliver S, Oakley L, Watson L. Interventions for promoting smoking cessation during pregnancy. *Cochrane Database Syst Rev* 2009;3:CD001055.

11. Kabir Z1, Daly S, Clarke V, Keogan S, Clancy L. Smoking ban and small-for-gestational age births in Ireland. *PLoS One* 2013;8:e57441.

Chapter 21 Anaemia

Will Lester

MRCOG standards

Relevant standard
Candidates are expected to understand the epidemiology, aetiology, pathophysiology, clinical characteristics, prognostic features and management of anaemia.

In addition, we would suggest the following.

Theoretical skills
• Revise the physiological changes of the blood in pregnancy.

Practical skills
• Interpret laboratory test results to determine cause and management of different types of anaemia in pregnancy

INTRODUCTION

Anaemia is the most common medical disorder of pregnancy.

Pre-existing bone marrow disorders and inherited haemoglobin (Hb) variants are discussed in Chapter 12. This chapter aims to revise the physiological changes in pregnancy, and discusses the maternal and fetal risks of anaemia, diagnosis and management.

PHYSIOLOGICAL CHANGES

• Plasma volume increases by 50 per cent.
• Red cell mass increases by up to 25 per cent.
• There is a consequent fall in Hb concentration, haematocrit and red cell count because of haemodilution.
• Mean cell volume (MCV) increases secondary to erythropoiesis.
• Mean cell Hb concentration (MCHC) remains stable.

• Serum iron and ferritin concentrations decrease secondary to increased utilisation and haemodilution
• Total iron-binding capacity increases.
• Iron requirements increase (due to expanding red cell mass and fetal requirements) from 2.5 mg/day in the first trimester to 6.6 mg/day in the third trimester (700–1400 mg total pregnancy).
• There is a moderate increase in iron absorption.
• Folate requirements increase in pregnancy (due to the fetus, placenta, uterus and expanded maternal red cell mass).
• There is no major effect on vitamin B_{12} stores, although cobalamin levels decrease (hormonal effects and active transport to the fetus).

DEFINITION

Anaemia is a pathological condition in which the oxygen-carrying capacity of red blood cells is insufficient to meet the body's needs.

Often the diagnosis is based on blood values, in particular Hb concentration. WHO recommends that the Hb concentration should not fall below 11 g/dL at any time during pregnancy,[1,2] but many clinicians use the figure of 10.5 g/dL as a cut-off after the first trimester, as recommended by the Centers for Disease Control and Prevention of the USA.[3,4] WHO defines postpartum anaemia as Hb <100 g/L.

INCIDENCE

Around 30–50 per cent of women become anaemic during pregnancy, with iron deficiency being responsible in more than 90 per cent of cases. The incidence of folate deficiency is around 5 per cent (though it is often underdiagnosed) and this is almost always the cause of megaloblastic anaemia in pregnancy, with vitamin B_{12} deficiency being rare.

CLINICAL FEATURES

Anaemia is very often asymptomatic in pregnancy, with the diagnosis being made on routine screening. Clinical features include tiredness, dizziness, palpitation and lethargy. Pallor may be apparent.

SCREENING

Anaemia is routinely screened for in pregnancy by estimating the Hb concentration by means of an FBC at pregnancy booking and again later in pregnancy, usually at 28 weeks. This lacks specificity but has the advantage of being cheap and simple to perform. The presence of a low Hb does not reveal the cause of the anaemia and a normal Hb does not exclude iron depletion.

IRON DEFICIENCY ANAEMIA

Aetiology

Iron deficiency is the most common cause of anaemia in pregnancy. There are significant iron demands during pregnancy, secondary to expanding red cell mass and fetal requirements, which can be met by only a limited increase in iron absorption, and by utilisation of iron stores. If iron stores are already depleted because of menstruation, recurrent pregnancies and poor intake, anaemia will develop rapidly. During pregnancy, the total iron-binding capacity (TIBC) increases secondary to the increased plasma volume, and serum iron falls. As iron demands exceed supply during pregnancy, ferritin levels fall. Decreased Hb concentration is a late event in iron deficiency.

Consequences

The evidence regarding the consequences of iron deficiency anaemia in pregnancy is conflicting. From the maternal perspective, as well as the clinical features described above, it has been suggested that impaired function of iron-dependent enzymes causes alterations in muscle function, neurotransmitter activity and epithelial changes throughout the body.[5] This has been used as the basis for the explanation for the apparent link between iron deficiency anaemia and preterm delivery, infection, medical intervention during labour and postpartum blood loss. It is clear that women with significant anaemia at the time of delivery will not tolerate blood loss as well, and are more likely to receive blood transfusion postnatally. From the fetal perspective, it is widely accepted that there is an increased risk of preterm delivery and IUGR; however, many of the studies have not controlled for other factors, such as smoking, that may be important.[6] There is also conflicting evidence regarding the neonatal iron status and cognitive development and behaviour of babies born to iron-deficient mothers.[7]

Diagnosis

Iron deficiency can be present in the absence of anaemia, and other parameters of the FBC that usually give a clue to this (reduced MCV, MCH and MCHC) are not as accurate during pregnancy (Table 21.1). As the MCV increases in pregnancy, an MCV well into the 'normal' range does not exclude iron deficiency as an underlying cause; however, a significantly elevated MCV (>106) should also trigger consideration of folate or vitamin B_{12} deficiency. It is also important that a microcytic anaemia is not automatically assumed to be caused by iron deficiency, as this may also be seen with beta-thalassaemia trait.

The diagnostic test for iron deficiency is a serum ferritin concentration. A concentration of <16 µg/L is highly sensitive for iron deficiency in terms of predicting absence of stainable iron in the bone marrow.[8] Unselected screening of ferritin is expensive, however, and is not generally recommended.

Treatment

Efficacy of treatment

Although it is clear that iron supplementation improves the haematological indices, there is little robust evidence to prove, especially in cases of mild anaemia in pregnancy with no complications, that such therapy improves clinical outcomes for these mothers or their babies; however, it is standard practice to offer iron supplements unless there is a contraindication.

It is not essential to delay oral iron therapy for anaemic women pending a ferritin result (unless there is an alternative explanation, e.g. beta-thalassaemia trait) and one strategy is a trial of treatment as a first-line diagnostic test, whereby an Hb increment demonstrated at 2 weeks is a positive result.[9]

The standard first-line treatment for iron deficiency is oral iron replacement [B], which is usually effective if there is enough time (maximum increase in Hb is 0.8 g/dL per week). The recommended dose is 100–200 mg of elemental iron per day. Ferrous salts are absorbed better than ferric salts [B] and should be used in preference. There is little to choose between the different ferrous salts in terms of absorption and

Table 21.1 Haematological values'

	Non-pregnant	Pregnant	Iron deficiency
Hb (g/dL)	12–15	11–15	<10.5
MCV (fL)	75–99	Increases	Decreases
TIBC (mmol/L)	45–72	Increases	Decreases by <15%
Serum iron (mmol/L)	13–27	Decreases	<12
Ferritin (mg/L)	15–300	Decreases	<12

- Hb, haemoglobin; MCV, mean cell volume; TIBC, total iron-binding capacity;

efficacy, and side effects are related to the amount of elemental iron contained. The choice of preparation should therefore be dictated by cost and patient tolerance, but it should be noted that a reduction in side effects is usually secondary to a reduction in the amount of elemental iron absorbed. Vitamin C taken simultaneously aids absorption [B], hence the common advice to take iron with fresh orange juice. There is, however, little to gain, other than increased cost, by using combination preparations with ascorbic acid included.

There is a 40 per cent risk of side effects with oral iron preparations, mainly gastrointestinal, and this can have a direct effect on tolerance and compliance. Slow-release preparations are often associated with a decrease in the incidence of side effects, but this is mainly secondary to decreased absorption of elemental iron, as most is not released from the preparation until it has passed through the first part of the duodenum, where iron absorption is optimal. For those with proven iron deficiency that cannot be managed with oral therapy because of lack of compliance, severe gastrointestinal side effects, continuing significant blood loss or malabsorption, parenteral preparations exist. It has been demonstrated that IV iron is most effective in improving the haematological indices, followed by intramuscular administration, with oral supplementation being least effective.[10]

However, this must be balanced against the invasiveness of administration and the possible adverse effects, which are mildest with oral supplementation and most severe with the IV route, including anaphylaxis. It is important that a diagnosis of iron deficiency anaemia is confirmed prior to parenteral treatment.

Intramuscular iron

Some parenteral iron preparations can be administered by deep intramuscular injection. It can be associated with pain at the time of injection and staining of the skin. The dose is calculated depending on the degree of anaemia and patient weight, but requires repeated injections, usually over the course of several weeks.

Intravenous iron

There are various IV iron preparations that are now available with significantly fewer side effects compared with historical iron dextran solutions. Parenteral iron can reduce the need for blood transfusion when oral therapy has failed as long as there are no contraindications. Parenteral iron should be avoided in the first trimester of pregnancy. Some preparations allow administration of a total body dose in a single infusion.

Blood transfusion

Towards the end of pregnancy there may not be the time available to increase the Hb with iron therapy, and blood transfusion may be indicated as well as iron therapy.

It should be borne in mind that blood transfusion is not without risk,[11] and effective screening programmes should detect anaemia early enough to allow iron therapy to be utilised. However, transfusion is the most rapid way to increase Hb concentration, but is a relatively slow way to increase iron stores.

Erythropoiesis stimulating agents

Recombinant human erythropoietin analogues are mainly used for the anaemia associated with erythropoietin deficiency in chronic renal failure, but can also be used to increase the autologous production of blood in normal individuals.

It has been used in cases of severe postpartum anaemia with success, and has been life saving in cases where blood transfusion is declined, for example Jehovah's witnesses. It has also been used during pregnancy in a small number of renal patients with no adverse maternal or perinatal complications.[12] Parenteral iron is usually given in addition to erythropoietin-stimulating agents to ensure effectiveness.

Prevention/prophylaxis

Prevention of iron deficiency is usually possible with a good balanced diet in the absence of ongoing blood loss. Identification and treatment of iron deficiency prior to pregnancy is optimal; however, many women enter pregnancy already iron deficient, or become so during pregnancy. Health education by the midwife regarding diet is therefore important.[13]

Guidelines produced by the British Committee for Standards in Haematology (BSCH)[9] recommend that ferritin should be checked in pregnancy in non-anaemic women at increased risk of iron depletion (eg. previous anaemia, multiple pregnancy, consecutive pregnancies with less than a year's interval and vegetarians), and also pregnant teenagers, women at high risk of bleeding and Jehovah's witnesses. If the ferritin is <30 µg/L, a dose of at least 65 mg elemental iron can be offered and the FBC and ferritin checked 8 weeks later.

These guidelines also recommend that women with a known haemoglobinopathy (eg. beta-thalassaemia trait, HbSS) should have serum ferritin checked and offered therapeutic iron if the ferritin is <30 µg/L.

There has been much work carried out on the role of routine iron supplementation in pregnancy, and this has been the subject of a Cochrane Review.[14] This meta-analysis of 40 trials including 12,706 women concluded that, although there is clear evidence of improvement in haematological indices in those women who receive iron supplements during pregnancy, there are not enough data to determine that routine supplementation with iron alone or in combination with folic acid has any substantial benefits or adverse effects on maternal

---

EBM

- Oral iron therapy with ferrous salts is the treatment of choice for iron deficiency anaemia in pregnancy [B].
- Vitamin C aids absorption but there is no evidence to support the use of combined preparations [B].
- There is insufficient evidence to recommend a policy of routine iron supplementation in pregnancy [A].

ANTENATAL OBSTETRICS

and fetal health and pregnancy outcomes (premature delivery and low birthweight) among populations in whom anaemia is common. The reviewers felt that there was not enough evidence to suggest a change in current recommended iron and folic acid doses with either modality of supplementation [A].

FOLATE DEFICIENCY

Aetiology

There is a significant increase in folate requirements during pregnancy because of the increased cell replication that takes place in the fetus, uterus and bone marrow (increase in red cell mass). Plasma folate concentrations decrease throughout pregnancy, reaching half the non-pregnant levels by term. The incidence of folate deficiency is higher in multiple pregnancies. Folate deficiency causes a megaloblastic anaemia, accounting for approximately 5 per cent of anaemia in pregnancy, although higher rates are found in other parts of the world and are thought to be secondary to poor diet. In the UK, many foods now have folate supplements added, making the recommended daily intake of 800 µg easier to achieve.

Consequences

There are clear links between periconceptual folate deficiency and neural tube defects,[15] as well as a suggested association with other anomalies,[16] hence the advice that all women planning a pregnancy should take 400 µg/day of folic acid and continue this for the first 12 weeks of pregnancy until the neural tube is closed [A]. From the maternal perspective, the consequences of folate deficiency are not just anaemia, but involvement of tissues with high rates of cell turnover, in particular mucous membranes; the effects of folate deficiency can thus be exacerbated by malabsorption if the gut mucosa is affected.

Diagnosis

During pregnancy a mild macrocytosis is often seen in the absence of folate or vitamin B_{12} deficiency and, conversely, a macrocytosis may be masked by coexisting iron deficiency leading to a reduced MCV. Red cell indices are therefore not necessarily helpful for diagnosis, although a significant macrocytosis should raise suspicion of possible folate or vitamin B_{12} deficiency. Examining the blood film may also be useful. Clinical suspicion is important and particular attention should be given to a dietary history which is typically low in fruit and vegetables.

Treatment

Severe folate deficiency is extremely rare, but, once megaloblastic haematopoiesis is established, treatment is impaired due to poor folate absorption from the affected gastrointestinal tract. In this situation, at least 5 mg oral folic acid daily is required.

Prevention/prophylaxis

The case for routine prophylaxis with 400 µg/day for the prevention of neural tube defects has already been discussed above. However, there are other situations in which folate prophylaxis is indicated. These include women taking anticonvulsant drugs [E] and those with haemolytic anaemias (see Chapter 27). In these situations, the recommended prophylactic dose is 5 mg/day throughout pregnancy.

VITAMIN B$_{12}$ DEFICIENCY

Vitamin B_{12} deficiency is rare during the reproductive years, and can be associated with infertility; therefore, vitamin B_{12} deficiency during pregnancy is uncommon. Absorption is unchanged by pregnancy, and vitamin B_{12} is actively transported across the placenta to the fetus. Serum cobalamin levels drop significantly during pregnancy despite normal tissue levels and so a standard vitamin B_{12} laboratory assay is of low diagnostic utility. The clinical history is therefore important (e.g. history of gastrectomy, Crohn's disease, vegan diet or a diet that suggests folate deficiency as the cause). There is some evidence that the holotranscobalamin assay is more specific in predicting genuine vitamin B_{12} deficiency but this assay is not currently widely available and requires further studies to evaluate its clinical utility as part of routine laboratory testing.[17]

Management

In cases of known vitamin B_{12} deficiency, treatment should be optimised prior to conception (and may be necessary to allow conception). Women on vitamin B_{12} replacement therapy should continue this as normal. Virtually all diets that contain animal products will supply enough vitamin B_{12} during pregnancy, although strict vegans may become deficient without supplements.

KEY POINTS

- Anaemia is the most common medical disorder of pregnancy, with iron deficiency being the most common underlying cause.
- Screening for anaemia in pregnancy is recommended in conjunction with dietary advice.
  * Be aware of how pregnancy can affect normal laboratory parameters, e.g. increasing MCV and reduced vitamin B_{12} levels.
- There is insufficient evidence to support routine iron prophylaxis in the absence of other risk factors.
- The role of periconceptual folate supplementation should be emphasised at pre-conceptual counselling.

ANTENATAL OBSTETRICS

Further Reading

Devalia V, Hamilton MS, Molloy AM; BCSH. Guidelines for the diagnosis and treatment of cobalamin and folate disorders. *Br J Haematol* 2014;166:496–513.

Pavord S, Myers B, Robinson S, Allard S, Strong J, Oppenheimer C; BCSH. UK guidelines on the management of iron deficiency in pregnancy. *Br J Haematol* 2012;156:588–600.

Key References

1. WHO. *Nutritional Anaemias.* Technical Report Series. Geneva: WHO, 1972.
2. WHO. *Iron Deficiency Anaemia, Assessment, Prevention, and Control: A guide for programme managers.* Available from: www.who.int/reproductive-health/docs/anaemia.pdf.
3. Centers for Disease Control. Current Trends: CDC criteria for anaemia in children and child-bearing age women. *Morb Mortal Wkly Rep* 1989;38: 400–4.
4. Ramsey M, James D, Steer P. *Normal Values in Pregnancy.* 2 edn. London: WB Saunders.
5. Finch CA, Cook JD. Iron deficiency. *Am J Clin Nutr* 1984;39:471–7.
6. Scholl TO, Hediger ML. Anemia and iron deficiency anemia: compilation of data on pregnancy outcome. *Am J Clin Nutr* 1994;59 (Suppl):492S–501S.
7. Walter T. Effect of iron-deficiency anaemia on cognitive skills in infancy and childhood. *Baillière's Clin Haematol* 1994;7:815–27.
8. Hallberg L, Bengtsson C, Lapidus L, Lindstedt G, Lundberg PA, Hultén L. Screening for iron deficiency: an analysis based on bone-marrow examinations and serum ferritin determinations in a population sample of women. *Br J Haematol* 1993;85:787–98.
9. Pavord S, Myers B, Robinson S, Allard S, Strong J, Oppenheimer C; BCSH. UK guidelines on the management of iron deficiency in pregnancy. *Br J Haematol* 2012;156:588–600.
10. Reveiz L, Gyte GML, Cuervo LG. Treatments for iron deficiency anaemia in pregnancy. *Cochrane Database Syst Rev* 2007;2:CD003094.
11. SHOT *Annual Report 2000/2001.* London: Serious Hazards of Transfusion Steering Group, 2002.
12. Breymann C, Major A, Richter C *et al.* Recombinant human erythropoietin and parenteral iron in the treatment of pregnancy anemia: a pilot study. *J Perinat Med* 1995;23:89–98.
13. Watson F. Routine iron supplementation – is it necessary? *Modern Midwife* 1997;7:22–6.
14. Pena-Rosasa JP, Viteri FE. Effects of routine oral iron supplementation with or without folic acid for women during pregnancy. *Cochrane Database Syst Rev* 2006;3:CD004736.
15. Lumley J, Watson L, Watson M, Bower C. Periconceptual supplementation with folate and/or multivitamins for preventing neural tube defects. *Cochrane Database Syst Rev* 2001;3:CD001056.
16. Elwood JM. Can vitamins prevent neural tube defects? *Can Med Assoc J* 1983;129:1088–92.
17. Devalia V, Hamilton MS, Molloy AM; BCSH. Guidelines for the diagnosis and treatment of cobalamin and folate disorders. *Br J Haematol* 2014;166:496–513.

Chapter 22 Abdominal pain

Clare L Tower

MRCOG standards

There is no specific established standard for this topic, but we would suggest the following points for guidance. Several of the many causes of abdominal pain can be found in core module 9, Maternal Medicine. A detailed discussion of every cause of abdominal pain in pregnancy is both impractical and cumbersome, and many of the disorders are discussed elsewhere in detail. Thus, this chapter aims to give an overview of the approach to abdominal pain in pregnancy, with a focus on differential diagnoses, and aspects of the approach that are specific to pregnant women.

INTRODUCTION

Abdominal pain is an extremely common complaint in pregnant women, with a majority of women experiencing it at some point during pregnancy. The vast majority is benign and self limiting. However, an approach to abdominal pain in pregnancy must enable identification of serious pathology to allow successful treatment to be implemented. There are many pitfalls in the assessment of pregnant women with abdominal pain and sadly several are found in the triennial maternal mortality report.[1] In particular, diagnosis of the 'acute abdomen', often defined as a collection of symptoms and signs of intraperitoneal disease best treated with surgery,[2] is notoriously difficult. The commonest surgical causes of the acute abdomen in pregnancy are appendicitis and cholecystitis.[3]

HISTORY AND EXAMINATION

In the same way as outside pregnancy, a systematic approach to the history and examination of the abdominal pain is required. A detailed outline of this can be found in many undergraduate textbooks. The gravid uterus and the physiological changes in pregnancy can mask some of the typical findings seen outside pregnancy. For example, the location of the appendix becomes displaced upwards as gestation increases. Therefore, whereas the appendix may lie at McBurney's point in the first trimester, by the late third trimester it may become located in the right hypochondrium, or be located behind the pregnant uterus. The enlarging uterus also separates the intra-abdominal organs from the parietal peritoneum with increasing gestation. Therefore, signs of peritonism may be masked as the inflamed abdominal organ no longer irritates the parietal peritoneum. Furthermore, many associated symptoms and signs can also be those common in a normal pregnancy, for example nausea and vomiting. A thorough but focused history and examination will usually suggest a short list of likely differential diagnoses (Table 22.1), thus guiding further investigation. Causes can be considered as either obstetric or non-obstetric, then within a systems review, e.g. gastrointestinal, renal and other. Involvement of other specialists, such as gastroenterologists, urologists or surgeons, may be indicated.

INVESTIGATIONS AND IMAGING

The list of possible differential diagnoses will guide suitable and targeted investigations (Table 22.1). Knowledge of how biochemical and haematological markers differ from the non-pregnant state is imperative in order to understand the significance of the results. White cell counts are typically increased during pregnancy, as is alkaline phosphatase due to placental production. Biochemical markers such as urea and creatinine fall. A summary of the variations seen in the commoner investigations performed during pregnancy is given in Table 22.2.

There has been much debate about the suitability of varying imaging modalities during pregnancy, largely due to concerns about the effect on the fetus. Ultrasound is considered safe and widely used, and can be useful in the diagnosis of, for example, appendicitis and renal tract obstruction. It is widely available, cheap and does not require the use of contrast medium or ionising radiation. However, the accuracy can be operator dependent and it may produce inconclusive results. Diagnosis of renal tract obstruction is a common example of how pregnancy causes difficulties in interpretation of

Table 22.1 Differential diagnoses, key findings and investigations

Disorder	Key clinical features	Specific investigations	Management
Obstetric – early pregnancy			
Miscarriage	Pain and bleeding	USS, hCG and progesterone levels	Expectant, medical or surgical
Ectopic pregnancy	Pain followed by a small amount of bleeding, peritonism, shoulder tip and rectal pain; may present with diarrhoea	USS, hCG and progesterone levels	Expectant, medical or surgical
Ruptured corpus luteal cyst	Signs of peritonism	USS	Analgesia ± laparoscopy
Adnexal torsion	Twisting pain, peritonism Commoner in first trimester and postpartum	USS	Analgesia ± laparoscopy
Obstetric – late pregnancy			
Round ligament pain	Bilateral, stitch like	None	Analgesia and reassurance
Braxton Hicks	Painful/painless tightenings not causing cervical dilatation	Vaginal examination to exclude labour	Reassurance
Labour	Painful contractions	Vaginal examination, CTG, etc.	Consider tocolysis and steroids if preterm
Placental abruption	Constant pain, rigid uterus, sometimes frequent and short-lasting contractions ± bleeding	Fetal assessment, bloods	Resuscitation, delivery
Pre-eclampsia	Epigastric, right upper quadrant	All pte-eclampsia investigations	Treat blood pressure, consider delivery
Polyhydramnios	Tight, distended abdomen, difficult to feel fetal parts	USS, exclude diabetes, infection (TORCH)	Detailed fetal scan, consider amnio-drainage
Adnexal torsion	Twisting pain, peritonism	USS	Analgesia ± laparoscopy
Fibroid degeneration	Constant localised pain, over the fibroid	USS to confirm fibroids; degenerative cystic changes may be present	Analgesia
Uterine rupture	Sudden-onset constant pain, haemodynamic collapse, vaginal bleed, haematuria	All bloods, cross-match, CTG	Resuscitate and surgery
Acute fatty liver	Epigastric/right upper quadrant pain, often associated with malaise, nausea and vomiting; may be jaundiced and have ascites	All pre-eclampsia investigations – may have hyperuricaemia, hypoglycaemia, deranged LFTs. USS/CT or MRI of liver	Stabilise and deliver
Urinary retention (retroverted uterus)	Unable to pass urine, palpable and uncomfortable bladder	Catheter; USS will help exclude other causes	Conservative management; usually resolves after 12 weeks
Physiological obstruction of ureters	Renal angle tenderness	USS to assess renal pelviectasis (2 cm normal)	Usually conservative; if significant, may require nephrostomy
Chorioamnionitis	Tender uterus, offensive discharge, systemic signs of sepsis, usually preceded by ruptured membranes	Blood cultures, inflammatory markers, speculum, CTG	Intravenous antibiotics, resuscitate and deliver

(continued)

Table 22.1 Differential diagnoses, key findings and investigations (*continued*)

Disorder	Key clinical features	Specific investigations	Management
Symphysis pubis dysfunction	Suprapubic tenderness, over bone; worse on movement and standing on one leg	Full physiotherapy assessment	Physiotherapy, analgesia
Rectus abdominis rupture	Sudden-onset pain, usually precipitated by cough or vomit; rare and usually in multiparous women; may have associated haematoma	Exclude other causes of abdominal pain	Analgesia; expanding haematoma may require surgical exploration
Non-obstetric			
Renal tract causes Urinary tract infection	Dysuria, frequency of micturition	Urine dipstick, urine for culture	Increase oral intake of fluid, antibiotics
Pyelonephritis	Loin pain (renal angle tenderness), radiating round to abdomen and into groin, rigors	Blood cultures, urine dipstick and culture, renal USS	Antipyretics, IV antibiotics, IV fluids
Renal calculi	Loin pain (renal angle tenderness), radiating round to abdomen and into groin, often colicky in nature	Urine dipstick (microscopic haematuria), urine for culture, renal USS	Conservative management with fluids and analgesia; involve urologists
Gastrointestinal tract causes Constipation	Constant or colicky abdominal pain; infrequent, hard stools		Dietary advice, stool softeners
Gastritis/peptic ulcer disease	Epigastric pain, often constant or burning; duodenal ulcers relieved by food, gastric ulcers made worse by food; may be associated with nausea, vomiting, haematemesis	Gastroscopy if severe; involve gastroenterologists	Antacids and ulcer-healing drugs – H_2-receptor antagonists/proton-pump inhibitors
Appendicitis	Pain, not always localised to right iliac fossa, especially in third trimester; signs of peritonism; associated anorexia, nausea, vomiting and pyrexia	Inflammatory markers (white blood cell count, C-reactive protein); USS of abdomen; pyuria may be present	Involve general surgeons, surgical management
Bowel obstruction	Colicky abdominal pain, associated with vomiting and nil passed per rectum; high-pitched or absent bowel sounds; usually have risk factors; perforation will cause signs of peritonism	Abdominal X-ray; involve general surgeons; colonoscopy	Conservative management – IV fluids, nasogastric tube; may require surgery
Cholecystitis/ cholelithiasis	Epigastric or right upper quadrant pain (colicky or stabbing); may radiate through to back and be associated with nausea and vomiting; intolerance of fatty food; tenderness and guarding	USS of gallbladder/liver, LFTs	Conservative management – analgesia, fluids, antibiotics if infected; surgery may be indicated (see text)
Pancreatitis	Epigastric pain, radiates through to back; associated with nausea and vomiting	USS of upper abdomen, CT scan, LFTs, amylase and lipase three times normal, calcium low, high blood glucose	Involve surgeons, conservative management; use of prognostic scoring systems
Gastroenteritis	Generalised, usually crampy abdominal pains, associated with diarrhoea and vomiting	Stool sample	Fluids; manage at home if possible
Hepatitis	Right upper quadrant/epigastric pain; may be associated with jaundice	USS of liver, LFTs, hepatits screen	Involve hepatologist, depends on underlying cause
Strangulated hernia	Peritonism, may be associated with bowel obstruction	Involve surgeons	Involve surgeons, treat bowel obstruction

(continued)

Table 22.1 Differential diagnoses, key findings and investigations (*continued*)

Disorder	Key clinical features	Specific investigations	Management
Inflammatory bowel disease	Generalised pain, associated diarrhoea, mucus and rectal bleeding, vomiting, weight loss	Inflammatory markers, sigmoidoscopy, colonoscopy	Involve gastroenterologists, steroids, mesalamine, other immune modulators such as azathrioprine
Other Abdominal bleeding	Very rare; ruptured liver capsule, splenic artery aneurysms, aortic aneurysms, cause haemorrhagic shock and abdominal pain	FBC, cross-match, assess fetal wellbeing with CTG	Resuscitate, surgical management
Pelvic vein thrombosis	Often thrombosis of right/left iliac vein, causing groin tenderness, leg swelling, sometimes pyrexia	Doppler ultrasound, venogram, thrombophilia screen	Anticoagulation using LMWH, involve haematologists; may require filter in inferior vena cava
Systemic causes, e.g. DKA, increased calcium, sickle cell crisis	Generalised abdominal pain, associated with being systemically unwell	Urea, electrolytes, blood glucose, bone profile	Treatment dependent on cause; involve the general physicians
Trauma – remember domestic violence	Associated with bruising; domestic violence commonly results in abdominal trauma during pregnancy	Assessment of fetal wellbeing, Kleihauer's test, particularly if rhesus negative; check for other injuries	Ensure safety, specialist midwifery service, social input
Pneumonia	Right lower-lobe pneumonia may cause right upper quadrant pain; associated with respiratory symptoms	Chest X-ray, blood gases, inflammatory markers, sputum cultures	Antibiotics, may require oxygen and high-dependency support if severe

TORCH, toxoplasmosis, rubella, cytomegalovirus, herpes simplex and HIV; USS, ultrasound scan.

Table 22.2 Biochemical and haematological variations in pregnancy

Investigation	Non-pregnant	Pregnant	Notes
Haemoglobin (g/dL)	12–15	11–14	Haemoglobin falls, to lowest at around 32 weeks
White cell count (x 10^9/L)	4–11	6–16	White cells increase; further increases in response to steroids when given for lung maturity, and in labour
Platelets (x 10^9/L)	150–400	Can fall by around 10% in pregnancy	
C-reactive protein (g/L)	Does not vary in pregnancy		
Urea (mmol/L)	2.7–7.5	<4.5	Falls with increasing gestation
Creatinine (µmol/L)	65–100	<75	
Amylase	Generally unchanged in pregnancy		
Uric acid (urate) (mmol/L)	0.18–0.35	Generally considered as 0.1 x no. of weeks' gestation, e.g. 0.35 at 35 weeks	
AST/ALT (IU/L)	<40	Both usually lower in pregnancy, with 30 as upper limit of normal	
Alkaline phosphatase (IU/L)	30–130	Increases with gestation, up to around 400	

scan findings. Physiological dilatation of the renal collecting system occurs in pregnancy due to a combination of compression and smooth muscle relaxation secondary to progesterone. A physiological dilatation of up to 2 cm is considered 'acceptable', and is often greater on the right. In physiological dilatation, the ureter will taper to a normal calibre as it crosses the pelvic brim, but, in pathological dilatation, this is lost. Also, ureteric 'jets of urine' entering the bladder can be seen in physiological dilatation, a phenomenon that is also lost in pathological dilatation.[4]

If ultrasound produces inconclusive findings, further imaging may be needed. Investigations involving ionising radiation have often been avoided during pregnancy due to concerns about the radiation effect on the fetus in terms of teratogenesis, pregnancy loss and future malignancy. However, the overall risks are very small. Fetal risks, thought to be maximal with exposure between 8 and 15 weeks, are not increased by exposures <5 rad. Risks of subsequent carcinogenesis are also small. It is estimated that a 1 to 2-rad exposure may increase the risk of leukemia from 1:3000 to 1:2000.[5] Table 22.3 gives

Table 22.3 Radiation doses[5]

Procedure	Fetal exposure mrad	Fetal exposure in dose equivalents
Chest X-ray (two views)	0.02–0.07 mrad	0.008 rem (0.08 mSv)
Abdominal X-ray	0.1 mrad	0.1 rem (1 mSv)
Intravenous urography	≥1 rad, depending on number of images	0.6 rem (6 mSv)
CT of the abdomen	3.5 rad	3 rem (30 mSv)

- Rad is the old non-SI unit of radiation; 1 rad = 0.01 gray in the SI system. As different types of radiation have a different impact on the human body, the dose equivalent is used in order to allow meaningful comparisons of damage. This incorporates a modifying factor (energy deposited per unit mass of tissue). The SI unit of this is the sievert (Sv), and the non-SI the rem.

approximate radiation doses of various types of investigation. For comparison, these are much lower than a long-haul intercontinental flight that provides a 15-mrem dose of radiation, and a short-haul flight that provides 6 mrem.[6] Thus, fetal risks are minimal and should not prevent an important investigation in pregnancy. However, CT scanning is uncommonly used, with the main indications for its use being trauma and renal stone pathology in the second and third trimesters.[7] There is growing interest and expertise in the use of MRI for the investigation of non-obstetric abdominal pain in pregnancy.[8] This is considered safe although there remains debate about the use of the usual MRI contrast agent, gadolinium.[9] This agent crosses the placenta and there are few data relating to safety in human pregnancy. Hence MRI in pregnancy should be without the use of intravenous contrast, although some authors consider oral use acceptable.[8]

DIFFERENTIAL DIAGNOSES

A list of specific differential diagnoses, investigations and management are given in Table 22.1. Several are discussed in other sections of the book. Hence, detailed descriptions are given only for significant conditions not discussed elsewhere.

Appendicitis

Appendicitis is the commonest cause of an acute surgical abdomen during pregnancy, with an incidence of 1 in 500–2000 pregnancies, and it accounts for 25 per cent of surgery conducted for non-obstetric indications. Diagnosis is often hampered due to the physiological effects of pregnancy. Ultrasound is useful, although less so during the third trimester, or if the appendix has perforated. As a result, approximately 5–50 per cent of pregnant patients who undergo appendectomy have a normal appendix.[3] Similarly, perforation is more common in pregnancy, and is associated with significant fetal and maternal mortality. Fetal loss rates of up to 20–35 per cent have been reported in older studies with more recent studies suggesting loss rates up to 8 per cent,[3] partly due to the high incidence of preterm labour secondary to peritonitis. Uncomplicated appendicitis without perforation has a low

fetal loss rate of around 2 per cent. Not surprisingly, maternal mortality increases in the third trimester.

Management of appendicitis is surgical, and involving general surgical colleagues early is recommended. Surgery can be open, using an incision over the point of maximal tenderness (may be right paramedian or midline in late pregnancy), or laparoscopic. Laparoscopic surgery is now considered acceptable during pregnancy, even during the third trimester.[10] A 15-mmHg pneumoperitoneum is well tolerated by the fetus. Reports in the literature describe Veress needle insertion either in the mid-clavicular line or 2 cm below the inferior costal margin, or with the open Hasson technique. The open Hasson entry technique is recommended as it avoids insufflation of the uterus which would be catastrophic to the fetus. In cases in which there is diffuse peritonitis, intravenous antibiotics are recommended preoperatively. Caesarean section may also need to be considered if the mother is severely unwell, particularly as gestation approaches term.

Acute cholecystitis

Acute cholecystitis is the second commonest surgical cause of an acute abdomen in pregnancy, predominantly caused by gallstones or biliary sludge. Gallstone formation is more likely in pregnancy as progesterone predisposes to increased bile stasis and high levels of oestrogen increase the cholesterol secretion. Although gallstones have been reported in 1–3 per cent of pregnant women, they are commonly asymptomatic as cholecystitis affects only 0.1 per cent.[3] This may increase as women continue to delay pregnancies until they are older. The signs and symptoms are largely the same as those found outside pregnancy and are summarised in Table 22.1. Serum levels of direct bilirubin and transaminases may be raised, and amylase may be raised. Alkaline phosphatase is of limited use due to placental production. Ultrasound will detect 95–98 per cent of gallstones, and, in acute cholecystitis, gallbladder thickening (>3 mm), pericholecystic fluid, sonographic Murphy's sign (focal tenderness under transducer when positioned over gallbladder), and dilatation of the intra- and extrahepatic ducts will be present.

Management can be medical or surgical. Until recently, medical management of hydration, analgesia and antibiotics was more common, with surgery being delayed until after delivery of the baby. However, reports have shown that delaying surgery is associated with a high recurrence rate, longer hospital stay, increased risk of gallstone pancreatitis, spontaneous miscarriage and preterm labour. Therefore, surgical management using laparoscopic or open cholecystectomy during pregnancy is growing in popularity. Endoscopic retrograde cholangiopancreatography (ERCP) can also be used during pregnancy, using techniques to reduce the fetal radiation dose.

Bowel obstruction

The incidence of bowel obstruction in pregnancy is around 1:2500 and in 60–70 per cent is caused by adhesions.[4] Volvulus occurs more commonly in pregnancy (25 per cent of bowel obstructions) and is believed to be due to the rapid change in size of the uterus having a physical influence on the surrounding mobile organs such as the caecum. Bowel obstruction has been associated with high maternal (6 per cent) and fetal (26 per cent) mortality rates, particularly in the third trimester, and the rates probably reflect delayed diagnosis.[11] Bowel surgeons should be involved in the management, and series have suggested that nearly a quarter of cases will require surgical resection.[11]

Pancreatitis

Acute pancreatitis has an incidence of 1 in 3000–4000 pregnancies, and occurs most often in the third trimester.[12] As in the non-pregnant state, the two most frequent causes are gallstones and alcohol. Symptoms, signs and management are the same as in non-pregnancy. Pancreatitis can range from mild disease (80 per cent) through to a severe necrotising form. Historically, the maternal and fetal mortality rate has been high in severe disease (up to 37 per cent), but improvements in diagnosis, treatment and neonatal care have reduced this in recent years to a maternal mortality rate of <1 per cent, and a perinatal mortality rate of up to 18 per cent.[12] Serum amylase and lipase are key in the diagnosis and will typically be three times the upper limit of normal. Lipase is more sensitive, and therefore is currently the recommended test.[13] Although these enzymes are useful for diagnosis, they do not aid in assessment of severity or prognosis. Prediction of which patients will progress to severe life-threatening disease is challenging. Therefore, there are several grading systems currently in use: Ranson's criteria, Glasgow score and the APACHE II (Acute Physiology and Chronic Health Evaluation II) assessment. Unfortunately, these systems are more complex to use in pregnancy as they do not account for the physiological effects of pregnancy on parameters such as white blood cell count. Therefore, management should involve surgical colleagues and is largely supportive with bowel rest, fluids, monitoring and analgesia. It has been suggested that pethidine and tramadol should be used as analgesia because they do not cause spasm of the sphincter of Oddi.[2] Women who are severely ill may require delivery of the baby.

Renal stones

Renal stones occur in approximately 1:200–1:2000 pregnancies, and may be associated with preterm labour.[10] Management should involve the urologists, and between 64 and 84 per cent will resolve with conservative management of fluids and analgesia.[14] Ultrasound is the initial investigation, but this may miss a partial blockage. Thus, an intravenous urogram (IVU) may be required. Outside pregnancy, unenhanced helical CT is the gold standard for diagnosis, and reports of use in pregnancy can be found in the literature. However, both these modalities involve a higher radiation dose. The presence of uncontrolled pain, sepsis, single kidney obstruction or preterm labour indicates that further interventions are required. Percutaneous nephrostomy, or a ureteric stent, can be used to temporarily relieve the obstruction. However, these may require replacing every 6–8 weeks. Ureteroscopy with a holmium laser is an option in pregnancy for stones smaller than 1 cm, and without sepsis.[15]

KEY POINTS

- Abdominal pain is very common in pregnancy.
- A systematic approach is required to identify serious from non-serious pathology.
- Differential diagnoses should be considered as pregnancy and non-pregnancy related.
- Diagnosis may be hampered by the physiological changes associated with pregnancy.
- Investigations should not be limited by pregnancy, particularly if the wellbeing of the mother may be adversely influenced.
- Appropriate involvement of other specialties is indicated.

References

1. CMACE. *Saving Mothers' Lives: Reviewing maternal deaths to make motherhood safer: 2006–2008*. The Eighth Report of the Confidential Enquiries into Maternal Deaths in the United Kingdom. *BJOG* 2011;118(Suppl 1):1–203.
2. Augustin G, Majerovic M. Non-obstetrical acute abdomen during pregnancy. *Eur J Obstet Gynecol Reprod Biol* 2007;131:4–12.
3. Gilo NB, Amini D, Landy HJ. Appendicitis and cholecystitis in pregnancy. *Clin Obstet Gynecol* 2009;52:586–96.
4. Glanc P, Maxwell C. Acute abdomen in pregnancy: role of sonography. *J Ultrasound Med* 2010;29:1457–68.
5. ACOG Committee Opinion. Number 299, September 2004 (replaces No. 158, September 1995). Guidelines for diagnostic imaging during pregnancy. *Obstet Gynecol* 2004;104:647–51.
6. Barish RJ. In-flight radiation exposure during pregnancy. *Obstet Gynecol* 2004;103:1326–30.

7. Wallace GW, Davis MA, Semelka RC, Fielding JR. Imaging the pregnant patient with abdominal pain. *Abdom Imaging* 2012;37:849–60.

8. Beddy P, Keogan MT, Sala E, Griffin N. Magnetic resonance imaging for the evaluation of acute abdominal pain in pregnancy. *Semin Ultrasound CT MR* 2010;31:433–41.

9. Tremblay E, Therasse E, Thomassin-Naggara I, Trop I. Quality initiatives: guidelines for use of medical imaging during pregnancy and lactation. *Radiographics* 2012;32:897–911.

10. Kilpatrick CC, Orejuela FJ. Management of the acute abdomen in pregnancy: a review. *Curr Opin Obstet Gynecol* 2008 Dec;20(6):534–9.

11. Perdue PW, Johnson HW Jr, Stafford PW. Intestinal obstruction complicating pregnancy. *Am J Surg* 1992;164:384–8.

12. Papadakis EP, Sarigianni M, Mikhailidis DP *et al.* Acute pancreatitis in pregnancy: an overview. *Eur J Obstet Gynecol Reprod Biol* 2011;159:261–6.

13. Rickes S, Uhle C. Advances in the diagnosis of acute pancreatitis. *Postgrad Med J* 2009 Apr;85(1002):208–12.

14. Srirangam SJ, Hickerton B, Van Cleynenbreugel B. Management of urinary calculi in pregnancy: a review. *J Endourol* 2008;22:867–75.

15. McAleer SJ, Loughlin KR. Nephrolithiasis and pregnancy. *Curr Opin Urol* 2004;14:123–7.

Chapter 23 Malignancy

Louise Kenny

Louise Kenny

MRCOG

The RCOG have issued a consensus view arising from the 55th Study Group on Cancer and Reproductive Health: http://www.rcog.org.uk/files/rcog-corp/uploadedfiles/roupConsensuViewsCancerandReproductiveHealth.pdf and a Green Top Guideline No.12 on Pregnancy and Breast Cancer: http://www.rcog.org.uk/files/rcog-corp/GTG12PregBreastCancer.pdf

Theoretical skills

- Recognise the influence that pregnancy has on the presentation and prognosis of malignant disease.
- Understand the need to balance benefit and harm to the fetus and the mother by delaying or proceeding with treatment.
- Know currently available evidence for guiding management and predicting outcomes for the more common cancers arising in pregnancy.

Practical skills

- Be able to manage a pregnancy with coexisting malignant disease.
- Be able to liaise with surgeons, oncologists, paediatricians and psychologists to create an individualised plan of care.
- Be able to manage a pregnancy complicated by an adnexal mass.
- Be able to manage a pregnancy with an abnormal cervical smear.

INTRODUCTION

Traditionally, the incidence of a new cancer diagnosis complicating pregnancy has been quoted as 1 in every 1000 pregnancies. However, there is evidence to suggest that the incidence is increasing, perhaps in part driven by the trend towards delaying childbirth and consequently increasing maternal age. In general, the distribution of cancers occurring in pregnancy mostly mirrors the distribution of cancers in young women. A recent Australian population cohort study found that estimates for the most common types of cancer in pregnancy were higher than the published international estimates: melanoma of skin (45.7 versus 8.7 per 100,000), breast cancer (28.8 versus 19.3 per 100,000) and thyroid cancer (17.4 versus 14.4 per 100,000), and lower for cervical (8.4 versus 12.0 per 100,000) and ovarian cancers (3.6 versus 5.2 per 100,000).[1] The overall distribution in this cohort partly arises from the predominance of melanoma, for which Australia has the highest incidence in the world.

Pregnancy does not affect the course of the cancer itself. However, diagnosis is often delayed as the presenting symptoms of malignancy may be confused with the common symptoms of pregnancy. Both the investigation and treatment of a malignancy may carry risks for the fetus, and serious conflict may occur between the desire to treat the mother appropriately while limiting harm to the pregnancy.[2] Future prospects for child-bearing may be subsequently limited by surgery, radiotherapy and chemotherapy. Psychological adjustment to a diagnosis of cancer is likely to be more difficult while pregnant.[3] Managing cancer during pregnancy therefore requires a multidisciplinary approach involving obstetricians, oncologists, paediatricians and counsellors. The role of an individual midwife or oncology nurse should not be underestimated [E].

EBM

Evidence to support management decisions in pregnancies complicated by cancer is derived mostly from retrospective uncontrolled studies [D]. Few case–control studies have been performed and the paucity of good-quality evidence must be made clear during patient counselling.

RADIOTHERAPY AND CHEMOTHERAPY DURING PREGNANCY

Fetal exposure to radiation and/or chemotherapeutic agents may potentially have a number of detrimental effects. These include:

- miscarriage and intrauterine fetal death;
- congenital anomalies;
- severe learning disability and microcephaly;
- prenatal and postnatal growth restriction;
- increase in the risk of childhood malignancy;
- infertility in the offspring;
- induction of germline genetic abnormalities.

Counselling couples about the fetal risks associated with cancer treatment is complicated by a lack of high-quality evidence. There have been no randomised trials, and publication and ascertainment bias skew the available data. Studies often involve small numbers, and are retrospective and unsystematic in their approach and follow-up. Chemotherapy and radiotherapy are often used in combination and the contributory effects of the illness itself on the pregnancy are impossible to isolate from other variables. Data are often out of date and irrelevant to newer management regimens. Experimental data from animal studies can be helpful, but there are marked interspecies differences and caution must be exercised in extrapolating directly to human pregnancies. Remember also that the background fetal anomaly rate is variably quoted as 3–6 per cent. All studies should be interpreted with this in mind.

Radiation exposure during pregnancy

Radiation dose is measured in grays and rads:

> 1 gray (1 Gy) = 100 rad
> 1 centi-gray (cGy) = 1 rad.

Calculating fetal exposure and radiation absorption during radiotherapy and radiological investigations is complicated and often imprecise. Although the primary radiation beam can be accurately directed and quantified, additional exposure occurs from leakage through the head of the linear accelerator, external scatter from beam modifiers and internal scatter within the patient. With appropriate shielding, fetal exposure can be reduced by as much as 50 per cent, although the effects of shielding can also be difficult to quantify. The gestation at which exposure occurs is also important for two reasons. Most importantly, fetal tissues show differential radiosensitivity throughout the course of the pregnancy (see below). Second, a larger fetus is more difficult to shield effectively and may lie closer to the irradiated field.

The effects of prenatal exposure to ionising radiation are described as either **deterministic** or **stochastic**. Deterministic effects are those where loss of function occurs due to cell destruction. The severity of the effect is dose related and a critical threshold exists below which the effect is not seen.

Miscarriage, intrauterine death, congenital anomalies and SMR are believed to follow this pattern. Stochastic effects are those where ionising radiation causes genetic cell modification and loss of cell-cycle control which, after a period of latency, leads to the development of cancer. Stochastic effects also demonstrate a dose–effect relationship, but without a threshold value.[4]

- Very early exposure to radiation during pregnancy (pre-implantation and early organogenesis; 0–2 weeks post-conception) will result in miscarriage or the pregnancy will continue unaffected.
- Mammalian animal experiments show that congenital abnormalities are more likely when exposure occurs during early organogenesis (3–7 weeks post-conception in a human pregnancy).
- Generalised growth and neurological development continue throughout normal pregnancy. Microcephaly, severe learning disability and permanent growth restriction remain potential risks for the fetus exposed during the remainder of the pregnancy. The 8- to 15-week period appears to be the time of highest risk and corresponds to a critical stage of cortical formation and organisation. There is minimal risk after 25 weeks, unless very high exposures occur.
- An increased predisposition to malignancy later in life appears to be a risk whatever the gestational age at which exposure occurs.

Evidence for the effects of radiation exposure during pregnancy is derived from three sources:

1. animal experiments;[5]
2. accidental human exposures;
3. the Japanese survivors of the atomic bomb.[6,7]

The high rate of fetal loss occurring with exposure during pre-implantation (conception to day 10) has been confirmed by rodent experiments and epidemiological data from Nagasaki and Hiroshima. Miscarriage and intrauterine death occur with a threshold of 10 cGy in these first few weeks; however, this increases steadily towards term, at which time the lower threshold for causing intrauterine death is estimated as >1 Gy.[4]

Animal experiments, mostly involving rodents, have shown that exposure during organogenesis causes a variety of congenital anomalies, notably involving the skeleton, eye and urinary tract. The threshold, extrapolating to humans, is possibly as low as 5 cGy, with a marked dose–response effect. However, human studies have failed to find this effect, with the exception of microcephaly. Teratogenesis should nevertheless remain a concern. It may be that the critically sensitive time in the human fetus is shorter, or that pregnancies with major anomalies abort spontaneously or have gone unrecorded.

Destruction of neural cells or failure of their migration may lead to microcephaly and/or learning disability. Data from Japan[7] has estimated a lower threshold for microcephaly of 10 rad (10 cGy), with the 8- to 15-week period being most crucial. The incidence of microcephaly was 40 per cent with exposures of 50 cGy or higher. Severe learning disability was also found more commonly in the offspring exposed between 8 and 25 weeks, with lower thresholds for severe learning disability of 6 cGy (8–15 weeks) and 28 cGy (16–25 weeks). Studies of IQ reflect these observations.[7]

There are fewer data on the effect of radiation exposure on developing germ cells. Delayed menarche has been observed in Japanese girls exposed to radiation *in utero* with a threshold of 25 cGy. No increase in the rates of infertility has yet been demonstrated.

A safe exposure limit of 5 cGy during pregnancy has been suggested. However, this does not take account of possible stochastic effects that do not show a lower threshold. An increase in childhood malignancies has been reported in a famous Oxford study of pelvimetry during pregnancy in which exposures were typically 1 cGY (the Oxford Survey of Childhood Cancers).[6,9] The background rate of childhood malignancy is 1 in 1300 before the age of 15. This study gave a relative risk of 1.4 for those offspring exposed *in utero* to pelvimetry. A pelvic CT scan typically exposes a fetus to approximately 2.5 cGy and this is thought to double the risk of a childhood malignancy. Clearly, setting a 5-cGy 'safe limit' may be considered simplistic, and the debate continues. Table 23.1 lists the mean fetal dose exposures predicted for various investigations. It is important to realise, however, that the actual dose is dependent on many factors and that the true value may be five-fold higher.

In practice, if cross-sectional imaging of the pelvis or abdomen is required during pregnancy, MRI is preferred over the use of CT scanning [E]. It is likely that single exposures carry greater fetal risk than divided doses, adding further to the difficulties in applying the available human data to real diagnostic and therapeutic scenarios [D].

Radiotherapy to the pelvis is contraindicated in pregnancy due to the effects on the fetus, which cannot be shielded. There are, however, situations in which radiotherapy remains a viable treatment modality in some cancers. Fortunately, shielding of the pelvis enables sufficient reduction in exposure to the fetus after the first trimester to allow the use of radiotherapy in the treatment of a number of cancers, e.g. breast cancer and lymphomas.

Table 23.1 Fetal radiation exposures during various radiological investigations[3]

Chest/skull X-ray	<0.001 cGy
Mammogram	0.0004 cGy
Ventilation–perfusion scan with ^{99m}Tc	<0.2 cGy
Abdominal X-ray	0.26 cGy
IVU/lumbar spine	0.32 cGy
Bone imaging with ^{99m}Tc	<0.5 cGy
Abdominal CT	0.8 cGy
Barium enema	1.6 cGy
Pelvic CT	2.5 cGy

KEY POINTS

- The dose required to induce embryonal lethality increases sharply during the first trimester from 0.1 cGy at day 1 to >1 Gy after the first trimester. The fetal effects of radiation include intrauterine death, congenital malformations, developmental or growth retardation and late malignancy.
- Within the first 2 weeks post-implantation, exposure to radiation is thought to be an all-or-nothing effect (resulting in fetal death if affected). Conversely, anomalies result from exposure (to doses >0.1 Gy) in the later weeks of the first trimester.
- Radiotherapy to the pelvis is contraindicated in pregnancy due to the effects on the fetus, which cannot be shielded. There are, however, situations in which radiotherapy remains a viable treatment modality in some cancers.

Chemotherapy and pregnancy

Prior to implantation, the blastocyst is immune to the effects of chemotherapy. The period of organogenesis between 5 and 10 weeks is, however, a critically sensitive time. Exposure to chemotherapy during this period may be associated with malformations in 10–20 per cent of cases [D].[10] After 12 weeks' gestation, malformations should be less common, although growth and neurological development remain potentially vulnerable throughout pregnancy.

A number of retrospective studies support these generalisations regarding the importance of the timing of chemotherapy during pregnancy. Congenital malformations seem no more likely if chemotherapy is given only during the second and third trimesters [D].[11] First-trimester exposure does indeed seem more hazardous, and this is somewhat dependent on the agents used [D].[10]

Antimetabolites carry the greatest risks to a first-trimester pregnancy. Although miscarriage is the most common outcome, aminopterin may cause neural tube, skeletal and clefting abnormalities. This anti-neoplastic agent has been replaced by methotrexate, which is structurally similar and has the same effects on the early fetus. Both should be avoided in the first trimester and later in the pregnancy where possible. A 14 per cent congenital anomaly risk has been quoted for **alkylating agents** (e.g. cyclophosphamide) if given in the first trimester. This risk falls to near background levels for administration in the second and third trimesters. The **antibiotics** such as doxorubicin and bleomycin do not have clear teratogenic effects, although they are still to be avoided in the first trimester where possible. **Vinca alkaloids**, such as vincristine and vinblastine, are harmful in animal pregnancies but this effect is not obvious in the few human pregnancies so far exposed in the first trimester [D]. Information is constantly updated with regard to the use of these drugs during pregnancy and it is wise to consult a drug information bureau before deciding management.

ANTENATAL OBSTETRICS

Other effects of fetal exposure to chemotherapy in the second and third trimesters are even less clear. Studies are conflicting with regard to prenatal and postnatal growth restriction, although one review concluded that intrauterine growth restriction occurred in 40 per cent of exposed pregnancies [D].[10]

The longer-term effects of fetal exposure to chemotherapy are also unclear. Survivors of cancer who received chemotherapy as children have been followed up closely with the assumption that late complications of treatment in this group might also be expected to occur in individuals exposed *in utero*. Investigators have looked for evidence of impaired intellect, reduced gonadal function (delayed puberty and reduced fertility), visceral damage and mutagenesis within germ cells. However, to directly apply these findings from individuals treated during childhood to those exposed to chemotherapy *in utero* makes the assumption that fetal cells behave in the same way as those of a child. This may not be the case, and fetal germ cells, for example, might be more susceptible to genetic damage than those of an older child.

However, there is currently no robust evidence to suggest that future fertility may be affected or to suggest any intellectual impairment or increase in the genetic problems in the next generation.

A more consistent effect of chemotherapy on the fetus is myelosuppression. A third of newborns delivered to women who received treatment for leukaemia during their pregnancy showed evidence of bone marrow suppression in one study [D].[12] Fortunately, this is rarely of clinical importance, and sepsis, serious anaemia and haemorrhage are uncommon in the neonate. However, it is good practice to avoid myelosuppressive agents in the 3 weeks prior to delivery, if possible [E].

Decisions regarding the timing of operative delivery should aim to avoid the increased susceptibility to maternal infection if performed within 2 weeks of a cycle of chemotherapy. Similarly, those prescribing chemotherapy need to be aware of the potentially dramatic dose changes required both during pregnancy and following delivery due to the attendant physiological changes.

Despite the lack of evidence for major harm from chemotherapy in the second and third trimesters, breastfeeding is usually discouraged if treatment continues into the puerperium [E]. This reflects unresolved uncertainties about the true safety of these agents and the knowledge that significant quantities do reach breast milk.

KEY POINTS

- Most cytotoxic chemotherapy molecules are small enough to cross the placenta and affect the fetus.
- The estimated risk of major teratogenicity in the first trimester is approximately 10–20 per cent. Use of combination agents increases the risk.
- Exposure during the second and third trimesters may give rise to growth restriction, prematurity and stillbirth, but are unlikely to be teratogenic.
- Delayed effects of exposure to chemotherapeutic agents appears to be rare. The currently available evidence suggests that there are no significant adverse effects on fertility or intellectual and neurological development in those exposed.
- Furthermore, no published data exists to suggest any increase in the rate of childhood malignancies in those subjected to chemotherapy *in utero*.
- Chemotherapy, where other treatment modalities are considered unsuitable, is therefore considered relatively safe in the second and third trimesters. Patients should be counselled regarding the increased risks of growth retardation (and consequent premature delivery) and stillbirth.
- There is no evidence to support using a reduced dose of chemotherapy in pregnancy [E].

SYMPTOM CONTROL IN THE PREGNANT PATIENT WITH CANCER

The symptoms of cancer and of normal pregnancy overlap and can easily be confused. Early satiety, nausea and vomiting, constipation, dyspnoea, fatigue and depression are all common during a normal pregnancy but can also be significant symptoms of malignancy. Every effort should be made to determine symptom aetiology when a known cancer coexists with pregnancy. Shortness of breath, for example, may simply be the effect of high progesterone levels and expanded tidal volume typical of the third trimester. However, in the cancer patient it may be a sign of pleural effusions, significant anaemia or lung metastases. Similarly, nausea and vomiting may have a more sinister cause, such as hypercalcaemia, electrolyte imbalance, uraemia and even intracranial metastases. Early advice from an oncologist should be sought when new symptoms arise.

Pain should be managed with paracetamol and opiates. NSAIDs are best avoided, especially in the third trimester. Tricyclic antidepressants can be safely used for neuropathic pain, but carbamazepine should not (see Chapter 27) [B].

Poor appetite may be secondary to depression, pain, and nausea and vomiting. Treatments for nausea include metoclopramide, prochlorperazine and cyclizine. Ondansetron and haloperidol can be used if necessary. Prednisone is effective for a number of symptoms, including nausea, anorexia and fatigue. Cannabis seems to be beneficial in a number of ways but is not advised during pregnancy [C]. Constipation is effectively treated with docusate, magnesium hydroxide and senna, all of which are safe in pregnancy.

The psychological adjustment to a diagnosis of cancer is always difficult, seldom more so than during pregnancy. Fears of limited life expectancy deprive couples of future hopes and plans for themselves and their family. Focusing on short-term goals and enjoying the present are so much harder to do during pregnancy. More specifically, there may be anxieties regarding the effect of the disease or its treatment on the fetus. The question of termination of a wanted pregnancy will be extremely distressing. There may be conflict over what is best for the woman herself and what will do least harm to the pregnancy. Concern for other children and anxieties about future fertility add further to the crisis. There is remarkably little research or evidence to guide practice, but the involvement of a mental health team or counselling service should be offered at the very least.

SPECIFIC EXAMPLES

Breast cancer

Breast cancer occurs in approximately 1 in 3000 pregnancies and approximately 10 per cent of women with breast cancer who are younger than 40 years will be pregnant at diagnosis. There is evidence to suggest there may be a transient increase in breast cancer during the first 3–4 years following pregnancy. In a population-based prospective study of 802,457 Norwegian women aged 20–56 years, a short-term increase in breast cancer after full-term pregnancy was observed, with a peak 3–4 years after the delivery.[13] Early menarche and late age at first pregnancy are also associated with an increased risk of breast cancer.

Pregnancy also increases the risk of breast cancer developing in carriers of *BRCA1* and *BRCA2* mutations. Carriers of these mutations who have children are significantly more likely to develop breast cancer by the age of 40 years than carriers who are nulliparous, with each pregnancy being associated with an increased risk of cancer. Having a baby at a young age does not appear to protect *BRCA1/BRCA2* carriers against subsequent development of breast cancer.

Stage for stage, the outcome is no different from that for breast cancers diagnosed outside pregnancy [B].[14] Continuing the pregnancy certainly does not seem to have a deleterious effect on outcome, and termination of pregnancy is not indicated for this reason [D]. However, at diagnosis, pregnancy-associated breast cancer tends to be larger in size, more advanced and more likely to have metastasised to local lymph nodes. This, in part, may be due to the 6-month average delay in its diagnosis. This is thought to increase the risk of nodal metastases by at least 10 per cent.

Breast masses are common in pregnancy. Lactational adenomas, galactoceles, mastitis and infarction of hypertrophied breast tissue are all benign pregnancy-induced breast lumps that may masquerade as malignancy. Breast enlargement, greater vascularity and increased tissue density add to the diagnostic difficulty. Mammography is safe with appropriate shielding but has a lower sensitivity in pregnancy. Fine-needle aspiration or excisional biopsy should be performed if there is any suspicion of malignancy. Once carcinoma has been diagnosed, a chest

X-ray may be needed for staging, and once again this is safe with shielding [E]. CT scanning for metastases should be replaced by ultrasound and MRI. If necessary, technetium bone scans can be employed, exposing the pregnancy to 0.5 cGy.

A common surgical option for breast cancer is lumpectomy followed by postoperative chest-wall radiotherapy to reduce local recurrence risks. Radiotherapy for breast cancer might typically be 50 Gy. With appropriate shielding, fetal exposure may be as little as 4 cGy at very early gestations (5 weeks), rising to 14–18 cGy in the second trimester when the uterus is larger. This is above the 'accepted' threshold of safety, and a modified radical mastectomy, which does not necessitate postoperative radiotherapy, should normally be advised during pregnancy instead [E]. The surgery itself carries minimal risk, if any, to the fetus. Conservative breast surgery can sometimes be performed in the third trimester, with adjunctive radiotherapy delayed until the puerperium.

Chemotherapy for breast cancer in the second and third trimesters is not associated with obvious fetal harm.[15] Where possible, the last dose should be given 3 weeks prior to delivery to limit the effects of fetal bone marrow suppression [E]. Tamoxifen use in pregnancy has previously been discouraged. Experiments in rodents have demonstrated anomalies similar to those found with *in utero* diethylstilbestrol (DES) exposure and an increased intrauterine fetal death rate. Although these effects appear to be species specific, there are only minimal human data testifying to the safety of tamoxifen in pregnancy and its use is not currently recommended. Trastuzumab, a monoclonal antibody targeted against the HER2/neu receptor, is contraindicated during pregnancy because of reported adverse fetal outcome. There are no data on other targeted therapies such as vascular endothelial growth factor antagonists, including bevacizumab.

Fetal surveillance by regular growth scanning is warranted, although a clear link with prenatal growth restriction has not been established. Placental metastases are found very rarely and there are no reports of breast cancer spreading to the fetus. Some authors suggest delivery at 34 weeks to limit the fetal exposure to chemotherapeutic agents. Others await spontaneous labour if fetal growth is normal. Neonatal blood sampling is necessary to exclude clinically relevant pancytopenia.

Pregnancy after breast cancer

With the high background incidence of breast cancer and progressive delay in child-bearing, it is not uncommon now to be asked for advice on this matter. Most studies have failed to show any effect on survival if pregnancy occurs after breast cancer [B].[16–19] Although it can be argued that women with a more favourable prognosis are more likely to consider a pregnancy, the survival among node-positive patients was not affected by pregnancy either. It has been suggested that becoming pregnant soon after breast cancer may affect long-term survival and that a delay should be advised. Studies that demonstrate a survival advantage with such a delay may simply be highlighting the improved prognosis for women who remain alive 2–5 years after the diagnosis. For younger women (who have a worse prognosis anyway), a delay of 2–5 years will have minimal impact on fertility. Allowing more time will help to give a more individualised prognosis. Such a delay may be more difficult to justify in women in their late 30s and 40s.

The use of tamoxifen during pregnancy is not recommended (see above). Breastfeeding is not contraindicated, but previous surgery and radiotherapy may impair subsequent lactation.

The following points are the recommendations given in the RCOG guideline:

- There is no indication that termination of pregnancy after diagnosis of breast cancer is necessary to improve the prognosis.
- Women planning pregnancy or who become pregnant after breast cancer should consult their clinical oncologist, surgeon and obstetrician.
- There is no evidence that the survival of women who have had breast cancer and subsequently become pregnant is compromised. However, an interval of at least 2 and preferably 3 years between treatment and conception is recommended.

Cervical cancer

The incidence of cervical disease in pregnancy is uncertain because reported series are retrospective. Some series include both pre-invasive and invasive lesions, whereas others include cases of cancer diagnosed during the pregnancy or during the postpartum period. The incidence of abnormal cervical cytological findings is estimated at 1–5 per cent of all pregnancies and the reported rate of cervical cancers ranges between 1 and 12 per 10,000 pregnancies. It commonly presents with vaginal bleeding but discharge and pain may also occur. A high proportion of cases are detected by cervical screening and are otherwise asymptomatic.

Cervical screening in pregnancy

False-positive cervical smears are more likely during pregnancy for a number of reasons:

- eversion of the squamocolumnar junction occurs as a consequence of high oestrogen levels and exposed columnar epithelium undergoes squamous metaplasia;
- cervical infiltration by leukocytes occurs in pregnancy;
- decidualisation of the cervix is a frequent finding;
- trophoblasts may be present in the cervical canal;
- relative immunosuppression may allow greater human papillomavirus (HPV) activity.

It is vital that the cytologist reading the smear is aware that it has been taken from a pregnant woman if false positives are to be kept to a minimum. In the UK it is not usual for routine cervical screening to be carried out in pregnancy, and smears are normally deferred until the postnatal appointment. However, if there is clinical concern regarding the cervix, or if it seems unlikely that the individual will return after the pregnancy for a smear to be carried out, there should be no hesitation in performing it while the woman is pregnant.

Most studies show a high degree of concordance between cytology (smears) and colposcopy [B][20] during pregnancy but the possibility of false-positive or false-negative results must always be considered.

Management of an abnormal smear in pregnancy

A reluctance to perform cervical smears during pregnancy may also arise from unfounded anxieties over the subsequent management of the abnormal smear. One study of colposcopy during pregnancy found concordance, overestimation and underestimation of the final diagnosis (based on cone histology) in 73 per cent, 17 per cent and 10 per cent, respectively, and this did not differ significantly from the non-pregnant control group.[21] Indeed, unsatisfactory colposcopy is less common during pregnancy due to eversion of the squamocolumnar junction. Squamous metaplasia is more common and the cervix will usually look larger and have increased vascularity. Colposcopy during pregnancy therefore requires experience and careful judgement. Hacker and colleagues demonstrated a 99.5 per cent diagnostic accuracy for colposcopy, with only a 0.5 per cent false-negative rate (with no missed invasive lesions) among 1064 pregnant women.[22]

If a smear taken in pregnancy has suggested low-grade cervical intraepithelial neoplasia (CIN) and the colposcopic impression agrees, these women can be managed by repeat colposcopy in each trimester, with a further evaluation in the postpartum period. There is no evidence that CIN progresses more rapidly in pregnancy, and indeed regression rates of 25–70 per cent have been documented for high-grade CIN first detected in pregnancy.[23]

If the colposcopic impression is of a higher-grade lesion, it is vital that micro-invasive and invasive cancers are excluded. Older studies recorded an unacceptably high rate of complications with knife conisation during pregnancy, principally a >500 mL blood loss in 7–13 per cent of cases (mostly in the third trimester).[22] Any causative association with miscarriage, preterm rupture of membranes, preterm delivery and chorioamnionitis remains uncertain, but concerns do exist. These concerns have seen a shift away from conisation in pregnancy towards the use of directed punch biopsies, which carry less morbidity. Concordance between directed biopsies and the final diagnosis is complete or within one degree of severity in over 95 per cent of cases [B].[19] Missed invasive lesions are extremely uncommon. Treatment of CIN II and III should be delayed to the postpartum period, but colposcopy every 8 weeks antenatally is advised to monitor for progression of the lesion [E].

If micro-invasive or invasive disease is suspected, conisation or a large-loop excision procedure should be done early in the pregnancy; the choice between these procedures depends on the size of the cervix, the clinical team's preference and the degree of suspicion.

Postpartum evaluation is extremely important for women who have antenatal colposcopy, even those who have undergone cone biopsy. Lesions may regress, persist or progress, and the diagnosis made during pregnancy may need to be upgraded. High rates of residual intraepithelial neoplasia and cytological abnormalities have been found following conisation, which should not necessarily be considered adequate treatment for CIN during pregnancy.[24]

Management of cervical cancer in pregnancy

Cervical cancer is normally staged clinically by chest X-ray, cystoscopy, urogram and fluorine-18-labelled fluorodeoxyglucose (^{18}FDG) CT scanning or MRI. Positron emission tomography (PET)-CT is not recommended in pregnancy because fetal absorption of the isotope exceeds recommendations. MRI is the investigation of choice for pelvic imaging during pregnancy.

Cervical cancer is usually treated surgically in its early stages. Chemoradiotherapy is reserved for more advanced disease due to the effects this treatment has on ovarian, bladder, bowel and sexual function. Knife conisation may be sufficient treatment for Ia1 (micro-invasive) cervical cancer outside pregnancy due to the low risk of recurrence or lymph node (LN) metastases. If this diagnosis is made during pregnancy and the cone biopsy margins are clear, the pregnancy should be allowed to continue, with vaginal delivery. However, the significant rate of positive margins and residual disease found with conisation in pregnancy makes further evaluation in the postpartum period imperative.[25] For women who have completed their families, a postpartum simple hysterectomy with ovarian conservation is recommended [E].

Higher-grade lesions (Ib1–IIa) are usually treated by simple or radical hysterectomy with LN sampling. Cancers presenting at less than 20 weeks' gestation have traditionally been treated immediately [E]. The hysterectomy can usually be performed with the fetus *in situ*; however, a hysterotomy, avoiding the lower part of the uterus, can be employed to remove the pregnancy and improve access if necessary. Delaying treatment until after delivery becomes an increasingly favourable option after 20 weeks' gestation for stage I cancers.[26] Nine studies involving 63 patients with stage I cervical cancer have examined the effect of a delay, varying between 1 and 32 weeks. Only one outcome was possibly affected by the delay. However, these studies are clearly non-randomised and the decision to delay should be made with oncologists and neonatologists after careful patient counselling. Steroids should be given to promote fetal lung maturation. Delivery at 32–34 weeks can now be justified with advances in the care of the preterm infant. Caesarean section is normally advised, due to theoretical concerns of haemorrhage from cervical lesions and increased malignant cell dissemination with vaginal delivery [E]. Local recurrence within episiotomy sites is well documented and is associated with a high mortality

rate. Radical hysterectomy at the time of caesarean section is associated with greater blood loss, but the rate of other complications is not increased [D].

Consideration should also be given to the use of neoadjuvant chemotherapy in the second and third trimesters. This may limit progression of disease and more confidently allow delay in surgical treatment, although its safety also remains in question.

Radiotherapy is employed with more advanced lesions (stage IIb and above) and usually takes the form of external beam *teletherapy* and intracavitary *brachytherapy*. The external beam alone employs 40–50 Gy. Most pregnancies will spontaneously abort after such high doses, usually within 5 weeks [D]. Occasionally, the fetus must be removed surgically. Preterm delivery of the fetus may be necessary at later gestations.

Where a lesion is very advanced, and the maternal prognosis poor, the woman may prefer to compromise her own treatment if this means limiting the risks to the fetus. Careful, sensitive counselling is clearly very important in this situation.

Ovarian cancer

The incidence of ovarian tumours in pregnancy is quoted as 1 in 1000 deliveries, although ovarian cancer is much less common (1 in 5000–18,000). Adnexal masses are found in approximately 1 in 100 pregnancies; 50 per cent measure <5 cm, 25 per cent are 5–10 cm and the remaining quarter are >10 cm in size. Box 23.1 lists various causes of adnexal mass found in pregnancy, in decreasing order of incidence.

There are various non-neoplastic ovarian lesions that are unique to pregnancy and that will resolve spontaneously after delivery. These include:

- luteoma of pregnancy;
- follicular cyst of pregnancy;
- hyperreactio luteinalis;
- granulosa cell proliferations;
- hilus cell hyperplasia;
- ectopia decidua.

With the extensive use of ultrasound for dating and assessing pregnancies, the recognition of adnexal masses in pregnancy has increased. Although most remain asymptomatic, 10–15 per cent will rupture, bleed or cause adnexal torsion [D], and

Box 23.1 The most common causes of adnexal mass in pregnancy

Functional cyst
Mature teratoma (dermoid)
Cystadenoma (serous and mucinous)
Para-ovarian cyst
Endometrioma
Leiomyoma
Malignancy (3–6 per cent of all cases)

these acute events are thought to increase the risk of miscarriage and preterm labour [D]. Occasionally, an ovarian mass may cause dystocia during labour or virilisation. As 1 in 20–50 ovarian lesions in pregnancy will be malignant[27] and as many as 1 in 6 may become symptomatic, a careful management decision has to be made when they are first recognised. Symptomatic adnexal lesions may need to be operated on immediately. Small (<6 cm) unilocular cysts are likely to resolve spontaneously before 16 weeks without causing harm and should be left alone [D].[28] A further ultrasound should be performed at 16 weeks' gestation. A persistent complex mass should prompt a laparotomy. Miscarriage is said to be less likely if intervention occurs at this point in the second trimester. Persistent simple cysts that are not associated with ascites and have no solid areas or thick septa within them can be treated conservatively. Dermoid cysts are often confidently diagnosed by ultrasound. These, too, can be left although the risk of a cyst accident must always be considered, as this may increase the risk of miscarriage. MRI may help with diagnosis in selected cases.

Tumour markers such as CA-125, AFP and hCG are helpful for diagnosis and treatment monitoring outside pregnancy. These substances may all be elevated during a normal pregnancy and do not usually feature in the diagnosis or management of the adnexal mass antenatally. Of note, however, an extremely high maternal serum AFP value, performed for fetal anomaly screening, has led to the diagnosis of endodermal sinus tumours on a number of occasions.

Surgery for an adnexal mass in pregnancy usually involves a lower midline incision, which allows adequate access with minimal uterine manipulation. Peritoneal washings should be taken and omental and peritoneal biopsies. Where appropriate, a simple cystectomy with ovarian conservation is attempted. Otherwise, a unilateral salpingo-oophorectomy should be performed. Frozen sections of the contralateral ovary can be taken to help intraoperative management, but bilateral oophorectomy should normally be avoided at the initial operation, as even malignant cases are usually early stage, chemosensitive or of low malignant potential. Para-aortic lymph node sampling and debulking should be considered in more complex cases, although it would be unusual for the uterus to need to be removed.

If an ovarian cyst is removed in the first trimester, it may have arisen from the corpus luteum and may have been providing hormonal support to the early pregnancy. It is accepted practice in this situation to provide progesterone supplementation until the second trimester is reached [D].

Management of ovarian cancer in pregnancy

The histopathological nature of ovarian cancer in pregnancy reflects the younger age of the affected population. Germ cell and epithelial cell cancers each account for 30–40 per cent of cases, but two-thirds of the epithelial group are of 'low malignant potential'. The remainder are mostly sex cord stromal tumours. Dysgerminomas are the most common malignant ovarian tumours found in pregnancy.

Stage I epithelial cancers, tumours of low malignant potential and stage Ia dysgerminomas do not require adjunctive treatment with chemotherapy. Other forms of germ cell tumour and more advanced epithelial cancers would normally be treated with chemotherapy postoperatively. Beyond the first trimester, the use of bleomycin, etoposide, cisplatin and vincristine/vinblastine has not been clearly linked with fetal harm, with a number of successful outcomes having been reported in the literature.[29] However, until more data have been collected, concerns will remain over the use of anti-neoplastic drugs during pregnancy, especially during the first trimester (see above).

Other malignancies

The principles of managing cancer in pregnancy can be illustrated by further examples:

- Older, uncontrolled studies suggested a poorer outcome stage for stage when melanoma presented during pregnancy. More recent, case–control studies show no difference in 3-year and 5-year survival rates [B].[30] Although melanoma is the malignancy most likely to metastasise to the placenta and fetus, this nevertheless rarely occurs. However, the placenta should be examined at delivery and sent for histopathology. The fetus will have metastases in 30 per cent of cases where placental involvement is found. Biopsy of the sentinel or draining node may be useful in predicting spread of malignant melanoma. A blue dye can be used to locate this lymph node, as an alternative to technetium-labelled sulphur colloid, avoiding fetal radiation exposure [D].
- Radiotherapy for head, neck and brain tumours usually carries a fetal dose exposure of <10 cGy due to the distance between the field and the uterus. Abdominal shielding can reduce this to <2 cGy.
- The treatment for Hodgkin's lymphoma and chronic myeloid leukaemia can often be delayed until after the pregnancy. Acute leukaemias and non-Hodgkin's lymphoma must be treated immediately, as the risks to the woman and her pregnancy from haemorrhage, anaemia and sepsis outweigh the possible fetal harm from chemotherapy, even in the first trimester [D].

KEY POINTS

- Pregnancy does not alter the course of cancer but may cause a delay in diagnosis.
- Sensitive methods of investigation can be safely employed during pregnancy.
- Safe treatments are available during pregnancy for dealing with all symptoms caused by cancer.
- Chemotherapy in the first trimester is associated with a significantly increased risk of fetal abnormalities. Treatment

during the second and third trimesters of pregnancy would seem to be safer, but the data are limited.

- Radiation exposure must be restricted to the very low levels found with investigative X-rays. Radiotherapy for pelvic, abdominal or chest malignancies usually carries excessive fetal risk, even with shielding.
- Management requires a multidisciplinary approach.

Key references

1. YY Lee, CL Roberts, T Dobbins *et al.* Incidence and outcomes of pregnancy-associated cancer in Australia, 1994–2008: a population-based linkage study. *BJOG* 2012;119:1572–82.

2. Iseminger KA, Lewis MA. Ethical challenges in treating mother and fetus when cancer complicates pregnancy. *Obstet Gynecol Clin North Am* 1998;25:273–85.

3. Schover LR. Psychosocial issues associated with cancer in pregnancy. *Semin Oncol* 2000; 27:699–703.

4. Fattibene P, Mazzei F, Nuccetelli C, Risica S. Prenatal exposure to ionising radiation: sources, effects and regulatory aspects. *Acta Paediatr* 1999;88:693–702.

5. Tribukait B, Cekan E. Dose–effect relationship and the significance of fractionated and protracted radiation for the frequency of fetal malformations following X-irradiation of pregnant C3H mice. In: *Developmental Effects of Pre-natal Irradiation*. Stuttgart: Gustave Fischer, 1982:29–35.

6. Muirhead CR, Kneale GW. Pre-natal irradiation and childhood cancer. *J Radiol Prot* 1989;9:209–12.

7. Otake M, Schull W. Radiation-related small head sizes among prenatally exposed A-bomb survivors. *Int J Radiat Oncol Biol Phys* 1992;63:255–70.

8. Mole RH. Irradiation of the embryo and fetus. *Br J Radiol* 1987;60:17–31.

9. Gilman EA, Kneale GW, Knox EG, Stewart AM. Pregnancy X-rays and childhood cancers: effects of exposure age and radiation dose. *J Radiol Prot* 1988;8:3–8.

10. Partridge AH, Garber JE. Long-term outcomes of children exposed to anti-neoplastic agents *in utero*. *Semin Oncol* 2000;27:712–26.

11. Doll DC, Ringenberg S, Yarbo JW. Anti-neoplastic agents and pregnancy. *Semin Oncol* 1989;16:337.

12. Reynosa E, Shepherd F, Messner H *et al.* Acute leukaemia in pregnancy: The Toronto Leukaemia Study Group experience with long-term follow-up of children exposed *in utero* to chemotherapeutic agents. *J Clin Oncol* 1987;5:1098–106.

13. Albreksten G, Heuch I, Kvale G. The short- and long-term effect of a pregnancy on breast cancer risk: a prospective study of 802,457 parous Norwegian women. *Br J Cancer* 1995;72:480–4.

14. Lethaby AE, O'Neill MA, Mason B *et al.* Overall survival from breast cancer in women pregnant or lactating at or after diagnosis. *Int J Cancer* 1996;67:751–5.

15. Berry DL, Theriault RL, Holmes FA *et al.* Management of breast cancer during pregnancy using a standardised protocol. *J Clin Oncol* 1999;17:855–61.

16. Harvey JC, Rosen PP, Ashikari R *et al.* The effect of pregnancy on the prognosis of carcinoma of the breast following radical mastectomy. *Surg Gynecol Obstet* 1981;153:723–5.

17. Mignot L, Morvan F, Berdah J *et al.* Pregnancy after breast cancer. Results of a case-control study. *Presse Med* 1986;15:1961–4.

18. Ariel I, Kempner R. The prognosis of patients who become pregnant after mastectomy for breast cancer. *Int Surg* 1989;74:185.

19. von Schoultz E, Johansson H, Wilking N, Rutquist LE. Influence of prior and subsequent pregnancy on breast cancer prognosis. *J Clin Oncol* 1995;13:430–4.

20. Guerra B, De Simone P, Gabrielli S, Falco P, Montanari G, Bovicelli L. Combined cytology and colposcopy to screen for cervical cancer in pregnancy. *J Reprod Med* 1998; 43:647–53.

21. Baldauf JJ, Dreyfus M, Ritter J, Philippe E. Colposcopy and directed biopsy reliability during pregnancy: a cohort study. *Eur J Obst Gynecol Reprod Biol* 1995;62:31–6.

22. Hacker NF, Berek JS, Lagasse LD *et al.* Carcinoma of the cervix associated with pregnancy. *Obstet Gynecol* 1982; 59:735–46.

23. Yost NP, Santoso JT, McIntire DD, Iliya FA. Postpartum regression rates of antepartum cervical intraepithelial neoplasia II and III. *Obstet Gynecol* 1999;93:359–62.

24. Hannigan EV, Whitehouse HH, Atkinson WD, Becker SN. Cone biopsy during pregnancy. *Obstet Gynecol* 1982;60:450–5.

25. Connor JP. Noninvasive cervical cancer complicating pregnancy. *Obstet Gynecol Clin North Am* 1998;25: 331–42.

26. Duggan B, Muderspach LI, Roman LD, Curtin JP, d'Ablaing G, Morrow P. Cervical cancer in pregnancy: reporting on planned delay in therapy. *Obstet Gynecol* 1993;82:598–602.

27. Creasman WT, Rutledge F, Smith JP. Carcinoma of the ovary associated with pregnancy. *Obstet Gynecol* 1971;38:111.

28. Thornton JG, Wells M. Ovarian cysts in pregnancy: does ultrasound make traditional management inappropriate? *Obstet Gynecol* 1987;69:717.

29. Boulay R, Podczaski E. Ovarian cancer complicating pregnancy. *Obstet Gynecol Clin North Am* 1998;25: 385–99.

30. MacKie RM, Bufalino R, Morabito A. Lack of effect of pregnancy on outcome of melanoma. *Lancet* 1991;337:653–5.

Chapter 24 Maternal infections in pregnancy

Tara Jayne Selman

MRCOG standards

- Conduct a booking visit including assessment of pre-existing infection and risk of infections.
- Formulate a management plan for treating and screening for infection.

Theoretical skills

- Have general knowledge of the immune system.
- Understand changes in the immune system and changes in pregnancy.
- Understand epidemiology, aetiology, signs/symptoms, investigation of infections in pregnancy.

Practical skills

- Recognise clinical presentation of the disease, performing necessary clinical investigations and treatment as part of a multidisciplinary team.
- Conduct pre-pregnancy counselling for women with pre-existing infection.

INTRODUCTION

The body has a natural resistance to infections with an ability to acquire resistance through natural exposure and vaccination. There are immune defences on the body's surface in the form of the epithelial skin barrier and IgA on mucosal membranes. The lymphatic system may trap organisms presenting them as targets for phagocytosis by macrophages. Those organisms that do enter the circulation can be destroyed by neutrophil or phagocytic cells. Acquired immune resistance is also present with the stimulation of antibody production (initially IgM) by plasma cells. Cell-mediated immunity also continues via the T lymphocytes. All of these systems remain in pregnancy; however, there are significant changes to tolerate the semi-allogenic fetus, resulting in a state of relative immunocompromise. These changes lead to an increase in the infectivity of certain infections such as cytomegalovirus (CMV) and herpes simplex virus (HSV). The changes in

maternal immune responses are also reflected by changes in autoimmune diseases: rheumatoid arthritis often ameliorates during pregnancy, although it can flare up.

This chapter covers infections that have significant impact on pregnant women's health or require significantly different treatment in pregnancy. Chapter 36 details those infections that have greater implications to the fetus.

VIRAL INFECTIONS

Rubella, parvovirus and CMV are all covered in Chapter 36, and the H1N1 virus in Chapter 65.

Herpes simplex virus

The virus is divided into two subgroups: type 1 associated with orofacial infections and encephalitis, and type 2 associated with genital infections, although there is a varying degree of overlap.[1]

Epidemiology and aetiology

HSV is transmitted through close physical contact with mucosal surfaces or abraded skin and during sexual intercourse. HSV type 1 is commonly contracted in childhood, resulting in up to 90 per cent of the adult population having positive serology. HSV type 2 is generally contracted from adolescence with the onset of sexual activity.

HSV remains latent in sensory neurons; the trigeminal nerve in type 1 and the sacral ganglia in type 2. Reactivation then occurs as a result of triggers such as trauma, fever, stress, menstruation and ultraviolet light. The antibodies to the subtypes are thought to offer some cross-protection.

Presentation and diagnosis

Primary facial herpes is classically asymptomatic, but when appearing the lesions can be seen in the oral mucosa, lips and eyes. In contrast primary genital herpes is usually severe with lesions that start with erythema, progressing to vesicles and then ulcers and finishing with crusting involving the vulva and cervix, and lasting 2 weeks. The ulcerations can result in associated lymphadenopathy, fever, malaise and retention of urine. Recurrent episodes tend to be less severe. Data from the USA suggests that 2 per cent of women acquire genital HSV in pregnancy, with the majority of cases being asymptomatic or not diagnosed correctly.[2]

Diagnosis is made initially by history and examination. In cases of suspected primary genital herpes a pregnant woman should be referred to a genitourinary physician for confirmation by viral polymerase chain reaction [C].[3]

Management

This chapter will concentrate on the management of genital herpes, which has major implications during pregnancy. Management is dependent both on gestation and on whether the episode is a primary or secondary occurrence.

All episodes of primary genital herpes should be managed jointly with genitourinary physicians. When primary genital herpes occurs in the first or second trimester management/treatment with aciclovir should commence without delay. This reduces the duration and severity of the symptoms and the duration of viral shedding. In the absence of disseminated disease oral treatment with 400 mg aciclovir three times a day for 5 days is appropriate. Women should be counselled that although not licensed in pregnancy aciclovir has been shown to be safe and well tolerated even when used in the first trimester.[4] Symptomatic relief may also be achieved with paracetamol and topical lidocaine gel. Provided that the woman does not go on and deliver in the next 6 weeks, then vaginal delivery is advocated and the woman can be reassured that there is no association with congenital abnormalities.[5] Evidence has shown that daily suppression with 400 mg aciclovir three times a day from 36 weeks should be recommended as it reduces the occurrences of HSV lesions and asymptomatic viral shedding [A].[3]

If primary genital herpes is suspected in the third trimester (from 28 weeks) then there are implications for mode of delivery. Elective caesarean section is recommended, especially if the lesions appear in the last 6 weeks of pregnancy, as the risk of neonatal transmission is then as high as 41 per cent [B].[6] If a woman is 'labouring' and decides to continue for a normal vaginal delivery there may be some benefit in treating her with IV aciclovir and avoiding invasive procedures (e.g. fetal blood sampling). As literature reports that up to 15 per cent of cases will actually be recurrent episodes, when presenting at this gestation consideration should be given to type -specific HSV antibody testing[C}. The maternal management of an episode in the third trimester is the same as in early gestation, although aciclovir therapy will usually occur until delivery. Parents should be told that the data suggesting poor outcomes in such pregnancies are conflicting,[8] with insufficient evidence to support the need for additional monitoring in pregnancy [B].

Women presenting at any stage of gestation with recurrent episodes are at low risk of neonatal infection. With lesions present at the time of delivery the risk of neonatal herpes is 0–3 per cent[3] and hence it is reasonable to advocate normal vaginal delivery, even if the woman has active lesions at the time of delivery. Although invasive procedures may increase the risk of neonatal transmission, as the background risk is low it is reasonable to perform these [C]. In those with recurrent episodes daily suppression with 400 mg aciclovir three times a day should be considered in the last 6 weeks of pregnancy [C].

In both primary and secondary outbreaks it is reasonable to expedite delivery when there are active lesions and pre-labour rupture of membranes at term. In primary herpes, when there is rupture of membranes in a preterm, pre-labour scenario, the decision for delivery or conservative management needs to be made by a multidisciplinary team. If a conservative approach is followed then the use of IV aciclovir should be considered. In the case of secondary herpes because the risk of transmission is low then the risks of prematurity prior to 34 weeks probably outweigh the advantages of delivery [C].

Those women with HIV co-infection should be treated in line with non-HIV-positive patients if the primary genital herpes occurs in the last trimester; however, there is some evidence to support a more aggressive approach for recurrent infection as there is evidence that the transmission risk to the neonate is higher. Therefore it is suggested that suppression therapy be commenced from 32 weeks. There is no evidence for the use of therapy in HSV-seropositive women without a history of genital herpes [C].[9]

KEY POINTS

- The management of women with genital herpes should be in conjunction with genitourinary medicine physicians.
- Aciclovir is considered safe to use in pregnancy, including the first trimester.
- If primary herpes occurs within 6 weeks of delivery elective caesarean section should be recommended.
- The risk of transmission of recurrent herpes to the neonate, even at term, is low and a normal vaginal delivery should be offered.
- Suppressive aciclovir should be considered in the last 6 weeks of pregnancy for those with a first- or second-trimester outbreak or recurrent episodes.

Varicella-zoster virus

The aetiology, presentation and diagnosis are covered in Chapter 36.

Prevention of chickenpox

Over 90 per cent of the antenatal population is seropositive for varicella-zoster virus(VZV) IgG antibody and hence primary infection in pregnancy is uncommon, occurring in approximately 3:1000 pregnancies. Prenatally vaccination of VZV IgG-seronegative women is possible and postpartum screening has been shown to be cost-effective; however, it is not currently routine practice.

At a booking visit if an antenatal women gives no past history of chickenpox she should be advised to avoid close contact with people with chickenpox or exposed shingles.

The incubation period is 1–3 weeks and the disease is infectious for 48 hours prior to the appearance of the rash until the vesicles have crusted over (usually 5 days). If it is suspected that a significant contact has occurred then serology should be performed and if the woman is not immune to VZV, due to the potentially serious effects of the virus in adulthood and the relative immunocompromised state in pregnancy, it is recommended that varicella-zoster IgG (VZIG) be given. Administration is effective up to 10 days after contact as it has been shown to prevent or reduce the severity of the condition [C].[9] Repeat dose of VZIG may be given if further exposure occurs 3 weeks or more after initial treatment. Women who have been treated with VZIG should be considered infectious for 8–28 days.

Treatment of chickenpox

Chickenpox in adulthood, although rare, can be associated with serious morbidity, with the development of pneumonia, hepatitis and encephalitis, and even mortality. These risks are increased in pregnancy with a five-times higher mortality rate of 3–24 per cent and with pneumonia occurring in 10 per cent of pregnant women with the disease. As a result of this it is recommended that a pregnant women who presents with chickenpox within the first 24 hours of a rash should be treated with oral aciclovir [C].[9]

Hospital management with a multidisciplinary team approach is obviously needed in cases where a woman develops any signs or symptoms that may indicate a serious complication. It is also recommended that hospital referral should be made if there is a history of lung disease, smoking or corticosteroid use, or if the pregnancy is in the later half.

If the infection occurs at the time of delivery then, if possible, delivery should be delayed for 5–7 days to allow for antibody transfer from mother to fetus, as the risk of neonatal VZV is high and this is a condition associated with high morbidity and mortality. Treatment with aciclovir is also recommended [C]. No specific treatment is required if the woman develops shingles as the fetus/neonate will be protected by maternal antibodies.

KEY POINTS

- If a suspected non-immune pregnant woman comes in contact with chickenpox then maternal serology to confirm status is recommended.
- Non-immune women with contact should be given VZIG up to 10 days after exposure.
- Oral aciclovir should be administered within 24 hours of the rash developing.
- Intravenous aciclovir, with hospital admission, should be considered for women presenting at 36 weeks' gestation and beyond, and those with complications.
- Delivery should be delayed until at least 7 days after the onset of the illness.

Postnatally, if a women develops chickenpox within 7 days of delivery then neonatal treatment with VZIG is recommended.

Human immunodeficiency virus

Epidemiology and aetiology

Infection with HIV occurs through sexual contact and contact with infected blood. The majority of HIV-positive women are from sub-Saharan Africa with a prevalence of 2–3 per cent; among UK-born women the prevalence, although increasing, is much lower at 0.3 per 1000.[10] In pregnancy one of the major concerns, both for women with pre-existing infection and for those with new diagnosis, is the risk of mother-to-child transmission (MTCT). The majority of management in pregnancy and delivery revolves around interventions to maintain a low MTCT rate. Prior to such management in the UK transmission occurred in 25 per cent of cases; in comparison now, in diagnosed cases optimally managed, the risk is estimated at just 0.57 per cent,[11] with an overall rate of 2 per cent when considering all exposed infants, i.e. those who have been born to diagnosed and non-diagnosed women.[12]

Despite HIV screening being routinely offered to all pregnant women a small proportion of those who are HIV positive will be missed, either because they decline screening or because they seroconvert during pregnancy. The National Screening Committee (NSC) does not recommend routine re-screening at 28 weeks' gestation; however, those who refused screening at their booking visit should routinely be re-offered it at this stage of gestation.

Management of HIV in pregnancy

The management of both the newly diagnosed and those with pre-existing disease needs to be as part of a multidisciplinary team.

Those with a new diagnosis should be advised to have sexual-health screening [B][13] and it is suggested that those with pre-existing infection consider this in pregnancy as well [C]. All women should obviously be offered their routine antenatal screening, with the addition of screening for hepatitis C. This should include screening for trisomy 21, although women should be counselled as to the increased risk of a false-positive test as significantly increased levels of beta-hCG and low levels of AFP have been reported in HIV-positive patients.[14] They also need to be counselled as to the risks of MTCT with chorionic villous sampling (CVS) and, to a lesser extent, amniocentesis. Any invasive prenatal testing should be delayed until the viral load is less than 50 HIV RNA copies/mL [C].

All pregnant women should be treated with combination antiretroviral therapy (cART) by week 24 of pregnancy [C][13] in order to limit MTCT, or prior to this if required for their own health. Those women who conceive on therapy should continue this. The type of therapy used and combinations should be guided by specialist physicians. There is increasing evidence that exposure to commonly used therapy, even in the first trimester, does not increase the risk of congenital malformations. Viral load is then measured throughout pregnancy with frequency depending on initial load and the gestation at which cART is commenced.

Without other obstetric indications the mode of delivery for women taking cART should be determined at 36 weeks and be dependent on the viral load. For women on cART with a viral load less than 50 HIV RNA copies/mL, a plan for vaginal delivery should be made [C].[13] When the viral load is 400 HIV RNA copies/mL or more at 36 weeks then delivery should be by planned caesarean section. For viral loads in between, the mode of delivery is unclear and should be guided by the actual viral load, the trend, additional obstetric factors and the views of the women [C]. A study of women delivered in the UK and Ireland with viral loads between 50 and 399 HIV RNA copies/mL showed an MTCT risk after caesarean section of 0.23 per cent compared with 1.06 per cent after planned vaginal delivery.[11]

Guidelines have been reviewed and it is now recommended that for those women having a planned vaginal delivery (i.e. viral load less than 50 HIV RNA copies/mL), delivery should follow the same management as for a non-HIV-positive woman [C].[13] Hence, as there is now thought to be little or no risk of MTCT, invasive procedures such as fetal blood sampling and the use of fetal scalp electrodes are no longer prohibited.

In women having planned elective caesarean section for a viral load >1000 HIV RNA copies/mL, treatment with IV zidovudine infusion should be commenced if they labour prior to section. This should also be used for those who present in labour with an unknown viral load.

In all cases of pre-labour spontaneous rupture of membranes after 34 weeks, delivery should be expedited [C].[13] The recommendations for mode of delivery will depend on the viral load and use of cART. For those on therapy with a viral load of less than 50 HIV RNA copies/mL without other factors, induction of labour would be appropriate as it is no longer thought that a prolonged rupture of membranes beyond 4 hours incurs a significant risk of MTCT. For pre-labour rupture of membranes before 34 weeks the timing of delivery needs to be decided on a case-by-case basis, after the use of intramuscular steroids and optimisation of viral load, and should be decided after multidisciplinary discussion.

Postnatally the need to continue cART therapy should be determined by the HIV physicians in line with national guidelines for non-pregnant women. All women, independent of treatment and viral load, should be advised not to breastfeed [A][13] and offered lactation suppression therapy.

Hepatitis B virus

Epidemiology and aetiology

Hepatitis B virus (HBV) is an extremely infectious double-stranded DNA virus that has three major structural antigens: surface antigen (HBsAg), core antigen (HBcAg) and e antigen (HBeAg). This blood-borne virus is transmitted sexually, vertically or by blood contamination. Carriage among pregnant women in the UK is estimated at 0.5 per cent, rising to 1 per cent in inner cities.

Diagnosis and management

Acute infection is often asymptomatic or associated with non-specific signs such as nausea, fatigue and vomiting. In IV drug users 30 per cent will develop jaundice. Physical examination may reveal hepatomegaly, splenomegaly or lymphadenopathy in 5 per cent of cases. The virus can go on to cause acute and chronic hepatitis. The acute condition is usually self-limiting with only 1 per cent of cases developing fulminating hepatic failure.

The diagnosis of the condition is made by the detection of HBsAg. The detection of HBeAg indicates active disease and the disappearance of HBsAg and the appearance of surface antibodies indicate disease resolution and these antibodies will provide immunity. Resolution usually occurs within 3 months, although a small number of those infected will continue to have viral replication for much longer.

All pregnant women are routinely offered screening for HBV. Those women who present for the first time in pregnancy or who have active disease should be managed as part of a multidisciplinary team. It is essential to ensure partner screening and testing for other STIs.

The risk of vertical transmission depends on the antigen status of the women. There is a 95 per cent transmission rate in the presence of both HBsAg and HBeAg, compared with 2–15% when HBeAg negative. Ninety-five per cent of cases of transmission occur at the time of delivery.

KEY POINTS

- HIV screening should be offered to all pregnant women routinely in the first trimester.
- All HIV-positive women should be managed by a multidisciplinary team and have commenced cART at 24 weeks.
- Normal vaginal delivery can be recommended if the detectable viral load is less than 50 HIV RNA copies/ml and labour should be managed as per guidelines for low risk women.
- Advice should be given not to breastfeed.

KEY POINTS

- New presentations of HBV in pregnancy should be managed as part of a multidisciplinary team and women should be screened for other sexually transmitted infections.
- Infectious status should be ascertained and the neonate treated according to maternal antigen status.
- Management of labour should include avoidance of invasive monitoring and fetal blood sampling.

Prevention of HBV infections of the neonate is achieved by avoiding fetal invasive procedures during labour and the administration of passive immunoglobulin in the first 24 hours to neonates of highly infectious mothers. Hepatitis vaccination is given to those born of low-infectivity mothers.

When a baby has been immunised there is no contraindication to breastfeeding.

Hepatitis C virus

Epidemiology and aetiology
Similar to HBV, hepatitis C virus (HCV) is transmitted sexually and via contaminated blood. In the UK it is most commonly seen in IV drug users. There is an 80 per cent chance of an IV drug user becoming HCV positive in the first year of drug use.[15] The overall adult prevalence of chronic HCV in western Europe is 0.5–2 per cent.

Diagnosis and management
HCV presents with non-specific symptoms associated with raised transaminase levels. Diagnosis should be made by identification of HCV RNA as antibodies are not detected until late in the disease. Early identification is essential as treatment with pegylated interferon and oral ribavirin can result in 50–80 per cent of those infected clearing the virus.[16] Without treatment 80 per cent of those infected will go on to develop chronic infection.

Currently routine screening of all antenatal patients is not recommended; however, it should be considered for high-risk groups. Women with a new diagnosis should be managed in conjunction with a hepatologist. The overall risk of MTCT is 5 per cent.[15] The likelihood of infection is linked to the presence of HCV RNA; with those pregnancies where the mother is HCV RNA negative, there is little or no chance of MTCT. Co-infection with HIV also increases the risk.

Currently intrapartum management should be the same as for HBV. There have been suggestions that elective caesarean section may prevent some MTCTs, however, the data are not conclusive and there are large studies that also refute this theory.

There is no evidence that avoiding breastfeeding reduces transmission. Currently there is no neonatal immunoprophylaxis available.

KEY POINTS

- Screening for HCV is recommend only for high-risk groups.
- MTCT is dependent on HCV RNA load.
- There is inconclusive evidence to support delivery by caesarean section.
- There is no contraindication to breastfeeding.

Hepatitis E and A viruses

Hepatitis E requires a special mention as pregnant women with acute infection have a risk of fulminant liver failure of 15 per cent, with a mortality rate of 5 per cent, which is above and beyond that seen outside pregnancy. The reason for this increased susceptibility is not clear. The virus is transmitted by the faecal–oral route and usually produces a self-limiting illness. The transmission route and self-limiting illness are similar to those seen in hepatitis A however, hepatitis A does not result in chronic illness or fulminant liver failure.

BACTERIAL INFECTIONS

Streptococcal A infection is covered in Chapter 65, UTIs in Chapter 13 and bacterial vaginosis and group B streptococci in Chapter 44.

Gonorrhoea

Epidemiology and aetiology
Gonorrhoea is caused by the Gram-negative intracellular diplococcus bacterium *Neisseria gonorrhoeae*. It is isolated from the epithelium of the genital tract, rectum, pharynx and eyes. Transmission is by direct inoculation of infected secretions from one mucous membrane to another. Ascending infection in women can result in uterine and tubal infection. It is most common among the younger age group (15–24 years) and is associated with multiple sexual partners, the presence of other STI and IV drug use.

Diagnosis and management
Between 30 per cent and 60 per cent of women will be asymptomatic. In those with symptoms the most common are increased or altered vaginal discharge (50 per cent of cases), lower abdominal pain (25 per cent of cases), bleeding during or after intercourse as a result of cervical infection, and dysuria. Rarely (less than 1 per cent of cases) disseminated infection resulting in fever, arthritis and skin disorders is seen, and these occur slightly more commonly in pregnancy.

Diagnosis can be made by several methods, none of which has 100 per cent sensitivity. Culture continues to offer a specific, sensitive and cheap diagnostic test at genital sites. It allows confirmatory identification and antimicrobial susceptibility testing, which is of increasing importance as antimicrobial resistance to *N. gonorrhoeae* continues to evolve. Selective culture media containing antimicrobials are recommended to reduce contamination [B][17]

Acute gonorrhoea in pregnancy has been associated with miscarriage, preterm labour, pre-labour rupture of membranes and an SGA fetus. If an acute infection occurs at the time of delivery or in association with ruptured membranes there is a 30–50 per cent risk of neonatal transmission. Neonatal infection presents in the first few days of life as bilateral purulent conjunctivitis. Prompt treatment with antibiotics is required to prevent blindness.

Pregnant women should be managed as per non-pregnant adult guidelines in conjunction with a genitourinary physician. Management includes screening for other STIs and advice on avoiding intercourse until the treatment has been completed and confirmed by repeat swabs. It is also important that the woman's partner has tested negative or been treated. Treatment is with 500 mg ceftriaxone intramuscularly as a single dose with 1 g azithromycin orally as a single dose [C].[17]

KEY POINTS

- Up to 60 per cent of infections will be asymptomatic.
- The most common symptoms are vaginal discharge or pelvic pain.
- Management should be as per non-pregnant adult guidelines in combination with a genitourinary physician.

Listeria monocytogenes

Epidemiology and aetiology
Up to 10 per cent of people carry *Listeria*, a Gram-positive bacterium, in their intestinal tract. The likelihood of infection depends on the strain of pathogen and the person's susceptibility. The majority of people will be unaware of the infection; however, pregnant women are among those vulnerable to the infection, hence the advice to avoid foods with an increased risk of contamination, such as raw meat, unpasteurised milk and raw unwashed vegetables.

Diagnosis and management
Listeria sp. can cause a range of non-specific symptoms including 'a flu-like illness' with fever, nausea and vomiting. In those that experience complications they can go on to develop septicaemia and meningo-encephalitis. It is also classically linked with the presence of meconium in very premature infants. The diagnosis is made by symptom-triggered culturing of the organisms from blood, stool sample or cerebrospinal fluid (CSF), or from serological testing.

KEY POINTS

- *Listeria monocytogenes* is found in up to 10 per cent of human intestinal tracts.
- Pregnancy increases a person's susceptibility to infection.
- Women should be advised to avoid foods that have an increased listeria contamination risk.

Treatment should be with penicillin as in the non-pregnant woman. Listeria infection has been linked to miscarriage, premature labour and stillbirth.

Chlamydia

Epidemiology and aetiology
Chlamydia trachomatis is the most common curable STI in Britain. Approximately 5–10 per cent of sexually active women under the age of 24 are infected with the serotypes D–K, responsible for 'occulogenital' transmitted strains of the disease. Risk factors for infection include age under 25 years, new sexual partner or more than one sexual partner in the past year (a new sexual partner being more important than the number of sexual partners), and lack of consistent use of condoms. *C. trachomatis* infection is frequently asymptomatic in both men and women, and ongoing transmission in the community is sustained by this unrecognised infection. In response to the evidence of high and increasing rates of infection, the Government has introduced a national chlamydia screening programme,[18,19] with recommendations that screening be offered to all sexually active women below the age of 25 years, and those over 25 years who had a new sexual partner or two or more partners in the last year. Screening is performed on first-catch urine samples by ligase reaction test.

Diagnosis and management
Symptomatic women may present with an abnormal vaginal discharge, dyspareunia, abdominal pain or dysuria. Untreated, it can result in pelvic inflammatory disease and perihepatitis. In pregnancy, as well as these symptoms, there have also been links to premature labour, premature rupture of the membranes and low birthweight. When the infection occurs at the time of delivery transmission to the neonate is possible. In untreated mothers 35–50 per cent will develop conjunctivitis and 11–20 per cent pneumonia.

Treatment in pregnancy differs from the standard, as tetracyclines are contraindicated. Instead a 7-day course of erythromycin is recommended. If not tolerated then a Cochrane review shows amoxicillin to be a suitable alternative in pregnancy [A].[20] Management should be, as with gonorrhoea, in conjunction with genitourinary physicians.

PROTOZOA

Trichomonas

Epidemiology and aetiology
Trichomonas vaginalis is a vaginal infection most commonly seen with co-infection with other STIs, in smokers and in women with decreased education level and increased sexual partners.

Diagnosis and management

Women typically present with an offensive, frothy, copious yellow–green discharge. Other symptoms include dyspareunia and vulvovaginal soreness. In pregnancy vaginal bleeding may also be associated. The diagnosis can be made by saline wet preparation identifying motile flagellated tichomonads, culturing, immunofluorescence and enzyme immunoassay techniques.

Management should be as per the non-pregnant woman including referral to a genitourinary physician and the use of metronidazole. It is uncertain if treatment reduces the association with preterm birth.

Toxoplasmosis and syphilis

These infections are covered in Chapter 36.

ACKNOWLEDGEMENTS

Joanna C Gillham, author of this chapter in the previous edition.

References

1. Whitley RJ, Roizman B. Herpes simplex virus infections. *Lancet* 2001;357:1513–18.
2. Arvin AM, Hendsleigh PA, Prober CG *et al.* Failure of antepartum maternal cultures to predict the infant's risk of exposure to herpes simplex virus at delivery. *N Engl J Med* 1986;315:796–800.
3. Foley E, Clarke E, Beckett VA *et al. Management of Genital Herpes in Pregnancy.* London:RCOG and BASHH, 2014.
4. Pasternak B, Hviid A. Use of acyclovir, valacyclovir and famciclovir in the first trimester of pregnancy and the risk of birth defects. *JAMA* 2010;304:859–66.
5. Acs N, Banhidy F, Puho E, Czeizel AE. No association between maternal recurrent genital herpes in pregnancy and higher risk of congenital abnormalities. *Acta Obstet Gynecol Scand* 2008;87:292–9.
6. Brown ZA, Vontver LA, Benedetti J *et al.* Effects on infants of a first episode of genital herpes during pregnancy. *N Engl J Med* 1987;317:1246–51.
7. Hensleigh PA, Andrews WW, Brown Z, Greenspoon J, Yasukawa L, Prober CG. Genital herpes during pregnancy: inability to distinguish primary and recurrent infections clinically. *Obstet Gynecol* 1997;89:891–5.
8. Brown ZA, Selke S, Zeh J *et al.* The acquisition of herpes simplex virus during pregnancy. *N Engl J Med* 1997;337:509–513.
9. Byrne BMP, Crowley PA, Carrington D. *Chickenpox in Pregnancy.* Green top guideline No.13. London: RCOG, 2007.
10. Health Protection Agency. *Data tables of the unlinked anonymous dried spot survey of newborn infants – prevalence of HIV in women giving birth.* Surveillance update, 2012.
11. Townsend C, Byrne L, Cortina-Borja M *et al.* Earlier initiation of ART and further decline in mother-to-child HIV transmission rates, 2000-2011. *AIDS* 2014;28:1049–57.
12. Health Protection Agency. *HIV in the United Kingdom: 2012 Report.* London: Health Protection Services, 2012.
13. De Ruiter A, Taylor G, Clayden P *et al.* British HIV association guidelines for the management of HIV infection in pregnant women 2012 (2014 interim review). *HIV Med* 2014;14:1–77.
14. Charlton TG, Franklin JM, Douglas M *et al.* The impact of HIV infection and anti-retroviral therapy on the predicted risk of Down syndrome. *Prenat Diag* 2014;34(2):121-7.
15. Maddrey WC. Update in hepatology. *Ann Intern Med* 2001;134:216–23.
16. Fischler B. Hepatitis C virus infection. *Seminars in Fetal and Neonatal Medicine* 2007;12:168–73.
17. Bignell C, FitzGerald M. *UK National Guideline for the Management of Gonorrhoea in Adults.* BASHH guideline. London: British Association for Sexual Health and HIV, 2011.
18. Department of Health. *National Chlamydia Screening Programme in England: Programme overview.* Department of Health 2004;(2).
19. Hamlyn C. *Roll out of the national Chlamydia screening programme (NCSP).* Department of Health 2005.
20. Brocklehurst P, Rooney G. Interventions for treating genital *Chlamydia trachomatis* infection in pregnancy. *Cochrane Database Syst Rev* 2000;(2):CD000054.

Chapter 25 Gestational diabetes

Clare L Tower

Clare L Tower

MRCOG standard

Core curriculum, Module 8 (Antenatal Care) and Module 9 (Maternal Medicine)

Knowledge criteria

Understand the purposes and practices of antenatal care including screening for abnormality and arrangements and conduct of booking and follow-up visits.

Understand the epidemiology, aetiology, pathophysiology, clinical characteristics, prognostic features and management of gestational diabetes:

- Impaired glucose tolerance and type 1 diabetes;
- Maternal, fetal and neonatal hazards;
- Ketoacidosis;
- Drugs (insulins and hypoglycaemic agents).

Be able to describe the natural history of diseases and illnesses that run a chronic course.

Have knowledge of long-term management plans for chronic conditions.

Clinical competency

Conduct a booking visit and arrange appropriate investigations. Understand the positive and negative effects of screening on the individual.

Diagnose, investigate and manage, with direct supervision, type 1 diabetes and impaired glucose tolerance.

INTRODUCTION

Gestational diabetes mellitus (GDM) is defined as impaired carbohydrate tolerance resulting in hyperglycaemia, which first develops or becomes diagnosed during pregnancy. Some of these women have previously undiagnosed diabetes, usually type 2. It is clinically important for the management of the pregnancy, but also because it significantly increases an individual's long-term risk of developing type 2 diabetes. Women developing GDM face similar increased risks as diabetic women in terms of macrosomia and its associated complications, neonatal hypoglycaemia and late pregnancy loss. Furthermore, their offspring are at increased risk of obesity and diabetes in the future.

PREVALENCE

The prevalence of GDM varies with the diagnostic criteria used (discussed below) and with ethnic group. The ethnic groups at particularly high risk are women from south Asia (India, Pakistan and Bangladesh) who have a relative risk 7.6- to 11-fold compared with white women and black Caribbean women (relative risk 3.1). Thus, the overall prevalence of GDM is between 1 and 5 per cent.[1]

EPIDEMIOLOGY

Studies investigating risk factors for development of GDM vary with the definition of the disorder used, which in turn is dependent on the type of testing (see below). Systematic reviews have suggested that the risk factors (Box 25.1) are obesity, advanced maternal age, previous gestational diabetes, family history of diabetes, specific ethnic groups as above, high weight gain in early adulthood and current smoking [A].

There has been much debate regarding the use of screening strategies to detect GDM, and studies have investigated the use of risk factors to guide screening. An RCT comparing risk-factor-based screening from the United States found positive predictive values for a first-degree relative with type 1 diabetes (15%), a first-degree relative with type 2 diabetes (6.7%), a previous baby >4.5 kg (12.2%), glycosuria (50%), current

Box 25.1 Risk factors for gestational diabetes[1]

Body mass index >30 kg/m^2

Previous macrosomic infant ≥4.5 kg

Previous gestational diabetes

First-degree relative with diabetes

Ethnic origin:
- South Asia (India, Pakistan, Bangladesh)
- Black Caribbean
- Middle Eastern (Saudi Arabia, United Arab Emirates, Iraq, Jordan, Syria, Oman, Qatar, Kuwait, Lebanon, Egypt).

suspected macrosomia and polyhydramnios (both 40%).[2] Other traditionally quoted risk factors for which less robust evidence exists include twin pregnancy, polycystic ovarian disease, parity (related to maternal age), previous congenital abnormality and previous stillbirth.

The risks of developing GDM in subsequent pregnancies are high, with recurrence rates between 30 and 84 per cent.[1] A systematic review found that the risk was highest in the ethnic groups at particular risk of an initial presentation of GDM.[1] Furthermore, women who have required insulin treatment for GDM in a previous pregnancy have a recurrence risk of 75%.

CAUSES

Pregnancy is a state of increased insulin resistance, secondary to the secretion of placental hormones such as progesterone, cortisol, placental lactogen, growth hormone and prolactin. This insulin resistance, evident by the second trimester, persists throughout the pregnancy and resolves with delivery of the placenta. Normal pregnant women demonstrate an increased pancreatic β-cell response and hyperinsulinaemia. This facilitates the supply of glucose to the fetus by altering maternal energy metabolism from carbohydrate to lipids. Women with GDM have an exaggeration of this insulin resistance, possibly due to a limited ability of the pancreatic β cells to increase insulin secretion. This may represent an early marker of deterioration in β-cell function. A subset (1–38%) of women with GDM have islet cell auto-antibodies, including insulin antibodies and glutamic acid decarboxylase antibodies. These women may be more likely to be of normal weight and are at increased risk of subsequent type 1 diabetes. A minority of women (<5%) have specific glucokinase mutation resulting in β-cell dysfunction and inability to compensate for the insulin resistance. During the third trimester, this impaired ability to compensate for the insulin resistance results in an increase in blood glucose levels in response to a glucose load. Although this may not be sufficient to cause symptoms, the excessive glucose load is able to exert an adverse effect on the fetus, through fetal hyperglycaemia and hyperinsulinaemia.

SCREENING AND DIAGNOSIS

There is now good evidence that the treatment of GDM improves pregnancy outcome and these women are at risk of type 2 DM in later life. Screening in pregnancy offers an opportunity for targeted surveillance and early intervention. Women with any of the risk factors listed in box 25.1 should be offered screening for GDM using the oral glucose tolerance test (OGTT) at 24-28 weeks.[1] This involves a fasting venous plasma glucose then ingesting a 75g glucose load and testing the venous plasma blood glucose at 2 hours (Table 25.1). In addition, women with more than 2+ glycosuria on a single urine dipstick, or + on 2 or more occasions should also be offered testing.[1] Fasting or random blood glucose, HbA1c or urinalysis should not be used for screening.

According to the NICE Diabetes in Pregnancy guidelines 2015, a diagnosis of GDM is made if the fasting plasma glucose is 5.6mmol/litre or more, or the two hour level is 7.8mmol/litre or more [A].[1] Women should be advised that a diagnosis of GDM will require increased monitoring and may lead to an increased risk of intervention during both pregnancy and labour prior to testing, to enable them to make an informed choice about screening. They should also be informed that whilst GDM can respond to diet and lifestyle changes some women need treatment with oral medications or insulin.

The optimal screening and diagnostic criteria for GDM have been hotly debated over the years. The NICE guideline 2015 changed the diagnostic criteria substantially from the previous 2008 guidelines which recommended the use of the WHO 1999 definitions.[1] Since that time, the evidence base has increased,[3] in particular with the publication of the Hyperglycaemia and Adverse Pregnancy Outcomes (HAPO) study.[4] This study conducted blind 2-hour 75 g OGTTs in over 23,000 non-diabetic women worldwide to examine the association between fasting, 1-hour and 2-hour plasma glucose levels and the primary outcomes of macrosomia (birthweight over the 90th centile), fetal hyperinsulinaemia and caesarean section rates. Plasma glucose levels were associated on a continuum with adverse outcomes and there was no threshold effect [B]. In 2010, the International Association of Diabetes and Pregnancy Study Groups (IADPSG) published a consensus document in an attempt to achieve universal agreement on diagnostic criteria for GDM.[5] Using the HAPO data, it developed a recommendation based on odds ratios of 1.75 for the risk of macrosomia, fetal hyperinsulinaemia and neonatal adiposity. It suggested universal screening of all pregnant women at 24–26 weeks, using a 2-hour OGTT, with a diagnosis of GDM if any glucose levels given in Table 25.1 are exceeded. If these criteria had been applied to the HAPO dataset, cumulatively 8.3 per cent of women would be diagnosed with GDM based on fasting levels, 14 per cent on 1-hour levels and 16 per cent on 2-hour levels. This has large implications for healthcare resources,[6] as it represents a substantial increase over the current rates of around 3.5 per cent.[3] These recommendations have been adopted by the American Diabetes Association but not the American College of Obstetricians and Gynecologists.

In addition to the HAPO data associating higher glucose with poor outcomes, there is now evidence that diet,

Table 25.1 Criteria for the 2-hour 75 g OGTT in the diagnosis of GDM at 24-28 weeks' gestation[3]

	IADPSG/SIGN	NICE[1]
	Venous plasma blood glucose (mmol/L)	Venous plasma blood glucose (mmol/L)
Fasting	≥5.1	≥5.6
1 hour	≥10	–
2 hours	≥8.5	≥7.8

lifestyle intervention and pharmacological therapies both lower maternal glucose and modify fetal growth in women with milder levels of hyperglycaemia (discussed below). The NICE guidelines 2015 acknowledge that the quality of evidence was low to moderate in terms of defining the diagnostic criteria, and a health economic analysis was also considered. Notably, the recommended diagnostic criteria differ from the WHO 2013 guidelines that adopted the IADPSG diagnostic thresholds. The guidelines therefore acknowledge that new evidence, including more robust health economic data will likely lead to a further review of these guidelines in the next 3-5 years.[1] The SIGN (2010) guidelines suggested a similar strategy to the IADPSG recommendations but based on risk factors (Table 25.2).[7]

Due to the high risk of recurrence, women who have had GDM in a previous pregnancy should be offered either early self monitoring of blood glucose or a 2 hour 75g OGTT as soon as possible after booking. If this test is normal, a repeat test at 24-28 weeks is recommended.[1]

MANAGEMENT

Congenital malformations

As expected from the pathogenesis, there is no excess risk of major congenital malformations in women developing GDM, as blood glucose would be expected to be normal during organogenesis. The exception to this is those women who have pre-existing diabetes would thus have had hyperglycaemia during the first trimester. Some UK centres have described 12–20 per cent of women with GDM as having persistently impaired glucose tolerance on postnatal testing, and are thus likely to have type 2 diabetes.

Antenatal care

After diagnosis, women should be offered a review in a Joint diabetic antenatal clinic within one week.[1] This will enable early discussion of the implications of GDM, and also the recommended management, which will include a discussion of diet and exercise. In addition, women should be taught how to self-monitor blood glucose and all women should be referred to a dietician. Antenatal care should be focused on reducing the risks of GDM, namely fetal macrosomia and the possible increased risk of pre-eclampsia.[6] Women benefit from a multidisciplinary management approach with access to obstetricians, diabetologists, dieticians, specialist nurses and midwives.

Glycaemic control

Several studies have now demonstrated the benefits of treating GDM. The Australian Carbohydrate Intolerance Study in Pregnant Women (ACHOIS) trial was published in 2005.[8] This study randomised 1000 women with impaired glucose tolerance, to routine care or diabetic care (diet, monitoring and insulin as appropriate). There was a lower rate of serious perinatal complications (defined as death, shoulder dystocia, fractures and nerve injury) in the 490 women in the intervention arm (1%), compared with 4% in the 510 women in the routine care group. More women in the intervention group underwent induction of labour and more babies were admitted to special care, but there was no increase in caesarean section rate and significantly fewer babies had macrosomia. The number of women needing treatment to prevent one adverse outcome was 34. A study using a similar design but more stringent thresholds for GDM diagnosis, with a fasting blood sugar of <5.3 mmol/L, showed a small reduction in birthweight in the treatment arm, a halving of

Table 25.2 SIGN (2010) criteria for diagnosis of GDM

Gestation	Test	Fasting glucose (mmol/L)	1-hour glucose (mmol/L)	2-hour glucose (mmol/L)	HbA1c (mmol/mol)	Diagnosis and action
Booking	Fasting sugar or HbA1c to all women with risk factors as in Box 25.1	≥7.0	–	≥11.1	≥48	Manage as pre-existing diabetes mellitus
		5.1-6.9	–	8.6-11	42-46	Intermediate levels; assess need for immediate home glucose monitoring or reassess using OGTT at 24-28 weeks
24–28 weeks	Low-risk women fasting blood sugar	As below	–	–	–	As below
	OGTT for women with risk factors as in Box 25.1	≥5.1	≥10	≥8.5	–	Diagnose GDM

the percentage of large-for-gestational-age infants and those weighing more than 4 kg, a reduction in risk of shoulder dystocia from 4 per cent to 1.5 per cent, and a reduction in risk of hypertensive disorders.[9] The primary goal of treatment is to achieve near-normal glycaemic control using blood glucose monitoring, diet and exercise, oral hypoglycaemic agents and insulin therapy, as studies have shown that women achieving lower glucose levels (fasting ≤4.9 mmol/L and 2-hour postprandial levels of 5.9–6.4 mmol/L) had the lowest complication rates.[10] NICE 2015 recommends that strategies to control blood glucose should be tailored to the individual woman, and her preferences should be considered in addition to her blood glucose monitoring profile.[1]

Diet and exercise

Lifestyle modifications, including dietary changes and exercise should be offered to all women diagnosed with GDM. Studies have shown that diets high in carbohydrates of low glycaemic index (GI) can improve overall glycaemic control and postprandial hyperglycaemia [A]. Several small observational studies have suggested that obese pregnant women with GDM may improve glycaemic control without any risks of ketonuria with a moderate (30%) reduction in calorie intake [C]. Increased exercise may also have beneficial effects, with several small studies showing improved glucose control and reduced need for insulin. Therefore, NICE guidelines suggest that women with GDM should choose diets containing low-GI carbohydrates and low-fat proteins. They should also be advised to undertake moderate exercise (30 minutes a day). Walking for 30 minutes after a meal may help improve blood glucose control.[1]

Diagnosis and recommended management as outlined in NICE guidelines 2015 are summarised in table 25.2 As an initial treament, women with a fasting plasma glucose at diagnosis of less than 7mmol/litre should be offered diet and exercise as a method of controlling blood sugar[1] as long as there are no other complications present such as polyhydramnios or macrosomia. They should be advised to test a fasting and a blood glucose one hour after a meal every day and that they should aim for the recommended target blood glucose levels stated in box 25.3.

Box 25.2 Targets for daily capiliary plasma glucose[1]

> Fasting less than 5.3mmol/l and
>
> 1 hour after meals less than 7.8 mmol/l or 2 hours after meals of less than 6.4mmol/l

If after 1-2 weeks of diet and exercise, blood glucose is not within these recommended levels, additional therapy should be offered.

Pharmacological treatments

Overall, 82–93 per cent of women with GDM will achieve glycaemic control with diet alone.[1] Poor control of blood glucose is associated with similar complications as for women with pre-existing DM (macrosomia, birth trauma, neonatal hypoglycaemia, perinatal death, induction of labour and caesarean section). Therefore, NICE guidance suggests that hypoglycaemic therapy should be considered if diet and exercise fail to achieve blood glucose targets over a period of 1–2 weeks.[1] Oral hypoglycaemic agents and insulin have been discussed in detail in Chapter 9. Options for treatment include oral hypoglycaemic agents (metformin or glibenclamide), regular insulin or insulin analogues. The choice is dependent on the particular patient and will depend on glucose control and acceptability. There are several studies demonstrating the clinical and cost-effectiveness of glibenclamide and metformin in GDM. A large Australian RCT comparing metformin with insulin in GDM randomised 363 women to receive metformin (46% required supplemental insulin) and 370 to receive insulin.[11] The primary outcome, a composite of neonatal outcomes including neonatal hypoglycaemia, respiratory complications, birth trauma, phototherapy, low Apgar scores and preterm birth, was the same (32%) in both groups. Interestingly, there was significantly less severe neonatal hypoglycaemia in the metformin group, but also a slightly higher rate of preterm birth less than 37 weeks. There was no difference in birthweight between the two groups, and women in the metformin group demonstrated lower weight gain (although the difference may not be clinically significant). Furthermore, metformin was more acceptable to patients.

Table 25.3 Recommended management of GDM at diagnosis (NICE 2015)

Fasting Plasma Glucose mmol/l at diagnosis	Complications	Management	Recommended pattern of blood glucose monitoring
<7	none	1-2 week trial diet and exercise	Fasting + 1 hour post meal daily
6.0–6.9	Polyhydramnios Macrosomia	Insulin ±Metformin in addition to diet and exercise	Oral therapy or single dose intermediate or long acting insulin: fasting and 1 hour post meal daily
≥7	-	Insulin ±Metformin in addition to diet and exercise	Multiple daily insulin doses: fasting, pre-meal, post-meal and bedtime daily

Therefore, it appears that metformin is a safe and acceptable treatment for women with GDM [B]. Therefore the current Scottish guidelines (SIGN 2010) recommend initial metformin or glibenclamide for women in whom lifestyle measures have two or more values above the following targets in a 2-week period.[7]

- ≥5.5 mmol/L pre-meal or ≥7.0 mmol/L 2 hours post-meal at ≤35 weeks
- ≥5.5 mmol/L pre-meal or ≥8.0 mmol/L 2 hours post-meal at >35 weeks
- Any post-meal levels >9.0 mmol/L.

NICE guidelines (2015) recommend metformin if blood glucose is not within the targets stated in box 25.2 within 1-2 weeks of diet and exercise intervention. In addition, women with polyhydramnios or macrosomia and a fasting plasma glucose of between 6-6.9mmol/l should be offered immediate treatment with insulin, with or without metformin. Similarly, if fasting blood glucose is 7.0mmol/l or more at diagnosis, insulin, with or without metformin should be offered as a treatment in addition to diet and exercise.[1] This, and the recommended daily monitoring regimen is summarized in table 25.2. If metformin is contraindicated or the woman finds the treatment unacceptable, then insulin therapy should be offered. Glibenclamide can be offered as an alternative to women who decline insulin, or in whom metformin cannot be tolerated.[1] HbA1c levels should not be used for monitoring blood glucose control routinely in the second or third trimesters of pregnancy in women with GDM.[1] However, it is recommended that HBA1c is tested at the time of diagnosis of GDM in order to exclude pre-existing type 2 diabetes.

Fetal monitoring

Women with GDM are at risk of developing fetal macrosomia. It has been suggested that this can be detected and predicted by the measurement of fetal abdominal circumference on ultrasound. A cohort study of 201 women with GDM reported the sensitivity of abdominal circumference at 30–33 weeks' gestation to predict macrosomia as 88 per cent, with a specificity of 83 per cent. The positive predictive value was 56 per cent and the negative predictive value 96 per cent.[12] One RCT of 141 women with GDM compared ultrasound at 28 and 32 weeks with 32 weeks alone.[13] Insulin therapy was commenced if the abdominal circumference was greater that the 75th percentile. This study found that there were more macrosomic babies in the group scanned only at 32 weeks. Thus, although there is a lack of robust evidence, NICE suggests that insulin therapy should be considered if macrosomia is present [C].[1] There are no studies clearly demonstrating benefits of particular monitoring regimens in terms of frequency of ultrasound scans. However, fetal monitoring should be conducted as for women with pre-existing DM (see Chapter 9).

Timing and mode of delivery

The majority of studies investigating timing and mode of delivery include women with pre-existing and gestational diabetes. This is discussed in Chapter 9. The timing and mode of delivery should be discussed with women, especially during the third trimester.

NICE recommends that pregnant women with uncomplicated GDM be offered elective birth no later than 40+6 weeks' gestation.[1] This represents a change from previous guidelines and the current Scottish guidelines (SIGN 2010) that suggest delivery between 38 and 40 weeks if parameters are normal.[7] Patient management should be individualised and timing and mode of delivery considered in the context of glycaemic control and fetal ultrasound findings. Women with complications should be electively delivered before this gestation but a woman with diet-controlled GDM, with good control and no evidence of macrosomia, does not need delivery before 40+6 weeks.[1]

Intrapartum care

Intrapartum maternal hyperglycaemia poses the same risks to the fetus of neonatal hypoglycaemia in GDM as in type 1 and type 2 diabetes. This is discussed in Chapter 9. Thus, blood glucose should be tested every hour and maintained between 4 and 7 mmol/L.[1] A sliding scale of intravenous insulin and dextrose should be instituted if blood glucose falls outside this range. However, this recommendation is based on a single study of 85 women with GDM [C]. Women who have not required treatment with insulin in the antenatal period are less likely to require IV insulin and dextrose. Similarly, women undergoing elective caesarean section are unlikely to require intraoperative insulin and dextrose infusions if they have not required antenatal insulin treatment. Women who require steroid treatment for lung maturity should be treated in the same way as women with pre-existing diabetes (see Chapter 9). In all cases, care of women should be individualised, and a jointly agreed care plan involving the obstetrician and diabetic team should be agreed antenatally and documented in the notes.

Postnatal care

Women with true GDM are unlikely to require insulin following delivery, so women with GDM should stop all hypoglycemic agents (oral or insulin) immediately after birth. In order to detect women with previously undiagnosed pre-existing diabetes, it is recommended that blood glucose monitoring be conducted in the early postnatal period.[1] NICE do not recommend a particular regimen for postnatal testing, but pre-meal and bedtime testing until blood glucose levels return to normal (4–6 mmol/L), then once daily while an inpatient, would be appropriate. Contraception should also be discussed prior to discharge. Women should be reminded of the symptoms of high blood glucose.

Future risks of developing DM

Women who have developed GDM are at increased risk of subsequent type 2 diabetes, with rates of progression within 5 years between 15 and 50 per cent [C].[14] Women should be advised of the symptoms of hyperglycaemia and advised that lifestyle or pharmacological modifications may reduce the likelihood of developing type 2 diabetes.[1,7] However, this advice is based on studies conducted on populations including older individuals and men. A systematic review and meta-analysis concluded that lifestyle interventions reduced the progression of impaired glucose tolerance to type 2 diabetes with a hazard ratio of 0.51 [A].[15] NICE guidelines (2015) therefore recommend that women undergo testing for diabetes between 6 and 13 weeks after birth [A].[1]

Prior to the 2008 NICE guidelines, the recommended test was the 75 g OGTT at 6 weeks postpartum and annually thereafter.[16] Subsequently a study suggested that a postnatal fasting plasma glucose of 6.0 mmol/L or more could be used to select women who should undergo a full glucose tolerance test.[17] In this study of 122 women tested 6 weeks postnatally, the fasting plasma glucose had a sensitivity of 100 per cent and a specificity of 94 per cent for identifying diabetes compared with a glucose tolerance test [D]. Thus, NICE suggested that changing from a glucose tolerance test to fasting plasma glucose could represent a cost saving to the NHS.[1] Current NICE guidelines recommend a fasting plasma glucose at 6-13 weeks, which may most conveniently be performed when the woman attends for her postnatal check.[1] If this is not possible or has not been performed, a fasting glucose or HbA1c should be offered after 13 weeks. The recommended actions based on this test is outlined in table 25.4. Ongoing management of women at moderate or high risk of developing type 2 DM is outlined in the NICE guideline on preventing type 2 DM.[12] The thresholds for defining moderate or high risk of type 2 DM differ in these guidelines compared to those used for women who have had GDM, in order to recognize population differences between studies. Women whose postnatal screening test is negative should be offered annual testing for diabetes. The 2010 SIGN guidelines recommend assessment at 6 weeks postnatally with a fasting blood glucose and then an OGTT if clinically indicated, followed by annual fasting blood glucose or HbA1c.[7]

KEY POINTS

- GDM is impaired carbohydrate tolerance that first develops during pregnancy.
- GDM is associated with increased risks of macrosomia and its associated complications, neonatal hypoglycaemia and late pregnancy loss.
- There are many well-defined risk factors, the main ones being ethnic origin, obesity and GDM in a previous pregnancy.
- There is current debate regarding screening and diagnostic testing for GDM. NICE guidelines recommend that women at risk should be tested using the 2-hour 75 g OGTT at 24-28 weeks' gestation.
- Women who have had GDM in a previous pregnancy should be offered early self-monitoring of blood glucose or an OGTT as soon as possible after booking and repeat at 24-28 weeks if normal.
- Diagnose GDM using a 75g 2 hour OGTT. Diagnosis should be made if the fasting plasma glucose is 5.6mmmol/l or more, or the 2 hour level is 7.8mmol/l or more.
- Treating GDM reduces the incidence of complications.
- Diet and lifestyle modifications should be offered to all women. Additional treatment with oral hypoglycaemic agents and/or insulin may also be needed.
- Pregnant women with GDM should be managed in a joint obstetric/diabetic clinic involving the input of obstetricians, diabetologists, dieticians, specialist nurses and midwives. Review should be offered within 1 week of diagnosis.
- Women should be taught how to self monitor plasma glucose
- The target for fasting plasma glucose is less than 5.3mmol/l.
- Postprandial levels should be less than 7.8 mmol/L.
- Women on insulin or glibenclamide should be advised to maintain plasma glucose above 4mmol/l.
- Women with GDM should be offered monitoring of fetal growth and wellbeing.
- Women with uncomplicated GDM should be offered elective delivery by 40+6 weeks gestation.. Care should be individualised, and will depend on glycaemic control and development of macrosomia.
- Women with macrosomia should have the risks and benefits of different modes of delivery discussed with them.

Table 25.4 Recommended postnatal testing and actions in women with GDM (1)

Fasting plasma glucose result	HbA1C Result	Recommended action
Less than 6.0mmol/l	Less than 39mmol/mol (5.7%)	Advise that there is a low chance of diabetes at present
		Continue with lifestyle advice as they have a moderate risk of developing type 2 DM (NICE guidelines for the prevention of Type 2 DM)12
		Recommend annual test for DM
Between 6-6.9mmol/l	Between 39 and 47mmol/mol (5.7-6.4%)	Advise that the woman is at high risk for developing type 2 DM.
		Offer advice and interventions in line with the (NICE guidelines for the prevention of Type 2 DM)12
7.0mmol/l or more	48mmol/mol (6.5%) or more	Type 2 DM is likely, offer diagnostic test (1)

- Maternal blood glucose should be monitored hourly during labour and be kept between 4 and 7 mmol/L during labour and delivery. Women who are diet controlled are unlikely to need any specific treatment during labour.
- Women GDM are unlikely to require insulin postnatally so should stop all hypoglycaemic agents immediately after birth.
- Women should undergo early postnatal glucose monitoring to ensure that their blood glucose is in the normal range.
- Women who have had GDM are at high risk of developing type 2 diabetes in the future. This risk can probably be reduced by lifestyle modifications.
- Women should be screened for diabetes at the 6-week postnatal check with a fasting plasma glucose and annually thereafter.
- All women should receive postnatal advice regarding contraception and planning their next pregnancy.

CONCLUSIONS

GDM is a common condition that is increasing in frequency, particularly in association with increasing obesity. If poorly controlled, as with pre-existing DM it is associated with increased maternal and fetal risks. There has been considerable debate regarding the best screening and diagnostic strategies. Women with a diagnosis of GDM require multidisciplinary management. Although most can be managed using lifestyle intervention, a significant proportion will require pharmacological measures. Fetal monitoring and delivery is largely similar to women with pre-existing DM. Women who develop GDM are at significant risk of subsequent development of type 2 DM, offering an opportunity for prevention in the form of diet and exercise.

References

1. *Diabetes in Pregnancy. Management of diabetes and its complications from preconception to the postnatal period.* NICE guideline. London: National collaborating Centre for Women's and Children's health 2015.
2. Griffin ME, Coffey M, Johnson H *et al.* Universal vs. risk factor-based screening for gestational diabetes mellitus: detection rates, gestation at diagnosis and outcome. *Diabet Med* 2000;17:26–32.
3. RCOG. Scientific Impact Paper No. 23. *Diagnosis and Treatment of Gestational Diabetes.* London: RCOG, 2011.
4. Metzger BE, Lowe LP, Dyer AR *et al.* Hyperglycemia and Adverse Pregnancy Outcome (HAPO) Study: associations with neonatal anthropometrics. *Diabetes* 2009;58:453–9.
5. Metzger BE, Gabbe SG, Persson B *et al.* International association of diabetes and pregnancy study groups recommendations on the diagnosis and classification of hyperglycemia in pregnancy. *Diabetes Care* 2010;33:676–82.
6. Coustan DR. Gestational diabetes mellitus. *Clin Chem* 2013;59:1310–21.
7. SIGN. *Management of Diabetes. A national clinical guideline.* Edinburgh: SIGN, 2010.
8. Crowther CA, Hiller JE, Moss JR *et al.* Effect of treatment of gestational diabetes mellitus on pregnancy outcomes. *N Engl J Med* 2005;352:2477–86.
9. Landon MB, Spong CY, Thom E *et al.* A multicenter, randomized trial of treatment for mild gestational diabetes. *N Engl J Med* 2009;361:1339–48.
10. Rowan JA, Gao W, Hague WM, McIntyre HD. Glycemia and its relationship to outcomes in the metformin in gestational diabetes trial. *Diabetes Care* 2010;33:9–16.
11. Rowan JA, Hague WM, Gao W *et al.* Metformin versus insulin for the treatment of gestational diabetes. *N Engl J Med* 2008;358:2003–15.
12. Bochner CJ, Medearis AL, Williams J, 3rd *et al.* Early third-trimester ultrasound screening in gestational diabetes to determine the risk of macrosomia and labor dystocia at term. *Am J Obstet Gynecol* 1987;157:703–8.
13. Rossi G, Somigliana E, Moschetta M *et al.* Adequate timing of fetal ultrasound to guide metabolic therapy in mild gestational diabetes mellitus. Results from a randomized study. *Acta Obstet Gynecol Scand* 2000;79:649–54.
14. Kim C, Newton KM, Knopp RH. Gestational diabetes and the incidence of type 2 diabetes: a systematic review. *Diabetes Care* 2002;25:1862–8.
15. Gillies CL, Abrams KR, Lambert PC *et al.* Pharmacological and lifestyle interventions to prevent or delay type 2 diabetes in people with impaired glucose tolerance: systematic review and meta-analysis. *BMJ* 2007;334:299.
16. Department of Heatlth. *National Service Framework for Diabetes: Standards.* London: Department of Health, 2002.
17. Holt RI, Goddard JR, Clarke P, Coleman MA. A postnatal fasting plasma glucose is useful in determining which women with gestational diabetes should undergo a postnatal oral glucose tolerance test. *Diabet Med* 2003;20:594–8.
18. *Type 2 diabetes: prevention in people at high risk.* NICE guideline. London: National collaborating Centre for Women's and Children's health 2012.

Chapter 26 Pre-eclampsia and non-proteinuric pregnancy-induced hypertension

Andrew Shennan

MRCOG standards

- Conduct pre-pregnancy counselling to a level expected in independent primary care.
- Manage severe pre-eclampsia/eclampsia.

In addition, we would suggest the following:.

Theoretical skills

- Distinguish between the different causes of hypertension in pregnancy.
- Understand the principles underlying the pathophysiology of pre-eclampsia.
- Describe and quantify the risk factors for pre-eclampsia.
- Know the principles of management of the woman who presents with pre-eclampsia.
- Advise a woman with a previous history of pre-eclampsia.

Practical skills

- Know how to manage the woman with severe pre-eclampsia; this will involve detailed knowledge of fluid management, hypertension control, anticonvulsant prophylaxis and anaesthetic issues.
- Be able to treat eclampsia.

INTRODUCTION

Women who are hypertensive and pregnant must be subdivided into those with:

- chronic hypertension (see Chapter 8);
- pregnancy-induced or gestational hypertension (PIH).

Women with PIH are subdivided further: the majority have non-proteinuric PIH, a condition associated with less maternal or perinatal mortality/morbidity, whereas a minority have the major pregnancy complication of pre-eclampsia.

It is imperative that every effort is made to accurately classify women with hypertension in pregnancy as having chronic hypertension, non-proteinuric PIH or pre-eclampsia. The aetiology and management of the three conditions are very disparate, as are implications for future pregnancies. The aetiology and management of chronic hypertension in pregnancy are discussed in Chapter 8. Women with non-proteinuric PIH need to be monitored to ensure that proteinuria does not develop and pre-eclampsia become apparent; non-proteinuric PIH is not an indication for admission unless there is severe hypertension, but induction of labour or antihypertensive treatment may be considered depending on gestation and blood pressure. This chapter focuses on pre-eclampsia.

Even in developed countries, women still die from pre-eclampsia and eclampsia, although most deaths are avoidable.[1] In the UK, fewer than ten women die each year. Eclampsia is now rarely associated with mortality, although severe hypertension and cerebral vascular accidents still occur.[2] Eclampsia has an estimated incidence in the UK of 26.8 cases per 100,000 maternities.[2] There were no maternal deaths in any eclamptic women, possibly attributed to the more judicious use of magnesium sulphate. Worldwide, however, maternal mortality from hypertensive disease accounts for approximately 60,000 deaths per year.

Because of concerns about the potential adverse effects of pre-eclampsia, many women who have a normal outcome require intensive surveillance; up to a quarter of antenatal admissions are as a direct result of monitoring and managing women with hypertension. Antenatal care is directed towards identifying women with hypertension and proteinuria. Day units reduce the need for inpatient management, but current methods for screening women at risk are poor and the onset and progression of the disease are unpredictable.

Perinatal mortality is also increased with pre-eclampsia. Pre-eclampsia is associated with IUGR, particularly when early in onset. Placental involvement also explains the association with placental abruptions. As delivery is the only cure, the hypertensive diseases of pregnancy have become the most common cause of iatrogenic preterm birth. They account for 15 per cent of all preterm births, but up to a quarter of very-low-birthweight infants. There is strong evidence linking size at birth to health in adulthood, i.e. there are fetal origins of adult disease.[3] Thus, the small babies resulting from pregnancies affected by pre-eclampsia have health implications in adult life, including an increased risk of hypertension, heart disease and diabetes when they become adults. Additional and significant longer-term health service resource implications result from subsequent learning disabilities and low IQ. Maternal disease severity and fetal involvement do not always correlate; for example, the babies of women who have eclampsia at term often have normal birthweight.[2]

CLASSIFICATION AND DEFINITION

The term 'pregnancy-induced hypertension' usually implies hypertension caused by, but unrelated to, other pathology associated with the pregnancy, a diagnosis that is difficult to make until after the pregnancy has ended.

Blood pressure and proteinuria define pre-eclampsia, but they are not fundamental to the aetiology and are more indicative of end-organ damage. In clinical practice, the threshold of abnormality is set low to identify at-risk cases, but this results in many women being identified with hypertension and/or proteinuria who are not at increased risk.

The International Society for the Study of Hypertension in Pregnancy (ISSHP), based on the recommendation of Davey and MacGillivray,[4] uses the term 'gestational hypertension' to include all women with PIH whether proteinuric or not, as long as they had been previously normotensive and not proteinuric. Once proteinuria has developed, this is assumed to be pre-eclampsia (Box 26.1).

If any organ system known to have the potential to be affected by pre-eclampsia is involved, the possibility of the disease must be suspected; hypertension and proteinuria cannot be relied upon to define the disease. However, for pragmatic reasons, these signs must remain hallmarks for definition. Tests for liver, kidney, blood and placental involvement should always be sought if pre-eclampsia is suspected (see below).

INCIDENCE

The prevalence of pre-eclampsia varies with the definition used and the population studied; however, pre-eclampsia occurs in less than 5 per cent of an average antenatal population. In some recent prospective studies, the incidence has been as low as 2.2 per cent, even in a primigravid population, in which the condition is known to have the highest prevalence.[5] The incidence of non-proteinuric PIH is approximately three times greater. Pre-eclampsia in women with a single risk factor is approximately 15 per cent.

Box 26.1 ISSHP classification (modified and abbreviated)

A. Gestational hypertension and/or proteinuria developing during pregnancy, labour or the puerperium in a previously normotensive non-proteinuric woman

1. Gestational hypertension (without proteinuria)
2. Gestational proteinuria (without hypertension)
3. Gestational proteinuric hypertension (pre-eclampsia)

B. Chronic hypertension (before week 20 of pregnancy) and chronic renal disease (proteinuria before week 20 of pregnancy)

1. Chronic hypertension (without proteinuria)
2. Chronic renal disease (proteinuria with or without hypertension)
3. Chronic hypertension with superimposed pre-eclampsia (new-onset proteinuria)

C. Unclassified hypertension and/or proteinuria

D. Eclampsia

Definitions

Hypertension in pregnancy:

- Diastolic BP >110 mmHg on any one occasion or
- Diastolic BP >90 mmHg on two or more consecutive occasions >4 hours apart

Proteinuria in pregnancy:

- One 24-hour collection with total protein excretion >300 mg/24 hours or
- Two 'clean-catch midstream' or catheter specimens of urine collected >4 hours apart with 2+ on reagent strip

AETIOLOGY

Although the primary events leading to pre-eclampsia are still unclear, it is now widely believed that a cascade of events leads to the clinical syndrome (summarised in Fig. 26.1). Although the inheritance of pre-eclampsia has yet to be characterised, there is a strong familial predisposition: a family history in either mother or sister increases the risk of pre-eclampsia four- to eight-fold. This genetic predisposition leads to a faulty interplay between the invading extravillous trophoblast cells (of fetal origin) and the maternal immunologically active decidual cells.

The faulty interplay results in a failure of trophoblast invasion into the myometrium and the maternal spiral arteries do not undergo their physiological vasodilatation.[6] Only the most superficial decidual portion of the spiral artery is invaded by the trophoblast. This inadequate trophoblast invasion is also seen in pregnancies complicated by fetal growth restriction (without pre-eclampsia), demonstrating that the maternal syndrome of pre-eclampsia must be related to additional factors.

ANTENATAL OBSTETRICS

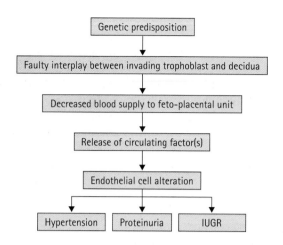

Fig. 26.1 Aetiology of pre-eclampsia. IUGR, intrauterine growth restriction

The diminished dilatation of the spiral arteries, associated increased resistance in the uteroplacental circulation and an impaired intervillous blood flow probably result in an inadequately perfused placenta. Ischaemia or ischaemia/reperfusion in the second half of gestation produces reactive oxygen species and oxidative stress in the placenta.

The placental hypoperfusion is also postulated to result in the secretion of a factor(s) into the maternal circulation that causes 'activation' of vascular endothelium.[7]

Endothelial cell activation explains the widespread manifestations of the disease, as the vascular endothelium trophoblasts regulate the remodelling of spiral arteries and enable normal vasculogenesis mediated through pro-angiogenic factors such as vascular endothelial growth factor (VEGF) and placental growth factor (PlGF). Soluble Fms-like tyrosine kinase 1 (sFLT-1) is a variant of the VEGF receptor, which is up-regulated in pregnancies with pre-eclampsia. It is known to antagonise VEGF and PlGF. Angiogenic factors are now increasingly used to predict[8] and aid in management (see below).

Endoglin (sEng) is associated with pre-eclampsia as early as 15 weeks. PlGF increases from the first trimester but less so in those destined to develop pre-eclampsia, while sFLT-1 will increase.

Many markers of endothelial damage are raised. Pre-eclampsia is associated with lipid changes (there is a two-fold increase in triacylglycerols and free fatty acids), and an increase in lipid peroxidation, both in the placenta and systemically, suggests that oxidative stress (an imbalance between free radical synthesis and antioxidant defence) may be involved in the endothelial cell changes.

MANAGEMENT

Screening for pre-eclampsia

History

More than a third of pre-eclampsia cases occur in women with risk factors; a careful history will allow the clinician to assess risk.

A family history in a first-degree relative increases the risk of pre-eclampsia four- to eight-fold, illustrating the strong genetic influence [D]. A woman has double the risk of pre-eclampsia if pregnant by a partner who had previously fathered an affected pregnancy [D].

An immunological element to the disease process is evidenced by the effect of exposure to the paternal antigen, via either the fetus or the partner. Pre-eclampsia occurs more commonly in first pregnancies; miscarriages or terminations of pregnancy provide some reduction in risk in subsequent pregnancies [D]. However, in women with chronic hypertension, a prior miscarriage is a risk factor for progression to pre-eclampsia. A new partner increases risk, whereas non-barrier methods of contraception and increased duration of sexual cohabitation reduce risk [D].

Exposure to a partner's 'foreign' antigens is common to these phenomena. Teenage mothers and pregnancies conceived by donor insemination have increased risk of pre-eclampsia, presumably due to the lack of exposure to such antigens [D].

Underlying medical disorders, particularly those involving vascular disease – such as chronic hypertension – increase the risk of pre-eclampsia (to over 20 per cent); this highlights the importance of the maternal susceptibility, as well as the placental aetiology in the disease process. All forms of glucose intolerance, including GDM, are associated with an increased risk [D]. This may be related to obesity, which is an independent risk factor.

Women with antiphospholipid syndrome and multiple pregnancies are at increased risk. Risk may be related to the size of the placenta; molar pregnancies have been associated with pre-eclampsia, as have pregnancies complicated by hydrops fetalis (mirror syndrome) or trisomy.

Women with a history of pre-eclampsia, particularly those requiring delivery before 37 weeks, all have about a 20 per cent chance of developing pre-eclampsia again [D].

Biophysical tests

The detection of raised blood pressure in early gestation is related to the subsequent risk of pre-eclampsia, even within the normal blood pressure range (i.e. the lower the blood pressure, the lower the risk). Automated blood pressure monitoring removes many of the errors of standard sphygmomanometry, but is only a weak indicator of risk, and these monitors may under-read in pre-eclampsia [D]. Two other biophysical tests have been investigated, but are not useful: isometric exercise testing and the roll-over test. Problems with reproducibility and poor predictor values mean that these have not been introduced into clinical practice. The angiotensin II sensitivity test, involving assessing the blood pressure response to infusion of the vasoconstrictor angiotensin II, has also shown poor predictor values in larger studies and is invasive, time-consuming and costly [B].

In contrast, Doppler analysis of the uterine artery waveform has reasonable sensitivity and specificity, and is relatively quick, non-invasive and relatively inexpensive if performed at the same time as other ultrasound scans. Poor placental perfusion is a characteristic feature of pregnancies destined to develop pre-eclampsia, and therefore it would seem logical to identify those women who have increased resistance in this circulation. In pregnancies at increased risk of pre-eclampsia, there is persistence of a relatively high-resistance circulation with a notch. The later this test is performed, the better the predictive values [D]. At 20 weeks' gestation in a low-risk population, approximately one in five women will develop pre-eclampsia if she has an abnormal waveform; the prediction value is considerably greater at 24 weeks [D]. This screening test does allow women to be targeted for increased surveillance and possible prophylactic therapies. The importance of screening tests will escalate if an adequate treatment to prevent pre-eclampsia is established.

Biochemical tests

The simple measurements of plasma volume, haemoglobin concentration and haematocrit all have a weak association with the development of pre-eclampsia, but poor prediction values [D]. Uric acid and platelets are sometimes measured in women with chronic hypertension to predict superimposed pre-eclampsia, but are lacking in sensitivity and specificity. The measurement of second-trimester hCG and maternal serum AFP is associated with a two-fold increase in pre-eclampsia, and is likely to reflect the disease process that occurs at the uteroplacental interface [D]. This may also explain why low pregnancy-associated plasma protein (PAPP-A) is associated with higher risks in later pregnancy. These increases in risk are not sufficient to alter clinical practice significantly. Many markers of endothelial activation have been shown to be increased in pre-eclampsia. Some will rise before the clinical manifestations of the disease, but there is invariably overlap between the women who are subsequently normal and those who develop pre-eclampsia, again limiting clinical usefulness. Urinary excretion of calcium, microalbuminuria and prostacyclin metabolites have been investigated, as well as urinary kallikrein:creatinine ratios, and further work may eventually establish a combination of tests that could be clinically useful, perhaps by combining endothelial and placental markers of the disease. More recently, sFLT-1 and PlGFs have been used as a ratio to enhance prediction with better prediction then previous tests, but these have not been adopted into clinical practice.

The role of prophylaxis

Surveillance and timely delivery are the essence of current antenatal management in order to prevent the consequences of pre-eclampsia. Preventing the manifestation of the disease would be highly preferred. There are a number of potential therapies that have been investigated in an effort to prevent the occurrence of pre-eclampsia. Aspirin, calcium and fish oils have gained the most focus in this regard, although other substances, such as magnesium, zinc and even rhubarb, have been investigated. Aspirin, a cyclooxygenase enzyme inhibitor, reverses the imbalance between the vasoconstrictor

thromboxane A_2 and the vasodilator prostacyclin that is known to occur in pre-eclampsia. In a meta-analysis of individual patient data (31 randomised trials and 32,217 women), the use of anti-platelet agents (particularly low-dose aspirin) resulted in a significant 10 per cent reduction in the relative risk of both pre-eclampsia and serious adverse outcome.[9] The number needed to treat in order to prevent pre-eclampsia was 114 and to prevent one serious adverse outcome was 51. Aspirin should be seriously considered in the management of very high-risk women and is likely to be safe. The dose, timing and the populations to be targeted are still being thoroughly investigated.

In a review of 12 RCTs in 15,206 women, calcium supplementation resulted in a significant reduction (52 per cent) in the relative risk of pre-eclampsia, with a higher effect in those at high risk (78 per cent) and with low calcium intake (64 per cent). Calcium supplementation may reduce parathyroid hormone release and intracellular calcium, leading to a reduction in smooth muscle contractility in women at risk of developing pre-eclampsia.[10] Calcium supplementation warrants further research.

Fish oils containing n-3 fatty acids are thought to inhibit platelet thromboxane A_2. However, the four trials that have investigated their use have not shown any reduction in pre-eclampsia [A].

Improvements in prediction now allow increased surveillance and possible prophylactic therapies to be targeted. The importance of these tests will escalate if an adequate treatment to prevent pre-eclampsia is established. The promise of angiogenic markers combined with clinical risk factors now provides a realistic strategy to target therapies.[8]

The potential role of oxidative stress in the aetiology of the maternal syndrome of pre-eclampsia has resulted in a number of studies on the supplementation of antioxidant vitamins C and E. However, none of these has shown benefit.

Maternal and fetal assessment

Before any management decisions are made, the first task is to confirm the diagnosis of pre-eclampsia (see above under Screening for pre-eclampsia), in order to ensure that iatrogenic morbidity does not ensue [E].

When women present with hypertension, both the gestational age and the previous pregnancy history are important factors in establishing risk of progression to pre-eclampsia: late-onset hypertension after 37 weeks' gestation rarely results in serious morbidity to mother or baby [D], but prophylactic delivery may be justified as maturity is likely and induction of labour does not result in increased risk of caeserean section [A]. However, hypertension that presents early, particularly before 28 weeks, will result in pre-eclampsia developing in almost half of women.

Care in assessing blood pressure will prevent misdiagnosis; blood pressure measurement is poorly performed in clinical practice, for example digit preference (the practice of rounding the final digit of the blood pressure to 0) occurs in more than 80 per cent of antenatal measurements. The antenatal population within the UK has a significant proportion of obese women. The standard bladder used in sphygmomanometer cuffs (23 × 12 cm) undercuffs about a quarter of the antenatal population, resulting in the overdiagnosis of hypertension, usually by more than 10 mmHg. Overcuffing underestimates measurements, but usually by less than 5 mmHg, and is preferable in cases of doubt. Keeping the rate of deflation during measurement to 2–3 mm/s will prevent overdiagnosing diastolic hypertension. A similar effect is achieved by using Korotkoff 5; fewer women will be diagnosed as hypertensive than when Korotkoff 4 is used. Korotkoff 4 is also less reproducible [C], and RCTs have confirmed that all healthcare providers should be using Korotkoff 5 when measuring blood pressure in pregnancy [B]. Repeating the blood pressure, or obtaining a series of readings in the day unit, will limit the overdiagnosis of hypertension [E].

Errors in the interpretation of proteinuria are also common with dipstick urine analysis, and 24-hour collections of urine are necessary to confirm the diagnosis [E]. More than 300 mg in 24 hours is considered abnormal. Newer automated devices that can be used by the bedside relate the proteinuria to creatinine, and closely equate to 24-hour collections. The point-of-care test for albumin:creatinine ratio has an overall sensitivity of 97 per cent, a specificity of 98 per cent, a positive predictive value of 92 per cent and a negative predictive value of 99 per cent, which is equally effective regardless of the time of testing.

Every effort should be made to identify women at risk of life-threatening complications. Most women who present with eclampsia will not have had a recent blood pressure or urine analysis that was sufficiently abnormal to have identified them as at risk. Only just over half of women who presented with eclampsia had had prior hypertension and proteinuria diagnosed together. Blood pressure and proteinuria cannot be relied upon alone. The syndrome of pre-eclampsia is multisystemic and it is the ease of measurements of hypertension and proteinuria that has led to their adoption in the diagnosis of pre-eclampsia. Other organ involvement must be considered, such as fetal involvement, or other signs, such as epigastric tenderness. For pragmatic reasons, other signs have not been introduced to define the disease, but they are equally important.

Management remote from term

Early onset pre-eclampsia is frequently associated with placental insufficiency, which can result in IUGR, abruption of the placenta and fetal death [C]. Fetal wellbeing must be carefully considered in all cases. A symphyseal–fundal height should be carefully measured in all women who present with pre-eclampsia, in addition to an enquiry as to fetal movements [E]. At early gestations, or in pregnancies with suspected IUGR, it is usual to confirm fetal growth with ultrasound, and to assess the amniotic fluid volume and umbilical artery Doppler waveform [E]. Suspected fetal compromise is a frequent cause for delivery in pre-eclampsia.

Involvement of other organ systems in the affected women must be sought.

- Platelets are consumed due to the endothelial activation. A platelet count $>50 \times 10^9$/L is likely to support normal haemostasis [E]; however, a falling platelet count, particularly to $<100 \times 10^9$/L, may indicate a need to consider delivery [E].
- Hypovolaemia results in an increased haematocrit and the haemoglobin may also be raised.
- If delivery or induction of labour is likely to be imminent, or if the platelet count is low, it is also sensible to screen for clotting abnormalities [E]. Pre-eclampsia can cause disseminated intravascular coagulation, and clotting must be adequate for regional anaesthesia.
- Uric acid, a measure of fine renal tubular function, is used to assess the disease severity, although severe disease can still occur with a normal uric acid level. Spuriously high levels of uric acid are associated with acute fatty liver of pregnancy.
- Raised urea and creatinine are associated with late renal involvement, but are not useful as an early indicator of disease severity (serial measurements may identify renal disease progression) [E].
- Pre-eclampsia can cause subcapsular haematoma, liver rupture and hepatic infarction, and liver transaminases should be measured. Aspartate transaminase (AST) and other transaminases indicate hepatocellular damage, and elevated levels may again indicate a need to consider delivery. It should be remembered that the normal range for transaminases is approximately 20 per cent lower than the non-pregnant range [C].

When liver involvement is associated with haemolysis and low platelets, this is known as HELLP (haemolysis, elevated liver enzymes and low platelet count) syndrome, which is a severe variant of pre-eclampsia. If proteinuria excretion is high (usually >3 g/24 hours), circulating albumin may fall, increasing the risk of pulmonary oedema. A raised AST can be associated with either haemolysis or liver involvement; lactate dehydrogenase levels are also elevated in the presence of haemolysis.

More recently it has been demonstrated that PlGF can be used in women with suspected disease to accurately determine who will require delivery in the short term (Chappell circulation).[11]

Corticosteroids should be given to enhance fetal lung maturity and are safe in pre-eclampsia [D]. Steroid therapy may assist in the recovery from the HELLP syndrome and has been used in the postpartum period. It is not unusual to see a slight improvement in biochemical parameters in the ante-natal period associated with corticosteroid use [D].

The treatment of moderate hypertension may be detrimental to fetal growth [D].[12] However, severe hypertension should be avoided, and blood pressures >150/110 mmHg require urgent therapy (see below) [E].[13]

In women with an established diagnosis of pre-eclampsia, delivery should be considered once fetal lung maturity is likely (approximately 32 weeks' gestation), particularly if either maternal multi-organ involvement or fetal compromise is apparent. However, women with pre-eclampsia presenting between 28 and 32 weeks can often be managed conservatively without substantial risk to the mother, as long as close inpatient supervision is maintained [E]. In such cases, conservative management reduces neonatal morbidity without significantly increasing maternal morbidity.

Maternal indications for delivery include an inability to control hypertension, deteriorating liver or renal function, a progressive fall in platelets or neurological complications. A non-reactive CTG with decelerations or a fetal condition that is clearly deteriorating often warrants delivery. It is now recognised that delivery at 37 weeks improves outcomes without detrimental effects on mode of delivery and the American College of Obstetricians and Gynaecologists recommends routine delivery even in women with hypertension without an established diagnosis of pre-eclampsia.[14]

Labour ward management of pre-eclampsia

A set protocol should be followed when a woman has severe pre-eclampsia [E].[13] All staff working on the labour ward must be familiar with the protocol in use. Typical entry criteria for such a protocol would be:

- eclampsia, or
- severe hypertension (>160/110 mmHg) with + or >1 g/24 hours proteinuria, or
- hypertension (>140/90 mmHg) with ++ or >3 g/24 hours proteinuria with an additional complication such as headache, visual disturbance, epigastric pain, clonus (more than three beats) or a platelet count <100 × 10⁹/L or AST >50 IU/L.

The two main reasons why women die, as demonstrated by the Confidential Enquiry, are cerebral haemorrhage and adult or acute respiratory distress syndrome,[1] and the two most important aetiological factors for these are severe hypertension and excess fluid intake. Control of blood pressure and fluid balance is therefore crucial.

Intrapartum blood pressure control

Blood pressure should be measured frequently (every 15 minutes) [E]. To facilitate this, automated sphygmomanometers may be used, but these oscillometric devices under-read the blood pressure in pre-eclampsia. Large changes in blood pressure should therefore be confirmed with a mercury sphygmomanometer [E].

As intracerebral haemorrhage complicates a significant proportion of deaths, mean arterial pressures (MAPs) are used to guide management, and most protocols recommend the instigation of IV anti-hypertensive therapy at MAP >125 mmHg [E]. Labetalol is now recommended as first-line treatment [C]. Regimens vary but NICE guidelines now recommend a standard approach to hypertensive management (Viscintin) (Box 26.2).

Box 26.2 NICE hypertension guidelines

- Labetalol: IV bolus of 20 mg if the MAP remains >125 mmHg, followed at 10-minute intervals by 40-, 80-, 80-mg boluses, up to a cumulative dose of 220 mg. Once MAP is <125 mmHg, an infusion of 40 mg/h is commenced, doubling (if necessary) at 30-minute intervals, until a satisfactory response or a dose of 160 mg/h is attained.

- If labetalol is ineffective, hydralazine can be used. Third-line agents include sodium nitroprusside and nifedipine.

Hydralazine: IV bolus of 5 mg if MAP remains >125 mmHg, followed by further boluses of 5 mg up to a cumulative dose of 15 mg. Once the MAP is <125 mmHg, an infusion of 10 mg/h is commenced, doubling (if necessary) at 30-minute intervals, until a satisfactory response or a dose of 40 mg/h is attained.

Colloid should be infused prior to treatment if the baby is undelivered, to protect the uteroplacental circulation and prevent hypotension and fetal distress [E].

Fluid management

As women with pre-eclampsia can have a reduced intravascular volume, leaky capillary membranes and low albumin levels, they are prone to pulmonary oedema. Renal failure is a rare complication of pre-eclampsia that usually follows acute blood loss, when there has been inadequate transfusion, or as a result of profound hypotension. Oliguria without a rising serum urea or creatinine is a manifestation of severe pre-eclampsia and not of incipient renal failure.

Administration of intravenous fluid in response to oliguria must be performed with caution [E].

Most protocols limit fluid intake (in the form of IV crystalloid) to approximately 1 mL/kg per h [E]. A Foley catheter should be inserted and fluid balance recorded.

In a well-perfused women, oliguria (<400 mL/24 h) requires no treatment as such. A low threshold for CVP assessment is recommended; in the absence of invasive monitoring, repetitive fluid challenges are to be avoided. If the CVP is high (>8 mmHg) with persistent oliguria, a dopamine infusion can be considered (1 µg/kg per min) [E]. If the creatinine or potassium rises, haemodialysis or haemofiltration may be necessary, and the advice of a renal physician should be sought. The administration of diuretics temporarily improves urine output, but further decreases the circulating volume and exacerbates electrolyte disturbances; furosemide should be given only if there are signs of pulmonary oedema [E]. In particularly difficult cases, pulmonary artery catheterisation should be considered.

Anticonvulsant therapy

Magnesium sulphate (up to 8 g) can be used to control an eclamptic fit. Alternatively, diazepam (10 mg) can be used [E], although its depressive properties are longer lasting than the anticonvulsant properties. An eclamptic fit is usually self-limiting, and prolonged fitting warrants a brain scan to rule out other pathology, such as an intracerebral bleed [E].

If an eclamptic fit occurs, magnesium sulphate is the prophylaxis of choice, as demonstrated by the Eclampsia Trial [B].[15] In addition to reducing the incidence of further fits, the benefits of magnesium sulphate over both diazepam and phenytoin include a significantly lower need for maternal ventilation, less pneumonia and fewer intensive care admissions. Magnesium sulphate acts as a membrane stabiliser and vasodilator and reduces intracerebral ischaemia. It is usually given as a 2 g IV loading dose and a maintenance infusion at 1–2 g/h. In cases of oliguria, care must be taken, as magnesium sulphate is renally excreted. Toxicity is detected by the absence of patellar reflexes, but ultimately respiratory arrest and muscle paralysis or cardiac arrest will occur. The antidote is 10 mL of 10 per cent calcium gluconate.

Even with severe pre-eclampsia, eclamptic fits are rare (<1 per cent). However, the Magpie Trial evaluated magnesium sulphate versus placebo in women with pre-eclampsia and demonstrated a clear benefit of prophylactic therapy [A]. Magnesium sulphate halved the risk of eclampsia and probably reduced the risk of maternal death. There did not appear to be any substantive harmful short-term effects to either the mother or baby.[15,16] Magnesium sulphate also reduces the risk of cerebral palsy in the fetus and is recommended for this reason alone in all premature deliveries prior to 32 weeks. The mother should receive the medication as per normal pre-eclamptic protocols.[17]

Anaesthesia

A general anaesthetic can be dangerous, as endotracheal intubation can cause severe hypertension. Regional blockade is the preferred method of analgesia for labour and of anaesthesia for operative deliveries [E], but a coagulopathy must be excluded. Platelet levels of $<80 \times 10^9$/L should ensure haemostasis, and most obstetric anaesthetists will insert a regional block under these circumstances. Care must be taken to avoid arterial hypotension (particularly following postpartum haemorrhage) in view of the vasoconstriction and reduced intravascular volume. A low threshold for central invasive monitoring is necessary in women who require a caesarean section [E].

Postpartum care

As a third of eclamptic fits occur postpartum, intensive monitoring is required, usually for 48 hours after delivery. Although eclampsia has been reported beyond this time, it is unlikely to be associated with serious morbidity. Blood pressure is frequently at its highest 3–4 days after delivery. Antihypertensive therapy may therefore need to be continued after discharge home; in the absence of fetal considerations, the most effective therapy can be used – and drugs such as methyl-dopa discontinued.

All women who have suffered severe pre-eclampsia should be reviewed at a hospital postnatal clinic 6–12 weeks after delivery [E]. In addition to blood pressure and urine testing, tests of renal and liver function should be instigated; residual disease may merit referral to a physician. Underlying predispositions to pre-eclampsia, such as an inherited thrombophilia or APS, should be excluded (multiparous women are more likely to have an underlying cause). The postnatal visit is also an excellent opportunity to discuss complications of the pregnancy and the planned management of any future pregnancy.

FUTURE CARDIOVASCULAR RISK

Women with pre-eclampsia have a four-fold increased risk of developing hypertension and nearly a two-fold increased risk of ischaemic heart disease, stroke and venous thromboembolism, even up to 14 years after the index pregnancy. Women who have early pre-eclampsia are at highest risk.[15] This reflects a possible common aetiology or a long-term effect on disease development and highlights the possible need for earlier cardiovascular risk assessment and the commencement of preventive therapies at an earlier age. It is plausible that active assessment of cardiovascular risk up to 6 months postpartum may lead to earlier identification of cardiovascular risk and the potential for lifestyle modification.[18]

KEY POINTS

- Pre-eclampsia is a multisystem disorder involving the placenta, liver, kidneys, blood, and neurological and cardiovascular systems; hypertension and proteinuria are diagnostic signs.
- Both maternal and fetal morbidity and mortality are more likely to occur with early onset disease.
- Despite the many tests being investigated, pre-eclampsia cannot be accurately predicted. An abnormal uterine artery Doppler at 20 weeks will increase risk approximately six-fold in both high- and low-risk women.
- Cerebral haemorrhage and adult respiratory distress are common causes of death in pre-eclampsia; therefore acute management focuses on controlling blood pressure and restricting fluid intake.
- The use of anti hypertensive therapy in moderately hypertensive women demonstrates a significant reduction in severe hypertension only; there are no other proven additional benefits.
- Low-dose aspirin in pregnancy results in a small (10 per cent) but significant reduction in pre-eclampsia; there is an associated reduction in preterm delivery.
- Magnesium sulphate is the anticonvulsant of choice following an eclamptic fit, resulting in fewer fits and less maternal morbidity compared with diazepam and phenytoin. There is also a clear benefit to prophylactic magnesium sulphate therapy – the risk of eclampsia is halved, and the fetus may have a lower risk of cerebral palsy.

Key References

1. Shennan AH, Redman C, Cooper C, Milne F. Are most maternal deaths from pre-eclampsia avoidable? *Lancet* 2012;379:1686–7.

2. Knight M. Eclampsia in the United Kingdom 2005. *BJOG* 2007;114:1072–8.

3. Barker DJP, Bull AR, Osmond C. Fetal and placental size and risk of hypertension in adult life. *BMJ* 1990;301:259–61.

4. Davey DA, MacGillivray I. The classification and definition of the hypertensive disorders of pregnancy. *Am J Obstet Gynecol* 1988;158:892–8.

5. Higgins JR, Walshe JJ, Halligan A *et al.* Can 24-hour ambulatory blood pressure measurement predict the development of hypertension in primigravidae? *Br J Obstet Gynaecol* 1997;104:356–62.

6. Brosens IA. Morphological changes in the uteroplacental bed in pregnancy hypertension. *Clin Obstet Gynecol* 1977;77:573–93.

7. Roberts JM, Taylor RN, Musci TJ *et al.* Pre-eclampsia: an endothelial cell disorder. *Am J Obstet Gynecol* 1989;161:1200–4.

8. Myers JE, Kenny LC, McCowan, LME *et al.* Angiogenic factors combined with clinical risk factors to predict preterm pre-eclampsia in nulliparous women: a predictive test accuracy study. *BJOG* 2011;120:1215–23.

9. Askie LM, Duley L, Henderson-Smart D *et al.* Antiplatelet agents for prevention of pre-eclampsia: a meta-analysis of individual patient data. *Lancet* 2007;369:1791–8.

10. Hofmeyr GJ, Duley L, Atallah A. Dietary calcium supplementation for prevention of pre-eclampsia and related problems: a systematic review and commentary. *BJOG* 2007;114:933–43.

11. Chappell LC, Duckworth S, Seed PT *et al.* Diagnostic accuracy of placental growth factor in women with suspected pre-eclampsia: a prospective multicenter study. *Circulation* 2013;128:2121–31.

12. Von Dadelszen P, Ornstein MP, Bull SB *et al.* Fall in mean arterial pressure and fetal growth restriction in pregnancy hypertension: a meta-analysis. *Lancet* 2000;355:87–92.

13. Visintin C, Mugglestone MA, Almerie MQ, Nherera LM, James D, Walkinshaw S; GuidelineDevelopment Group. Management of hypertensive disorders during pregnancy: summary of NICE guidance. *BMJ* 2010;341:c2207.

14. Hypertension in pregnancy. Report of the American College of Obstetricians and Gynecologists' Task Force on Hypertension in Pregnancy. *Obstet Gynecol* 2013, 122:1122–31.9.

15. Which anticonvulsant for women with eclampsia? Evidence from the Collaborative Eclampsia Trial. *Lancet* 1995;345:1455–63.

16. The Magpie Collaborative Group. Do women with pre-eclampsia, and their babies, benefit from magnesium sulphate? The Magpie Trial: a randomised placebo-controlled trial. *Lancet* 2002;359:1877–90.

17. Bellamy L, Casas JP, Hingorami AD, Williams DJ. Pre-eclampsia and risk of cardiovascular disease and cancer in later life: systematic review and meta-analysis. *BMJ* 2007;335:974. Doyle LW, Crowther CA, Middleton P, Marret S, Rouse D: Magnesium sulphate for women at risk of preterm birth for neuroprotection of the fetus. *Cochrane Database Syst Rev* 2009;1:CD004661.

18. Magee L, von Dadelszen P. Pre-eclampsia and increased cardiovascular risk. *BMJ* 2007;335:945–6.

Chapter 27 Medication in pregnancy

Clare L Tower

MRCOG standards

There is no specific established standard for this topic, but we would suggest the following points for guidance. A good understanding of prescribing principles is necessary as this has relevance to the large majority of core modules.

INTRODUCTION

As around a third of pregnancies are unplanned, pregnant women conceive while taking a wide variety of both prescription and over-the-counter medications. It is reported that approximately 50 per cent of women will take medication during pregnancy.[1] Many pregnant women require medication for specific pregnancy- and non-pregnancy-related conditions. Therefore, a broad understanding of the impact of pregnancy on drug pharmacokinetics (drug handling) and pharmacodynamics (drug actions) is required. Furthermore, the large majority of drugs cross the placenta, and some drugs have significant fetal effects. For this reason, most drugs are not licensed for use in pregnancy, thus prescribing in pregnancy often lies outside licensed indications. A detailed discussion of all drugs is beyond the scope of this book. Therefore, this chapter will review the general principles and provide examples. A detailed discussion of prescribing for particular disorders during pregnancy can be found in the relevant sections of this book.

PRE-CONCEPTION COUNSELLING

Encountering women of reproductive age with significant medical problems, for which they are taking prescribed medications, is becoming increasingly common. It is beneficial for many of these women to be seen pre-conceptually for several reasons. First, it allows optimisation of therapy such that pregnancy can be commenced with the lowest achievable risks. Typical examples of this include optimisation of glycaemic control in diabetic women and the prescription of high-dose (5 mg) folic acid to women at particular risk, such as those with epilepsy. Second it allows drugs with potentially

teratogenic effects to be changed to a safer alternative. There is also the opportunity to discuss particular risks and concerns, of both the medical problem itself and the medications that will be prescribed during pregnancy. Pregnant women often worry about the effects of medications on an unborn baby, and it is usual for them to put the unborn baby's needs above their own. Thus, women may suddenly stop drugs in early pregnancy that may have a significant impact on their own health. Discussions in the pre-conception period will prevent such non-compliance in early pregnancy of important medications, such as antiepileptics or immunosuppressants.

EFFECTS OF PREGNANCY ON PHARMACOKINETICS AND PHARMACODYNAMICS

Absorption

Pregnancy is associated with a reduction in gastric motility and an increase in gastric pH, but studies have demonstrated that pregnancy has no measurable affect on drug bioavailability via these mechanisms.[2] Nausea and vomiting are probably of more importance in reducing drug absorption during pregnancy.[3]

Distribution

The volume of distribution is defined as the volume in which an amount of drug would need to be distributed to produce a particular blood concentration. Therefore, for drugs that are highly bound in the tissues, e.g. basic drugs such as amphetamines, the volume of distribution is large but the plasma concentration is low. For acidic drugs, such as warfarin, which are highly protein bound, the volume of distribution is relatively low, but the plasma concentration high. Therefore, volume of distribution is dependent upon plasma volume, tissue volume, and the amount of binding of a drug in the tissues and in plasma proteins. Pregnancy causes an increase in plasma volume that reaches a peak of 50 per cent at around 32 weeks' gestation. In addition, the concentrations of the two main drug-binding proteins, albumin and α_1-acid glycoprotein, fall during pregnancy to around 70–80 per cent of pre-pregnancy levels by term. Therefore, pregnancy results in an increase in volume of distribution (due to increased plasma volume) and an increase in the fraction of a drug that is unbound, or active, in the plasma (due to a fall in plasma proteins). Thus, measurements of total drug concentration, which are used for medications such as phenytoin and sodium valproate, underestimate the corresponding unbound or active concentrations. This may result in prescribing higher doses than necessary, which is particularly important as the teratogenicity of both these drugs is reported in registries to be dose dependent [D]. Thus, measurement of unbound concentrations should be used wherever possible. This is of particular relevance to drugs with a narrow therapeutic window.

Metabolism

Following oral ingestion, drugs are absorbed by the gut and undergo first-pass metabolism in the liver by numerous enzymes. Although the liver smooth endoplasmic reticulum is the main site of enzymatic metabolism, virtually all cells have the ability to metabolise drugs to some degree, with other main sites being the epithelial cells of the gut, kidney, lung and skin. There are many enzymes involved and their activity is modified by pregnancy. Furthermore, there may be an increase in hepatic blood flow in pregnancy.[4]

The cytochrome P450 (CYP) system is a major enzymatic system involved in drug metabolism, of which there are now 57 human genes and 59 pseudogenes described, divided into 18 classes. Not only does pregnancy alter the activity of these enzymes, but it also varies with gestation, drug interactions (e.g. enzyme inducers) and genotype. Different genotypes at CYP loci result in an individual being a poor metaboliser or an extensive metaboliser for a particular enzyme. The uridine 5'-diphosphate glucuronosyltransferase (UGT) is a further enzyme system demonstrating modification during pregnancy. Changes in drug metabolism can have a significant effect on active drug levels. Enzymes demonstrating increased activity will result in reduced plasma levels of a drug, requiring an increase in dose, and vice versa. Thus, variation of drug metabolism with pregnancy is complex and, although the

majority of enzymes increase in activity, some decrease. The overall effect is further compounded by genetic variation and the effect of plasma volume and plasma proteins described above. Table 27.1 illustrates this with examples of drugs in which variation in metabolism is observed. This should be considered when prescribing in pregnancy and, since there are so many unknown factors, clinicians must be guided by the overall clinical affect of a drug.

Renal clearance

Pregnancy causes an increase in renal blood flow and glomerular filtration rate of more than 50 per cent, which can have a significant effect on drugs that are predominantly excreted by the kidneys. Thus, the clearance of β-lactam antibiotics such as penicillins and cephalosporins is increased during pregnancy [C]. Although there may be lower plasma levels as a result, levels in urine may be higher, which may be a desired effect for treating UTIs. LMWHs, such as dalteparin and enoxaparin, also demonstrate increased renal clearance during pregnancy, which may require dose adjustments [C].[5] Thus, a 20–65 per cent increase in dose for drugs that are renally excreted may be needed to maintain therapeutic levels [E].[4]

Drug transfer across the placenta

The majority of drugs are able to cross the placenta to the fetus to some degree, and there are very few that demonstrate no placental transfer. Transfer of drugs across the placenta can occur by passive transfer, active transport, facilitated diffusion, phagocytosis and pinocytosis.[6] By far the commonest method is passive diffusion, or movement of a molecule down a concentration gradient, and this is determined by the lipid solubility, polarity and molecular mass of the drug. Therefore, small, unionised lipid-soluble drugs are able to cross at the fastest rate. This can be influenced by the degree of plasma protein binding, and by placental metabolism. Drugs with a molecular mass <500 daltons (DA), which is the large majority, are able to cross the placenta by passive diffusion. Heparin (both unfractionated and low molecular weight) is

Table 27.1. Examples of modification of enzyme activity with pregnancy[4]

Enzyme	Change	Drug	Effect
CYP1A2	↓	Caffeine, clozapine, olanzapine	Increased half-life, increased unbound and active drug
CYP2A6	↑	Nicotine	Lower levels
CYP2C9	↑	Phenytoin, losartan, NSAIDs	Reduced levels
CYP2C19	↓	Proguanil, PPIs	Higher plasma levels
CYP2D6	↑	>40 drugs, e.g. β blockers, SSRIs, anti-arrhythmics	Reduced levels
CYP3A4	Variable	>50% drugs, e.g. nifedipine	Variable effects
UGT	↑↑	Lamotrigine, zidovudine, morphine	Increased clearance, thus reduced levels

● PPIs, proton-pump inhibitors such as omeprazole; SSRIs, selective serotonin reuptake inhibitors such as fluoxetine.

the most well-known drug that is unable to cross the placenta due to its high molecular mass of between 3000 and 5000 Da, depending on the preparation.

Whilst it is generally considered that facilitated diffusion, phagocytosis and pinocytosis play little significant role in drug transfer, there is growing interest in placental active transport, utilising energy-requiring drug transporters. Energy is usually derived from adenosine triphosphate (ATP), or from electrochemical gradients. All these transporters work against a concentration gradient, and several have now been described within the placenta. These include: P-glycoprotein (multidrug-resistant gene *MDR-1* product) that is able to transport digoxin and dexamethasone; MDR proteins 1–3, able to transport methotrexate and ampicillin; and the monocarboxylate and sodium/multivitamin transporters, able to transport valproate and carbamazepine.[7]

Placental drug metabolism

There is growing evidence that the placenta expresses many of the enzymes able to metabolise drugs. These include many of the CYP enzymes, UGT, glutathione *S*-transferase and sulphotransferases. The study of the clinical effects of many of these enzymes is in its infancy. However, it is known that for some enzymes it varies with gestation, and the activity of many is altered by alcohol and cigarette smoking. Drugs that undergo metabolism in the placenta include steroids, such as dexamethasone, and alcohol.[6]

A better understanding of placental transfer and metabolism of individual drugs may help in the development of fetal therapy. For example, transplacental passage of anti-arrhythmic drugs has been used to treat fetal supraventricular tachycardias since the first report in 1980.[8] The success rate of monotherapy is of the order of 50 per cent.[9]

Transfer of digoxin across the placenta is complex, involving both passive diffusion and active transport via P-glycoprotein. Co-administration of other antiarrhythmic drugs has been suggested to improve success by modifying P-glycoprotein transport of digoxin.[6]

Teratogenicity

A teratogen is an agent that is able to permanently alter the development, growth, structure or function of a developing embryo or fetus. The effect of drugs in the pre-implantation period (fertilisation to implantation) is often considered to be an 'all-or-nothing' phenomenon.[10] In other words, a drug will result in injury to a large number of cells, causing complete loss, or only a few cells are affected and the remaining cells can compensate at this early stage, resulting in no malformation. The period of organogenesis (embryonic phase, weeks 2–8 post-conception) is the most critical. Within this period, each structure has a period of maximal vulnerability and, usually, the earlier the insult the more severe the resulting malformation. Some structures that have initially formed during embryogenesis are still vulnerable to effects in the fetal period of development (9 weeks to term). For example,

failure of neural tube closure arises during days 17–30 post-fertilisation to cause anencephaly and neural tube defects, but encephaloceles have also been described post-closure during the fetal period.[10] Drugs that have an effect in this period are described as fetotoxic. Unfortunately, the teratogenicity of most drugs is established only after initial drug licensing, as pregnant women are excluded from human trials of new drugs. The classic and most famous example of this is thalidomide, which was introduced as an antiemetic in the 1950s and was subsequently withdrawn when it was found to cause phocomelia. Determining whether a particular drug is teratogenic is difficult, as there is a background population risk of major malformations of around 2 per cent, and data rely on retrospective reporting rather than robust RCTs.[1] This is particularly true for newer medications where data availability is limited.[11]

Lactation

The principles of drug transfer from the maternal circulation into breast milk are the same as those across any membrane, and thus will depend on the lipophilic properties, degree of ionisation and plasma protein binding of the drug. The amount of drug that the infant is exposed to will be dependent upon volume of milk ingested, maternal plasma levels and infant excretion (which probably varies with age, and is less with increasing immaturity). Plasma protein binding has been shown to have a significant impact on levels in breast milk. Drugs that are highly protein bound result in less infant exposure via breast milk. Measurable infant levels were found only for drugs with less than 70 per cent plasma protein binding.[4] Unfortunately, there are very few good data available on the drug exposure to infants via breast milk for the large majority of drugs, thus a risk–benefit analysis must be conducted on an individual basis. However, there are very few drugs for which breastfeeding is contraindicated.[10] In general terms, the lowest effective dose should be used and, if there are concerns (or if there are no data about a drug), timing breastfeeds to avoid times of peak maternal plasma levels should be recommended [E].

Specific drug considerations in pregnancy

Prescribing during pregnancy requires careful consideration of the risks and benefits, in discussion with the woman herself. In general, use of the lowest number of drugs (monotherapy where possible) and the lowest effective dose are recommended, remembering the effects of pregnancy on plasma levels of a drug [E]. For some drugs, e.g. lithium and lamotrigine, therapeutic drug monitoring is recommended.[3] Table 27.2 shows examples of the key considerations, applying the above principles, for particular drug classes during pregnancy and lactation. For obvious reasons, this is in no way exhaustive and more detailed discussions can be found in the literature referenced at the end of this chapter, or in the relevant sections of this book.

Table 27.2 Examples of drug-prescribing considerations during pregnancy

Drug	Pre-conception	Effects of pregnancy	Fetal considerations	Lactation
Cardiovascular system				
ACE inhibitors, ARBs	Should be changed to alternative if possible	Avoid – use only if no alternative with fetal monitoring of growth and liquor volume; stop if oligohydramnios [D, E]	Teratogenic in first trimester; renal and cardiac problems in late gestation [D, E]	Considered compatible
Antihypertensives	Optimise blood pressure control	Nifedipine may demonstrate increased clearance in third trimester [D, E]	Beta blockers associated with fetal growth restriction (less so with labetalol); IV doses should be given with fetal monitoring	Present in breast milk (except nifedipine, which is >90% protein bound); infants reported normotensive, so considered safe
Statins	–	–	Usually stop as may adversely affect placental development; studies ongoing	Considered compatible
Antibiotics				
Penicillins/ cephalosporins	–	Increased renal excretion, lower plasma levels	Cross placenta, considered safe	Small amounts in breast milk; safe
Tetracyclines	–	–	Increased risk of NTD, cleft palate and cardiovascular effects (not doxycycline); tooth discoloration [D, E]	Found in breast milk; concerns about effects on teeth
Ciprofloxacin	–	–	Only small amounts cross placenta but has been associated with bone/ cartilage problems; however, few data	Concentrated in breast milk; neonatal *Clostridium difficile* has been reported [D]
Analgesics				
Paracetamol	–	–	Safe	Safe
NSAIDs	–	–	Premature closure of ductus and kidney dysfunction >32 weeks [A]	Considered safe
Codeine	–	–	Has been inconsistently associated with respiratory tract malformations but considered safe for short-term use; may cause neonatal withdrawal	MHRA advise avoidance as may cause high levels of morphine in fast metabolisers, thus risk of cardiorespiratory depression in neonates [E]
Opiates	–	–	No major effects known, fetal dependence and withdrawal [D]	May improve fetal withdrawal symptoms; similar concerns regarding metabolism as for codeine but not subject to MHRA advice at time of writing [D]

(continued)

Table 27.2 Examples of drug-prescribing considerations during pregnancy (*continued*)

Drug	Pre-conception	Effects of pregnancy	Fetal considerations	Lactation
Gabapentin/ Pregabalin	–	–	UKTIS state no increased risk for gagapentin but limited data; pregabalin has shown teratogenicity and fetotoxicity at high doses in animals	Gabapentin present in breast milk, effects unknown; no data for Pregabalin so advise avoidance
Immunosuppressants				
Steroids	–	Usual maternal side effects; risk–benefit analysis to continuing treatment	Weak association with cleft lip; placenta metabolises 90% of prednisolone; association with reduced fetal weight [C]	Unknown levels in breast milk, but usually considered safe
Azathioprine	Counsel safe [D, E]	Considered safe [D, E]	Fetal liver lacks enzyme to convert to active metabolite (6-mercaptopurine)	Low concentrations of metabolites in breast milk; however, theoretically cause immunosuppression, thus usually not recommended for breastfeeding [E]
Cyclosporin	Counsel safe [D, E]	Counsel safe [D, E]	Increased risks of fetal growth restriction [D, E]	As above
Hydroxychloroquine	Counsel safe [D, E]	Counsel safe [D, E]	Counsel safe	Limited data but no reports of adverse effects; consider safe
Psychiatric drugs				
SSRIs	Consider changing to ones with lowest association with abnormalities (i.e. change from paroxetine); discuss risks and benefits	May require increased dose [D, E]	Paroxetine and sertraline associated with teratogenicity, such as cardiac defects, omphalocele (risk low approx. 2/1000); fluoxetine crosses placenta but not considered a teratogen [D, E]	Present in breast milk; avoid feeding at times of peak plasma levels; sertraline SSRI of choice[1] [E]
Lithium	Risk–benefit analysis involving psychiatrist	Risk–benefit analysis involving psychiatrist; some suggest reducing/stopping just prior to delivery [D, E]	Cardiovascular malformations, floppy infant, neonatal arrhythmias, hypoglycaemia, thyroid dysfunction [D]	Found in breast milk; breastfeeding generally avoided as neonatal clearance slower than adult [E]
Tricyclic antidepressants	Consider safe	Risk–benefit analysis	May cause neonatal withdrawal, possible risk of miscarriage and growth restriction; not associated with malformations	Probably safe

ANTENATAL OBSTETRICS

Drug	Pre-conception	Effects of pregnancy	Fetal considerations	Lactation
Diazepam	Risk–benefit analysis involving psychiatrist; do not stop abruptly	Risk–benefit analysis involving psychiatrist; do not stop abruptly	Possible association with orofacial clefts and cardiovascular malformations; neonatal withdrawal, respiratory depression and 'floppy infant' syndrome [D]	Excreted in breast milk; causes sedation, lethargy; advise avoid [E]
Antiepileptics				
Sodium valproate	Optimise treatment on lowest dose; avoid if possible	Total concentrations fall, but more so than the unbound concentrations; as teratogenicity is dose dependent, need to measure unbound levels [D, E]	Teratogen that is rapidly transported to fetus; associated with 'valproate syndrome', developmental delay [D, E]	Enters breast milk; neonatal serum levels <10% of maternal levels [D, E]
Carbamazepine	Obtain control on lowest dose possible		Associated with facial dysmorphism, developmental delay, NTD, phalanx and nail hypoplasia [D, E]	Probably safe in breastfeeding [D, E]
Phenytoin	Obtain control on lowest dose possible	Total concentrations fall, but more so than the unbound concentrations; as teratogenicity is dose dependent, need to measure unbound levels [D, E]	Associated with congenital heart defects and cleft palate [D, E]	Low transfer in breast milk; considered safe [D, E]
Lamotrigine	Obtain control on lowest dose possible	Increased clearance due to increased UGT activity [D, E]	Crosses placenta, limited data as newer drug [D, E]	Low transfer in breast milk, therefore considered safe [D, E]
Anticoagulants				
Warfarin	Discuss risks, and make plan for pregnancy; depends on indication for anticoagulation	Depends on reason for use: in general, avoid use at period of greatest teratogenicity and after 36 weeks; may be safe to use heparin as alternative throughout pregnancy, but for women with metal valves this may not provide sufficient anticoagulation [E]	Teratogen; exposure between 6 and 10 weeks associated with embryopathy; higher dose (>5 mg/day) associated with higher fetal risk [D, E]	Does not enter breast milk as highly protein bound [D]
Heparin	Reassure safe in pregnancy	Safe in pregnancy; increased renal clearance, may require increased dose; monitoring of factor Xa levels if therapeutic (rather than prophylaxis is required) [D, E]	Does not cross placenta due to molecular size	Safe in breastfeeding

- ACE, angiotensin-converting enzyme; ARB, angiotensin type 1 receptor blocker; MHRA, Medicines and Healthcare products Regulatory Agency; NTD, neural tube defect; SSRIs, selective serotonin reuptake inhibitors; UKTIS, UK Teratology Information Service.

ANTENATAL OBSTETRICS

KEY POINTS

- Pre-conception counselling offers an opportunity to optimise drug therapy, change medications with teratogenic potential and discuss compliance of important medications.
- Absorption of drugs is not significantly altered by pregnancy.
- Pregnancy is associated with increased plasma volume and reduced levels of plasma-binding proteins, which results in an increased unbound, or active, drug concentration.
- Pregnancy alters the activity of many of the enzymes involved in drug metabolism. Effects vary with enzyme, gestation, genotype and other prescribed drugs, and thus are often difficult to predict.
- Renal clearance of drugs increases during pregnancy, resulting in lower plasma levels of drugs that are predominantly excreted via this route.
- Drugs cross the placenta predominantly by passive diffusion and there is growing interest in the active transporters. Thus, small, lipid-soluble, non-ionised drugs cross at the highest rate.
- The embryonic period of human gestation (weeks 2–8 post-fertilisation) is the period of greatest vulnerability to the teratogenic effect of drugs.
- Transfer of drugs into breast milk is determined by lipophilic properties of a drug, molecular size and polarity. Highly plasma-bound drugs (>70%) do not cross into breast milk.
- In general, drugs in pregnancy and breastfeeding should be used at the lowest effective dose, using the lowest number of drugs (monotherapy where possible).

Key References

1. Henderson E, Mackillop L. Prescribing in pregnancy and during breastfeeding: using principles in clinical practice. *Postgrad Med J* 2011;87:349–54.
2. Loebstein R, Lalkin A, Koren G. Pharmacokinetic changes during pregnancy and their clinical relevance. *Clin Pharmacokin* 1997;33:328–43.
3. Matsui DM. Therapeutic drug monitoring in pregnancy. *Ther Drug Monit* 2012;34:507–11.
4. Anderson GD. Using pharmacokinetics to predict the effects of pregnancy and maternal–infant transfer of drugs during lactation. *Expert Opin Drug Metab Toxicol* 2006;2:947–60.
5. Ensom MH, Stephenson MD. Pharmacokinetics of low molecular weight heparin and unfractionated heparin in pregnancy. *J Soc Gynecol Investig* 2004;11:377–83.
6. Syme MR, Paxton JW, Keelan JA. Drug transfer and metabolism by the human placenta. *Clin Pharmacokin* 2004;43:487–514.
7. Ganapathy V, Prasad PD, Ganapathy ME, Leibach FH. Placental transporters relevant to drug distribution across the maternal-fetal interface. *J Pharmacol Exp Ther* 2000;294:413–20.
8. Kerenyi T, Gleicher N, Meller J. Transplacental cardioversion of intrauterine supraventricular tachycardia with digitalis. *Lancet* 1980;ii:393–4.
9. Ito S. Transplacental treatment of fetal tachycardia: implications of drug transporting proteins in the placenta. *Semin Perinatol* 2001;25:196–201.
10. Buhimschi CS, Weiner CP. Medications in Pregnancy and Lactation. Part 1. Teratology. *Obstet Gynecol* 2009;113:166–88.
11. Rasmussen SA. Human teratogens update 2011: can we ensure safety during pregnancy? *Birth Defects Res A Clin Mol Teratol* 2012;94:123–8.

Chapter 28 Maternal mortality

James Drife

INTRODUCTION

Maternal death is still common in many parts of the world but has become rare in developed countries. In the UK its infrequency means that when a maternal death does occur it can be a shattering experience for everyone involved. Lessons for prevention are best learned by aggregating cases nationally. The CEMD operated continuously in the UK for over 60 years and their methods have been emulated in many countries across the world. They are now being run by MBRRACE-UK (Mothers and Babies: Reducing Risk Through Audits and Confidential Enquiries –UK), which also undertakes surveillance of infant deaths and maternal and perinatal morbidities.

INCIDENCE

Worldwide

The WHO estimates that in 2010 there were 287,000 maternal deaths –a decline of 47 per cent from levels in 1990 –and that the global maternal mortality rate (MMR) is now 210/100,000 live births, down from 400/100,000.[1] Sub-Saharan Africa and southern Asia accounted for 85 per cent of the global burden in 2010, with one-third of the world's maternal deaths occurring in two countries, India and Nigeria. Of the 40 countries that still have an MMR of over 300/100,000, all but four are in sub-Saharan Africa, where 10 per cent of maternal deaths are due to HIV (Fig. 28.1). Elsewhere, MMRs over 300/100,000 are found in Laos, Afghanistan, Haiti and Timor-Trieste. When a high MMR is combined with a high fertility rate, the result is disastrous. In Chad, for example, a girl has a 1 in 15 chance of dying as a result of pregnancy or delivery, and in Afghanistan the chance is 1 in 30.

The UK

In the UK, maternal death occurs in around 1 in 10,000 pregnancies. The MMR rose from 9.9/100,000 pregnancies in 1985–7 to 13.9/100,000 in 2003–5, partly (but not entirely) due to more complete reporting of *indirect* deaths, which now outnumber *direct* deaths[2] (Table 28.1). In 2006–8, however, there was a statistically significant fall in the MMR to 11.39/100,000, and the downward trend included both black African and white ethnicities.

Incomplete reporting of maternal deaths occurs in all countries. Death certificate data are inadequate and if the UK relied only on these, the MMR would be 6.76/100,000 – around 60 per cent of the true rate. Instead, the UK makes strenuous efforts to ascertain as many of the deaths as possible. This has involved computer linkage of birth and death registration, and a long tradition of reporting maternal deaths to the national CEMD. The high ascertainment in the UK makes comparisons with other countries potentially misleading.

Confidential enquiries into maternal deaths

Since 1952, every maternal death in England and Wales has been the subject of a detailed enquiry, conducted by

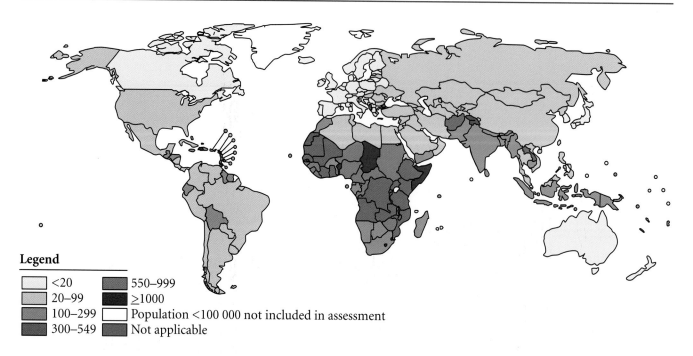

Legend

<20	550–999
20–99	≥1000
100–299	Population <100 000 not included in assessment
300–549	Not applicable

Fig. 28.1 World map of maternal mortality (From the WHO[1])

Table 28.1 Number of maternal deaths notified to the UK Confidential Enquiry

	1994-6	1997-9	2000-2	2003-5	2006-8
Direct	134	106	106	132	107
Indirect	134	136	155	163	154
Coincidental	36	29	36	55	50
Late direct	4	7	4	11	9
Late indirect	32	39	45	71*	24**
Total	340	317	346	432	344

*This increase in late indirect deaths was due to improved ascertainment.

**This reduction was due to a change in data collection: only deaths within 6 months of delivery were included.

clinicians –doctors and, nowadays, midwives. Any death during pregnancy or within a year after delivery is reported to the CEMD, which was initially run by the Ministry of Health and latterly by CMACE. In January 2013 the enquiry became part of MBBRACE-UK (the acronym means 'Mothers and Babies: Reducing Risk through Audits and Confidential Enquiries across the UK'), which is part of the National Perinatal Epidemiology Unit, based in Oxford.[3] The methodology is similar to that used by CMACE. Forms requesting all relevant details are sent to all clinicians involved in the case, and the completed forms are reviewed by national assessors in obstetrics, pathology, midwifery and, if appropriate, anaesthetics, general medicine, intensive care, and psychiatry (Fig. 28.2).

Cases are anonymised, so that those involved can comment frankly and make their own suggestions for improvements, and no blame is attached to individuals. MBRRACE-UK covers England, Scotland and Wales, and a similar system

exists in Northern Ireland. Reports will be published annually. They are UK wide, making the identification of individual cases more difficult, and they make recommendations for improving practice.

DEFINITIONS

The definitions given here are those used by CEMD:

- *Maternal death*: death of a woman while pregnant or within 42 days of termination of pregnancy, from any cause related to or aggravated by the pregnancy or its management, but not from accidental or incidental causes.
- *Direct death*: death resulting from obstetric complications of the pregnant state (pregnancy, labour and puerperium), from interventions, omissions, incorrect treatment or a chain of events resulting from any of the above.

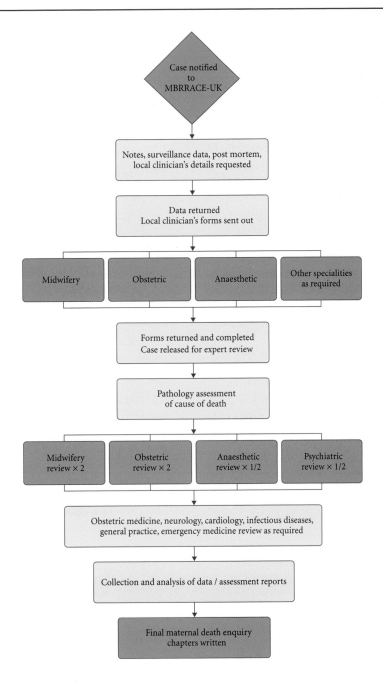

Fig. 28.2 MBRRACE-UK maternal death enquiry[4]

- *Indirect death*: death resulting from previous existing disease or disease that developed during pregnancy and was not due to direct obstetric causes, but was aggravated by the physiological effects of pregnancy.
- *Late death*: death occurring between 42 days and 1 year after abortion, miscarriage or delivery, due to 'direct' or 'indirect' maternal causes.
- *Coincidental death*: death from an unrelated cause which happens to occur in pregnancy or the puerperium.
- *Maternal mortality rate*: this is expressed in the UK as the number of deaths per 100,000 maternities. A 'maternity' is a clinical pregnancy ending in livebirth, stillbirth, miscarriage or abortion.

- The WHO, however, defines the maternal mortality *rate* as 'the number of maternal deaths per 100,000 women of reproductive age', and the maternal mortality *ratio* as 'the number of maternal deaths per 100,000 live births'. Close attention needs to be paid to definitions and denominators.

AETIOLOGY

The causes of maternal mortality are similar all over the world, although overall rates and the relative contribution of each cause vary from country to country.

Worldwide

The leading causes of direct death according to global estimates (Table 28.2) –haemorrhage, hypertensive disorders and sepsis – are largely treatable conditions.[5] The underlying causes in many developing countries include lack of access to contraception, unsafe abortion, lack of primary care or transport facilities, and inadequate equipment and staffing in district hospitals. In 1990 only 55 per cent of deliveries in developing regions were attended by skilled health personnel, but in 2009 this proportion had risen to 65 per cent. There are wide disparities between regions: for example, in eastern Asia, which has experienced the greatest MMR decline, the contraceptive prevalence rate is now 84 per cent, compared with 22 per cent in sub-Saharan Africa, the region with one of the lowest MMR declines.[1]

Education of women is important. In India, the states with high rates of female literacy also have high rates of contraceptive use and low MMRs. In all countries, safer care could be provided to illiterate women if there were the political will to do so.

Table 28.2 Global causes of maternal death[5]

Haemorrhage	22.9%
Hypertensive disorder	18.5%
Abortion	14.5%
Hepatitis	12.5%
Other infectious diseases	12.5%
Sepsis or infection	8.6%
Syphilis	6.2%
Obstructed labour	4.3%

The UK

The specific causes of maternal death in the UK are shown in Table 28.3. The number of direct deaths has changed little in the last 12 years but the number of indirect deaths has steadily increased.

Direct deaths

THROMBOEMBOLISM

This was the leading direct cause of maternal death in the UK from 1985 to 2005, but the number fell dramatically to 18 in 2006–8, the first full triennium after the publication of a new RCOG guideline on thromboprophylaxis. This total was equally divided between antepartum and postpartum deaths. Three occurred before 12 weeks of pregnancy.

HYPERTENSIVE DISEASE

When the Enquiry began in 1952–4, there were 246 deaths from hypertensive disease in England and Wales. In 2006–8 in the UK, the total was 19. The condition is no less common, but care is now better. Of the 19 deaths in 2006–8, 9 were from intracranial haemorrhage.

HAEMORRHAGE

Haemorrhage is treated well in the UK. Out of over 2 million pregnancies in the triennium 2006–8, there were only 9 deaths from this cause. Two were from placenta praevia and two from abruption. Postpartum haemorrhage (PPH) caused five deaths. Two of the cases of PPH involved genital tract tears. Until 2000–2 a separate chapter was devoted to genital tract trauma but the reduction in deaths from this cause made this unnecessary.

Table 28.3 Causes of maternal deaths in the UK 2003-8[2]

Cause	2003-5	2006-8
Direct		
Thromboembolism	41 (19)	18 (6)
Pre-eclampsia/eclampsia/acute fatty liver	19 (9)	22 (14)
Haemorrhage/genital tract trauma	17 (10)	9 (4)
Amniotic fluid embolism	17 (6)	13 (2)
Early pregnancy deaths	14 (10)	11 (6)
Genital tract sepsis	18 (12)	26 (12)
Anaesthetic	6 (6)	7 (3)
Total direct deaths	132 (72)	107* (47)
Indirect		
Cardiac	48 (15)	53 (13)
Psychiatric	19 (3)	13 (6)
Cancer	10 (2)	3 (0)
Other indirect	86 (25)	85 (28)
Total indirect deaths	163 (45)	154 (47)

- Figures are numbers of cases. (Figures in parentheses are cases with major substandard care.)
* Includes one case of choriocarcinoma that was classified as direct.

AMNIOTIC FLUID EMBOLISM

Formerly, amniotic fluid embolism (AFE) was diagnosed only when the pathologist confirmed fetal squames in the lungs. From 1991 to 1993, clinically obvious cases have also been included, but only after assiduous assessment to rule out misclassification. There were 13 deaths from AFE in 2006–8 and the diagnosis was confirmed at autopsy in 11. The number of histologically confirmed cases has remained around 8–10 per triennium for over 20 years.

EARLY PREGNANCY DEATHS

This category covers deaths before 24 weeks' gestation (formerly the upper limit was 20 weeks). In 2006–8 six were from ectopic pregnancy (out of an estimated 32,000 cases), and five were from miscarriage. There were two deaths from sepsis after legal termination of pregnancy. Before the Abortion Act of 1967, there were around 30 deaths every year from criminal abortion, most of them being due to sepsis.

SEPSIS

Until 1935, streptococcal puerperal sepsis was the leading cause of maternal death in the UK, causing hundreds of deaths each year. Within 50 years this cause was eliminated and in the 1982–4 report a modest sentence – 'No deaths could be directly attributed to puerperal sepsis' –marked one of the great medical achievements of the twentieth century. Since 1985, however, there has been a small but steady rise in the number of deaths from sepsis to 18 in 2003–5 and then, worryingly, to 29 in 2006–8 (including 3 late deaths). Of the 29 deaths 13 were due to group A streptococcus, which is widely carried in the throat. All 13 women had, or worked with, small children. Nine of the women presented with septic shock after rapid progression of the illness.

ANAESTHESIA

Despite the rising caesarean section rate, the number of maternal deaths from anaesthesia fell steadily from 37 in 1970–2 to only one in 1994–6. Since then the number has risen to seven in 2006–8. This illustrates the need to maintain vigilance –then as now, the main lesson is that trainees must know the limits of their competence.

Indirect deaths

The 154 indirect deaths in 2006–8 were divided into 53 cardiac and 13 psychiatric cases, 3 cases of malignancy possibly affected by pregnancy and 85 'others'.

CARDIAC DISEASE

The total of 53 deaths made this the leading cause of maternal death in 2006–8. Formerly, the major cardiac problem was rheumatic heart disease, as it still is in many developing countries, but there were no deaths from this cause in 2006–8. The leading causes were cardiomyopathy and sudden adult death syndrome and the full list is shown in Table 28.4. The steady increase in deaths from heart disease is linked with increasing obesity, increasing age at child-bearing and the continuing high rate of smoking among women in the UK.

PSYCHIATRIC

In 2006–8, four women committed suicide in pregnancy and nine within 6 weeks of delivery. Another 16 suicides were late indirect deaths, between 6 weeks and 6 months after delivery. Most of the methods were violent, such as hanging or jumping from a height. There were a further 38 cases in which psychiatric disorder caused or contributed to the death. In the past, not all psychiatric deaths were reported, but, after the enquiry highlighted the problem in the 1990s, case ascertainment improved and the extent of the problem of psychiatric disorders in pregnancy was at last recognised.

CANCER

In most countries, death from cancer during pregnancy is classed as 'coincidental' but, in the UK, deaths from cancer are classed as indirect if it appears that the pregnancy may have masked the disease or affected the diagnosis or outcome. CNS tumours in particular fall into this category.

OTHER INDIRECT DEATHS

There were 85 'other indirect' deaths in 2006–8. The main causes were diseases of the CNS (36 deaths), among which 14 deaths were due to epilepsy and 11 to subarachnoid or intracerebral haemorrhage. There were seven deaths from infectious diseases, two of which were due to HIV.

Coincidental deaths

The 50 coincidental deaths included 9 cases of neoplasia unaffected by the presence of pregnancy, 17 road traffic accidents and 11 cases of homicide –in seven cases by the woman's partner or close relative. Domestic violence, or intimate partner violence, is now a major concern to the maternity services and a chapter in the 2006–8 report is devoted to this problem. A further 34 women who died from other causes were known to be subject to domestic abuse.

Table 28.4 Deaths from cardiac disease in the UK, 2006-8[2]

Aortic dissection	7
Myocardial infarction	6
Ischaemic heart disease	5
Sudden adult death syndrome (SADS)	10
Cardiomyopathy (including peripartum)	13
Myocarditis or myocardial fibrosis	4
Thrombosed aortic or tricuspid valve	2
Infectious endocarditis	2
Ventricular hypertrophy/heart failure	1
Congenital heart disease	3
Total	**53**

ANTENATAL OBSTETRICS

PREVENTION

Worldwide

Almost 200 countries signed up to the eight Millennium Development Goals (MDGs) agreed at the UN Millennium Summit in 2000. MDG 5 is a 75 per cent reduction in the global MMR from its 1990 level by the year 2015. Various institutions including the WHO and the World Bank have supported work towards this target and substantial, but varied, progress has been made (Table 28.5).[6] Several countries, such as South Africa and Malaysia, have set up confidential enquiries similar to the UK model. Enquiries can identify the major problems, but implementing their recommendations requires commitment from politicians, doctors, other healthcare workers and the population as a whole.

Postpartum haemorrhage can be reduced by routine oxytocics at delivery, and unsafe abortion by contraceptive services and legal termination of pregnancy. Otherwise, the main need is less for prevention than for prompt treatment of pregnancy complications. This requires transport, trained healthcare workers, drugs and equipment. The importance of medical care in pregnancy and childbirth was underlined two decades ago by a comparative study in the USA, which showed that a religious group that had good general health but refused all modern medical care had a maternal mortality rate similar to those in developing countries.[3]

Past experience in the UK

Until 1935, the UK's MMR was around 400/100,000 (one death in 250 births), but it fell steadily between 1936 and 1985 (Fig. 28.2). Other indicators of public health, such as infant mortality, fell slowly and steadily during the twentieth century, but maternal mortality fell rapidly during and after the Second World War, when social conditions could hardly be

Table 28.5 Global changes in maternal mortality, 1980–2008

Maternal mortality ratio per 100,000 livebirths by region	1980	1990	2000	2008
Asia				
Pacific	28	14	10	8
Central	105	72	60	48
East	162	86	55	40
South	788	560	402	323
South-east	438	248	212	152
Australasia	9	7	6	6
Caribbean	426	348	323	254
Europe				
Central	47	34	18	13
Eastern	54	43	41	32
Western	16	10	8	7
Latin America				
Andean	326	229	156	103
Central	125	85	70	57
Southern	76	54	44	41
Tropical	150	113	71	57
North Africa/Middle East	299	183	111	76
North America	12	11	13	16
Oceania	517	416	329	279
Sub-Saharan Africa				
Central	711	732	770	586
East	707	690	776	508
Southern	242	171	373	381
West	683	582	742	629

- From: Hogan *et al.*, *Lancet* 2010;375:1609–23.

said to be improving. This strongly suggests that the fall was due to specific factors, such as:

- antibiotics: sulfonamides were introduced in 1937 and penicillin in 1944; death rates from puerperal sepsis quickly fell;
- blood transfusion became safe during the 1940s;
- ergometrine, for the treatment and prevention of PPH, was introduced in the 1940s;
- better training of midwives and obstetricians: Midwives Acts were passed in 1902 and 1936, and the RCOG was founded in 1929;
- reduced parity: the average family size began to fall long before the pill was introduced in 1961;
- legalisation of abortion in 1967 was followed by elimination of criminal abortion as a cause of maternal death (Fig. 28.3).

The current picture in the UK

Preventing maternal deaths involves identifying the women most at risk and providing them with appropriate care. Using denominator data collected by the Office for National Statistics and, combining these with findings from the Confidential Enquiry, general risk factors can be identified.

General risk factors

- *Age.* The MMR begins to rise around the age of 35 and rises more sharply after 40. In 2006–8, the MMR was 8.2 in the 20–24 age group and 29.2 among women aged over 40. In the past the 'grande multipara' was recognised as a high-risk case, but age and parity go together and, as high parity became rare in the UK, the importance of maternal age became clearer.
- *Ethnicity.* A higher risk among black women compared with white women was documented in the UK for the first time in 1994–6 and has been found in many countries including the USA, France and the Netherlands. Although

in the UK the MMR in both black and white women has recently fallen, this disparity persists (Table 28.6). In 2006–8 black African and black Caribbean women were almost four times more likely to die than white women. Of the 28 black African women who died, only 9 were UK citizens, most of the others being recently arrived immigrants, refugees or asylum seekers. Black Caribbean women are much less likely to have language difficulties but are more likely than white women to be poor attenders for antenatal care. Social factors, such as communication problems, are important but a survey by UKOSS showed that severe maternal morbidity was 2.4 times higher in black African and black Caribbean women than in white women, and the increased risk persisted after adjustment for factors such as socio-economic status.

- *Social class.* The huge effect of social class was shockingly illustrated in the 1997–9 report, which showed that the MMR among the lowest social class in Britain was 135/100,000 –similar to that in a developing country – and that 97 of the 242 maternal deaths occurred in social class 9. This group includes itinerant people ('travellers'), who tend to turn up at the wrong time or day at the antenatal clinic or fail to keep appointments. It is all too easy to overlook such people's needs in a service that caters mainly to the wishes of more articulate and better organised women. Such detailed data are no longer available but the 2006–8 report shows that women whose husbands or partners were unemployed were nearly six times more likely to die than women with employed partners.
- *Obesity.* It is estimated that 25 per cent of women in the UK aged 16 or over are obese. In 2006–8, the BMI was available for 87 per cent of the women who died: almost 50 per cent were overweight or obese, with the figure rising to 78 per cent among deaths from thromboembolism and 61 per cent among deaths from cardiac disease. A UKOSS survey of morbid obesity (BMI 50 or over) showed increased risks of severe morbidity including a 4.5-fold increase in the risk of pre-eclampsia, and a 6-fold increase in the chance of requiring general anaesthesia.

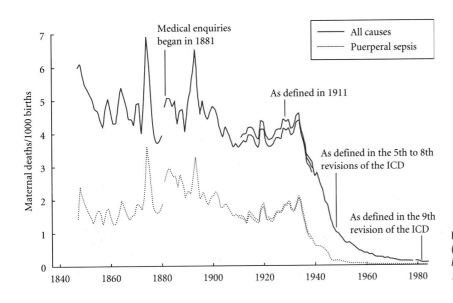

Fig. 28.3 MMR in England and Wales, 1847–1984 (reproduced from *Report on Confidential Enquiries into Maternal Deaths in England and Wales 1982–84*, published by HMSO, 1989)

- *Assisted conception.* Eight of the women who died in 2006–8 were known to have undergone assisted reproduction techniques (ARTs) including IVF. In the previous triennium, 2003–5, the total was nine, and four of those deaths were due to ovarian hyperstimulation syndrome. Multiple pregnancy is associated with a doubling of the risk of maternal death.

Substandard care

CEMD also identifies substandard care. Standards are rising all the time and the proportion of cases in which care falls below current standards has not changed over the years. Substandard care may involve only a minor aspect of the treatment and does not necessarily mean that the death could have been avoided. Nevertheless, in 2006–8 major substandard care was identified in 44 per cent of direct deaths and 31 per cent of indirect deaths. Examining these cases gives an insight into the challenges of real-life medical practice and helps to indicate how deaths may be avoided. Guidelines and protocols are everywhere but they can save lives only if they are understood and implemented. An example of their success is given in the next section, on thromboembolism.

Direct deaths

THROMBOEMBOLISM

In 2006–8 care was substandard in 10 of the 18 deaths from thromboembolism. Seven women received inadequate thromboprophylaxis, and in six cases there was a failure to investigate chest symptoms in at-risk women, sometimes even after repeated presentation. Nevertheless, the main message in this triennium was the sharp fall in deaths from thromboembolism. This was due to better awareness of the condition, which meant few instances of unnecessary delay in treatment and few cases in which risks were ignored.

The reduction in deaths from thromboembolism since the 1990s occurred in two phases, each linked to an RCOG guideline. In 1995, the RCOG produced recommendations on thromboprophylaxis after caesarean section. Deaths after caesarean section fell dramatically in the next triennium (1997–9) whilst deaths after vaginal delivery did not change (Table 28.7). In 2004 the RCOG produced a guideline for thromboprophylaxis during pregnancy and after vaginal delivery,[8] and a statistically significant fall in antepartum deaths and deaths after vaginal delivery followed in the next triennium (2006–8).

This is a good illustration of the close relationship between the Enquiry and a professional body whose guidelines are respected by clinicians. The thromboprophylaxis guideline was subsequently refined, with weight-specific dosage advice on LMWH, but the basic principles remain the same. Risk factors such as obesity and a personal or family history of thromboembolism should be identified as early as possible in pregnancy, and vigilance is needed for new risk factors during pregnancy, such as immobilisation or long-haul air travel. And, of course, symptoms must be promptly investigated.

Table 28.6 Ethnicity and maternal mortality in the UK, 2006–8[2]

Ethnic group	Direct and indirect deaths	MMR/100,000 maternities	Relative risk*
White	156	8.5	1.0
Mixed	2	6.1	0.7
Black African	25	32.8	3.9
Black Caribbean	8	31.9	3.8
Indian	8	12.5	1.5
Pakistani	13	14.3	1.7
Bangladeshi	2	6.1	0.7
Chinese/other Asian	2	15.1	1.8
Other	8	8.0	0.9
Total	233	13.5	

*Compared with white.

Table 28.7 Deaths from thromboembolism

Mode of delivery	1994–6	1997–9	2000–2	2003–5	2006–8
Antepartum*	18	17	9	18	8
Vaginal delivery	10	10	7	8	2
Caesarean section	15	4	9	7	6
Total	46**	31	25	33	16

*Includes deaths after miscarriage/ectopic, deaths in labour and deaths followed by postmortem CS.

**Includes three deaths whose timing was not recorded.

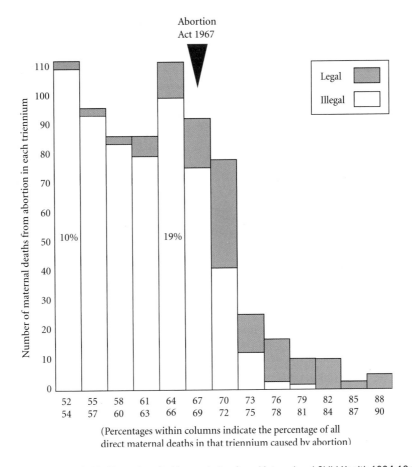

Fig. 28.4 Maternal deaths from abortion, 1952–90. (Reproduced with permission from *Maternal and Child Health* 1994;19:348.)

HYPERTENSIVE DISEASE

A depressing feature of recent reports has been the unchanging number of deaths from hypertensive disease. In 2006–8 there were 19 deaths from pre-eclampsia/eclampsia, 9 of which were due to intracranial haemorrhage. An encouraging feature of recent reports, however, is the lack of deaths due to pulmonary oedema caused by fluid overload during treatment: in 1994–6 this was the cause of eight deaths but fluid balance protocols have improved greatly since then.

It is frustrating that intracranial haemorrhage due to inadequate antihypertensive therapy continues to be a leading cause of death. A decade ago it became clear that systolic blood pressure was often being ignored while attention was focused on the diastolic, and the reports have repeatedly recommended urgent treatment of severe hypertension. The 2006–8 report recommends: 'Systolic blood pressures of 150 mmHg, or above, require effective antihypertensive treatment' and 'If systolic pressure is >180 mmHg, this is a medical emergency'. These simple recommendations are too often ignored, perhaps because they are not incorporated into local protocols.

HAEMORRHAGE

Major obstetric haemorrhage occurs in about 1 in 250 births, according to the Scottish Confidential Audit of Severe Maternal Morbidity. This means around 8000 cases of severe haemorrhage in the UK in 2006–8, and it is an indicator of the quality of emergency care that there were only 9 deaths from this cause – a fall from 14 in the previous triennium. Five of the nine deaths were due to PPH.

Substandard care was noted in six cases, and a major failure in three of the cases of PPH was a lack of routine observation in the postpartum period, or a failure to appreciate that bleeding was occurring. The 2003–5 report recommended the use of colour-coded 'MEOWS' (Modified Early Obstetric Warning Sign) charts to help alert staff to warning signs such as an increasing pulse rate, and these have been widely adopted, but, as the 2006–8 report points out, 'They are only useful if observations are made and abnormal readings acted upon'.

Two deaths were associated with placenta praevia accreta, which has become a concern because the rising caesarean section rate has led to more cases of placenta praevia implanted over a uterine scar. Key recommendations in previous reports have included the need to warn women about the future risks of caesarean section, and the need for placental localisation in women with a previous caesarean section. The reports have repeatedly stated that caesarean section for placenta praevia must be carried out by an experienced surgeon. Recent reports have stressed the importance of multidisciplinary planning when problems are anticipated and have recommended calling a second consultant when severe haemorrhage occurs. The fall in deaths suggests that these recommendations have been heeded.

ANTENATAL OBSTETRICS

Nevertheless, it is worth remembering that deaths from haemorrhage have fallen to single figures in the past, once in the 1980s and once in the 1990s. The cyclical rise and fall in deaths from this cause suggests that lessons are easily forgotten, and underlines the need for constant vigilance. The incidence of severe haemorrhage does not change.

AMNIOTIC FLUID EMBOLISM

Deaths from AFE have remained fairly constant in number, and in 2006–8 there were 13 deaths from this cause. In five of these cases there was no substandard care and, indeed, in two of these cases there was exemplary care, including prompt perimortem caesarean section. Substandard care in the remaining cases included poor organisation of transfer facilities, delay in contacting the consultant obstetrician and delay in communicating with relatives.

AFE used to be regarded as a condition with an almost 100 per cent mortality rate but important lessons have been learned from national surveillance conducted by UKOSS since 2005. A similar international registry has recently been established in the USA.[9] UKOSS data showed a constant incidence of 2 per 100,000 pregnancies and an overall mortality rate of 16.5 per cent. It appears that high-quality supportive care can result in good outcomes for mother and baby, and the 2006–8 report concluded: 'Amniotic fluid embolism, particularly if the collapse occurs in a well-equipped unit, should now be considered a treatable and survivable event in the majority of cases.'

EARLY PREGNANCY DEATHS

Substandard care was present in the majority of deaths in early pregnancy in 2006–8. There were six deaths from ectopic pregnancy –the lowest number for 20 years –and substandard care included failure to consider the diagnosis in a woman who presented with diarrhoea, vomiting and abdominal pain, despite previous reports drawing attention to gastro-intestinal symptoms as the sole presentation of ectopic pregnancy. A woman diagnosed with 'pregnancy of unknown location' in an early pregnancy assessment (EPA) unit received inadequate follow-up and died of an ectopic pregnancy. Five women died after spontaneous miscarriage –the highest number for 15 years. The introduction of EPA units has been associated with more conservative management of non-continuing pregnancies but their protocols must be meticulously followed and persistent bleeding needs to be recognised as an indication for prompt surgical intervention.

SEPSIS

Sepsis is now the leading cause of direct death in the UK. Death and serious illness from pregnancy-related sepsis are still very rare, however, which means that many healthcare workers will never have seen a case, making it difficult for them to recognise the earliest signs and symptoms. Streptococci can produce overwhelming sepsis in a frighteningly short time, but infection is often insidious in onset and may not reveal itself for several days postpartum, when the woman has gone home. The first presentation may be to a midwife, GP or junior doctor in the emergency department, and the main message of the 2006–8 report is 'Be aware of sepsis – beware sepsis'.

Among the 29 women who died in 2006–8, the fatal outcome was inevitable in many cases but might have been different in 12 if the infection had been diagnosed and treated more promptly. The first sign may be tachycardia. Tachypnoea is sepsis until proved otherwise. Immediate aggressive antibiotic treatment in the first 'golden hour' offers the best hope of recovery, and high-dose broad-spectrum IV antibiotic treatment must be started immediately without waiting for microbiology results.

Streptococci are transferred by droplet spread, and puerperal women should be advised to wash their hands before going to the toilet or changing sanitary towels. Women may make light of the initial symptoms and public awareness of the condition needs to be increased.

GENITAL TRACT TRAUMA

Death from genital tract trauma is now so rare that the 2006–8 report did not include a chapter on this cause, though genital tract tears were implicated in two deaths from PPH. Difficult forceps deliveries are rarely if ever attempted nowadays, though the resultant increase in the caesarean section rate has brought its own problems.

ANAESTHESIA

Of the seven deaths attributed to anaesthesia in 2006–8, three had major and three had minor substandard care. Two deaths were the result of failure to ventilate the lungs, one after induction of general anaesthesia and the other when a tracheostomy tube came out in a critical care ward. In 1967–9 there were 32 such deaths, and this was a major reason for the move to regional anaesthesia in obstetrics. Today general anaesthesia is infrequently used and the management of failed intubation needs to be rehearsed and assessed regularly. Anaesthetists have been assiduous in learning lessons from the successive reports of the CEMD.

Indirect deaths

Table 28.3 shows that although the proportion of cases with substandard care is lower among indirect deaths than among direct deaths, one-third of the indirect deaths were associated with major substandard care and, unlike direct deaths, the proportion did not fall in 2006–8.

CARDIAC DISEASE

There was major substandard care in 13 of the 53 deaths from cardiac disease in 2006–8, and there were lessons to be learned from another 14 cases. Failure to consider acute coronary syndrome was a repeated finding. ECGs can be normal between episodes of angina, and a single ECG does not exclude ischaemia. Failure to investigate chest pain was also a factor in four of the seven deaths from aortic dissection. It is gratifying that awareness of thromboembolism has increased but it is now necessary to remind clinicians that 'not all chest pain in pregnancy is the result of pulmonary emboli'. Aortic dissection is not confined only to women with Marfan's syndrome, and chest pain severe enough to require opiate analgesia needs full investigation. Cardiomyopathy may present up to 6 months after delivery, and women with known cardiomyopathy need referral to specialist units where obstetricians and cardiologists work together.

PSYCHIATRIC DISEASE

The 2006–8 report found that psychiatric care was less than optimal for 69 per cent of women known to be involved with psychiatric services in their current pregnancy. In most women the psychiatric team had not appreciated the severity of the woman's illness. Suicide risk must not be equated with social deprivation: over half of the maternal suicides were married, employed, living in comfortable circumstances and aged 30 or over.

Morbid fear of having their child removed was a feature in some cases. Referral to safeguarding teams should not be routine when mothers develop a mental illness but should take place as a result of risk assessment. When referral is necessary to safeguard the child, extra vigilance and care are required.

Most women who suffer maternal death from suicide have a past history of serious affective disorder. Women with a past history of severe mental illness complicating pregnancy have a 33–55 per cent chance of recurrence. All women should be routinely asked in early pregnancy about current and previous mental health problems. Questioning should be sensitive but explicit. Each unit should have a protocol for the management of women at high risk, and specialist perinatal psychiatric services, both inpatient and community, should be available.

In some deaths, physical symptoms and agitation were wrongly attributed to psychiatric disorder, leading to delay in diagnosis and treatment. This is particularly risky when a woman has no previous history of psychiatric disease or when she does not speak English or comes from an ethnic minority.

OTHER INDIRECT DEATHS

Of the 36 women who died from neurological conditions, 11 had major substandard care, and of the other 52 deaths from indirect causes 17 women had major substandard care. Only 6 of the 14 women with epilepsy had received pre-pregnancy counselling and in most of the cases of epilepsy the woman had not been referred for review by a neurologist despite her known history. This meant the opportunity was lost to consider adjusting the anticonvulsant dose or check drug levels if necessary. Women with epilepsy are still unaware of the rare but real risk of drowning while bathing unattended. A shower is preferable and the bathroom door should remain unlocked.

Five women died of asthma –a similar number to those in previous reports –and none had had specialist care in pregnancy, despite three having brittle asthma or multiple hospital admissions. Women often withhold or decrease their medication in pregnancy for fear of harming the fetus, and specialist referral can reassure them about this.

Coincidental deaths

ROAD TRAFFIC ACCIDENTS

Pregnancy is not a contraindication to the use of seat belts, and women should be advised that the belt is placed 'over and under the bump'.

DOMESTIC VIOLENCE

The 2006–8 report emphasises the importance of 'Asking the question' at some opportune point during the antenatal period. If abuse is disclosed on such routine questioning, this must be recorded in a way that protects the woman from further violence and there must be local strategies for referral to a support network. If the woman chooses midwifery-led care, the midwife should receive support from an experienced colleague. Women who are known to suffer domestic abuse should not be regarded as 'low risk'.

Domestic violence may be the reason for late booking or poor attendance, or conversely for repeated attendance with minor injuries or non-existent complaints. Other warning signs include drug or alcohol abuse, or the constant presence of a partner at examinations. Every woman should be seen on her own at least once during the pregnancy. Staff must adopt a non-judgemental and supportive attitude[10] and should remember that health professionals, too, may be victims of abuse.

THE FUTURE

Over the past 20 years, interest has been growing in 'near misses' –incidents that might have resulted in a maternal death but for prompt and effective treatment. These incidents occur more frequently than maternal deaths and in countries with a low MMR analysis of near misses should provide a more representative picture to allow policy guidance. One problem with this approach has been the wide variation in criteria for identifying cases,[11] but the WHO has developed a set of unified criteria along with a set of indicators for identifying quality of care.[12] Some of these criteria are laboratory based and questions have been raised about their practical value in low-resource settings, where the need is greatest.[13]

In the UK, a continuous audit of severe maternal morbidity in Scotland has been running since 2003, collecting data on consistently defined events in all consultant-led maternity units in Scotland.[14] In 2006–8 1025 women experienced 1237 events, giving a rate of severe maternal morbidity of 5.88 per 1000 births. There were 13 direct and indirect maternal deaths in the same period, giving a mortality/morbidity ratio of 1 in 79. By far the commonest morbidity was major obstetric haemorrhage, defined as an estimated blood loss of 2.5 litres or more, which occurred in 4.5/1000 births. In 2011 the rate of morbidities except haemorrhage declined, but the rate of major obstetric haemorrhage increased, affecting 1 in 170 births. The rate is not affected by social class, except that the most affluent quintile were more likely to experience morbidity. There was a significantly higher rate of major obstetric haemorrhage in women with a BMI over 35.

Perhaps the most valuable lesson from audits of severe maternal morbidity is that even when the MMR is very low the risks of pregnancy have not gone away. The low rates of maternal mortality in developed countries are not due to improved health of the population but to effective intervention when problems occur. The rates of severe morbidity today, around 4/1000, are similar to the MMR in the UK before 1935 (Fig. 28.1), and to the MMRs in parts of Africa today.[1]

Audits of morbidity and confidential enquiries into mortality are complementary. Aggregation of deaths classified by cause teaches lessons that cannot be learned by looking at each of these rare events in isolation. In 2006–8 the reports of local investigations into individual deaths were available to the national assessors, who found that their quality was extremely variable. It is very difficult for a hospital to investigate such a rare and upsetting event without outside support, and a national perspective is essential.

- Risk factors for maternal death include age, obesity, low social class and black ethnicity.
- Most of the deaths worldwide, and many in the UK, are preventable

SUMMARY

The worldwide total of maternal deaths has fallen to under 300,000 per year, but still represents a largely preventable tragedy. We know how to treat the conditions that cause these deaths. Ensuring that treatment reaches the women who need it is a matter of political will, and obstetricians have a duty to act as advocates for the women at risk.

In the UK, the maternity services have been successful in making pregnancy safe for most women but substandard care still occurs. Women from ethnic minorities are at increased risk, as are the most deprived sections of the community. The Confidential Enquiry led the way in revealing these disturbing facts, and others such as the risks associated with psychiatric disease, domestic violence and, today, obesity. The purpose of the enquiry is to save lives, and its recommendations are always firmly based on its findings. The importance of this process is increasingly recognised in the UK and worldwide.

One final point: although knowledge of the most recent report is essential, lessons of previous reports must also be remembered, and this may become even more important in the future when annual reports are published. To quote from the last of the triennial reports,[2] 'Experience has taught us that old messages need repeating, especially as new cadres of healthcare workers join the service, and there are always new and unexpected challenges'.

KEY POINTS

- Maternal death is the death of a woman while pregnant or within 42 days after the end of pregnancy. *Direct* deaths result from obstetric complications and *indirect* deaths from disease aggravated by, but not directly due to, pregnancy.
- Across the world the average MMR is now 210 per 100,000. Of the estimated global total of 287,000 maternal deaths every year, the vast majority are in developing regions.
- In developed countries the MMR is around 10 per 100,000 maternities. In Britain between 1936 and 1985 the MMR fell steadily due to antibiotics, blood transfusion, ergometrine, better training of midwives and obstetricians and the 1967 Abortion Act.
- Direct deaths in the UK fell in 2006-08, but it remains to be seen if that fall will be sustained. The leading cause of direct death is no longer thromboembolism, but sepsis.
- Indirect deaths in the UK outnumber direct deaths. The leading cause is cardiac disease.

Key References

1. WHO. *Trends in maternal mortality: 1990 to 2010. WHO, UNICEF, UNFPA and The World Bank estimates.* Geneva: WHO, 2012.
2. CMACE. *CEMACH: Saving mothers' lives: reviewing maternal deaths to make motherhood safer –2006–2008. The Eighth Report on Confidential Enquiries into Maternal Deaths in the United Kingdom. BJOG* 2011;118(Suppl 1):1–203.
3. Knight M. How will the new confidential Enquiries into Maternal and Infant Death in the UK operate? The work of MBRRACE-UK. *Obstetrician & Gynaecologist* 2013;15:65.
4. MMBRACE Newsletter, Issue 4. September 2013. www.npeu.ox.ac.uk/mbrrace-uk.
5. Bhutta ZA, Black RE. Global maternal, newborn and child health –so near and yet so far. *N Engl J Med* 2013;369:2226–35.
6. Hogan MC, Foreman KJ, Naghavi M *et al.* Maternal mortality for 181 countries, 1980–2008: a systematic analysis of progress towards Millennium Development Goal 5. *Lancet* 2010;375:1609–23.
7. Kaunitz AM, Spence C, Danielson TS, Rochard RW, Grimes DA. Perinatal and maternal mortality in a religious group avoiding obstetric care. *Am J Obstet Gynecol* 1994; 150:826–31.
8. RCOG Guidelines and Audit Committee. *Thromboprophylaxis during pregnancy. labour and after vaginal delivery. Guideline no 37.* London: RCOG, 2004.
9. Clark SL. Amniotic fluid embolism. *Obstet Gynecol* 2014;123:337-48.
10. Aston G, Bewley S. Abortion and domestic violence. *Obstetrician & Gynaecologist* 2009;11:163–8.
11. Tuncalp O, Hindin MJ, Souza JP, Chou D, Say L. The prevalence of maternal near-miss: a systematic review. *BJOG* 2012;119:653–61.
12. Souza JP, Say L, Pattinson R, Gulmezoglu AM *et al. Evaluating the quality of care for severe pregnancy complications: the WHO near-miss approach for maternal health.* Geneva: WHO, 2011.
13. Spector J. Practical criteria for near-miss needed for low-income settings. *Lancet* 2013;282:504–5.
14. Healthcare Improvement Scotland. *Scottish Confidential Audit of Severe Morbidity: reducing avoidable harm.* 9th Annual report (Data from 2011). Healthcare Improvement Scotland, 2013.

SECTION THREE

Fetal Conditions

Chapter 29 Biochemical screening

Michele P Mohajer

INTRODUCTION

Over the last 50 years, many biochemical substances produced by the fetoplacental unit have been identified in maternal serum. A number of these have been found to be associated with certain fetal conditions and have been incorporated into national screening programmes. This section aims to describe those programmes, along with their advantages and disadvantages.

In 1956, the first biochemical marker identified in maternal serum was alpha-fetoprotein (AFP); the association between a raised serum AFP and open spina bifida was not demonstrated until 1974.[1]

BIOCHEMICAL SCREENING FOR NEURAL TUBE DEFECTS

AFP is produced by the fetal liver. It crosses into the maternal serum from the amniotic fluid or via the placenta. Maternal serum AFP (MSAFP) rises throughout most of pregnancy (from 12 weeks to 32 weeks), hence accurate determination of gestational age is mandatory. To allow for the increase in concentration in the second trimester, it is convenient to express all AFP values as a multiple of the normal median (MoM) at the relevant gestational age. The separation between the distribution of MSAFP levels in pregnancies with open fetal defects and that in normal pregnancies is greatest at 16–18 weeks' gestation, and therefore screening is optimum at this stage.

AFP screening was intended for the detection of open spina bifida, and not closed spina bifida. Using a cut-off level of 2.5 MoM, 79 per cent open spina bifida and 88 per cent anencephaly can be detected [C]. If all neural tube defects (NTDs) are considered, the detection rate is 72 per cent, with a false-positive rate of 0.001 per cent.[2]

Raised MSAFP is also associated with other fetal malformations or conditions, including:

- multiple pregnancy;
- abdominal wall defects (gastroschisis, exomphalos, bladder extrophy):
  - congenital nephrosis;
- spontaneous fetal loss.

There is also some degree of association between a raised MSAFP and the following conditions:

- pre-eclampsia;
- preterm delivery
  - low birthweight;
  - underestimated gestation;
  - low maternal weight;
  - African-Caribbean ethnic origin;
  - male fetus;
  - raised MSAFP in a previous pregnancy;
- smoking.

Levels of MSAFP may be lowered in association with other conditions, including:

- Down's syndrome (trisomy 21);
- Edward's syndrome (trisomy 18);
- type 1 diabetes;
- overestimated gestation;
- high maternal weight.

AFP screening now has a minor role in the detection of fetal defects due to the widespread use of sophisticated ultrasound techniques. Using ultrasound to demonstrate the characteristic cranial signs of spina bifida (the 'lemon and banana' sign), the detection rate of all NTDs is 81 per cent [C], with a false-positive rate of 0.0003 per cent.[3] This detection rate exceeds that of AFP screening programmes.

The role of amniocentesis in MSAFP screening

Prior to high-resolution ultrasound, amniocentesis was routinely performed to detect increased levels of AFP and acetylcholinesterase (AChE) in the amniotic fluid in an attempt to diagnose open fetal defects. The risk of fetal loss may be eight times higher when amniocentesis is performed in these circumstances [A], and it therefore should not be performed as an initial investigation.[4]

Many more biochemical substances have been identified that are produced during pregnancy. Many of these have been investigated for their usefulness in detecting pregnancy complications. Two notable hormones, human placental lactogen (hPL) and oestriol (E_3), were used widely to assess placental function. These have now been abandoned due to the development of better biophysical methods.

BIOCHEMICAL SCREENING FOR DOWN'S SYNDROME

The main area of development of other biochemical markers in pregnancy has been in screening for Down's syndrome (trisomy 21).

Down's syndrome is still the commonest cause of severe learning disability. The natural birth prevalence increases with maternal age, from 1 in 1500 under the age of 25, to 1 in 1000 at age 30, and to 1 in 100 at age 40. The overall incidence of the condition has increased due to women having their babies at an older age.

In the early 1980s, antenatal screening relied on identifying women above a specified age (e.g. 35 years) and offering them amniocentesis. In 1984, low MSAFP levels in the mid-trimester were found to be associated with Down's syndrome.[5] Later, hCG was found to be raised in Down's syndrome, and unconjugated oestriol (uE_3) was found to be reduced. Division of hCG into its free subunits (alpha-hCG and beta-hCG) provided additional value in screening. More recently, a fourth biochemical marker, inhibin-A, has been found to be raised in Down's syndrome pregnancies.[6]

Subsequently, measurement of biochemical substances in the first trimester of pregnancy has also demonstrated an association with Down's syndrome. The two markers used are free beta-hCG and PAPP-A.

Accurate gestational age assessment is vital to the utility of these biochemical markers. Biochemical screening is applicable only to singleton pregnancies, so ultrasonic assessment is again mandatory. All markers vary with gestation, and so MoMs are used to determine abnormal values.

First-trimester screening

Two biochemical markers, namely free beta-hCG and PAPP-A, when measured between 8 and 14 weeks in combination with maternal age, can detect 62 per cent of Down's syndrome pregnancies, with a 5 per cent false-positive rate.[8] These serum markers, when combined with maternal age and NT measurement, comprise a combined test, which has an estimated detection rate of 85 per cent for a 5 per cent false-positive rate.[9] This test is usually performed in a single visit, which reduces the anxiety of waiting for a result.

First-trimester screening provides the opportunity to establish a diagnosis in early pregnancy (if CVS is utilised). This method of national screening requires substantial financial support for the training and education of health professionals, the provision of information and counselling services, and the expansion of expertise in diagnostic ultrasound and invasive tests such as CVS [C].

Second-trimester screening

Second-trimester screening is carried out between 15 and 20 weeks of pregnancy. Serum screening programmes incorporate:

- two components (MSAFP and total hCG or free beta-hCG): the double test;
- three components (MSAFP, hCG and uE_3): the triple test; or
- four components (MSAFP, hCG, uE_3 and inhibin): the quadruple test.

The screening performance of these markers improves with the addition of markers, such that, for a false-positive rate of 5 per cent, the detection rates for the double, triple and quadruple tests are 59 per cent, 69 per cent and 76 per cent, respectively.[7] However, the extra cost of using additional serum markers must be considered.

Certain factors can influence serum markers:

- Type 1 diabetes and increased maternal weight lower all markers.
- Twin gestation produces approximately twice the level of all serum markers.
- Minor variations occur with ethnic differences and in smokers.
- Other conditions in which serum screening may be unreliable include maternal renal failure and severe dehydration (e.g. severe hyperemesis gravidarum).

The aim of screening is to maximise the detection rate with a low false-positive rate, in order that invasive testing is minimised.

Integrated/hybrid screening

Simultaneously using markers from both trimesters yields a better screening performance than using markers in either trimester alone. Thus, if the first-trimester triple test is combined with the second-trimester quadruple test, the detection rate for Down's syndrome has been estimated at 94 per cent for a 5 per cent false-positive rate.[10] If the false-positive rate is fixed at 1 per cent, the detection rate will be 85 per cent. This approach therefore yields a higher detection rate than any other screening test at a given false-positive rate. The SURUSS (serum, urine and ultrasound screening study) report showed that, if the risk cut-off level is fixed at 1:200, the detection rate is 89 per cent for a 2.4 per cent false-positive rate. The FASTER (First- and Second-Trimester Evaluation of Risk) trial showed comparable results.[12] However, the logistics of introducing such a screening system need to be considered. The result of the first-trimester screen would need to be concealed from the woman, and thus would negate the advantage of early prenatal diagnosis. If ultrasound facilities are not sufficiently developed to perform reliable NT measurement, the full, integrated test cannot be provided. In the absence of NT, the detection rate for the integrated test is 85 per cent for a 5.5 per cent false-positive rate.[10] In addition, the infrastructure necessary for the organisation and counselling of integrated/hybrid screening far exceeds that required for the present screening programmes. Nevertheless, the enormous financial and emotional advantage of a test with a 1 per cent false-positive rate cannot be denied.

National recommendation for Down's syndrome screening

Current recommendations state that all pregnant women should be offered first-trimester screening (by 13 weeks and 6 days), but that provision should be made to allow for later screening (as late as 20 weeks 0 days).[13] Ideally the combined test (NT +beta-hCG+PAPP-A) should be offered between 11 weeks and 13 weeks 6 days. For women who book later in pregnancy, the most clinically effective serum screening (triple or quadruple test) should be offered between 15 weeks 0 days and 20 weeks 0 days.

The NSC recommendations specified that, by 2008, all trusts should offer Down's syndrome screening to all pregnant women with the aim to improve detection to >/= 90% with a screen positive rate (SPR) <2%.

BIOCHEMICAL SCREENING FOR OTHER ABNORMALITIES

A number of other chromosomal abnormalities have been shown to be associated with biochemical markers:

- *Trisomy 18/trisomy 13*. These are the next most common aneuploidies surviving to birth. There is evidence to support serum screening for these, but it is not sufficiently robust to introduce into the NHS fetal anomaly screening programme at present. The mid-trimester anomaly scan is more sensitive and specific.[14]
- *Triploidy*. This chromosomal abnormality is inconsistent with survival. Affected pregnancies may be identified in the mid-trimester, as there are very high or very low levels of AFP and hCG, and low levels of E_3.
  - *Turner's syndrome (45,X)*. In Turner's syndrome associated with hydrops, the serum markers show a pattern similar to that of Down's syndrome pregnancies. In those without hydrops, the hCG level is low.
  - *Smith–Lemlie–Opitz syndrome*. This is an autosomal recessive condition associated with moderate-to-severe learning disability. In these pregnancies, uE_3 is very low or undetectable, and MSAFP and hCG tend to be low. The risk of a pregnancy affected with this condition can thus be calculated, and the diagnosis is confirmed by measuring 7-dehydrocholesterol (7-DHCO) in the amniotic fluid.

Adverse pregnancy outcome. Low markers in the first trimester (hCG and PAPP-A) and elevated mid-trimester MSAFP and inhibin are associated with preterm birth, fetal loss, growth restriction, placental abruption and pre-eclampsia.[15]

HEALTH ECONOMICS OF SCREENING

A major challenge in the delivery of Down's syndrome screening services is the need to set up an adequate organisational structure. This not only means dedicated laboratory facilities with computer-assisted test interpretation and expertise to provide invasive prenatal testing, but also a team of experienced coordinators to undertake the enormous workload of counselling. This counselling is essential, both prior to undertaking the test and in the event of a screen-positive result when invasive testing is contemplated. It is this last service provision that has poor structure in many screening programmes, and fiscal implications are generally underestimated. In the ideal structure, each unit should have a clear screening policy agreed centrally. A screening coordinator is responsible for reporting results to women and coordinating the local screening service. A local director of screening, of consultant status, guides and supports the service, and is attentive to advances in screening and their controlled introduction into practice.

EBM

- High-resolution ultrasound has a better detection rate for open fetal defects than a high MSAFP [C].
- With accurate ultrasound dating, second-trimester biochemical screening using four markers can detect 76 per cent of Down's syndrome pregnancies [B].
- First-trimester serum screening is as effective as mid-trimester serum screening [B].

KEY POINTS

- A raised MSAFP has good sensitivity but poor specificity for open fetal defects; mid-trimester ultrasound scan is considered superior with a greater sensitivity and specificity.
- Mid-trimester serum screening for Down's syndrome is widely available in the UK.
- Detection rates vary depending on the number of markers used.
- A dating scan must be performed prior to Down's syndrome screening.
- Combined (first-trimester) screening is the recommended method and should be offered to all pregnant women.
- Counselling before and after testing accounts for the bulk of the workload.

Published Guidelines

Grudzinskas JG, Ward RHT (eds). *Screening for Down's syndrome in the first trimester. Recommendations arising from the Study Group.* London: RCOG Press, 1997.

NHS Fetal Anomaly Screening Programme. *Screening for Down's syndrome: UK NSC recommendations 2011–2014 Model of Best Practice.* Exeter: UK National Screening Committee.

NICE Clinical Care Guideline 62: *Antenatal Care.* London: NICE, 2008.

RCOG. *Antenatal screening for Down's syndrome.* London: RCOG Press, July 2003.

Key References

1. Wald NJ, Brock DJH, Bonnar J. Prenatal diagnosis of spina bifida and anencephaly by maternal serum alpha-fetoprotein measurement. A controlled study. *Lancet* 1974;i:765–7.

2. Report of UK Collaborative Study on Alpha-fetoprotein in relation to neural tube defects. Maternal serum alpha-fetoprotein measurement in antenatal screening for anencephaly and spina bifida in early pregnancy. *Lancet* 1977;i:1323–32.

3. Papp Z, Toth-Pal E, Papp CS, Torok O. Impact of prenatal mid-trimester screening on the prevalence of fetal structure anomalies: a prospective epidemiological study. *Ultrasound Obstet Gynecol* 1995;6:320–6.

4. Morrow RJ, McNay MB, Whittle MJ. Ultrasound detection of neural tube defects in patients with elevated maternal serum AFP levels. *Obstet Gynecol* 1991;78:1055–7.

5. Cuckle HS, Wald NJ, Lindenbaum RH. Maternal serum alpha-fetoprotein measurement. A screening test for Down's syndrome. *Lancet* 1984;i:926–9.

6. Wald NJ, Densem JW, George L, Muttukrishna S, Knight PG. Prenatal screening for Down's syndrome using Inhibin-A as a serum marker. *Prenat Diagn* 1996;16:143–53.

7. Wald NJ, Densem JW, Smith D, Klee GG. Four marker serum screening for Down's syndrome. *Prenat Diagn* 1994;14:707–16.

8. Wald NJ, George L, Smith D, Densem JW, Petterson K, on behalf of the International Prenatal Screening Group. Serum screening for Down's syndrome between 8 and 14 weeks of pregnancy. *Br J Obstet Gynaecol* 1996;103:407–12.

9. Wald NJ, Hackshaw AK. Combining ultrasound and biochemistry in first trimester screening for Down's syndrome. *Prenat Diagn* 1997;17:821–9.

10. Wald NJ, Watt HC, Hackshaw AK. Integrated screening for Down's syndrome based on tests performed during the first and second trimesters. *N Engl J Med* 1999;341:461–7.

11. Wald NJ, Rodeck C, Hackshaw AK, Walters J, Chitty L, Mackinson AM. First and second trimester screening for Down's syndrome: the results of the serum, urine and ultrasound screening study (SURUSS). *J Med Screen* 2003;10:56–104.

12. Malone FD, Canick JA, Ball RH *et al.* First trimester screening or second trimester screening, or both, for Down's syndrome. *N Engl J Med* 2005;353:2001–11.

13. NICE. Clinical Care Guideline No. 62: *Antenatal Care* London: NICE, 2008.

14. Screening for Down's syndrome: UK NSC recommendations 2011–2014 Model of Best Practice.

15. Gagnon A, Wilson RD, Audibert F *et al.* Obstetrical complications associated with abnormal maternal serum marker analytes. *J Obstet Gynaecol Can* 2008;10:918–49.

Chapter 30 Ultrasound Screening

Michele P Mohajer

INTRODUCTION

The incidence of major structural abnormality is 2–3 per cent, and far exceeds all chromosomal abnormalities or single-gene defects. As a result of the technological development in high-resolution ultrasound equipment, the prenatal diagnosis of most major structural malformations is possible. As a consequence, there has been a significant fall in perinatal mortality rates due to the termination of affected fetuses. In addition to this role, ultrasound scanning is vital in determining gestation, viability and number of fetuses. The advent of such technological development has provided the foundation for the subspecialty of fetal medicine.

WHAT IS SCREENING?

The purpose of screening for fetal malformation is not simply to terminate the fetus prior to viability in order to reduce perinatal mortality rates. Although screening does reduce perinatal mortality rates, the identification of fetal malformation allows parents to make informed choices regarding their pregnancy. This facilitates physical and psychological preparation for the delivery of an infant with a birth defect, which may even take place in another centre. In addition, identification of certain abnormalities may allow parents to avail themselves of *in-utero* treatments that can improve the infant's condition prior to birth. Ultrasound screening can also be used to identify some fetuses with chromosomal disease, in which case invasive diagnostic procedures can be performed.

WHO SHOULD BE SCREENED?

Certain conditions increase a woman's chance of having a malformed fetus. So-called 'high-risk' groups can be identified, such as women with type 1 diabetes, maternal drug ingestion (e.g. anticonvulsants, warfarin) or a positive family history. However, 95 per cent of abnormalities occur in fetuses born to mothers who have no risk factors at all.[1] Therefore, routine ultrasound scanning of all pregnancies is the preferred method to identify structural malformations [A]. However, vast differences exist in detection rates, ranging from 16 per cent to 85 per cent.[2-4]

The reasons for these differences are unclear. The skill and training of the operator are important, but perhaps an important variable is the gestational age at which the scan is done. The optimum time for the identification of structural fetal anomalies is 18–21 weeks [B].[5,6] Prior to performing the ultrasound scan, it is vital that the parents understand the objectives, the limitations and also the detection rates for the major malformations.[6] This is ideally done by the provision of information leaflets [C].

TIMING OF SCREENING

The detailed fetal anomaly scan at 18–21 weeks

The scan initially checks viability and number of fetuses, as well as placental site and amniotic fluid volume. Standard views of the fetus are then taken.[18] These are:

1 transverse section through the fettle head, assessing head shape and internal structures;
2 face: lips;
3 fetal spine: sagittal, coronal and transverse views;
4 fetal abdomen: longitudinal and transverse; identifying intra-abdominal organs: stomach, kidneys, bladder and ventral wall integrity and cord insertion;
5 transverse section through fetal thorax to examine four-chamber view of the heart and outflow tracts;
6 Limbs: identify three long bones in each limb, hands and feet.

Inability to obtain the standard images may occur due to fetal position or maternal size.

MAJOR STRUCTURAL MALFORMATIONS

CNS malformations

Many major structural defects of the CNS may be identified at the 20-week scan, and certain malformations can be identified at earlier gestations.

Neural tube defects

These malformations occur when there is a failure of dorsal fusion in early embryological life, such that neural tissue is exposed. NTDs (anencephaly, cephalocele and spina bifida) are the commonest CNS malformations in the UK, and much attention has been applied to the screening and prevention of these anomalies. Anencephaly is characterised by the absence of the cerebral hemispheres and cranial vault, and can be identified from as early as 11–12 weeks. The prognosis is uniformly fatal within the first hours or days of life. Cephalocele is a protrusion of the intracranial contents through a bony defect of the skull. These contents may include only meninges (cranial meningocele) or brain tissue (encephalocele). Ultrasound examination can identify a solid or cystic paracranial mass. The prognosis depends on the presence of brain tissue within the sac and other associated intracranial features. Spina bifida, in which the defect exists in the vertebral fusion, is the commonest CNS malformation. Demonstration of the lesion itself by ultrasound may be difficult. However, the intracranial signs associated with spina bifida, the Arnold–Chiari malformation (herniation of the cerebellum and brain stem through the foramen magnum), are more easily identifiable.[7] This demonstration of the 'lemon and banana' sign has displaced MSAFP as the main screening test for spina bifida

in many units. The detection rate for open spina bifida on ultrasound screening is 81 per cent, with a false-positive rate of 0.0003 per cent.[8]

Hydrocephalus

This condition arises when there is an abnormal accumulation of CSF, resulting in enlargement of the ventricular system. It is commonly associated with other intracranial and extracranial abnormalities. Diagnosis on ultrasound examination is achieved by demonstration of enlarged lateral ventricles and anterior displacement of the choroid plexus. The three major forms are aqueduct stenosis, communicating hydrocephalus and the Dandy–Walker syndrome. This last syndrome is characterised by the addition of a cyst in the posterior fossa and defect in the cerebellar vermis, both of which are detectable on ultrasound. The prognosis is variable, again depending on the severity of the hydrocephalus and the presence of additional malformations.

Other less common CNS malformations may be identified on ultrasound. These include holoprosencephaly, iniencephaly, arachnoid cysts, porencephalic cysts, agenesis of the corpus callosum, hydrancephaly, microcephaly, intracranial tumours and aneurysm of the vein of Galen.

Cardiac malformations

Systematic examination of the fetal heart has enabled the prenatal diagnosis of many congenital heart defects. Since the fetal heart is almost horizontal, a transverse section through the fetal chest will demonstrate a four-chamber view. This standard view provides information about the position and size of the fetal heart, the cardiac chambers and the atrioventricular connections. Congenital heart abnormalities associated with an abnormal four-chamber view include:

- hypoplastic left heart;
- hypoplastic right heart;
- atrioventricular canal defect;
- large ventricular septal defect;
- large atrial septal defect;
- single ventricle;
- valve stenosis or atresia;
- Ebstein's anomaly;
- cardiac tumour;
- cardiac situs abnormalities.

However, there is a wide variation in the ability of ultrasound screening for cardiac abnormalities, with detection rates varying from 6 per cent to 77 per cent.[1,4] These differences may be related to the gestational age at which the scan is performed, the type of congenital heart abnormality and the experience of the operator. Several cardiac defects are associated with a normal standard four-chamber view. These include:

- tetralogy of Fallot;
- transposition of the great arteries;
- small atrial and ventricular septal defects;

FETAL CONDITIONS

- mild pulmonary or aortic valve stenosis;
- mild coarctation of the aorta.

With the improvements in paediatric cardiac surgery, prenatal diagnosis of cardiac conditions has become much more important. Parents can make informed choices, if given the realistic expectations of the problem.

Thoracic malformations

By obtaining transverse and longitudinal views of the fetal chest, space-occupying lesions, solid or cystic, may be diagnosed. The fetal lungs are uniformly echogenic. Fluid within the pleural cavity (pleural effusions) may be identified as a result of certain fetal conditions. Chylothorax, a relatively common cause of pleural effusion in neonatal life, is an accumulation of chyle in the pleural cavity. Bronchogenic cysts may appear as sonolucent areas within the fetal chest.

Congenital cystic adenomatous malformation of the lung (CCAML) is a condition whereby there is overgrowth of terminal bronchioles at the expense of saccular spaces. The ultrasound appearance varies according to the type: either macrocystic, with large cystic structures within the chest, or microcystic, where there is increased echogenicity of the lung tissue. Lung sequestrations may also appear as an echogenic mass. Cystic structures within the chest may also be demonstrated in the fetus with congenital diaphragmatic hernia. When there is a defect, the stomach or other abdominal contents may be demonstrated above the level of the diaphragm.

Gastrointestinal and abdominal wall malformations

Demonstration of the integrity of the abdominal wall is made on transverse and longitudinal views. Ventral wall defects, gastroschisis and exomphalos may be identified.

Gastroschisis is a para-umbilical defect, and can be diagnosed by the presence of herniated organs floating freely within the amniotic cavity. An exomphalos is a central defect surrounded by a membrane on which the umbilical cord is inserted. These defects may also be associated with an elevated MSAFP. In isolation, the prognosis for both of these malformations is good with surgical correction, but karyotyping should be considered in the case of exomphalos, as an association with aneuploidy exists. Rarer defects in the abdominal wall may be diagnosed, known as bladder and cloacal extrophy.

Intra-abdominal pathology may be diagnosed on ultrasound such as:

- fetal ascites;
- small and large bowel obstruction;
- meconium peritonitis;
- mesenteric, omental and retroperitoneal cysts.

Many of the obstructive malformations may be associated with polyhydramnios.

Urogenital malformations

The fetal kidneys and bladder are relatively easily identified structures in the mid-trimester. Many fetal renal problems are associated with a disturbance in amniotic fluid volume. By 16 weeks, the majority of the amniotic fluid is produced by the fetal kidneys. If oligohydramnios is diagnosed in the mid-trimester, in the absence of a history of ruptured membranes, fetal renal malformation must be suspected.

Renal agenesis may be bilateral or unilateral. If bilateral, there is associated anhydramnios, and the condition is fatal. Visualisation of the fetal kidneys in this situation is difficult due to loss of the acoustic window and may be facilitated by an amnio-infusion.

Infantile polycystic kidney disease is an autosomal recessive disease. Ultrasound diagnosis is made by the demonstration of bilateral, enlarged, hyperechogenic, fetal kidneys, absent fetal bladder and associated oligohydramnios. The prognosis is poor.

Obstructive uropathy may occur due to an obstruction at the urethra or ureter. Urethral obstruction, due either to urethral atresia or posterior urethral valves, may be demonstrated by the presence of a distended fetal bladder, hydroureter and hydronephrosis. Ureteric obstruction, which may be unilateral or bilateral, can be diagnosed by ultrasound by the demonstration of hydronephrosis.

In multicystic dysplastic kidney disease (MDKD), ultrasound examination of the fetal kidneys shows the presence of multiple cysts, and increased echogenicity of the surrounding parenchyma. The kidneys are enlarged and, where there is bilateral disease, the prognosis is fatal.

Tumours of the kidney and adrenal gland, if present in fetal life, can also be diagnosed on ultrasound scans.

Skeletal malformations

Diagnosis of skeletal abnormalities requires a full examination of the fetus, with a skeletal survey. This involves both morphological and biometric examination of the skull, vertebrae, ribs, long bones, and digits of the hands and feet. Measurement of the femur length at a dating scan may be the first clue to a skeletal problem.

Skeletal malformations may affect the whole skeleton and may be lethal, such as:

- achondrogenesis;
- thanatophoric dysplasia;
- short-rib polydactyly syndromes;
- fibrochondrogenesis;
- homozygous achondroplasia;
- osteogenesis imperfecta (perinatal type);
- hypophosphatasia (perinatal type).

Lethality is usually dependent on thoracic cage involvement and subsequent development of pulmonary hypoplasia.

Other skeletal problems, such as radial anomalies, talipes equinovarus, femoral hypoplasia, facial clefts and digital anomalies, may be identified and may form part of another syndrome, including chromosome anomalies.

The prognosis depends on the involvement of other, non-skeletal, malformations.

The overall detection rate of skeletal problems is 90 per cent.[9]

Hydrops fetalis and cystic hygroma

This is a condition in which fluid accumulates within the body cavities and soft tissues of the fetus. The aetiologies of this condition are numerous (see Chapter 40).[10] Visualisation of fluid within the fetus is relatively easy, and the commonest area of fluid accumulation is at the fetal neck, the cystic hygroma. This is usually due to lymphatic obstruction, and is recognised as a cystic structure adjacent to the fetal neck. Cystic hygromas are frequently associated with chromosomal abnormalities. Smaller degrees of fluid in this area are referred to as nuchal oedema or nuchal translucency. As detailed below, it is this latter anomaly that has been identified at earlier gestations (11–14 weeks), and has now been incorporated into screening programmes for aneuploidy.

SCREENING FOR CHROMOSOMAL DISEASE

Many structural malformations identified on scan may be associated with chromosomal disease, such as:

- cystic hygroma;
- cardiac defects;
- exomphalos;
- holoprosencephaly;
- microcephaly;
- diaphragmatic hernia;
- oesophageal/duodenal atresia;
- renal anomalies;
- radial aplasia;
- micrognathia;
- clinodactyly of the fifth finger;
- polydactyly;
- talipes;
- facial clefts.

At the time of the 20-week scan, minor ultrasound abnormalities may be seen that may also be associated with aneuploidy. These are known as 'soft markers'. They may not constitute a structural defect, but, when seen along with another risk factor for chromosomal disease, karyotyping may be considered. Soft markers include:

- nuchal oedema;
- mild renal pyelectasis;
- hyperechogenic bowel;
- echogenic intracardiac foci;
- strawberry-shaped skull;
- mild ventriculomegaly;
- shortened long bones;
- choroid plexus cysts;
- clenched fists;
- rocker-bottom feet;
- sandal gap;
- single umbilical artery.

These soft markers have been included in some screening programmes for Down's syndrome. However, apart from nuchal oedema, there is no strong evidence at present that the other soft markers are helpful in identifying Down's syndrome [A].[11]

A recent NHS fetal anomaly screening programme has refined recommendations such that only the following markers should be referred for further management:

- Nuchal oedema (>6 mm);
- Ventriculomegaly (atrium 10 mm or greater);
- Echogenic bowel;
- Renal pelvic dilatation (>7 mm AP);
- Small measurements compared with the dating scan (<3rd centile);
- Facial clefting.

Choroid plexus cysts, head shape, cisterna magna (in the absence of brain abnormality), echogenic foci and two-vessel cord should not be recorded or referred, and should be considered as 'normal variants'.[12]

FIRST-TRIMESTER SCREENING

Ultrasound scanning in the first trimester was primarily introduced for viability and accurate dating. With improved resolution, a number of fetal defects may also be seen, such as:

- anencephaly;
- holoprosencephaly;
- encephalocele;
- Dandy–Walker syndrome;
- cardiac anomalies;
- gastroschisis;
- exomphalos;
- megacystis;
- diaphragmatic hernia;
- multidysplastic kidney;
- some skeletal dysplasias.

Using a combination of transabdominal and transvaginal ultrasound, up to 59 per cent of major structural defects may be diagnosed at the 11- to 14-week scan.[12,13]

An important component of the first-trimester scan is the NT measurement, which is the maximum thickness of the subcutaneous translucency between the skin and the soft tissue overlying the cervical spine. It has not only been shown to be an effective screening test for aneuploidy, but also may identify a fetus at risk of cardiac defects, skeletal dysplasias and genetic syndromes.[14] There are sufficient data to show that NT screening for Down's syndrome at 10–14 weeks is superior to serum screening with multiple markers at 15–20 weeks' gestation [A]. Assessment of the fetal nasal bone during the first trimester may improve the detection of Down's syndrome. However, studies of general population screening have not been able to support this.[14]

First-trimester combined screening (nuchal translucency + hCG + PAPP-A) is now the recommended screening test for Down's syndrome (see Chapter 29). The counselling, expertise and training required to successfully implement such a national screening test have been challenging.

HAZARDS OF THE ULTRASOUND SCAN

Many epidemiological and laboratory studies have been performed to search for evidence of the possible biological effects of diagnostic ultrasound. Childhood cancer, dyslexia, non-right-handedness, delayed speech development and reduced birthweight have all been implicated, but as yet there is no good evidence to establish a firm link between ultrasound and these end-points.[1]

Although a sophisticated investigation, there are limitations to ultrasound. Adequate visualisation of the fetal anatomy may not be possible due to the fetal position or maternal habitude. In situations of gross maternal obesity, confirmation of fetal viability may be extremely difficult.

Visual confirmation of fetal normality appears to promote a positive attitude towards the pregnancy, with improved compliance on healthcare issues such as smoking and alcohol.[15] However, the detection of fetal defects and, in particular, soft ultrasound markers may generate immense anxiety and rejection, even if the subsequent invasive testing proves that the fetus is healthy. Hence, for the successful maintenance of ultrasound screening programmes, a framework of skilled midwives, sonographers and counsellors is necessary. This is not only to deal with parents in whom a fetal abnormality has been diagnosed, but also to ensure that, prior to the ultrasound scan, women have a clear idea about what the test is likely to achieve and its reliability in doing so.

Perhaps the greatest hazard of ultrasound is misdiagnosis.

EBM

- Screening the whole population rather than selective scanning is the most reliable way to identify a fetal abnormality [A].
- A scan undertaken between 18 and 21 weeks is the most effective method to identify a wide range of fetal abnormalities [B].
- Screening for fetal abnormality reduces the perinatal mortality rates through identification and termination of affected pregnancies [A].

KEY POINTS

- Detailed ultrasound at 18–21 weeks is an important screening examination in which most life-threatening malformations can be diagnosed.
- Pregnant women should receive clear information regarding the objectives of the ultrasound examination and the likelihood of finding an abnormality.
- The success of the ultrasound examination depends on the operator, the ultrasound equipment, the fetal position and the maternal habitude.
- When an abnormality is detected on ultrasound, the parents should have ready access to skilled counsellors who are able to provide them with full information, options and support in order to allow them to make an informed choice.

Published Guidelines

Grudzinskas JG, Ward RHT (eds). itals*Recommendations arising from the Study Group on Screening for Down's Syndrome in the First Trimester*. London: RCOG Press, 1997.

NICE. Clinical Care Guideline No. 62; *Antenatal Care. Routine care for the healthy pregnant woman*. London: NICE 2008.

UK National Screening Committee. *Fetal Anomaly Ultrasound screening Programme. 18^{+0} to 20^{+6} weeks Fetal Anomaly Scan National Standards and Guidance for England.* Exeter: UK National Screening Committee, 2010.

Key References

1. Whittle M. *Ultrasound Screening for Fetal Abnormalities*. Report of the RCOG Working Party. London: RCOG Press, 1997.

2. Crane JP, LeFevre ML, Winborn RC *et al.* and the RADIUS Study Group. A randomized trial of prenatal ultrasonographic screening: impact on the detection, management and outcome of anomalous fetuses. *Am J Obstet Gynecol* 1994;171:392–9.

3. Luck C. Value of routine ultrasound scanning at 19 weeks: a four year study of 8849 deliveries. *BMJ* 1992;304:1474–8.

4. Carvalho JS, Mavrides E, Shinebourne EA *et al.* Improving the effectiveness of routine prenatal screening for major congenital heart defects. *Heart* 2002;88:387–91.

5. Drife JO, Donnai D (eds). *Antenatal Diagnosis of Fetal Abnormalities*. London: RCOG Press, 1991, 354–5.

6. NICE. Clinical Care Guideline No. 62; *Antenatal Care. Routine care for the healthy pregnant woman*. London: NICE 2008.

7. Nicolaides KH, Campbell S, Gabbe SG, Guidetti R. Ultrasound screening for spina bifida: cranial and cerebellar signs. *Lancet* 1986; ii:72–4.

8. Papp Z, Toth-Pal E, Papp CS, Torok O. Impact of prenatal mid-trimester screening on the prevalence of fetal structure anomalies: a prospective epidemiological study. *Ultrasound Obstet Gynecol* 1995;6:320–6.

9. Whittle MJ. *Routine Ultrasound Screening in Pregnancy.* Report of the RCOG Working Party. London: RCOG Press, 2000: 7–12.

10. James D. Fetal hydrops. In: *The Yearbook of Obstetrics and Gynaecology*, Vol. 9. London: RCOG Press, 2001: 277–87.

11. Smith-Bindman R, Hosmer W, Feldstein VA, Deeks JJ, Goldberg JD. Second-trimester ultrasound to detect fetuses with Down's syndrome. A meta-analysis. *JAMA* 2001;285:1044–55.

12. UK National Screening Committee. Fetal Anomaly Ultrasound Screening Programme. *Soft Marker screening policy.* Exeter: UK NSC, 2009.

13. Whitlow BJ, Chatzipapas IK, Lazanakis ML, Kadir RA, Economides DL. The value of sonography in early pregnancy for the detection of fetal abnormalities in an unselected population. *Br J Obstet Gynaecol* 1999;106:929–36.

14. Reading AE, Campbell S, Cox DN, Sledmere CM. Health beliefs and healthcare behaviour in pregnancy. *Psychol Med* 1982;12:379–83.

15. Malone FD, Ball RH, Nyberg DA *et al.* First trimester nasal bone evaluation for aneuploidy in the general population. *Obstet Gynecol* 2004;104:1222–8.

16. Nicolaides KH, Heath V, Liao AW. The 11–14 week scan. *Clin Obstet Gynaecol* 2000;14:581–94.

17. Souka AP, Pilalis A, Kavalakis I *et al.* Screening for major structural abnormalites at the 11-14 week ultrasound scan. *Am J Obstet Gynecol* 2006;194:393–396.

18. NHS Fetal Anomaly Ultrasound screening Programme. (NHS FASP). 18^{+0} to 20^{+6} weeks Fetal Anomaly Scan National Standards and Guidance for England. Exeter: UK NSC, 2010.

FETAL CONDITIONS

Chapter 31 Invasive and non-invasive prenatal diagnosis

Michele P Mohajer

MRCOG standards

Theoretical skills

- Understand the indications for an invasive test.
- Know the advantages and disadvantages of each test.

Practical skills

- Be able to counsel a woman about the procedure and its risks.
- Have observed other procedures such as chorionic villous sampling, placental biopsy, cordocentesis, intrauterine transfusion.

INTRODUCTION

High-resolution ultrasound has enabled direct access to the different constituents of the gestational sac from the middle of the first trimester of pregnancy. An ever-increasing range of invasive techniques is being developed to facilitate the diagnosis of chromosomal and single-gene defects, metabolic disorders, intrauterine infection, fetal anaemia, thrombocytopenia and some structural problems.

All invasive procedures carry a small risk of fetal loss. Early prenatal testing provides the opportunity for surgical termination of the pregnancy if required, but the earlier invasive testing tends to increase the fetal loss rate. Non-invasive techniques for identifying fetal cells in maternal blood and cervical mucus have been the focus of much research.[1] This technique of non-invasive prenatal diagnosis (NIPT) using free fetal DNA (cfDNA) with detection rates of >99 per cent has now become incorporated into clinical use[15] but is not currently available within the health service in the UK. Developments in techniques employing multiplex PCR have enabled reliable prenatal diagnosis of fetal blood groups[2] and fetal aneuploidy.[3]

The routinely used invasive procedures are amniocentesis, CVS and fetal blood sampling (FBS).

AMNIOCENTESIS

Amniocentesis involves the aspiration of amniotic fluid from the amniotic sac via a needle inserted through the maternal abdomen. It is the commonest prenatal diagnostic procedure in the UK. It was first introduced in 1966 for the diagnosis of genetic disease.[4] It was subsequently used to confirm open NTDs by measurement of liquor alpha feto protein in the presence of a raised MSAFP (see Chapter 29).[5] It is usually performed between 15 and 16 weeks' gestation.

Method

Using an aseptic technique, a 22-gauge needle is inserted through the maternal abdomen under direct real-time ultrasound control with continuous needle-tip visualisation. This method is more successful than blind techniques [B]. Fluid (15–20 mL) containing fetal cells is aspirated into a syringe and sent to the genetics laboratory for testing.

Indications for amniocentesis

The main indication for amniocentesis is for fetal karyotyping. In view of the risk of miscarriage, the procedure is offered when there is an increased risk of aneuploidy, such as for:

- women with positive screening for Down's syndrome;
- women of advanced maternal age (traditionally 35 years);
- ultrasound detection of an abnormality or soft markers;
- parental balanced translocation;
- a previous history of chromosomal abnormality.

One of the major disadvantages for the woman has been the long wait for the result, which may take from 2 weeks to 4 weeks. Molecular genetics has developed two techniques, which have permitted the rapid diagnosis of the many major chromosomal abnormalities. These two tests, fluorescence *in-situ* hybridization (FISH) and quantitative fluorescence polymerase chain reaction (QF-PCR), can provide results in 24–48 hours.[6] FISH relies on the unique ability of a portion of single-stranded DNA (known as a probe) to hybridise with its complementary target DNA sequence. By attaching a fluorescent label to the appropriate probe, diagnosis of autosomal trisomies for chromosomes 13, 18 and 21, and X and Y chromosomes can be made in 6–8 hours by direct fluorescent microscopy. QF-PCR uses highly polymorphic small tandem repeat markers, which allow distinction between normal and trisomic DNA samples. Diagnosis of the major chromosomal abnormalities (trisomies 13, 18, 21 and sex chromosome copy number abnormalities) can be performed in 24–48 hours. Both techniques share the same diagnostic dilemma in that conventional chromosomal analysis is required to detect other chromosomal disorders. However, as a result of its reliability, rapidity and relatively low cost, QF-PCR has been introduced in most laboratories as an adjunct to long-term culture.[7] Where the indication for amniocentesis is a screen-positive result, QF-PCR may be the only technique offered.

Amniocentesis is also used for the diagnosis of single-gene disorders. However, culture of the cells and extraction of the DNA often means a significant delay in receiving the result.

Using PCR techniques, amniocentesis can also be used to facilitate the diagnosis of certain congenital infections (see Chapter 36), such as cytomegalovirus and toxoplasmosis.

Amniocentesis no longer has a role to play in isoimmunised pregnancies. The absorbance difference at the wavelength 450 nm provided an indirect measurement of the bilirubin in amniotic fluid. However, in view of the increased likelihood of further sensitisation, other non-invasive methods for estimating the degree of fetal anaemia are now in routine use (fetal, middle cerebral artery, Doppler peak systolic velocity).[8]

Amniocentesis is also no longer used to estimate the AFP and AChE for the diagnosis of NTDs. Amniocentesis performed in the presence of raised MSAFP is associated with a significant increase in fetal loss [A].

Complications

The fetal loss rate from the procedure varies, but the only RCT of low-risk women reports a rate of 1 per cent [A].[9] Many units report their own miscarriage rate based on their own individual audit data. Operator experience has been shown to be important [B]. Adequate levels of training (30 procedures per year) are necessary to maintain success and reduce complications, although postgraduate training is moving towards a competency-based rather than a numerical goal. Cell culture may fail in 0.5 per cent of amniocenteses, necessitating a further invasive test.

Early amniocentesis

Owing to the relative ease of the procedure, amniocentesis at earlier gestations was performed in order to provide women with the advantages of early prenatal diagnosis. Early amniocentesis can be performed from 10 weeks' gestation. However, the technique is considered unsafe prior to 14 weeks as it carries a higher fetal loss rate (7.6 per cent), increased fetal talipes

and respiratory morbidity, and reduced amniocyte culture rate compared with other procedures [A].[10]

CVS AND PLACENTAL BIOPSY

These procedures refer to the sampling of placental tissue. Placental biopsy is the term used when the procedure is performed after the first trimester. Placental tissue can be obtained by catheter, needle aspiration or biopsy forceps. Transabdominal and transcervical methods are both used. The procedure can be performed from 10 weeks' gestation. Early diagnosis allows the woman the option of termination before 13 weeks' gestation.

Transabdominal CVS

Using aseptic techniques, an 18- to 20-gauge needle is inserted through the maternal abdomen to the placental site under direct ultrasound guidance. Placental tissue is aspirated into a syringe attached to the needle. Similarly, a fine biopsy forceps can be used through an outer guide needle. If the placenta is completely posterior and low lying, access via the transabdominal route may not be possible.

Transcervical CVS

This method is ideal for the posterior low-lying placenta. The cervix and vagina are visualised through a speculum and cleaned with sterile solution. Transabdominal ultrasound is performed to visualise the cervical canal. The needle, catheter or biopsy forceps is then introduced through the cervix towards the placenta under ultrasound guidance, and a sample is taken.

The choice of a transabdominal or a transcervical approach should be dependent on operator experience, the placental site and the axis of the uterus. Transcervical CVS is associated with less discomfort than the transabdominal approach, but there may be concern regarding the potential risk of infection with the transcervical route. However, several randomised trials show almost identical miscarriage rates with the two routes [A].[16]

Indications for CVS

CVS has the advantage of yielding a large amount of tissue and is therefore the method of choice when large amounts of DNA are required in the diagnosis of monogenic disorders. With the increasing use of early screening tests for Down's syndrome, and with high-resolution ultrasound detecting abnormalities in the first trimester, CVS is more frequently requested.

Although direct chromosome preparations and other rapid cell culture techniques have allowed rapid karyotyping, QF-PCR is now widely used for rapid test reporting.[7] This is advantageous to parents who do not wish to wait for results and who wish to avail themselves of early termination if an affected fetus is found.

Complications

The fetal loss rate has always been considered to be higher with CVS than with amniocentesis. Second-trimester amniocentesis is safer than early amniocentesis or transcervical CVS, and is the procedure of choice in the second trimester [A]. CVS should be regarded as the procedure of choice when testing is required before 15 weeks' gestation. The procedure-related loss above the individual background risk is considered to be 1 per cent.[11]

Placental mosaicisms can occur in about 2 per cent of cases. This presents counselling difficulties and necessitates further invasive testing to obtain fetal cells.

There has been concern regarding the association of CVS and limb defects. This complication appears to be related to the procedure being performed at earlier gestations. Subsequent studies have shown no association when the procedure is performed after 10 weeks.[12]

FETAL BLOOD SAMPLING

Sampling of blood from the fetal circulation has now been used for a variety of diagnostic purposes. It requires expertise, and should be performed by clinicians with extensive experience in all other ultrasound-guided procedures.

Method

The procedure can be performed from 16 to 18 weeks' gestation onwards. However, before 20 weeks it carries increased risk of cord accidents. A 20-gauge needle is introduced through the maternal abdomen under direct ultrasound control. Fetal blood can be aspirated from either the placental insertion or the fetal insertion of the umbilical cord. Cardiac puncture or intrahepatic vessels may also be sampled.

Indications for FBS

Rapid high-quality karyotyping can be obtained with this method within 48–72 hours. This is particularly useful when an abnormality is detected late in the pregnancy.

FBS is also vital in the diagnosis of fetal haematological problems such as anaemia and thrombocytopenia. It has also been used to assess the acid–base status of the fetus in growth restriction, but non-invasive biophysical methods and Doppler studies are more routinely used.

Complications

Bleeding at the site of the needle and fetal bradycardia may occur as a result of the procedure, especially in association with the umbilical artery site. The overall procedure-related fetal loss is 1–2 per cent. Introduction of infection may occur

and, more importantly, if the mother is carrying HIV or other viruses, transmission to the fetus may occur.[13]

FETOSCOPY

With improvement in fibreoptic technology, direct *in-utero* visualisation of the fetus can now be achieved. This may be useful for identifying small structural abnormalities and facilitating direct organ biopsy, such as skin and muscle biopsy. Organ biopsy can also be performed under ultrasound control. This is used only in specialist centres and >80% of indications is for the treatment of severe twin-to-twin transfusion syndrome.

COUNSELLING

The decision as to which invasive test is required must be tailored to the individual mother. It is imperative that she is given full details of the range of tests available, the procedures, advantages and disadvantages, and risk of fetal loss or damage. This information should be given well before the procedure is attempted, allowing her to make her decision, and should be non-directive. The discussion should be followed up with written information.[14]

CONCLUSIONS

These invasive procedures allow the diagnosis and assessment of a large number of abnormalities, so that parents can make choices about the continuation or otherwise of their pregnancies. Early diagnostic procedures provide the advantage of early termination, if sought, but must be balanced against the increased fetal loss, or the possibility of terminating a fetus that may have miscarried spontaneously. Rapid molecular tests have improved the waiting time for results but have limitations. Further developments in the identification of fetal cells in maternal tissues will inevitably reduce the necessity of invasive diagnostic tests.

EBM

- The rate of miscarriage following amniocentesis is approximately 1 per cent [A].
- Early amniocentesis has a higher complication rate than CVS and mid-trimester amniocentesis [A].
- Amniocentesis performed under direct ultrasound visualisation is associated with higher rates of success [B].

KEY POINTS

- Amniocentesis is the most commonly performed prenatal diagnostic procedure.
- CVS should not be performed at less than 10 weeks' gestation because of the association of limb defects.
- Most invasive tests other than amniocentesis are generally performed in a tertiary referral centre.
- The specific invasive test should be tailored to the individual woman's circumstances and wishes.
- A team of specialist counsellors should be available for the parents both before and after invasive techniques are performed.

Published Guidelines

Alfirevic Z, Walkinshaw SA, Kilby MD. *Amniocentesis and chorion villus sampling.* RCOG 'Green Top' Guideline No. 8. London: RCOG Press, 2010.

RCOG. Amniocentesis Consent Advice: Setting standards to improve women's health. London: RCOG Press, 2006.

Key References

1. Lamvu G, Kuller JA. Prenatal diagnosis using fetal cells from the maternal circulation. *Obstet Gynaecol Surv* 1997;52:433–7.

2. Daniels G, Finning K, Martin P, Massey E. Non-invasive prenatal diagnosis of fetal blood group phenotypes: current practice and future prospects. *Prenatal Diagn* 2009;29:101–7.

3. Lo YM. Non-invasive prenatal detection of fetal chromosome aneuploidies by maternal plasma nucleic acid analysis: a review of the current state of the art. *BJOG* 2009;116:152–7.

4. Steele MW, Breg WR. Chromosome analysis of human amniotic fluid cells. *Lancet* 1966;i:383–5.

5. Bennet MJ. Fetal loss after second trimester amniocentesis in women with raised serum alpha-fetoprotein. *Lancet* 1978;ii:987.

6. Thein AT, Abdel-Fattah SA, Kyle PM, Soothhill PW. An assessment of the use of interphase FISH with chromosome specific probes as an alternative to cytogenetics in prenatal diagnosis. *Prenat Diagn* 2000;4:275–80.

7. Cirigliano V, Voglno G, Marongiu A *et al.* Rapid prenatal diagnosis by QF-PCR: evaluation of 30,000 consecutive clinical samples and future applications. *Ann NY Acad Sci* 2006;1075:288–98.

8. Oepkes D, Seward PG, Vandenbussche FP *et al.* Doppler ultrasonography versus amniocentesis to predict fetal anaemia. *N Eng J Med* 2006;355:156–64.

9. Tabor A, Philip J, Madsen M, Bang J, Obel EB, Norgaard-Pederson B. Randomised controlled trial of genetic amniocentesis in 4606 low-risk women. *Lancet* 1986;i:1287–93.

10. Nicolaides K, Brizot MdeL, Patel F, Snijders R. Comparison of chorionic villus sampling and amniocentesis for fetal karyotyping at 10–13 weeks' gestation. *Lancet* 1994;344:435–9.

11. Alfirevic Z, Mujezinovic F, Sundberg K. Amniocentesis and chorion villus sampling for prenatal diagnosis. *Cochrane Database System Reviews* 2009;3:CD003252.

12. Froster UG, Jackson L. Limb defects and chorion-villus sampling: results from an international registry, 1992–94. *Lancet* 1996;347:489–94.

13. Workman MR, Philpott-Howard J. Risk of fetal infection from invasive procedures. *J Hosp Infect* 1997;35:169–74.

14. NHS Fetal Anomaly Screening Programme. *Amniocentesis and Chorion Villus Sampling. Policy, standards and protocols.* Exeter:UK NSC, 2008.

15. Song K, Musci TJ, Caughey AB. Clinical utility and cost of non-invasive prenatal testing with cfDNA analysis in high-risk women based on a US population. *J Matern Fetal Neonatal Med* 2013;26:1180–5.

16. Jackson L, Zachary J, Fowler S *et al.* A randomised comparison of transcervical and transabdominal chorionic villus sampling. *N Engl J Med* 1992;327:594–8.

Chapter 32 Understanding genetics and genetic tests

Fiona Mackie and Denise Williams

MRCOG standards

Theoretical skills

Genetic modes of inheritance, common genetic conditions, the importance of screening and the diagnosis thereof.

- Modes of inheritance (Mendelian, multifactorial)
- Cytogenetics
- Phenotypes of common aneuploidies (Down's syndrome, Edward's syndrome, Patau's syndrome, Turner's syndrome, Klinefelter's syndrome, triple X, multiple Y)
- Translocation
- Molecular genetics (DNA transcription, DNA translation, DNA blotting techniques, gene amplification techniques, principles of gene tracking)

Pre-conception care

- Principles of inheritance of disease

Practical skills

- Counsel about genetic disease
- History taking and pedigree analysis
- Demonstrate an ability to explain correctly and place in context for the women: genetic disorders and their inheritance with examples such as Tay-Sachs disease, cystic fibrosis and thalassaemia

INTRODUCTION

Genetic factors are known to contribute to the majority of human diseases, so information about an individual's genetic make-up may be important to their clinical care and that of their family. In this chapter we describe the basic genetic mechanisms and provide relevant information to help identify patients with, or at risk of, a genetic condition, so that they can be counselled appropriately. This will include information about genetic testing, recognising its uses and limitations, and understanding which patients should be referred to specialist clinical genetics services.

Our understanding of genetics is growing rapidly and exciting developments both in laboratory techniques and computer science mean that an increasing number of genetic diagnoses are now possible. However, the disadvantages of this expanding field include the creation of ethical dilemmas and detection of conditions for which there is no cure.

CLASSIFICATION OF GENETIC DISORDERS

Genetic disorders are classified into:

- multifactorial
- chromosomal
- single gene
- mitochondrial
- somatic mutations.

Most conditions seen by healthcare professionals are multifactorial. In multifactorial inheritance, a condition occurs as the result of a combination of environmental factors such as obesity or smoking, and numerous genetic factors. More rarely a condition occurs because of an alteration to the number or structure of a chromosome, or a mutation in an individual gene. It is important that these 'chromosomal' and 'single-gene' disorders are recognised as they may have significant implications to the wider family. Mitochondrial disorders always show maternal inheritance and, as they are rare, will not be discussed further. Disorders due to somatic mutations are unlikely to be encountered in obstetric practice, but are extremely common and play an important role in the development of many cancers. A few conditions may be the result of environmental factors alone, e.g. fetal anticonvulsant syndrome. These environmental conditions are also not discussed here.

CHROMOSOMAL DISORDERS

Chromosomal disorders are very common and are estimated to affect at least 7.5 per cent of all conceptions. However, they usually result in a non-viable pregnancy, so the liveborn frequency is 0.6 per cent. About 60 per cent of early spontaneous miscarriages have a chromosomal abnormality, 5 per cent of late spontaneous miscarriages and 4–5 per cent of stillbirths. The clinical features that suggest a chromosomal disorder in a child are:

- multiple congenital anomalies;
- short stature including IUGR;
- learning difficulties;
- microcephaly;
- dysmorphism.

There are two main types of chromosome abnormality: numerical and structural. These are associated with an error during meiosis.

Numerical abnormalities: aneuploidy describes a chromosome problem that is caused by an extra or missing chromosome. The most common examples of aneuploidy are Down's syndrome, which is caused by an extra copy of chromosome 21 (trisomy 21) and Turner's syndrome (monosomy X, X0) (Table 32.1). The exact mechanisms causing aneuploidy are not known, but generally they are more likely to happen at an advanced maternal age. If a couple has a baby with a numerical chromosome abnormality, they are at higher risk of having another baby with aneuploidy compared with the general population, irrespective of maternal age (with some exceptions).

Structural abnormalities: these result from chromosome breakage, followed by abnormal repair. The most common structural abnormalities are translocations, inversions, deletions and duplications. A detailed knowledge about chromosome structure, meiosis and mitosis is required to understand the aetiology of these abnormalities, and referral to a clinical geneticist is recommended.

Translocations occur when there is breakage of two different (i.e. non-homologous) chromosomes which then exchange fragments. This can either be balanced or unbalanced:

- A translocation is balanced if there is an even swap of genetic material between the two chromosomes – no net loss or gain of any chromosome material; there is the correct amount of material present, but in a different order. The individual is clinically normal, but is said to be a 'carrier' of the balanced translocation. A balanced

Table 32.1 Common aneuploidy (numerical) chromosome conditions

Condition	Genetic error	Features
Down's syndrome	Trisomy 21 (95%) Robertsonian translocation of Ch 14:21 (3%) Mosaicism (1%)	- Learning disabilities - Hypotonia - Cardiac abnormalities: ASDs, VSDs, AVSDs most common - Gastrointestinal abnormalities: Hirschsprung's disease, duodenal atresia, imperforate anus - Dysmorphic features: upslanting palpebral fissures, speckling of the iris (Brushfield's spots), flat facial profile, brachycephaly - Single palmar crease - Subfertility - Increased risk of: acute myeloid/lymphoblastic leukaemia, Alzheimer's disease, hypothyroidism
Edward's syndrome	Trisomy 18	- Low birthweight - Cardiac abnormalities: ASDs, valvular abnormalities - Abdominal abnormalities: exomphalos, inguinal/diaphragmatic hernia, renal malformations - Facial clefts - Spina bifida - Severe-to-profound developmental delay - Microcephaly - Dysmorphic features: prominent occiput, simple ears, over-riding fingers, rocker-bottom feet - 90–95% die <1 year old

Condition	Genetic error	Features
Patau's syndrome	Trisomy 13	• Low birthweight • Holoprosencephaly • Cardiac abnormalities: VSDs, ASDs • Abdominal abnormalities: omphalocele, renal malformations • Microphthalmia/anophthalmia • Cleft lip +/− palate • Post-axial polydactyly • Dysmorphic features: hypotelorism, scalp defects • Microcephaly • Severe to profound developmental delay • 90–95% die <1 month old
Turner's syndrome	Monosomy X (XO)	• Proportionate short stature • Lymphoedema • Congenital heart disease; coarctation of the aorta, ASDs • Horseshoe kidney • Gonadal dysfunction; 'streak ovaries' • Webbed neck (redundant neck skin due to resolving cystic hygroma) • Cubitus valgus • Intelligence normal • >99% of affected pregnancies will spontaneously miscarry.
Klinefelter's syndrome	XXY	• Tall stature • Male karyotype • Infertility • Hypogonadotrophic hypogonadism • Small testes, poorly developed secondary sexual characteristics, gynaecomastia
Triple X syndrome	XXX	• Normally clinically normal, so often not diagnosed • Tall stature • Mild learning disabilities in 15–25%
Multiple Y syndrome	XYY	• Normal phenotype, often not diagnosed • Tall stature

ASD, atrial septal defect; AVSD, atrioventricularseptal defect; VSD, ventricular septal defect.

translocation is important because of the risk of producing chromosomally 'unbalanced' products. This may cause a chromosomally abnormal baby presenting with multiple congenital anomalies including learning difficulties, stillbirth, miscarriage or subfertility.

• A translocation is unbalanced if there is an uneven swap of genetic material between the non-homologous chromosomes. This results in both extra and missing chromosome material, which is nearly always clinically significant. The unbalanced translocation may arise for the first time in an individual, or may have been inherited from a parent with the 'balanced' form of the translocation. Two main types of translocation exist: reciprocal

and Robertsonian translocations. Reciprocal translocations may involve any of the chromosomes, including the sex chromosomes, whereas Robertsonian translocations involve only chromosomes 13–15, 21 and 22. A relatively frequent translocation is the Robertsonian 14;21 translocation which predisposes to Down's syndrome (Fig. 32.1). It is important to note that the other possible outcomes demonstrated in Fig. 32.1 (monosomy 14, monosomy 21, and translocation trisomy 14) are not viable, and will miscarry.

Inversions occur when a single chromosome breaks in two places, then the segment of genetic material between the

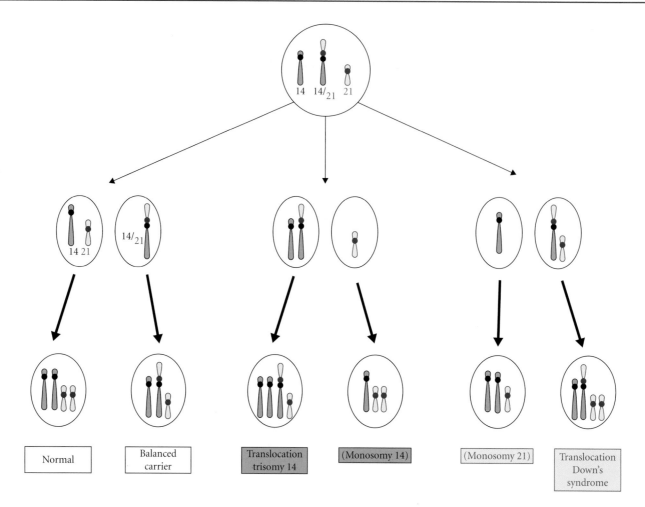

Fig. 32.1 Robertsonian translocation

breaks turns through 180° and rejoins. As with translocations an inversion may be balanced or unbalanced. A carrier of a balanced inversion will be healthy; the medical significance is the increased risk of producing unbalanced gametes. Unbalanced inversions present in the same way as unbalanced translocations. There are two types of inversion: paracentric (excluding the centromere) and pericentric (including the centromere). With few exceptions the unbalanced products of a paracentric inversion are not compatible with viability.

Deletions occur when there is loss of any part of a chromosome. If a large amount of genetic material is lost this will usually produce a non-viable pregnancy. If only a small amount of genetic material is lost, the pregnancy may be viable, but result in physical abnormalities and learning difficulties in the child. Two common examples are DiGeorge's syndrome (22q11.2 gene deletion), and cri-du-chat syndrome (deletion of the short arm of chromosome 5) (Table 32.2).

Duplications occur when there are two copies of a segment of a chromosome, thus resulting in extra genetic material. Duplications are more common than deletions and are normally less harmful. A duplication of the long arm of chromosome 15 is relatively frequent, though the phenotypic effect can be difficult to interpret, particularly when the diagnosis is made antenatally.

Chromosomal mosaicism

Another occurrence to be familiar with is that of chromosomal mosaicism. Chromosomal mosaicism refers to the presence of two or more cell lines in an individual, which differ from each other in chromosome number or structure. Although the individual has developed from a single fertilised egg, the two cell lines means that they have two different genotypes. Mosaicism commonly results from errors in cell division during mitosis, but other explanations exist. Mosaicism in chromosomal disorders is well known. For example, about 1 per cent of patients with trisomy 21 mosaic for cell lines with two copies of chromosome 21 and cell lines with three copies of chromosome 21 (Fig. 32.2).

The presence of a normal cell line in mosaicism tends to improve the clinical outcome for some patients. In conditions where a chromosomal abnormality is known to result in miscarriage, mosaicism for the same abnormality can be seen in children.

A well-known mosaic condition is the Pallister–Killian syndrome which is caused by the presence of an abnormal extra chromosome called an isochromosome 12p in a proportion of body cells.

Table 32.2 Deletion syndromes

Condition	Genetic error	Features
DiGeorge's syndrome	22q11.2 deletion New (90–95%) Familial (5–10%)	• Congenital heart disease, especially tetralogy of Fallot • Cleft lip +/− palate • Hypocalcaemia/hypoparathyroidism • Hypoplastic thalamus, thus prone to infections • Learning disabilities in some
Cri-du-chat syndrome	Deletion of short arm of chromosome 5 New (85–90%) Unbalanced product of familial translocation (10–15%)	• Characteristic cry like a meowing kitten • Feeding problems • Hypotonia • Cardiac abnormalities: ASDs, VSDs, PDAs, tetralogy of Fallot most common • Dysmorphic features: down-slanting palpebral fissures, strabismus, flat nasal bridge, micrognathia • Single palmar crease • Microcephaly • Severe cognitive, speech and motor delay • Behavioural problems

PDA, patent ductus arteriosus.

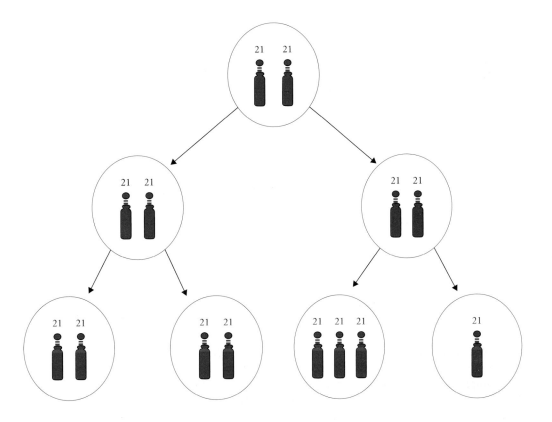

Fig. 32.2 Chromosomal mosaicism

Placental mosaicism

The finding of a mosaic karyotype following CVS or amniocentesis is extremely difficult and needs to be interpreted in the context of the pregnancy as a whole. Referral to the clinical genetics service is essential, but it may still be difficult to provide a clear prognosis. Mosaicism can also be restricted to the placenta so-called confined placental mosaicism (CPM). When mosaicism is detected following CVS, an amniocentesis or FBS is usually recommended so that further chromosome analysis can be performed. Most pregnancies that are diagnosed with CPM continue to term with no complications and the children develop normally. However, some pregnancies with CPM are complicated by IUGR and the pregnancy loss rate is higher than among pregnancies without CPM. This means that once CPM is diagnosed a pregnancy needs to be monitored closely.

SINGLE-GENE DISORDERS

Single-gene (or Mendelian) disorders (Table 32.3) are caused by mutations in a single gene. They are described as autosomal (the mutation is in a gene on the non-sex chromosomes, 1–22) or X-linked (the mutation occurs in a gene on the X-chromosome). Three main types of single gene disorders exist:

- autosomal dominant;
- autosomal recessive;
- X-linked recessive.

Although the individual disorders are rare, there are over 6500 disorders listed as single-gene disorders, so collectively these types of condition are relatively common.[5] The family tree can provide useful information about how a condition runs in the family (see Fig. 32.3a for an example).

Mosaicism may also occur with single-gene disorders and there are many examples of this in clinical practice. A parent who appears to have a mild condition may in fact be mosaic. Their children will be more severely affected if they receive a germ cell with the mutant allele, as this will then be present in every cell in their body.

Some autosomal dominant and X-linked recessive disorders can occur anew. This means that the mutation has arisen for the first time in that individual, i.e. it has not been inherited and the parents are unaffected. Recurrence risks are small, but increased above the general population risk due to the possibility of mosaicism in the germ cells (so-called germline mosaicism).

Autosomal dominant conditions

An individual is affected by an autosomal dominant condition if that condition manifests in heterozygotes, i.e. an individual with one normal and one mutant copy of the relevant gene (Fig. 32.3b).

The main points about autosomal dominant conditions are:

- Each child of an affected parent has a 50 per cent chance of inheriting the condition.
- Males and females are equally affected.
- Males and females can both transmit the disorder.
- There may be variable expression – the severity of the disorder in the offspring may be similar/more severe/less severe than in the parent.
- There may be clinical variability of a condition due to reduced or incomplete penetrance. Penetrance refers to the proportion of individuals with a particular genetic mutation who are affected. If some people with a mutation do not develop the condition during their lifetime,

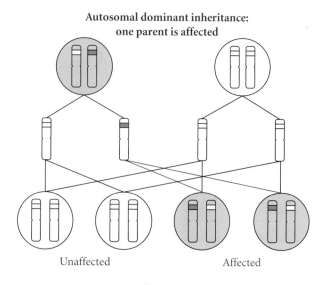

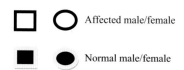

Fig. 32.3a Example of family tree, specifically for a autosomal dominant disorder

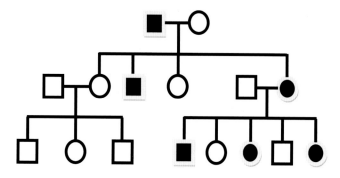

Fig. 32.3b Example of autosomal dominance inheritance

the condition shows reduced or incomplete inheritance. Inherited breast and ovarian cancer due to *BRCA1* and *BRCA2* mutations shows incomplete penetrance, as not everyone with the mutation will develop cancer.

Autosomal recessive conditions

An individual is affected by an autosomal recessive condition if that condition only manifests in homozygotes or compound heterozygotes i.e. an individual in which there is a mutation in both copies of the relevant gene (Figs 32.4a and 32.4b).

The main points about autosomal recessive conditions are:

- The risk that carrier parents will have an affected child is 25 per cent (1 in 4).
- Males and females are equally affected.
- Healthy siblings of an affected individual have a two-thirds risk of being a carrier.
- All children of an affected individual whose partner is not a carrier will be obligate carriers.
- Consanguinity increases the risk of serious congenital and genetic disorders, most commonly autosomal recessive conditions. The birth prevalence is approximately double that for children of unrelated parents.

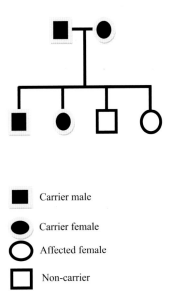

Fig. 32.4a Example of a family tree, specifically for an autosomal recessive disorder

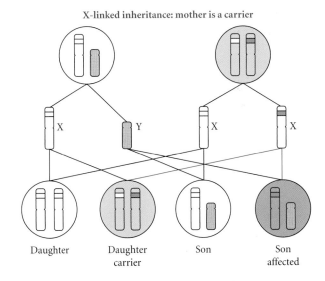

Fig. 32.5a Example of X-linked recessive inheritance where mother is a carrier

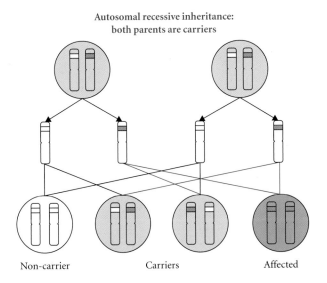

Fig. 32.4b Example of autosomal recessive inheritance

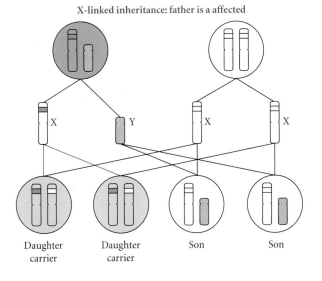

Fig. 32.5b Example of X-linked recessive inheritance where father is affected

Table 32.3 Common single-gene conditions

Condition	Genetic error	Features
Achondroplasia	Autosomal dominant *FGFR3* gene; chromosome 4 99% of affected individuals have one of two mutations	• Most common cause of disproportionate short stature • Normal life expectancy in the majority; a minority have hydrocephalus, obstructive sleep apnoea or middle-ear dysfunction • 75% due to new mutation, with parents of normal stature • Antenatal diagnosis may detect short limbs, but often not until third trimester • Gene testing routinely available
Huntington's disease	Autosomal dominant Huntington gene; chromosome 4 Caused by expansion in 'CAG' triplet repeat	• Peak age of onset 40–45 years • Chorea • Neuropsychiatric disturbance • Dementia • Age-dependent penetrance
Inherited breast (and ovarian) cancer	Autosomal dominant Two major genes: *BRCA1*: chromosome 17 and *BRCA2*: chromosome 13 Numerous mutations	• <5% of breast cancer in UK population is due to an inherited predisposition • The family tree suggests familial breast cancer when several women have had breast cancer on one side of the family, the diagnosis is made at a young age, an individual has had breast cancer more than once or has had early onset breast and ovarian cancer, a male with breast cancer in the family, along with other affected females • Women with mutations in *BRCA1* and *BRCA2* have a significantly increased lifetime risk of developing breast and ovarian cancer and should be offered additional screening
Sickle cell anaemia	Autosomal recessive Beta-globin gene; chromosome 11 One mutation	• Causes episodes of pain, chronic haemolytic anaemia and severe infections, usually from early childhood • Target cells and Howell–Jolly bodies seen on blood film • Sickle-shaped red blood cells, often precipitated by infection, can lead to vaso-occlusive/splenic sequestration/aplastic/haemolytic crises • Heterozygotes have partial protection against malaria • Included in NHS newborn blood spot screening programme
β-Thalassaemia	Autosomal recessive Beta-globin gene; chromosome 11 More than 200 different mutations identified Heterozygotes may have a mild anaemia and are said to have thalassaemia trait or thalassaemia minor	• Group of inherited conditions; beta-thalassaemia major is the most common • There is a reduced rate of synthesis of the beta-haemoglobin chain • Skeletal deformities if diagnosis made late • Haemochromatosis • Healthy at birth • Severe hypochromic, microcytic anaemia between 3 months and 1 year. Blood film shows target cells and fragmented RBCs • For children born in UK, near normal life expectancy
Cystic fibrosis	Autosomal recessive *CFTR* gene; chromosome 7 Δ-F508 (c.1521_1523delCTT) most common mutation, but >1000 different mutations identified. Mutations differ in different ethnic groups	• There is viscous mucus production due to problem with a chloride ion protein involved in anion transport • Recurrent chest infections • Pancreatitis • Malabsorption • Subfertility • Meconium ileus • Can present antenatally with hyperechogenic bowel • Included in NHS newborn blood spot screening programme

Condition	Genetic error	Features
Infantile Tay-Sachs disease (hexosaminidase A deficiency)	Autosomal recessive *HEXA* gene; chromosome 15	• Progressive neurodegeneration, seizures, blindness and deafness from 3–6 months of age • Most die <4 years old • Common in Jews of Ashkenazi ancestry
Duchenne muscular dystrophy	X-linked recessive Dystrophin gene familial (66%) new (33%)	• Delayed motor and speech milestones • Progressive proximal muscle weakness, initially lower limbs, then ascending upwards and resulting in muscle wasting and fibrosis • Cardiomyopathy • Specialist care from a multidisciplinary team dramatically improves quality of life • Average life expectancy: 25 years

X-linked recessive conditions

X-linked recessive conditions are seen in males when a mutation is present in the relevant gene on their only copy of the X-chromosome. Females have two X-chromosomes and are said to be carriers if they have one normal copy and one 'mutant' copy of the relevant gene. Female carriers of X-linked recessive conditions rarely show any features of the condition (Figs 32.5a and 32.5b).

The main points about X-linked recessive conditions are:

• The mutant genes are on the X-chromosome.
• All males who inherit the mutation are affected.
• Carrier females are unaffected.
• When a carrier female has a pregnancy there are four possible outcomes, all equally likely: affected son, unaffected son, carrier (unaffected) daughter, non-carrier daughter. Put another way, sons of carrier females have a 50 per cent chance of being affected, and daughters of carrier females have a 50 per cent chance of being unaffected carriers.
• When an affected man has children, all of his daughters will be carriers; none of his sons will be affected. This means that the family tree will not show male-to-male transmission. However, many X-linked conditions are so severe that affected males do not reproduce.

MULTIFACTORIAL CONDITIONS

Most conditions seen by healthcare professionals are multifactorial. In multifactorial inheritance, a condition occurs when 'environmental' influences, such as diet, act on a genetic predisposition to develop a condition. Examples of such adult-onset conditions include type 1 diabetes and asthma. Common birth defects, such as cleft lip +/− palate and NTDs are also inherited in this way.

Knowledge about the environmental factors predisposing to the condition can help reduce the risk of developing these conditions. For congenital malformations, the best example of this is the use of periconceptual folic acid to prevent NTDs.

GENETIC TESTING

Genetic tests may be used to detect, confirm or rule out a genetic condition. During pregnancy these tests provide parents with information so that they may avoid the birth of a baby with a serious genetic condition, or it may start discussions about coping with a child with that condition. A directory of genetic tests available in NHS laboratories is available on the UK Genetic Testing Network (UKGTN) website.[10] The UK National Screening Committee provides recommendations to Public Health England for the Fetal Anomaly Screening Programme (FASP) in the UK.[11] The most common laboratory techniques for investigating an individual for a possible chromosomal or single-gene disorder are shown in Table 32.4.

New methods of genetic testing

More powerful methods of genetic testing are now possible, but are not yet routinely available in NHS laboratories, though they are being used in many research projects, including in prenatal settings. These are known as exome and genome sequencing.[7] Both techniques are an extension of next generation sequencing and enable the entire genetic make-up of an individual to be analysed. Their potential is enormous, allowing genetic diagnoses to be made when this was not possible previously.[2] However, for each patient a large amount of data is generated and interpretation of results can be extremely challenging. Such techniques are not undertaken without full understanding and consent from the patient.

FETAL CONDITIONS

Table 32.4 Common laboratory testing techniques for various genetic disorders

Technique	Application	Reporting time from sample receipt in laboratory
Karyotyping; routine chromosome testing	Counts the number of chromosomes and looks for structural changes in the chromosomes. Most commonly performed on blood (WBC), amniotic fluid cells, placenta, skin and bone marrow, but almost any tissue can be used. Unlike other methods of genetic testing, karyotyping will detect balanced chromosomal rearrangements and is the preferred method for investigating couples who have experienced recurrent miscarriages	14-21 calendar days
PCR	A laboratory technique used to increase the amount of DNA in a sample by several orders of magnitude	3 working days
QF-PCR	A method combining PCR and the labelling of chromosomes 13, 18, 21 and each sex chromosome with 'fluorescent' markers which allows the number of copies of each chromosome to be assessed. Used mainly as a rapid prenatal test for these common trisomies	3 working days
Multiplex ligation-dependent probe amplification (MLPA)	Detects deletions or duplications of part of a gene or whole chromosome. Used in many clinical settings; e.g. in prenatal diagnosis for the detection of common aneuploidies; in oncology clinics for the detection of deletions of the *BRCA1* and *BRCA2* genes	3 working days
FISH	Detects the presence or absence of a specific DNA sequence on the chromosomes. FISH uses a fluorescent probe which attaches itself to the exact part of the DNA that a scientist wishes to visualise. Most commonly used to detect deletions such as 22q11.2 deletion. increasingly replaced by microarrays	Antenatal results reported simultaneously with routine choromosome testing
Microarray-based comparative genomic hybridisation (array CGH); 'microarrays'	Relatively new method of looking for subtle chromosome imbalances. The technique compares a sample of patient DNA with a control sample which has no known genetic alterations, so allowing the detection of loss or gain of genetic material. The deletions and duplications (copy number variants [CNVs]) detected by this method are much smaller than those possible by routine karyotyping and are often referred to as microdeletions and microduplications. Array CGH may benefit families as it may provide a diagnosis, when this was not possible previously. However, some chromosome and DNA alterations have not previously been reported and their significance is not known. This can make results difficult to interpret	14-21 calendar days
DNA (Sanger) sequencing	Checking for alterations in the order of bases in the genetic code. The method used to determine the exact order of the bases (C, G, A and T) in a particular gene. Interpreting the results requires expert knowledge as a variation in the 'sequence' will be significant and cause genetic disease only if the function of the protein it produces is affected. Results of uncertain significance may be found. Only possible antenatally if mutation in family is known.	10 working days
Next generation sequencing (NGS)	There are several different NGS methods which allow large-scale DNA sequencing in a single test. Often used to sequence a subset of genes that predispose to a group of conditions, e.g. inherited cancer syndromes. Generates an enormous amount of data requiring expert interpretation	No time frame, not yet used in clinical practice

Another exciting prospect is the recent development of non-invasive prenatal diagnosis for aneuploidy using cell-free fetal DNA (cffDNA),[13] which is known to be present in small quantities in maternal plasma, thus allowing the diagnosis of fetal genetic disorders from peripheral maternal blood samples and avoiding the risks associated with CVS and amniocentesis. Testing for aneuploidy by cffDNA is in the initial stages of being introduced into UK clinical practice,[1,14] and is already in use in the USA. Non-invasive prenatal diagnosis for other genetic disorders is much more difficult technically, but it is these families who will benefit most as they have the greatest risk of recurrence. Testing for one or two conditions, most notably achondroplasia and thanatophoric dysplasia, already exists. A number of research projects in this area are ongoing and hope to develop reliable techniques which can be translated into clinical practice. This is an area of rapid development and advice from the local clinical genetics service is recommended.

COUNSELLING ABOUT GENETIC DISEASE

Genetic counselling advises patients at risk of a potentially hereditary disorder about the consequences of the disorder, the probability of developing or transmitting it and the ways in which this may be prevented, avoided or ameliorated. Ideally couples should receive counselling prior to conception, but this is possible only if factors known to increase the risk of genetic disorder have been identified before pregnancy. Such factors include a previous child with, or a family history of, a single-gene disorder, a parent having a chromosome anomaly, advanced maternal age, parental consanguinity, ethnic origin and population carrier screening. For many families a genetic condition becomes apparent during pregnancy only after an abnormal ultrasound scan or after biochemical screening test results. This is extremely stressful. Further prenatal genetic testing may be helpful in providing additional information about the aetiology of the problems, which can help couples make more informed choices. This is most likely to be by an invasive diagnostic test such as CVS or amniocentesis. These tests do carry a small risk of miscarriage (1–2 per cent) but often provide useful information, particularly about the fetal karyotype. Couples should be given the opportunity to understand the nature of the problems seen and the different options available to them, before making a decision about the management of the pregnancy. This may include referral to other specialists including neonatologists, paediatric cardiologists, neurologists or surgeons. Decisions people make are very personal; some couples accept the risk and have no further testing, others choose to refine the risk with further tests, whilst some may choose to terminate the pregnancy. Many factors are considered before making a decision including the prognosis for the child, the impact of the disorder on the family, financial considerations and religious beliefs. Patient support groups such as Antenatal Results and Choices (ARC)[3] and Unique[15] can provide valuable support to families at this difficult time. It is important that we give couples as much information as possible in order to facilitate the tough decisions surrounding further management of their pregnancy.

Ongoing follow-up and support are essential and needs to include information about the likelihood of the same problem occurring again and risks to other family members. Couples who have a high chance of having a further affected pregnancy should have the opportunity to discuss the different options available to them. This may include undertaking a further pregnancy (accept risk, prenatal diagnosis or preimplantation genetic diagnosis if available, donor egg or sperm), postpone pregnancy hoping that prenatal testing will become available in the future, adoption or choose to have no further children.

KEY POINTS

- Taking a detailed family history can help identify patients with, or at risk of, a genetic condition.
- The majority of conditions are inherited. The most common modes of inheritance are chromosomal, single gene and multifactorial. Single-gene disorders show autosomal dominant, autosomal recessive and X-linked recessive inheritance.
- It is essential to have a definitive diagnosis in order to give precise information about the condition including accurate recurrence risks. If a diagnosis has been made by another healthcare professional, seek confirmation of that diagnosis whenever possible. Genetic testing can provide useful information that may contribute to the clinical care for some patients and families. Genetic tests are permanent (unlike a patient's Hb result). It is therefore important to recognise its uses and limitations.
- Genetic diseases are rare, but collectively common (around one person in every 17). They are most appropriately managed by a team of specialists and referring patients to local genetics services can facilitate this.
- It is important to be aware of the ethical dilemmas surrounding genetic testing in families.

Published Guidelines

There are no NICE or RCOG Greentop Guidelines on prenatal genetic testing, although ACOG has published a variety of committee opinions on genetic testing and the RCOG has published a Scientific Impact Paper on non-invasive prenatal testing.

Key References

1. American Congress of Obstetricians and Gynecologists. *Committee Opinions.* Cell-free DNA screening for fetal aneuploidy https://www.acog.org/Resources-And-Publications/Committee-Opinions/Committee-on-Genetics/Cell-free-DNA-Screening-for-Fetal-Aneuploidy (accessed 05 August 2015).
2. American Congress of Obstetricians and Gynecologists. *Committee Opinions.* The use of chromosomal microarray analysis in prenatal diagnosis https://www.acog.org/Resources-And-Publications/Committee-Opinions/Committee-on-Genetics/The-Use-of-Chromosomal-Microarray-Analysis-in-Prenatal-Diagnosis (accessed 05 August 2015).
3. Antenatal Results & Choices ARC. *ARC.* http://www.arc-uk.org/ (accessed 20 January 2014).
4. Clarke A. *Harper's Practical Genetic Counselling.* 8th ed. London: Hodder Arnold, 2014.
5. Donaldson L. *Rare is Common in: 2009 Annual Report of the Chief Medical Officer.* London: Department of Health; 2010: p39 -45.

6. Firth HV, Hurst JA, Hall JG. *Oxford Desk Reference – Clinical Genetics.* Oxford: Oxford University Press, 2005.

7. Hillman SC, McMullan DJ, Hall G, Togneri FS, James N, Maher EJ, et al. Use of prenatal chromosomal array: prospective 41(6): 610-20

8. Johns Hopkins University. *OMIM: Online Mendelian Inheritance in Man.* http://omim.org/ (accessed 20 January 2014).

9. NHS. *NHS National Genetics and Genomics Education Centre.* http://www.geneticseducation.nhs.uk/ (accessed 20 January 2014).

10. NHS. *UK Genetic Testing Network.* http://ukgtn.nhs.uk/ (accessed 20 January 2014).

11. NHS Screening Programmes. *Fetal Anomaly Screening Programme Standards 2015-2016.* version 0.8. London: Crown, 2015.

12. Pagon RA, Adam MP, Bird TD, Dolan CR, Fong C-T, Smith RJH, Stephens K. *Gene Reviews.* http:// www.ncbi.nlm.nih.gov/books/NBK1116/ (accessed 20 January 2014).

13. Soothil PW, Lo YMD Non-invasive prenatal testing for chromosomal abnormality using maternal plasma DNA https://www.rcog.org.uk/globalassets/documents/guidelines/sip_15_04032014.pdf (accessed 05 August 2015).

14. The NHS RAPID Project: Reliable Accurate Prenatal Diagnosis. Available at: http://www.rappid.co.uk/ (accessed 20 January 2014)

15. The Rare Chromosome Disorder Support Group. *Unique.* http://www.rarechromo.co.uk/html/home.asp (accessed 20 January 2014).

Chapter 33 Management of fetal anomalies

Michele P Mohajer

INTRODUCTION

The management of the pregnancy in which an abnormal fetus is identified involves a whole multidisciplinary team of specialists. This team comprises the sonographer, fetal medicine specialist, geneticist, neonatologist and paediatric surgeon, along with the nurse specialists within each team. When the diagnosis is made, clear information should be made available to the parents regarding the condition, prognosis and level of disability, should the baby be born alive. This may be very difficult to achieve. Many conditions have such a wide variation in outcome (e.g. Down's syndrome and spina bifida) that accurate prediction may not be possible. When given an adverse prenatal diagnosis, parents are deeply shocked and experience acute grief. They may not be able to take in the information given to them. Written information, contact numbers and support groups are important, but parents may have great difficulty reaching a decision, especially one that results in the termination of the pregnancy. Therefore, management includes not only the practical aspect of the specific disorder, but also the psychological support for the parents and family involved in the pregnancy.

PRACTICAL MANAGEMENT

Termination of pregnancy

When parents are told of a fetal abnormality, they must make decisions, the most important being whether to continue or terminate the pregnancy. The response to diagnosis will be tempered by the options available to the parents, including *in-utero* treatment, postnatal treatment or termination. If the condition is lethal, the decision to terminate may be easier, but, more often than not, the condition carries a risk of physical or mental impairment, which is difficult to quantify. Once a serious abnormality has been diagnosed, evidence shows that the parents will terminate the pregnancy in 80–90 per cent of cases.[1]

Conditions that are considered lethal include:

- anencephaly;
- bilateral renal agenesis;
- lethal skeletal dysplasias;
- some severe complex cardiac defects;
- triploidy;
- trisomies 18, 13 and 15.

Other conditions are not lethal, but are well documented as being associated with long-term handicap, and include:

- spina bifida;
- trisomy 21 and other chromosomal abnormalities;
- cardiovascular abnormalities;
- muscular dystrophies;
- phocomelia.

If the decision to terminate is reached, the methods available and associated risks must be discussed with the parents.

METHODS OF TERMINATION

Surgical termination

Surgical termination may be performed by vacuum aspiration or dilatation and evacuation. Vacuum aspiration or suction curettage is the method used until the end of the first trimester. Dilatation of the cervix prior to surgery is achieved by passing graduated metal dilators or inserting vaginal prostaglandin preparations. Abortion is then performed by the use of a Perspex suction tube connected to vacuum apparatus. The inherent risk associated with abortion relates to the use of general anaesthesia and the invasive nature of the procedure – with complications of haemorrhage, uterine perforation and infection. The incidence of haemorrhage is 1.5/1000, uterine perforation 1–4/1000 and of cervical trauma 1 per cent. Post-abortion infection occurs in up to 10 per cent of cases and is significantly reduced if prophylactic antibiotics are given [B]. Suction curettage has been shown to produce lower risks of these complications than sharp curettage.[2] Complications are lessened the earlier the gestation.[11] Couples should also be informed of the risk of failed abortion, which occurs in 2.3/1000 surgical terminations.

Dilatation and evacuation is performed in some areas up until 20 weeks' gestation. Mechanical dilatation of the cervix to 14 mm is performed, and fetal parts are extracted with the use of appropriate instruments. This may be done under ultrasound control. Cervical dilatation may be complicated by cervical tears, uterine perforation and the creation of false passages. The use of cervical priming agents such as mifepristone, misoprostol and gemeprost has improved the safety of the procedure [B].[3] It is a very distressing procedure, but safe and effective when undertaken by specialist practitioners with a sufficiently large caseload [A]. However, it is not widely available. It also prevents a full postmortem examination of the fetus being carried out in order to confirm any ultrasound diagnosis.

Medical termination

Medical termination of pregnancy has been revolutionised by the introduction of prostaglandins and the antiprogesterone mifepristone.

Gestations of 9 weeks (63 days) or less can be successfully terminated with mifepristone 600 mg, followed 48 hours later by a prostaglandin (gemeprost or misoprostol). Less than 0.5 per cent will fail to respond to this regimen,[4] which should be the method of choice at these gestations [A]. However, the diagnosis of fetal abnormality is extremely rare by 9 weeks' gestation and so medical termination is usually performed in the second trimester. Medical termination has the additional advantage of allowing the opportunity for a postmortem examination. Pre-treatment with mifepristone (200 mg) sensitises the myometrium to prostaglandin agents and so reduces the induction–abortion interval [B]. Misoprostol is the prostaglandin of choice as it requires specific conditions for storage and transfer. The risk of failure to terminate the pregnancy is 6/1000.

The standard regimen is: mifepristone 200 mg orally, followed 36–48 hours later by misoprostol 800 mg vaginally, then misoprostol 400 mg orally to a maximum of four oral doses.

Third-trimester termination and intrauterine fetocide

Since 1990, termination of pregnancy after 24 weeks has become legal if there is a lethal abnormality or sufficient evidence that the infant will be born with serious mental or physical disability.[5] This is an extremely distressing situation to all involved, including the parents, obstetricians and midwives. The safety of medical termination has made late termination much safer, but the law states that the fetus must not be born alive. This requires intrauterine fetocide – which is achieved by fetal intracardiac injection of potassium chloride (KCl) via a 20-gauge transabdominal needle under ultrasound control. This procedure should be performed by an operator experienced in invasive fetal procedures. Fetal sedation may be necessary prior to the fetocide. This is achieved by the administration of diazepam or pethidine into the fetal circulation. An ultrasound should be performed 1 hour after the injection of KCl to ensure cessation of fetal heart pulsation.

When the abnormality is incompatible with survival, fetocide is not mandatory, but the delivery management should be carefully discussed with the parents and health professionals involved and a care plan agreed. If the condition is not lethal, fetocide should be offered after 21^{+6}. Failure to do so contradicts the intention of the abortion.[10]

The assessment of the level of disability is an extremely difficult area. Although the outcome of some abnormalities is well documented, an accurate prognosis of many prenatally detected anomalies is not possible. Advice from genetic specialists, counsellors and support groups may be sought, but ultimately the decision to terminate the pregnancy will rest with the parents. Consideration should be given to karyotyping the fetus by sending a fetal blood sample (and banking DNA) for cytogenetic analysis (with informed consent).

The postmortem examination

Parents may find the prospect of a postmortem examination of their baby very distressing, but it is a vital part of the management. Although high-quality ultrasound provides an accurate diagnosis of major fetal pathology, postmortem examination provides more detail, identifies abnormalities that permit a more specific diagnosis and modifies genetic counselling. Important diagnostic refinements are identified in up to 40 per cent of cases.[6]

The issue of postmortem examination has become further complicated by the legal requirement of consent. Consent is now required for the postmortem examination of fetuses at all gestations and, additionally, if tissues or organs are retained for later study or research. If parents do not consent to a postmortem examination, it is important to request photographs, X-rays and a sample of tissue (skin or placenta) for cytogenetic studies, which may provide additional information.

THE CONTINUING PREGNANCY

The pregnancy may continue for many reasons. For example, the condition may be amenable to postnatal treatment. This particularly applies to structural malformations that can be surgically corrected, such as:

- gastroschisis;
- exomphalos;
- diaphragmatic hernia;
- duodenal atresia;
- some cardiac defects (Fallot's tetralogy, ASDs, VSDs, transposition of the great vessels);
- posterior urethral valves;
- cleft lip.

It is important that parents receive full information regarding the treatment and long-term outcome of the condition; this is preferably provided by the surgeon performing the procedure. Certain conditions such as gastroschisis will require continued fetal surveillance throughout pregnancy, as there may be growth problems or loops of bowel may become obstructed. Most pregnancies will also require continued surveillance for psychological support. Even though parents have been given optimistic expectations of the outcome, they will be anxious throughout, and need constant reassurance from all members of the team. If paediatric surgical teams are not within the hospital, parents may have to travel to a main centre to receive both prenatal counselling and delivery if their neonatal unit is unable to cope with their situation.

Certain fetal conditions are amenable to intrauterine therapy.

Hydrops fetalis is discussed in Chapter 40. Cases secondary to fetal anaemia may respond to intrauterine fetal blood transfusion. Fetal tachydysrhythmias may also result in fetal hydrops. Maternal administration of antiarrhythmic drugs (digoxin, flecainide, amiodarone) is effective in converting the fetal rate to sinus rhythm and also reversing the hydrops.[7]

If fluid is in a particular cavity, for example a pleural effusion, its presence may compromise normal lung development. Pleural drainage may be performed, as both a diagnostic and a therapeutic procedure. If the fluid accumulates, a pleuro-amniotic shunt can be inserted. This shunt procedure can be applied to other conditions. In the case of posterior urethral valves, outflow obstruction can be so severe as to cause bilateral hydronephrosis and irreversible renal damage. A vesico-amniotic shunt can be inserted into the fetal bladder and so bypass the urethral obstruction.

Sophisticated techniques to perform intrauterine surgery have been developed. If a diaphragmatic hernia is present early in pregnancy, the presence of a mass in the fetal chest compromises fetal lung development such that the infants often die of pulmonary hypoplasia. *In-utero* endoscopic placement of a balloon in the fetal trachea may improve outcome.[8]

Parents may elect to proceed with the pregnancy because there is not enough certainty or evidence that the malformation will result in a significant degree of mental or physical disability. This decision will vary among individuals and depend on their own particular circumstances, for example an infertile couple with a long-awaited pregnancy may accept the risk of potential handicap more than a multigravid mother for whom the risk of a handicapped child may compromise the wellbeing of her existing family.

Examples of such abnormalities include:

- Dandy–Walker malformation;
- agenesis of the corpus callosum;
- distal limb abnormalities;
- some cardiac defects.

Finally, parents may not want termination, even if the condition has a 100 per cent mortality rate, because of religious or moral beliefs. These wishes must be respected.

The management of these continuing pregnancies requires skilled, personalised care. There are few published data that consider the psychological impact of continuing the pregnancy with a prenatally diagnosed abnormality. There are reasons to hypothesise that women who elect to continue a pregnancy may experience a better psychological outcome than women who terminate: such women are thought to be spared the guilt associated with decision-making. However, some reports suggest that these women would seek early prenatal diagnosis in a subsequent pregnancy. Management of continuing pregnancies includes communication between hospital and community health workers, continuity of care with the same personnel, adequate time and repeated counselling (outside routine clinic hours), written information and contacts with support groups.[9] Serial ultrasound scans may be requested to provide reassurance that the baby is still alive and growing.

The management of the pregnancy with a malformation requires additional considerations as well as emotional support. Parents need to be prepared for:

- how, where and when their baby will be delivered;
- what their baby will look like;
- what will happen to their baby after delivery.

There may also be practical difficulties if delivery is to take place in a tertiary centre. The costs of transport, childcare and subsistence must be considered.

Discussion needs to occur with other healthcare professionals as to the timing and appropriate place of delivery of the fetus.

PLANNING FOR THE FUTURE

Once the pregnancy is over, carefully planned follow-up is an essential part of the management. In the case of termination or death of the infant, time for grieving must be allowed. Grief reactions will vary among individuals depending on different circumstances. Some couples want intensive counselling and contact with the medical team, whereas others want time away from what has become an emotionally painful environment. Postmortem results may provide additional information as to the precise diagnosis. This could influence the management of a subsequent pregnancy and the choice of a prenatal test.

Referral to a genetic specialist may be required in order to assess the risk of recurrence and possibly to investigate other family members. Follow-up with the paediatric or neonatal team involved is an important part of the bereavement counselling.

Parents will require information on the availability of early, reliable prenatal diagnosis if another pregnancy is contemplated.

Couples may require more than one bereavement counselling session, either because the results are incomplete or because they wish it. Sensitivity to the individual's needs is essential in this situation.

Finally, a letter summarising the discussion should be sent to the parents. This provides documentation and also allows the information to be assimilated at a later date, away from the hospital environment.

EBM

- Termination of pregnancy is more likely if the diagnosis is made earlier in gestation [C].
- The risks of termination of pregnancy are reduced if abortion is performed at earlier gestations [B].
- Psychological stress is high after termination, with 40 per cent of women showing symptoms of psychiatric morbidity [B].

KEY POINTS

- Parents must have as much access to information as possible before making a choice.
- Referral to a tertiary centre may be necessary for further investigation or treatment.
- Psychological morbidity is high following termination for fetal abnormality using either surgical or medical methods.
- Whether or not they continue the pregnancy, the parents will need long-term support from both hospital specialists and the community.

Published Guidelines

NICE. *Fetal vesico-amniotic shunt for lower urinary tract outflow obstruction.* NICE interventional procedure guidance 202. 2006.

Penney G. *The Care of Women Requesting Induced Abortion.* Evidence-Based Clinical Guidelines No. 7. London: RCOG Press, 2004.

RCOG. *Termination of Pregnancy for Fetal Abnormality in England, Scotland and Wales.* London: RCOG Press, 2010.

Key References

1. RCOG. *Ultrasound Screening for Fetal Abnormalities.* Report of the RCOG Working Party. London: RCOG Press, 1997, 2–3.
2. Edelman DA, Brener WE, Berger GS. The effectiveness and complications of abortion by dilatation and vacuum aspiration versus dilatation and rigid metal curettage. *Am J Obstet Gynecol* 1974;119:473.
3. Schulz KF, Grimes DA, Cates W. Measures to prevent cervical injury during suction curettage abortion. *Lancet* 1983;i:1182–4.
4. UK Multicentre Trial. The efficacy and tolerance of mifepristone and prostaglandin in first trimester termination of pregnancy. *Br J Obstet Gynaecol* 1990;97:480–6.
5. Gevers S. Third trimester abortion for fetal abnormality. *Bioethics* 1999;13:306–13.
6. Clayton-Smith J, Farndon PA, McKeown C, Donnai D. Examination of fetuses after induced abortion for fetal abnormality. *BMJ* 1990;300:295–7.
7. van Engelen AD, Weijtens O, Brenner J et al. Management outcome and follow-up of fetal tachycardia. *J Am Coll Cardiol* 1994;24:1371–5.
8. Doné E, Gucciardo L, Van Mieghem T et al. Prenatal diagnosis, prediction of outcome and in utero therapy of isolated congenital diaphragmatic hernia. *Prenat Diagn* 2008;28:581–91.
9. Chitty LS, Barnes CA, Berry C. Continuing with pregnancy after a diagnosis of lethal abnormality: experience of five couples and recommendations for management. *BMJ* 1996;313:478–80.
10. RCOG. *Termination of Pregnancy for Fetal Abnormality in England, Scotland and Wales.* London: RCOG Press, 2010.
11. Department of Health. *Abortion Statistics, England and Wales: 2008.* Statistical bulletin 2009/1. London: DH, 2009.

Chapter 34 Previous history of fetal loss

Abi Merriel and Arri Coomarasamy

MRCOG standards

Theoretical skills

- Understand the epidemiology, aetiology and pathogenesis of fetal loss.
- Understand the indications and limitations of investigations (endocrine, anatomical, immunological, genetic, radiological and bacteriological).

Practical skills

- Be able to manage subsequent pregnancies in women with a history of late fetal loss/stillbirth.

INTRODUCTION

An estimated 2.64 million stillbirths occurred in 2009.[1] Approximately 98 per cent of this burden lies in low- and middle-income countries.[2] The global stillbirth rate is approximately 18.9 per 1000 total births, whereas in high-income settings, the rate is 3.1 per 1000 total births.[1] In the UK, 1 in 200 babies is born dead, with 3558 stillbirths (4.9/1000 total births) occurring in 2012.[3] Each family that experiences a stillbirth encounters their own personal response to their loss and healthcare staff may be among a small group of people with whom they can talk openly.[4] Many parents will have questions about their possible future pregnancies in terms of timing, risks, care during pregnancy and chances of having a healthy baby.[4] Given their past loss, for many couples another pregnancy may be an 'emotional rollercoaster'.[4] Many women with a history of pregnancy loss have increased risks for future pregnancy loss and other obstetric complications.[5] Therefore, expert support is often required and this should be provided by staff who have the right attitude, training, knowledge and skills.[4]

DEFINITIONS

In the UK, a fetal loss up to 24 completed weeks of gestation is defined as a miscarriage. A *late* fetal loss is defined as *in-utero* death delivering between 22^{+0} and 23^{+6}. A stillbirth is defined as a baby delivering with no signs of life after 24 completed weeks of pregnancy. These definitions are not universal. According to the International Classification of Diseases, a stillbirth is defined as a baby born at 22 completed weeks of pregnancy or weighing at least 500 g. However, in order to allow international comparisons, the WHO recommends reporting babies born dead from 28 completed weeks gestation or 1000 g or more as a stillbirth.[6] For the purposes of this chapter, we have grouped late fetal losses and stillbirths and will refer to them as intrauterine fetal deaths (IUFDs).

CAUSES OF IUFD

Placental pathology contributes to over half of IUFDs.[7] Placental abruption accounts for a population-attributable risk for stillbirth of 15 per cent.[5] In addition, placental insufficiency contributes to fetal growth restriction, which is identified in 40–60 per cent of stillbirths.[7] One large cohort study showed that there were 12 times higher odds of a growth-restricted fetus being stillborn compared with a normally grown baby.[8]

Infection contributes to approximately 12 per cent of IUFDs. Its burden seems to be more in IUFDs of earlier gestations (less than 28 weeks) in the context of chorioamnionitis and preterm pre-labour rupture of membranes.[7] Infective agents contributing to IUFDs include parvovirus, cytomegalovirus, toxoplasmosis and *listeria*.[8] Chronic infections should also be excluded, e.g. syphilis.[9]

Umbilical cord accidents or abnormalities such as true cord knots may contribute to (8 per cent) or cause (9 per cent) IUFDs.[7]

Medical and pregnancy disorders contribute to nearly 25 per cent of cases, and are causal in 7 per cent of cases. Diabetes and hypertensive disorders are the most important conditions leading to this burden.[7] Other diseases can also have a significant effect on a pregnancy, for example Antiphospholipid Syndrome (APLS) (especially with renal involvement) and thrombophilias.[8] Although most high-income settings have rhesus disease prophylaxis, the contribution of red cell antibodies to fetal demise continues to exist.[8]

Intrapartum deaths contribute to approximately 14 per cent of third-trimester IUFDs in high-income settings; however, in parts of sub-Saharan Africa and Asia over 50 per cent of these deaths are intrapartum.[6] In high-income settings, one series has suggested that, whilst 9 per cent of stillbirths were intrapartum, only 3 per cent of these were attributable to intrapartum events.[7]

Congenital abnormalities are associated with 6–12 per cent of stillbirths.

Unexplained causes are assigned to up to 60 per cent of IUFDs.[8] However, much of the published literature suggests that, when IUFDs are fully investigated, only one in four IUFDs still remains unexplained.[10] Fig. 34.1 illustrates the causes of stillbirth in the UK in 2009.

RISK FACTORS FOR IUFDS AND STILLBIRTH

Several important and potentially modifiable risk factors have been identified across numerous studies and have been summarised in a meta-analysis: maternal weight, maternal smoking, maternal age, parity, SGA, placental abruption, and pre-existing maternal diabetes or hypertension.[5] These risk factors may exist alone or may combine, for example, in women delaying child-bearing in high-income settings. The most important of these modifiable risk factors is maternal weight.

The IUFD rate among multiple gestations is four times higher than for singletons. This is particularly important to consider in the context of the use of assisted reproductive technologies.[11] Alcohol and illicit drug use may serve to increase the risk of an IUFD.[11]

Other-well documented risk factors for IUFDs include lack of access to antenatal care,[5] educational attainment of the mother,[5] ethnic origin[11] and socio-economic status.[5,11]

INVESTIGATION AND RISK ASSESSMENT

Some of the factors involved in fetal loss have a clear causal link, such as an abruption or a cord event, whilst others may have a contributory role, e.g. obesity. Some losses may be associated with multiple aetiologies, e.g. a fetal loss could be directly linked to an abruption, but the woman may have risk factors such as APLS and pre-eclampsia. In order to provide the parents with as much information as possible they should be offered investigations to determine the reason for the death of their baby. This will aid accurate risk prediction and allow planning of risk modification.[12] If writing to another hospital, it is prudent to request copies of the original investigation reports. The RCOG recommends that the investigations in

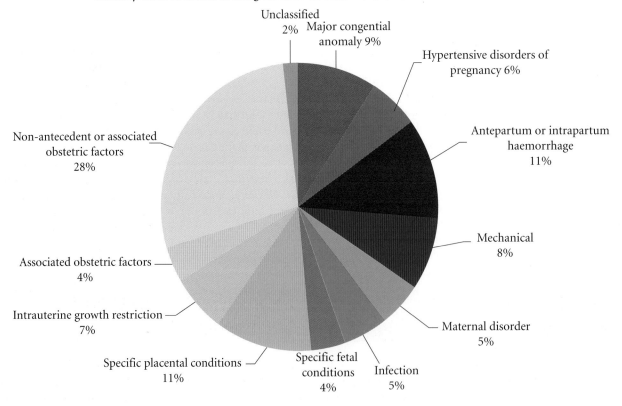

Primary cause of Stillbirth using the CMACE maternal and Fetal Classification

Unclassified 2%
Major congential anomaly 9%
Hypertensive disorders of pregnancy 6%
Antepartum or intrapartum haemorrhage 11%
Mechanical 8%
Maternal disorder 5%
Infection 5%
Specific fetal conditions 4%
Specific placental conditions 11%
Intrauterine growth restriction 7%
Associated obstetric factors 4%
Non-antecedent or associated obstetric factors 28%

Fig. 34.1 Causes of stillbirths in the UK in 2009[14]

Table 34.1 Adapted from RCOG Guideline on Late IUFD and Stillbirth[12]

Test to be considered	Reasons for test
Maternal standard haematological tests including CRP and bile salt	Pre-eclampsia and its complications
	Multi-organ failure in sepsis or haemorrhage
	Obstetric cholestasis
Maternal coagulation times and plasma fibrinogen	DIC
Kleihauer Disseminated intravascular coagulation	Lethal fetomaternal haemorrhage
	To decide level of requirement for anti-RhD gamma-globulin
Maternal, fetal and placental bacteriology (blood cultures (maternal and fetal), midstream urine, vaginal and cervical, fetal and placental swabs)	Suspected maternal bacterial infection
Maternal serology (viral screen, syphilis, tropical infections)	Occult maternal–fetal infection
Maternal random blood glucose and HbA1c	Occult maternal DM or GDM
Maternal thyroid function	Occult maternal thyroid disease
Maternal thrombophilia screen	Maternal thrombophilia
Anti-red cell antibody serology	Immune haemolytic disease
Maternal anti-Ro and anti-La antibodies	Occult maternal autoimmune disease
Maternal alloimmune antiplatelet antibodies	Alloimmune thrombocytopenia
Parental bloods and fetal and placental tissues for karyotyping	Parental balanced translocation/mosaicism
	Aneuploidy, single-gene disorders
Maternal urine for cocaine metabolites	Occult drug use
Postmortem examination may be full or limited at the request of the parents (external, autopsy, microscopy, X-ray, placenta and cord) by a specialised perinatal pathologist	To attempt to explain the cause of the fetal death

Table 34.1 are considered in the event of a late pregnancy loss.[12]

Once a cause and/or associated risk factors have been established, an attempt should be made to estimate the risk of adverse obstetric outcomes, particularly IUFDs, for the specific woman.

For many couples with a previous pregnancy loss, risk identification, future risk estimation and future pregnancy management plans may have been discussed in the follow-up consultation(s) after their previous loss. Generally, such plans should be adhered to, unless there are clear reasons to deviate. If changes are necessary, it is important to explain to the couple the need for the changes.

95 per cent reduction in stillbirths from Rh isoimmunisation.[8] In order to develop targeted interventions it is vital that the causes of IUFDs are appropriately identified. One of the biggest challenges with this is the number of different classification systems (over 35) and the fact that they are not all applicable across different healthcare settings.[6] Some of the contemporary internationally accepted systems include: Amended Aberdeen, Extended Wigglesworth, PSANZ-PDC, ReCoDe, Tulip and CODAC.[13] In January 2008, a new Perinatal Death Notification (PND) form, including a new classification of cause of death, was introduced by CEMACH. This tool has enabled a reduction in the number of unexplained IUFDs from approximately 50 per cent to 28 per cent in the report published in 2011.[14]

CLASSIFICATION OF IUFDS AND STILLBIRTH

The previous successes in improving outcomes in IUFDs have largely been due to the specific targeting of appropriate interventions, e.g. rhesus immune prophylaxis resulted in a

CONSIDERING A SUBSEQUENT PREGNANCY

For couples planning another pregnancy following an IUFD, the timing of the pregnancy and the likelihood of recurrence of pregnancy loss are important concerns. SANDS

Guidelines for Professionals[4] suggest the following approach in helping couples planning to have a baby after a previous pregnancy loss:

1 Offer parents time to discuss their ideas, concerns, expectations and feelings, together as a couple and individually, to help reach a decision about timing of pregnancy.
2 Offer parents the opportunity to discuss the specific individualised risks for the mother and baby in a future pregnancy.
3 Reassure parents that there is no specific right time for them to try for a baby.
4 Encourage the parents to look after and look out for each other physically and emotionally, particularly focusing on ways of reducing their anxiety (e.g. with the use of relaxation techniques).
5 Offer pre-conception advice to reduce or manage risks, e.g. cessation of smoking and weight reduction.
6 Offer and organise referral to other specialists as appropriate, e.g. geneticists and, if the parents wish, a counsellor.
7 Acknowledge that a future pregnancy is likely to be stressful, but emphasise that there will be support to ensure the couple's and baby's health.

IUFD recurrence

Several cohort studies have been undertaken to investigate the likelihood of recurrence of IUFDs. Each of these studies has its limitations; one of the more recent ones based on a Scottish database suggested an increased risk of IUFDs in a subsequent pregnancy with an adjusted OR of 1.96 (99% CI 1.60, 2.41). However, this study was unable to adjust for cause of first stillbirth.[15] In an earlier Australian study, limited to unexplained IUFDs, there was no statistically significant increase in IUFDs in a subsequent pregnancy (OR 1.62; 95% CI 0.63, 4.20).[16] What the various studies agree on is that the increased risk of a subsequent IUFD for a woman where no cause has been determined is small. However, there does tend to be increased obstetric intervention leading to prematurity, emergency caesarean section and PPH.[9]

Pre-pregnancy management strategies

If a woman is diagnosed with a treatable condition that may have contributed to her previous IUFD, e.g. diabetes, thyroid disease or chronic renal disease, this disorder must first be optimised. Most infections are acute, but it is still important to exclude and treat chronic infections, e.g. syphilis, prior to embarking on another pregnancy.[2] Periodontal disease should also be identified and treated as chronic disease has been linked to worsened perinatal outcomes.[9]

It is important, as with any pregnancy, to optimise the woman's health prior to a pregnancy. This can be targeted around addressing the key modifiable risk factors: obesity and smoking.[5] In addition to this, ensuring that women are taking the appropriate supplements of folic acid and vitamin D is prudent.

Couples may have questions about the optimum interval between their IUFD and becoming pregnant again. This may be particularly important considering the psychological implications of an IUFD. Mothers may experience more anxiety with a short inter-pregnancy interval, whereas partners may suffer more with a delay in conception.[12] Short inter-pregnancy intervals of less than 6 months are associated with increased risk of adverse perinatal outcomes;[17] however, this risk remains low.[12]

Antenatal care

The antenatal period may be a time of significant stress for a woman with a previous IUFD. Women often request increased surveillance and testing in a subsequent pregnancy.[18]

Initially, accurate dating and availability of combined screening will provide the opportunity to offer testing for aneuploidies, as trisomies 21, 18 and 13 are the commonest conditions associated with fetal death.

Consultant-led care should be recommended to women who have had a previous IUFD.[12] This approach will offer the opportunity to arrange regular antenatal visits, which can provide reassurance to the woman. In addition serial assessment of fetal growth, plotted on customised charts, can be initiated where appropriate.[9,12]

All women with an unexplained IUFD should be offered screening for GDM.[12] One intervention of proven benefit is to offer women heparin when medically indicated (e.g. APLS, inherited thrombophilias, cardiac disease requiring anticoagulation).[2]

For patients who travel to or live in malaria-endemic areas the use of insecticide-treated nets during pregnancy is essential.[2]

Delivery planning

Women with previous IUFDs who are at high risk due to contributing factors or who have had an unexplained stillbirth should be advised to deliver at an obstetric unit.[12] Many couples are extremely anxious and may request to be delivered early.[18] No studies have adequately investigated the effects of scheduled induction of labour on the fetus; however, what is known is that the higher rates of induction of women with previous IUFDs is coupled with an increase in instrumental deliveries and caesarean sections.[12] Many clinicians consider delivery by 39 weeks to be an important intervention for women with previous unexplained IUFDs.[9] The psychological benefits of elective induction should be weighed against the risk of respiratory distress syndrome (albeit small) and risks of induction (e.g. abnormal CTG, uterine hyperstimulation and instrumental deliveries).

KEY POINTS

- The stillbirth rate in the UK is 4.9/1000.
- Of all stillbirths, 98 per cent occur in the developing world.
- Several different classification systems exist for identifying causes of IUFDs; a new perinatal death reporting system in the UK has resulted in fewer unexplained IUFDs – approximately one in four is unexplained.
- Risk factors for stillbirths include: maternal weight, smoking and age, parity, SGA, placental abruption, pre-existing maternal diabetes mellitus and hypertension.
- Risk evaluation should include a careful review of past history, notes and investigation results, and assessment for current risk factors (e.g. smoking and BMI).
- Timing of pregnancy and likelihood of another pregnancy loss are major issues to couples with previous fetal loss; SANDS provides guidelines to counsel such couples.
- Recurrence of IUFDs following unexplained IUFDs may be slightly increased, but is still very small.
- In future pregnancies, fetal growth evaluation, ideally using a customised growth chart reference, is important, especially in a previous IUFD with a normally formed SGA baby.
- Induction of labour by 39 weeks is preferred by many couples with a past history of stillbirth, and endorsed by most obstetricians.

Postnatal care

A previous IUFD makes a woman vulnerable to depression, especially if the inter-pregnancy interval is short.[19] Vigilance and appropriate management are necessary.

References

1. Cousens S, Blencowe H, Stanton C et al. National, regional, and worldwide estimates of stillbirth rates in 2009 with trends since 1995: a systematic analysis. *Lancet* 2011;377:1319–30.
2. Bhutta ZA, Darmstadt GL, Haws RA, Yakoob M, Lawn JE. Delivering interventions to reduce the global burden of stillbirths: improving service supply and community demand. *BMC Pregnancy Childbirth* 2009;9(Suppl 1):S7.
3. Office for National Statistics. Statistical Bulletin: *Childhood, Infant and Perinatal Mortality in England and Wales, 2012.* London: Office for National Statistics, 2014:1–16.
4. Schott J, Henley A, Kohner N. *Pregnancy Loss and the Death of a Baby: Guidelines for professionals* 3rd edn. London: Sands, 2007.
5. Flenady V, Koopmans L, Middleton P et al. Major risk factors for stillbirth in high-income countries: a systematic review and meta-analysis. *Lancet* 2011;377:1331–40.
6. Lawn JE, Blencowe H, Pattinson R et al. Stillbirths: Where? When? Why? How to make the data count? *Lancet* 2011;377:1448–63.
7. Flenady V, Middleton P, Smith GC et al. Stillbirths: the way forward in high-income countries. *Lancet* 2011;377:1703–17.
8. Fretts RC. Etiology and prevention of stillbirth. *Am J Obstet and Gynecol* 2005;193:1923–35.
9. Robson SJ, Leader LR. Management of subsequent pregnancy after an unexplained stillbirth. *J Perinatology* 2010;30:305–10.
10. Measey MA, Charles A, d'Espaignet ET, Harrison C, deKlerk N, Douglass C. Aetiology of stillbirth: unexplored is not unexplained. *Aust NZ J Public Health* 2007;31:444–9.
11. Fretts R. Stillbirth epidemiology, risk factors, and opportunities for stillbirth prevention. *Clin Obstet Gynecol* 2010;53:588–96.
12. RCOG. *Late Intrauterine Fetal Death and Stillbirth.* London: RCOG, 2010:1–33.
13. Flenady V, Frøen JF, Pinar H et al. An evaluation of classification systems for stillbirth. *BMC Pregnancy Childbirth* 2009;9:24.
14. CMACE. *Perinatal Mortality 2009: United Kingdom.* London: CMACE, 2011:1–100.
15. Bhattacharya S, Prescott GJ, Black M, Shetty A. Recurrence risk of stillbirth in a second pregnancy. *BJOG* 2010;117:1243–7.
16. Robson S, Chan A, Keane RJ, Luke CG. Subsequent birth outcomes after an unexplained stillbirth: preliminary population-based retrospective cohort study. *Aust N Z J Obstet Gynaecol* 2001;41:29–35.
17. Conde-Agudelo A, Rosas-Bermúdez A, Kafury-Goeta AC. Birth spacing and risk of adverse perinatal outcomes. *JAMA* 2006;295:1809–23.
18. Robson SJ, Leader LR, Dear K, Bennett MJ. Women's expectations of management in their next pregnancy after an unexplained stillbirth: an internet-based empirical study. *Aust NZ J Obstet and Gynaecol* 2009;49:642–6.
19. Hughes PM, Turton P, Evans CD. Stillbirth as risk factor for depression and anxiety in the subsequent pregnancy: cohort study. *BMJ* 1999;318:1721–4.

Chapter 35 Multiple pregnancy

Bill Martin

MRCOG standards

Theoretical skills

- Understand the different forms of twins and their risks.
- Understand the potential problems of multiple pregnancies and the general principles of management.

Practical skills

- Be able to discuss with a patient the differences between monochorionic and dichorionic placentation.
- Be able to discuss the general complications of multiple pregnancies.
- Be able to discuss the increased perinatal risk of multiple pregnancies.

INTRODUCTION

Dizygous pregnancy rates vary with maternal age, race, nutrition and geography. The highest rates are reported in sub-Saharan Africa (Nigeria – 40/1000 births) and the lowest in the Far East (Japan – 6.7/1000 births)[1]. Monozygous twinning rates are, however, fairly constant, at 3–5/1000 births, although there is some anecdotal evidence that the incidence is also increasing. Multiple pregnancies have increased in the UK from 11.1/1000 maternities in 1988 to 15.9/1000 maternities in 2012.[2] On average, 1 in 5 IVF pregnancies results in multiple births compared with 1 in 80 for women who conceive naturally. With approximately 13,000 IVF babies being born each year this contributes significantly to the multiple birth rate.[3] Though predominantly dizygotic, pregnancies that result from assisted conception techniques are at greater risk of monozygotic division than those spontaneously conceived. In 2009, the Human Fertilisation and Embryology Authority (HFEA) launched the elective single embryo transfer (eSET) policy, which allowed centres to develop their own eSET strategy, with the aim of reducing the UK IVF multiple pregnancy rate to 10 per cent over a period of years.[3]

MATERNAL RISKS

The mother is at increased risk for several pregnancy complications, including miscarriage, hyperemesis gravidarum, premature labour and delivery, anaemia, pre-eclampsia, antepartum and postpartum haemorrhage, polyhydramnios, operative delivery and increased stay in hospital. Women who have twins are also at increased risk of having problems with breastfeeding and developing postnatal depression.

FETAL RISKS

Multiple pregnancies are associated with an increase in fetal and neonatal mortality compared with singleton pregnancies. The perinatal morbidity and mortality increase with increasing order of multiple pregnancy. The majority of perinatal deaths are associated with preterm birth and IUGR[4] (discussed further below). The stillbirth rate for twin births is 2.5 times that for singleton births, and the stillbirth rate for triplet and higher-order births is 3.1 times that for singleton births. The neonatal death rate for twin births is 6.7 times that for singleton births with the neonatal death rate for triplet and higher-order births being 14.8 times higher.[4] Monochorionic (MC) twins have an increased loss rate (14.2 per cent) compared with dichorionic (DC) twins (2.6 per cent), mainly due to losses before 24 weeks. The differential loss rate is mainly the result of twin–twin transfusion syndrome (TTTS) which accounts for 20 per cent of stillbirths in multiple pregnancies.[5]

Preterm labour

Twins are five times more likely to be born preterm compared with singletons,[6] and delivery before 32 weeks is approximately twice as common in MC compared with DC twins.[6] Nearly 27 per cent of triplets deliver prior to 32 weeks.

IUGR

Growth restriction of one or more of the fetuses in a multiple pregnancy is very common. The aetiology is not well understood, but (in the absence of TTTS) occurs in one twin in 10 per cent of MC and DC twins.[5] Twin birthweight discordance has been demonstrated to be a risk factor for preterm birth and adverse perinatal outcome. The NICE guideline recommends using a 25 per cent discordancy to identify a clinically important indicator of IUGR that merits referral for a tertiary fetal medicine opinion.[4] The presence of discordant growth in twins presents difficulties in management, more so in MC compared with DC due to the presence of vascular anastomoses in the former.

Single fetal death

This may occur either early in gestation or later as the pregnancy progresses. Fetal death after 24 weeks' gestation is relatively uncommon, occurring in 1.1 per cent and 3.6 per cent of dichorionic diamniotic (DC/DA) and monochorionic diamniotic (MC/DA) twin pregnancies, respectively.[7] Morbidity to the surviving fetus depends on the chorionicity of the pregnancy. When one MC twin dies *in utero*, there is a 12 per cent risk of death and an 18 per cent risk of neurological damage. The same figures for DC twins are 4 per cent and 1 per cent.[5] These complications are usually as a consequence of severe hypotension occurring during the death of the other twin.

The risk of cerebral palsy is increased in the surviving twin after a co-twin death, and same-sex twins are at greater risk than unlike-sex twins. The likely cause, in addition to the consequences of prematurity, is twin–twin transfusion problems associated with monochorionicity.

TTTS

TTTS is a condition that complicates up to 15 per cent of MC twin pregnancies.[5] It is characterised by haemodynamic imbalances caused by unidirectional deep arterio-venous anastomotic vessels (AVA) and a relative lack of superficial vascular anastomoses (arterio-arterial [AAA] and veno-venous [VVA] anastomatoses) which have bidirectional potential and can, if present, protect against those imbalances. TTTS can occur in MC/MA twins but is rarer, possibly because of the presence of protective AAAs.[5] In 5 per cent of cases TTTS can reverse with the donor becoming the recipient and vice versa (twin anaemia polycythaemia sequence or TAPS). This can occur after treatment with amnioreduction or laser.

The diagnosis requires the ultrasound demonstration of polyhydramnios around one twin (the recipient) and oligohydramnios around the other twin (the donor), with the separating membrane completely covering this fetus (stuck twin). The recipient twin is usually appropriately grown for gestational age, has a large distended bladder and may, if severely compromised, be hydropic. Recipient fetuses may also develop cardiac dysfunction and neonatal hypertension.

The donor twin, on the other hand, is frequently severely growth restricted, with abnormal umbilical artery Doppler waveforms. If untreated, the perinatal mortality rate of TTTS is extremely high (>90 per cent). Although twin–twin transfusion is usually a gradual process, it can happen suddenly with the death of one twin, usually the recipient.

Twin reversed arterial perfusion (TRAP) sequence

This complication occurs in approximately 1 per cent of MC pregnancies. It is characterised by an acardiac twin, which receives its blood supply via a large AAA from a normal co-twin (known as the 'pump' twin). This results in absent or rudimentary development of the upper body structures as the acardiac twin is supplied with deoxygenated blood. The perinatal mortality of the pump twin is considerable, with death usually occurring through complications of high-output cardiac failure leading to hydrops fetalis or polyhydramnios-induced preterm delivery.

Congenital anomalies

There is an excess of malformations in twins compared with singleton pregnancies.[4] These include malformations arising from the process of development and are often midline structural anomalies (e.g. NTDs, cardiac and cleft lip anomalies). An extreme example is the development of conjoined twins. Other malformations occur through disruption in a previously normally formed fetus. Disruptions are more common in MC pregnancies and consist of predominantly vascular-type lesions (e.g. hydrancephaly, porencephaly, small bowel atresia). A further mechanism leading to maldevelopment is the constraint of sharing the uterine cavity (e.g. talipes, congenital dislocation of the hip).

Other fetal risks

There are complications that usually arise in the third trimester and in particular in the intrapartum period. These include: intrapartum hypoxaemia through entanglement (interlocking twins); umbilical cord accidents such as cord prolapse which are more likely in multiple pregnancy due to an increased frequency of malposition; and cord entanglement in monoamniotic (MA) twins.[5]

KEY POINTS

- Preterm labour and delivery are the biggest cause of adverse perinatal outcome in multiple pregnancy [B].
- Maternal risks relate mainly to increased uterine distension and the development of pre-eclampsia [B].
- An excess of congenital malformations means that examination of multiple pregnancies by detailed ultrasound scanning is mandatory [B].

MANAGEMENT

Diagnosis and determination of chorionicity

Dizygous twins are always DC/DA. The chorionicity of monozygotic twins depends on the timing of embryo splitting after fertilisation. They may be:

- DC/DA, if <3 days;
- MC/DA, 4–7 days;
- MC/MA, 8+ days.

The early establishment of chorionicity is crucial to management of twins.[5] Complications are greater in MC compared with DC twins. Twenty per cent of twins are MC but such pregnancies are associated with an almost 26 per cent risk of perinatal mortality.

In the first trimester, chorionicity may be determined with nearly 100 per cent accuracy. In contrast, mid-trimester assessment is only 80–90 per cent accurate. If two placentae are visualised or if the fetuses are discordant for gender, the pregnancy must be DC. Visualisation of the *twin-peak* or *lambda* sign is also useful in the diagnosis of dichorionicity; however, the absence of this sign is not as reliable in the confirmation of monochorionicity. Membrane thickness has also been used to assign chorionicity. In difficult cases, zygosity studies may need to be performed, but there is no evidence that this approach improves overall outcome in MC twins.

Screening for aneuploidy and prenatal diagnosis

Serum screening in multiple pregnancies is not as reliable as in singletons. Therefore the screening method of choice is combined screening employing NT scanning plus biochemical tests – PAPP-A and β-hCG. This allows screening in the first trimester with calculation of a risk for each fetus.[8] Before any invasive procedure is undertaken for karyotyping, careful ultrasound mapping of the different placentae and gestational sacs is important to assist in subsequent management when the karyotype results are available. The pregnancy loss rates for genetic amniocentesis in twins are considered similar to those seen in singletons. No data exist on loss rates with amniocentesis for higher-order multiples. CVS is also possible in multiple pregnancies. Although CVS carries a higher loss rate, it has the advantage of being performed earlier, but may be less reliable than amniocentesis as up to 4 per cent of CVS samples show evidence of co-twin contamination.

Monitoring of fetal growth

Serial growth scans should be performed to evaluate fetal growth velocity and to detect any abnormalities in umbilical/fetal artery Doppler waveform analysis and amniotic fluid volume. In DC twins, 4-weekly scans from 24 weeks should be employed to try to identify growth restriction, with more frequent scans if growth appears suboptimal. MC pregnancies should be monitored fortnightly from 16 weeks.[4,5]

The management of growth restriction in twin pregnancies needs to consider the risks to both the fetuses. Severe growth restriction in one fetus in a DC pregnancy might warrant a conservative approach (even allowing the growth-restricted fetus to succumb *in utero*), thus sparing the healthy fetus the risks of iatrogenic prematurity. This situation is more complicated in MC pregnancy due to the presence of vascular anastamoses which could lead to damage/demise of the co-twin under these circumstances (see below).

Multifetal pregnancy reduction (MFPR)

In higher multiple pregnancy, with expectant management (i.e. non-reduction), 17 per cent and 28 per cent deliver at less than 29 weeks with triplets and quadruplets, respectively. In addition triplets and quadruplets have higher rates of other adverse outcomes including increased perinatal death, major anomalies, need for neonatal intensive care, respiratory distress syndrome, intrauterine growth restriction and serious neurological morbidity. Due to these issues and the additional increased maternal risk (e.g. pre-eclampsia), there is a consensus that multifetal pregnancy reduction at approximately 12 weeks should be offered to women with triplets (and higher multiples) to lower the incumbent risks.

With increasing experience, post-procedure miscarriage rates are now <10 per cent, such that reductions from triplets to twins and from quadruplets to twins carry outcomes as good as those of unreduced twin gestations, and the chance of taking home a live baby increases from 80 per cent to 90 per cent.

Preterm labour

Prediction of preterm labour in twin pregnancies is as difficult as in singleton pregnancies. Cervical assessment has been suggested as one method to evaluate the risk of preterm labour. However, the frequency of monitoring/assessment of the cervix is unclear. In singleton pregnancy a cervical length of 15 mm is predictive of preterm labour. In twin pregnancies, the mean cervical length is similar to that of singletons (38 mm), but a cervical length of 25 mm at 23 weeks' gestation predicts about 80 per cent of women who deliver spontaneously at <30 weeks, with a false-positive rate of approximately 11 per cent.[9]

Home uterine monitoring, fetal fibronectin estimation, prophylactic cervical cerclage, progesterone supplementation and tocolysis have not been shown to reduce the incidence of preterm labour in twin pregnancies[4] and have largely been abandoned.

There is currently not enough evidence to support a policy of routine hospitalisation for bed rest in multiple pregnancies. No reduction in the risk of preterm birth or perinatal death is evident, although there is a suggestion that fetal growth is improved. Indeed, in uncomplicated twin pregnancies, there is a suggestion that bed rest may be harmful in that the risk of very preterm birth is increased.

Antenatal steroids

The 2011 NICE guidelines[4] recommend the use of corticosteroids in a targeted way, i.e. where preterm delivery is considered likely. Untargeted (prophylactic) steroids are not recommended. Steroids should be offered in MC twin pregnancies as part of a planned delivery after 36 weeks, and similarly in triplet pregnancy as part of planned delivery after 35 weeks (see below).

Treatment of TTTS and TRAP

Treatment options for pregnancies affected by TTTS and TRAP have included serial amnioreduction, septostomy, selective feticide and laser ablation of the communicating anastomoses. A recent Cochrane Review (2014)[10] concluded that although, compared with amnioreduction, laser does not appear to improve survival significantly, it remains the treatment of choice due to the significant reduction in long-term neurological morbidity. Amnioreduction continues to have a place where laser therapy is not available or where TTTS occurs late in pregnancy (>26 weeks' gestation). The RCOG Guideline[5] concludes that TTTS before 26 weeks should be treated at regional fetal medicine centres by laser ablation. In advanced TTTS where one of the twin pair is *in extremis*, selective feticide is an option, allowing the survival of one twin with an 85 per cent success rate. Current management of TTTS therefore favours amnioreduction or expectant management for stage 1, laser ablation for stages 2–4, and selective reduction if imminent fetal demise of one twin threatens the co-twin.

A rare complication of MC twin pregnancy, with or without TTTS and which may occur following seemingly successful laser therapy, is TAPS. There may be no discordance in liquor volume but there is a large difference in Hb level. Severe sequelae may result including hydrops fetalis and fetal death. Optimal treatment is unclear but these cases require tertiary-level management.

In cases of TRAP, disruption of the acardiac twin's cord or intrafetal vessel ablation with laser, diathermy or the more recently available radiofrequency interstitial thermal ablation (RITA) are the available treatments with survival reported in >70 per cent of pump twins.

Treatment of co-twin death

In DC pregnancies, expectant management is indicated. Regular assessment of the pregnant woman's coagulation status is necessary in order to detect changes in the coagulation system that may occur. In both MC and DC pregnancies, if one twin dies there is risk of death or neurological damage in the surviving twin (see above).[5] Management depends upon the gestation and on the elapsed time since the fetal death. When death has occurred within 24–36 hours at an early gestation, fetal blood sampling with rescue transfusion may be considered if the surviving fetus is anaemic as indicated by middle cerebral artery Doppler (TAPS). At later gestations, delivery may be more appropriate if there are significant concerns regarding the wellbeing of the survivor. But caution must be exercised as any damage is likely to have occurred and delivery may only add risks of prematurity and not improve outcome.

If a co-twin death has occurred some time previously, consideration should be given to appropriate imaging of the surviving fetus's brain with either ultrasound or MRI to detect cystic changes. If these changes are apparent, offering termination of the pregnancy is an option.

Labour and delivery

The NICE guidance[4] suggests the following approach.

Women with uncomplicated MC twin pregnancies should be informed that elective birth from 36 weeks 0 days does not appear to be associated with an increased risk of serious adverse outcomes. For women with uncomplicated DC twin pregnancies the equivalent gestation is 37^{+0} weeks.

Both MC and DC twins should be informed that continuing uncomplicated twin pregnancies beyond 38 weeks 0 days increases the risk of fetal death.

Women with triplet pregnancies should be informed that continuing uncomplicated triplet pregnancies beyond 36 weeks 0 days increases the risk of fetal death.

Thus women with uncomplicated MC twin pregnancies should be offered elective birth from 36 weeks 0 days (after antenatal corticosteroids). DC twin pregnancies should be offered elective birth from 37 weeks 0 days and triplet pregnancies should be offered elective birth from 35 weeks 0 days, after a course of antenatal corticosteroids has been offered.

If elective birth is declined, appointments with a specialist obstetrician should be made with weekly ultrasound assessment of wellbeing and fortnightly fetal growth scans.

If there is evidence of TTTS or other complications, timing of delivery must be individualised.

The mode of delivery is decided based on the presentation of the first twin. Vaginal delivery is preferred in vertex–vertex presentations. The optimal mode of birth for the second twin presenting as non-vertex is unknown, with retrospective reviews in the literature providing support for both caesarean birth and vaginal birth for the second non-vertex twin.

For the very-low-birthweight infant (1500 g), opinion is divided as to the optimal mode of delivery. Whereas some advocate caesarean delivery in all cases, there is little evidence that caesarean section improves perinatal outcome.

For MC/MA twins delivery should be around 32 weeks and be by caesarean section [C].[4] Although some authors suggest that triplets and higher-order multiples may be safely delivered vaginally despite the obvious difficulties in monitoring, caesarean section is the more usual mode of delivery.

KEY POINTS

- Determination of chorionicity is important to allocate pregnancy risk [B].
- Combined screening is the method of choice for aneuploidy screening [B].
- Prenatal diagnosis using amniocentesis or CVS is suitable in multiple pregnancy [B].
- Ultrasound assessment should be carried out every 4 weeks from 20 weeks in DC twins and every 2 weeks from 16 weeks in MC twins (good practice point) (RCOG).[5]
- The management of TTTS and TRAP necessitates referral to an appropriate fetal medicine unit [B,D]. Such conditions carry high perinatal mortality, even with treatment.
- Optimal treatment of TTTS is laser ablation [A].
- Cervical length measurement may be useful in predicting preterm birth in multiple pregnancy [B].
- Uncomplicated MC twins aim to deliver vaginally by 36-37 weeks (good practice point) (RCOG).[5]
- Uncomplicated DC twins aim to deliver vaginally by 37-38 weeks (good practice point) (RCOG).[5]

CONCLUSIONS

The management of a multiple pregnancy is a major challenge for obstetricians. These pregnancies are at increased risk of maternal and fetal complications that require specialised management. There is an increasing vogue to manage these patients in specialised multiple pregnancy clinics, with access to a fetal medicine specialist with a special interest in multiple pregnancy.

Key References

1. Dodd JM, Grivell RM, Crowther CA. Multiple pregnancy. In: James DK, Steer PJ, Weiner CP, Crowther CA, Gonik G (eds). *High Risk Pregnancy: Management options.* 4th edn. Edinburgh: Elsevier Saunders, 2010.
2. Office for National Statistics. *Birth statistics.* 2012 series FM1. London: ONS, 2013.
3. Human Fertilisation & Embryology Authority. Multiple births and single embryo transfer review. London: HFEA, 2013. Available at http://www.hfea.gov.uk/Multiple-births-after-IVF.html.
4. NICE. Clinical Guideline No. 129. *Multiple pregnancy: the management of twin and triplet pregnancies.* London: NICE, 2011.
5. RCOG. Guideline No. 51. *Management of Monochorionic Twin Pregnancy.* London: RCOG, 2009.
6. Sebire NJ, Snijders RJ, Hughes K, Sepulveda W, Nicolaides KH. The hidden mortality of monochorionic twin pregnancies. *Br J Obstet Gynaecol* 1997;104:1203–7.
7. Lee YM, Wylie BJ, Simpson LL, D'Alton ME. Twin chorionicity and the risk of stillbirth. *Obstet Gynecol* 2008;111(2 Pt 1):301–8.
8. NHS Fetal Anomaly Screening Programme. *Down's Syndrome Screening: UK NSC Policy Recommendations 2011-2014: Model of best practice.* Exeter: UK NSC, 2013.
9. Souka AP, Heath V, Flint S, Sevastopoulou I, Nicolaides KH. Cervical length at 23 weeks in twins in predicting spontaneous preterm delivery. *Obstet Gynecol* 1999; 94:450–4.
10. Roberts D, Neilson JP, Kilby MD, Gates S. Interventions for the treatment of twin-twin transfusion syndrome. *Cochrane Database Sys Rev* 2014 1:CD002073.

Chapter 36 Fetal infections

Tara Jayne Selman

MRCOG standards

Theoretical skills

- Knowledge of the most common maternal infections that can result in fetal morbidity and mortality.
- Understand the maternal and fetal tests that can determine *in-utero* infection.
- Appreciate the long-term implication of fetal infection.
- Understand the treatment and preventive measures.

Practical skills

- Be able to counsel pregnant women with regard to the risk of fetal infection, diagnostic methods, treatments and pregnancy options, and refer appropriately those at risk of fetal infection to a fetal medicine unit.

BACKGROUND

The majority of common maternal infections acquired during pregnancy are of little or no consequence to the fetus; however, there are some important infections that have significant sequelae for the fetus and may result in anything from fetal demise through to structural difference and neuro-development delay. The effect on the fetus is dependent on not only the type of infection but also the gestation acquired. Prenatal diagnosis is usually initiated as a result of routine screening at booking, a history of exposure of the mother to infectious contacts or differences seen on ultrasound scan. Independent of the infection type, management always requires a multidisciplinary team approach including microbiologists, obstetricians, fetal medicine experts and paediatricians. This team is responsible for confirming maternal infection and determining, with potential confirmation of, the risk of fetal infection. For those with an infected fetus careful and empathetic counselling is then necessary covering any intrauterine treatment, fetal surveillance and in some situations the possibility of termination of pregnancy.

This chapter will concentrate on the prenatal diagnosis and management of some of the more common or serious fetal infections.

RUBELLA

Introduction

The rubella virus (formerly known as German measles as it was described first by two German physicians) is found only in humans and is transmitted by aerosol via the respiratory tract, with close contact usually required for transmission.

The national immunisation programmes in many countries have made this disease increasingly rare as a result of herd immunity; however, one should have a high index when seeing immigrants to the UK. Studies in the UK from antenatal screening results have shown that 4–8 per cent of immigrant women, but less than 2 per cent of UK-born women, are susceptible to rubella infection.[1]

Rubella is normally a mild disease, especially in children, although it can cause more severe symptoms in adults. There is an incubation period on average of 14 days (12–23 days) prior to the development of the classic non-confluent maculo-papular rash seen first on the face then spreading to the trunk. There is often a lymphadenopathy, most commonly suboccipital, post-auricular and cervical, prior to and lasting after the disappearance of the rash. These signs are often accompanied by a prodromal phase with malaise and low-grade fever and also headache, sore throat and cough. In 20–50 per cent of cases the entire infection may be subclinical. In adults the most common complications are arthralgia and arthritis; rarely post-infection encephalopathy (1:6000) and thrombocytopenia (1:3000) are seen. The viraemia occurs for 7 days prior to the rash developing and for 7–12 days after the onset of the rash, hence a person is infectious for over 2 weeks.[2]

Maternal diagnosis

Laboratory confirmation of rubella infection is required as the condition frequently is subclinical or has associated signs and symptoms that are indistinguishable from other infections such as parvovirus B19 and group A streptococcus.[3] An acute infection may be diagnosed by isolation of the virus from throat swabs, but it is more common for an acute rubella-specific immunoglobulin (IgM) response to be isolated [C] using fluorescent immunoassay techniques. The presence of rubella-specific IgG indicates previous infection or immunisation and immunity is normally lifelong.

Fetal infection

There are few prospective studies using sensitive laboratory techniques to accurately determine the rate of fetal infection. The most vulnerable gestation for transplacental infection is in the first trimester, occurring in approximately 80 per cent of cases. Of these, congenital defects occur in about 85 per cent, with multiple defects common if the infection was in the first 8 weeks of gestation, and in 20 per cent of cases in this gestation range the infection results in miscarriage.[4,5] After 12 weeks the risk to the fetus declines rapidly to somewhere in the region of 25 per cent in the early second trimester.

Fetal rubella infection can result in a number of abnormalities referred to collectively as congenital rubella syndrome. These classic abnormalities are heart defects (patent ductus arteriosis, pulmonary stenosis, pulmonary arterial hypoplasia), eye defects (cataracts, microphthalmos, retinopathy), CNS problems (mental and psychomotor delay, speech and language delay), microcephaly and sensorineural deafness.[5] Fetal infections later in the pregnancy may result in isolated deafness. There is emerging evidence to suggest that *in-utero* exposure to rubella may have long-term mental health sequelae with individuals being at higher risk of schizophrenia in adulthood. The virus is thought to prevent maturation of critical brain structural and functional components implicated in the aetiology of the disorder.[6]

The exact pathogenesis of congenital rubella infection is not fully understood. One hypothesis is that the virus crosses the fetus via the chorion in the first trimester and virus-infected desquamated epithelial cells are transported to the fetal circulation and fetal organs. In early pregnancy the fetal immune response has not developed and fetal damage may be by viral retardation of division, induced apoptosis of essential cells, or interference with the cell cycle and tissue necrosis.[7,8]

Diagnosis in the fetus and management

When primary infection has occurred in the first 12 weeks of pregnancy a woman should be counselled that the risk of congenital defects is very high and some women may wish to terminate the pregnancy.

The rate of infection declines rapidly between 12 and 18 weeks and is almost zero after 20 weeks,[2] hence counselling at this gestation is inevitably more focused on prenatal diagnosis. Fetal blood sampling to measure levels of rubella-specific IgM can be performed and rubella-specific RNA identified using reverse-transcriptase polymerase chain reaction (RT-PCR) [C,D].[9] The risk of false-negative results and the uncertainty over the effects on the fetus of infection should be discussed with the woman prior to testing.

Treatment and prevention

In the absence of an antiviral drug to treat rubella or prevent transmission, the cornerstone of prevention is childhood vaccination. Primary rubella vaccination failure is rare, with many studies showing a 100 per cent seroconversion rate. Vaccination programmes have been shown to be cost-effective in both developing and developed countries if coverage rates of more than 80 per cent are achieved. Pre-pregnancy counselling should include evidence of immunity, with vaccination offered to susceptible women [C]. There is insufficient evidence to support rescreening of previously seropositive women and no data to support or refute the principle of offering rubella vaccination to women who have low titres. In the UK the vaccine, which contains attenuated rubella virus, is usually given in combination with measles and mumps vaccines as the MMR. The vaccine is contraindicated in pregnancy and pregnancy should be avoided for 1 month afterwards.

KEY POINTS

- Maternal infection in the first trimester results in an extremely high rate of fetal transmission and subsequent congenital rubella syndrome [C].
- Termination of pregnancy should be discussed as part of counselling when the infection has occurred in the first trimester due to the high risk of congenital malformations [C].
- Prenatal diagnosis should be considered when maternal infection has occurred in the second trimester as the risk to the fetus declines rapidly between 12 and 18 weeks' gestation.

CYTOMEGALOVIRUS

Introduction

Cytomegalovirus (CMV) is a ubiquitous double-stranded DNA virus that belongs to the herpes virus family. It is one of the most common congenital infections, with the prevalence of congenital CMV at birth in the region of 1 per cent. The reported incidence of primary maternal infection in pregnancy is 0.7–4.1 per cent, with transmission to the fetus occurring in approximately one-third of cases.[10]. Approximately 50–70 per cent of pregnant women show serological evidence of previous infection. Although recurrent infection can lead to fetal infection the risk of transmission is much lower (1–3 per cent), as is the severity of fetal infection.

Almost all CMV infections in non-immunosuppressed pregnant women are asymptomatic with only a small proportion (up to 5 per cent) displaying a mononucleosis-like syndrome.[11] Transmission of the virus requires close contact between individuals though contaminated urine, saliva, semen, cervical secretions and breast milk.

Maternal diagnosis

Due to the asymptomatic nature of the condition laboratory testing is relied upon for maternal diagnosis. CVM IgG has a high sensitivity and specificity as a sign of a past or recent infection. Seroconversion from two samples will provide the most accurate and reliable diagnosis of a primary infection. Although CMV IgM is suggestive of a recent or ongoing infection with a high sensitivity, its specificity is low. If a sample has both CMV IgM and IgG, comparison with a sample early in pregnancy can aid in diagnosis. Alternatively CMV IgG avidity testing can be performed. This test will examine the binding capacity of CMV IgG antibodies which is low early after infection.[12]

Fetal infection

Eighty to ninety per cent of neonates with congenital CMV infection are asymptomatic in the neonatal period. On ultrasound the fetus may exhibit IUGR, microcephaly, cerebral atrophy, ventriculomegaly, intracranial calcification and/or fetal hydrops. The presence of fetal abnormalities on ultrasound worsens the prognosis. The likelihood of CMV having an effect on the fetus is not gestation dependent, but the sequelae differ. In early infection fetal brain anomalies are more frequently seen and the neonate is more likely to be symptomatic in comparison to later infection where hepatitis and thrombocytopenia are more common. Congenital CMV infection is the most common cause of deafness and learning disabilities in the UK, as rubella, measles and mumps have become much rarer due to vaccination. The outcome for the 10 per cent of neonates who are clinically affected at birth is poor. There is an associated mortality rate of 30 per cent and 90 per cent will have severe neurological sequelae. Of those asymptomatic at birth 10–15 per cent will develop long-term sequelae.

Diagnosis in the fetus and management

The diagnosis of fetal infection may be suggested by maternal serology and ultrasound findings. Women with CMV infection in pregnancy should be offered fetal diagnosis which is usually by quantitative PCR on the amniotic fluid, although it is possible from CVS and fetal blood [C].[13] The diagnostic sensitivity is high if the sample is taken after week 21 of pregnancy (once fetal diuresis is established) and 6 weeks after maternal serum is positive [B]. A negative result still has to be treated with caution as it can be falsely negative due to CMV levels

being too low to detect. As the fetus may still be affected in the absence of ultrasound findings, termination of pregnancy should be discussed alongside serial ultrasound surveillance.

Treatment and prevention

There is no vaccination for CMV, although research has shown CMV glycoprotein B vaccine may potentially reduce the incidence of maternal and congenital CMV infection, with a suggested 50 per cent vaccination efficacy rate; phase 3 trials are awaited.[14] There is also no effective fetal therapy. Ganciclovir can transiently reduce viral shedding and may reduce the audiological consequences of CMV in some infected infants [C,D].

KEY POINTS

- Pre-pregnancy immunity to CMV is in the range of 55–85 per cent.
- Primary infection rate in pregnancy is 1–4 per cent with an approximate 40 per cent fetal transmission rate [C].
- Congenital CMV incidence is between 0.3 and 3 per cent [C].
- Ten per cent of neonates with congenital CMV will be symptomatic at birth. There is a poor prognosis in this group with a 30 per cent mortality rate, and in survivors up to 90 per cent have neurodevelopmental delay and 60 per cent hearing loss.

TOXOPLASMOSIS

Introduction

Toxoplasmosis is a unicellular protozoan that is found worldwide, although it is more common in tropical areas. Seroprevalence in Europe is high: up to 54 per cent in southern European countries, decreasing with increasing latitude to 5–10 per cent in northern Sweden and Norway. The cat is the definitive host and produces oocysts and sporozoites. Ingestion leads to the formation of tachyzoites; these cause parasitaemia and further dissemination in subsequent bradyzoites which lead to latent infection with the formation of tissue cysts in the skeletal muscle, heart muscle and CNS tissue. Toxoplasmosis can be transmitted to pregnant women through ingestion of tissue cysts in raw or inadequately cooked meat, or in uncooked foods that have been in contact with contaminated meat. It can also be transmitted through inadvertent ingestion of oocysts and sporozoites in cat faeces and contaminated surface water.[15] It is not possible to confirm the source of infection; however, there is a wide consensus among experts that acquiring toxoplasmosis is often associated with unsafe eating habits. In adults the infection is usually asymptomatic, although they may develop a mild malaise, lethargy and lymphadenopathy.

Maternal diagnosis

As with rubella and CMV the diagnosis of maternal infection is usually a serological one. When IgM and IgG are identified conversion from a seronegative sample taken at booking is helpful in accurately confirming the diagnosis. Without such a sample interpretation is more difficult as low levels of CMV IgM can be found for up to several years after an acute infection.[16] Presumed positive testing can be confirmed in laboratories using specific and sensitive ELISA testing [C].

Fetal infection

Congenital toxoplasmosis has a classic triad of chorioretinitis, intracranial calcifications and hydrocephalus. The likelihood of fetal infection and the severity are gestation dependent. In the first trimester fetal infection will often result in miscarriage; if miscarriage does not occur maternal infection is less likely to result in congenital infection; however, if it does occur the differences are usually more severe. As pregnancy progresses the likelihood of transplacental passage increases but fetal injury is less likely.[17]

Diagnosis in the fetus and management

Fetal infection can be identified by PCR of amniotic fluid [C].[18] When counselling a woman the gestation that the infection is likely to have occurred (if known) should be taken in to account as well as the parasitic load of the amniotic fluid, with infections acquired before 20 weeks' gestation and a parasite load of 1100 parasites/mL amniotic fluid, and women with fetal anomalies shown on ultrasound, having a poor prognosis. In such pregnancies termination should be discussed with the parents.

Treatment and prevention

On confirmation of maternal infection recommendations are still that spiramycin should be commenced to reduce the likelihood of fetal transmission [C];[18] however, a Cochrane review of treatment of toxoplasmosis infection in pregnancy failed to identify studies to support this.[19] It is thought that, for an effect to be seen on clinical outcome (reduction in neurological symptoms rather than in chorioretinitis), treatment needs to be commenced within 4 weeks of infection [C]. Hence spiramycin should be commenced before PCR results from amniocentesis and continued even if this is negative, due to the theoretical risk of later infection from the placenta infected earlier in pregnancy. Some recommend that, with a positive PCR from amniotic fluid from 18 weeks, combination therapy of pyrimethamine (avoided in the first trimester due to potential teratogenicity risk) and sulfadiazine be used.

Due to the potential ineffectiveness and risks of treatment, prevention is of primary importance. This requires prenatal education on the importance in pregnancy of handling and cooking meat correctly, wearing gloves to handle cat litter and avoiding contact with objects that are potentially contaminated with cat faeces.

KEY POINTS

- In the UK it is felt that the risk of congenital toxoplasmosis is low and routine screening of pregnant women would not be cost-effective [C].
- Public education is needed to prevent infection during pregnancy.
- It is possible that early maternal treatment may reduce transmission or at least reduce neurological sequelae.
- Fetal risk is gestation dependent. Severe congenital disease occurs in up to 25 per cent of fetuses infected in the first and second trimesters.

PARVOVIRUS B19

Introduction

Parvovirus B19, also commonly referred to as fifth disease or erythema infectiosum, is a small single-stranded DNA virus that at least 50 per cent of pregnant women are seropositive for and hence immune to. The virus is often asymptomatic in adults, although they may initially present with symptoms similar to a common cold followed by the classic slapped-cheek rash. Adults who are symptomatic will often experience a polyarthropathy syndrome. The virus is spread via aerosol route and those infected are contagious for 5–10 days prior to the rash developing. Significant contact is required to contract the virus. This is defined as being in the same room as the infected person for over 15 minutes, or face-to-face contact. The infection is usually seen in epidemics.

Maternal diagnosis

The diagnosis is again a serological one which is triggered by a history of significant contact with an infected party (usually a child) or due to fetal finding. A positive serological diagnosis is made in the presence of parvo-specific IgM antibodies. These usually appear 2–3 days after an acute infection and may persist up to 6 months. The presence of specific IgG is seen a few days after the development of IgM and usually remains lifelong, and hence is evidence of previous infection and confers lifelong immunity. If viral exposure was recent then it is possible that it is still within the incubation period and it is suggested that if a women is seronegative she be re-tested 2–4 weeks later.[20]

Fetal infection

The virus itself is not thought to be teratogenic [D]; however, the effects of transmission to the fetus can be serious and fatal. The risk of transplacental infection increases with gestation, from 15 per cent until 15 weeks to 25 per cent thereafter and up to 70 per cent towards term. In early pregnancy (first and early second trimester) there is a 9 per cent fetal loss rate. After this gestation the risk to the fetus is of developing hydrops secondary to fetal anaemia or cardiac dysfunction from acute myocarditis [C,D]. The virus has a predilection for erytopoietic cells which leads to a transient but severe pancytopenia.[21] There is in the region of a 3–10 per cent risk of developing hydrops following infection and once present a 50 per cent risk of fetal demise.

Diagnosis and management

Diagnosis is made either as a result of isolation of the virus from PCR at amniocentesis or from fetal blood sample performed as part of the investigation of fetal hydrops [C]. Fetal hydrops usually occurs 2–4 weeks after the acute fetal infection. A fetus potentially identified as being at risk due to maternal serology, but not showing signs of infection, should be monitored by ultrasound weekly for up to 8 weeks after maternal exposure for signs of fetal hydrops, and with middle cerebral artery, peak systolic velocity measurements to predict fetal anaemia. A fetus with either hydrops or anaemia requires management at a tertiary fetal medicine centre. The management is controversial as 30 per cent of cases of hydrops will resolve spontaneously due to the self-limiting nature of the virus, however there are no robust methods to determine in which fetus this will occur and hence active management of all cases usually occurs. A fetal blood sample (via cordocentesis or intrahepatic umbilical vein) is taken to confirm the underlying diagnosis of fetal anaemia and its cause, and intrauterine transfusion is given [C].[22]

KEY POINTS

- There is a 1:5 risk of transplacental infection of the fetus in non-immune pregnant women [C].
- The risk of fetal infection is gestation dependent.
- The time interval between maternal infection and fetal consequence is 4-5 weeks.
- Fetal consequences of infection can be self-limiting and treatable. Management should be in a tertiary referral fetal medicine centre capable of performing intrauterine transfusion [C,E].

SYPHILIS

Introduction

Syphilis is caused by the spirochaete *Treponema pallidum.* Often women infected with syphilis are not aware of their condition, with the primary painless genital sores going unnoticed. Secondary syphilis presents several weeks or months later with cutaneous, mucosal and sometimes systemic symptoms. It is

at this stage that syphilis is most contagious and it can last up to a year. Finally the infection enters a latent stage which may have an absence of clinical manifestations, but can still result in transplacental fetal infection.[23] Worldwide this is a common cause of both fetal growth restriction and fetal hydrops.

Maternal diagnosis

Screening of antenatal patients for syphilis is part of the national screening programme. Unlike most common bacterial infections *T. pallidium* cannot be cultured rapidly or cheaply. There are several serological tests that are used such as VDRL (Venereal Disease Reference Library), RPR, FTA-abs (fluorescent treponemal antibody absorption test), MHA-TP (Microhemagglutination assay) or TPI assay (Triose Phosphate isomerase assay).

Fetal infection

Spirochaetes can cross the placenta from 14 weeks' gestation, with the risk of fetal infection increasing with gestational age.[24] During the first 4 years of acquiring syphilis an untreated pregnant woman will have a 70 per cent chance of transmitting the infection to the fetus. The results for an infected fetus are profound and range from spontaneous miscarriage and stillbirth through to non-immune hydrops, growth restriction and preterm delivery. About two-thirds of liveborn infants with congenital syphilis are asymptomatic at birth and later are affected with deafness, neurological impairment and bone deformities.

Diagnosis and management

Fetal infection can be diagnosed by serology from fetal blood sample, detecting syphilis-specific IgM antibodies (maternal IgM does not cross the placenta), or alternatively *T. pallidium* DNA can also be detected using PCR techniques with amniotic fluid [C].[25] Ultrasound features which are suggestive of infection may also be seen e.g. fetal hydrops, hepatomegaly, placentomegaly and small bowel dilation. Hepatomegaly appears to be the most sensitive ultrasound marker [D].

There is no treatment for an infected fetus and as with all serious fetal infections discussion around termination of pregnancy is appropriate.

Treatment and prevention

The use of penicillin has formed the long-stay treatment for syphilis and remains so, as unlike other sexually transmitted infections (STIs) it has not yet developed a resistance to this. When syphilis is diagnosed in pregnancy a penicillin regimen appropriate for the stage of disease should be used [C], with monthly serology titres allowing evaluation of the adequacy of treatment. In theory penicillin treatment will prevent the transplacental passage of the pathogen; however, as many as

KEY POINTS

- Worldwide congenital syphilis is still a major cause of perinatal morbidity and mortality.
- The risk of transplacental transmission is greatest within the first year of untreated maternal syphilis.
- If untreated, of those pregnancies infected 30 per cent of fetuses will die *in utero* and 30 per cent in the early neonatal period, with the others developing late congenital symptoms.

14 per cent of women, despite the recommended treatment, will have a fetal death or deliver a neonate with congenital syphilis [C].[26,27]

VARICELLA

Introduction

Varicella-zoster virus (VZV) is a highly contagious DNA virus of the herpes family. It is transmitted by respiratory droplets and by direct personal contact with vesicle fluid. The primary infection is characterised by fever, malaise and a pruritic rash. During pregnancy the illness tends to be more severe than in childhood and it can result in maternal pneumonia, encephalitis or myocarditis. The incubation period is 7–21 days and a person is infectious 48 hours before the rash appears and continues to be infectious until the vesicles crust over, typically 5 days. Over 90 per cent of the antenatal population in the UK are seropositive for VZV-specific IgG antibody, so infection is uncommon, affecting 1 in 1000 pregnancies. Following primary infection the virus remains dormant in sensory nerve root ganglia and can become reactivated to give a vesicular erythematous skin rash in a dermatome distribution, i.e. shingles. It is possible to acquire the infection from exposed sites.[28]

Maternal diagnosis

For a woman with no previous history of chickenpox and a significant history of exposure the risk to the woman can be determined by looking for serological evidence of VZV IgG. The diagnosis itself is made from examination of the classic rash. Although treating seronegative women with significant contact with varicella-zoster immunoglobulin, and those with active disease with aciclovir, is important for maternal health, there is no evidence to prove that it reduces the risk of transmission of VZV to the fetus.[28]

Fetal infection

The effect of VZV on the fetus is gestation dependent. In the first trimester fetal infection may lead to spontaneous miscarriage. From as early as 3 weeks until 28 weeks' gestation it is possible for the fetus to develop fetal varicella syndrome (FVS), although the risk overall is small: 1–2 per cent until 20 weeks, with most cases occurring after the first trimester[29] and rapidly declining towards 28 weeks with no cases reported after 28 weeks.[30] Fetal varicella syndrome consists of limb deformity, microcephaly, hydrocephaly, soft tissue calcification and IUGR.

Diagnosis and management

Diagnosis of fetal infection can be made by ultrasound findings. There is usually a time lag of at least 5 weeks after the primary infection before fetal differences are seen.[28] Amniocentesis may be performed to confirm the diagnosis with PCR identification of VZV DNA. In the absence of ultrasound scanning finding a positive amniocentesis has a high sensitivity but low specificity for the development of VZV. If the PCR is positive but the ultrasound normal at 17–21 weeks the risk of FVS (fetal varicella syndrome) is low; if repeat ultrasound scanning at 24 weeks is also normal then the risk of FVS is almost zero. The risk, conversely, is very high if there are ultrasound features and positive PCR [D].

Treatment and prevention

There is no intrauterine treatment currently available. For women known to be seronegative varicella vaccine can be administered. This is a live attenuated vaccine and hence pregnancy should be avoided for 1–3 months after administration.

ACKNOWLEDGEMENTS

Dr Sailesh Kumar, author of this chapter in the previous edition.

References

1. Tookey PA, Cortina-Borja M, Peckham CS. Rubella susceptibility among pregnant women in North London. *J Public Health Med* 2002;24:211–6.
2. Best JM. Rubella. *Semin Fetal and Neonatal Med* 2007;12:182–92.
3. Daffos F, Forestier F, Grangeot-Keros L *et al.* Prenatal diagnosis of congenital rubella. *Lancet* 1984;ii:1–3.
4. Mellinger AK, Cragan JD, Atkinson WL *et al.* High incidence of congenital rubella syndrome after rubella outbreak. *Pediatr Infect Dis J* 1995;14:573–8.
5. Miller E, Cradock-Watson JE, Pollock TM. Consequences of confirming maternal rubella at successive stages of pregnancy. *Lancet* 1982;ii:781–4.
6. Brown AS, Susser ES. In utero infection and adult schizophrenia. *Mental Retard Dev Disabil Res Rev* 2002;8:51–7.
7. Banatvala JE, Brown DWG. Rubella. *Lancet* 2004;363:1127–37.
8. Lee J-Y, Bowden DS. Rubella virus replication and links to teratogenicity. *Clin Microbiol Rev* 2000;13:571–87.

9. Bosma TJ, Corbett KM, O'Shea S *et al*. PCR for detection of rubella virus RNA in clinical samples. *J Clin Microbiol* 1995;33:1075–9.

10. Kenneson A, Cannon MJ. Review and meta-analysis of the epidemiology of congenital cytomegalovirus infection. *Rev Med Virol* 2007;17:355–63.

11. Zanghellini F, Boppana SB, Emery VC, Griffiths PD, Pass RF. Asymptomatic primary cytomegalovirus infection: virologic and immunologic features. *J infect Dis* 1999;180:702–7.

12. Malm G, Engman M-L. Congenital cytomegalovirus infections. *Semin Fetal Neonatal Med* 2007;12: 154–9.

13. Enders G, Bader U, Lindemann L *et al*. Prenatal diagnosis of congenital cytomegalovirus infection in 189 pregnancies with known outcome. *Prenat Diag* 2001;21:362–77.

14. Pass RF, Zang C, Evan A *et al*. Vaccine prevention of maternal cytomegalovirus infection. *N Engl J Med* 2009;360:1191–9.

15. Dubey JP. Sources of toxoplasma gondii infection in pregnancy. Until rates of congenital toxoplasmosis fall, control measures are essential. *BMJ* 2000;321: 127–8.

16. Patersen E. Toxoplasmosis. *Semin Fetal Neonatal Med* 2007;12:214–23.

17. Sever JL, Ellenberg JH, Ley AC et al. Toxoplasmosis: maternal and pediatric findings in 23,000 pregnancies. *Pediatrics* 1988;82:181-92,

18. Hohlfeld P, Duffos F, Costa JM *et al*. Prenatal diagnosis of congenital toxoplasmosis with polymerase-chain-reaction test on amniotic fluid. *N Engl J Med* 1994;331:695–9.

19. Dunn D, Wallon M, Peyron F *et al*. Mother to child transmission of toxoplasmosis: risk estimates for clinical counselling. *Lancet* 1999;353:1829–33.

20. Rodis JF. Parvovirus infection. *Clin Obstet Gynecol* 1999;42:107–20.

21. Ismail K, Kilby MD. Human parvovirus B19 and pregnancy. *Obstet Gynecol* 2003;5:4–9.

22. Agrawal P, Gillham J. Fetal infection: a pragmatic approach to recognition and management. *Obstet Gynaecol Repro Med* 2009;20:22–6.

23. Walker GJA, Walker DG. Congenital syphilis: A continuing but neglected problem. *Semin Fetal Neonatal Med* 2007;12:198–206.

24. Goldenberg RL, Thompson C. The infectious origins of stillbirth. *Am J Obstet Gynecol* 2003;189:861–73.

25. Zoechling N, Schluepen EM, Soyer HP *et al*. Molecular detection of *Treponema pallidum* in secondary and tertiary syphilis. *Br J Dermatol* 1997;136:683–6.

26. McFarlin BL, Bottoms SF, Dock BS, Isas NB. Epidemic syphilis: maternal factors associated with congenital infection. *Am J Obstet Gynecol* 1994;170:535–40.

27. Conover CS, Rend CA, Miller GB, Schmid GP. Congenital syphilis after treatment of maternal syphilis with penicillin regimen exceeding CDC guidelines. *Inf Dis Obstet Gynecol* 1998;6:134–7.

28. Byrne BMP, Crowley PA, Carrington D. *Chickenpox in pregnancy*. Green-top Guideline No. 13. London: RCOG, 2007.

29. Patuszak AL, Levy M, Schick B *et al*. Outcome after maternal varicella infection in the first 20 weeks of pregnancy. *N Engl J Med* 1994;330:901–5.

30. Tan MP, Koren G. Chickenpox in pregnancy revisited. *Repro Toxicol* 2005;21:410–20.

FETAL CONDITIONS

Chapter 37 Tests of fetal wellbeing

Alexander Heazell

INTRODUCTION

Tests of fetal wellbeing in the antenatal period aim to reduce perinatal morbidity and mortality and infant morbidity by correctly identifying fetal compromise *in utero* so that appropriate intervention (usually delivery) can be instigated. To achieve the desired clinical impact a test must have sufficient sensitivity and specificity and be coupled to an effective intervention. For example, a perfectly predictive test with sensitivity and specificity of 100 per cent will have no clinical value if there is no intervention to prevent the outcome. In practical terms no such perfect test exists; tests must be sufficiently sensitive to predict or identify a compromised fetus but must also be specific to prevent unwarranted intervention and parental anxiety.

Development of tests that can achieve the required sensitivity and specificity is challenging as the poor outcomes they aim to detect and prevent are comparatively rare, increasing the likelihood of a false-positive result. The comparative rarity of stillbirth or severe neonatal morbidity means that studies to test these interventions need to be very large and are thus expensive and difficult to undertake. Therefore, current practice is often based on a lower quality of evidence than one would hope for.

FETAL COMPROMISE

Fetal compromise has no widely accepted definition. However, in practice fetal compromise usually describes a series of events culminating in fetal hypoxia which in turn leads to acidaemia. If the cause persists then the fetus is at risk of severe morbidity (e.g. cerebral palsy) or will ultimately die. Potential causes of fetal compromise may be acute or chronic and include: impaired maternal nutrient or oxygen supply, uteroplacental dysfunction, impaired blood supply to the fetus (e.g. cord accident) and fetal anaemia (e.g. fetomaternal haemorrhage). Of these, placental dysfunction is the most frequent cause of antepartum fetal compromise. It is important to note that placental dysfunction can occur as the end-point of various pathological processes (e.g. abnormal development, infarction, inflammation, infection), the discussion of which is beyond the scope of this chapter.

In the presence of nutrient and oxygen deprivation secondary to placental dysfunction, the fetus initially responds by reducing its growth rate (Fig. 37.1).[1] Persistent nutrient and oxygen deprivation may lead to further adaptations, including reduction in fetal movements and redistribution of fetal blood flow. Changes to fetal and placental blood flow may occur which can be detected using Doppler ultrasound of the umbilical artery, middle cerebral artery and ductus venosus. Changes to the fetal heart rate trace are a late sign of fetal compromise and are regarded as a pre-terminal event. Therefore, signs of fetal compromise and tests to detect it may detect problems at different stages of its development. Consequently, each strategy to evaluate fetal wellbeing has the potential for false-positive and false-negative results depending on the timing of that investigation and the cause of fetal compromise.

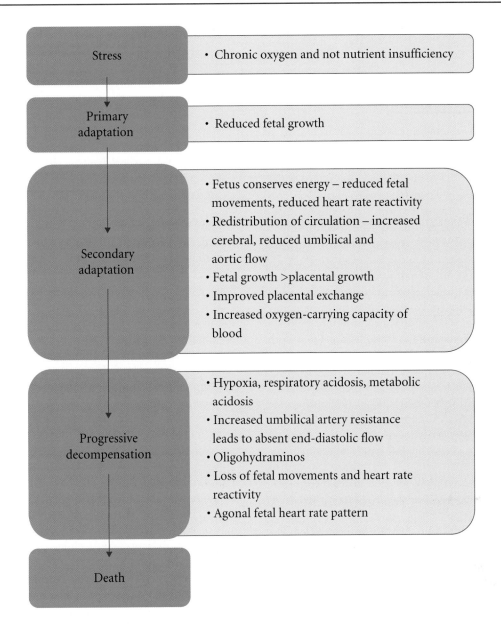

Fig. 37.1 The proposed fetal response to stress that results in adaptations to fetal growth, altered fetal movements, altered fetal blood flow and ultimately changes to the fetal heart rate. (Reproduced with permission from Warrander *et al. Medical Hypotheses* 2011;76(1):17–20)

TESTS OF FETAL WELLBEING

Tests of fetal wellbeing can be grouped by method into biochemical tests of placental function, evaluation of fetal activity/fetal movements, ultrasound-based techniques including Doppler ultrasound and evaluation of fetal heart rate traces.

Biochemical tests of placental function

Since fetal wellbeing is to a large extent dependent on placental function, one way of evaluating fetal wellbeing is to assess placental function. Prior to the advent of ultrasound in obstetrics various biochemical tests were employed to assess placental and fetal wellbeing including measurement

of E_3, hPL and hCG in maternal plasma, serum and urine.[2] The utility of these markers was not robustly assessed prior to a switch to ultrasound evaluation of fetal wellbeing from the mid-1970s onwards. A systematic review found only one study of 622 women with high-risk pregnancies comparing women who had E_3 measured with those who did not [A].[3] This showed no difference in perinatal mortality or rates of planned delivery between the groups. Recently, interest in biochemical markers of placental function has increased again. One small study found that in pregnancies before 35 weeks' gestation measurement of PlGF was able to differentiate placental fetal growth restriction from constitutionally small fetuses with 86 per cent specificity and 100 per cent sensitivity [C].[4] Another report of 625 women with suspected pre-eclampsia found that a measurement of

PlGF <5th centile is more accurate than currently used tests to diagnose pre-eclampsia with a sensitivity of 98 per cent [B].[5]

Fetal movement counting

Maternal perception of fetal movement (FM) is defined as a swish, roll or kick and is usually perceived after 20 weeks' gestation, increasing to a maximum around 32 weeks which plateaus until term.[6,7] There should be no reduction in FM until the onset of labour. There have been several attempts to numerically define normal FM and reduced FM (RFM) but few studies have been devised and validated in women with low-risk pregnancies.[8] No numerical definition (e.g. <10 movements in 12 hours) has been shown to be superior to maternal perception of RFM.[8] Thus, the current definition is based on the subjective maternal perception of RFM. Presentation with RFM is common (approximately 5 per cent of pregnancies) and RFM occurs before stillbirth in 55% of cases.[9] Importantly, women who present with RFM and who have a live baby at presentation are at a 2 to 3-fold increased risk of stillbirth.[10] RFM is associated with altered placental structure and function which adds biological plausibility to the link between RFM and stillbirth [C].[11]

Structured fetal movement counting (FMC), when mothers are asked to count baby's movements, does not reduce perinatal mortality [A],[12] although this may reflect an incorrect alarm limit (e.g. 10 movements in 12 hours) or a lack of intervention. This meta-analysis was dominated by one large RCT of 68,000 women which showed no reduction in perinatal mortality in women assigned to count fetal movements.[13] Importantly, the perinatal mortality rate in all women in this study was very low, suggesting that awareness of FM and the need to present with RFM may be more important. A large case–control study in Norway found a significant reduction in perinatal mortality following the introduction of information to increase maternal awareness of FM and RFM, combined with standardised management including an ultrasound scan to detect SGA fetuses [B].[14] This approach is currently being tested in a stepped-wedge cluster trial in the UK (AFFIRM study; NCT01777022).

A systematic review found no trials specifically addressing the management of RFM.[15] Current management of women presenting with RFM after 28 weeks' gestation is to perform a CTG to exclude fetal compromise and consider performing an ultrasound scan for fetal biometry, liquor volume and umbilical artery Doppler if risk factors for fetal growth restriction are present. Current guidance recommends that these tests be performed in all women who present with RFM on two or more occasions as they have an increased risk of fetal growth restriction and stillbirth [B].[16] If these investigations are abnormal then appropriate intervention should be initiated. If the investigations are normal then women should be reassured but encouraged to present if they have further concerns regarding RFM.[16]

Ultrasound assessment of fetal biometry and Doppler ultrasound

This is covered in more depth in the chapter on fetal growth restriction (Chapter 38). For the purposes of this chapter the role of these techniques in identifying fetal compromise will be considered. Ultrasound scanning has been used to measure fetal size for many years. In late pregnancy this usually involves measuring the biparietal diameter (BPD), head circumference (HC), abdominal circumference (AC) and femur length (FL) using a standardised approach. The AC or a combination of these measurements can be used to give an estimated fetal weight (EFW) using a variety of formulae.[17] The individual parameters or combined EFW can be plotted against normal ranges; ideally these should be customised for maternal physical characteristics (height, weight, ethnicity, parity).[18] A systematic review and meta-analysis of 8 trials involving 27,024 participants found that routinely performing ultrasound fetal biometry in the third trimester does not reduce perinatal mortality [A].[19] However, the studies included in the review were largely completed before 2000, and did not all combine intervention following the ultrasound scan and are also underpowered to show a difference in perinatal mortality in a low-risk population.

Blood flow through various fetal and maternal vessels can be evaluated by application of Doppler ultrasound. Doppler assessment of blood flow through the umbilical cord is thought to reflect downstream placental resistance to flow. The clinical utility of umbilical artery Doppler depends on the population to which it is applied; in high-risk pregnancies measurement of umbilical artery Doppler is associated with a significant reduction in perinatal mortality [A].[20] In contrast, its measurement in low-risk pregnancies has no beneficial effect on outcome [A].[21] Measurement of flow in other vessels such as the middle cerebral artery and ductus venosus has been assessed in smaller trials. The results of the TRUFFLE study, which compared standard monitoring based on umbilical artery Doppler alone, computerised CTG and ductus venosus Doppler, are awaited.[22]

Ultrasound biophysical profile

The ultrasound biophysical profile (BPP) describes an ultrasound-based assessment of fetal wellbeing over a 30-minute period which involves observation of fetal breathing movements, limb/body movements, fetal tone and posture, estimation of amniotic fluid volume and fetal heart reactivity determined by CTG (Table 37.1) [C].[23] Each component is scored as normal (2) or abnormal (0) with scores under 8 regarded as abnormal. A retrospective analysis of 86,955 BPP recordings demonstrated a very high negative predictive value of 99.9 per cent, but a lower positive predictive value of 35 per cent [C]. Systematic review and meta-analysis of 5 trials including 2,974 participants showed no significant reduction in perinatal mortality following the use of BPP in women with high-risk pregnancies comparing BPP vs conventional monitoring [A].[24]

Ultrasound grading of placenta

Grannum *et al.* described a subjective assessment of placental echo-texture in an attempt to sonographically identify placental dysfunction.[25] Due to its subjective nature this approach is complicated by high intra- and inter-observer variability and a lack of understanding about what placental echogenicity actually measures [C].[26,27] Nevertheless, one clinical trial of 2,000 women showed a reduction in perinatal mortality [B].[28] More recent studies have reported that a 'jelly-like' placenta and focal echogenic cystic lesions (ECLs) are related to intervillous thrombosis and fibrin deposition [C].[29,30] Although the presence of ECLs is associated with a poor prognosis in fetuses with severe growth restriction, there have been no studies to determine whether this approach reduces perinatal mortality or morbidity.[31]

CTG and computerised CTG

CTG is used to assess the fetal heart rate (FHR) before and during labour. Before labour this is sometimes referred to as a non-stress test (NST) in contrast to a stress test when Syntocinon or nipple stimulation is used to induce contractions and their effect on the FHR is observed. The NST-CTG pattern can be analysed manually or automatically by a computer algorithm. Manual assessment involves assessment of the baseline rate, variability, accelerations and decelerations to form an overall impression (Fig. 37.2A). The baseline describes the average FHR and baseline variability describes the fluctuations in baseline FHR or the 'bandwidth' of the trace. The baseline variability reflects the balance between the sympathetic and parasympathetic nervous systems and is reduced in fetal compromise. Accelerations are transient increases of FHR >15 beats/min for >15 seconds and are thought to be associated with fetal activity and indicate fetal wellbeing. Whilst the absence of accelerations in labour is of uncertain significance, absence of accelerations for a period >40 minutes would be abnormal. Decelerations describe a decrease of the FHR of >15 beats/min from the baseline FHR for >15 seconds. The presence of decelerations in an antepartum CTG is abnormal. An example of a normal and abnormal antepartum NST-CTG is shown in Figs 37.2B and 37.2C. Despite a relationship between the features of an NST-CTG and fetal compromise the efficiency of NST to predict perinatal morbidity and mortality is <40 per cent.[32] Therefore, it is unsurprising that a systematic review and meta-analysis of 6 studies of 2,105 women showed no reduction in perinatal mortality. There was no increase in obstetric intervention [A].[33]

It is well recognised that there is a large intra- and inter-observer variation in manual interpretation of NST-CTG. Computerised algorithms have been developed to increase the objective nature of NST-CTG assessment and detect subtle changes missed by clinicians. The most widely accepted are the Dawes Redman criteria developed in Oxford, UK (Box 37.1).[34] This approach emphasises the importance of variability, particularly short-term variability (STV) of 3.75-second epochs. The STV is a better predictor of fetal compromise than accelerations or decelerations [C].[35] A systematic review and meta-analysis of two studies of 469 women demonstrated that computerised assessment vs traditional assessment of NST-CTG found a significant reduction in perinatal mortality to 0.9 per cent compared with 4.2 per cent, although this was not statistically significant for preventable deaths [A].[33]

The NST-CTG may be augmented by vibro-acoustic stimulation (VAS), when a probe is held over the maternal abdomen and a sound is transmitted to the fetus via the maternal abdomen. This is thought to be safe for the baby but may precipitate increased fetal movements. Systematic review and meta-analysis of 12 trials including 6,822 women showed that VAS reduced the incidence of non-reactive antenatal CTG tests by 38 per cent compared with no stimulation [A]. In addition, VAS increased fetal movements.[36]

Table 37.1 Individual components of the biophysical profile score[23]

Component	Definition of normal (score 2)
Fetal breathing movements	More than one episode of >30 seconds duration within a 30-minute time frame
Limb/body movements	Four or more discrete body movements (including fine motor movements)
Fetal tone and posture	Active extension and return to flexion, opening and closing of mouth and hands
Amniotic fluid volume estimation	Maximum pool depth >3 cm
FHR reactivity	Normal NST-CTG over 20 minutes

A

	Reassuring	Non-reassuring	Abnormal
Baseline	110–160	100–109 161–180	<100 >180 Sinusoidal pattern >10 min
Variability	≥5 beats/min	<5 for 40–90 min	<5 for 90+ min
Accelerations	Present	The absence of accelerations in an antenatal CTG is non-reassuring	
Decelerations	None	Typical variable decelerations Single prolonged deceleration for up to 3 min	Atypical variable decelerations of late decelerations for 30+min Single prolonged deceleration for >3 min

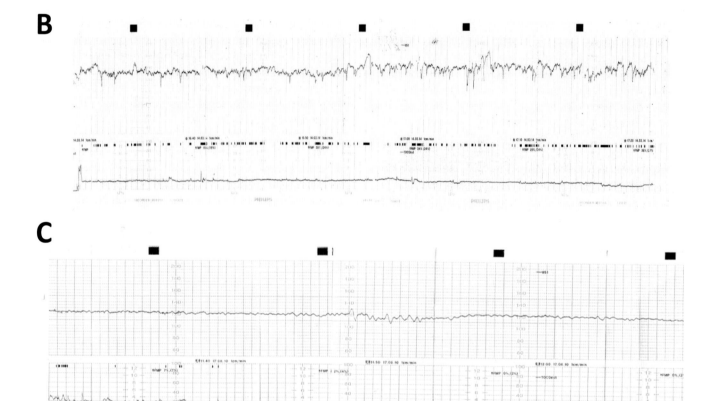

Fig. 37.2 (A) Protocol for assessing antepartum non-stress test cardiotocograph (NST-CTG). (B) Normal antenatal NST-CTG showing a normal baseline, variability and presence of two accelerations during the duration of the recording. (C) Abnormal antepartum NST-CTG showing reduced variability and no accelerations; this infant was born by emergency caesarean section with evidence of severe acidosis.

Box 37.1 Dawes Redman criteria for a normal computerised CTG recording[34]

> Baseline heart rate between 116–160 beats/min. Slightly lower or higher may be acceptable after 30 minutes if all other parameters are normal.
>
> No evidence of sinusoidal fetal heart rhythm.
>
> Long-term variation (mean range of variation around baseline for 1 minute >1st centile for gestation.
>
> Short-term variation should be ≥3 ms.
>
> More than one FM or three accelerations.
>
> No large decelerations ≥20 beats.
>
> No errors or decelerations at the end of the recording.

SUMMARY

Evidence regarding the tests to confirm fetal wellbeing or suspect fetal compromise is of variable quality. There is reliable evidence for the use of umbilical artery Doppler in high-risk pregnancies and computerised NST-CTG. Likewise, evidence suggests that routine measurement of fetal size by ultrasound scan and umbilical artery Doppler in low-risk pregnancies is not associated with a reduction in perinatal mortality, although there are issues with underpowered analyses. The value of other methods to assess fetal wellbeing has not been assessed by rigorous trials.

KEY POINTS

- Manual interpretation of NST-CTG does not improve pregnancy outcome.
- Computerised CTG assessment is more effective than conventional NST-CTG interpretation.
- Biochemical assessment of placental function does not improve pregnancy outcome.
- Maternal awareness of FM is associated with fetal wellbeing.
- After maternal perception of RFM, fetal wellbeing should be assessed by NST-CTG and consideration given to ultrasound assessment of fetal growth.
- Current evidence does not support the routine use of ultrasound measurement of fetal growth after 24 weeks' gestation.
- Umbilical artery Doppler reduces perinatal mortality in high-risk pregnancies but not in low-risk populations.
- Ultrasound BPP does not improve pregnancy outcome compared with NST-CTG and may increase obstetric intervention.
- Placental echogenicity assessed by ultrasound is complicated by wide variation in measurements, but one trial found a reduction in perinatal mortality.

References

1. Maulik D. Doppler velocimetry for fetal surveillance: adverse perinatal outcome and fetal hypoxia. In: Maulik D, ed. *Doppler Ultrasound in Obstetrics and Gynecology.* New York: Springer-Verlag, 1997.
2. Greene JW, Jr, Duhring JL, Smith K. Placental function tests. A review of methods available for assessment of the fetoplacental complex. *Am J Obstet Gynecol* 1965;92:1030–58.
3. Neilson JP. Biochemical tests of placental function for assessment in pregnancy. *Cochrane Database Syst Rev* 2012;8:CD000108.
4. Benton SJ, Hu Y, Xie F *et al.* Can placental growth factor in maternal circulation identify fetuses with placental intrauterine growth restriction? *Am J Obstet Gynecol* 2012;206(2):163.e1–7.
5. Chappell LC, Duckworth S, Seed PT *et al.* Diagnostic accuracy of placental growth factor in women with suspected pre-eclampsia: a prospective multicenter study. *Circulation* 2013;128:2121–31.
6. Natale R, Nasello-Paterson C, Turliuk R. Longitudinal measurements of fetal breathing, body movements, heart rate, and heart rate accelerations and decelerations at 24 to 32 weeks of gestation. *Am J Obstet Gynecol* 1985;151:256–63.
7. Froen JF, Heazell AE, Tveit JV, Saastad E, Fretts RC, Flenady V. Fetal movement assessment. *Semin Perinatol* 2008;32:243–6.
8. Heazell AE, Froen JF. Methods of fetal movement counting and the detection of fetal compromise. *J Obstet Gynaecol* 2008;28:147–54.
9. Efkarpidis S, Alexopoulos E, Kean L, Liu D, Fay T. Case-control study of factors associated with intrauterine deaths. *Med Ged Med* 2004;6:53–8.
10. O'Sullivan O, Stephen G, Martindale EA, Heazell AE. Predicting poor perinatal outcome in women who present with decreased fetal movements - a preliminary study. *J Obstet Gynaecol* 2009;29:705–10.
11. Warrander LK, Batra G, Bernatavicius G *et al.* Maternal perception of reduced fetal movements is associated with altered placental structure and function. *PLoS One* 2012;7:e34851.
12. Mangesi L, Hofmeyr GJ. Fetal movement counting for assessment of fetal wellbeing. *Cochrane Database Syst Rev* 2007;1:CD004909.
13. Grant A, Elbourne D, Valentin L, Alexander S. Routine formal fetal movement counting and risk of antepartum late death in normally formed singletons. *Lancet* 1989;2:345–9.
14. Tveit JV, Saastad E, Stray-Pedersen B *et al.* Reduction of late stillbirth with the introduction of fetal movement information and guidelines - a clinical quality improvement. *BMC Pregnancy Childbirth* 2009;9:32.

FETAL CONDITIONS

15. Hofmeyr GJ, Novikova N. Management of reported decreased fetal movements for improving pregnancy outcomes. *Cochrane Database Syst Rev* 2012;4:CD009148.

16. RCOG. *Management of Reduced Fetal Movements.* London: RCOG, 2011.

17. Hadlock FP, Harrist RB, Sharman RS, Deter RL, Park SK. Estimation of fetal weight with the use of head, body, and femur measurements: a prospective study. *Am J Obstet Gynecol* 1985;151:333–7.

18. RCOG. *The Investigation And Management Of The Small-For-Gestational-Age Fetus.* London: RCOG, 2013.

19. Bricker L, Neilson JP, Dowswell T. Routine ultrasound in late pregnancy (after 24 weeks' gestation). *Cochrane Database Syst Rev* 2008:CD001451.

20. Alfirevic Z, Stampalija T, Gyte GM. Fetal and umbilical Doppler ultrasound in high-risk pregnancies. *Cochrane Database Syst Rev* 2010:CD007529.

21. Alfirevic Z, Stampalija T, Gyte GM. Fetal and umbilical Doppler ultrasound in normal pregnancy. *Cochrane Database Syst Rev* 2010:CD001450.

22. Lees C, Marlow N, Arabin B *et al.* Perinatal morbidity and mortality in early-onset fetal growth restriction: cohort outcomes of the trial of randomized umbilical and fetal flow in Europe (TRUFFLE). *Ultrasound Obstet Gynecol* 2013;42(4):400–8.

23. Manning FA, Baskett TF, Morrison I, Lange I. Fetal biophysical profile scoring: a prospective study in 1,184 high-risk patients. *Am J Obstet Gynecol* 1981;140:289–94.

24. Lalor JG, Fawole B, Alfirevic Z, Devane D. Biophysical profile for fetal assessment in high risk pregnancies. *Cochrane Database Syst Rev* 2008;1:CD000038.

25. Grannum PA, Berkowitz RL, Hobbins JC. The ultrasonic changes in the maturing placenta and their relation to fetal pulmonic maturity. *Am J Obstet Gynecol* 1979;133:915–22.

26. Moran M, Ryan J, Higgins M, Brennan PC, McAuliffe FM. Poor agreement between operators on grading of the placenta. *J Obstet Gynaecol* 2011;31:24–8.

27. Cooley SM, Donnelly JC, Walsh T, McMahon C, Gillan J, Geary MP. The impact of ultrasonographic placental architecture on antenatal course, labor and delivery in a low-risk primigravid population. *J Matern Fetal Neonatal Med* 2011;24:493–7.

28. Proud J, Grant AM. Third trimester placental grading by ultrasonography as a test of fetal wellbeing. *BMJ (Clin Res Ed)* 1987;294:1641–4.

29. Jauniaux E, Ramsay B, Campbell S. Ultrasonographic investigation of placental morphologic characteristics and size during the second trimester of pregnancy. *Am J Obstet Gynecol* 1994;170(1 Pt 1):130–7.

30. Proctor LK, Whittle WL, Keating S, Viero S, Kingdom JC. Pathologic basis of echogenic cystic lesions in the human placenta: role of ultrasound-guided wire localization. *Placenta* 2010;31:1111–5.

31. Viero S, Chaddha V, Alkazaleh F *et al.* Prognostic value of placental ultrasound in pregnancies complicated by absent end-diastolic flow velocity in the umbilical arteries. *Placenta* 2004;25:735–41.

32. Devoe LD, Castillo RA, Sherline DM. The non-stress test as a diagnostic test: a critical reappraisal. *Am J Obstet Gynecol* 1985;15:1047–53.

33. Grivell RM, Alfirevic Z, Gyte GM, Devane D. Antenatal cardiotocography for fetal assessment. *Cochrane Database Syst Rev* 2012;1:CD007863.

34. Dawes GS, Moulden M, Redman CW. System 8000: computerized antenatal FHR analysis. *J Perinat Med* 1991;19:47–51.

35. Dawes GS, Moulden M, Redman CW. Short-term fetal heart rate variation, decelerations, and umbilical flow velocity waveforms before labor. *Obstet Gynecol* 1992;80:673–8.

36. Tan KH, Smyth RM, Wei X. Fetal vibro-acoustic stimulation for facilitation of tests of fetal wellbeing. *Cochrane Database Syst Rev* 2013;12:CD002963.

Chapter 38 Small for gestational age and intrauterine growth restriction

Jennifer A Tamblyn and R Katie Morris

INTRODUCTION

Intrauterine growth restriction (IUGR) is a major cause of perinatal mortality and morbidity[1] [B]. Antenatal awareness that the fetus is not growing well is an essential quality indicator of maternity care.

The definition of small for gestational age (SGA) for a fetus *in utero* is an estimated fetal weight (EFW) that measures <10th percentile on ultrasound (US). This diagnosis does not necessarily imply pathological growth abnormalities, and may simply describe a fetus at the lower end of the normal range. Fetal AC or EFW <10th centile can be used to diagnose an SGA fetus, and severe SGA is classified as an EFW or AC <3rd centile.

IUGR is not synonymous with SGA. It denotes a pathological process in which a fetus does not attain its biologically determined growth potential. It is necessary to differentiate growth restriction from SGA, since this modified intrauterine growth pattern can cause significant fetal compromise in addition to the complications associated with SGA. Serial US growth measurements identify IUGR, which is defined by a reduction in AC and/or EFW growth velocity when measured at least 3 weeks apart.[2] Since an objective definition of reduced growth velocity remains undefined at present, visual assessment of AC and EFW growth trajectory remains standard clinical practice. As outlined below, abnormal placental artery Doppler studies also reflect the presence of placental vascular pathological mechanisms, and importantly identify those pregnancies at increased risk of perinatal mortality. Identification of SGA remains important since the likelihood of IUGR is significantly higher in severe cases.

PHYSIOLOGY OF FETAL GROWTH

The regulation of fetal growth is complex and is based upon maternal, placental and fetal interactions. The primary determinants are nutrient and oxygen placental transfer, which are dependent upon the interaction of genetic determinants, endocrine signalling and substrate supply. Approximately 40 per cent of fetal growth is determined by genetic factors that influence production of growth factors, e.g. insulin growth factor 1 (IGF-1) and IGF-2, transplacental substrate transport and the rate of tissue formation.[3] The remaining 60 per cent is determined by the fetal *in-utero* environment, which in turn primarily reflects maternal physiology and placental function.

In normal fetal development, exponential growth reaches maximum velocity during the third trimester. At this time there is a significant increase in total fetal body fat mass.[4] To facilitate increased nutrient transport and fetal growth, functional maturation of the placenta progressively occurs across gestation.[4]

Placental nutrient transport is reliant upon placental surface area, protein transporter concentration and transporter binding affinity for essential nutrients such as glucose, amino acids and fatty acids.[5] Placental oxygen diffusion is determined by fetal–placental surface area, and placental fetomaternal blood flow. Maternal cardiac output, which increases by 30–40 per cent during normal pregnancy, increases uterine perfusion from 50 ml/min in week 10 to 1300 ml/min at term. This large increase in uterine perfusion exceeds the minimal requirements for fetal oxygenation, and serves to protect against acute variations in perfusion.[5]

Regarding the fetal circulation, one-third of total cardiac output is directed to the placenta during mid-gestation and one-fifth at term.[6] Towards the end of pregnancy there is also an increase in recirculation of umbilical blood in the fetal body. Fetal circulatory adaptations exist to ensure preferential distribution of blood flow, first to the liver (70–80 per cent), followed by the heart where there is streaming of nutrient-rich blood within the right atrium to supply the myocardium and brain. Finally, the ductus venosus (DV) shunts oxygenated umbilical blood directly to the heart, bypassing the liver, to maintain adequate blood flow to the cerebral, cardiovascular and adrenal systems for fetal growth and function.[5]

A major, final, non-genetic factor determining fetal size in all pregnancies is 'maternal constraint'. This refers to a set of poorly defined physiological processes by which maternal and uteroplacental factors act to limit the growth of the fetus and influence its predetermined growth trajectory.[3]

Clearly the regulation of fetal growth is complex and as outlined is dependent upon maternal, placental and fetal interactions. Abnormalities may involve any of these compartments, resulting in a complex multisystem disorder as outlined below.

AETIOLOGY OF SGA

The aetiologies of IUGR are diverse, involving multiple complex mechanisms. Approximately one third is determined by genetic factors, while two thirds are environmental.

The most common cause of IUGR (80–90 per cent) is placental insufficiency. Abnormal invasion of fetal trophoblast cells for implantation and vascular remodelling is hypothesised causative and is associated with smaller placentae and reduced nutrient exchange.[4] There is also abnormal uterine and umbilical artery (UA) perfusion on both sides of the placenta, and disproportional or reduced placental perfusion subsequently results in both inefficient oxygen and nutrient maternofetal exchange. Unlike acute hypoxia, in chronic deficiency the FHR is maintained until late fetal decompensation ensues. This reflects preferential redistribution of blood flow to the cerebral, cardiovascular and adrenal systems which serves to preserve fetal growth and function within the adverse setting.[6]

In general, most placental causes of IUGR involve maternal vascular compromise resulting in placental ischaemia, such as pre-eclampsia.[7] Growth restriction is normally asymmetrical in this setting, characterised at birth by reduced AC, length and weight, with preserved fetal HC.[8] A prior history of placenta-mediated disease is also a risk factor for a subsequent SGA neonate. This includes pre-eclampsia and prior stillbirth;[7] in particular those with a history of previous, preterm, unexplained stillbirth, due to its association with SGA.[9] Regardless of cause, women who have previously had an SGA neonate have a 3.9 (2.14–7.12)-fold increased risk of a subsequent SGA (birthweight [BW] <10th centile).[7] This risk is increased further following two SGA births, or if another risk factor for SGA, such as maternal hypertension, coexists.[10] Placental abruption and unexplained antepartum haemorrhage are also risk factors for restricted fetal growth.[11,12]

There are numerous underlying aetiologies of IUGR which are not caused primarily by placental insufficiency, but indirectly lead to it. This includes other maternal medical conditions that lead to reduced uteroplacental blood flow, reduced maternal blood volume and/or oxygen-carrying capacity, or decreased nutrition to the fetus; namely diabetes with vascular disease,[13] renal disease[14] and APLS.[15] SLE[16] and certain cardiac conditions, in particular cyanotic congenital heart disease,[17] present an increased risk.

There are certain non-modifiable maternal factors associated with IUGR which are not disease related. These include ethnicity (Indian/Asian),[18] nulliparity,[19] maternal SGA[20] and maternal age ≥35 years (higher for women ≥40 years),[21] a low maternal pre–pregnancy weight,[22] and a short (<6 months) or long (>60 months) inter–pregnancy interval,[23] and are thus also implicated in IUGR.

Considering other non-placental causes of IUGR, restriction is often symmetrical at birth and is frequently caused by an early fetal insult. Several maternal exposures have a seemingly causative relationship with an SGA infant, including moderate alcohol intake,[24] drug abuse (cocaine, a potent vasoconstrictor, being the most significant),[25] cigarette smoking[26] and caffeine consumption ≥300 mg/day in the third trimester.[27]

Genetic diseases of the fetus constitute 5–20 per cent of causes of IUGR,[28] with a higher incidence in more severe cases. The commonest chromosomal defects are triploidy (total 69 chromosomes) and trisomy 18, both of which are often severe and present as early as the first trimester. Trisomies 13 and 21 are also causative and are similarly associated with early onset growth restriction. Trisomy 16, which is usually lethal in the non-mosaic state, can cause growth restriction when occurring as confined placental mosaicism. Up to 16 per cent of cases of IUGR have been associated with confined placental mosaicism. Partial deletions of chromosomes such as 4q (Wolf–Hirschhorn syndrome), and 5q (cri-du-chat syndrome), as well as complete deletion of a sex chromosome in Turner's syndrome (45X), have been linked. Finally, a number of single gene disorders and uniparental disomy chromosomal aberrations are also associated with IUGR.[28]

In the absence of identifiable congenital defects, inborn errors of metabolism and structural malformations, in particular congenital heart disease, diaphragmatic hernia, abdominal wall defects, and anencephaly have also been identified as associated with IUGR.[28]

Fetal infections implicated in SGA include rubella, CMV, HIV, toxoplasmosis, malaria and VZV.[28] The most common pathogens reported are CMV and toxoplasmosis, which should be tested for most frequently. Rubella is less of a threat due to vaccination. Syphilis is still encountered in pregnancy both in developed and developing countries, and testing should be offered in those considered at risk.[29] Malaria is the predominant infectious cause in endemic regions such as Africa and south-east Asia. Women considered at risk should again be advised to have testing.[28]

In multiple pregnancies IUGR is also more common, in particular MC gestations. Twin gestations physiologically decrease their growth rate after about 28 weeks of gestation. Discordant growth of multiples is usually defined as a

20 per cent reduction in EFW of the smaller compared with the larger fetus.[28] If less than 30 weeks, this may represent TTTS; it may also be a marker of structural or genetic anomalies, infection or placental insufficiency as for singleton births. Importantly, the risk of mortality or neonatal morbidity is higher among neonates in SGA-discordant twins than in appropriate-for-gestational-age (AGA)-discordant twins (20 per cent versus 6 per cent).[30]

At present there is insufficient evidence to determine how these risk factors relate to each other, and consequently how they should be managed. The most recent RCOG guidance does aid clinicians by stratifying each risk factor for SGA into 'minor' and 'major' categories based upon the most current evidence.[2] As discussed below, the investigation and management of SGA and IUGR are also guided by this classification.

DIAGNOSIS OF SGA

SGA is diagnosed ultrasonographically and is defined as a fetal AC or EFW <10th centile. Severe SGA is classified as an EFW or AC <3rd centile. Antenatal detection of SGA is important since there is an increased risk of perinatal mortality and morbidity. However, US assessment of growth velocity is superior to single estimates of final AC or EFW in the prediction of suboptimal perinatal outcomes.[31] It is therefore important to differentiate SGA from IUGR, given the higher prevalence of adverse outcomes. To accurately assess a change in fetal size (AC or EFW), two measurements of AC or EFW at least 3 weeks apart are required.[32] In current clinical practice this is subjectively assessed by visual interpretation of the customised growth chart. Whether a more objective, standardised measure of FGR should be used is contentious. More frequent measurements of fetal size are appropriate only where BW prediction is relevant outside the context of diagnosing SGA/IUGR.

A major challenge in obstetrics is the accurate and timely detection of SGA. Despite increased awareness, a significant proportion of cases are still undetected antenatally. The reported accuracy of the symphysio-fundal height (SFH) measurement alone to detect SGA is highly variable (average sensitivity 65 per cent, 50 per cent false-positive rate)[B].[33] Furthermore, in a low-risk population, the sensitivity for SGA has been found to be as low as 21 per cent [C].[34]

Effective screening for IUGR is therefore essential and begins by accurate pregnancy dating. In all cases of suspected SGA the mother's menstrual history, relevant assisted reproductive technology information, and either a first-trimester or an early second-trimester dating US should be reviewed carefully. Crown–rump length (CRL) may be used to date a pregnancy up to 13 weeks. CRL should not be used later than this due to increased fetal flexion. As an alternative, biparietal diameter and/or HC is used; some units include femur length measurement.[35] Recalculating dates in a first-trimester small baby should not be routinely performed,

as this may represent early onset growth restriction. Smith *et al.*, who investigated the association between low BW and fetal size in the first trimester (4229 pregnancies), found that when the CRL was 2–6 days smaller than expected there was a significantly increased risk (compared with normal or larger expected CRL) of BW <2500 g at term (RR 2.3; 95% CI 1.4–3.8), and BW <5th centile for gestational age (GA) (RR 3.0; 95% CI 2.0–4.4). The data suggest that suboptimal first-trimester growth may be associated with SGA.[36] In cases for which the last menstrual period is unknown and there are no US data prior to 13 weeks, US may calculate GA to within 7–10 days up until 20 weeks. However a high index of suspicion for SGA should be maintained, and beyond this limit US should not be used to adjust the estimated due date.

At each antenatal visit, women receive an SFH measurement. This should ideally be plotted on a customised centile chart since this improves accurate SGA detection.[37,38] Taking account of maternal characteristics (height, weight, parity and ethnic group), as well as GA at delivery and infant sex, improves identification of neonatal SGA babies at high risk of morbidity and mortality compared with the prior population centiles.[37] Pathological factors such as smoking and hypertension are excluded to predict the optimum weight a baby can achieve at term.[38] The use of customised growth charts also improves the predictive accuracy of adverse prenatal outcome in the setting of SGA: specifically threatened preterm labour, antepartum haemorrhage, PIH, pre-eclampsia, stillbirth and early neonatal death [C].[22] Importantly, individual growth velocities of low-risk fetuses with a normal outcome are less likely to cross beneath the 10th centile when using customised reference standards (reduced false-positive rate).[39]

A single SFH that plots below the 10th centile or serial measurements that demonstrate slow or static growth (i.e. they cross centiles in a downward direction) should prompt immediate referral for sonographic assessment. For low-risk pregnancies in the UK, SFH currently represents the primary mode of surveillance, even though it is not highly predictive of SGA: sensitivity 27 per cent and specificity 88 per cent.[40] Since the standard measurement of fetal AC or EFW in the third trimester of low-risk pregnancies is not found to significantly reduce the incidence of neonatal SGA, or improve perinatal outcome, routine fetal biometry is not currently justified.[41] Only in women for whom SFH measurement is likely to be inherently inaccurate (BMI >35, large fibroids, polyhydramnios, multiple pregnancy) is serial biometry routinely performed.[33]

In view of the above, a comprehensive antenatal booking assessment to identify women at risk of developing SGA is vital to ensure identification of those women requiring sonographic surveillance. All women with one major risk factor for SGA (Table 38.1) are advised to receive serial US assessment of fetal size at 26–28 weeks.[2] They should also receive an assessment of wellbeing with UA Doppler from this point since in high-risk populations this is found to reduce overall perinatal morbidity and mortality[A].[42,43] An abnormal result reflects the presence of placental vascular pathological

FETAL CONDITIONS

Table 38.1 Summary of risk factors for an SGA neonate

A. Available From History at Booking		
Risk Category	**Risk**	**Minor or Moderate**
Maternal risk factors		
Age	Maternal age >/=35 years	Minor
	Maternal age >40 years	Moderate
Parity	Nulliparity	Minor
BMI	BMI <20	Minor
	BMI 25-29.9	Minor
	BMI ≥30	Minor
Maternal substance exposure	Smoker	Minor
	Smoker 1–10 cigarettes per day	Minor
	Smoker ≥11 cigarettes per day	Moderate
	Cocaine	Moderate
IVF	IVF singleton pregnancy	Minor
Exercise	Daily vigorous exercise	Moderate
Diet	Low fruit intake pre-pregnancy	Minor
Previous pregnancy history		
Previous SGA	Previous SGA baby	Moderate
Previous Stillbirth	Previous stillbirth	Moderate
Previous pre-eclampsia	Pre-eclampsia	Minor
Pregnancy Interval	Pregnancy interval <6 months	Minor
	Pregnancy interval ≥60 months	Minor
Maternal medical history		
SGA	Maternal SGA	Moderate
Hypertension	Chronic hypertension	Moderate
Diabetes	Diabetes and vascular disease	Moderate
Renal disease	Renal impairment[15]	Moderate
APLS	Antiphospholipid syndrome	Moderate
Paternal medical history		
SGA	Paternal SGA	Moderate
B. Current Pregnancy Complications		
Threatened miscarriage	Heavy bleeding similar to menses	Moderate
Fetal anomaly	Echogenic bowel	Moderate
Pre-eclampsia	Pre-eclampsia	Moderate
Pregnancy induced hypertension	Mild	Minor
	Severe	Moderate
Placental abruption	Placental abruption	Minor
Unexplained APH	Unexplained APH	Moderate
Weight gain	Low maternal weight gain	Moderate
Exposure	Caffeine ≥300 mg/dy in third trimester[40]	Moderate
Down's syndrome marker	PAPP-A <0.4 MoM	Moderate

BMI body mass index; IVF in-vitro fertilisation; SGA small for gestational age; APLS antiphospholipid APH ante-partum haemorrhage; PAPPA pregnancy associated plasma protein A

mechanisms and identifies pregnancies at increased risk for perinatal mortality, without increasing the rate of inappropriate obstetric intervention. Again reviews of the clinical utility of UA Doppler strongly suggest that this should not be used as a routine screening modality for women at 'low risk' of SGA.[44]

Women who have multiple minor risk factors for SGA are currently referred for a UA Doppler assessment at 20–24 weeks of gestation.[2] If abnormal (mean pulsatility index [PI] >95th centile [bilaterally] and/or 'notching'), serial US measurements and UA Doppler from 26–28 weeks of pregnancy are advised since persistence after 24 weeks has a moderate predictive value for a severely SGA neonate [A].[45] In the third trimester, UA Doppler has limited predictive accuracy for adverse outcomes in SGA and is therefore not routinely used. It is also not performed in women with a major risk factor for SGA since the negative likelihood ratio (predictive strength of a normal result) is not sufficient to negate the risk of SGA [A].[42]

Serial US measurement of fetal size and assessment of wellbeing with UA Doppler is also routinely advised following detection of an echogenic fetal bowel or when first-trimester levels of PAPP-A are low (<0.415 MoM). The reasons for this are beyond the scope of this chapter; however, both are independently associated with neonatal SGA and fetal mortality [C].[46,47]

In the first-trimester UA Doppler studies are not currently recommended since low end-diastolic velocities and an early diastolic notch are considered normal.[2] However, recent evidence from a large systematic review (55,974 women) suggests that there may be value clinically in the setting of IUGR. The sensitivity and specificity of abnormal flow velocity waveforms (resistance index [RI] or PI ≥90th centile and 'notching') for early-onset fetal growth restriction were 39.2 per cent (95% CI 26.3–53.8) and 93.1 per cent (95% CI 90.6–95.0) respectively. These findings suggest that, in high-risk women, UA Doppler studies performed at initial dating may aid detection of early onset IUGR [A].[48]

INVESTIGATION AND SURVEILLANCE OF THE SGA FETUS

Following antenatal diagnosis of SGA, investigations are required to identify a potential underlying cause. Comprehensive reassessment for any potential SGA risk factors (Table 38.1) that may have been overlooked at booking, and/or developed during the antenatal period, is particularly important following detection. Any changes in personal or socio-economic circumstances may be contributory and should also be explored. Comprehensive re-evaluation of fetal anatomy and uterine/UA Doppler studies is essential for identifying a potential underlying cause and for the assessment of fetal wellbeing. Determining whether SGA is symmetrical or asymmetrical is of less importance clinically

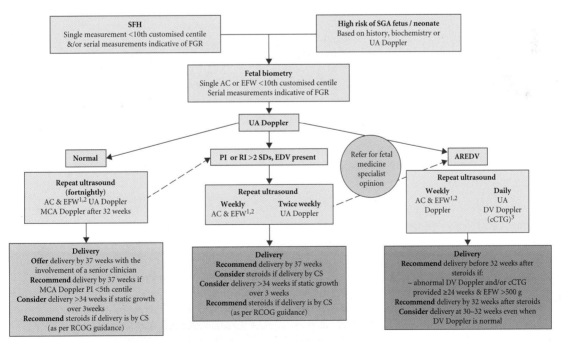

[1] Weekly measurement of fetal size is valuable in predicting birthweight and determining size for gestational age
[2] If two AC/EFW measurements are used to estimate growth, they should be at least 3 weeks apart
[3] Use cCTG when DV Doppler is unavailable or results are inconsistent – recommend delivery if STV <3 ms.
AREDV, absent/reversed end–diastolic velocity; cCTG, computerised cardiotography; EDV, end–diastolic velocity; FGR, fetal growth restriction; MCA, middle cerebral artery; STV, short-term variation; SFH, symphysis–fundal height.

Fig. 38.1 The management of the SGA fetus. (Reproduced with kind permission from RCOG[2])

since asymmetrical IUGR may progress to generalised growth restriction in particularly severe cases.

The extent of investigation is in part determined by the GA of onset severity. All women diagnosed with SGA should receive more regular blood pressure and urine surveillance for the presence of pre-eclampsia. If severe SGA is identified at the mid-trimester anomaly scan, a detailed fetal anatomical survey and UA Doppler by a fetal medicine specialist may be required. Karyotyping may also be offered in this setting, particularly for women with structural anomalies, GA <23 weeks, a high Down's syndrome screening risk (>1 in 150), or polyhydramnios. This may be particularly relevant when Doppler studies are normal since a placental pathology is less likely [C].[49,50]

Considering aberrant liquor volume, albeit strongly associated with SGA and adverse perinatal outcome, the predictive strength of the amniotic fluid index (AFI) in this setting is limited by its poor predictive accuracy (LR 2.77 [1.93, 3.96] and LR 0.58 [0.48, 0.69]), and significant heterogeneity. Thus, oligohydramnios should be used in conjunction with other prognostic factors and should not be used as an independent diagnostic or surveillance tool in the setting of SGA [A].[51]

As the IUGR fetus is at increased risk of mortality, as well as hypoxia and metabolic acidosis during labour, meticulous surveillance of fetal growth and wellbeing is essential for the SGA fetus (Fig. 38.1). When Doppler flow indices are normal it may be reasonable to repeat surveillance every 14 days [B].[52] The relationship between increased placental vascular impedance and the shape of the UA velocity waveform is not entirely linear, however; as the placental abnormality expands the likelihood of adverse fetal outcome increases. At least a 50 per cent reduction of terminal placental vessels is required before the PI becomes abnormal.[44] An increasing RI is also strongly correlated with adverse fetal outcome.[53] When UA Doppler flow indices are abnormal therefore (PI >+2 standard deviations above mean for GA) and delivery is not indicated, surveillance is required twice weekly if end-diastolic velocities remain present [C].[54,2] Doppler abnormalities such as absent or reversed end-diastolic flow (AREDV) are significantly associated with suboptimal fetal outcome and daily Doppler indices are required unless delivery is imminent [C][54] (summarised in Fig. 38.1).

Further investigation of the fetal circulatory system by Doppler examination of the MCA, DV and umbilical vein (UV) may be considered in certain instances such as AEDFV. This should be a consultant-based decision by a professional with significant fetal medicine expertise.

A decrease in the Doppler indices of the MCA (reduced MCA PI or MCA PI/umbilical artery PI [cerebroplacental ratio]) signifies 'brain sparing' and cerebral vasodilatation. The predictive accuracy of MCA Doppler for SGA is, however, limited and should not be used as a 'high-risk' screening test like UA Doppler [A].[55] However, in view of its association with adverse fetal outcomes, if MCA Doppler is abnormal, delivery should be delayed no later than 37 weeks of gestation. In the term SGA fetus with normal UA Doppler, an abnormal MCA

Doppler (PI <5th centile) has a moderate predictive value for acidosis at birth and is therefore used to guide timing of delivery.[56] In the preterm SGA fetus, MCA Doppler has limited accuracy and is not used to time delivery.[57]

DV Doppler also has a moderate predictive value for acidaemia and adverse fetal outcome and is considered a late sign of severe IUGR.[58] Chronic hypoxia causes increased blood flow through the DV (cardiovascular diversion), with a concomitant reduction in hepatic blood flow via the UV. In severe IUGR, decreased or absent DV flow may be observed and has a moderate predictive accuracy for compromise of fetal/neonatal wellbeing overall and perinatal mortality in high-risk pregnancies with placental insufficiency. As such, DV Doppler is used for surveillance in the preterm SGA fetus with abnormal UA Doppler and subsequently used to inform decisions regarding delivery [A].[58]

Controversially, recent findings from the Prospective Observational Trial to Optimise Paediatric Health in IUGR (PORTO) study, which evaluated multi-vessel Doppler in 1116 non-anomalous IUGR fetuses, raise important questions regarding the usefulness of multi-vessel Doppler assessment with regard to fetal surveillance and timing of delivery. Although they confirmed that the classic pattern of progression from abnormal UA to MCA to DV was evident, this occurred no more frequently than the multiple other potential patterns of Doppler deterioration. Importantly UA and MCA Doppler remained the most useful and practical tool for identifying fetuses at risk of adverse perinatal outcome, identifying 88 per cent of all adverse outcomes [C].[59]

MANAGEMENT OF SGA

Significant challenges exist regarding both the prevention and the management of SGA. At present no proven preventive or therapeutic strategies other than delivery truly exist. This in part reflects both the diverse range of maternal, fetal and placental aetiologies, and their poorly understood pathogenic associations with SGA. Furthermore, in many cases the underlying cause remains unknown even in those women for whom pathologically restricted growth is identified.

Timely detection of SGA remains crucial since this will inform both the clinician and the mother that the pregnancy is at increased risk, and also enable more detailed investigation to inform timing for delivery. Introduction of a structured antenatal surveillance programme is also found to significantly reduce the risk of adverse fetal outcomes, such as stillbirth and neonatal mortality secondary to preterm birth, compared with cases of SGA fetuses that failed to be detected antenatally.[38,54]

The antenatal interventions that may improve perinatal outcomes in SGA prior to delivery are limited. For women at high risk of pre-eclampsia antiplatelet agents (e.g. aspirin) may be effective in preventing SGA birth. Although the effect size is small, a systematic review which included 1317 women with abnormal UA Doppler has concluded that aspirin if started before 16 weeks of pregnancy reduces the incidence of both pre-eclampsia and neonatal SGA. Aspirin started after 20 weeks is not, however, effective in reducing the risk of an SGA infant and is therefore not of value [A].[60] NICE recommends that women either at high risk of PET or with more than one moderate risk factor take 75 mg aspirin daily from 12 weeks' gestation until birth.[61]

A single course of antenatal corticosteroids is also given to any woman diagnosed with an SGA fetus between 24[+0] and 35[+6] weeks of gestation, if delivery is considered imminent. This serves to promote fetal lung maturation and reduce neonatal death and morbidity. Appropriate timing of delivery is determined by the gestational age and fetal condition, and the presence of fetal lung maturity in a preterm fetus will help facilitate this decision.[62]

There is also evidence to suggest that magnesium sulphate before birth may be neuroprotective for the fetus and may reduce the incidence of cerebral palsy among preterm infants. A recent Cochrane systematic review (including five eligible trials of women threatening or likely to give birth at less than 37 weeks (6145 babies)) concluded that a significant neuroprotective effect is observed. The number of women who need to be treated to benefit one baby by avoiding cerebral palsy is 63. A significant reduction in the rate of substantial gross motor dysfunction is also achieved [A].[63]

Interventions to promote smoking cessation may prevent delivery of an SGA infant and improve birthweight. The overall health benefits of smoking cessation certainly support intervention, and all women who are pregnant and smoke should be offered this option [A].[64]

TIMING OF DELIVERY IN SGA

One of the most important aspects of SGA management is an understanding of the decisions relevant to delivery. The main consideration needs to be appropriate timing, as the balance between the risks of iatrogenic morbidity due to prematurity and continued exposure to an unfavourable intrauterine environment requires careful evaluation.

Since delivery outcomes for SGA fetuses with an AREDV in the UA primarily follow caesarean section, the risks associated with induced/spontaneous labour are uncertain. For this reason any SGA fetus diagnosed with AREDV in the UA after 32 weeks is normally delivered by caesarean section before 37 weeks [C].[65] Delivery may, however, be considered promptly following detection of AREDV if determined safer by a senior obstetrician. For those SGA fetuses at or near term without an AREDV on UA, induction of labour with continuous FHR monitoring may be offered by a senior obstetrician.[66] However, women should be aware that the risk of pathological decelerations in labour, emergency caesarean section for suspected fetal compromise, and metabolic acidaemia at delivery are higher compared with an appropriate-for-gestational-age (AGA) grown fetus [C].[65] If the growth velocity is normal the

RCOG recommend that delivery should still be considered by 37 weeks due to the stronger association with adverse perinatal outcome compared with those with AGA [C].[65,2]

The randomised, multicentre Growth Restriction Intervention Trial (GRIT) compared the effects of early and delayed delivery for such babies. The study included 587 babies and the median time-to-delivery intervals were 0.9 and 4.9 days for the immediate and delayed groups respectively. Mortality prior to discharge was not significantly different (10 per cent immediate group, 9 per cent delay group [OR 1.1, 95% CI 0.61–1.8]). Although in the delay group a higher stillbirth rate was observed, an almost equal number of additional perinatal deaths occurred in the earlier delivery group. As expected this group also had more acutely ill babies at delivery, who required increased mechanical ventilator support, and suffered major complications such as intraventricular haemorrhage and necrotising enterocolitis. Whether these babies would have died *in utero* had intervention been delayed is unknown [B].[1] Given the significant risk of neonatal morbidity and mortality, particularly among those born very preterm, a senior obstetrician should be responsible for ensuring that a comprehensive, individualised surveillance and delivery plan is made in close consultation with both the parents and the neonatal team.

For the preterm SGA fetus with AREDV detected prior to 32 weeks' gestation, delivery is appropriate if the DV Doppler becomes abnormal or umbilical vein pulsations appear, provided that the fetus is viable and received steroids. Even when the DV Doppler is normal, delivery should still be strongly considered before 32 weeks since early delivery in this setting is not shown to significantly increase overall perinatal mortality or long-term neurodevelopmental outcomes [B].[1,67]

SGA PROGNOSIS

Low BW remains a major cause of morbidity and mortality in early infancy and childhood [B, C].[1,68] It is important to recognise the clinical significance of SGA and IUGR independently, as most adverse outcomes are concentrated in the growth-restricted group, and the majority of term SGA infants have no appreciable morbidity or mortality [D].[69] For IUGR, the overall perinatal mortality rate has improved to approximately 8 per cent, with 70 per cent surviving without severe neonatal morbidity [B].[70]

More reliable distinction of IUGR has also enabled the inclusion of growth restriction into the 'Classification of stillbirth by relevant condition at death' (ReCoDe) system. The study included 2625 stillbirths and 451,197 total births, representing an average stillbirth rate of 5.82 per 1000. Using the ReCoDe classification only 398 cases (15.2 per cent) remained unclassified as 'no relevant condition identified', with the largest category of stillbirths 'fetal growth restriction' (43.0 per cent) [C].[9] The significance of this is clear and renews focus towards antenatal identification of IUGR in the prevention of stillbirth.[38]

Prematurity is an additional factor that significantly contributes to this risk of morbidity and mortality in IUGR [B].[1, 8] GA is by far the most powerful predictor of survival to term in very preterm babies of 22–31 weeks. However, weight also has a powerful, non-linear effect on survival (*P*=0.006) [C].[70] The recent prospective multicentre randomised management study of fetal growth restriction (Trial of Randomised Umbilical and Fetal Flow in Europe or TRUFFLE) investigated perinatal morbidity and mortality rates following early onset IUGR. The study group comprised 503 women with a singleton fetus of 26–32 GA, AC <10th centile and UA Doppler PI >95th centile. Overall, 81 per cent of deliveries were indicated by fetal condition and 97 per cent were by caesarean section. Of the 490 liveborn babies with follow-up data, 27 (5.5 per cent) deaths occurred with 118 (24 per cent) suffering severe morbidity [B].[71]

The acute neonatal complications of SGA and growth restriction include an increased risk of hypothermia, hypoglycaemia, respiratory distress and birth hypoxia, hypocalcaemia, polycythaemia, intraventricular haemorrhage and necrotising enterocolitis [C].[68] Cerebral palsy (CP) is also more common in term babies whose BW is low for their GA at delivery. A comparison of 10 European registers for 4503 singleton children with CP was examined. They identified that babies of 32–42 weeks' gestation with a BW for GA <10th percentile were four to six times more likely to have CP than children between the 25th and 75th percentiles. In babies of less than 32 weeks' gestation, the relationship between weight and risk was less clear due to the adverse outcomes associated with early preterm birth [C].[72]

At-2 year follow-up the GRIT Study reported no overall difference in the rate of death or severe disability between the immediate or deferred delivery group (19% vs 16%). Despite adjustment for GA and UA Doppler category, the OR (95% CI) remained 1.1 (0.7–1.8). Importantly, their results do not support early delivery as a useful measure to prevent terminal hypoxaemia and improve long-term brain development. An extremely fine balance between the risk of *in-utero* death and stillbirth does, however, clearly exist, and decisions regarding timing of delivery should be judged on an individual case basis by an expert obstetrician [B].[67]

Regarding childhood and long-term sequelae, IUGR is thought to elicit a fetal programming process that has long-term implications. The neurodevelopmental deficits are often mild, such as changes in muscle tone, coordination deficits, visual deficits, lower verbal skills and intellectual competence, attention disorders and emotion regulation difficulties. An increased risk for learning disability is also noted [C].[73] Neurodevelopmental outcome is mediated primarily by growth catch-up velocity.[74] Those without catch-up in height and/or head circumference have the worst outcome [C].[73]

Children born SGA are also shorter during childhood and as adults, with heights on average 1 standard deviation below the population mean. Those born very prematurely and with more severe degrees of growth restriction are less likely to achieve a stature within the normal range. Endocrine and metabolic disturbances in the SGA child are also recognised, but there is no evidence to recommend routine investigation of all SGA children [C].[75]

The 'developmental origins of adult disease' hypothesis states that adverse influences early *in utero* can result in permanent changes in physiology and metabolism, which result in increased disease risk in adulthood. This hypothesis originally evolved from observations by Barker and Osmund:[76] the 'Barker hypothesis' which reported that in England those regions with the highest rates of infant mortality also had the highest mortality rates from coronary heart disease. Since low BW was the commonest cause of infant death, they postulated that those babies who survived were at increased risk of coronary heart disease later in life.[76] Epidemiological studies have since demonstrated this and further relationships between BW and type 2 diabetes, insulin resistance, hypertension and cerebrovascular disease. A modest positive association between BW and subsequent BMI and waist circumference is also reported.[77] The most widely accepted theory underlying the developmental origins hypothesis is programming, which is the process whereby a stimulus or insult during a sensitive or critical period has irreversible long-term effects on development.[78] Potential mechanisms include altered fetal nutrition and increased glucocorticoid exposure. Changes in the intrauterine environment, including nutrient availability, may also alter gene expression via alterations in DNA methylation, and thereby increase susceptibility to chronic disease in adulthood. Moreover, such epigenetic changes, if they do occur in the gametes, may be heritable. This 'intergenerational effect' may account for the association between maternal and paternal SGA and subsequent second-generation SGA.[2,79]

CONCLUSION

The accurate and timely detection of SGA remains a significant challenge in obstetrics. Differentiation of IUGR is particularly important given the increased associated perinatal morbidity and mortality. As a consequence of the diverse range of underlying pathogeneses, current proven strategies to prevent and treat SGA are limited. Timely delivery therefore remains at the forefront of SGA management, with accurate detection and comprehensive fetal surveillance fundamental to reducing perinatal morbidity and mortality. Given the consequences of severe IUGR and preterm birth, and furthermore the implications for future antenatal care, postnatal follow-up is essential.

References

1. GRIT Study Group. A randomised trial of timed delivery for the compromised preterm fetus: short-term outcomes and Bayesian interpretation. *BJOG* 2003;110:27–32.

2. RCOG. *Small-for-Gestational-Age Fetus, Investigation and Management.* Green-top Guideline No. 31. London: RCOG, 2013:1–34. http://www.rcog.org.uk.

3. Gluckman P, Hansonb M. Maternal constraint of fetal growth and its consequences. *Semin Fetal Neonatal Med* 2004; 9:419–25.

4. Pardi G, Marconi A, Cetin I. Placental-fetal interrelationship in IUGR fetuses: a review. *Placenta* 2002;23 (Suppl A):S136–41.

5. Sankaran S, Kyle P. Aetiology and pathogenesis of IUGR. *Best Pract Res Clin Obstet Gynaecol* 2009;23:765–77.

6. Kiserud T, Ebbing C, Kessler J, Rasmussen S. Fetal cardiac output, distribution to the placenta and impact of placental compromise. *Ultrasound Obstet Gynecol* 2006; 28:126–36.

7. Ananth C, Peltier M, Chavez M, Kirby R, Getahun D, Vintzileos A. Recurrence of ischemic placental disease. *Obstet Gynecol* 2007;110:128–33.

8. Pallotto E, Kilbride H. Perinatal outcome and later implications of intra-uterine growth restriction. *Clin Obstet Gynecol* 2006;49:257–69.

9. Gardosi J, Kady S, McGeown P, Francis A, Tonks A. Classification of stillbirth by relevant condition at death (ReCoDe): population-based cohort study. *BMJ* 2005;331:1113–17.

10. Voskamp B, Kazemier B, Ravelli A, Schaaf J, Mol BW, Pajkrt E. Recurrence of small-for-gestational-age pregnancy: analysis of first and subsequent singleton pregnancies in the Netherlands. *Am J Obstet Gynecol* 2013;208:374.e1–6.

11. Jaquet D, Swaminathan S, Alexander GR *et al.* Significant paternal contribution to the risk for small for gestational age. *BJOG* 2005;112:153–9.

12. Costa S, Proctor L, Dodd J *et al.* Screening for placental insufficiency in high-risk pregnancies: is earlier better? *Placenta* 2008;29:1034–40.

13. Howarth C, Gazis A, James D. Associations of type 1 diabetes mellitus, maternal vascular disease and complications of pregnancy. *Diabet Med* 2007;24:1229–34.

14. Fink J, Schwartz M, Benedetti T, Stehman–Breen C. Increased risk of adverse maternal and fetal outcomes among women with renal disease. *Paediatr Perinat Epidemiol* 1998;12:277–87.

15. Yasuda M, Takakuwa K, Tokunaga A, Tanaka K. Prospective studies of the association between anticardiolipin antibody and outcome of pregnancy. *Obstet Gynecol* 1995;86:555–9.

16. Yasmeen S, Wilkins E, Field N, Sheikh R, Gilbert W. Pregnancy outcomes in women with systemic lupus erythematosus. *J Matern Fetal Med* 2001;10:91–6.

17. Drenthen W, Pieper P, Roos-Hesselink J *et al.* Outcome of pregnancy in women with congenital heart disease: a literature review. *J Am Coll Cardiol* 2007;49:2303–11.

18. Alexander G, Wingate M, Mor J, Boulet S. Birth outcomes of Asian–Indian–Americans. *Int J Gynaecol Obstet* 2007;97:215–20.

19. Shah P. Knowledge Synthesis Group on Determinants of LBW/PT Births. Parity and low birth weight and preterm birth: a systematic review and meta–analyses. *Acta Obstet Gynecol Scand* 2010;89:862–75.

20. Shah S, Shah V, Knowledge Synthesis Group on Determinants of LBW/PT Births. Influence of maternal birth status on offspring: a systematic review and meta–analysis. *Acta Obstet Gynecol Scand* 2009;88:1307–18.

21. Odibo A, Nelson D, Stamilio D, Sehdev H, Macones G. Advanced maternal age is an independent risk factor for intra-uterine growth restriction. *Am J Perinatol* 2006;23:325–8.

22. Gardosi J, Francis A. Adverse pregnancy outcome and association with small for gestational age birthweight by customized and population-based centiles. *Am J Obstet Gynecol* 2009;201:1–8.

23. Conde–Agudelo A, Rosas–Bermúdez A, Kafury–Goeta A. Birth spacing and risk of adverse perinatal outcomes: a meta-analysis. *JAMA* 2006;295:1809–23.

24. Jaddoe V, Bakker R, Hofman A *et al.* Moderate alcohol consumption during pregnancy and the risk of low birth-weight and preterm birth. The generation R study. *Ann Epidemiol* 2007;17:834–40.

25. Gouin K, Murphy K, Shah PS, Knowledge Synthesis Group on Determinants of LBW/PT Births. Effects of cocaine use during pregnancy on low birthweight and preterm birth: systematic review and meta-analyses. *Am J Obstet Gynecol* 2011;204:340:1–12.

26. McCowan L, Roberts C, Dekker G *et al.* Risk factors for small-for-gestational-age infants by customised birthweight centiles: data from an international prospective cohort study. *BJOG* 2010;117:1599–607.

27. CARE Study group. Maternal caffeine intake during pregnancy and risk of fetal growth restriction: a large prospective observational study. *BMJ* 2008;337:a2332.

28. Hendrix N, Berghella V. Non-placental causes of intra-uterine growth restriction. *Semin Perinatol* 2008;32:161–5.

29. Sheffield J, Sanchez P, Wendel G *et al.* Placental histopathology of congenital syphilis. *Obstet Gynecol* 2002;100:126–133.

30. Yinon Y, Mazkereth R, Rosentzweig N *et al.* Growth restriction as a determinant of outcome in preterm discordant twins. *Obstet Gynecol* 2005;105:80–84.

31. Chang T, Robson S, Spencer J, Gallivan S. Prediction of perinatal morbidity at term in small fetuses: comparison of fetal growth and Doppler ultrasound. *BJOG* 1994;101:422–7.

32. Mongelli M, Sverker E, Tambyrajia R. Screening for fetal growth restriction: a mathematical model of the effect of time interval and ultrasound error. *Obstet Gynecol* 1998;92:908–12.

33. Morse K, Williams A, Gardosi J. Fetal growth screening by fundal height measurement. *Best Pract Res Clin Obstet Gynaecol* 2009;23:809–18.

FETAL CONDITIONS

34. Bais J, Eskes M, Pel M, Bonsel G, Bleker O. Effectiveness of detection of intra-uterine growth retardation by abdominal palpation as screening test in a low risk population: an observational study. *Eur J Obstet Gynecol Reprod Biol* 2004;116:164–9.

35. RCOG. *Ultrasound Screening*. London: RCOG, 2000. http://www.rcog.org.uk/womens-health/clinical-guidance/ultrasound-screening#intro.

36. Smith G, Smith M, McNay M, Fleming J. First-trimester growth and the risk of low birth weight. *N Engl J Med* 1998;339:1817–22.

37. de Jong C, Francis A, Van Geijn H, Gardosi J. Customised fetal weight limits for antenatal detection of fetal growth restriction. *Ultrasound Obstet Gynecol* 2000;15:36–40.

38. Figueras F, Gardosi J. Intra-uterine growth restriction: new concepts in antenatal surveillance, diagnosis, and management. *Am J of Obstet Gynecol* 2011;204:288–300.

39. Gardosi J, Francis A. Controlled trial of fundal height measurement plotted on customised antenatal growth charts. *Br J Obstet Gynaecol* 1999;106(4):309–17.

40. Persson B, Stangenberg M, Lunell NO, Brodin U, Holmberg NG, Vaclavinkova V. Prediction of size of infants at birth by measurement of symphysis fundus height. *Br J Obstet Gynaecol* 1986;93:206–11.

41. Neilson JP. Symphysis–fundal height in pregnancy. *Cochrane Database Syst Rev* 2000;2:CD000944.

42. Alfirevic Z, Stampalija T, Gyte G. Fetal and umbilical artery Doppler ultrasound in normal pregnancy. *Cochrane Database of Syst Rev* 2010:8:CD001450.

43. Morris R, Malin G, Robson S, Kleijnen J, Zamora J, Khan K. Fetal umbilical artery Doppler to predict compromise of fetal/ neonatal wellbeing in high–risk population: systematic review and bivariate meta–analysis. *Ultrasound Obstet Gynecol* 2011;37: 135–42.

44. Divon M. Umbilical artery Doppler velocimetry: Clinical utility in high-risk pregnancies. *AJOG* 1996;174:10–14.

45. Cnossen J, Morris R, ter Riet G *et al.* Use of uterine artery Doppler ultrasonography to predict pre-eclampsia and intra-uterine growth restriction: a systematic review and bivariable meta-analysis. *CMAJ* 2008;178:701–11.

46. Mailath-Pokorny M, Klein K, Klebermass-Schrehof K, Hachemian N, Bettelheim D. Are fetuses with isolated echogenic bowel at higher risk for an adverse pregnancy outcome? Experiences from a tertiary referral center. *Prenatal Diagnosis* 2012;32:1295–9.

47. Carbone, J, Tuuli, M, Bradshaw, R, Liebsch J, Odibo, A. Efficiency of first-trimester growth restriction and low pregnancy-associated plasma protein-A in predicting small for gestational age at delivery. *Prenatal diagnosis* 2012;32: 724–9.

48. Velauthar L, Plana M, Kalidindi M *et al.* Uterine artery Doppler in the first trimester as a risk factor for adverse pregnancy outcomes: A meta-analysis involving 55,974 women. *Ultrasound Obstet Gynecol* 2014;43:500–507.

49. Snijders R, Sherrod C, Gosden C, Nicolaides K. Fetal growth retardation: associated malformations and chromosomal abnormalities. *Am J Obstet Gynecol* 1993;168:547–55.

50. Anandakumar C, Chew S, Wong Y, Malarvishy G, Po L, Ratnam S. Early asymmetric IUGR and aneuploidy. *J Obstet Gynaecol Res* 1996;22:365–70.

51. Morris R, Meller C, Tamblyn J *et al.* Association and prediction of amniotic fluid measurements for adverse pregnancy outcome: systematic review and meta-analysis. *Br J Obstet Gynaecol* 2014;121:686-99.

52. McCowan L, Harding J, Roberts A, Barker S, Ford C, Stewart A. A pilot randomized controlled trial of two regimens of fetal surveillance for small-for-gestational-age fetuses with normal results of umbilical artery Doppler velocimetry. *Am J Obstet Gynecol* 2000;182:81–6.

53. Seyam Y, Al-Mahmeid M, Al-Tamimi K. Umbilical artery Doppler flow velocimetry in intra-uterine growth restriction and its relation to perinatal outcome. *Int J Gynecol Obstet* 2002;77:131–7.

54. Lindqvist P, Molin J. Does antenatal identification of small-for-gestational age fetuses significantly improve their outcome? *Ultrasound Obstet Gynecol* 2005;25:258–64.

55. Morris R, Say R, Robson S, Kleijnen J, Khan K. Systematic review and meta-analysis of middle cerebral artery Doppler to predict perinatal wellbeing. *Eur J Obstet Gynecol Reprod Biol* 2012;165:141–55.

56. Cruz–Martinez R, Figueras F, Hernandez–Andrade E, Oros D, Gratecos E. Fetal brain Doppler to predict caesarean delivery for non-reassuring fetal status in term small-for-gestational-age fetuses. *Obstet Gynecol* 2011;117:618–26.

57. Baschat A, Cosmi E, Bilardo C *et al.* Predictors of neonatal outcome in early-onset placental dysfunction. *Obstet Gynecol* 2007;109:253–61.

58. Morris R, Selman T, Verma M, Robson S, Kleijnen J, Khan K. Systematic review and meta-analysis of the test accuracy of ductus venosus Doppler to predict compromise of fetal/neonatal wellbeing in high-risk pregnancies with placental insufficiency. *Eur J Obstet Gynecol Reprod Biol* 2010;152:3–12.

59. Unterscheider J, Daly S, Geary MP *et al.* Predictable progressive Doppler deterioration in IUGR: does it really exist? *Am J Obstet Gynecol* 2013;209:539.e1–7.

60. Bujold E, Morency AM, Roberge S, Lacasse Y, Forest JC, Giguere Y. Acetylsalicylic acid for the prevention of pre-eclampsia and intra-uterine growth restriction in women with abnormal uterine artery Doppler: a systematic review and meta–analysis. *J Obstet Gynecol Can* 2009;31:818–26.

61. National Collaborating Centre for Women's and Children's Health. *Hypertension in pregnancy: the management of hypertensive disorders during pregnancy.* NICE Clinical guideline. London: RCOG Press, 2010.

62. RCOG. *Antenatal Corticosteroids to Prevent Neonatal Morbidity and Mortality.* Green-top Guideline No. 7. London: RCOG, 2010.

63. Doyle L, Crowther C, Middleton P, Marret S, Rouse D. Magnesium sulphate for women at risk of preterm birth for neuroprotection of the fetus. *Cochrane Database Syst Rev* 2009;1:CD00461.

64. Lumley J, Chamberlain C, Dowswell T, Oliver S, Oakley L, Watson L. Interventions to promote smoking cessation during pregnancy. *Cochrane Database Syst Rev* 2009;3:CD001055.

65. Karsdrop V, van Vugt J, van Geijn H *et al.* Clinical significance of absent or reversed end diastolic waveforms in umbilical artery. *Lancet* 1994;344:1664–8.

66. Li H, Gudmundsson S, Olofsson P. Prospect of vaginal delivery of growth restricted fetuses with abnormal umbilical artery blood flow. *Acta Obstet Gynecol Scand* 2003;82:828–33.

67. Thornton JG, Hornbuckle J, Vail A, Spiegelhalter DJ, Levene M; GRIT study group. Infant wellbeing at 2 years of age in the Growth Restriction Intervention Trial (GRIT): multicentred randomised controlled trial. *Lancet* 2004;364:513–20.

68. Bernstein I, Horbar J, Badger G, Ohlsson A, Golan A. Morbidity and mortality among very-low-birth-weight neonates with intra-uterine growth restriction. The Vermont Oxford Network. *Am J Obstet Gynecol* 2000;182:198–206.

69. Jones R, Roberton N. Small for dates babies: are they really a problem? *Arch Dis Child* 1986;61:877–80.

70. Cole T, Hey E, Richmond S. The PREM score: a graphical tool for predicting survival in very preterm births. *Arch Dis Child Fetal Neonatal Ed* 2010;95:F14–19.

71. Lees C. Marlow N, Arabin B *et al.* Perinatal morbidity and mortality in early-onset fetal growth restriction: cohort outcomes of the trial of randomized umbilical and fetal flow in Europe (TRUFFLE). *Ultrasound Obstet Gynecol* 2013;42:400–8.

72. Jarvis S, Glinianaia S, Torrioli M, Platt M, Miceli M, Jouk P. Cerebral palsy and intra-uterine growth in single births: European collaborative study. *Lancet* 2003;362:1106–11.

73. Sommerfelt K, Markestad T, Ellertsen B. Neuropsychological performance in low birth weight preschoolers: a population-based, controlled study. *Eur J Pediatr* 1998;157:53–8.

74. Geva R, Leitner Y, Harel S. Children born with intra-uterine growth restriction: neurodevelopmental outcome. Preedy V (ed.), In: *Handbook of Growth and Growth Monitoring in Health and Disease.* New York: Springer, 2012:193–208.

75. Karlberg J, Albertsson-Wikland K. Growth in full term small-for-gestational-age infants: from birth to final height. *Pediatr Res* 1995;38:733–739.

76. Barker D, Osmond C. Infant mortality, childhood nutrition, and ischaemic heart disease in England and Wales. *Lancet* 1986;i:1077–81.

77. Rogers I, EURO-BLCS Study Group. The influence of birthweight and intra-uterine environment on adiposity and fat distribution in later life. *Int J Obes Relat Metab Disord* 2003;27:755–77.

78. De Boo H, Harding J. The developmental origins of adult disease (Barker) hypothesis. *Austr and NZ J Obstet Gynaecol* 2006;46:4–14.

79. Waterland RA, Jirtle R. Early nutrition, epigenetic changes at transposons and imprinted genes, and enhanced susceptibility to adult chronic diseases. *Nutrition* 2004;20:63–8.

Chapter 39 Aberrant liquor volume

Jennifer A Tamblyn and R Katie Morris

MRCOG curriculum (antenatal care module 8)

- Understand the epidemiology, aetiology, pathogenesis, diagnosis, prevention, management, delivery and complications of aberrant amniotic fluid volume (polyhydramnios, oligohydramnios).
- Trainees should demonstrate that they can competently manage oligohydramnios and polyhydramnios.

INTRODUCTION

Amniotic fluid (AF) is essential for appropriate fetal growth and development. It provides a 'low resistance' environment for the fetus, allowing freedom of movement and hence musculoskeletal development while providing protection from external forces and infection. Any disruption in AF homeostasis will lead to either insufficient (oligohydramnios) or excess (polyhydramnios) AF. A finding of abberant liquor volume (LV) on US is associated with increased perinatal morbidity and, in the case of oligohydramnios, increased perinatal mortality. In order to systematically investigate and manage pregnancies complicated by aberrant liquor volume, a broad understanding of AF dynamics is required.

AMNIOTIC FLUID HOMEOSTASIS

The total amniotic fluid volume (AFV) is the sum of the inflow and outflow into the amniotic space, reflecting total extracellular fetal fluid balance. Up until approximately 33 weeks AF production increases at a non-linear rate. For each week of gestation, a wide variation in AFV can be seen.[1] From 36 weeks, a reduction in total AFV is observed, with a particularly rapid decline from 41 weeks. Quantitatively, at 22 weeks the median AFV is approximately 600 mL, reaching 800 mL at its peak, before declining to 700 mL by 40 weeks.[2] Importantly, from approximately 22–39 weeks, the AFV remains unchanged despite a significant gain in fetal weight. Clearly a fine balance exists to regulate AFV, particularly in late gestation when approximately 1000 mL fluid flows into and out of the amniotic compartment daily.[1] If abnormalities in flow continue over a prolonged period of time then this will result in abnormal LVs.

The mechanism underpinning AF regulation is not fully elucidated, and during early gestation the exact source of production and composition of AF remain unclear. Before 16 weeks, AF has the same osmolality as maternal plasma and it is most likely to be a transudate that passes from the maternal circulation. Since coelomic fluid is similar to maternal plasma and is located within the extra-coelomic space alongside the amniotic sac, this is the probable solute source during early development. Fetal urine is present in the amniotic space from 8–11 weeks but only becomes a major contributor in the latter half of pregnancy, reaching 1000–1200 mL/day at term.[3] This fundamental source of AF is demonstrated by the almost complete lack of AF in fetuses with renal agenesis.[4] Respiratory tract secretions, transfer of fluid across the chorionic plate and umbilical cord, and direct movement of fluid from maternal blood across the wall of the uterus into the amniotic cavity also contribute to AF production.

Maintaining AFV requires removal of AF and the fetal skin provides a major osmotic pathway for AF shifts until it becomes keratinised after 22–25 weeks.[5] After this time oral and nasal mucosae continue to exchange fluid but this is no longer a major source of AFV regulation.[5] Other mechanisms of removal include fetal swallowing, removing 200–1500 mL/day,[6] and intramembranous transport (exchange between AF and fetal blood across the fetal placental surface) responsible for 200–500 mL/day. Transmembranous flow, which is the exchange between AF and maternal blood within the uterine wall, also contributes to this process (10 mL/day).[6]

AFV ASSESSMENT

Clinical assessment of AFV by palpation is unreliable. As such, AFV measurements have become standard in fetal surveillance, especially in the evaluation of high-risk pregnancies.

Due to its three-dimensional (3D) structure, absolute AFV is not routinely measured. Instead two-dimensional (2D) prenatal US is used and surrogate measures are employed to assess AF levels. However, it is recognised that these measures have a poor correlation with actual AFV, as determined by the 'gold-standard' dye-dilution method, due to the influences of fetal position, transducer pressure, maternal hydration status and observer inconsistency. More sophisticated methods include dye-dilution tests, 3D magnetic resonance imaging and 3D US; these are rarely performed outside the research setting due to their invasive nature (dilution techniques), being technically time-consuming by nature and high cost.[7]

Four principle sonographic methods are used to define AF levels with 2D ultrasound: subjective assessment, 2×2 measurement, single deepest pocket (SDP) and amniotic fluid index (AFI). SDP represents the deepest pocket measured vertically in the anterior–posterior plane at any location in the amniotic cavity as long as the umbilical cord or fetal parts are excluded. This parameter is also recognised as the 'deepest vertical pocket' (DVP), 'maximum pocket depth' (MPD) or 'maximum vertical pocket' (MVP). AFI is measured after 20 weeks by dividing the amniotic cavity into four quadrants using the maternal linea nigra as the midline. The DVP without fetal parts or cord is ascertained for each quadrant and then the four measurements are summed. For clinical purposes a single set of cut-offs for abnormal AFVs is used throughout pregnancy. To determine the threshold for normal and abnormal LVs, normograms with 5th and 95th percentile cut-offs have been defined for AFI, SDP, 2D pocket and dye-directed techniques across individual gestational ages.

Despite multiple studies and trials, no single sonographic method has emerged as superior in predicting adverse pregnancy outcome.[8] In fact, it has been suggested that AFI may characterise more women as having oligohydramnios, leading to an increase in obstetric interventions without a concomitant measurable improvement in pregnancy outcome.[9] Since effectiveness evidence supports the use of MVP, this is recommended until more robust evidence is available [A].[8] In the case of a twin pregnancy, MVP is the preferred technique since AFI measurements for each individual fetal amniotic sac can be technically difficult and inaccurate, particularly in the case of MC multiple pregnancies [C].[10]

POLYHYDRAMNIOS

Any increase in the AFV surrounding the fetus is termed 'hydramnios'. Once a pre-defined sonographic value has been exceeded this is classified as 'polyhydramnios', which effects approximately 1–2 per cent of pregnancies.[11] In late second and third trimester for both singleton and multiple pregnancies, an MPD >8 cm, AFI $\geq$25 cm, or above the 95th centile for gestational age, is diagnostic of polyhydramnios. Further sub-categorisation to mild (MVP 8–12cm, AFI >24 cm and <30 cm), moderate (MVP 12–15cm, AFI $\geq$30 cm and <35 cm), and severe (MVP >15 cm, AFI $\geq$35 cm) may be of

value with regard to the investigation and management of polyhydramnios. Initial suspicion of polyhydramnios in low-risk women may be achieved clinically following identification of a discordantly high SFH. Additional symptoms and signs include a distended, uncomfortably tense abdomen, difficult palpation of fetal parts, and excessive FM. Despite its own inherent inaccuracies, 2D US detection of polyhydramnios is, however, more reliable, and as such represents the primary diagnostic modality.

Causes of polyhydramnios

Excess AFV results from either an increase in AF production or abnormal AF regulation and removal. Consequently, a diverse range of maternal and fetal conditions may adversely disturb fluid balance (Table 39.1). One of the most common causes is poorly controlled maternal diabetes mellitus, with the excess fluid most probably developing secondary to osmotic diuresis and fetal polyuria. Rarer causes of fetal polyuria include TTTS and Barter's syndrome.[3,12]

Table 39.1 Causes of polyhydramnios

Maternal disease	Diabetes mellitus
Fetal	TTTS (increased amniotic fluid in the recipient twin and decreased amniotic fluid in the donor twin)
	Barter's syndrome
Structural	Tracheal atresia
	Duodenal and oesophageal atresia
	Mediastinal/thoracic mass
	Diaphragmatic hernia
Neuromuscular	Anencephaly
	Muscular dystrophy
	Fetal akinesia
Genetic	Chromosomal anomalies (aneuploidy [trisomies 21, 18 and 13])
	Non-immune hydrops
Cardiac failure	Sacrococcygeal teratoma, vein of Galen aneurysm, fetal anaemia, maternal alloimmunisation, glucose-6-phosphatase deficiency, alpha-thalassaemia, fetomaternal haemorrhage
Infectious	Congenital syphilis
	Viral hepatitis
Idiopathic	

Decreased AF absorption results from either a failure of fetal swallowing and/or intestinal reabsorption, e.g. tracheal atresia, intestinal obstruction (oesophageal or duodenal atresia), extrinsic intestinal compression (diaphragmatic hernia or masses within the thorax and mediastinum) and neurological disorders (anencephaly, muscular dystrophy, fetal akinesia syndrome). In the presence of additional complications such as fetal growth restriction, an underlying chromosomal aberration such as aneuploidy (trisomies 18 and 21) should be considered.[3,12] Other important causes of increased AFV include non-immune hydrops and cardiac failure, which may occur secondary to underlying reduced fetal vascular resistance (sacrococcygeal teratoma, vein of Galen aneurysm) or fetal anaemia (maternal alloimmunisation).[3,12] Parvovirus B19, CMV[13] [D], congenital syphilis[14] and viral hepatitis infection[15] should be included in the differential diagnoses for polyhydramnios only when there is clinical suspicion or other suggestive sonographic findings such as non-immune hydrops.

As the liquor volume increases so does the likelihood of an underlying congenital anomaly. In severe polyhydramnios (AFI ≥35 cm) almost 80 per cent of pregnancies were found to be associated with a prenatally diagnosed structural fetal anomaly.[11] This was also the case in a retrospective cohort study of 672 singleton pregnancies with hydramnios (P<0.001), which also found that 11 per cent of neonates had one or more congenital anomalies (US anomaly detection was 79 per cent). In those with a normal US evaluation, the risk of a major anomaly was 1 per cent in mild cases, 2 per cent with moderate and 11 per cent with severe hydramnios (P<0.001). Of those anomalies eluded, cardiac septal defects, cleft palate, imperforate anus, and tracheo-oesophageal fistula were the most common.[16]

The timing of sonographic detection of polyhydramnios may also be useful in predicting fetal outcome. In 138 cases with polyhydramnios presenting prior to 26 weeks' gestation (21 severe, 18 moderate and 92 mild do not = 131); congenital abnormalities were noted in 86 per cent of severe, 72 per cent of moderate and 17 per cent of mild polyhydramnios cases. In the cases of mild polyhydramnios with no associated anomalies, in 91 per cent the polyhydramnios resolved but for those with associated anomalies there was resolution in only 13 per cent. For moderate polyhydramnios the corresponding figures were 80 per cent resolved and 0 per cent if associated with other anomalies or maternal conditions. No cases of severe polyhydramnios resolved. Thus second-trimester polyhydramnios that persists is associated with an increased risk of congenital anomaly [D].[17]

In a large proportion of cases the cause of polyhydramnios however, remains idiopathic. A prospective case–control study which included 6492 pregnant women diagnosed polyhydramnios in 251 (3.9 per cent) cases: 81.5 per cent mild and 18.5 per cent moderate. Of the 231 pregnancies for which complete follow-up data were available, idiopathic (no evidence of congenital or placental abnormalities, diabetes mellitus or isoimmunisation) polyhydramnios occurred

in 65.4 per cent. Diagnosis of idiopathic polyhydramnios occurred any time between 20 and 40 weeks' gestation (mean 33 weeks). Of these cases, most were mild (AFI >24 cm); (81.5 per cent) with only 18.5 per cent classified as moderate (AFI ≥30 cm)[18] [C].

Investigation of polyhydramnios

The investigation of cases of polyhydramnios should be individualised based on gestational age, polyhydramnios severity, and maternal and past obstetric history. A detailed review of maternal history, with an emphasis upon maternal symptoms and potential risk factors for increased AFV, such as diabetes, should initially be performed. Serological testing to exclude underlying alloimmunisation and a 75-g glucose tolerance test (repeated if completed previously) should be routinely performed. In those cases in which an underlying infectious aetiology is suspected, specific serological testing may be indicated.

Sonographic evaluation of the fetus will in the first instance include fetal number, chorionicity, severity of hydramnios and fetal growth. It would seem appropriate that a case of polyhydramnios diagnosed at <30 weeks' gestation should be referred to a fetal medicine unit for assessment for structural and chromosomal anomalies. For those diagnosed after 30 weeks consideration should be given to other risk factors for congenital or structural anomaly (e.g. previous obstetric and family history, findings at the detailed US, risk factors for karyotypic anomaly) when deciding whether a fetal medicine referral is necessary [C].[11] This, however, remains contentious and certainly more clear guidance regarding the indications for more detailed investigation of polyhydramnios is warranted.

Complications of polyhydramnios

The maternal complications of polyhydramnios relate primarily to excessive uterine distension, and as such are determined by the extent and rate of AF accumulation. In mild cases, minimal maternal symptoms such as general abdominal discomfort and slight dyspnoea may develop. In moderate-to-severe polyhydramnios marked respiratory distress and severe abdominal symptoms may ensue. An increased risk of preterm rupture of membranes and labour is also observed [C].[19] Interestingly the underlying cause (increased in those with an underlying congenital anomaly and maternal diabetes), as opposed to the severity of aberrant AFV, appears significant with regard to the timing of preterm labour onset [C].[19] The incidence of placental abruption and cord prolapse also appears higher when there is sudden uterine decompression following membrane rupture; the exact risk of this, however, remains unknown [C].[20] Postnatally, the incidence of maternal haemorrhage secondary to uterine atony is also significantly higher in those women with pregnancies complicated by polyhydramnios.[21]

Operative delivery rates are higher when polyhydramnios exists due to labour dystocia secondary to excessive uterine size and poor contraction quality[22] [C] and an increased risk of unstable lie [C].[20] Associations between idiopathic polyhydramnios and perinatal morbidity are poor apart from a strong positive association between polyhydramnios and birthweight >90th centile. The predictive ability of aberrant AFV to predict outcome is generally poor due to its poor sensitivity [A].[8]

A prospective study examining fetal outcomes in 200 pregnancies complicated by aberrant AFV found the perinatal mortality rate (PMR) (42.25 per cent) to be significantly higher compared with both the normal and the low AFV groups ($P<0.001$). It was concluded that a higher rate of congenital anomalies was primarily responsible [C].[23] Again these findings are not supported after systematic review of the literature demonstrated no association between idiopathic polyhydramnios and fetal mortality (total of 144,681 fetuses). Whether this discrepancy is due to the inclusion of mild and moderate polyhydramnios is, however, uncertain and requires further clarification [A].[8]

Management of polyhydramnios

Management should be guided by the underlying cause of the polyhydramnios and the severity of maternal symptoms. In those cases secondary to maternal diabetes, polyhydramnios is associated with poor glycaemic control, and increased birthweight [C].[24] Importantly, aberrant AF has been shown to improve in response to optimisation of glycaemic control with oral/subcutaneous anti-diabetic therapy. Women with a pregnancy affected by diabetes should be under the care of a joint obstetric/diabetic team to optimise outcome for mother and baby. The management of specific disorders such as TTTS, and maternal diabetes, are discussed in greater detail in their relevant chapter.

Considering idiopathic polyhydramnios, mild asymptomatic cases may be managed expectantly. No proven benefits for fluid and salt restriction or diuretic agents have been reported, and are not routinely advised.[12] If moderate-to-severe polyhydramnios results in pronounced maternal distress (in the setting of an appropriately grown, sonographically normal fetus) a more aggressive approach may be indicated. Decisions regarding induction of labour and delivery should be made by a senior obstetrician taking into account aetiology, gestation and maternal considerations, and in an environment with the facilities to manage the potential complications relating to sudden uterine decompression, including abruption, fetal malposition, umbilical cord prolapse and PPH.

In those cases for which the risks of preterm delivery are too high, active treatment may be required, particularly in the setting of significant maternal compromise (respiratory or uterine activity). Treatment should be guided by the underlying aetiology and may include amnio-reduction and indometacin. Therapeutic amnio-reduction involves trans-abdominal aspiration of AF under indirect sonographic vision and is reported

to prolong gestation and improve perinatal outcomes [D].[25] However, significant risks, which develop in 2–3 per cent of pregnancies, include preterm pre-labour rupture of membranes, infection, placental abruption and membranous detachment [C].[26] Furthermore, re-accumulation may develop rapidly and serial re-treatments may be indicated up to every 2–3 days. For these reasons amnio-reduction should be reserved for only particularly severe cases of polyhydramnios, and should be performed only in a centre with sufficient expertise to perform the procedure safely, and only when prolongation of gestation is required [C].

Indometacin, a prostaglandin synthetase inhibitor, may also be considered as a treatment for severe polyhydramnios at less than 32 weeks to reduce maternal symptoms and prolong gestation [D].[27] Albeit more widely recognised for its role as a tocolytic in the prevention of preterm labour, it also reduces fetal urine production and subsequent AFV. The dose required is determined according to total AFV, ranging from 50 mg/day to 200 mg/day. Since there is a potential delay in treatment onset (4–20 days), therapy is often commenced after an initial amnio-reduction, but subsequently avoids the need for serial invasive procedures.[3] This has also been successfully utilised in twin gestations (not TTTS) to successfully reduce AFV.[28] The main fetal risks of treatment include premature closure of the ductus arteriosus, intraventricular haemorrhage and renal failure. Prior to 34 weeks, the effect on the ductus is usually not significant. Meta-analyses within the setting of preterm labour have found that indometacin treatment at <34 weeks' gestation for tocolysis does not increase the risk of PDA. Treatment should be used with caution and once AFV has returned to the upper range of normal, treatment is to be stopped immediately [B].[3,29]

KEY POINTS

- Polyhydramnios prevalence is 1–2 per cent.
- For late second to early third trimester, MPD >8 cm, AFI ≥25 cm, or >95th centile for gestational age is diagnostic.
- Idiopathic polyhydramnios remains the most common aetiology.
- Polyhydramnios is positively associated with an increased fetal birthweight.
- Maternal complications relate primarily to excessive uterine distension.
- Polyhydramnios severity is positively associated with an increased risk of an underlying congenital anomaly.

OLIGOHYDRAMNIOS

An aberrantly low AFV surrounding the fetus is termed 'oligohydramnios'. Typically, diagnosis usually occurs at the second-trimester anomaly scan, a fetal growth US scan in the setting of high-risk pregnancy surveillance or following an acute clinical presentation such as reduced fetal movements.

Quantitatively, oligohydramnios may be defined as an MVP <2 cm. An AFV <200 mL or 500 mL,[5] AFI <5 cm, or an AFI below the 5th percentile for gestational age, or a subjectively low AFV is also diagnostic.[6]

Importantly, oligohydramnios is associated with a number of adverse antepartum, intrapartum and perinatal pregnancy outcomes. This has led to an almost uniform recommendation for delivery following its diagnosis at term.[6] Albeit more common in the third trimester, aberrantly low AFV may occur at any stage of pregnancy. Furthermore, the earlier oligohydramnios develops the more severe both fetal morbidity and mortality outcomes become.[30] As discussed below, the decisions regarding antenatal management are therefore also more complex.

Causes of oligohydramnios

Oligohydramnios may result from excessive AF loss, underproduction or excretion. Consequently, a diverse range of maternal and fetal conditions may again adversely disturb fluid balance (Table 39.2). The exact cause is often gestational dependent; however, a significant proportion remains idiopathic. In some cases oligohydramnios may be a transient finding, simply reflecting maternal dehydration.[6]

Persistent AF underproduction may be secondary to absent or dysfunctional kidneys, or urinary tract obstruction. Congenital abnormalities of the fetal urinary tract such as bilateral renal agenesis, lower urinary tract obstruction, cystic dysplasia, Meckel–Gruber syndrome or VACTERL (vertebral,

anal, cardiac, tracheo-oesophageal, renal, limb association) may be responsible.[3,12] In a structurally normal fetus, oligohydramnios may reflect impaired uteroplacental blood flow and be associated with IUGR or fetal hypoxia. Central redistribution of oxygenated fetal blood towards essential organs while there is a concomitant reduction in peripheral renal perfusion and total urine output is one mechanism by which the fetus adapts to chronic hypoxia.[6] Maternal disease, e.g. hypertension and chronic kidney disease, and iatrogenic causes, e.g. angiotensin-converting enzyme inhibitors and prostaglandin synthase inhibitors, may result in oligohydramnios for this reason. Other causes of low AFV include preterm premature rupture of the membranes (PPROM), spontaneous rupture of the membranes (SROM), TTTS, CMV infection and post-dates maturity (>42 weeks).[3,12,31]

The commonest cause of oligohydramnios is PPROM, which complicates 1–2 per cent of pregnancies and is associated with 30–40 per cent of preterm births (<37 weeks), and 18–20 per cent of perinatal deaths [A].[32] Sonographic detection of oligohydramnios in second-trimester PPROM is associated with a particularly poor prognosis and as such is recognised as a predictor of poor fetal survival [D].[33] The management of PPROM is discussed in the relevant chapter.

Investigation of oligohydramnios

Given the range of potential diagnoses prior to term, the detection of persistent oligohydramnios should prompt detailed review of maternal history, sonographic assessment

Table 39.2 Causes of oligohydramnios

Maternal disease	Hypertension
	Chronic kidney disease
	Diabetes insipidus
	Maternal dehydration
Pregnancy complications	Spontaneous membrane rupture
	Preterm pre-labour rupture of membranes
	Post-dates (>42 weeks)
Fetal	IUGR
	TTTS
Structural	Bilateral renal agenesis or dysplasia
	Urethral obstruction
	Cystic dysplasia
	Meckel–Gruber syndrome
	VACTERL
Uteroplacental insufficiency	
Infectious	Congenital viral infection – CMV
Iatrogenic	Angiotensin-converting enzyme inhibitors
	Prostaglandin synthase inhibitors
Idiopathic	

for evidence of membrane rupture, anatomical evaluation of the renal system and bladder, and assessment of placental function and fetal growth. The extent of investigation is in part guided by the gestational age of detection since, in those near term, induction of labour is indicated. Given the range of maternal and fetal conditions associated with low AFV, however, the validity of oligohydramnios as a diagnostic tool for PPROM is restricted by its poor sensitivity.[31] In part this is because US is unlikely to detect minor leakages in AFV. As such within this setting AFV should be interpreted in collaboration with maternal history and clinical findings.[31]

Complications of oligohydramnios

Classically, oligohydramnios is considered an indicator of adverse perinatal outcome. Regardless of underlying aetiology, the earlier oligohydramnios develops the poorer the prognosis. As reported by Shipp et al., who evaluated the significance of severe oligohydramnios and anhydramnios in 250 singleton pregnancies between 13 and 42 weeks, second-trimester-onset oligohydramnios compared with third-trimester onset was associated with a significantly increased rate of congenital anomalies (50.7 per cent vs 22.1 per cent) and poorer fetal survival (10.2 per cent vs 85.3 per cent) [D].[30] In part this is due to its association with lethal conditions including renal agenesis and early IUGR, but also reflects an increased severity of pulmonary hypoplasia, limb malformations and poor fetal growth. A significant association of oligohydramnios and poor fetal growth (birthweight <2500 g and <10th centile), neonatal death and perinatal mortality is also demonstrated [A].[8]

AF is critical for the canalicular phase of lung development occurring between 17 and 26 weeks. Severe oligohydramnios in early pregnancy results in underdevelopment of this fetal lung tissue and can result in fetal lung hypoplasia. Kilbride et al.[34] prospectively investigated whether sequential US assessment of AFV (<1 cm vertical pocket) could predict the occurrence of pulmonary hypoplasia and neonatal mortality in pregnancies complicated by second-trimester PROM. They found that both the duration of severe oligohydramnios and the timing of PROM were independent significant predictors of increased neonatal risk. In cases of severe oligohydramnios greater than 14 days following PROM at <25 weeks' gestation, the predicted neonatal mortality was in excess of 90 per cent [C].[34]

Maternal implications depend on aetiology with chorioamnionitis secondary to PPROM being the most serious. Perinatal morbidity is not shown to be increased once congenital anomalies have been excluded [A].[35]

Management of oligohydramnios

Oligohydramnios is not routinely treated during pregnancy and decisions regarding management are often dependent upon gestational age at diagnosis. A key priority is first to identify the underlying aetiology, since within the context of fetal growth restriction or maternal disease, severe oligohydramnios is considered an indication for delivery if >37 weeks. In uncomplicated post-dates pregnancies (>40 weeks) delivery is also advisable; whether a significant improvement in perinatal outcome is achieved however is contentious.[36] In those women less than 37 weeks, the frequency and intensity of fetal surveillance and management should principally be guided by the underlying aetiology, gestational age and aberrant AFV severity.

Specifically considering the SGA fetus, the use of umbilical artery Doppler has been shown to reduce perinatal morbidity and mortality and is therefore the recommended primary surveillance tool [A].[37] Further management of the SGA fetus is discussed in Chapter 38.

There is some evidence that maternal hydration can temporarily increase AFV; however, the actual clinical benefits of this are not determined [A].[38] Within the context of PPROM, amnio-infusion has been described as a method of temporarily reversing low AFV. The procedure involves infusion of isotonic fluid by a needle inserted into the uterine space surrounding the fetus, thus directly increasing AFV. Current evidence regarding the safety and efficacy of therapeutic amnio-infusion is presently insufficient and is therefore not routinely recommended in women with PPROM. For those cases determined appropriate for amnio-infusion, therefore, this must be performed in a specialist fetal medicine centre within the context of a multidisciplinary team [A].[31,39] The recently published prospective multicentre amnioinfusion in preterm premature rupture of membranes (AMIPROM) RCT compared short- and long-term outcomes for participants with very early rupture of membranes (between 16+0 and 19+6 weeks' gestation and 20+0 and 23+6 weeks' gestation) randomised to either serial amnio-infusion (MPD <2 cm) or expectant management until 37 weeks. It found no significant differences in maternal, perinatal or pregnancy outcomes. A larger definitive study to evaluate amnio-infusion for improvement in healthy survival is still required since only 56 pregnancies were reviewed (28 serial amnio-infusion, 28 expectant management) [B].[40]

When there is isolated oligohydramnios in the presence of an AGA non-compromised fetus with no evidence of maternal disease, guidance regarding appropriate management is uncertain. Currently a propensity towards antenatal fetal surveillance and induction of labour is observed. A randomised case–control study has concluded that increased AFV surveillance in low-risk pregnancies at late gestation does not significantly improve perinatal outcome [B].[41] Further research is required in this area.

KEY POINTS

- Oligohydramnios is defined as MVP <2 cm, AFV <200 mL or 500 mL, AFI <5 cm, or AFI <5th centile for gestational age.
- Detailed review of maternal history, fetal sonographic assessment for membrane rupture, anatomical evaluation, placental function and fetal growth is routinely performed.
- Oligohydramnios duration and severity are independent predictors of increased neonatal mortality secondary to pulmonary hypoplasia in the setting of PROM.

FETAL CONDITIONS

- Oligohydramnios is associated with poor fetal growth, neonatal death and perinatal mortality.
- Management is primarily determined by the underlying aetiology.
- At <37 weeks the frequency and intensity of fetal surveillance and management are guided by aetiology, gestational age at onset and severity.

CONCLUSION

Sonographic detection of aberrant liquor volume is a common situation. Understanding gestation-dependent AFV dynamics is empirical given the numerous causes of both low and high AFV. Given the associated morbidity and mortality associated with certain aetiologies, comprehensive, informed investigation and subsequent parental counselling are essential in this setting. What remains to be ascertained is the clinical significance of idiopathic, uncomplicated, aberrant AFV. At present it is therefore essential that AFV measures are considered within the clinical context and in conjunction with other investigations.

References

1. Brace R. Physiology of amniotic fluid volume regulation. *Clin Obstet Gynecol* 1997;40:280–9.
2. Brace R, Wolf E. Normal amniotic fluid volume changes throughout pregnancy. *Am J Obstet Gynecol* 1989;161:382–8.
3. Mahon A, Kalache K. Amniotic fluid. *In*: Rodeck C, Whittle M, eds. *Fetal Medicine: Basic Science and Clinical Practice*. 2 edn. Washington: Churchill Livingstone Elsevier, 2009, 642–8.
4. Sivit C, Hill M, Larsen J, Kent S, Lande I. The sonographic evaluation of fetal anomalies in oligohydramnios between 16 and 30 weeks gestation. *Am J Roentgenol* 1986;146:1277–81.
5. Magann E, Sandlin A, Ounpraseuth S. Amniotic fluid and the clinical relevance of the sonographically estimated amniotic fluid volume: oligohydramnios. *J Ultrasound Med* 2011;30:1573–85.
6. Sherer D, Langer O. Oligohydramnios: use and misuse in clinical management. *Ultrasound Obst Gyn* 2001;18:411–19.
7. Chauhan S, Magann E, Morrison J, Whitworth N, Hendrix N, Devoe L. Ultrasonographic assessment of amniotic fluid does not reflect actual amniotic fluid volume. *Am J Obstet Gynecol* 1997;177:291–6.
8. Morris R, Meller C, Tamblyn J *et al.* Association and prediction of amniotic fluid measurements for adverse pregnancy outcome: systematic review and meta-analysis. *BJOG* 2014;121:686-99.
9. Magann E, Chauhan S, Doherty D, Magann M, Morrison J. The evidence for abandoning the amniotic fluid index in favor of the single deepest pocket. *Am J Perinatol* 2007;24:549–55.
10. Magann E, Chauhan S, Whitworth N, Klausen J, Nevils B, Morrison J. The accuracy of the summated amniotic fluid index in evaluating amniotic fluid volume in twin pregnancies. *Am J Obstet Gynecol* 1997;177:1041–5.
11. Pri-Paz S, Khalek N, Fuchs K, Simpson L. Maximal amniotic fluid index as a prognostic factor in pregnancies complicated by polyhydramnios. *Ultrasound Obst Gynecol* 2012;39: 648–53.
12. Taylor M, Fisk N. Hydramnios and Oligohydramnios. In: James D, Steer J. Weiner G, Gonik B, eds. *High Risk Pregnancy. Management Options* 3rd edn. Pennsylvania: Saunders Elsevier, 2005:272–90.
13. Greenough A. The TORCH screen and intrauterine infections. *Arch Dis Child Fetal Neonatal Ed* 1994; 70:F163–5.
14. Levine Z, Sherer D, Jacobs A, Rotenberg O. Nonimmune hydrops fetalis due to congenital syphilis associated with negative intrapartum maternal serology screening. *Am J Perinatol* 1998;15:233–6.
15. Leikin E, Lysikiewicz A, Garry D, Tejani N. Intrauterine transmission of hepatitis A virus. *Obstet Gynecol* 1996;88(4 Pt 2):690–1.
16. Dashe J, McIntire D, Ramus R, Santos-Ramos R, Twickler D. Hydramnios: anomaly prevalence and sonographic detection. *Obstet Gynecol* 2002;100:134–9.
17. Hendricks S, Conway L, Wang K *et al.* Diagnosis of polyhydramnios in early gestation: indication for prenatal diagnosis? *Prenat Diagn* 1991;11:649–54.
18. Panting-Kemp A, Nguyen T, Chang E, Quillen E, Castro L. Idiopathic polyhydramnios and perinatal outcome. *Am J Obstet Gynecol* 1999;181(5 Pt 1):1079–82.
19. Many A, Hill L, Lazebnik N, Martin J. The association between polyhydramnios and preterm delivery. *Obstet Gynecol* 1995;86:389–91.
20. Dilbaz B, Ozturkoglu E, Dilbaz S, Ozturk N, Sivaslioglu A, Haberal A. Risk factors and perinatal outcomes associated with umbilical cord prolapse. *Arch Gynecol Obstet* 2006;274:104–7.
21. Joseph K, Rouleau J, Kramer M, Young D, Liston R, Baskett T. Investigation of an increase in postpartum haemorrhage in Canada. *BJOG* 2007;114:751–9.
22. Magann E, Doherty D, Lutgendorf M, Magann M, Chauhan S, Morrison J. Peripartum outcomes of high-risk pregnancies complicated by oligo- and polyhydramnios: a prospective longitudinal study. *J Obstet Gynaecol Res* 2010;36:268–77.
23. Guin G, Punekar S, Lele A, Khare S. A prospective clinical study of feto-maternal outcome in pregnancies with abnormal liquor volume. *J Obstet Gynaecol India* 2011;61:652–5.
24. Vink J, Poggi S, Ghidini A, Spong C. Amniotic fluid index and birth weight: is there a relationship in diabetics with poor glycemic control? *Am J Obstet Gynecol* 2006;195:848–50.
25. Piantelli G, Bedocchi L, Cavicchioni O *et al.* Amnioreduction for treatment of severe polyhydramnios. *Acta Biomed* 2004;75 (Suppl 1):56–8.

26. Leung W, Jouannic J, Hyett J, Rodeck C, Jauniaux E. Procedure-related complications of rapid amniodrainage in the treatment of polyhydramnios. *Ultrasound Obstet Gynecol* 2004;23:154–8.

27. Cabrol D, Jannet D, Pannier E. Treatment of symptomatic polyhydramnios with indomethacin. *Eur J Obstet Gynecol Reprod Bio* 1996;66:11–15.

28. Rosen D, Rabinowitz R, Beyth Y, Fejgin M, Nicolaides K. Fetal urine production in normal twins and in twins with acute polyhydramnios. *Fetal Diagn Ther* 1990;5:57–60.

29. Abou-Ghannam G, Usta I, Nassar A. Indomethacin in pregnancy: applications and safety. *Am J Perinatol* 2012;29:175–86.

30. Shipp T, Bromley B, Pauker S, Frigoletto F, Benacerraf B. Outcome of singleton pregnancies with severe oligohydramnios in the second and third trimesters. *Ultrasound Obstet Gynecol* 1996;7:108–13.

31. RCOG. *Preterm Prelabour Rupture of Membranes*. Green-top Guideline No. 44. London: RCOG, 2006. http://www.rcog.org.uk

32. Buchanan S, Crowther C, Levett K, Middleton P, Morris J. Planned early birth versus expectant management for women with preterm pre-labour rupture of membranes prior to 37 weeks' gestation for improving pregnancy outcome (Review). *Cochrane Database Syst Rev* 2010;3:CD004735.

33. Hunter T, Byrnes M, Nathan E, Gill A, Pennell C. Factors influencing survival in pre-viable preterm premature rupture of membranes. *J Matern Fetal Neonatal Med* 2012;25:1755–61.

34. Kilbride H, Yeast J, Thibeault D. Defining limits of survival: lethal pulmonary hypoplasia after midtrimester premature rupture of membranes. *Am J Obstet Gynecol* 1996;175:675–81.

35. Rossi A, Prefumo F. Perinatal outcomes of isolated oligohydramnios at term and post-term pregnancy: a systematic review of literature with meta-analysis. *Eur J Obstet Gynecol Reprod Biol* 2013;169:149–54.

36. Gibb D, Cardozo LD, Studd J, Cooper D. Prolonged pregnancy: is induction of labour indicated? A prospective study. *Br J Obstet Gynaecol* 1982;89:292–5.

37. RCOG. *Small-for-Gestational-Age Fetus, Investigation and Management*. Green–top Guideline No. 31, 2nd edn. London: RCOG, 2013:1–34.

38. Hofmeyr G, Gülmezoglu A, Novikova N. Maternal hydration for increasing amniotic fluid volume in oligohydramnios and normal amniotic fluid volume. *Cochrane Database Syst Rev* 2002;1:CD000134.

39. NICE. Therapeutic amnio-infusion for oligohydramnios during pregnancy (excluding labour). *Interventional Procedures* IPG192 2006. http://www.nice.org.uk

40. Roberts D, Vause S, Martin W *et al*. Amnio-infusion in very early preterm premature rupture of membranes – pregnancy, neonatal and maternal outcomes in the AMIPROM randomised controlled pilot study. *Ultrasound Obstet Gynecol* 2014; 43:490–9.

41. Zhang J, Troendle J, Meikle S, Klebanoff M, Rayburn W. Isolated oligohydramnios is not associated with adverse perinatal outcomes. *BJOG* 2004;111:220–5.

Chapter 40 Fetal hydrops

Caroline Fox and Sailesh Kumar

MRCOG standards

Epidemiology, aetiology, pathogenesis, diagnosis, prevention, management, delivery, complications, prognosis with regard to the following:

Fetal haemolysis
- Relevant antigen–antibody systems
- Prevention
- Fetal pathology
- Diagnosis
- Assessment of severity
- Intrauterine transfusion (indications, techniques, referral)
- Delivery (timing, method)
- Counselling

Non-haemolytic hydrops fetalis
Demonstrate an ability to explain correctly and place in context for the woman: effects upon fetus and neonate of infections during pregnancy, including HIV, measles, chickenpox, rubella, cytomegalovirus, parvovirus and toxoplasmosis.

INTRODUCTION

The term 'fetal hydrops' describes the accumulation of fluid in two or more serous cavities, e.g. pericardium, pleura, abdomen or subcutaneously, and may also be associated with poly-hydramnios.[1] It represents a non-specific, end-stage disorder of a broad range of conditions, where there is an imbalance in fluid movement between the interstitial and vascular spaces.[2] Fetal hydrops can be better understood by first dividing it into its traditional classification of immune hydrops (IH), i.e red cell alloimmunisation involving fetal haemolysis, or non-immune hydrops (NIH). As fetal hydrops represents a significant degree of fetal compromise it is associated with high rates of perinatal morbidity and mortality, although these will be discussed further as, not unsurprisingly, the outcome is variable depending on the aetiology.[3] However, rates are usually higher (up to 98 per cent)[3] in NIH than in IH (25 per cent).[4]

PREVALENCE AND EPIDEMIOLOGY

Fetal hydrops affects approximately one in 3000 pregnancies.[1] In the past IH, predominantly due to rhesus isoimmunisation, was a major contributor; however, since the introduction of effective rhesus prophylaxis in the 1970s there has been a significant decline in its prevalence.[5] Currently 90 per cent of all fetal hydrops cases are NIH. A recent systematic review reported the following associations with NIH, in order of frequency of occurrence:[6]

- Cardiovascular, e.g. structural anomalies, arrhythmias, tumours – 21.7%
- Chromosomal abnormalities or syndromes – 17.8%
- Haematological, e.g. haemoglobinopathies, congenital leukaemia/transient myeloproliferative disorders, red cell aplasia – 10.4%
- Infection, e.g. toxoplasmosis, rubella, CMV, herpes simplex, enterovirus, syphilis, varicella zoster, Lyme disease (*Borrelia burgdorferi*), HIV, parvovirus B19 – 6.7%
- Thoracic, e.g. cystic adenomatoid malformation, extrapulmonary sequestration, diaphragmatic hernia, hydro-chylothorax, mediastinal tumours, lethal skeletal dyplasias – 6.0%
- Lymphatic dysplasia – 5.7%
- Placental, e.g. TTTS, umbilical/chorionic vein thrombosis, placental chorioangioma – 5.6%
- Urinary tract abnormalitie, e.g. structural anomalies, tumours – 2.3%
- Inborn errors of metabolism, e.g. lysosomal or glycogen storage disorders – 1.1%
- Extra-thoracic tumours, e.g. sacrococcygeal teratomas – 0.7%
- Gastrointestinal, e.g. duodenal/jejunoileal atresia, volvulus, meconium peritonitis – 0.5%

- Miscellaneous, e.g. maternal non-steroidal use – 3.7%
- Idiopathic, 17.8%.

This illustrates the wide range of disorders that can present with hydrops and reinforces the message that hydrops is a non-specific symptom rather than a diagnosis in itself.

CAUSES

Fluid movement across the vascular and interstitial spaces is regulated by their relative hydrostatic and osmotic pressures, as well as by the permeability of the intervening capillary wall. According to the Starling equation, fluid movement will occur when the hydrostatic pressure gradient across the capillary wall is greater than the osmotic pressure gradient. Therefore any mechanism that results in increased hydrostatic pressure, e.g. increased central venous pressure due to outflow tract obstruction as seen in pulmonary stenosis, or decreased osmotic pressure, e.g. decreased hepatic production of proteins in infection-induced liver dysfunction, can result in the accumulation of fluid in the interstitial space and thus fetal hydrops.[2] The other element that can contribute to increased interstitial fluid accumulation is reduced lymph flow. This is because lymph usually returns albumin to the circulation, thereby reducing the osmotic pressure of the interstitial space, but if this flow is reduced then excess fluid can also accumulate in tissues.[7] Although lymph flow can be disturbed in isolation, as occurs in lymphatic dysplasia, it is more common for this to be a repercussion of an increase in central venous pressure, where a slight increase can result in a marked decrease in lymphatic flow.[2] The pathophysiology resulting in fetal hydrops therefore can be summarised to include conditions resulting in congestive heart failure, which would include all cases of immune hydrops, conditions with obstructed lymphatic flow, and conditions characterised by decreased plasma osmotic pressure or increased capillary permeability, but may represent a combination of these.[2]

COMMON CONDITIONS CAUSING FETAL HYDROPS

Immune hydrops

The rhesus blood group consists of five major antigens, D, C, c, E and e, although in total more than 50 different red cell antigens have been associated with haemolytic disease of the fetus or newborn.[8] However only three antibodies seem to be associated with severe disease, namely anti-RhD, anti-Rhc and anti-Kell.[8] Rhesus disease may occur when fetal red cells enter the maternal circulation via a fetomaternal haemorrhage, known as maternal sensitisation or alloimmunisation. However, the sensitising event in relation to other antibodies, i.e. Kell may not be pregnancy related but occur at the time of a previous blood transfusion,[8] making Kell typing of blood transfusions for women of reproductive age very important. Where the antigens displayed by the maternal and fetal erythrocytes differ, e.g. a mother is RhD negative but her fetus is RhD positive, then the mother will produce antibodies to the fetal genotype. In general this first alloimmunised pregnancy involves minimal fetal or neonatal disease; however, subsequent pregnancies are associated with worsening haemolytic anaemia.[9] This occurs when maternal IgG crosses the placenta and binds to the fetal erythrocytes, which are then sequestered in the fetal spleen and undergo haemolysis. The fetal liver responds to this increased red cell turnover by stimulating erythropoiesis, leading to hepatomegaly, but where demand outstrips supply the fetus will become severely anaemic and will develop cardiac failure and hydrops. Kell sensitisation is thought to differ slightly from other red cell alloimmunisation in that fetal anaemia is exacerbated by erythropoietic suppression from the outset.[8]

Although fetal haemolysis is thought to be associated predominantly with anti-RhD, anti-Rhc and anti-Kell, numerous other antibodies including anti-k, anti-RhcE, anti-Fya, anti-Jka, anti-CCw, anti-RhE and anti-Rhe can be associated with a need for *in-utero* transfusion.[8] However, the majority of these other antibodies are more commonly associated with haemolytic disease of the newborn rather than the fetus.[8] This is significant because these babies need monitoring after birth as they can develop increasingly severe hyperbilirubinaemia, requiring exchange transfusion to prevent bilirubin encephalopathy (kernicterus).

The widespread use of anti-D immunoglobulin has resulted in a major reduction in the incidence of RhD alloimmunisation. In the UK, the introduction of postnatal immunoprophylaxis with anti-D in 1969, which has since been extended to include anti-D use for any potentially sensitising event, has led to a fall in the number of deaths attributable to RhD alloimmunisation from 46/100,000 births in 1969 to 1.6/100,000 in 1990.[5] However, full coverage of immunoprophylaxis has not been achieved, and no such prophylaxis exists for the other red cell antibodies, therefore maternal alloimmunisation continues to contribute to perinatal mortality and morbidity.

Non-immune hydrops

Cardiovascular anomalies

Cardiovascular anomalies are the most frequent cause of NIH. The mechanism for this is most commonly congestive heart failure leading to increased central venous pressure. This can occur due to: obstructed outflow tracts, e.g. in pulmonary or aortic stenosis; diverted blood flow, e.g. transposition of the great arteries; abnormal venous return, e.g. in anomalous pulmonary venous return; abnormal ventricular filling, e.g. hypoplastic left heart; decreased ionotropic force, e.g. fetal arrhythmias; and reversed flow in the inferior vena cava, e.g. seen in atrial tachycardias such as atrial flutter.

Cardiac dysrhythmias, both tachyarrhythmias, i.e. supraventricular tachycardia, and bradyarrhythmias, i.e. complete heart block, are associated with fetal hydrops through disturbance of the cardiac diastolic function but also by the effect of hypoxia directly on the myocardium.

Placental anomalies such as chorioangioma, sacrococcygeal teratomas and vein of Galen aneurysms can act as a large peripheral arteriovenous shunt and induce hydrops by decreasing peripheral vascular resistance and therefore cardiac afterload.

Chromosomal and genetic disorders

Chromosomal and genetic disorders are strongly associated with hydrops, particularly if this is diagnosed prior to 24 weeks when they account for 45 per cent,[3] in either the presence or absence of coexistent structural anomalies. Turner's syndrome and trisomy 21 account for the majority of cases, although genetic syndromes and in-born errors of metabolism can also present in this way.[3,6] Karyotyping is therefore indicated in the initial investigation of hydropic fetuses, with more detailed genetic testing if indicated from the history. The diagnosis should be considered based on ultrasound findings and family history. It is important to make the diagnosis as many of these conditions carry a significant recurrence risk, and genetic counselling is needed.

Haematological disorders

On some continents, such as south-east Asia, haemoglobinopathies and particularly alpha-thalassaemia zero are the most common cause of fetal hydrops; however, these causes are unusual in most other populations.[10] Haematological causes in general result in fetal anaemia and pregnancy can therefore be prolonged with *in-utero* transfusion, although this cannot be viewed as curative.[3]

Infection

A multitude of viruses can be associated with fetal infection by causing dysfunction of bone marrow, myocardium and vascular endothelium leading to the development of fetal hydrops.[6] In practice the most common causative organism is parvovirus B19 (also known as slapped cheek syndrome or erythema infectiosum).[3] Transplacental infection of the fetus occurs in approximately 35 per cent, usually 1–3 weeks after maternal infection, and may resolve spontaneously but is also associated with inhibition of erythropoeisis and therefore fetal anaemia.[11] This is due to the presence of cellular receptors and co-receptors for parvovirus on erythroid progenitor cells, allowing them to be infected with parvovirus, as is also the case in fetal endothelial and myocardial cells.[11] The risk of hydrops after parvovirus infection ranges from 3.9 per cent to 12 per cent, with the risk being highest during the hepatic stage of haematopoeitic activity, between 8 and 20 weeks' gestation.[12] The interval between infection and hydrops is usually 2–6 weeks; however, intervals of 10–12 weeks and even 20 weeks have been reported.[12]

Thoracic anomalies

Any disorder that causes increased intrathoracic pressure, such as a space-occupying lesion in the fetal thorax, e.g. diaphragmatic hernia, cystic adenomatoid malformation, chylothorax or rarely mediastinal teratoma, or that limits the space the usual organs have to occupy, e.g. skeletal dysplasias, can result in hydrops.[2] This is because venous return will be impaired, as may fetal swallowing if the oesophagus is compressed, resulting in increased central venous pressure with eventual hydrops and polyhydramnios respectively.

Other causes of NIH

TTTS complicates 10–15 per cent of MC/DA twin pregnancies and if this is severe (stage IV), hydrops will be evident in the recipient twin due to high-output cardiac failure.

Structural anomalies of the urinary tract (i.e. urethral atresia) more commonly cause isolated ascites, due to bladder or renal pelvis rupture, rather than true hydrops although this has been reported.

MATERNAL RISKS AND COMPLICATIONS

'Mirror' syndrome can be associated with fetal hydrops in association with oedema of the placenta. It is characterised by an unusual form of pre-eclampsia, which can be extremely quick to develop and deteriorate. For this reason mothers with hydropic fetuses require regular review for their own health as well as that of their fetus. An increased risk of PPH and amniotic fluid embolus has also been reported.[13]

MANAGEMENT

Immune hydrops

Red cell alloimmunisation remains an important problem but due to its infrequent occurrence there is a lack of RCT evidence, so management is based largely on expert opinion. Thus although the RCOG and NICE guidelines,[5,14] as well as a Health Technology Assessment systematic review and economic evaluation,[15] exist on routine immunoprophylaxis for women who are RhD negative, these do not include management advice for affected pregnancies. The general principles, however, include routine testing for red cell antibodies associated with haemolytic disease of the fetus and newborn in all pregnant women. The further principles outlined below are taken from a recent systematic review of cohort studies of red cell alloimmunisation in pregnancy and recommend that management is undertaken by maternal–fetal medicine specialists [C].[9] If antibodies are detected the titre should be calculated and then repeated, usually monthly to 24–28 weeks and then every 2 weeks thereafter. If the titre always remains low, e.g. less than 16, then the pregnancy can be allowed to progress to 38 weeks. However, if the titre is above a critical value, usually taken as 32 for antibodies other than Kell, or 8 for Kell, then surveillance for fetal anaemia in the form of MCA Doppler scans is indicated every week or fortnight. If the peak systolic velocity of the MCA is indicative of fetal anaemia (≥1.5 MoM) then fetal blood sampling to determine fetal haematocrit is warranted with intrauterine transfusion (IUT) if fetal anaemia is confirmed. IUT has not only dramatically improved survival for fetuses affected by IH, to in excess of 90 per cent,[16,17] but also reduced the occurrence of neurological morbidity in survivors,[9] although experts agree that it is likely the best outcome will be achieved by avoiding hydrops in the first place [E].[16] Timing of delivery is based on the level of antibody titres and fetal wellbeing but for any pregnancy with significant antibody titres delivery would be expected to be by 34–35 weeks' gestation if IUT has been needed [E].[18]

If the patient has had a previously affected pregnancy titres are not necessarily predictive of the degree of fetal anaemia, which is known to worsen in subsequent pregnancies.[9] Therefore MCA scanning to detect likely recurrence of fetal anaemia is required. Where fetal anaemia presents in the early second trimester perinatal mortality is much higher and intravascular transfusion is not feasible, but management can involve intraperitoneal transfusion as well as IV immunoglobulin and plasmapharesis.[9,16,17]

Treatment advances have made a vast difference to the prognosis of red cell alloimmunised pregnancies but the other area of significant advance has been the advent of non-invasive prenatal diagnosis of RhD status by analysis of cffDNA.[9] It is now possible to reliably determine the fetal RhD genotype in the late first or early second trimester for both male and female fetuses (sensitivity 100 per cent, specificity 98.3 per cent)[19] and hopefully non-invasive testing for other red cell antigens will soon be possible.

Non-immune hydrops

General management

Patients whose fetuses are affected with hydrops should be referred to a fetal medicine centre where the necessary expertise and experience are available [E]. A detailed ultrasound scan, including Doppler insonation of the fetal cerebral vasculature and liquor volume, is mandatory [C]. The ultrasound scan must also include careful evaluation of the fetal anatomy and, particularly if skeletal dysplasia is suspected, all the long bones, hands, feet, skull shape and thoracic circumference must be examined.[20] Fetal echocardiography should also be performed, to exclude cardiac malformations, and noting normal atrial and ventricular rate and rhythm. Some indication of the cause of hydrops may be obtained from the sites of fluid collection, e.g. parvovirus usually presents with cardiomegaly and ascites.

Karyotyping should be offered in all cases. Samples should be sent for cytogenetics and infection screen. The placenta and umbilical cord should be carefully examined to exclude

a chorioangioma or other vascular abnormalities. More recently, the finding that fetal anaemia can be predicted with up to 100 per cent sensitivity using the peak systolic velocity in the middle cerebral artery has significantly improved the assessment of these fetuses.[21] Invasive fetal assessment in hydrops almost always involves fetal blood sampling [C]. This enables fetal blood to be obtained for a variety of investigations (FBC, karyotype, virology, enzyme studies, liver function tests, acid–base status and protein concentrations). The volume of blood required for these tests is small and should not compromise the fetus. Some of the investigations, such as karyotype or viral studies, can also be carried out on amniotic fluid or chorionic villi; however, fetal blood is preferable for complete haematological, biochemical and metabolic information. The risks of fetal blood sampling in a hydropic fetus are significantly greater than in the non-hydropic state. However, this risk must be balanced against the high mortality inherently associated with fetal hydrops [E].

Maternal blood should also be checked for atypical antibodies (indirect Coombs' test), FBC and Hb electrophoresis, viral serology and, in selected cases, glucose-6-pyruvate dehydrogenase (G6PDH) and pyruvate kinase carrier status. Other tests, such as for the presence of anti-Ro and anti-La antibodies, should be performed if the hydropic fetus is severely bradycardic. Many of the tests are selected depending on the clinical picture and family history. If more evidence emerges of unusual viral infections causing hydrops, specific tests to detect these organisms may be necessary.

Fetal anaemia is treated by *in-utero* intrauterine transfusions, irrespective of the cause of hydrops. Fetal tachyarrhythmias can be treated by administering specific cardiotrophic drugs either indirectly to the mother or directly to the fetus [C,E]. Although the transfer of drugs through an oedematous placenta is believed to be impaired, cardioversion is certainly possible in many instances.[22] Hydrops secondary to fetal bradyarrhythmias is frequently associated with structural heart abnormalities. The mortality in this group of fetuses is significantly worse.[23]

Pleural effusions can be treated by pleuroamniotic shunting [C] and large fetal tumours can be treated either fetoscopically *in utero* or occasionally by open surgery [C,E]. Hydrops in the recipient fetus in stage IV TTTS may be treated with fetoscopic laser ablation, or less commonly serial amnioreduction [E].[24] As fetal hydrops in this setting may be a pre-terminal event selective feticide may be the only option if the co-twin donor is to survive [C].

Human parvovirus B19

Maternal infection is diagnosed by the detection of parvovirus IgM and IgG antibodies, although neither is detectable for the first week, with IgM antibodies detectable first at about 7–10 days. IgM antibodies peak at 10–14 days and then decline within 2–3 months. Conversely IgG antibodies start to increase from 14 days, then reach a peak at about 6 weeks, after which they plateau, but are thought to persist to provide lifelong immunity.[12] Antibody levels are usually detected by enzyme immune assays but these can be falsely negative so if there is a high clinical index of suspicion either these can be repeated after 14 days or PCR analysis can be requested for parvovirus DNA as well.[12] Fetal ultrasound to assess for signs of fetal anaemia or hydrops, in the context of maternal diagnosis, is usually sufficient to support the diagnosis of fetal parvovirus infection.[12] However, to provide definitive diagnosis of fetal infection parvovirus DNA detection from either amniotic fluid or fetal blood sampling is required.[12] If maternal infection is confirmed then regular, for example weekly fetal surveillance with ultrasound including MCA Doppler, is required for at least 12 weeks but possibly even 20 weeks. Where fetal anaemia and hydrops do develop these can be treated with IUT and, in contrast with IH-related anaemia, because the infection is transient one IUT is often sufficient, although less commonly the fetus may remain hydropic, and there is still a risk of neurological damage in survivors, making it important to follow these babies up.[12]

OUTCOME

Overall, the perinatal mortality rate in cases of NIH is high (>98 per cent)[3] despite improvements in diagnosis and management. Early development of hydrops has a particularly poor prognosis. The mortality rate is highest among neonates with congenital anomalies (60 per cent) and lowest among neonates with congenital chylothorax (6 per cent). Mortality is higher in premature infants and those delivered in poor condition (lower 5-minute Apgar scores, higher levels of inspired oxygen support, and more often treated with high-frequency ventilation during the first day after birth). Once the diagnosis is made, urgent referral to a fetal medicine unit is essential.

The outcome in cases of IH treated by serial intrauterine transfusions is much better (>90 per cent survival).[16,17] In severe TTTS the outcome is poor, especially in stage IV disease when the recipient is hydropic.[24]

KEY POINTS

- Fetal hydrops represents an accumulation of interstitial fluid that is a symptom of an underlying disorder rather than a diagnosis in itself.
- Fetal hydrops carries a high rate of perinatal morbidity and mortality, so referral to a maternal-fetal medicine specialist is advised [E].
- Non-immune hydrops accounts for 90 per cent of all cases of fetal hydrops.
- Immune hydrops is most commonly related to anti-D, anti-C and anti-K antibodies, but all pregnant women should have red cell antibody detection undertaken routinely and if antibodies are detected should be monitored with serial titres and recourse to MCA Doppler and *in-utero* transfusion if indicated [A].

- Management of non-immune hydrops is dependent on the cause, but is largely supportive; however, if fetal anaemia is present *in-utero* transfusion is indicated [C].
- Timing of delivery is based on the degree of fetal compromise and the risks of prematurity but patients should be in a unit with level 3 neonatal care [E].

References

1. Warsof SL, Nicolaides KH, Rodeck C. Immune and non-immune hydrops. *Clin Obstet Gynecol* 1986;29:533–42.
2. Bellini C, Hennekam RCM. Non-immune hydrops fetalis: A short review of etiology and pathophysiology. *Am J Med Genet* 2012;158A:597–605.
3. Sohan K, Carroll SG, De La Fuente S, Soothill P, Kyle P. Analysis of outcome in hydrops fetalis in relation to gestational age at diagnosis, cause and treatment. *Acta Obstet Gynecol Scand* 2001;80:726–30.
4. Schumacher B, Moise KJ, Jr. Fetal transfusion for red blood cell alloimmunization in pregnancy. *Obstet Gynecol* 1996;88:137–50.
5. RCOG. *The Use of Anti-D Immunoglobulin for Rhesus D Prophylaxis*. Green-top Guideline No. 22. London: RCOG, 2011.
6. Bellini C, Hennekam RCM, Fulcheri E *et al*. Etiology of nonimmune hydrops fetalis: A systematic review. *m J Med Genet* 2009;149A:844–51.
7. Brace RA. Effects of outflow pressure on fetal lymph flow. *Am J Obstet Gynecol* 1989;160:494–7.
8. Moise KJ. Fetal anemia due to non-Rhesus-D red-cell alloimmunization. *Semin Fetal Neonatal Med* 2008;13:207–14.
9. Moise KJ, Argoti PS. Management and prevention of red cell alloimmunization in pregnancy. A systematic review. *Obstet Gynecol* 2012;120:1132–39.
10. Santo S, Mansour S, Thilaganathan B *et al*. Prenatal diagnosis of non-immune hydrops fetalis: what do we tell the parents? *Prenat Diagn* 2011;31:186–95.
11. Broliden K, Tolfvenstam T, Norbeck O. Clinical aspects of parvovirus B19 infection. *J Intern Med* 2006;260(4):285–304.
12. Dijkmans AC, de Jong EP, Dijkmans BAC *et al*. Parvovirus B19 in pregnancy: prenatal diagnosis and management of fetal complications. *Curr Opin Obstet & Gynecol* 2012;24:95–101.
13. Ismail KM, Martin WL, Ghosh S, Whittle MJ, Kilby MD. Etiology and outcome of hydrops fetalis. *J Matern Fetal Med* 2001;10:175–81.
14. NICE. *Routine Antenatal Anti-D Prophylaxis for Women who are Rhesus D Negative (TA156)*. London: NICE, 2008.
15. Pilgrim H, Lloyd-Jones M, Rees A. Routine antenatal anti-D prophylaxis for RhD-negative women: a systematic review and economic evaluation. *Health Tech Assess* 2009;13:iii, ix–x1,1–103.

16. Lindenburg ITM, van Kamp IL, van Zwet EW, Middeldorp JM, Klumper F, Oepkes D. Increased perinatal loss after intrauterine transfusion for alloimmune anaemia before 20 weeks of gestation. *BJOG* 2013;120:847–52.

17. Papantoniou N, Sifakis S, Antsaklis A. Therapeutic management of fetal anemia: review of standard practice and alternative treatment options. *J Perinat Med* 2013;41:71–82.

18. Brennard J, Cameron, A. Red cell alloimmunisation. In: Kilby MD, Johnson A, Oepkes DE, eds. *Fetal Therapy.* Cambridge: Cambridge University Press, 2012.

19. Bombard AT, Akolekar R, Farkas DH *et al.* Fetal RHD genotype detection from circulating cell-free fetal DNA in maternal plasma in non-sensitized RhD negative women. *Prenat Diagn* 2011;31:802–8.

20. Saltzman DH, Frigoletto FD, Harlow BL, Barss VA, Benacerraf BR. Sonographic evaluation of hydrops fetalis. *Obstet Gynecol* 1989;74:106–11.

21. Mari G, Deter RL, Carpenter RL *et al.* Noninvasive diagnosis by Doppler ultrasonography of fetal anemia due to maternal red-cell alloimmunization. Collaborative Group for Doppler Assessment of the Blood Velocity in Anemic Fetuses. *N Engl J Med* 2000;342:9–14.

22. van Engelen AD, Weijtens O, Brenner JI *et al.* Management outcome and follow-up of fetal tachycardia. *J Am Coll Cardiol* 1994;24:1371–5.

23. Lopes LM, Tavares GM, Damiano AP *et al.* Perinatal outcome of fetal atrioventricular block: one-hundred-sixteen cases from a single institution. *Circulation* 2008;118:1268–75.

24. Roberts D, Gates S, Kilby M, Neilson JP. Interventions for twin-twin transfusion syndrome: a Cochrane review. *Ultrasound Obstet Gynecol* 2008;31:701–11.

Chapter 41   Malpresentation

Alexander M Pirie

MRCOG standards

Module 1: Clinical skills
- Communicate effectively.
- Take notes concisely and accurately.

Module 5: Core surgical skills
- Demonstrate an understanding of the issues surrounding informed consent, including knowledge of complication rates, risks and likely success rates of different operations.

Module 8: Antenatal care
- Demonstrate skill in listening and conveying complex information (e.g. concerning risk).
- External cephalic version.

Modules 10 and 11: Management of labour and management of delivery
- The exam may test certain aspects of practical skill relating to normal and abnormal delivery.

(MRCOG syllabus 2013)

INTRODUCTION

In cases of tragic outcome, junior obstetricians cast a shadow of suspicion upon themselves when their witness statements mix up the specific obstetric terms *presentation*, *position* and *lie*. This is usually by referring to the *breech position* rather than the correct *breech presentation*. This is not mere pedantry, but vital clear thinking which defines the baby's *presentation* as being the leading part of the baby which is lowest in the birth canal.[1,2]

- *Presentation* is most commonly *cephalic, breech, face, brow, arm, shoulder, foot* or *compound*.
- *Position* refers to the relationship of the denominator of the presenting part to the maternal pelvis. So for cephalic presentations, the denominator is the occiput, and the positions can be *occipito-anterior, occipito-posterior, occipito-lateral*. For a breech presentation, the denominator

is the sacrum, so the positions can be *sacro-lateral, sacro-anterior, sacro-posterior*, etc.
- *Lie* refers to the relationship between the long axis of the baby and the long axis of the mother. So lie can either be *longitudinal, transverse, oblique* or *unstable*.
- A *malpresentation* is any presenting part which is not cephalic. Breech is the commonest malpresentation, followed by the much rarer face, brow and compound. The MRCOG candidate should know that malpresentation has its own specific complications and traditional management strategies. Other than for breech presentation, evidence quality to guide management for face and brow is low, partly because these are relatively uncommon.

BREECH PRESENTATION

This is the commonest malpresentation, which affects 3 per cent of babies at term. There is extensive evidence, debate and technique regarding breech presentation which is fully covered in Chapter 57.

FACE PRESENTATION

Prevalence and causes

The prevalence of face presentation is generally quoted at around 1 in 500–1250;[3-5] it will vary with the local population as it relates to parity, prematurity and uterine obstructions such as fibroids and placenta praevia. The use of mid-trimester anomaly scanning probably decreases the term frequency of face presentation by reducing anomalies associated with the face such as anencephaly and iniencephaly. Macrosomia and polyhydramnios are also associated with face presentation, and so it may be commoner in obese populations with more diabetes. Seventy-five per cent of face presentations are mento-anterior position.[2]

Clinical examination

The diagnosis should always be suspected with premature labour, failed induction or slow progress. Vaginally, the bony landmarks of the chin, malar and orbital ridges can be felt, and the soft opening of the mouth and nares. It is rarely confused with a vertex but more commonly confused with a breech. It is important to distinguish between mento-anterior and mento-posterior positions of the face, as the latter is less likely to deliver vaginally.

Abdominally, with a vertex presentation there is a smooth curved line between the fetal back and the occiput, with very little depression between them. With a face presentation, however, the extended head can be felt as a deep depression between the back and the head.

Management

- Explanation to the patient of need for further assessment and her consent.
- Discussion of risks and options including risks of facial oedema impairing initial feeding and also risk of contusions or lacerations to the face.
- Ultrasound and notes review to exclude placental, uterine or fetal anomaly.
- If mento-anterior position and pelvis feels adequate (see Chapter 57 for clinical pelvimetry), the deep curve of the sacrum allows the head to flex forwards and vaginal delivery is possible. This can be assisted with forceps and appropriate analgesia.
- If mento-posterior, unless baby is small or premature, vaginal birth is less likely as the full length of the mento-vertical diameter descends. If after a full discussion the mother is keen to try for vaginal birth, sometimes the mento-posterior face rotates to mento-anterior in the second stage of labour and then flexes for vaginal birth.
- The maternal risks include perineal injury with the larger diameters and also second-stage caesarean section.[6]

BROW PRESENTATION

Prevalence and causes

The prevalence of brow was found to be 1 in 775 in a modern series,[5] but older estimates quote figures of 1 in 1500–3500.[1-4] As with face presentation, there is a causal link with prematurity, contracted pelvis and fetal anomalies (such as fetal goitre). The incidence can also appear variable because there is no clear distinction of when a 'deflexing brow' becomes a face presentation. Increasing rates of caesarean section for slow progress will also mask a number of brow presentations.

Clinical examination

Brow presentation tends to be a labour phenomenon rather than an antenatal finding. The clinician may be surprised by the relatively high station of the head abdominally, as well as the deep depression between occiput and fetal back, rather than the usual smooth curved line. Vaginally, the supraorbital ridges are felt and the frontal bones with anterior fontanelle. However, a deep caput succedaneum can mask the landmarks in later labour.

Management

- Brow is the least favourable of cephalic presentations because the full mento-vertical diameter of 13–14 cm presents to the birth canal.
- Full discussion with the woman regarding risks and options will help determine how to proceed.
- If the woman values vaginal birth over caesarean section, a short trial of further labour with appropriate fetal monitoring may allow spontaneous correction, either by flexion or further deflexion to a mento-anterior face presentation.
- Beware the growing *caput succedaneum* as this can become very deep with a brow presentation and give the impression that the head is lower than it really is.
- Uterine rupture has been described with brow presentation, particularly if oxytocin is used.
- Ultimately caesarean section is performed with due attention to the particular risks of second-stage caesarean section.[5]

TRANSVERSE LIE, OBLIQUE LIE AND UNSTABLE LIE

Prevalence and causes

Transverse, oblique and unstable lie are essentially the same thing, and probably most accurately referred to as oblique lie. The prevalence has been variously quoted at 1 in 150–350 births.[1,2] Oblique lie has a strong association with prematurity, multiparity, polyhydramnios, placenta praevia, multiple pregnancy and uterine or fetal anomaly and so the prevalence will vary with the availability of mid-trimester scanning and population characteristics.

Clinical examination

When the Leopold manoeuvres are performed abdominally, the pelvis will feel empty, with the head high or in one of the iliac fossae. Vaginally, the pelvis will feel empty, or a presenting part may be felt bouncing at the very tip of a long finger. Care must be taken not to precipitate a cord prolapse.

Complications

- Cord prolapse at membrane rupture;
- Arm prolapse or compound presentation at membrane rupture;
- Difficulty delivering the baby at caesarean section.

FETAL CONDITIONS

Management

- Ultrasound to exclude placenta praevia, lower pole fibroids, fetal anomaly, polyhydramnios, etc.
- Full discussion with woman, explanation of risks of cord prolapse etc. and support informed choice.
- Explanation of 'First Aid' measures in event of spontaneous rupture of membranes and cord prolapse.
- Explain all-fours position with bottom up, call 999, keep bladder full, stay in position until delivery.
- Give information letter for ambulance crew or family with above information.
- Many obstetricians recommend admission to hospital from 37 weeks until delivery, although there are arguments for and against (see below) and documentation of informed choice is essential.
- At term, 'stabilising induction' can be performed where patient is taken to theatre, clinical pelvimetry, prepared for caesarean section and membranes undergo controlled rupture with view to immediate caesarean section if cord prolapses, or proceed to immediate oxytocin and careful maternal positioning after amniotomy, followed by continuous electronic fetal monitoring.
- If caesarean section is performed, transverse lie is one of the indications for classical caesarean section (with a vertical uterine incision but low transverse skin incision). Otherwise, the inexperienced obstetrician sometimes enters the lower segment to find an empty cavity with the baby being high above and impossible to bring down. If a lower-segment approach is possible, then a hand should be inserted in the uterus, then a foot grasped and checked for a heel to confirm it is a foot, and then gentle traction will usually bring the baby as a uterine breech extraction.
- The above advice is based on opinion, experience and small historical cohort studies, but there is no high-quality trial evidence to guide practice beyond this.

HOSPITAL VERSUS HOME MANAGEMENT FOR UNSTABLE LIE

An unstable lie is defined as the lie being mobile after 37 weeks. Many obstetricians recommend hospital admission from that gestation until delivery because of the small risk of cord prolapse. Planned caesarean section or stabilising induction is usually delayed until 39 weeks to promote fetal lung maturity.

Many of these women have an unstable lie because of their high parity, and therefore have children at home. The benefits of minimising the harms of cord prolapse by recommending hospital admission have to be balanced against the emotional and financial harms of being in hospital for a fairly long time and having to arrange alternative childcare. Ideally this question could be answered in part by comparative cohort studies, or by a randomised trial to include cost effectiveness and patient-reported outcomes.

Whether home or hospital management is decided, an honest discussion of the risks is required using the 'three-domain' decision model (see Chapter 57 for details) where the woman's values, intuition and understanding of risks can be evaluated to enable skilful support and informed choice. This must be documented in detail.

I will leave the reader with a legal case in England for reflection. In *Loraine versus Wirral University Teaching Hospital NHS Trust*, Lord Justice Plender was asked to determine liability where the claimant had an unstable lie due to a fibroid, but was not admitted to hospital.[7] The debate for most obstetricians would be whether home management risks a cord prolapse. However, in this case, the patient didn't have a cord prolapse, but sadly had a placental abruption at home with ongoing consequences for her son. Although the Court accepted that the abruption was not related to the unstable lie and high head, it was argued that had she been admitted for the high head, then the abruption would have happened in hospital with a probable better outcome with more rapid caesarean section.

The Judge explains that he is being asked to find on a difficult point of law on causation:

'I must determine whether the Defendant, and any other person in a similar position, is liable to compensate an individual who suffers an unforeseeable manifestation of a foreseeable danger arising from a breach of a duty of care owed to such an individual.'

The Judge found as follows:

'Even in the absence of such complicating factors as an obstructing fibroid and footling presentation, the leading medical textbooks in circulation at the time indicated that hospital admission might be an appropriate course for a lady at this advanced stage of her pregnancy. Turnbull's Obstetrics 1995 at 263 stated "Many units will feel happier if they can admit her [the mother] two or three weeks before term for daily observation." Dewhurst's Textbook of Obstetrics and Gynaecology, 1999 at 288 stated "Patients with transverse lie should not be allowed to labour because of the risks of uterine rupture and cord prolapse ... Recurrent unstable lie justifies hospital admission at 37 weeks to await labour." Steer's High Risk Pregnancy, 1999 at 305 stated "This approach [i.e. the interventionist approach] involves hospital admission from 37 weeks onwards."'

On that argument, the Judge determined that the Claimant should have been admitted to hospital for the unstable lie and, had that happened, the entirely unfortunate coincidence of the placental abruption would probably have had a better outcome for her son, and so the case was settled against the hospital.

As a practising obstetrician in one of the largest maternity units in Europe, I am not sure that all experienced obstetricians interpret the quotes from those textbooks to mean that every patient with an unstable lie MUST be admitted to hospital. Rather, we would interpret those textbooks to mean that we should give serious consideration to hospital admission for such a patient, and discuss (and document) the pros and cons on an individual basis, empowering each woman to a personal choice. But we must defer to the fact that case law is made by the Courts and not by doctors. On that sobering note, I will close this chapter with the words of the Glasgow hands-on obstetrician who pioneered obstetric ultrasound; he began his trusty old obstetric textbook with the humbling dedication:

> '*To all who have known doubt, perplexity and fear as I have known them, to all who have made mistakes as I have, to all whose humility increases with their knowledge of this most fascinating subject…I dedicate this work*'[1]

References

1. Donald I. *Practical Obstetric Problems.* London: Lloyd-Luke Ltd, 1974.
2. Chassar Moir J, Myerscough PR. *Munro Kerr's Operative Obstetrics.* 8th edn. London: Balliere, Tindall and Cassell, 1971.
3. Duff P. Diagnosis and management of face presentation. *Obstet Gynecol* 1981;57(1):105–12.
4. Benedetti TJ, Lowensohn RL, Tuscott AM. Face presentation at term. *Obstet Gynecol* 1980;55(2):199–202.
5. Bhal PS, Davies NJ, Chung T. A population study of face and brow presentation. *J Obstet Gynecol* 1998;18(3):231–5.
6. Murphy DJ, Liebling RE, Verity L, Swingler R, Patel R. Early maternal and neonatal morbidity associated with operative delivery in second stage of labour: a cohort study. *Lancet* 2001;358(9289):1203–1207.
7. *Loraine versus Wirral University Teaching Hospital NHS Foundation Trust*; Citation Number [2008] EWHC 1565 (QB) Case Ni: 6MA90744.

Chapter 42 Prolonged pregnancy

Devender Roberts and Rajeshwari Myagerimath

Standards

The recommendations on prolonged pregnancy from NICE guidelines 62, Induction of labour and 70, Antenatal care are summarised below:

- At the 38-week antenatal visit, all women should be offered information about the risks associated with pregnancies that last longer than 42 weeks, and their options should be discussed.
- Women should be informed that membrane sweeping makes spontaneous labour more likely, and therefore reduces the need for formal induction of labour to prevent prolonged pregnancy.
- Women with uncomplicated pregnancies should usually be offered induction of labour between 41^{+0} and 42^{+0} weeks. The exact timing should take into account the woman's preferences and local circumstances.
- Women who decline induction of labour from 42 weeks should be offered increased antenatal monitoring consisting of at least twice-weekly CTG and US estimation of the maximum amniotic pool depth.

INTRODUCTION

Prolonged pregnancy is defined as a pregnancy that continues beyond 42 weeks (294 days),[1,2] the gestational age having been established by an ultrasound scan in the first trimester (or no later than 16 weeks of gestation).[1] This is the standard international definition accepted by WHO and FIGO. The terms *prolonged pregnancy* and *post-term pregnancy* are often interchanged but refer to the same condition.[3]

EPIDEMIOLOGY

Prevalence and incidence

The prevalence of prolonged pregnancy varies depending on population characteristics and local management practices.

Population characteristics that affect prevalence include: the percentage of primigravidas in the studied population, the prevalence of obesity, the number of women with a prior prolonged pregnancy and the number of women with a genetic predisposition.[4] The proportion of women with pregnancy complications and the frequency of spontaneous preterm labour also influence the rate of prolonged pregnancy. Some studies have looked at the link between ethnicity and overall duration of pregnancy, but it is not well established.[5,6] Local management practices such as scheduled induction of labour (IOL), differences in the use of early ultrasound for pregnancy dating, and elective caesarean section rates will affect the overall prevalence of prolonged pregnancy.[7]

Incidence of prolonged pregnancy occurs in 5–10 per cent of all pregnancies.[8] The use of ultrasound in early pregnancy for precise dating significantly reduces the number of prolonged pregnancies compared to dating based on the last menstrual period and/or second-trimester ultrasound.[9–12]

Causes and risk factors

The most common cause of prolonged pregnancies is inaccurate dating.[13,14] When prolonged pregnancy truly exists the cause is usually not clear. It may represent simple biological variation. Prolonged pregnancy is common in primigravidas. Women with a single previous prolonged pregnancy have a 27 per cent chance of recurrence and those with two prior prolonged pregnancies a 39 per cent chance.[15] Male fetuses, hormonal factors, genetic predisposition and obesity are all associated with increasing the risk for a prolonged pregnancy.[10,16]

Fetal adrenal insufficiency and fetal adrenal hypoplasia are associated with prolonged pregnancies. This is thought to be secondary to their effect on circulating hormones that play a role in spontaneous labour. Similarly, placental sulphatase deficiency, a rare X-linked recessive disorder, can prevent spontaneous labour due to a defect in placental sulphatase activity and the resulting decreased oestriol (E3) levels.[10]

There is evidence to suggest that genetic factors may have a role i.e. women who themselves were results of a prolonged pregnancy are at higher risk of prolonged pregnancy (relative risk is 1.3).[17] Twin studies also support a genetic predisposition. Rates of prolonged pregnancy are increased in women whose twin sister has had a previous prolonged pregnancy.

This association is greater in monozygotic than in dizygotic twins.[18]

In a retrospective cohort study of 29,224 deliveries over four years, it was found that high pre-pregnancy BMI is associated with an increase in the prevalence of prolonged pregnancy. Prolongation of pregnancy was seen in 30 per cent of women with BMI 30–34.9 kg/m^2 compared to 22.3 per cent of normal-weight women, and women with BMI 35–39.9 kg/m^2 and >40 kg/m^2 had further increased incidence of prolonged pregnancy (32.4 and 39.4 per cent respectively) [C].[19,20] The association of obesity with prolonged pregnancy, but not pre-term labour, implied that obesity is associated with uterine quiescence or a suppression of myometrial activity. This study adds to the previously reported findings of an association between obesity and reduced myometrial contractility by both clinical and laboratory markers.[21] However, the lack of association between increasing BMI and length of first and second stages of labour, higher caesarean section for failure to progress and higher incidence of retained placenta miti-gates against an underlying aetiology of poor myometrial contractility in obese women with prolonged pregnancy in established labour. Hence the suggestion is that the effect of obesity on myometrial activity is more important in delay-ing the onset of labour than in reducing myometrial function once labour is established.[19]

Diets rich in n-3-polyunsaturated fatty acids (PUFA) are thought to be associated with a higher incidence of pro-longed pregnancy by interfering with uterine production of prostaglandins, possibly by inhibiting the production of dienoic prostaglandins, primarily PGF2α and PGE2, which are mediators of uterine contractions and cervical ripening. An RCT by the Danish group on the effect of fish-oil sup-plementation in the third trimester showed prolongation of pregnancy by an average of 4 days (95% CI 1.5 to 6.4 days p=0.006) when compared to olive oil or placebo, without any detrimental effect on the growth of the fetus or on the course of labour.[22]

FETAL AND NEONATAL RISKS OF PROLONGED PREGNANCIES

Continuation of pregnancy beyond 41 weeks increases the risk of adverse outcomes for the woman and the fetus. Prolonged pregnancy is associated with post-maturity syndrome. In this syndrome there is IUGR, association with meconium-stained amniotic fluid, oligohydramnios and fetal distress, evidence of loss of subcutaneous fat and dry cracked skin reflecting placental insufficiency.[23] Approximately 20 per cent of post-term fetuses have fetal post-maturity syndrome. It is apparent that not every prolonged pregnancy is complicated by post-maturity syndrome, but it is likely that the majority of morbidity and mortality associated with prolonged pregnancies arises because of post-maturity.

A retrospective study of over 170,000 singleton births demonstrated a 6-fold increase in stillbirth rates in prolonged pregnancies, from 0.35 at 37 weeks to 2.12 per 1000 ongo-ing pregnancies at 43 weeks.[23] The perinatal mortality rate at 42 weeks' gestation is twice as high as that at 40 weeks, 4-fold at 43 weeks and 5–7-fold at 44 weeks. There is evidence that when calculated per 1000 ongoing pregnancies, perinatal mortality rates increase sharply after 40 weeks.[10,11,23,24]

A number of key morbidities are greater in infants born beyond 41 weeks' gestation including meconium aspiration, neonatal acidaemia, low Apgar scores, fetal macrosomia and shoulder dystocia with resultant risks of orthopaedic or neu-rological injury.[11,25,26] Prolonged pregnancy is an independ-ent risk factor for low umbilical artery pH at delivery and low 5-minute Apgar scores, neonatal encephalopathy, and infant death in the first year of life. Meconium aspiration syndrome is seen at higher rates in post-term neonates.[16,23,27-30]

While preterm delivery is a well-established risk factor for cerebral palsy, a population-based follow-up study from 1967–2001 in Norway suggested that delivery at 42 weeks or later is also associated with increased risk of moderate to severe cerebral palsy, requiring entitlement to benefit for dis-ability (RR 2.4, 95% CI 1.1 to 5.3) when compared to delivery at 40 weeks' gestation.[31]

MATERNAL RISKS OF PROLONGED PREGNANCY

The maternal risks of prolonged pregnancy are often underestimated. These include an increase in labour dysto-cia (9–12 per cent vs 2–7 per cent at 40 weeks), an increase in severe perineal injury (3 and 4 degree perineal lacera-tions) related to macrosomia (3.3 per cent vs 2.6 per cent at 40 weeks) and operative vaginal delivery, and a doubling in the rate of caesarean delivery (14 per cent vs 7 per cent at 40 weeks).[30, 32-34] These risks are even higher in obese women with prolonged pregnancies.[19] In addition to the medical risks, the emotional impact (anxiety and frustration) of car-rying a pregnancy 1–2 weeks beyond the estimated due date should not be underestimated.

MANAGEMENT

Accurate dating of pregnancy

Accurate pregnancy dating is crucial in the diagnosis and management of prolonged pregnancy.[35] Routine ultrasound examination for pregnancy dating demonstrated a reduc-tion in the rate of false-positive diagnosis and thereby the overall rate of prolonged pregnancy from 10–15 per cent to approximately 2–5 per cent, and thereby minimised unnec-essary intervention.[3,6] Due to the lower margin of error first-trimester ultrasonography seems to be superior to mid-trimester ultrasound for pregnancy dating.[35]

Prevention of prolonged pregnancy

Several minimally invasive interventions have been recommended to avoid formal induction and encourage spontaneous onset of labour at term. This includes membrane sweeping, unprotected sexual intercourse, nipple stimulation and acupuncture.

Sweeping of the membranes, also named stripping of the membranes, is a relatively simple technique usually performed in an outpatient setting. It has the potential to initiate labour by increasing local production of prostaglandins and, thus, reduce pregnancy duration. Sweeping the membranes at or beyond 40 weeks appears to significantly reduce not only the incidence of prolonged pregnancy but also the frequency of using other methods for induction of labour. There is no evidence that sweeping the membranes increases the risk of maternal and neonatal infection, or of premature rupture of the membranes. However, women's discomfort during the procedure and other side effects must be balanced with the expected benefits before submitting women to sweeping of the membranes.[1,36-38]

A systematic review evaluating interventions aimed at prevention, or improvement of outcomes of delivery beyond term, showed sweeping the membranes performed as a general policy from 38 to 40 weeks onwards decreased the frequency of prolonged pregnancy: pregnancy continuing beyond 42 weeks (RR 0.28, 95% CI 0.15 to 0.50, NNT 11) and beyond 41 weeks (RR 0.59, 95% CI 0.46 to 0.74, NNT 9). Sweeping the membranes in women at term generally reduces the delay between randomisation and spontaneous onset of labour, or between randomisation and delivery, by a mean of three days. It increased the likelihood of either spontaneous labour within 48 hours (RR 0.77, 95% CI 0.70 to 0.84) or of delivery within one week (RR 0.71, 95% CI 0.65 to 0.78). A reduction in the frequency of using other methods to induce labour ('formal induction of labour') in women allocated to sweeping was reported in most trials (RR 0.60, 95% CI 0.51 to 0.71). The overall risk reduction was 14 per cent. About eight women need to have sweeping of membranes to avoid one formal induction of labour [A].[38]

Membrane sweeping is the only evidence-based intervention known to reduced prolonged pregnancy.

Cochrane reviews on the role of other interventions designed to reduce the incidence of prolonged pregnancy, including sexual intercourse, nipple stimulation and acupuncture, are uncertain and that further studies of sufficient power are needed to assess their value.[14,39-41]

Induction of labour

The data from 22 RCTs comparing elective IOL were analysed in a systematic review, which has governed policy for many units in the UK over the past decade.[14,42] The conclusions of the analysis favoured a policy of IOL at 41 completed weeks and beyond, to reduce perinatal mortality, decrease meconium staining of the amniotic fluid and cause a small decrease in caesarean section, compared to conservative management. [A]

Compared with a policy of expectant management, a policy of labour induction was associated with fewer (all-cause) peri-natal deaths; 17 trials, 7407 women (RR 0.31, 95% CI 0.12 to 0.88). There was one perinatal death in the labour induction policy group compared with 13 perinatal deaths in the expectant management group. The number needed to treat to benefit (NNTB) with IOL in order to prevent one perinatal death was 410 (95% CI 322 to 1492). For the primary outcome of perinatal death and most other outcomes, no differences between timing of induction subgroups were seen; the majority of trials adopted a policy of induction at 41 completed weeks (287 days) or more. Fewer babies in the labour induction group had meconium aspiration syndrome (RR 0.50, 95% CI 0.34 to 0.73; eight trials, 2371 infants) compared with a policy of expectant management. There was no statistically significant difference between the rates of NICU admission for induction compared with expectant management (RR 0.90, 95% CI 0.78 to 1.04; 10 trials, 6161 infants). For women in the policy of induction arms of trials, there were significantly fewer caesarean sections compared with expectant management in 21 trials of 8749 women (RR 0.89, 95% CI 0.81 to 0.97).[42]

The recommendations of the Society of Obstetricians and Gynaecologists of Canada for management of pregnancy at 41 to 42 weeks are broadly in agreement with these findings.[11]

The American College of Obstetricians and Gynecologists recommendations on management of prolonged pregnancy also support a policy of IOL.

While much of the work has been conducted in prolonged pregnancies, evidence from one of the retrospective cohort study showed that some of the fetal risks such as presence of meconium, increased risk of neonatal acidaemia and even stillbirth have been described as being greater at 41 weeks and even at 40 weeks as compared with 39 weeks of gestation.[43,44] In addition to stillbirth being increased prior to 42 weeks, another retrospective cohort study found that the risk of neonatal mortality also increases beyond 41 weeks' gestation.[45] Thus, 42 weeks does not represent a threshold below which risk is uniformly distributed. Indeed, neonatal morbidity (including meconium aspiration syndrome, birth injury and neonatal acidaemia) appears to be lowest at around 38 weeks and increase in a continuous fashion thereafter.[46] Similar to neonatal outcomes, maternal morbidity also increases in term pregnancies prior to 42 weeks' gestation. Complications such as chorioamnionitis, severe perineal lacerations, caesarean delivery rates, PPH and endomyometritis all increase progressively after 39 weeks of gestation.[35,44,47-50]

Current guidance for the management of prolonged pregnancy in the UK is based on NICE guidelines on induction of labour and antenatal care.[1,2] Based on the evidence from epidemiological data, trial data and health economic analysis, the guideline development group (GDG) reached a consensus that, on balance, induction of labour should be offered from 41^{+0} weeks onwards. The guideline found that IOL became more acceptable to women as gestation advanced (45 per cent wanted expectant management at 37 weeks vs 31 per cent at 41 weeks, p <0.05).[51]

There is evidence to suggest that this policy is acceptable to women. In a Scandinavian RCT of women at 41 weeks' gestation, 74 per cent of women who were induced desired the same management, whereas only 38 per cent of women with serial antenatal monitoring desired the same management.[52]

One of the common dilemmas in the management of the obese pregnant woman with prolonged pregnancy is how to balance the maternal risks of IOL, including caesarean section and PPH, with the fetal risks of perinatal morbidity and mortality associated with prolonged gestation. A retrospective (historical) cohort study looked at the effect of higher maternal BMI on delivery outcome following induction for prolonged pregnancy and demonstrated that IOL for these women was associated with increased rates of caesarean section delivery (28.4 per cent for obese women compared with 18.9 per cent for normal-weight women). Although this 28.4 per cent caesarean section rate is high, it is also important to realise that over 70 per cent of obese pregnant women with prolonged pregnancy delivered vaginally, and with rates of labour and neonatal complications also comparable to normal-weight women. The results of this study suggest that IOL in obese women with prolonged pregnancy is a reasonable and safe management option.[19]

Monitoring prolonged pregnancy

The NICE antenatal guideline recommends increased antenatal fetal surveillance consisting of at least twice-weekly CTG and US estimation of maximum amniotic pool depth in women who decline induction of labour. These recommendations are supported by both the American College of Obstetricians and Gynecologists and the Society of Obstetricians and Gynaecologists of Canada, despite lack of evidence that it improves perinatal mortality. This recommendation is based on the evidence that perinatal morbidity and mortality increase as gestational age advances.

It has been suggested that AFI is preferable to MPD liquor volume assessment in these pregnancies. However, there is still debate about what constitutes the best cut-off values for both measurements, as liquor volumes fall after term. An RCT comparing the two methodologies showed that use of AFI did not improve perinatal outcomes but was associated with an increase in the intervention rate. Thus MPD is probably the tool of choice for assessing liquor in these prolonged pregnancies [B].[53,54] More complex fetal monitoring with a formal biophysical scoring system has been suggested, but an RCT shows that it holds no advantage over simple monitoring with NST-CTG and liquor assessment [B].[55]

CTG monitoring is usually applied on the basis of observational data, although it is of no proven benefit [C].[56]

It has been suggested that computerised CTG may be superior to conventional CTG, but this has yet to be tested in clinical trials. The use of Doppler analysis of various fetal arterial systems has also been advocated in the assessment of prolonged pregnancies, but again this has not been evaluated by RCT. In addition, complex arterial Doppler assessment is not suitable as a screening tool in standard practice. The use of umbilical artery Doppler is claimed to be of benefit; however, the alterations in the waveforms are subtle.[57]

In a prospective questionnaire-based survey, only 31 per cent of women at 41 weeks' gestation opted for conservative management despite this being the unit's policy [C].[51] Many women will see induction as interference with a natural process, and loss of maternal choice is a major determinant of maternal dissatisfaction with the management of pregnancy and labour. It is therefore vital that each woman is treated on an individual basis and counselled regarding the risks of prolonged pregnancy, to allow her to make her own decision about induction of labour.[3]

KEY POINTS

- Prolonged pregnancy is a condition associated with increased risk of stillbirth, post-maturity syndrome and perinatal mortality and morbidity.
- Induction of labour should be offered between 41 and 42 weeks.
- Women who opt for conservative management beyond 42 completed weeks should have fetal surveillance with twice-weekly CTG and US measurement of the MPD.

CONCLUSIONS

- The use of early ultrasound dating reduces the incidence of prolonged pregnancy [A].
- Induction of labour after 41 weeks reduces perinatal mortality rates without increasing caesarean section rates. Nevertheless some will opt for conservative management with fetal surveillance [A].
- Sweeping the membranes significantly reduces the incidence of prolonged pregnancy and the need for other methods of induction of labour, with no evidence of increase in the risk of maternal or neonatal adverse outcomes [A].
- No clear evidence exists to support the hypothesis that fetal monitoring can reduce the perinatal mortality in prolonged pregnancy but it is suggested as good practice by the NICE antenatal guideline. Therefore IOL seems the best policy to avoid perinatal risks [C].
- Lower-grade evidence [B,C] supports the use of NST-CTG and liquor assessment using MPD in monitoring prolonged pregnancy.

FETAL CONDITIONS

References

1. National Collaborating Centre for Women's and Children's Health. NICE. *Antenatal Care: Routine care for the healthy pregnant woman*. London: RCOG Press, 2008.

2. National Collaborating Centre for Women's and Children's Health. *Induction of labour*. London: NICE, 2008 July; 32.

3. Caughey AB, Snegovskikh VV, Norwitz ER. Post-term pregnancy: how can we improve outcomes? *Obstet Gynecol Surv* 2008;63:715–24.

4. Galal M, Murray H, Petraglia F, Smith R. Post-term pregnancy. *ObGyn* 2012;4:175–87.

5. Collins JW. Post-term delivery among African Americans, Mexican Americans and Whites in Chicago. *Ethn Dis* 2001;11: 181–7.

6. Caughey AB, Stotland NE, Washington AE, Escobar GJ. Who is at risk for prolonged and postterm pregnancy? *Am J Obstet Gynecol* 2009;200:683.e1–5.

7. Martin JA, Hamilton BE, Sutton PD *et al*. Births: final data for 2005. *Natl Vital Stat Rep* 2007;56:1–103.

8. Shea KM, Wilcox AJ, Little RE. Post-term delivery: a challenge for epidemiologic research. *Epidemiology* 1998;9:199–204.

9. Tunon K. A comparison between ultrasound and a reliable last menstrual period as as predictors of the day of delivery in 15,000 examinations. *Ultrasound Obstet Gynecol*. 1996;8:178–85.

10. Doherty L, Norwitz ER. Prolonged pregnancy: when should we intervene? *Curr Opin Obstet Gynecol* 2008;20:519–27.

11. Delaney M, Roggensack A, Leduc DC *et al*. Guidelines for the management of pregnancy at 41^{+0} to 42^{+0} weeks. *J Obstet Gynaecol Can* 2008;30:800–23.

12. Bennett KA, Crane JM, O'Shea P, Lacelle J, Hutchens D, Copel JA. First-trimester ultrasound screening is effective in reducing post-term labor induction rates: a randomized controlled trial. *Am J Obstet Gynecol* 2004;190:1077–81.

13. Neilson JP. Ultrasound for fetal assessment in early pregnancy. *Cochrane Database Syst Rev* 2000:Cd000182.

14. Crowley P. Interventions for preventing or improving the outcome of delivery at or beyond term. *Cochrane Database Syst Rev* 2000:CD000170.

15. Kistka ZA, Palomar L, Boslaugh SE, DeBaun MR, DeFranco EA, Muglia LJ. Risk for post-term delivery after previous post-term delivery. *Am J Obstet Gynecol* 2007;196:241.e1–6.

16. Eik-Nes SH, Grottum P. ACOG Practice Bulletin. Clinical management guidelines for. *Ultrasound Obstet Gynecol* 2004;104:639–46.

17. Mogren I, Stenlund H, Hogberg U. Recurrence of prolonged pregnancy. *Int J Epidemiol* 1999;28:253–7.

18. Laursen M, Bille C, Olesen AW, Hjelmborg J, Skytthe A, Christensen K. Genetic influence on prolonged gestation: a population-based Danish twin study. *Am J Obstet Gynecol* 2004;190:489–94.

19. Arrowsmith S, Wray S, Quenby S. Maternal obesity and labour complications following induction of labour in prolonged pregnancy. *BJOG* 2011;118:578–88.

20. Djelantik AA. Contribution of overweight and obesity to the occurrence of adverse pregnancy outcomes in a multi-ethnic cohort: population attributive fractions for Amsterdam. *BJOG*. 2012;119:283-90.

21. Zhang J, Bricker L, Wray S, Quenby S. Poor uterine contractility in obese women. *BJOG* 2007;114:343–8.

22. Olsen SF, Sorensen JD, Secher NJ *et al*. Randomised controlled trial of effect of fish-oil supplementation on pregnancy duration. *Lancet* 1992;339:1003–7.

23. Hilder L, Costeloe K, Thilaganathan B. Prolonged pregnancy: evaluating gestation-specific risks of fetal and infant mortality. *Br J Obstet Gynaecol* 1998; 105:169–73.

24. Costeloe K, Thilaganathan B, Cotzias CS. Prospective risk of unexplained stillbirth in singleton pregnancies at term. *Br J Obstet Gynaecol* 1999;319:287–8.

25. Spellacy WN, Miller S, Winegar A, Peterson PQ. Macrosomia: maternal characteristics and infant complications. *Obstet Gynecol* 1985;66:158–61.

26. Rosen MG, Dickinson JC. Management of post-term pregnancy. *N Engl J Med* 1992;326:1628–9.

27. Gulmezoglu AM. Induction of labour for improving birth outcomes for women at or beyond term. *Cochrane Database Syst Rev*. 2012:Cd004945.

28. Kitlinski ML, Kallen K, Marsal K, Olofsson P. Gestational age-dependent reference values for pH in umbilical cord arterial blood at term. *Obstet Gynecol* 2003;102:338–45.

29. Badawi N. Antepartum risk factors for newborn encephalopathy: the Western Australian case-control study. *BMJ* 1998;317:1549-53.

30. Rand L, Robinson JN, Economy KE, Norwitz ER. Post-term induction of labor revisited. *Obstet Gynecol* 2000;96:779–83.

31. Moster D, Wilcox AJ, Vollset SE, Markestad T, Lie RT. Cerebral palsy among term and postterm births. *JAMA* 2010;304:976–82.

32. Campbell MK, Ostbye T, Irgens LM. Post-term birth: risk factors and outcomes in a 10-year cohort of Norwegian births. *Obstet Gynecol* 1997;89:543–8.

33. Alexander JM. Forty weeks and beyond: pregnancy outcomes by week of gestation. *Obstet Gynecol* 2000;96:291–4.

34. Treger M, Hallak M, Silberstein T, Friger M, Katz M, Mazor M. Post-term pregnancy: should induction of labor be considered before 42 weeks? *J Matern Fetal Neonatal Med* 2002;11:50–3.

35. Mandruzzato G, Alfirevic Z, Chervenak F *et al*. Guidelines for the management of post-term pregnancy. *J Perinat Med* 2010;38:111–9.

36. Yildirim G, Gungorduk K, Karadag OI, Aslan H, Turhan E, Ceylan Y. Membrane sweeping to induce labor in

low-risk patients at term pregnancy: a randomised controlled trial. *J Matern Fetal Neonatal Med* 2010;23:681–7.

37. de Miranda E, van der Bom JG, Bonsel GJ, Bleker OP, Rosendaal FR. Membrane sweeping and prevention of post-term pregnancy in low-risk pregnancies: a randomised controlled trial. *BJOG* 2006;113:402–8.

38. Boulvain M, Stan C, Irion O. Membrane sweeping for induction of labour. *Cochrane Database Syst Rev* 2005:Cd000451.

39. Schaffir J. Survey of folk beliefs about induction of labor. *Birth* 2002;29:47–51.

40. Smith CA, Crowther CA, Grant SJ. Acupuncture for induction of labour. *Cochrane Database Syst Rev* 2013;8:Cd002962.

41. Kavanagh J, Kelly AJ, Thomas J. Breast stimulation for cervical ripening and induction of labour. *Cochrane Database Syst Rev* 2005:Cd003392.

42. Gulmezoglu AM, Crowther CA, Middleton P, Heatley E. Induction of labour for improving birth outcomes for women at or beyond term. *Cochrane Database Syst Rev* 2012;6:Cd004945.

43. Caughey AB, Washington AE, Laros RK, Jr. Neonatal complications of term pregnancy: rates by gestational age increase in a continuous, not threshold, fashion. *Am J Obstet Gynecol* 2005;192:185–90.

44. Caughey AB, Musci TJ. Complications of term pregnancies beyond 37 weeks of gestation. *Obstet Gynecol* 2004;103:57–62.

45. Bruckner TA, Cheng YW, Caughey AB. Increased neonatal mortality among normal-weight births beyond 41 weeks of gestation in California. *Am J Obstet Gynecol* 2008;199:421.e1–7.

46. Nicholson JM, Kellar LC, Kellar GM. The impact of the interaction between increasing gestational age and obstetrical risk on birth outcomes: evidence of a varying optimal time of delivery. *J Perinatol* 2006;26:392–402.

47. Caughey AB, Stotland NE, Washington AE, Escobar GJ. Maternal and obstetric complications of pregnancy are associated with increasing gestational age at term. *Am J Obstet Gynecol* 2007;196:155.e1–6.

48. Caughey AB, Nicholson JM, Cheng YW, Lyell DJ, Washington AE. Induction of labor and cesarean delivery by gestational age. *Am J Obstet Gynecol* 2006;195:700–5.

49. Yoder BA, Kirsch EA, Barth WH, Gordon MC. Changing obstetric practices associated with decreasing incidence of meconium aspiration syndrome. *Obstet Gynecol* 2002;99:731–9.

50. Heimstad R, Romundstad PR, Eik-Nes SH, Salvesen KA. Outcomes of pregnancy beyond 37 weeks of gestation. *Obstet Gynecol* 2006;108:500–8.

51. Roberts LJ, Young KR. The management of prolonged pregnancy: an analysis of women's attitudes before and after term. *Br J Obstet Gynaecol* 1991;98:1102–6.

52. Heimstad R, Romundstad PR, Hyett J, Mattsson LA, Salvesen KA. Women's experiences and attitudes towards expectant management and induction of labor for post-term pregnancy. *Acta Obstet Gynecol Scand* 2007;86:950–6.

53. Crowley P, O'Herlihy C, Boylan P. The value of ultrasound measurement of amniotic fluid volume in the management of prolonged pregnancies. *Br J Obstet Gynaecol* 1984;91:444–8.

54. Alfirevic Z, Luckas M, Walkinshaw SA, McFarlane M, Curran R. A randomised comparison between amniotic fluid index and maximum pool depth in. *Br J Obstet Gynaecol* 1997;104:207–11.

55. Alfirevic Z, Luckas M, Walkinshaw SA, McFarlane M, Curran R. A randomised controlled trial of simple compared with complex antenatal fetal. *Br J Obstet Gynaecol* 1995;102:638–43.

56. Fleischer A, Schulman H, Farmakides G, Perrotta LA, McGovern G, Katz N. Antepartum non-stress test and the postmature pregnancy. *Obstet Gynecol* 1985;66:80–3.

57. Fischer RL, Kuhlman KA, Depp R, Wapner RJ. Doppler evaluation of umbilical and uterine-arcuate arteries in the postdates pregnancy. *Obstet Gynecol* 1991;78:363–8.

Chapter 43 Routine intrapartum care: an overview

Mary Higgins

Definitions

Dystocia: Failure to progress within any stage of labour based on either total time or rate of progress based on a partogram.
Lie: Orientation of the fetal long axis with respect to the long axis of the mother (longitudinal, oblique or transverse).
Malpresentation: Any position of the fetus other than occiput anterior.
Normal birth: A birth without surgical intervention, use of instruments, induction, epidural or general anaesthesia.
Partogram: A graph demonstrating the dilatation of the cervix as a function of time – can also record station, maternal vital signs and fetal heart rate.
Position: The position of the fetal presentation in relation to the maternal pelvis (occiput anterior, posterior, transverse; mento anterior or posterior, sacrum anterior posterior or transverse).
Presenting part: Fetal part at the pelvic outlet (cephalic, breech, compound).
Stages of labour:

First stage: Time from diagnosis of labour to full dilatation of the cervix.
Second stage: Time from full dilatation of cervix to delivery of the fetus.
Passive second stage: Full dilatation of the cervix prior to or in the absence of involuntary expulsive contractions.
Active second stage: Full dilatation with expulsive contractions, baby visible, active maternal effort following confirmation of full dilatation of the cervix in the absence of expulsive contractions.
Third stage: Time from delivery of the fetus to delivery of the placenta.

Station: Relationship between the presenting part and the ischial spines. May be described either based on centimetres or 'thirds', or based on distance from lowermost portion of the presenting part or bi-parietal diameter.

INTRODUCTION

Just under half of the 729,624 births in the UK in 2012 were normal – that is, without surgical intervention, use of instruments, induction, epidural or general anaesthesia.[1] If one includes the women who had epidural anaesthesia but a normal vaginal delivery then this percentage increases. Ninety percent of women in the UK will give birth to a single baby, presenting head first, after 37 weeks' gestation, and most women (75 per cent) will go into labour spontaneously. If the delivery and birth progress normally these women will not need the support of the obstetric team, other than as a supportive service to the midwifery team should problems arise. It is important that obstetricians be aware of the physiological processes of normal labour and delivery, both as a method of early recognition of pathology and in acknowledgement of the stellar work of midwifery staff. Recognition by obstetricians and midwives of early problems can prevent emergencies happening in women who were previously deemed normal – a central theme in the Active Management of Labour,[2] and a key responsibility of the consultant on call.[3]

ONSET OF LABOUR

Aristotle proposed that labour began once the infant had outgrown maternal supplies and therefore needed to be able to function independently of its parent. More recent theories include changes in the progesterone-to-oestrogen ratio, or in the sensitivity of progesterone receptors, secretion of steroids from the fetus and changes in the uterine wall tension as well as changes in cytokines. Prostaglandins and inflammatory markers may play a part. The complexity of possible causes is shown in Fig. 43.1.

DIAGNOSIS OF LABOUR

Internationally there are several different definitions of when to make a diagnosis of labour, from cervical effacement with pains[2] to cervical dilatation greater than 6 cm.[4] In the UK, labour is defined as either latent (painful contractions and some cervical change up to 4 cm dilatation) or established (regular painful contractions and progressive cervical dilatation from 4 cm).

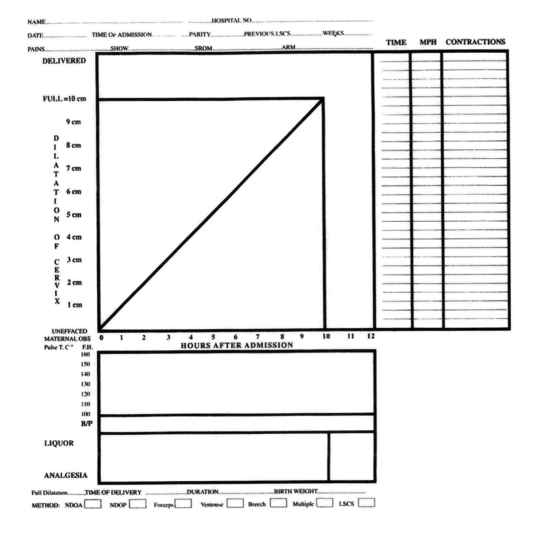

Fig. 43.1 Partogram

LABOUR IN PRIMIPAROUS WOMEN COMPARED TO LABOUR IN MULTIPAROUS WOMEN

The differences between first and subsequent labours are so significant that in our unit, like many others, two different colour partograms are used to distinguish between the two [E]. In a first labour a woman, no matter how well informed, has yet to experience the emotional and physical experience of labour. With this in mind the care and experience of her healthcare provider are invaluable to provide her with the support she requires at this, one of the most profoundly emotional experiences of her lifetime. It is continuously astonishing how acutely women and their partners remember everything that happens to them and everything that is said to them at this time. As first-time labours are often longer and more uncertain of outcome as the functional capacity of the pelvis is unknown, this highlights the need for high standards of care and attention. In contrast, labour in a multiparous woman is different: the pelvis has been tested, the uterus is more efficient, labour is normally shorter and the woman has personal experience to give her confidence in her own ability. One major concern is the risk of uterine rupture and the need for great caution in the use of oxytocin as a result; though the labour is different, excellent midwifery and obstetric care are still required.

CARE OF THE WOMAN IN LABOUR

Place of birth

In the UK, women may choose to deliver at home, in a midwife-led unit or in an obstetric-led unit (Box 43.1).

Box 43.1 Recommendations regarding place of birth (adapted from the NICE Guidelines on Intrapartum Care)

Home/Midwife-led Unit

Advantages: Higher likelihood of a normal delivery without intervention.

Disadvantages: If something does go unexpectedly wrong during labour the outcome may be worse than in an obstetric-led unit.

Women choosing to labour at home or in a midwifery-led unit should be informed of the locally available services, the likelihood of being transferred into the obstetric unit and the time this may take.

Obstetric-led Unit

Advantages: Immediate access to obstetricians, anaesthetists, neonatologists and other specialist care including epidural anaesthesia; women with a pre-existing medical condition or previous complicated birth should be advised to give birth in an obstetric-led unit.

Disadvantages: More likely to have intervention.

The NICE Guidelines on Intrapartum Care[5] outline medical conditions and other factors indicating increased risk and suggesting planned delivery in an obstetric unit as well as conditions and factors indicating individual assessment when planning place of birth. Should an obstetric opinion be required, either by the woman or her midwife, regarding the place of birth this should be obtained from a consultant obstetrician and clearly documented in the hand-held maternity notes. Examples of conditions or factors suggesting delivery in an obstetric unit include: diabetes, BMI >35 at booking, epilepsy, multiple birth, recurrent antepartum haemorrhage, previous obstetric complication (including retained placenta requiring removal in theatre), anaemia (Hb <8.5 g/dL at onset of labour), SGA infant or previous myomectomy. Individual assessment can be used for women with conditions such as ulcerative colitis, hepatitis B or C with normal liver function tests, previous intrauterine death due to a non-recurrent cause, age over 40 at booking or BMI between 30 and 34 or single antepartum haemorrhage of unknown origin [D].

In labour, circumstances may change so that consideration may be given to transferring the woman from her home or midwifery unit to an obstetric unit. In making this decision, the clinicians need to bear in mind the likelihood of birth during transfer. Such indications include need for electronic fetal monitoring, delay in first or second stage of labour, maternal request for epidural, obstetric emergency, retained placenta, maternal pyrexia or hypertension, significant meconium-stained liquor or malpresentation first diagnosed at the onset of labour. Twenty-five per cent of intended home deliveries required hospital delivery in 2012, of which half of the transfers occurred prior to the onset of labour.[1]

There is not enough information on the possible risks to the woman or her baby relating to the planned place of birth – a recent Cochrane Review identified only two small randomised trials, of which only one (involving 11 women) contributed data to the review [A].[6]

Communication in labour

A woman in labour should be treated with respect and be involved in what is happening to her – this includes establishing her wants and expectations for labour, supporting her in one-on-one care, and only offering clinical intervention when it is warranted. One-on-one care does not merely mean a physical presence, but also requires the emotional support of a trained companion – especially valuable in first labours. Lack of such support can significantly affect both the morale of the woman and her confidence in her care provider [D,E], best described as follows:

'As human consciousness is seldom more open to impression than during the momentous hours of labour, a casual approach to just another routine assignment may leave a mother with a burning sense of resentment. Apparently trivial episodes such as a curt tone of voice, a bloodstained glove, a mindless exposure in the lithotomy position or a failure to convey the result of pelvic examination,

though not seemingly of great consequence in themselves, still portray an often deplorable lack of sensitivity in professional staff who should know a great deal better.'2

When additional expertise is being requested, such as when a midwife requests the opinion of an obstetrician, the woman should be involved in this and the obstetrician should be of sufficient expertise to provide that opinion.

In order to continue with efficient communication the woman should be greeted with an introduction of who the person is and what their role is in her care. Knocking and waiting prior to entering her room shows respect for her personal space and should be standard in all but the most pressing emergencies.

Different women need different approaches to labour – some require quiet support and others boisterous encouragement. Therefore the clinicians and attendants need experience and sensitivity to match the type of support they give to the needs of the mother;[7] often the partner (usually forgotten) can advise on this.

If the woman has a written birth plan it is important to read it and discuss it with her. Despite popular opinion in obstetrics, women with written birth plans do not have an increased rate of episiotomy or delivery by caesarean section, and may have a decreased incidence of epidural use [C].[8]

In the case of an acute emergency it is even more necessary that staff maintain a calm and confident approach so that the woman is reassured of their support.

Pain relief in labour

Pain relief in labour has proven to be one of the most controversial areas of labour management, with women themselves being divided between 'natural' and 'medicalised' labour. While a low-risk woman is unlikely medically to need regional anaesthesia (compared to a woman requiring a caesarean delivery where it would be inhumane to deny regional or general anaesthesia to her) it is nearly universally recognised that women should have several options available to them in labour so that they can choose, in discussion with their care provider, what form of pain relief they may wish. Thousands of studies have been published on options for pain relief for parturients, the reviews of which are beyond the scope of this chapter.

What is obvious is that options other than regional analgesia alone are reasonable and may work perfectly well for some women, especially if their labour is progressing normally. Women choosing to use breathing or relaxation techniques should be supported in their choice, and the playing of music of their choice should be supported. Aromatherapy may be used for pain relief, though a review of two trials showed no difference in pain intensity or the rate of subsequent use of epidural anaesthesia [A].[9] The opportunity to labour in water is recommended for pain relief, as it has been shown to significantly reduce the rate of analgesia (OR 0.84, 95% CI 0.7 to 0.98) without increasing the rate of maternal infection [A].[10]

Other options for pain relief include:

- Transcutaneous electrical nerve stimulation (TENS): research is inconsistent whether TENS will reduce pain scores, but many women said that they would use it again in future labours and no obvious harm has been identified. NICE guidelines suggest TENS should not be offered in established labour. Given the limited evidence base and absence of adverse events, midwifery literature has recently supported offering women in labour the choice of TENS [A].[11]

- Inhalational analgesia (e.g. Entonox) should be made available as it reduces pain intensity and gives pain relief during labour. Flurane derivatives appear to cause more drowsiness and nitrous oxide more nausea [A].[12] As an example of cultural differences in labour ward management, inhalational analgesia tends to be used in Western Europe for management of pain relief in early labour, and only used in advanced labour in North America.

- Intramuscular or intravenous opioids provide some relief from pain in labour but the effect appears to be moderate and is associated with a higher rate of maternal nausea, vomiting and drowsiness [A].[13]

- Remifentanil patient-controlled analgesia provides a superior analgesia and patient satisfaction compared to pethidine but lower pain relief compared to epidural [A].[14] One-on-one midwifery care, appropriate monitoring and experience in both the medication and its possible complications are required in order to maintain patient safety when administering remifentanil due to the serious complications that have been described with its use [E].[15]

- Regional anaesthesia: while epidural (or combined spinal epidural) analgesia appears to be effective in reducing pain in labour there is an increased risk of instrumental delivery (A, RR 1.42).[16] Before choosing epidural anaesthesia, the risks and benefits should be explained as well as the implications of epidural anesthesia for labour.[5]

Eating and drinking in labour

Following Mendelson's work in the 1940s (showing an increased risk of aspiration in those who had recently eaten and then underwent general anaesthesia) oral intake has been restricted in labouring women. Since that time, however, anaesthesia has improved considerably with increased rates of regional anesthesia. A recent Cochrane review of 3130 women over five trials concluded that there are no benefits or harm in restricting foods and fluids to women at low risk of anesthesia; no studies were identified investigating women at higher risk of anaesthesia [A].[17] Women in low-risk established labour should be encouraged to eat a light diet and drink isotonic drinks, unless they have been administered opioids or developed risk factors making general anesthesia more likely.

PROGRESS IN LABOUR

One of the most common questions asked by labouring women is at what point should they deliver. It is recommended that women should be told that first-time mothers deliver, on average, within 8 hours (rarely past 18 hours) and subsequent labours last on average 5 hours (rarely past 12 hours). This knowledge is important for the woman's psychological well-being as well as for decisions she may make about analgesia in labour.

The diagnosis of delay in labour is more than a simple line on a partogram. While delay in the first stage of labour is based on cervical dilatation less than 2 cm in 4 hours (or slowing of progress in non-primiparous women), other factors such as strength, duration and frequency of contractions as well as descent and rotation of the fetal head may play a part. As an example, a multiparous woman whose cervical dilatation increases from 2 cm to 3 cm may be considered to have delay in labour, but if the fetal position has changed from OP to OA and from station minus 3 to the spines, with an increase in strength and frequency of contractions, then this is more reassuring of normal labour and therefore care may be individualised to whether amniotomy or oxytocin is truly required in her case, rather than patience.

It is recommended that a partogram should be used when labour is established. Various types of partograms have been published in the literature, and no one type has been exclusively recommended within the UK. At its simplest, a partogram is a graph demonstrating the dilatation of the cervix as a function of time, though many also report fetal position, station, FHR and maternal vital signs. The classic Friedman curve was said to be developed by Friedman in the 1950s as he sat in a hospital waiting room anticipating the birth of his first child – as information was relayed to him on the progress of his wife in labour he drew a graph on mathematical paper in order to predict when the delivery would occur. Friedman went on to develop a graph based on nulliparous[18] and multiparous[19] women. The partogram was further adapted to add an 'action line' in order to determine either when a woman needed to be transferred to an obstetric unit[20] [D] or else have some intervention aimed to correct dystocia [B].[21] The value of Friedman's work is that

he introduced the concept of latent and active phases of labour, and gave an intellectual approach to labour which went on to inform both the Active Management of Labour and modern care of the labouring woman.

One concern is the applicability of the Friedman curve to the modern care of the parturient – of the 100 women studied initially,[18] four underwent induction of labour, 68 were delivered by forceps and one by caesarean section. Cervical assessment was performed at the peak of a contraction (only 22 received 'caudal anaesthesia' – mostly for delivery) and examinations were performed *per rectum* rather than vaginally. With this in mind, other partograms have been developed, some using similar populations to Friedman but different statistical methods[22] and others using modern populations of parturians [C].[20,21] Interestingly, partograms have also been developed based on individual patient factors: the influence of the fetal gender on progress in labour[25] (male fetus increasing the active first phase by 0.6 hours), and the influence of maternal BMI[26,27] (with average length of labour increasing by 1.7 hours in women with a BMI >30) [C].

No one partogram is recommended for use in the UK, and it is advisable that clinicians be aware of which partogram is in use in their unit. It is recommended that if an action line is to be used [E], it should be the WHO action line, which is set at 4 hours to the right of the alert line.[28]

FETAL MONITORING

Intermittent auscultation, whether by handheld Doppler or Pinard, is recommended for every low-risk woman in spontaneous labour. Admission CTG is not recommended as it is associated with a higher rate of continuous electronic fetal monitoring (CEFM), fetal blood sampling and delivery by caesarean section [A].[29]

The frequency of fetal monitoring as recommended is outlined in Table 43.1. Monitoring of the FHR should be converted to CEFM when an abnormal heart rate is auscultated, there is meconium staining of liquor, maternal pyrexia or fresh bleeding or oxytocin is required. CEFM can also be used if the mother requests it. Otherwise intermittent auscultation

Table 43.1 Recommendations regarding maternal and fetal observations in labour (adapted from the NICE Guidelines on Intrapartum Care)

First stage of labour	
Maternal observations	**Fetal observations**
• 4-hourly temperature and BP	• Fetal heart rate auscultation after every contraction
• Hourly pulse rate	• At least every 15 minutes
• Half-hourly documentation of frequency of contractions	• Lasting at least 1 minute
• Frequency of emptying of bladder	• Fetal descent, station, position
• Vaginal examination offered every 4 hours, or if concerns regarding progress, or in response to the woman's wishes	• Liquor

(continued)

Table 43.1 Recommendations regarding maternal and fetal observations in labour (adapted from the NICE Guidelines on Intrapartum Care) (*continued*)

Second stage of labour	
Maternal observations	**Fetal observations**
• 4-hourly temperature • Hourly pulse rate and BP • Half-hourly documentation of frequency of contractions • Frequency of emptying of bladder • Vaginal examination offered every hour (active stage), or in response to the woman's wishes	• Fetal heart rate auscultation after every contraction • At least every 5 minutes • Lasting at least 1 minute • Fetal descent, station, position • Liquor
Third stage of labour	
Maternal observations	**Neonatal observations**
• Based on her general physical condition and degree of blood loss	• Apgars recorded at 1 and 5 minutes routinely • Minimal separation from the mother within the first hour: encourage skin to skin • Head circumference, birthweight and temperature after 1 hour

should be used as a preference in low-risk women as CEFM increases the risk of instrumental and caesarean delivery [A].[30]

Should there be abnormalities on the CTG suggestive of fetal distress, there are a number of options available. Further information may be obtained either by fetal blood (scalp) sampling (measuring either fetal pH or fetal lactate, which requires smaller blood volumes than pH) or STAN monitoring (monitoring elevation of the ST segment of the ECG, requiring specialist equipment not universally available in the UK). Options also include changing clinical circumstances (stopping oxytocin, change of maternal position, amnio-infusion) or consideration of delivery. Each of these options can be considered in the context of the individual situation, available equipment and the wishes of the parents to be, but should be discussed with senior obstetric and midwifery personnel.

Other maternal and fetal monitoring recommendations are shown in Table 43.1.

CAUSES OF DYSTOCIA

The mnemonic of the '3 Ps' relates to the relative incidence of the common causes of dystocia in labour. The first P (**powers**) relates to uterine contractions, or inefficient uterine activity, and may be corrected using amniotomy or oxytocin. Inefficient uterine action rarely occurs in a multiparous woman in spontaneous labour and therefore great care needs to be taken when considering the use of oxytocin to correct slow progress in labour, especially in the second stage of labour. The obstetrician would be wise to consider why a woman would not make progress in the second stage

when her pains have been sufficient until then to achieve full dilatation.

The second (**passenger**) relates to the position of the fetus, with an OP position being a relatively common cause of delay in both the first and second stage. Correction of malposition needs to be individualised to both the type of malposition and the individual patient, and to the experience of the clinician. Recently there have been several papers published assessing the use of ultrasound to diagnose malposition in labour, especially as part of the assessment for instrumental delivery.

The final P refers to the **passage** – or the relationship of the fetus to the pelvis. Only when both the powers and the passenger have been corrected can the diagnosis of dystocia due to the passage (or cephalo-pelvic disproportion, CPD) be made. In the National Maternity Hospital in Dublin great care is taken to make the correct indication for delivery so as not to over-diagnose CPD due to the possible implications for further deliveries. Here a woman being delivered by CS for 'dystocia – unable to treat' (as oxytocin caused decelerations on the CTG) is different to the woman delivered by CS for 'dystocia – unsuccessful treatment' (following a full course of oxytocin in an infant with an OA position), and as such would receive different recommendations regarding future deliveries.

A fourth P can be added to the mnemonic to consider a cause of slow progress in the second stage – the **perineum**.

DELIVERY

The NICE Guidelines distinguish between a passive and active second stage of labour and recommend that birth should take place within 3 hours of start of the active second stage

(2 hours in multiparous women). Prolongation of the second stage of labour is associated with increased maternal and neonatal morbidities. Interestingly, prolongation of the active second stage, but not the passive stage, is associated with an increased risk of PPH (adjusted OR 10.6 compared to baseline <10 minutes) [C].[31] Prolongation of the second stage is also associated with a higher risk of long-term complications such as urinary incontinence[32] and cervical insufficiency in a future pregnancy (OR 24.9) [C].[33]

It is recommended that a diagnosis of delay in the second stage should be made when it lasts more than 2 hours (1 hour in multiparous women) and the woman transferred to the care of a healthcare professional who is competent in performing an instrumental delivery [E]. Once the decision is made that an instrumental delivery may be required, the decision itself does not protect against the risks of an unintentional further prolonged labour, with one study showing that 74 per cent of prolonged second stages occurred while waiting after a decision had been made to perform an instrumental delivery [C].[34]

Women may choose to labour in the second stage in a supine, lateral, upright or 'all-fours' position. A systematic review showed several benefits (reduction in assisted births, episiotomies and abnormal FHR patterns) to women labouring upright but a possible increase in blood loss >500 mL. As the methodological quality of the papers varied the authors recommended that the results be interpreted with caution[35] [A] but that at present women should be allowed to make choices about which birth position they assume, which in turn can affect the woman's sense of control during labour [D].[36]

POSTNATAL CARE

Active management of the third stage of labour involves administration of prophylactic uterotonic, early cord clamping and controlled cord traction for delivery of the placenta. Active management reduces the risk of PPH, the need for further uterotonics and the need for blood transfusion[37] [A] but increases maternal vomiting after birth, after-pains and use of analgesia.

One area of active management of the third stage causing much recent controversy relates to the timing of cord clamping. Advocates of delayed cord clamping cite increased birthweight and neonatal Hb due to the placental transfusion of blood after delivery, whereas others have concerns regarding the risk of maternal haemorrhage. Assessment of late clamping (>1 minute after birth or after the cord has stopped pulsating) as an individual component of the active management of the third stage showed no difference in the rate of severe PPH in early versus late clamping, with increased neonatal Hb and iron stores, and an increased requirement for phototherapy for jaundice in the late group [A].[38]

Following delivery, it is recommended that observations be based on the woman's general physical condition and her degree of blood loss. This is based on a lack of high-level evidence on maternal observations in the third stage of labour, but lack of evidence does not imply lack of effect. At least one set of vital observations should be taken in this time so as to provide objective measurement of maternal wellbeing, especially when there has been an abnormality detected in the first or second stage of labour [E].

CONCLUSION

The majority of women will conceive spontaneously, have a normal pregnancy and deliver vaginally without incident. Despite this normality, labour and delivery are among the most profound physical and emotional times in a womans life, and it is our privilege to work as a team in caring for women and their families at this time.

References

1. Office for National Statistics. Births in England and Wales, 2012. http://www.ons.gov.uk/ons/rel/vsob1/birth-summary-tables--england-and-wales/2012/stb-births-in-england-and-wales-2012.html, 2013.
2. O'Driscoll K, Boylan D. *Active Management of Labour - The Dublin Experience*. 3rd ed. London: Mosby, 1999.
3. RCOG. Good Practice No 8. *Responsibility of the Consultant on Call*. 2009.
4. Higgins MFD. Assessment of Labor Progress. *Expert Review of Obstetrics and Gynecology* 2013;8(1):83–95.
5. National Collaborating Centre for Women's and Children's Health. Intrapartum care of healthy women and their babies during childbirth. Commissioned by the National Institute for Health and Clinical Excellence, editor. London: RCOG Press, 2007.
6. Olsen O, Clausen JA. Planned hospital birth versus planned home birth. *Cochrane Database of Systematic Reviews* (Online) 2012;9:CD000352.
7. Steer P, Flint C. ABC of labour care: physiology and management of normal labour. *BMJ* (Clinical research ed.) 1999;318(7186):793–6.
8. Deering SH, Zaret J, McGaha K, Satin AJ. Patients presenting with birth plans: a case-control study of delivery outcomes. *The Journal of Reproductive Medicine* 2007;52(10):884–7.
9. Smith CA, Collins CT, Crowther CA. Aromatherapy for pain management in labour. *Cochrane Database of Systematic Reviews* (Online) 2011:CD009215.
10. Cluett ER, Burns E. Immersion in water in labour and birth. *Cochrane Database of Systematic Reviews* (Online) 2009:CD000111.
11. Bedwell C, Dowswell T, Neilson JP, Lavender T. The use of transcutaneous electrical nerve stimulation (TENS) for pain relief in labour: a review of the evidence. *Midwifery* 2011;27(5):e141–8.

12. Klomp T, van Poppel M, Jones L, Lazet J, Di Nisio M, Lagro-Janssen AL. Inhaled analgesia for pain management in labour. *Cochrane Database of Systematic Reviews* (Online) 2012;9:CD009351.

13. Ullman R, Smith LA, Burns E. Mori R, Dowswell T. Parenteral opioids for maternal pain relief in labour. *Cochrane Database Systematic Reviews.* 2010;Sep 8;(9):CD007396.

14. Schnabel A, Hahn N, Broscheit J, Mullenbach RM, Rieger L, Roewer N, Kranke P. Remifentanil for labour analgesia: a meta-analysis of randomised controlled trials. *Eur J Anaesthesiolog* 2012;29(4):177-85.

15. Kranke P, Girard T, Lavand'homme P, Melber A, Jokinen J, Muellenbach RM, Wirbelauer J, Honig A. Must we press on until a young mother dies? Remifentanil patient controlled analgesia in labour may not be suited as a "poor man's epidural". *BMC Pregnancy Childbirth* 2013;13:139.

16. Anim-Somuah M, Smyth RM, Jones L. Epidural versus non-epidural or no analgesia in labour. *Cochrane Database of Systematic Reviews* (Online) 2011(12):CD000331.

17. Singata M, Tranmer J, Gyte GM. Restricting oral fluid and food intake during labour. *Cochrane Database of Systematic Reviews* (Online) 2013;8:CD003930.

18. Friedman EA. Primigravid labor; a graphicostatistical analysis. *Obstetrics and Gynecology* 1955;6(6):567–89.

19. Friedman EA. Labor in multiparas; a graphicostatistical analysis. *Obstetrics and Gynecology* 1956;8(6):691–703.

20. Philpott RH. Obstructed labour. *Clinics in Obstetrics and Gynaecology* 1982;9(3):625–40.

21. O'Driscoll K, Foley M, MacDonald D. Active management of labor as an alternative to cesarean section for dystocia. *Obstetrics and Gynecology* 1984;63(4):485–90.

22. Zhang J, Troendle J, Mikolajczyk R, Sundaram R, Beaver J, Fraser W. The natural history of the normal first stage of labor. *Obstetrics and Gynecology* 2010;115(4):705–10.

23. Zhang J, Troendle JF, Yancey MK. Reassessing the labor curve in nulliparous women. *American Journal of Obstetrics and Gynecology* 2002;187(4):824–8.

24. Lavender T, Hart A, Walkinshaw S, Campbell E, Alfirevic Z. Progress of first stage of labour for multiparous women: an observational study. *BJOG: an international journal of obstetrics and gynaecology* 2005;112(12):1663–5.

25. Cahill AG, Roehl KA, Odibo AO, Zhao Q, Macones GA. Impact of fetal gender on the labor curve. *American Journal of Obstetrics and Gynecology* 2012;206(4):335 e1–5.

26. Norman SM, Tuuli MG, Odibo AO, Caughey AB, Roehl KA, Cahill AG. The effects of obesity on the first stage of labor. *Obstetrics and Gynecology* 2012;120(1):130–5.

27. Vahratian A, Zhang J, Troendle JF, Savitz DA, Siega-Riz AM. Maternal pre-pregnancy overweight and obesity and the pattern of labor progression in term nulliparous women. *Obstetrics and Gynecology* 2004; 104(5 Pt 1):943–51.

28. World Health Organization partograph in management of labour. World Health Organization Maternal Health and Safe Motherhood Programme. *Lancet* 1994;343(8910):1399–404.

29. Devane D, Lalor JG, Daly S, McGuire W, Smith V. Cardiotocography versus intermittent auscultation of fetal heart on admission to labour ward for assessment of fetal wellbeing. *Cochrane Database of Systematic Reviews* (Online) 2012;2:CD005122.

30. Alfirevic Z, Devane D, Gyte GM. Continuous cardiotocography (CTG) as a form of electronic fetal monitoring (EFM) for fetal assessment during labour. *Cochrane Database of Systematic Reviews* (Online) 2013;5:CD006066.

31. Le Ray C, Fraser W, Rozenberg P, Langer B, Subtil D, Goffinet F. Duration of passive and active phases of the second stage of labour and risk of severe postpartum haemorrhage in low-risk nulliparous women. *European Journal of Obstetrics, Gynecology, and Reproductive Biology* 2011;158(2):167–72.

32. Brown SJ, Gartland D, Donath S, MacArthus C. Effects of prolonged second stage, method of birth, timing of caesarean section and other obstetric risk factors on postnatal urinary incontinence: an Australian nulliparous cohort study. *BJOG* 2011;118(8): 991-1000.

33. Vyas NA, Vink JS, Ghidini A *et al.* Risk factors for cervical insufficiency after term delivery. *American Journal of Obstetrics and Gynecology* 2006;195(3):787–91.

34. Bleich AT, Alexander JM, McIntire DD, Leveno KJ. An analysis of second-stage labor beyond 3 hours in nulliparous women. *American Journal of Perinatology* 2012;29(9):717–22.

35. Gupta JK, Hofmeyr GJ, Shehmar M. Position in the second stage of labour for women without epidural anaesthesia. *Cochrane Database of Systematic Reviews* (Online) 2012;5:CD002006.

36. Nieuwenhuijze MJ, de Jonge A, Korstjens I, Bude L, Lagro-Janssen TL. Influence on birthing positions affects women's sense of control in second stage of labour. *Midwifery* 2013;29(11):e107–14.

37. Begley CM, Gyte GM, Devane D, McGuire W, Weeks A. Active versus expectant management for women in the third stage of labour. *Cochrane Database of Systematic Reviews* (Online) 2011(11):CD007412.

38. McDonald SJ, Middleton P, Dowswell T, Morris PS. Effect of timing of umbilical cord clamping of term infants on maternal and neonatal outcomes. *Cochrane database of systematic reviews* (Online) 2013;7:CD004074.

SECTION FOUR

Late Pregnancy and Intrapartum Events

Chapter 44 Preterm labour

Myles Taylor and Stuart Rundle

INTRODUCTION

There are two major clinical subtypes of preterm births. *Indicated preterm deliveries*, undertaken for maternal or fetal reasons, make up approximately one third of all such births. The remaining two thirds are classified as *spontaneous preterm births* and have two subdivisions: spontaneous preterm labour and preterm pre-labour rupture of the membranes (PPROM).

DEFINITION

In the UK, preterm birth includes all deliveries between 24^{+0} and 36^{+6} weeks. Many developed countries now officially register all deliveries with a birthweight above 500 g. In 2011, 7.1 per cent of UK livebirths were preterm with 5.6 per cent of singletons and 53.1 per cent of multiple pregnancies delivering before 37 completed weeks of gestation. For reasons related to aetiology, outcome and recurrence risk, the WHO divides preterm deliveries into three gestational periods:

- moderate to late preterm births at 32^{+0} to 36^{+6} weeks (incidence 5.5 per cent);
- very preterm births at 28^{+0} to 31^{+6} weeks (incidence 0.7 per cent);
- extreme preterm births at 24^{+0} to 27^{+6} weeks (incidence 0.4 per cent).

Significantly higher rates of preterm birth of up to 12 per cent are reported from the United States. Conversely, many Nordic countries quote rates below 5 per cent. This must reflect differing aetiological, socio-economic and cultural factors.

NEONATAL OUTCOMES

Survival

When counselling parents, doctors must use perinatal statistics that are up to date and, where possible, reflect local outcomes. The UK Office for National Statistics (ONS) produces an annual report providing accurate, high-quality and up-to-date data regarding gestation-specific neonatal and infant mortality in England and Wales. In 2011, the overall infant mortality for preterm babies born between 24 and 37 weeks of gestation was 25.4 deaths per 1000 livebirths, compared with 1.5 deaths per 1000 livebirths for babies born at term, though the rates of mortality for preterm births are not linear (Fig. 44.1). Predicted survival can be modified by accurate estimates of fetal weight or antenatal assessments of fetal wellbeing.

Morbidity

The risks of later neurodevelopmental impairment, disability and handicap are especially significant within the 24–26-week gestational window. The UK-based EPIcure Study reported that 50 per cent of the survivors at 23–25 weeks' gestation were impaired, half with severe disability.[1] In another study, up to 40 per cent of survivors born before 26 weeks' gestation were found to have a head circumference below the third centile at two years of age, after which little 'catch-up' growth is possible.[2] Follow-up of very-low-birthweight children to school age has also shown later educational difficulties.[3] Additional concerns relate to social behaviour, as well as subsequent influences on adult health.

AETIOLOGY AND PATHOGENESIS

Several mechanisms are described for the pathogenesis of preterm birth. With the possible exception of true cervical weakness or incompetency, these mechanisms seem to share a final common pathway that involves up-regulation of prostaglandin production and the production of uterotonic agents and enzymes that weaken the fetal membrane and degrade cervical stroma. Activation of the fetal hypothalamic–pituitary–adrenal axis, long hypothesised as a potential initiating mechanism in normal labour, may also be implicated in preterm labour.

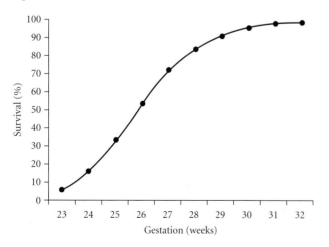

Fig. 44.1 Percentage predicted survival for European infants known to be alive at the onset of labour

Infection

Subclinical infection of the choriodecidual space and amniotic fluid is the most widely studied aetiological factor underlying spontaneous prematurity. Many indirect lines of evidence support the role of subclinical infection in human preterm labour, including the following:

- Vaginal colonisation with a variety of micro-organisms has been associated with an increased risk of spontaneous prematurity. However, it is plausible that the presence of such pathogens may simply be markers for other socio-economic, sexual or behavioural factors that ultimately lead to preterm labour.
- If an amniocentesis is performed in preterm labour with intact membranes, 10–15 per cent of amniotic fluid samples result in positive cultures.
- Histological chorioamnionitis is much more common after spontaneous preterm birth, with lower gestational ages having a higher likelihood of infection [A]. Of note, most cases are subclinical, with only 10 per cent of histologically proven cases of chorioamnionitis having overt clinical signs of infection.

Vascular

Spontaneous prematurity has been associated with an increase in membrane haemosiderin deposits, thought to reflect decidual haemorrhages. The link between placental abruption and either uterine activity or PPROM is well recognised.

Uterine over-distension

Multiple pregnancy and polyhydramnios are the most common causes of uterine distension. Myometrial stretch has been shown to result in up-regulation of oxytocin receptors and prostaglandin production. Stretch of the fetal membranes may also result in the formation of prostaglandins and other cytokines that are key to the initiation of labour.

Multiple pregnancy

In 2011, 1.6 per cent of all maternities in the UK involved multiple pregnancies, mostly twin pregnancies. The median gestation at delivery for twins is approximately 35 weeks and for triplets 33 weeks. Presently, assisted reproduction techniques (ART) are responsible for up to one third of twin pregnancies and three quarters of triplets, leading to an increasing burden of preterm births. The UK HFEA has strategies in place for reducing the number of multiple pregnancies resulting from ART to no more than 15 per cent of assisted conceptions. In those pregnancies affected by higher-order multiples, multifetal reduction has been shown to reduce the risk of preterm birth and should always be considered.

outcome for babies. It should certainly be considered where neonatal stabilisation would be difficult or impossible. It may also help to keep mother and baby together where transfer of the mother after delivery is likely to be difficult. All units should have guidelines for referral and communication.

FETAL ASSESSMENT

Maternal steroid therapy can suppress both fetal activity and heart rate variability. Umbilical artery Doppler studies can also be influenced. In fetuses with absent/reversed end diastolic flow (EDF), a short-term return of EDF is commonly observed.

When labour has started or is thought to be imminent:

- Whenever possible, the presentation in preterm labour should be confirmed by ultrasound, as clinical palpation is notoriously unreliable;
- An accurate estimated fetal weight, particularly below 28 weeks, can aid parental counselling.

There are considerable difficulties surrounding the interpretation of the FHR in preterm infants, particularly at extremely early gestations. Simply applying the criteria used at term is inappropriate. Some work has suggested that the baseline rate is more important than either decelerations or variability. Of note, RCTs have failed to show any benefit from continuous as opposed to intermittent monitoring in moderately preterm births [B].[26] Decisions regarding monitoring in labour at very preterm gestations must be discussed with parents. Intervention on the basis of FHR monitoring may not be justifiable near the limits of viability.

MODE OF DELIVERY

Many clinicians feel that fetal morbidity and mortality, the difficulty in diagnosing intrapartum hypoxia/acidosis and the maternal risk do not justify caesarean section for fetal indications below 26 weeks. At this early gestation, intrapartum caesarean section has not been shown to improve neonatal outcomes. As gestation advances, both neonatal outcomes and the ability to diagnose fetal compromise improve, and intervention for fetal reasons becomes universally appropriate. The safety of breech vaginal delivery is often questioned based on observational data suggesting an increased mortality and morbidity in the preterm breech born vaginally. However, there are recent similar studies that conclude the opposite.[27] Although the obstetric community agreed on the need for a well-conducted RCT to answer this question, this was not translated into recruitment when trials were attempted. A careful attempt at vaginal breech delivery, preferably under epidural analgesia, is not absolutely contraindicated [C].

Type of caesarean section

At the earliest gestations, the lower segment is poorly formed, often leading to vertical uterine incisions. A classical uterine incision carries up to a 12 per cent risk of uterine rupture in subsequent pregnancies, some of which will occur antenatally. The modified DeLee vertical lower segment incision does not appear to carry any greater risk than a conventional transverse incision and should be used in preference [D]. Alternatively, it is often possible to perform an en-caul delivery through a transverse incision if the membranes are left intact.

ANALGESIA

In terms of intrapartum analgesia, the use of epidural anaesthesia is frequently advocated. There has been little research on the subject. Postulated benefits include avoiding expulsive efforts before full dilatation or a precipitous delivery, a relaxed pelvic floor and perineum, and the ability to proceed quickly to abdominal delivery. Concerns are often expressed about the prolonged effects of narcotic analgesia on a preterm infant with limited metabolic capacity.

COMMUNICATION

There are two vital areas of communication in the management of women with threatened preterm labour:

1 communication with the woman and her family and
2 communication with the neonatal paediatricians.

Where possible, a clear management plan should be discussed with the parents. This should include monitoring in labour, potential interventions and what will happen to the baby afterwards. Involvement of the neonatal paediatricians is helpful, especially where there are difficult issues to cover, such as the management of an extremely preterm infant. Even when resuscitation would not be appropriate, parents often appreciate the opportunity to have discussed the care of their baby with the paediatricians. When labour does occur, it is vital to alert the neonatologists. Outcomes in very preterm infants have been shown to be improved if there is a senior paediatrician present at delivery. This can usually only be accomplished with some advanced warning.

SUMMARY

- Oral metronidazole significantly lowers the risk of preterm birth, by 60 per cent in high-risk women positive for bacterial vaginosis.
- Asymptomatic bacteriuria carries an increased risk of preterm birth; the risk is reduced by appropriate antibiotic treatment.

- Intrapartum antibiotics should be offered to women who are known to be colonised with GBS. Antenatal screening or treatment is not recommended.
- When based on historical factors alone, cervical cerclage improves outcomes only in women with three or more previous very early deliveries.
- Hospitalisation for bed rest leads to an increase in preterm births.
- Tocolytics have no significant benefit on perinatal mortality or the prolongation of pregnancy to term, but do reduce the number of women delivering within 48 hours by 40 per cent.
- A single course of maternal steroids given between 26 and 34 weeks' gestation and received within 7 days of delivery results in markedly improved neonatal outcomes.
- Maternal magnesium sulphate is beneficial in reducing the risk of cerebral palsy due to very or extreme preterm birth.
- There is no evidence of benefit and some evidence of harm associated with the use of antibiotics in uncomplicated preterm labour with intact membranes.

KEY POINTS

- Beneficial antenatal treatments for high-risk women include metronidazole for bacterial vaginosis, antibiotics for asymptomatic bacteriuria, cerclage for three or more second-trimester losses or very preterm births and progesterone supplementation.
- In symptomatic women, the following factors are associated with a high risk of delivery within 7 days: cervical dilatation >3 cm, ruptured membranes or any vaginal bleeding.
- A single course of corticosteroids should be given when delivery before 34 weeks is likely within the next 7 days. In general, repeat courses should be avoided, as they may carry risk without conferring benefit.
- Fetal fibronectin and cervical-length scanning can aid decision making in determining appropriate timing of maternal corticosteroid administration.
- After the diagnosis of preterm labour is confirmed, consideration should be given to the issues of neonatology consultation, fetal monitoring, mode of delivery and intrapartum antibiotics if a known GBS carrier, as well as administration of maternal magnesium sulphate.

Published Guidelines

American College of Obstetricians and Gynaecologists Practice Bulletin. Prediction and Prevention of Preterm birth. *Obstet Gynecol* 2012;120:964–73.

Australian National Health and Medical Research Council Clinical Practice Guideline. *Antenatal Magnesium Sulphate Prior to Preterm Birth for Neuroprotection of the Fetus, Infant and Child.* 2010. http://www.nhmrc.gov.au/guidelines/publications/cp128.

Position Statement of the Fetus and Newborn Committee, Canadian Paediatric Society. *Counselling and management of anticipated extremely preterm birth.* Oct 2012. http://www.cps.ca/en/documents/position/management-anticipated-extremely-preterm-birth.

RCOG. Scientific Impact Paper. *Magnesium Sulphate to Prevent Cerebral Palsy Following Preterm Birth.* London: RCOG Press, Sept 2011. www.rcog.org.uk.

RCOG. Clinical Guideline. *Preterm labour: tocolyhtic drugs.* London: RCOG Press, Feb 2011. www.rcog.org.uk.

RCOG. Clinical Guideline. *Antenatal Corticosteroids to Prevent Neonatal Morbidity.* London: RCOG Press, Oct 2010. www.rcog.org.uk.

RCOG. Clinical Guideline. *Cervical Cerclage.* London: RCOG Press, May 2011. www.rcog.org.uk.

Key References

1. Wood NS, Marlow N, Costeloe K, Gibson AT, Wilkinson AR. Neurologic and developmental disability after extremely preterm birth. EPICure Study Group. *N Engl J Med* 2000;343(6):378–84.
2. Bohin S, Draper ES, Field DJ. Health status of a population of infants born before 26 weeks' gestation derived from routine data collected between 21 and 27 months post-delivery. *Early Hum Dev* 1999;55(1):9–18.
3. Mercer BM, Goldenberg RL, Moawad AH *et al.* The preterm prediction study: effect of gestational age and cause of preterm birth on subsequent obstetric outcome. National Institute of Child Health and Human Development Maternal-Fetal Medicine Units Network. *Am J Obstet Gynecol* 1999;181:1216–21.
4. Rafael TJ, Hoffman MK, Leiby BE, *et al.* Gestational age of previous twin preterm birth as a predictor for subsequent singleton preterm birth. *Am J Obstet Gynecol* 2012;206:156.e1–6.
5. Schaaf J, Hof M, Mol B, Abu-Hanna A and Ravelli A. (2012), Recurrence risk of preterm birth in subsequent twin pregnancy after preterm singleton delivery. *BJOG* 2012;119:1624–9.
6. Kyrgiou M, Koliopoulos G, Martin-Hirsch P *et al.* Obstetric outcomes after conservative treatment for intraepithelial or early invasive cervical lesions: systematic review and meta-analysis. *Lancet* 2006; 367:489–98.
7. Hauth JC, Goldenberg RL, Andrews WW *et al.* Reduced incidence of preterm delivery with metronidazole and erythromycin in women with bacterial vaginosis. *N Engl J Med* 1995;333:1732–6.
8. Heath VC, Southall TR, Souka AP *et al.* Cervical length at 23 weeks of gestation: prediction of spontaneous preterm delivery. *Ultrasound Obstet Gynecol* 1998;12:312–17.
9. Medical Research Council/RCOG. Final report of the Medical Research Council/RCOG multicentre randomised trial of cervical cerclage. MRC/RCOG Working Party on Cervical Cerclage. *Br J Obstet Gynaecol* 1993;100:516–23.

10. Dodd JM, Jones L, Flenady V, Cincotta R, Crowther CA. Prenatal administration of progesterone for preventing preterm birth in women considered to be at risk of preterm birth. *Cochrane Database of Systematic Reviews* 2013;7:CD004947. DOI: 10.1002/14651858.CD004947. pub3.

11. ACOG Committee Opinion No. 419 October 2008. Use of progesterone to reduce preterm birth. *Obstet Gynecol* 2008;112:963–5.

12. Abdel-Aleem H, Shaaban OM, Abdel-Aleem MA. Cervical pessary for preventing preterm birth. *Cochrane Database of Systematic Reviews* 2013;5:CD007873. DOI: 10.1002/14651858.CD007873.pub3.

13. Goldenberg RL, Iams JD, Mercer BM *et al.* The preterm prediction study: the value of new vs standard risk factors in predicting early and all spontaneous preterm births. NICHD MFMU Network. *Am J Public Health* 1998; 88:233–8.

14. Iams JD, Casal D, McGregor JA *et al.* Fetal fibronectin improves the accuracy of diagnosis of preterm labor. *Am J Obstet Gynecol* 1995;173:141–5.

15. Abbott DS, Radford SK, Seed PT *et al.* Evaluation of a quantitative fetal fibronectin test for spontaneous preterm birth in symptomatic women. *Am J Obstet Gynecol* 2013;208:122.e1–6.

16. Rizzo G, Capponi A, Arduini D *et al.* The value of fetal fibronectin in cervical and vaginal secretions and of ultrasonographic examination of the uterine cervix in predicting premature delivery for patients with preterm labor and intact membranes. *Am J Obstet Gynecol* 1996;175:1146–51.

17. Wapner RJ, Sorokin Y, Mele L *et al.* Long-term outcomes after repeat doses of antenatal corticosteroids. *N Engl J Med* 2007;357:1190–8.

18. Murphy KE, Hannah ME, Willan AR *et al.* Multiple courses of antenatal corticosteroids for preterm birth (MACS): a randomised controlled trial. *Lancet* 2008;372:2143–51.

19. Banks BA, Cnaan A, Morgan MA *et al.* Multiple courses of antenatal corticosteroids and outcome of premature neonates. North American Thyrotropin-Releasing Hormone Study Group. *Am J Obstet Gynecol* 1999;181:709–17.

20. Doyle LW, Crowther CA, Middleton P, Marret S, Rouse D. Magnesium sulphate for women at risk of preterm birth for neuroprotection of the fetus. *Cochrane Database of Systematic Reviews* 2009;1: CD004661. DOI: 10.1002/14651858.CD004661.pub3.

21. Australian Research Centre for Health of Women and Babies. Antenatal Magnesium Sulphate Prior to Preterm Birth for Neuroprotection of the Fetus, Infant and Child – National Clinical Practice Guidelines. Adelaide. ARCH; 2010 [www.adelaide.edu.au/arch/].

22. The Canadian Preterm Labor Investigators Group. Treatment of preterm labor with the beta-adrenergic agonist ritodrine. *N Engl J Med* 1992;327:308–12.

23. Kenyon SL, Taylor DJ, Tarnow-Mordi W. Broad spectrum antibiotics for spontaneous preterm labour: the ORACLE II randomised trial. ORACLE Collaborative Group. *Lancet* 2001;357:989–94.

24. Kenyon S, Pike K, Jones DR *et al.* Childhood outcomes after prescription of antibiotics to pregnant women with spontaneous preterm labour: 7-year follow-up of the ORACLE II trial. *Lancet* 2008;372:1319–27.

25. Kenyon S, Pike K, Jones DR *et al.* Childhood outcomes after prescription of antibiotics to pregnant women with preterm rupture of the membranes: 7-year follow-up of the ORACLE I trial. *Lancet* 2008;372:1310–18.

26. Shy KK, Luthy DA, Bennett FC *et al.* Effects of electronic fetal-heart-rate monitoring, as compared with periodic auscultation, on the neurologic development of premature infants. *N Engl J Med* 1990;322:588–93.

27. Wolf H, Schaap AH, Bruinse HW *et al.* Vaginal delivery compared with caesarean section in early preterm breech delivery: a comparison of long-term outcome. *Br J Obstet Gynaecol* 1999;106:486–91.

Chapter 45 Pre-labour rupture of the membranes

Myles Taylor and Stuart Rundle

MRCOG standards

- Candidates should be able to diagnose and manage rupture of the membranes in term and preterm pregnancies.

In addition, we would suggest the following:

Theoretical skills

- Understand the changes in amniotic fluid volume at different gestational ages.
- Understand the physical and biochemical properties of amniotic fluid that can be used diagnostically.
- Be aware of the risks associated with pre-labour rupture of the membranes (PROM), both at term and preterm.
- Have a thorough knowledge of the management options for PROM at term.
- Know the organisms likely to cause chorioamnionitis along with their appropriate antibiotic therapies.

Practical skills

- Be able to confirm membrane rupture using clinical history, examination and specialised tests.
- Assess amniotic fluid volume using ultrasound.
- Be able to diagnose clinical chorioamnionitis by examination and additional testing.

INTRODUCTION

PROM is a common clinical problem, and the assessment of women with possible membrane rupture is a management issue faced in everyday practice. When PROM occurs, the fetus loses the relative isolation and protection afforded within the amniotic cavity. In general, PROM refers to rupture of the membranes with leakage of amniotic fluid in the absence of uterine activity. Pre-term PROM (PPROM) occurs when rupture of membranes occurs before 37 weeks' gestation. At term, approximately 75 per cent of women will labour within 24 hours of membrane rupture. The latency period tends to be longer with decreasing gestational age: at 26 weeks, only half of women are in labour within 1 week; at 32 weeks, half will labour within 24–48 hours.

INCIDENCE

PROM occurs in approximately 8 per cent of term pregnancies and complicates 2–3 per cent of pregnancies that have not reached 37 weeks' gestation. PPROM is associated with approximately one third of all deliveries before 37 weeks' gestation. It is important to make a distinction between term PROM and PPROM, as the conditions have different aetiologies, risks and recommended management plans.

AETIOLOGY

The pathophysiology of PROM is not well understood but probably includes a variety of mechanical, infective and constitutional mechanisms.[1] The main risk factors for PPROM include a history of PPROM in a previous pregnancy, genital tract infection, antepartum bleeding and smoking.[2]

Term PROM

Rupture of the membranes at term usually reflects physiological (as opposed to pathophysiological) processes. Apoptosis (programmed cell death) refers to the natural deterioration and breakdown of cells and cellular structure over time. The role of apoptosis in PROM has attracted considerable research interest. As term approaches, uterine activity is known to increase and Braxton–Hicks contractions are prominent. Such repetitive stretching of the membranes may lead to weakening via several mechanisms. First, it induces focal thinning of the membranes. Second, it leads to strain hardening, a biomechanical phenomenon associated with materials becoming less elastic and less able to withstand stress. Such stretch-induced weakening will be most likely at the internal cervical os, where physiological ripening of the cervix will allow a degree of membrane prolapse.

PPROM

In contrast to the 'natural' phenomenon occurring at term, PPROM usually has pathological origins. Ascending infection appears to be one of the major causes and appears to be a more frequent aetiology than in preterm labour with intact membranes. That chorioamnionitis can be associated with preterm PROM is easily understood. As with preterm labour, the majority of these infections are subclinical and give few signs or symptoms until fluid loss has occurred.

Another factor strongly linked with PPROM is antepartum haemorrhage, particularly when it occurs recurrently. A weak cervix can also predispose to early membrane rupture. It will fail as a barrier to ascending infection and, by allowing membrane prolapse, will allow localised biomechanical weakening, as described for term PROM.

There is a strong epidemiological link between maternal smoking and PPROM, which is dose dependent. As smoking is a modifiable behaviour and a reduction in smoking has been shown to reduce risk, this should be pointed out to women, particularly those with a history of PPROM in a previous pregnancy.

CLINICAL ASSESSMENT

The correct diagnosis of PROM, either preterm or at term, is crucial. Many interventions will be based upon the diagnosis. If undertaken unnecessarily, these interventions will undoubtedly increase maternal and fetal morbidity.

History

A history from the mother of 'a gush of fluid' followed by recurrent dampness will correctly identify over 90 per cent of cases of pre-labour membrane rupture.[3]

Examination

PROM should be confirmed by a sterile speculum examination, performed after the mother has rested supine for 20–30 minutes. Amniotic fluid can be seen pooling in the posterior fornix, either spontaneously or after fundal pressure. The presence of meconium should be noted. At preterm gestations, meconium is suggestive but not diagnostic of intra-amniotic infection; at term, it is a relative contraindication to expectant management. The absence of any pooling is an equally important finding. The cervix can usually also be seen, allowing assessment of length and dilatation.

A digital examination must be avoided unless the patient is thought to be in established labour, as it is known to increase the incidence of:

- chorioamnionitis;
- postpartum endometritis;
- neonatal infection.

A digital examination also decreases the length of the latent period before the onset of labour, with the greatest decreases seen at the earliest gestations.[4]

Point-of-care testing

Concern about the consequences of misdiagnosing true PROM has led investigators to seek secondary tests that can be used at presentation. Two common tests use either nitrazine sticks (relying on the higher alkaline pH of amniotic fluid) or the ferning pattern seen when amniotic fluid is dried onto a glass slide and then viewed under a microscope. Importantly, neither of these tests has been shown to be more reliable than a basic history and examination.[3] Both have appreciable false-positive and false-negative rates, which appear to be further increased in women with prior negative speculum examinations. While potentially useful as an adjunct in the diagnosis of PROM in resource-poor settings, their use has largely been superseded by the introduction and commercial availability of more specialised and technologically advanced tests that are rapidly able to detect amniotic fluid proteins present in cervico-vaginal discharge at the point of presentation.

The two most commonly used bedside tests able to detect the presence of amniotic fluid proteins utilise the high concentration of either insulin-like growth factor binding protein-1 (IGFBP-1) or placental alpha micro-globulin-1 (PAMG-1) within amniotic fluid compared to other body fluids. Both tests have appreciably lower false-positive and false-negative rates than that achievable with history and examination alone. A recent meta-analysis of prospective cohort studies comparing IGFBP-1 and PAMG-1 in the diagnosis of PPROM reported a sensitivity and specificity of 96.0 per cent and 98.9 per cent respectively for the PAMG-1 test.[5]

Fetal fibronectin is a protein found at the chorio-decidual junction rather than being found in high concentration in amniotic fluid. Testing for presence of fFN is commonly used to determine the risk of preterm labour in women with intact membranes and has been postulated for use in the diagnosis of PROM. fFN testing has been shown to become negative in some women after membranes have been ruptured for more than 12 hours if liquor is not seen on speculum examination. It should be noted that none of these technologically advanced tests for the detection of PROM have been evaluated against the true gold standard for the detection of PROM: the amnio-dye test.

If diagnostic uncertainty remains following presentation, clinical assessment and point-of-care testing, repeated dry pads argue against the diagnosis while the use of pads which change colour when in contact with fluids with a pH >5.2 are now available.[6]

Ultrasound

Amniotic fluid volume can be assessed by ultrasound. Even at term, the normal variation in directly measured AFV is considerable, ranging from 250 to 1200 mL, making ultrasound diagnosis of reduced AFV a non-specific test for the detection of PROM. As the variation in AFV can be much greater in preterm gestations, the diagnostic role of ultrasound in PPROM is very limited. Despite this, the ultrasound assessment of AFV has been reported to correlate with latency in PPROM and with neonatal mortality and morbidity in mid-trimester PROM.

Misdiagnosed PROM

The improvement in detection of PROM in clinically equivocal cases brought about by specialised bedside tests is likely to result in a fall in the incidence of misdiagnosed PROM. Ladfors *et al.*[7] have studied the outcome of women presenting with possible PROM after 34 weeks' gestation in whom amniotic fluid could not be seen on speculum examination. Vaginal samples were taken and blindly analysed later for diamine oxidase, an enzyme that is absent from urine or vaginal secretions but present in large amounts in amniotic fluid. Of the women with negative speculum examinations, 12 per cent tested positive for diamine oxidase. Nearly 90 per cent of these diamine oxidase-positive women went into labour within 48 hours, compared to only 45 per cent of the diamine oxidase-negative women. Crucially, no difference in maternal or neonatal outcome was seen between the two groups. This suggests that a delay in the diagnosis of PROM in women with an initially negative speculum examination is of no clinical consequence [C].

CLINICAL MANAGEMENT

Term PROM

A clinician with experience of diagnosing membrane rupture should assess women reporting a history suggestive of PROM at or beyond 37 completed weeks of gestation. Whether this assessment should take place immediately or after a suitable delay, in which labour may establish, has not been the subject of extensive research. The predominant risk to the fetus after PROM at term is ascending infection. The risks to the mother are of uterine infection, via either chorioamnionitis or postpartum endometritis.

A 2006 systematic review of 12 randomised or quasi-randomised trials of women with term PROM compared immediate intervention to expectant management[8] and found that the former was associated with a reduction in the rate of maternal infection and neonatal unit admission without an increase in the risk of caesarean section or operative vaginal delivery [A]. The results were limited by the heterogeneity of the included studies, the largest of which was the Canadian TERMPROM Study.[9] This study and subsequent secondary analyses[10-14] have provided considerable evidence to share with prospective parents.

The trial compared four management policies, namely immediate induction with intravenous oxytocin, immediate induction with vaginal prostaglandins, expectant management for up to 4 days followed by induction with oxytocin, or expectant management followed by induction with vaginal prostaglandins. The absolute risks associated with any policy were found to be small. Table 45.1 outlines the differences in labour outcome among the four management policies. None reached statistical significance. In Table 45.2, the risks of maternal and neonatal infection are reviewed. Although clear trends are obvious in these tables, readers are referred to the original publication for tests of significance. Four points from the original trial are worthy of separate mention.

Table 45.1 Delivery outcomes after membrane rupture at term, TERMPROM Study[9]

	Immediate induction		Expectant management	
	Oxytocin (%)	Prostaglandin (%)	Oxytocin (%)	Prostaglandin (%)
C-sect (overall)	10.1	9.6	9.7	10.9
C-sect (multiparous)	4.3	3.5	3.9	4.6
C-sect (nulliparous)	14.1	13.7	13.7	15.2
C-sect (nulliparous, unfavourable cervix)	14.8	14.1	15.0	14.9
SVD, nulliparous	60.8	60.8	58.0	58.9
Use of oxytocin	91.9	43.1	49.9	43.8
PROM–delivery interval	17.2 hours	23.0 hours	33.3 hours	32.6 hours

- C-sect, caesarean section; SVD, spontaneous vaginal delivery; PROM, pre-labour rupture of membranes.

Table 45.2 Perinatal infectious morbidity after membrane rupture at term, TERMPROM study[9]

	Immediate induction		Expectant management	
	Oxytocin (%)	Prostaglandin (%)	Oxytocin (%)	Prostaglandin (%)
Fever before or during labour	3.8	5.8	8.7	6.7
Antibiotics before or during labour	7.5	9.0	11.9	11.6
Postpartum fever	1.9	3.1	3.6	3.0
Neonatal infection	2.0	3.0	2.8	2.7
Neonatal antibiotics	7.5	10.9	13.7	12.2
NICU stay >24 hours	6.6	9.2	11.6	10.2

- NICU, neonatal intensive care unit.

1 The use of prostaglandins did not reduce the subsequent need for oxytocin; this was no different between the two groups randomised to prostaglandins and the expectantly managed group randomised to induction with oxytocin.

2 Only a minority of women (approximately 18 per cent) randomised to expectant management waited 4 days before induction.

3 The four babies that unexpectedly died in the trial were all in the expectant management arms. Two were antepartum stillbirths and two were related to fetal distress in advanced labour, both of which started spontaneously.

4 The views of the women participating in the trial showed a preference for immediate induction, as opposed to expectant management.

A more recent, large retrospective cohort study[15] examining dichotomised time thresholds for significant increases in the risk of infective sequelae of PROM at term found that a latency of greater than 12 hours was associated with a significantly increased risk of chorioamnionitis (OR 2.3, 95% CI 1.1–4.4); however, once again it should be emphasised that the absolute risk remained small (1.3% incidence before 12 hours vs 3.3% after). Similar small risk increases were demonstrated for maternal endometritis at a threshold of 16 hours and PPH at a threshold of 8 hours.

Later publications from the TERMPROM investigators showed that the least expensive policy was immediate induction of labour using oxytocin.[14] In terms of where to undertake expectant management, the evidence suggested an increased risk of infection and caesarean section when women were allowed home. If this was translated into clinical practice, and women needed to remain in hospital, it would clearly increase the cost of expectant management further. In contrast, maternal satisfaction, particularly amongst multiparous women, was greater with management at home.[12]

Regardless of whether a policy of immediate induction or expectant management is pursued, factors linked with perinatal infection include an increasing number of vaginal examinations after membrane rupture, an increasing interval between membrane rupture and labour onset, and an increasing duration of active labour.[10,11] There is also clear evidence that immediate induction of labour using oxytocin should be recommended for women who are known to be colonised with GBS [B].[13] Expectant management in this situation was associated with a 3–4-fold increase in risk of neonatal infection, and even immediate induction with prostaglandins failed to lower this.

In general, the evidence suggests that immediate induction is associated with less maternal and neonatal infection and a shorter interval from membrane rupture to delivery [A] but given the small risk differences personal preference should be given considerable influence. There is no evidence that mode of delivery is influenced by induction of labour in the context of term PROM. When oxytocin is used initially, healthcare costs are lower and the interval to delivery is shortest. However, meta-analysis has suggested that the use of epidural analgesia is increased [A]. When prostaglandins are used initially, infection risks may be marginally greater, the interval to delivery slightly increased, and oxytocin required subsequently in nearly half of the women [A].

Preterm PROM

The major risks in preterm PROM are:

- chorioamnionitis;
- abruption;
- preterm delivery.

Other risks include cord prolapse and operative delivery. Many tests have been used to predict chorioamnionitis, which is usually subclinical. Serum markers, such as white cell count and C-reactive protein, have a poor predictive ability and should principally be used to support a clinical diagnosis. Oligohydramnios, as assessed by ultrasound, can select a group at higher risk of infection and/or earlier delivery, but again is not diagnostic. Amniocentesis can give valuable information but remains technically difficult when little amniotic fluid remains and is not recommended practice in the UK.

In contrast to preterm labour with intact membranes, transvaginal ultrasound measurements of cervical length are not predictive of early delivery. As well as PPROM being a common sequela of antepartum haemorrhage, early membrane rupture carries a 5 per cent risk of subsequent abruption. However, this risk varies inversely with gestational age and is reportedly as high as 50 per cent below 24 weeks.[16]

Although neonates born after PPROM are reported to have lower incidences of respiratory distress syndrome when compared to preterm labour without PROM, maternal steroids still appear to reduce the risk further [A]. There does not appear to be any significant increase in maternal sepsis after single steroid courses. Despite the fetal and maternal risks associated with PPROM there is evidence that intentional delivery prior to 34 weeks of gestation does not reduce maternal or neonatal morbidity and may be associated with additional risks to the fetus.[17] Tocolytics are relatively contraindicated in this situation and are known to be less effective.

Antibiotic therapy for PPROM

The UK ORACLE I Trial demonstrated a role for oral erythromycin in PPROM.[18] In this study, women with PPROM were randomised to one of four oral regimes:

1 Erythromycin (250 mg qds);
2 Co-amoxiclav (325 mg qds);
3 Both erythromycin (250 mg qds) and co-amoxiclav (325 mg qds);
4 Placebo.

The antibiotics were taken for 10 days. In singleton pregnancies, erythromycin alone was associated with a significant reduction (from 14.4 to 11.2 per cent) in the composite primary outcome, a measure of neonatal mortality and major morbidity [B]. The reductions with either co-amoxiclav or both antibiotics failed to reach significance. Unfortunately, the 10-day course of co-amoxiclav led to a significant increase in proven neonatal necrotising enterocolitis, from 0.5 to 1.9 per cent. Once again, antibiotics have been demonstrated to have the potential for harm. In contrast to those in preterm labour with intact membranes, 7-year follow-up of those children prescribed antibiotics for PPROM in the Oracle I Trial did not show any functional impairment.[19] Thus the prophylactic use of erythromycin is currently recommended when PPROM is diagnosed (RCOG guideline number 44).

Chorioamnionitis remains a notoriously difficult diagnosis. For research purposes, it requires:

- maternal pyrexia (>38°C), and at least two of either:
- maternal tachycardia >100 bpm;
- fetal tachycardia >160 bpm;
- uterine tenderness;

- raised C-reactive protein;
- offensive vaginal discharge.

When clinically suspected, delivery is almost always appropriate, as antibiotic therapy is rarely curative. Based on the culture results after amniocentesis in PPROM, anaerobes are the most common isolate, followed by GBS and then other streptococci.

The care of women known to be GBS carriers has been simplified by the ORACLE Trial, as the organism is usually sensitive to erythromycin. After completion of a 10-day course, further antibiotics should probably be withheld until labour starts.

There are two gestational age ranges that require special consideration.

Pre-viable PROM below 23–24 weeks' gestation

Lung development has reached a critical stage and appears to be at least partly reliant on normal amniotic fluid volumes. There are significant risks of lethal pulmonary hypoplasia, a condition that cannot be reliably predicted on prenatal ultrasound. These risks are highest early in the mid-trimester and when severe oligohydramnios is found on serial ultrasound monitoring. As there are additional risks of chronic pulmonary morbidity, fetal limb contractures and extreme preterm birth with consequent co-existent morbidity and mortality, many parents will opt for termination of pregnancy.

Researchers have investigated the role of minimally invasive surgery and membrane sealants in this situation, as the prognosis is otherwise very poor, but results have proved disappointing.

PPROM at 34–37 weeks' gestation

This is another controversial area. Randomised trials have failed to reach a consensus on whether a policy of IOL versus expectant management may lead to fewer adverse pregnancy outcomes such as hospitalisation, perinatal infection and neonatal morbidity. A 2010 Cochrane review concluded that there was insufficient evidence to guide practice on the benefits and harms of immediate delivery versus expectant management in late preterm PROM.[20] Two recent large randomised trials have sought specifically to address the question of IOL versus expectant management between 34 and 37 weeks' gestation. The Dutch PPROMEXIL (PPROM Expectant Management versus IOL) trial group failed to show a reduction in adverse neonatal outcome following IOL versus expectant management between 34 and 37 weeks' gestation.[21] The international multicentre PPROMT (Preterm Pre-labour Rupture of Membranes Close to Term) trial has yet to report its findings.

Inpatient versus outpatient care

For some women who rupture membranes early, without immediately ensuing labour, the dilemma of best place of management must be considered. There are no good trials to inform practice. As it is recognised that 48–72 hours is a critical time during which many women will labour or develop clinical chorioamnionitis, it is recommended that all women with PPROM be managed as inpatients during this time. After this, a decision to change to outpatient management must be taken at consultant level. Women must know the potential risks and be educated in measurement of their temperature and signs and symptoms of developing chorioamnionitis. It is suggested that women measure their temperature twice daily (RCOG guideline 44).

Neither umbilical artery Doppler analysis nor biophysical testing has proven effective at early identification of the infected fetus. However, given that PPROM is associated with growth restriction, monitoring of fetal growth by ultrasound seems reasonable.

ACKNOWLEDGEMENT

This chapter has been revised and updated. The authors and editors acknowledge the contribution of Griff Jones to the chapter on this topic in a previous edition of the book.

KEY POINTS

- At term, the outcomes for women with PROM are as good in women induced immediately as in those managed conservatively. Where possible, women should be offered the choice.
- At term, women known to be colonised with GBS should be encouraged to allow immediate induction of labour using oxytocin after PROM.
- At term, early induction using oxytocin appears to reduce perinatal infection and shorten hospital stay without increasing operative intervention. It should be strongly recommended to women known to be GBS positive.
- Immediate induction is associated with increased use of epidural analgesia.
- Maternal steroid use in PPROM reduces the risk of respiratory distress syndrome.
- Erythromycin used for 10 days after PPROM is associated with a significant reduction (from 14.4 per cent to 11.2 per cent) in neonatal mortality and major morbidity.
- Co-amoxiclav when used for PPROM leads to a significant increase in proven neonatal necrotising enterocolitis, from 0.5 per cent to 1.9 per cent.
- Term PROM is usually a reflection of normal physiology, whereas pathological processes, such as infection and antepartum haemorrhage, often underlie PPROM.

- Accurate diagnosis of membrane rupture is essential and can usually be achieved by simple history and speculum examination alone.
- Diagnostic uncertainty following clinical examination can be resolved with the use of specialised bedside tests that detect amniotic fluid proteins in cervico-vaginal secretions.
- A digital vaginal examination should always be avoided after PPROM unless advanced labour is suspected.

Published Guidelines

NICE, CG70. *Induction of Labour.* London: RCOG, July 2008.
RCOG Evidence-based Clinical Guideline Number 44. *Preterm pre-labour rupture of membranes.* London: RCOG, November 2006 (Minor amendment October 2010).

Key References

1. French JI, McGregor JA. The pathobiology of premature rupture of membranes. *Semin Perinatol* 1996;20(5):344–68.
2. Harger JH, Hsing AW, Tuomala RE *et al.* Risk factors for preterm premature rupture of fetal membranes: a multicenter case-control study. *Am J Obstet Gynecol* 1990;163(1 Pt 1):130–7.
3. Friedman ML, McElin TW. Diagnosis of ruptured fetal membranes. Clinical study and review of the literature. *Am J Obstet Gynecol* 1969;104(4):544–50.
4. Lewis DF, Major CA, Towers CV, Asrat T, Harding JA, Garite TJ. Effects of digital vaginal examinations on latency period in preterm premature rupture of membranes. *Obstet Gynecol* 1992;80(4):630–4.
5. Ramsauer B, Vidaeff AC, Hosli I *et al.* The diagnosis of rupture of fetal membranes (ROM): a meta-analysis. *J Perinat Med* 2013 May; 41(3):233–40.
6. Mulhair L, Carter J, Poston L, Seed P, Briley A. Prospective cohort study investigating the reliability of the AmnioSense method for detection of spontaneous rupture of membranes. *BJOG* 2009;116(2):313–8.
7. Ladfors L, Mattsson LA, Eriksson M, Fall O. Is a speculum examination sufficient for excluding the diagnosis of ruptured fetal membranes? *Acta Obstet Gynecol Scand* 1997;76(8):739–42.
8. Dare MR, Middleton P, Crowther CA, Flenady V, Varatharaju B. Planned early birth versus expectant management (waiting) for premature membrane rupture at term (37 weeks or more). *Cochrane Database Syst Rev* 2006;CD005302.
9. Hannah ME, Ohlsson A, Farine D *et al.* Induction of labor compared with expectant management for prelabor rupture of the membranes at term. TERMPROM Study Group. *N Engl J Med* 1996;334(16):1005–10.
10. Seaward PG, Hannah ME, Myhr TL *et al.* International Multicentre Term Prelabor Rupture of Membranes Study:

evaluation of predictors of clinical chorioamnionitis and postpartum fever in patients with prelabor rupture of membranes at term. *Am J Obstet Gynecol* 1997;177(5):1024–9.

11. Seaward PG, Hannah ME, Myhr TL *et al.* International multicenter term PROM study: evaluation of predictors of neonatal infection in infants born to patients with premature rupture of membranes at term. Premature Rupture of the Membranes. *Am J Obstet Gynecol* 1998;179(3 Pt 1):635–9.

12. Hannah ME, Hodnett ED, Willan A, Foster GA, Di Cecco R, Helewa M. Prelabor rupture of the membranes at term: expectant management at home or in hospital? The TermPROM Study Group. *Obstet Gynecol* 2000;96(4):533–8.

13. Hannah ME, Ohlsson A, Wang EE *et al.* Maternal colonization with group B *Streptococcus* and prelabor rupture of membranes at term: the role of induction of labor. TermPROM Study Group. *Am J Obstet Gynecol* 1997;177(4):780–5.

14. Gafni A, Goeree R, Myhr TL *et al.* Induction of labour versus expectant management for prelabour rupture of the membranes at term: an economic evaluation. TERMPROM Study Group. Term Prelabour Rupture of the Membranes. *CMAJ* 1997;157(11):1519–25.

15. Tran SH, Cheng YW, Kaimal AJ, Caughey AB. Length of rupture of membranes in the setting of premature rupture of membranes at term and infectious maternal morbidity. *Am J Obstet Gynaecol* 2008;198:700.e1–700.e5

16. Holmgren PA, Olofsson JI. Preterm premature rupture of membranes and the associated risk for placental abruption. Inverse correlation to gestational length. *Acta Obstet Gynecol Scand* 1997;76(8):743–7.

17. Al-Mandeel H Alhindi MY, Suave R. Effects of intentional delivery on maternal and neonatal outcomes in pregnancies with preterm prelabour rupture of membranes between 28 and 34 weeks of gestation: a systematic review and meta-analysis. *J Mater Fetal Neonatal Med* 2013;26:83–9.

18. Kenyon SL, Taylor DJ, Tarnow-Mordi W. Broad-spectrum antibiotics for preterm, prelabour rupture of fetal membranes: the ORACLE I randomised trial. ORACLE Collaborative Group. *Lancet* 2001;357(9261):979–88.

19. Kenyon S, Pike K, Jones DR *et al.* Childhood outcomes after prescription of antibiotics to pregnant women with preterm rupture of the membranes: 7-year follow-up of the ORACLE I trial. *Lancet* 2008;372(9646):1310–18.

20. Buchanan SL, Crowther CA, Levett KM, Middleton P, Morris J. Planned early birth versus expectant management for women with preterm pre-labour rupture of membranes prior to 37 weeks' gestation for improving pregnancy outcome. *Cochrane Database Syst Rev* 2010;CD004735.

21. van der Ham DP, van der Heyden JL, Opmeer BC *et al.* Management of late-preterm premature rupture of membranes: the PPROMEXIL-2 trial. *Am J Obstet Gynecol* 2012;207:276.e1–10.

Chapter 46 Antepartum haemorrhage

Lucy Kean

INTRODUCTION

Definitions

Antepartum haemorrhage (APH) is variously described as bleeding from the genital tract in pregnancy before the onset of labour at gestations from 20 to 24 weeks. Between 20 and 24 weeks management may be broadly the same, except delivery will rarely be expedited. The recent guideline produced by the RCOG uses 24 weeks as a starting gestation.[1] For the purposes of this chapter, the threshold of 20 weeks will be used, as this is often the gestation at which women will be admitted to the labour suite rather than the gynaecology ward.

APH is one of the commonest reasons for admission in pregnancy. It affects approximately 4 per cent of all pregnancies and is associated with increased rates of fetal and maternal morbidity and mortality.

Minor bleeding is defined as less than 50 mL that has settled; major bleeding is 50–1000 mL with no sign of clinical shock; massive haemorrhage is blood loss of >1000 mL and/or signs of clinical shock.

Recurrent APH is bleeding on more than one occasion.

Aetiology

The causes of APH can be divided into three main groups:

- Placenta praevia;
- Placental abruption;
- Local causes:
  - friable cervical ectropion/cervical trauma
  - local infection of the cervix/vagina
  - genital tract tumours
  - varicosities;
- Others:
  - marginal placental bleeding
  - show
  - vasa praevia;
- Undetermined.

Placenta praevia and abruption together account for 50 per cent of bleeding and represent the greatest threat to the fetus and mother. However, despite the other causes appearing to be more minor (with the exception of vasa praevia) these carry an increased perinatal mortality of at least 3 per cent, and must therefore represent a group of pathological conditions. When the cause is unexplained, there remains an increased risk of fetal growth being poorer. Thus all APH must be fully investigated and evaluated.

PLACENTA PRAEVIA

The incidence of placenta praevia is variable depending on the population and background caesarean section rate, with rates from 0.4 to 0.8 per cent reported. In the UK rates are rising as the CS rate rises and the age of mothers increases.[2]

Definitions

Placenta praevia is defined as a placenta partially or wholly situated in the lower uterine segment. It is most usefully graded as minor or major depending on whether the placenta covers the internal os or not.

- Grade 1: the placental edge is in the lower segment but does not reach the internal os.
- Grade 2: the placental edge reaches but does not cover the internal os.

  These grades represent a minor degree of placenta praevia.

- Grade 3: the placenta covers the internal os and is asymmetrically situated.
- Grade 4: the placenta covers the internal os and is centrally situated.

  These grades represent a major placenta praevia.

Aetiology

Uterine surgery

Placenta praevia is strongly associated with previous uterine surgery. Its incidence increases with the number of procedures performed (Table 46.1) [C].[2]

Women with two or more previous abortions have a 2.1 (95% CI 1.2–3.5)-times increased risk of subsequently developing placenta praevia. Other procedures such as curettage and submucous myomectomy also increase the risks of praevia.

Maternal age

Placenta praevia increases dramatically with advancing maternal age, with women older than 40 years having a nearly 9-fold greater risk than women under the age of 20, after adjustment for potential confounders, including parity [C].

Smoking

The relationship between smoking and placenta praevia is not clear but there does appear to be a small but significant increase in risk in smokers.

Assisted conception

The risk is significantly higher in assisted-conception pregnancies with an odds ratio of 5.6 (95%CI 4.4–7) reported [C].[3]

Multiparity appears to increase the risk, as does a multiple pregnancy.

Associations

- Fetal abnormality: the rate of fetal abnormality is approximately doubled in women with placenta praevia [C].
- IUGR is common in women with multiple bleeds from a placenta praevia. The overall rate is 15 per cent [C].
- Ten per cent of women with a bleeding placenta praevia will have a coexistent abruption [C].

Diagnosis

- In most women, the placental site will have been determined at the anomaly scan, and may be known to be low-lying at the time of bleeding. Placenta praevia usually presents with painless bleeding (though 10 per cent will have concurrent abruption).
- Often a small bleed or number of small bleeds will precede a much larger one (though this is not always the case).
- The presenting part is usually high, being prevented from engaging by the placenta lying in the lower segment.
- The fetal condition generally remains good until the maternal blood loss causes compromise, or an abruption coexists.

It is difficult to diagnose a placenta praevia until the lower segment begins to form at about 28 weeks; however, a low-lying placenta can cause bleeding from the second trimester onwards.

Placental-site location is now a recommended part of the fetal anomaly screening examination in the UK, and cases are now detected on routine ultrasound at 18–21 weeks. Five per cent of women have ultrasound evidence of a low placenta at 16–18 weeks, but only 0.5 per cent have a placenta praevia at delivery. Transabdominal ultrasound is usually the test first performed, although it can be very difficult to determine the placental edge with a posterior placenta.

Table 46.1 The relationship between placenta praevia and caesarean section

Number of previous caesarean sections	Incidence of placenta praevia (%) [total 0.3%]	Incidence of placenta accreta in those with placenta praevia (%)	Overall risk of placenta accreta (%)
0	0.26	5	0.01
1	0.65	24	0.16
2	1.8	47	0.85
3	3	40	1.2
4	10	67	6.7

Transvaginal imaging is better and the woman does not need a full bladder, thus avoiding maternal discomfort. Also there is less distortion of the anatomy of the lower uterine segment and cervix. Transvaginal ultrasound (TVS) does not appear to provoke vaginal bleeding [B].[2] TVS should be performed at the routine anomaly scan at 18–21 weeks as it will reduce the need for third-trimester repeat scanning in 20–60 per cent of women.

MRI has also been used to identify placenta praevia, though it is expensive and not superior to TVS performed by an experienced person.

The following factors on second-trimester ultrasound are associated with the persistence of a placenta praevia in the third trimester:

- The placenta covers the internal os with an overlap of more than 1.5 cm [C].[4]
- The leading edge of the placenta is thick [C].[5]
- The placenta is posterior.
- There is a uterine scar.

Morbidly adherent placenta

Morbidly adherent placentae occur in approximately 1 in 200–400 deliveries in the USA and 1 in 800 deliveries in the UK. The major risk factor is uterine scarring, and thus the incidence is increasing with the increasing caesarean section rate. However, prior manual removal, submucous myomectomy or uterine curettage may also cause scarring and an increase in risk. A short caesarean section-to-conception interval has also been causally related.

Three degrees of adherence have been described: accreta, increta and percreta, where the placenta adheres to or invades into or through the uterine wall because of abnormal development of the decidua basalis.

Accreta is the most common, comprising 80 per cent. PPH will occur in most cases, particularly if the accreta is partial, where non-contracted portions of myometrium are adjacent to adherent placenta. Diagnosis in an increasing number of cases is made antenatally[6] but still many are only diagnosed in the third stage. Antenatal diagnosis using colour flow or power Doppler ultrasound and MRI has been described. It is important to determine whether an accreta is present in women at most risk (previous caesarean section with an anterior placenta praevia), as it is crucial in forward planning and discussion of options with the woman.

The NPSA in conjunction with RCOG have formulated a patient safety bundle that lists the requirements for good management of a potential placenta accreta. All women undergoing caesarean section at high risk of placenta accreta should be managed in line with this care bundle. This will include:

- Women with one or more previous caesarean sections and placenta praevia.
- Women with a previous scar where imaging of placental localisation has found the placenta to be lying over the previous scar, even if it is well clear of the internal cervical os.

The elements of the care bundle are:

1 Consultant obstetrician planned and directly supervising delivery.
2 Consultant obstetric anaesthetist planned and directly supervising anaesthesia at delivery.
3 Blood and blood products available on site.
4 Multidisciplinary involvement in pre-operative planning.
5 Discussion and consent includes possible interventions (such as hysterectomy, leaving placenta in situ, cell salvage and interventional radiology).
6 Local availability of level 2 critical care bed.

NICE guidance also recommends having a senior haematologist available for discussion.

Imaging modalities for placenta accreta include ultrasound and MRI.

Ultrasound imaging using greyscale, colour and power Doppler entails looking for loss of the usual sonolucent zones between the placenta and myometrium and between the myometrium and bladder, evidence of placenta within the bladder and abnormal vascular patterns. MRI features are of uterine bulging, placental bands on T2 weighted images and signal heterogeneity within the placenta.

Positive predictive values of 75–88 per cent have been reported. However, these are research studies, and in clinical practice there is often less experience with both ultrasound and MRI, such that the positive and negative predictive values are likely to be less. NICE recommend both ultrasound and MRI for suspected accreta. However, in the end the diagnosis is always made surgically.

MANAGEMENT OF PLACENTA PRAEVIA

Management of the woman who does not bleed or in whom bleeding is minor and settled

Maternal risks

Bleeding

APH is the cardinal sign of placenta praevia and it is unusual for a woman with placenta praevia to reach the late third trimester without vaginal bleeding. Bleeding becomes more likely as the frequency and strength of contractions increase, causing shearing of the placenta at the level of the internal os. The bleeding is said to be painless, though a considerable number (10 per cent) of women who bleed from a placenta praevia will have a coexistent abruption. It is also reported that most women experience a minor bleed before any major bleeding. Whilst this is true for many women, some will have a significant haemorrhage as their first event.

Hospitalisation

There are few data on which to base the management of placenta praevia. One reasonably large observational study involving 161 women demonstrated that the risk of bleeding was not related to the degree of praevia.[7] Only one small randomised study has been performed which showed only reduced hospital stay in the home care arm.[8]

Management decisions regarding women who have not bled are difficult and must be made individually. Important factors may include:

- where the woman lives in relationship to the hospital and whether she has an adult with her at home;
- other factors that may make a placenta praevia more difficult to manage, such as a scarred uterus.

Because there have been no trials on this aspect of management, the decision to manage as an outpatient must be made at a senior level and fully discussed with the woman and her partner. It is important to remember that long-term hospitalisation carries significant financial and psychological implications for women and their families and may not be justified for women who have never bled.

For women who have had bleeding, most obstetricians would recommend inpatient management from 34 weeks. However there may be exceptions, such as a placenta that migrates enough for vaginal delivery to become an option. Women who are managed as inpatients show a trend towards later delivery.

Recent transfusion guidance in the UK means that blood can only be cross-matched on a sample that is less than 72 hours old. This may pose particular problems for women with complex cross-matching, such as those with multiple antibodies. Where this situation exists, close communication with the transfusion laboratory is essential.

Surveillance

The rate of fetal abnormality is approximately double the background rate in women with placenta praevia. When a diagnosis of placenta praevia is made, a careful reassessment of the fetal anatomy must be undertaken.

There is a considerable false-positive rate of diagnosis of low-lying placenta at 18–20 weeks using transabdominal (TA) scanning. A repeat transvaginal (TV) scan at 20–24 weeks will reduce the number of women who require follow-up and minimise anxiety for these women. Where the placenta appears to cover the internal os, a re-scan at 32 weeks is recommended as these women have a lower chance of placental migration, and require more careful management in the third trimester.[2] In women with a minor praevia, a full assessment should take place at approximately 36 weeks. If the placenta is >2 cm from the os a vaginal delivery is more often achieved. The thickness of the placental edge is also important; a thin leading edge is a more favourable finding for vaginal delivery. If the placenta is still low, a further scan in a week or two may show some changes as the lower segment continues to develop.

Tocolysis

Tocolysis for the treatment of uterine activity has been used to good effect in some studies [C].[9] It appears to be safe to use, gaining on average 13 days when compared to women in whom it was not used. It must be used judiciously to settle uterine activity that is causing bleeding. It must never be considered in women who show signs of cardiovascular instability or where there is evidence of fetal compromise. Studies have mainly used beta-sympathomimetics, which have a physiological disadvantage. Where tocolysis is considered agents other than beta-agonists should be considered first. Given the lack of cardiovascular side effects, an oxytocic antagonist would probably be the first choice.

Planning for delivery

In the woman who has not bled or in whom bleeding has been minor, there are a number of factors that need to be taken into account. These include:

- making a final decision about how to deliver for women with minor praevia;
- timing in relationship to the gestation of the pregnancy;
- ensuring a fully experienced and prepared team is assembled for delivery.

Deciding when to attempt a vaginal delivery

There has been much debate about when a vaginal delivery can be expected and when it is unlikely to occur. RCOG guidelines suggest that the decision regarding mode of delivery should be made on clinical grounds, supplemented by sonographic assessment.[2]

One large observational study has shown that if the placenta is within 2 cm of the internal os, the vast majority of women will require caesarean section [C].[10] This is therefore accepted as a reasonable cut-off for expecting to need to perform a caesarean section. However, where the leading edge of the placenta is thick, the placenta may still have an impact at this distance. Once the placenta is more than 4.5 cm from the internal os, it is unlikely to be problematic. The grey area of 2–4.5 cm must be managed clinically and will depend on features such as the station of the fetal head and the position of the placenta (anterior or posterior, anterior being slightly less problematic as the anterior lower segment tends to retract more in labour).

Ideally all women will have had a planned third trimester with repeat scanning, admission where necessary and plans made for delivery if this occurs earlier than anticipated. Where plans have been made for vaginal delivery, but heavy bleeding occurs in labour, the situation must be evaluated clinically as CS may be required.

If a woman presents in late pregnancy either for planned CS or in labour with the head engaged, it is reasonable to scan transvaginally to reassess the relationship between the placenta edge and head. A decision to proceed to vaginal birth must then be based on the relationship between the head and placenta and the wishes and expectations of the woman. If a vaginal delivery occurs, uterotonics may be needed to ensure adequate uterine contraction for a few hours.

PLANNED CAESAREAN SECTION FOR PLACENTA PRAEVIA

Timing of caesarean section

Pre-labour CS carries an increased risk of respiratory complications in the newborn. Occasionally these are severe enough to require intensive intervention. Table 46.2 shows the incidence of respiratory morbidity for each week of gestation in babies delivered prior to labour from 37 to 41 weeks [D].[11]

It has also been noted that the incidence of respiratory distress syndrome is higher amongst infants born to mothers delivered by elective CS for placenta praevia and relates to lower cortisol levels in these infants [C].[12] This suggests that the maturing processes in these infants are not accelerated. The RCOG guideline 'Antenatal Corticosteroids to Reduce Neonatal Morbidity and Mortality' (2010) states that antenatal corticosteroids should be given to all women for whom an elective CS is planned prior to 38[+6] weeks of gestation [A].

When bleeding is occurring, the risks and benefits of delivery versus conservative management can only be assessed on an individual basis. However, there is often pressure to deliver earlier because of hospital inpatient management. If there are no compelling medical reasons for delivery before 38 weeks, the risks to the fetus must be fully discussed with the mother before delivery.

Planning the caesarean section

The degree of technical difficulty of CS for placenta praevia will be related to:

- gestation;
- the degree of praevia;
- whether the praevia is anterior;
- the presence of other risk factors making a morbidly adherent placenta more likely;
- the sonographic or MRI appearances of the placenta;
- previous abdominal procedures, which may make access to the uterus more difficult;
- morbid obesity.

Where placenta accreta is suspected, planning using the NPSA care bundle is vital.p

Table 46.2 Respiratory morbidity amongst infants delivered by elective caesarean section

Gestation	Respiratory morbidity per 1000 (95% CI)	Odds ratio compared to vaginal delivery at term (95% CI)
37 1 0–37 1 6	73.8 (49.1–106.1)	14.3 (8.9–23.1)
38 1 0–38 1 6	42.3 (31.1–56.2)	8.2 (5.5–12.3)
39 1 0–39 1 6	17.8 (8.0–33.5)	3.5 (1.7–7.1)

Autologous blood transfusion is not recommended in the management of placenta praevia, as when blood is needed it is often required in very large amounts.[2] Haemoglobin should be optimised before delivery. Cell salvage should be considered. Where blood or blood products are declined thorough discussion of the available options such as cell salvage must be undertaken and full informed consent gained as far in advance as possible.

Discussion regarding the prophylactic placement of uterine artery embolisation catheters should take place in advance where an accreta is suspected. Women who have declined the use of blood or blood products should be delivered in a unit where interventional radiology is available.

A planned CS must enlist the help of all those thought to be necessary. This will include at the very least:

- senior obstetrician;
- senior anaesthetist;
- experienced midwives, anaesthetic assistants and theatre staff.

Where a morbidly adherent placenta is a strong possibility, discussion with a surgical/urological team may be necessary as bladder involvement is not uncommon. Because of the risk of ureteric injury when a hysterectomy is required for an accreta, ureteric stent placement has been suggested prior to CS, as this reduces the risk of ureteric damage; this should be evaluated on a case-by-case basis.

When a CS is likely to involve significant haemorrhage, the haematology staff (medical and laboratory) should be alerted. The appropriate amount of blood should be cross-matched in advance, with cryoprecipitate and fresh frozen plasma urgently available. The laboratory should be warned if there is likely to be a need for more blood or blood products.

Consent

It is important that the potential outcomes are discussed with the mother before delivery. This must include a discussion of management in the presence of continued or heavy bleeding and the possibility of the need for hysterectomy or other techniques.

Type of anaesthetic

The type of anaesthesia used is the ultimate responsibility of the anaesthetist. The final decision can only be made when the anaesthetist has all the facts at his or her disposal. Good communication before the delivery is vital.

There is evidence that blood loss at CS for placenta praevia is less when regional anaesthesia is used and that this does not compromise mothers [C].[13] (Elective delivery is different from delivery of the cardiovascularly unstable woman with acute bleeding, as discussed below.) When procedures are likely to take slightly longer, a combined spinal–epidural approach may be undertaken. If a hysterectomy is required many women will require conversion to general anaesthesia.

Surgery

Accountability

The surgery must be performed or supervised by an experienced obstetrician. The CEMD in the UK 1994–1996 recommended that a consultant be present during surgery for a placenta praevia. The main reason for this recommendation is that a decision to proceed to life-saving hysterectomy is likely to be made earlier by a senior person. Death of a woman from haemorrhage at elective CS has been defined by the NPSA as a 'never event'. This excludes women who have declined blood products and in whom a placenta accreta is found, but does include death after major placenta praevia.

The surgeon must avail him/herself of all the available information before commencing the CS. It is prudent to try to plan how the uterine incision will relate to the placenta before starting. Careful ultrasound mapping of the placental site prior to operation will help the surgeon to know where the placenta lies and the best route to deliver the baby.

It is also the responsibility of the surgeon to ensure that appropriate consent has been gained, that all the team members are aware the procedure is about to commence, and that the blood is available in theatre. These vital steps should not be delegated to anyone else in an elective situation and should form part of the usual WHO safe-surgery checklist undertaken before surgery commences. The surgeon should have a clear idea of the views of the woman regarding management in the face of haemorrhage with regard to uterine preservation or hysterectomy. Uterine artery catheter placement will be more advantageous where uterine preservation is important.

Technique

Uterine incision

Caesarean section is usually performed through a transverse skin incision and through the lower segment of the uterus, but if there is an anterior placenta praevia, the vessels may cover the entire anterior lower segment and the placenta will be encountered underneath the uterine incision. Some authors have recommended a classical CS in this situation, but this may make any repeat CS even more hazardous, and lower segment bleeding can be difficult to see and secure in this case. In cases of a centrally implanted praevia with the potential for an accreta, an upper segment incision, avoiding the placenta entirely with the aim of leaving the placenta in-utero or performing a planned hysterectomy, can be considered [D].

Delivery

The baby may be delivered by the obstetrician passing a hand round the margins of the placenta, or by incising the placenta. It is often easier to bring down one of the baby's feet and perform breech extraction than to try to deliver a very high head past the placenta that occupies the uterine incision. Prolonged delay in delivery can lead to fetal exsanguination if the placenta has been cut. Some authors have recommended clamping the cord as soon as the uterine incision is made, to prevent fetal bleeding if the placenta is cut. However, in many cases this is not easy and can add unnecessary delay.

Third stage

Oxytocics should be administered (5 units syntocinon IV) as soon as the baby is delivered. An oxytocin infusion or long-acting oxytocin analogue should then be commenced to continue uterine contraction. The uterine angles should be secured with Green–Armytage clamps before delivery of the placenta, and any large bleeding venous sinuses in the incision can also be secured.

The placenta should be delivered by controlled cord traction.

If the placenta does not separate, there are different choices depending on whether the accreta is total or partial. If the whole placenta is adherent, bleeding is usually minimal. The placenta can be left *in situ* and the uterus closed. This carries future risks of sepsis, haemorrhage or need for placental removal, but successful cases of placental passage followed by a future pregnancy have been described. Using methotrexate does not speed the passage of the placenta. The safest option is hysterectomy. Where this is chosen the uterus should be closed and then removed.

If the placenta is partially adherent (the more common scenario in a scarred uterus), the issue is usually that the non-adherent parts separate, but the adherent parts prevent efficient contraction, and so heavy bleeding ensues. The options are to a) perform a hysterectomy (safest) or b) remove the separated parts and attempt to control the bleeding. Various strategies have been described, including over-sewing of bleeding areas, re-section of the placenta and the portion of uterine segment it adheres to (possible if this is a small portion of lower segment scar), removal of as much placenta as possible then using brace sutures, or radiological embolisation techniques to reduce blood flow to bleeding areas.

In all strategies successful pregnancies afterwards have been reported, but also ultimate recourse to hysterectomy is often required.

If the placenta separates the lower segment must be examined. Delivery of the uterus may improve visualisation. Bleeding with a placenta praevia at this stage is most troublesome from the lower segment as this contracts poorly. Various strategies have been employed to improve haemostasis. These include:

- over-sewing individual bleeding sinuses;
- packing the uterine cavity;
- siting a balloon device, which can be inflated to provide uterine compression and removed later per vaginum;
- extra ecbolics, including prostaglandin PGF2α, intramyometrial vasopressin, misoprostol;
- radiographic embolisation techniques;
- uterine or internal iliac artery ligation.

What is most important is that if haemorrhage is continuing and excessive, early recourse to hysterectomy is the safest strategy and the abdomen should not be closed until haemostasis is assured.

Post-delivery monitoring

Women delivered with a major placenta praevia or who have had significant intra-operative haemorrhage must be carefully monitored in a high-dependency setting until continuing loss has been excluded.

The management of major PPH is discussed in Chapter 64. Again it is vital that if haemorrhage is continuing, early recourse to hysterectomy is undertaken.

If all or part of the placenta is retained, follow-up with weekly serum hCG and interval ultrasound (determined by clinical features) should be undertaken.

Postnatal counselling

When haemorrhage has been severe, women will need the opportunity to go through events with the senior member of the team. The anaesthetist may wish to be involved. It is important that women understand what implications there may be for future deliveries, especially where there has been particularly difficult surgery.

The management of women with severe antepartum bleeding with placenta praevia utilises the steps above. Further management of the woman with severe bleeding is discussed below.

VASA PRAEVIA

Vasa praevia (VP) occurs when fetal vessels cross or run within the membranes between the amnion and chorion close to the internal cervical os, and are thus at risk of rupture during labour, either as a result of shearing at membrane rupture or from compression from the fetal head. It has been variously reported as occurring in 0.015–0.04 per cent of all pregnancies and has a high perinatal mortality. If the diagnosis is made antenatally the perinatal loss rate is substantially reduced. The presentation is usually bleeding at the time of membrane rupture, followed by fetal bradycardia. The two main types of VP occur when:

1 The umbilical cord inserts directly into the membranes rather than the placenta (a velamentous insertion) (Type I);
2 There is an additional separate (succenturiate) placental lobe with vessels crossing over from one portion of the placenta to the other (Type II).

Risk factors for vasa praevia are:

- Bilobed placenta or succenturiate lobe;
- Velamentous insertion;
- Low-lying placenta in the second trimester;
- Multiple pregnancy;
- In-vitro fertilisation.

Placenta praevia, low-lying placenta and bilobed or succenturiate placenta account for 89 per cent of pregnancies complicated by VP. Antenatal diagnosis is usually only made if there is the suspicion of a higher risk and TVS performed.

If an antenatal diagnosis is made, delivery by elective CS is recommended, though the timing of delivery is not based on evidence. Delivery is recommended between 35 and 37 weeks following a course of steroids for fetal lung maturation [D].[2] Whether admission prior to this is needed is debatable and each case should be individually assessed.

VP does not form part of the National Screening programme in the UK at present. A recent re-evaluation of the available evidence by the NSC suggested that women with identifiable risk factors should undergo TVS after the 20-weeks scan, repeated later if VP is suspected. However, this has not yet been fully evaluated from either a feasibility or cost perspective.[14] The review also noted that many practitioners did not consider themselves experienced enough to know what is abnormal. It is likely that the NSC will eventually recommend some form of screening for VP. In the meantime, it seems reasonable to consider a TV ultrasound after the 18–20-weeks scan if there is a bilobed or succenturiate placenta, and if a velamentous insertion is noted, and perhaps to offer women who have more than one of the other risk factors a scan. As RCOG recommend that TV ultrasound should be done to reduce the need for follow-up for women with a low-lying placenta at the detailed scan, then this whole group could be screened for VP with no extra effort. That would leave the last two risk groups. Perhaps it would be reasonable to consider TV scanning all women with IVF multiple pregnancies. It would not be many women and these women will be attending for additional ultrasound anyway, so the increase in workload is likely to be small.

PLACENTAL ABRUPTION

Definition

Abruption is defined as bleeding following premature separation of a normally sited placenta.

It occurs in as many as 5 per cent of pregnancies, though the majority of these are small and only visible on placental examination after delivery. It can most easily be graded as follows.

Grade 0: An asymptomatic retroplacental clot seen after placental delivery.
Grade 1: Vaginal bleeding and uterine tenderness; visible retroplacental clot after delivery.
Grade 2: Revealed bleeding may or may not be present but placental separation is significant enough to produce evidence of fetal compromise and retroplacental clot visible after delivery.
Grade 3: Revealed bleeding may or may not be seen but there are significant maternal signs (uterine tetany, hypovolaemia, abdominal pain), with late-stage fetal compromise or fetal death. Thirty per cent of these women will develop disseminated intravascular coagulopathy (DIC).

Abruption has historically been associated with very poor fetal and maternal outcomes. Perinatal mortality rates vary widely as the diagnostic criteria are generally clinical and broad. The minimal perinatal mortality rate is at least 4 per 1000 and maternal mortality continues to be a risk.

Aetiology and associations

The aetiology of placental abruption is unclear, but there are a number of recognised associations.

The risk factors for abruption include:

- previous abruption;
- family history of abruption;
- fetal abnormality;
- rapid uterine decompression (rupture of membranes with polyhydramnios);
- trauma;
- chorioamnionitis/premature rupture of membranes;
- smoking/illicit drug use (cocaine and amphetamines especially);
- abnormal placentation (circumvallate placenta etc.);
- pre-eclampsia;
- underlying thrombophilia;
- first-trimester bleeding (especially if a haematoma is seen).

Women with a low BMI, who have undergone assisted reproductive techniques, multiparous and older women are also at increased risk.

A history of previous abruption carries the greatest risk, with an increase in risk of about 8 times above the background rate. Women who have a sister who has had a significant abruption are at increased risk themselves (odds ratio 2).[15]

Debate surrounding the role of thrombophilia continues. There does appear to be an increased risk in women who are heterozygous for factor V Leiden or the prothrombin gene.[16] What is as yet unproven is whether there are any effective interventions to prevent abruption in women with underlying thrombophilia.

Given that placental abruption is associated with disturbed placentation, any factor seen in these cases will be associated with an increased risk of abruption. These include pre-eclampsia, growth restriction, oligohydramnios, fetal abnormality (especially aneuploidy) and pregnancies with abnormal umbilical artery Doppler velocities.

Diagnosis

The diagnosis of placental abruption is primarily a clinical one. There may or may not be revealed bleeding. The woman may have had pain preceding or during the bleed and the uterus may be irritable; alternatively, if a large abruption is present, the uterus may be hard and tender.

In grades 2 and 3, the clinical picture is usually clear and the management will be dictated by the fetal and maternal condition. Grades 0 and 1 may be much more difficult to diagnose. There will be much overlap between women with marginal bleeding and bleeding due to other causes. This is largely irrelevant clinically, as all women with APH represent a high-risk group for whom surveillance in pregnancy needs to be increased.

Ultrasonography is not a good method of diagnosing placental abruption. Small areas are difficult to visualise and, in the acute phase and in large abruptions, can be isoechoic and look like placenta. When an abruption is clinically suspected, it is prudent to manage with that as the diagnosis. Ultrasound should be used to:

- confirm fetal viability;
- assess fetal growth;
- measure liquor volume;
- perform umbilical artery Doppler velocities;
- confirm fetal normality as far as possible;
- exclude placenta praevia.

Kleihauer testing should be performed in women who are rhesus negative. This will ensure that an appropriate dose of anti-D is given should a large fetomaternal haemorrhage be detected. Kleihauer testing as a diagnostic tool has not been shown to be of clinical value in determining whether pain or bleeding is secondary to abruption.[17]

Management specific to abruption

When to deliver

The main management decision to be made with abruption is whether to deliver the fetus. This will of course depend on the clinical picture and the gestation. Approximately 50 per cent of women who abrupt will present in labour, and the decision then must be how to deliver the fetus.

When fetal compromise is confirmed at viable gestations, the aim should be to deliver the fetus. Studies comparing neonatal outcomes at gestations of viability suggest that CS is a better choice for the fetus; however, even when CS is performed, perinatal mortality rates of 15–20 per cent are reported in this group. At very low gestations, a vaginal delivery should be the aim. Labour is often quick and although prostaglandins and oxytocin can be used, they are rarely needed.

It is important when performing CS to alert the haematology laboratory and to arrange to have blood cross-matched as soon as possible (see below). Whether there is time to delay to await the results of clotting screens and cross-matching will depend on the degree of maternal bleeding and the condition of the fetus.

It is important to:

- remember that there may already be considerable unrevealed bleeding which may increase the blood loss well above that which has been revealed;
- be as prepared as possible;
- seek senior help if this is thought likely to be necessary;
- expect heavy postpartum bleeding.

If the fetus is already dead, a vaginal delivery should be the expectation. At least 30 per cent of women will develop DIC with placental abruption and delivery should be expedited. The management is discussed further below.

The time taken to achieve delivery will depend entirely on the rate of bleeding, the rate of change in the clotting studies and the clinical condition of the mother. Fortunately, delivery is usually rapid and after delivery the DIC will usually begin to resolve.

If the abruption is small, the fetus uncompromised and the mother well, a conservative approach may be utilised. There can only be gains for the mother and fetus if there are benefits in terms of maturity and the option to give steroids. If abruption is thought to be the diagnosis and the fetus is mature, delivery in a controlled manner is probably the best management plan. After 38 weeks in most cases of suspected abruption, delivery should be considered. Between 34 and 38 weeks, cases must be managed on an individual basis. When a conservative approach is undertaken, increased surveillance is essential. In the acute phase, a period of inpatient management with twice-daily CTG until stability is confirmed is warranted. Fetal growth must be serially assessed, and umbilical artery Doppler waveform analysis is also helpful.[18]

Bleeding of other causes

The group of other causes comprises a wide range of conditions. As a group, these causes carry an approximately 5-fold increased risk of perinatal mortality and therefore warrant careful consideration.

Management will depend on the individual cause, but there are some general principles:

- It is preferable to err on the side of caution, and safer to increase surveillance rather than to assume that the cause must be benign.
- There is no evidence to support a policy of delivery at term in the well fetus, but steps to ensure fetal wellbeing must be continued if a conservative approach is adopted.

MANAGEMENT OF THE WOMAN PRESENTING WITH ANTEPARTUM HAEMORRHAGE

Management at initial presentation

A rapid assessment of the condition of both the mother and the fetus is a vital first step.

A clinical history can be quickly taken in an acute situation. A more detailed history can be taken once the immediate clinical picture is established. When taking the initial history, questions should be asked regarding:

- dates by previous scan;
- amount of bleeding;
- associated or initiating factors;
- abdominal pain;
- coitus;
- trauma;

- leakage of fluid;
- previous episodes of bleeding;
- previous uterine surgery (including induced abortions and surgically managed miscarriages);
- smoking and use of illegal drugs (especially cocaine);
- fetal movements;
- blood group;
- position of the placenta, if known from a previous scan.

Smoking increases the risk of placenta praevia, placental abruption and marginal bleeding. This is a dose-dependent effect. Fetal growth restriction is associated with both marginal placental bleeding and placental abruption. The mother may have noticed a reduction in fetal movements. The use of cocaine and crack cocaine is strongly associated with placental abruption.

Maternal assessment
In the initial stages, this should include:

- pulse;
- blood pressure;
- uterine palpation for size, tenderness, presenting part.

A vaginal examination must not be performed until a placenta praevia has been excluded.

Fetal assessment
It should be established whether a fetal heart can be heard, making sure it is fetal not maternal (the mother may be very tachycardic). If a fetal heart is heard and the gestation is estimated to be 26 weeks or more, FHR monitoring should be commenced.

These initial steps take very little time. Following this initial assessment, women will fall into one of two categories.

1 The bleeding is minor or settling and neither the mother nor fetus is compromised.
2 The bleeding is heavy and continuing and the mother or fetus is or soon will be compromised.

Group 1: bleeding is minor or settling and neither the mother nor fetus is compromised
This is the most common group. It is usually clearly apparent that neither mother nor fetus is in danger on admission. Time can then be taken to conduct a full and thorough history and examination.

Once it is clear that the placenta is not low, a vaginal examination can be undertaken with the following aims:

- to assess the degree of bleeding;
- to ascertain cervical changes, which may be indicative of labour;
- to assess local causes of bleeding (trauma, polyps, cervical lesions, etc.);
- to take bacteriological samples if infection is suspected (high vaginal and endocervical swabs, urine PCR or endocervical swabs for chlamydia, plus viral swabs if herpes is suspected).

After a careful history and examination, it should be possible to use selected investigations to help establish a diagnosis.

Further investigations

- Full blood count.
- Kleihauer testing in women known to be rhesus negative or in women with unknown blood group.
- Grouping and saving of serum, with blood cross-matched if there is continuing or severe bleeding.
- Clotting screen in cases of suspected abruption or heavy bleeding.

Ultrasound is useful for:

- measurement of fetal size;
- assessment of liquor volume;
- location of the placenta in relation to the internal cervical os;
- establishment of fetal wellbeing:
  – biophysical profile;
  – umbilical artery Doppler velocimetry.

Ultrasound is not generally helpful in diagnosing abruption. Acute abruptions can be difficult to see as they may have the same echogenicity as placenta. It should be made clear that the ultrasound examination is primarily to assess the position of the placenta and the wellbeing of the fetus. Women are often disappointed if they have been led to believe the ultrasound will identify the cause of the bleeding.

If the source of bleeding is fetal, the fetus is usually quickly compromised. This may present with a fetal tachycardia progressing rapidly to a sinusoidal CTG and finally a terminal bradycardia. Point-of-care testing is usually too slow to be helpful in these cases.

A Kleihauer test is mandatory for all rhesus-negative women. All RhD-negative women will require 500 IU anti-D (unless they are already sensitised). The Kleihauer test must be done to determine whether there has been a large fetomaternal haemorrhage, in which case more anti-D will be needed.

The Kleihauer is not a useful test to differentiate small abruptions from bleeding of other causes [C].[17] Fetal cells may appear in the maternal circulation in as many as 15 per cent of women at some time in pregnancy, and a lack of fetal cells in the maternal circulation does not preclude an abruption.

When any pregnant woman complains of episodes of vaginal bleeding in pregnancy, other than confirmed causes of haemorrhage, cervical cancer must be excluded by direct observation of the cervix and a cervical smear taken. This should be undertaken irrespective of her past medical history or reports of normal past cervical smears [E].

Surveillance after a limited APH

Although some units admit women who have had APH for 24 hours, there is no evidence to suggest that this improves outcome once fetal and maternal wellbeing has been established [D]. Management must be individualised, taking into account the suspected cause of bleeding, gestation, fetal assessment and continuing maternal risk factors.

The following must be borne in mind.

- No bleeding, however light, should be dismissed without full investigation.
- Once APH has occurred, the pregnancy becomes high risk, and a management plan for ongoing fetal surveillance must be formulated and discussed with the mother.
- Women must be advised to watch for warning signs such as a decrease in the frequency of fetal movements, further bleeding or pain, and should be assessed again should any of these occur.

Planning for the rest of pregnancy

If bleeding settles and the mother is discharged, a clear plan for the remainder of the pregnancy should be made. Even if the cause is thought to be minor, extra fetal surveillance is needed as a higher fetal mortality rate is seen compared with background. Fetal surveillance for growth and wellbeing should be instituted, as guided by the clinical picture. If all remains well, induction of labour at term is not needed, but the degree of surveillance after the due date may need to be increased.

Group 2: severe ongoing bleeding, compromised mother and/or fetus

Delivery must be expedited if the mother is compromised. If the fetus is compromised, the decision to deliver will be based on the gestational age. In most cases, delivery will be indicated.

The method of delivery will be determined by the cause and severity of the bleeding, the fetal gestation and status. Women with major haemorrhage from a placenta praevia will need delivery by CS.

Placental abruption causing maternal or fetal compromise necessitates delivery. If the fetus is already dead, vaginal delivery after stabilisation of the mother is usually the safest option. However, if the bleeding continues, and the mother's condition cannot be stabilised, delivery should be achieved by the quickest method, which may be CS. Coagulopathy will only begin to resolve once the placenta is delivered, and may be severe enough to warrant replacement with FFP, cryoprecipitate and platelets. These women usually labour very quickly. Epidural or spinal anaesthesia must not be used if the clotting studies are abnormal or not available. CVP lines can be useful, but should be sited through an antecubital long line, and not sited or removed until clotting is normal.

It can be difficult to measure antepartum blood loss accurately, as the loss may be concealed (placental abruption) or diluted by amniotic fluid.

Major haemorrhage can be defined by blood loss and/or vital signs:

- blood loss >1000 mL;
- disturbance of conscious state;
- systolic pressure <100 mmHg;
- blood pulse >120 bpm;
- reduced peripheral perfusion.

Disturbances of coagulation due to loss or consumption of platelets and clotting factors may occur during haemorrhage. DIC is the coagulation problem most often encountered in obstetric patients. This and the other complications – fetal or maternal death, adult respiratory distress syndrome, renal and hepatic failure – are more likely to occur if adequate replacement of blood volume is not instigated rapidly.

Aims of treatment of major haemorrhage

- Rapid restoration of the circulating blood volume and oxygen-carrying capacity.
- Cessation of further blood loss.
- Restoration/maintenance of normal blood coagulation.
- Delivery of the live fetus (where appropriate).

Resuscitation should aim to keep the Hb concentration above 8 g/dL, the pulse rate below 100 bpm, and the systolic blood pressure above 100 mmHg. Four units of cross-matched blood should be available at all times. BCSH recommend aiming to keep the platelet count above 75×10^9, the prothrombin and activated prothrombin times $<1.5 \times$ mean control, and fibrinogen >1 g/L [E].[17]

The success of treatment is dependent on careful organisation as well as prompt treatment and the use of appropriate blood products and non-blood volume expanders. The patient, her partner and relatives must be kept fully informed.

When major haemorrhage is identified

1. Call for help. The immediate team will consist of:
   - the obstetric specialist registrar;
   - the obstetric senior house officer;
   - the anaesthetic registrar;
   - the senior midwife.

   The consultant obstetrician and anaesthetist should be informed.

   A member of staff should be nominated to run samples and record events.

2. Start facial oxygen 10–15 L/min (hypoxia will reduce uterine contractions).

3. Insert two intravenous cannulae (14 gauge brown/orange), one into each antecubital fossa.

4. Take 30 mL of blood for:
   - FBC;
   - clotting screen (including fibrinogen and fibrin – degradation products or D-dimers if DIC is suspected);
   - cross-match 6 units;
   - urea and electrolytes, liver function.

5. Commence the following infusions:
   - up to 2 L 0.9% saline/Hartmann's solution;
   - colloid (up to 1.5 L);
   - uncross-matched Rh-negative blood or group-specific blood (if clinical condition is critical);
   - cross-matched blood as soon as available.

Cross-matched blood is the ideal but crystalloid first and colloid second should be used until blood is available. Group O RhD-negative blood should only be used as a last resort, but can be life saving when haemorrhage is severe. Group O RhD-negative blood **must not** be given to patients known to have anti-c antibodies from their antenatal records [E].

Fluids should be warmed, as cold injury exacerbates DIC.

6. Site an indwelling catheter to monitor urine output and aim to keep output above 30 mL/h.

7. One member of staff should be assigned to record the following:
   - pulse;
   - blood pressure;
   - CVP (half-hourly) if a line is present (see below);
   - continuous FHR (where appropriate);
   - fundal height (abruption/PPH);
   - any drug administration (time, type, dose);
   - measured blood loss.

8. The senior obstetrician present should coordinate and manage the clinical situation i.e. prompt treatment of the cause of haemorrhage, adequate fluid replacement and regular checking of FBC and clotting status in order to prevent and treat DIC.

A major haemorrhage box is an asset on any acute unit. It should contain everything needed for the initial resuscitation (fluids, cannulae, tourniquet, blood bottles and forms, oxytocics, etc., Fig. 46.1).

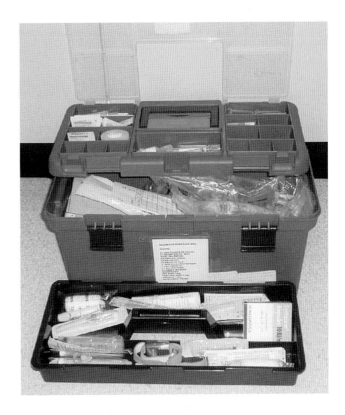

Fig. 46.1 A major haemorrhage box

BLOOD TRANSFUSION CONSIDERATIONS

The goals of haematological management are to maintain:

- Hb above 80 g/L;
- Platelet count >75 × 10⁹/L;
- Prothrombin time <1.5 × control mean;
- Activated prothrombin times <1.5 × control mean;
- Fibrinogen >1 g/L (remembering that 4 g/L is the lower limit of normal in pregnancy).

Packed cells and stored blood lack platelets and clotting factors. Fresh whole blood is not available because of potential hazards of viral transmission. FFP and sometimes cryoprecipitate are usually necessary to compensate after transfusion of 4–6 units. Stored blood also is a source of thromboplastins and can lead to or exacerbate DIC when large amounts are transfused. In most units, up to 4 units of FFP may be issued before the coagulation screen result is known for a patient in critical condition (usually 6 units already transfused and blood loss continuing), provided that coagulation studies are being processed.

Thrombocytopenia can also occur during massive transfusion, but in DIC a platelet transfusion is rarely required unless the platelet count falls below 50 × 10⁹ and there is continued blood loss.

Blood should be administered through blood-warming equipment and rapid administration of warmed fluid should be achieved by the use of a compression cuff on the infusion bag. The use of a blood filter is not necessary. Cold injury increases the risk of DIC.

Extra blood and products should be ordered early – the amount of each will depend on the clinical situation and FBC and coagulation screen results. In established DIC, extra FFP or cryoprecipitate and platelets may be needed, according to instructions from the haematologist.

Recombinant factor VIIa (NovoSeven) has been used in cases of severe continuing haemorrhage. It does not work where there is hypofibrinogenaemia or thrombocytopenia (fibrinogen <1 g/L, platelets less than 20 × 10⁹) so should be given after cryoprecipitate and platelets if needed in cases where continued bleeding is thought to be secondary to thrombostatic failure [C].[19] The prothrombotic properties of recombinant factor VIIa necessitate careful postnatal precautions for thromboembolism deterrence. In the immediate post-haemorrhage period, good hydration and compression devices should be used, with heparin added when clinically safe.

Once bleeding has been stopped, the patient should be managed in an obstetric high-dependency setting or adult intensive therapy unit.

Central venous pressure monitoring

CVP monitoring can be helpful where there has been massive haemorrhage, concealed blood loss or when blood loss is continuing.

A long line should be used if there are concerns regarding clotting.

A pressure between 3 and 7 cmH$_2$O, using the angle of Louis as the reference zero, should be established.

- Ensure that the rate of transfusion at least equals the rate of continuing blood loss and is, in addition, adequate to replace the loss already measured.
- Do not over-transfuse the patient with cell-free colloid as this will result in a severely anaemic patient, with a high CVP, preventing further blood transfusion.
- Do not exceed a CVP of 7 cmH$_2$O (this leads to a high risk of pulmonary oedema due to low colloid oncotic pressure).
- Do not use or rely on increasing the CVP excessively to correct oliguria.
- Consider using a fluid challenge test if you are unsure of the adequacy of fluid replacement:

Infuse 250 mL Hartmann's or 0.9% saline rapidly (2 minutes). Observe the CVP changes over the following 5–10 minutes.

- *Hypovolaemia*: rapid rise and fall back to previous CVP level.
- *Isovolaemia*: rise and fall back to slightly higher CVP level.
- *Hypervolaemia*: rise to higher CVP level sustained for more than 10 minutes.

MAJOR HAEMORRHAGE AND SPECIFIC ANTEPARTUM CONDITIONS

Placenta praevia

It is unusual for the placental site to be unknown, as most women have a detailed fetal anomaly scan. Bleeding significant enough to cause maternal hypotension requires delivery.

If the placenta is known to be praevia, delivery by CS is needed. If the placental site is unknown, the following strategy is helpful.

- Is the presenting part engaged? If so, a placenta praevia is less likely.
- Ultrasound scan can be performed to confirm the leading edge of the placenta, but only if the practitioner is trained to do so.
- If the presenting part is high and delivery is needed, an examination in theatre should be considered if the diagnosis is still unclear.
- The consultant must be informed prior to delivery and should be present for delivery or as soon as possible.

Major abruption

Large abruptions can lead on to DIC in 30 per cent of women. Management must be directed at ensuring the safety of the mother and fetus. Abruption is associated with a high risk for PPH.

- Usually presents with pain and vaginal bleeding with a woody, hard, tender uterus.
- If fetal heart is detected, continuous monitoring is needed.
- Vaginal examination should be performed with due caution.
- Follow the guidelines for massive obstetric haemorrhage, above.
- Prevent PPH and monitor for renal failure.
- Discuss with consultant haematologist.
- If no fetal heart is detected, ultrasound confirmation should be performed, membranes should be ruptured and syntocinon commenced to empty the uterus.
- FBC and clotting must be monitored at least 4-hourly as these can deteriorate quickly.

DIC

This is defined as inappropriate activation of the clotting cascade, leading to widespread coagulation, increased fibrinolysis and end-organ failure.

The obstetric causes can be divided into three areas.

1   Injury to vascular endothelium:
   – pre-eclampsia;
   – hypovolaemic shock;
   – septicaemia;
   – cold injury (large amounts of cold fluid).
2   Release of thrombogenic tissue factors:
   – placental abruption;
   – amniotic fluid embolism;
   – prolonged intrauterine fetal death.
3   Production of procoagulant phospholipids:
   – incompatible blood transfusion;
   – septicaemia.

Disseminated intravascular coagulation represents a cascade of events which can vary in severity, and range from a compensated state with only laboratory evidence of increased coagulation and fibrinolytic factor turnover, through to massive uncontrollable haemorrhage with very low concentrations of plasma fibrinogen, raised fibrin degradation products (FDPs) and thrombocytopenia. The evolution of events leading to DIC is shown in Fig. 46.2. End-organ damage is caused by hypotension, fibrin–platelet clump deposition in small vessels, and persisting endothelial damage leading to increased vascular permeability.

The following organs are most susceptible to damage.

- Kidneys:
   – acute tubular necrosis;
   – glomerular damage.
- Lungs:
   – pulmonary oedema;
   – adult respiratory distress syndrome/systemic inflammatory response syndrome.

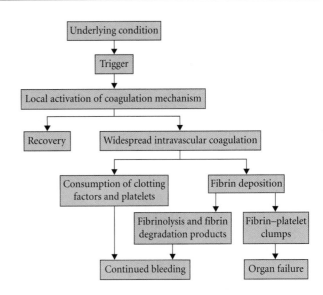

Fig. 46.2 Evolution of disseminated intravascular coagulation

- Central nervous system:
   – infarcts;
   – cerebral oedema.

The principles of management are:

- maternal resuscitation;
- treatment of the cause;
- replacement of blood and clotting factors;
- intensive monitoring until resolution.

Prompt and aggressive fluid replacement will limit damage to the endothelium and allow rapid clearance of fibrin–platelet clumps.

A full coagulation screen should be obtained for any patient at risk of DIC (this should include FDPs or D-dimers and fibrinogen; a thrombin time is useful if fibrinogen testing cannot be done). In DIC, all aspects of the routine clotting study are deranged (activated partial thromboplastin time, partial thromboplastin time and thrombin time). In pregnancy, the normal range for fibrinogen is increased, with the lower limit of normal being 4 g/L. In any woman in whom the fibrinogen falls to 1 g/L, a cryoprecipitate infusion (which is rich in fibrinogen) should be considered. Measurement of fibrin degradation products can be useful; D-dimers that are more specific may also be measured when other indices of coagulation are abnormal.

Management of DIC

Senior haematological advice should always be sought if DIC is suspected. The mainstay of the management of massive haemorrhage is to stop further loss of blood and resuscitate with appropriate blood products. Mild DIC may be controlled by adequate transfusion with stored blood and FFP. More FFP will be required in severe cases. FFP provides factors V and VIII, other labile coagulation factors and some antithrombin IIIa and fibrinogen. Cryoprecipitate (with a higher concentration of fibrinogen) and platelets may also be needed.

After initial resuscitation, management will be dependent on repeated checks of the haemoglobin, platelet count and coagulation status.

- Remember that stored blood contains thromboplastins and can exacerbate DIC once 6 units have been given.
- Remember the fibrinogen reference range in pregnancy is >4 g/L. Any woman with a fibrinogen of <1 g/L requires cryoprecipitate if there is active bleeding.

Treatment of the cause

DIC will not settle until the cause resolves. The urgency of treatment will be determined by the severity of the DIC and other factors such as maternal and fetal condition.

In general, following abruption and intrauterine fetal death, vaginal delivery should be the aim. Usually this will be accomplished within 4–6 hours. If DIC becomes uncontrollable during this time, more rapid delivery will be needed. Although it is considered that transfusion of replacement clotting factors may add fuel to the fire of DIC, it is recommended that replacement is aggressively pursued whilst delivery is being accomplished.

After delivery, steps to avoid PPH should be instituted.

Post-delivery surveillance

The aims are to:

- ensure adequate blood and clotting factor replacement;
- prevent further bleeding;
- monitor renal function and urine output until resolution;
- be vigilant for signs of impending lung involvement.

Fortunately, most women make a rapid recovery following delivery. It is important to ensure that the patient and her partner have the opportunity for a full debriefing.

SUMMARY

Antepartum haemorrhage increases the risk of perinatal death regardless of the cause. All women with APH therefore warrant careful fetal and maternal evaluation. In many cases a cause cannot be found, but the increase in perinatal mortality requires careful fetal surveillance for the remainder of all such pregnancies. Abruption carries the largest fetal and maternal risk. Women with underlying placental disease carry the highest risk for abruption.

Placenta praevia is becoming increasingly prevalent. As repeated caesarean sections are performed, the risk of a placenta praevia with a morbidly adherent placenta increases. A multidisciplinary approach is needed to ensure good maternal outcomes in the most difficult cases.

- Transvaginal ultrasound provides the most information and is safe in the diagnosis of placenta praevia.
- The risk of placenta praevia and accreta increases with each subsequent caesarean section.

- Regional anaesthesia for elective caesarean section for placenta praevia is safe and is associated with less maternal bleeding than general anaesthesia.

KEY POINTS

- The major causes of APH are abruption, placenta praevia and a mixed category of other causes.
- APH of any cause carries an increase in the risk of perinatal death for that pregnancy.
- Maternal deaths related to abruption and placenta praevia continue to be reported. Senior involvement is needed in the delivery of women with placenta praevia.
- Placenta praevia and accreta are likely to become more common as the CS rate rises.
- Increased surveillance is required for all ongoing pregnancies complicated by APH.
- Large abruptions carry a high risk of DIC and require a multidisciplinary approach to optimise care.

Key References

1. RCOG. *Antepartum haemorrhage.* Green-top Guideline No. 63 1st edn. November 2011.
2. RCOG. *Placenta praevia, placenta praevia accreta and vasa praevia: diagnosis and management.* Green-top Guideline No. 27. January 2011.
3. Romundstad LB, Romundstad PR, Sunde A, von Düring V, Skjaerven R, Vatten LJ. Increased risk of placenta previa in pregnancies following IVF/ICSI; a comparison of ART and non-ART pregnancies in the same mother. *Hum Reprod* 2006 Sep;21(9):2353–8.
4. Becker RH, Vonk R, Mende BC, Ragosch V, Entezami M. The relevance of placental location at 20–23 gestational weeks for prediction of placenta previa at delivery: evaluation of 8650 cases. *Ultrasound Obstet Gynecol* 2001;17:496–501.
5. Ghourab S. Third-trimester transvaginal ultrasonography in placenta previa: does the shape of the lower placental edge predict clinical outcome? *Ultrasound Obstet Gynecol* 2001;18:103–8.
6. Eller AG, Porter TF, Soisson P, Silver RM. Optimal management strategies for placenta accreta. *BJOG* 2009;116:648–54.
7. Love CD, Fernando KJ, Sargent L, Hughes RG. Major placenta praevia should not preclude out-patient management. *Eur J Obstet Gynaecol Repr Biol* 2004;117:24–9.
8. Wing DA, Paul RH, Millar LK. Management of the symptomatic placenta praevia: a randomized, controlled trial of inpatient versus outpatient expectant management. *Am J Obstet Gynecol* 1996;175:806–11.
9. Besinger RE, Moniak CW, Paskiewicz LS, Fishes SG, Tomich PG. The effect of tocolytic use in the management

of symptomatic placenta praevia. *Am J Obstet Gynecol* 1995;172:1770–8.

10. Oppemheimer LW, Farine D, Knox Ritchie JW *et al.* What is a low-lying placenta? *Am J Obstet Gynecol* 1991;165:1036–8.

11. Morrison JJ, Rennie JM, Milton PJ. Neonatal respiratory morbidity and mode of delivery at term: influence of timing of elective caesarean section. *Br J Obstet Gynaecol* 1995;102:101–6.

12. Bekku S, Mitsuda N, Ogita K, Suehara N, Fujimura M, Aono T. High incidence of respiratory distress syndrome (RDS) in infants born to mothers with placenta previa. *J Matern Fetal Med* 2000;9:110–13.

13. Parekh N, Husaini SWU, Russell IF. Caesarean section for placenta praevia: a retrospective study of anaesthetic management. *Br J Anaesth* 2000;84:725–30.

14. NSC. *Vasa praevia and placenta praevia screening in pregnancy. External review against programme appraisal criteria for the UK National Screening Committee (UK NSC).* NSC, April 2013.

15. Rasmussen S, Irgens LM. Occurrence of placental abruption in relatives. *BJOG* 2009;116:693–9.

16. Robertson L, Wu O, Langhorne P *et al.* Thrombophilia in pregnancy: a systematic review. *Br J Haematol* 2006;132(2):171–96.

17. Emery CL, Morway LF, Chung-Park M, Wyatt-Ashmead J, Sawady J, Beddow TD. The Kleihauer–Betke test. Clinical utility, indication, and correlation in patients with placental abruption and cocaine use. *Arch Pathol Lab Med* 1995;119:1032–7.

18. Morris R, Malin G, Robson S, Amora J. Fetal umbilical artery Doppler to predict compromise of fetal/neonatal wellbeing in a high-risk population: systematic review and bivariate meta-analysis. *Ultrasound Obstet Gynecol* 2011;37:135–42.

19. RCOG. *Postpartum Haemorrhage: prevention and management.* Green-top Guideline No. 52. London: RCOG, 2009.

LATE PREGNANCY AND INTRAPARTUM EVENTS

Chapter 47 Intrauterine fetal death

Lucy Kean

INTRODUCTION

Intrauterine fetal death or stillbirth is variously defined in different countries, by gestation or birthweight. In England and Wales, stillbirth is defined as a baby delivered with no signs of life known to have died after 24 completed weeks of pregnancy. This definition allows fetuses known to have died before this time, but not expelled from the uterus until after 24 weeks, to be categorised as fetal losses or miscarriages. Therefore parents are not required to notify the registrar of births and deaths of these earlier losses. Most of these are co-twin deaths, which remain in-utero. The WHO uses birth after 28 weeks, or of a baby weighing 1000 g or more. This definition is most useful for international comparisons.

Globally, stillbirth affects 2.6 million families each year, with 98 per cent occurring in low- and middle-income countries. Stillbirth reduction remains a global challenge, with many countries not recording stillbirths at all.[1]

There has been much recent criticism of the lack of progress in reducing the rate of stillbirth in the United Kingdom. In 2011 the stillbirth rate rose slightly to 5.2 per thousand total births from 5.1 in 2010, as rates in the rest of Europe appear to be falling. However, recent data produced from areas with a high uptake of the use of customised growth charts has demonstrated a clear fall in the rates of stillbirth, though recognising that these areas often had higher rates of loss prior to intervention. However, a clear downward trend in these areas has been matched by no movement in other areas without the intervention.[2] The rationale is that early recognition of small babies or those with plateauing growth allows for intervention before catastrophic placental failure. These data have led to the recommendation that customised fetal growth charts are used in the routine antenatal care of women (RCOG Investigation and management of the SGA fetus 2013) [C].

For the purposes of this chapter, fetal death after 20 weeks' gestation is taken as the focus, as these women are generally managed on the labour ward.

STILLBIRTH CLASSIFICATION SYSTEMS

The ability to determine the cause of an IUFD will be related to the rate of uptake of postmortem (PM) examination, the quality of the examination and the experience of the examiner.

Various methods of designation and classification of stillbirth have been used. The aims of each system are to retain important information towards understanding the causes of stillbirth, to be easy to apply and have high inter-observer agreement. There are six contemporary systems, the Extended Wrigglesworth and Amended Aberdeen systems, CODAC (Cause of Death and Associated Conditions), PSANZ-PDC (Perinatal Society of Australia and New Zealand – Perinatal Death Classification), ReCoDe (Relevant Conditions at Death) and Tulip. Recent studies have suggested that the two older systems (Wrigglesworth and Aberdeen) perform less well in terms of the proportion of unexplained stillbirths and inter-observer agreement. Wrigglesworth and Aberdeen systems lead to a higher proportion of unexplained stillbirths (52 and 44 per cent) with CODAC and Tulip having the lowest rate of unexplained stillbirth (9.5 and 10 per cent). ReCoDe and PSANZ-PDC report unexplained loss rates of 15 and 14 per cent. It can be seen, therefore, that the ability to determine a cause of death will be at least in part related to the system that is used to analyse the pathology.

At present there is no international consensus on the best system to use and so causes of stillbirth will remain difficult to compare. The RCOG guideline of 2010[3] still states that parents should be told that no specific cause is found in almost half of stillbirths, a fact that we can see is now no longer the case if newer methods of pathological classification are used.

Box 47.1 Causes of IUFD

> **Fetal**
> - Cord accidents
> - Feto–fetal transfusion
> - Feto–maternal haemorrhage
> - Chromosomal and genetic disease
> - Structural abnormality
> - Infection
> - Anaemias of fetal origin e.g. alpha-thalassaemia
>
> **Direct maternal effects**
> - Obstetric cholestasis
> - Metabolic disturbance e.g. diabetic ketoacidosis
> - Reduced oxygen states e.g. cystic fibrosis, obstructive sleep apnoea
> - Uterine abnormalities e.g. Ashermann's syndrome
> - Antibody production e.g. rhesus disease, platelet alloimmunisation, congenital heart block
>
> **Maternal placental effects**
> - Pre-eclampsia
> - Renal disease
> - Antiphospholipid syndromes
> - Thrombophilia
> - Smoking
> - Drug abuse e.g. cocaine
>
> **Primary placental disease**
> - Placental villous dysmaturity (Stallmach changes)

CAUSES

The causes of fetal death are many (Box 47.1). An understanding of the aetiology and associations can better direct investigations.

These individual conditions and the fetal effects they cause are discussed in greater detail in the relevant chapters.

ASSOCIATIONS

It is recognized that IUFD is more common amongst certain groups, though the exact aetiology for the increase in risk is uncertain. Advanced maternal age, obesity, advanced gestation and social deprivation are all associated with increased risk. Non-white ethnic origin and booking after 12 weeks are also associated with higher risk [C]. Multiple pregnancies have an increased risk, as do women with diabetes and hypertension. Women who experience intimate partner violence have an increased risk of stillbirth and miscarriage. Reducing the disparity in stillbirth rates between disadvantaged groups and more affluent populations remains a major goal for developed countries.

The contribution of each of the above factors to fetal death may be variable. Many of these diseases or conditions are common and yet fetal death is uncommon. It is vitally important not to ascribe causation to associations without investigation, as this may lead to important further information being missed and may inappropriately ascribe causation. Although abruption may lead to fetal demise, it may not be the whole story, as abruption is commoner with fetal abnormality, thrombophilia, growth restriction, smoking and illicit drug use. Equally, thrombophilia is common (affecting more than 5 per cent of the population), and whilst some types have been shown to contribute to fetal death in some women, they may also be an incidental finding after a fetal death of another cause. There is still much controversy regarding the role of thrombophilia in stillbirth. Large randomised trials of management have not been performed and thrombophilia is not a single entity. Association is strongest amongst women who deliver a very growth-restricted baby, but there is little guidance on future interventions to reduce risk, though increased surveillance will obviously be important.

Diabetes is associated with stillbirth as gestation increases. Current guidance advises delivery at or after 38 weeks in women with diabetes A].[4]

Obstetric cholestasis (OC) is discussed further in Chapter 15. The association with fetal death once the condition is recognised is probably small, with rates similar to the background rate of 5.7/1000 being reported in recent studies. That OC is associated with higher rates of meconium passage, fetal compromise in labour and CS shows that there is an association with reduced fetal resilience. It is a difficult diagnosis to make at PM, as the features are very non-specific in the fetus (generally just an anoxic mode of death). Direct questioning about itching may point to the diagnosis, which can be confirmed by measurement of maternal bile acids.

Cord accidents are often attributed as the cause of death, as the finding of a cord knot or tight nuchal cord is easily seen at delivery and is often seen as a clear demonstration of the cause of death which parents can understand. However, it is rare for knots or cord entanglement to cause antepartum stillbirth, though these may be implicated intrapartum. These findings are seen as often in pregnancies resulting in live births. Only if pathological confirmation is obtained should these be deemed causal. Many parents decline PM because causation is erroneously ascribed to a cord accident.

MANAGEMENT

Diagnosis of the death

IUFD presents with decreased fetal movement in as many as 50 per cent of cases. Others present with an unexpected finding at a routine ultrasound or antenatal visit or with signs of an acute event such as abruption, ruptured membranes or the onset of labour. In the developing world, intrapartum stillbirth accounts for nearly half of all losses, with 1.2 million babies being lost each year.[1]

When an IUFD is suspected, it is vitally important to establish the diagnosis as soon as possible. It is natural for parents to cling on to every shred of hope for as long as possible, and delay in diagnosis can lead to a false elevation of hope.

Fetal death must be diagnosed by ultrasound. CTG and auscultation can be very misleading. The heart rate tracing of an anxious mother can be identical to that of a fetus. Even heart rate tracings achieved by scalp electrode can record the maternal heart rate when the fetus is dead.

The ultrasound must be performed by a trained practitioner and a second opinion is recommended if practicably possible. Colour-flow mapping can be very useful, especially in the obese woman. It is sometimes, but not always, helpful for the parents to be shown the still fetal heart.

Ultrasound can also confirm features that may be helpful in further investigation. There may be:

- Spalding's sign (overlapping of the fetal skull bones when the fetus has been dead for some time);
- oligohydramnios;
- signs of fetal hydrops;
- intrafetal gas.

Once the ultrasound has confirmed fetal death, it is very important that the news is given to the parents in an unambiguous and sensitive way. Phrases such as 'I cannot see a fetal heartbeat' can be taken by parents to mean that the operator cannot be sure or is not sufficiently trained. It is much better to explain that the baby has died and to express your sorrow.

Offer to call a supporter (partner, friend) if the woman has attended unaccompanied. It may be necessary to repeat the scan when the partner arrives. It is also worthwhile doing a repeat scan if the woman reports passive fetal movement, as many do, as this can be important for the parents in knowing that the diagnosis is correct.

The initial reaction of parents will vary according to their prior suspicions, and many parents will initially feel anger. It is helpful for parents to be able to express their distress freely and without interruption. Do not try to challenge anger expressed against medical or midwifery staff at this time. If the pregnant woman has family with her, they should be allowed time together to come to terms with the findings.

All units should have a clear protocol for the management and investigation of women with fetal death. It should encompass lines of responsibility so that steps are not inadvertently omitted or repeated.

It is important to establish the events leading up to the fetal death, as there may be factors that will impact on the next pregnancy. It does not take long to take a history of events, and mothers may forget important factors later. It is an important process for the mother; she may feel the need to go through events preceding the admission. Although some of the information that parents volunteer is not relevant, it should be listened to sympathetically and never dismissed as irrelevant.

Establishing the safety of the mother and providing choice

At this point it is important to accede to mothers' choices in regard to management and to carefully advise if her choices may compromise safety. Empathy, choice and continuity of carer are three of the most valued aspects that parents report. The provision of written information is also helpful, as parents remember little of what they are told in the acute period.

Measurement of blood pressure and urinalysis should be undertaken to rule out significant pre-eclampsia. Where the fetal death is due to an abruption, clinical signs are usually apparent from the outset. If it is felt that the fetus has been dead for some time, a clotting screen should be performed to ensure that there is no coagulopathy (unlikely if the fetus is recently demised, but a 30 per cent risk after 4 weeks). Signs of maternal infection should also be recorded, as the presence of chorioamnionitis will alter management [C].

PREVENTION OF RHESUS (D) ISOIMMUNISATION

Massive fetomaternal haemorrhage is one cause of fetal death and may have occurred hours or even days before clinical presentation. If the woman is RhD negative, blood for Kleihauer testing should be taken soon after the diagnosis for an estimation of the volume of fetal–maternal transfusion. Anti-RhD immunoglobulin should be given as soon as possible after presentation and not delayed. Delivery may not occur until after the 72-hour watershed beyond which immunoprophylaxis is less effective. A further dose of anti-RhD immunoglobulin might be necessary once the Kleihauer result is known and clearance of fetal cells should be rechecked at 48 hours where a large fetomaternal haemorrhage has been encountered. If it is deemed important to know the fetal blood type and this cannot be ascertained from a fetal blood sample after birth, testing of the rhesus status can be undertaken by using free fetal DNA analysis from a maternal sample. This result will not usually be available within the 72 hours required for anti-D prophylaxis, and so all rhesus-negative women should receive at least a standard dose of anti-D when the fetal blood type is unknown [C].

HOW TO DELIVER

If the mother is well, the next step is to decide how and when to deliver her. Many women are horrified that a vaginal delivery is often recommended. This must be approached in a sympathetic manner. Most women will understand that a straightforward vaginal delivery will minimise the length of postnatal inpatient time and speed their general recovery. There may be circumstances in which CS has to be considered. These will include women for whom this management was previously planned, women with a major placenta praevia and women who simply cannot bear the concept of a vaginal delivery. There can be no set rules and each case must be individually managed. There have been no studies that have assessed the psychological impact of different delivery strategies in this context [D].

TIMING OF DELIVERY

Women should be offered the choice of when they would like to deliver. Clearly if there are conditions that pose a risk to maternal safety (abruption, pre-eclampsia, infection) then advice on expediting delivery needs to be given.

The risk of coagulation problems secondary to a retained dead fetus is small. Estimated risk is 30 per cent if the fetus has been retained for 4 weeks. Therefore, given that over 85 per cent of women will deliver spontaneously within 3 weeks following IUFD, conservative management is an option that can be offered, though testing for DIC twice weekly is recommended. Prolonged time before delivery will limit PM evaluation in some cases. Some women will want to spend time at home before commencing induction and others will want to start the process as soon as possible.

Women should be cared for within an environment that allows for supporters to stay but in which maternal safety is not compromised. In many units, a dedicated room is set aside for their management. Experienced midwifery care should be provided.

Women should have full access to analgesia as required. Diamorphine or morphine is a better option in this setting (compared to pethidine) as both have a longer half-life. Epidural analgesia should be available for women with normal clotting, and patient-controlled analgesia may be useful for those who cannot receive epidural analgesia.

INDUCTION OF LABOUR

If the woman appears to be physically well, her membranes intact and there is no evidence of infection or bleeding, she should be offered a choice of immediate IOL or expectant management. If there is evidence of ruptured membranes, infection or bleeding, immediate IOL is the preferred management option.

There are various strategies that have been used for IOL after fetal death. Whichever method is used, it is important to remember that complications such as uterine rupture and shoulder dystocia can occur and management must be safe. Until relatively recently, third-trimester induction was generally achieved with standard prostaglandin E2 preparations. This was because of their safety profile in relation to uterine rupture. Now, the combination of the anti-progesterone mifepristone and the prostaglandin analogue misoprostol is recommended. The advantage of this protocol is that the induction to delivery time is shorter (median 8.5 hours, and about 7 hours shorter than if mifepristone is not used). However, in order for the process to work efficiently, the mifepristone needs to be given 24–48 hours before starting misoprostol [B]. Although this time can be spent at home, many women do not wish to delay starting. Higher rates of anxiety have been reported in women in whom the diagnosis to commencement of induction time is greater than 24 hours. In women who do not wish to wait, misoprostol alone or prostaglandin E2 may be used. There is usually a longer time from induction to delivery in these cases. Misoprostol is not licensed for this indication and informed consent should be documented.

A standard protocol for mifepristone/misoprostol induction is shown below.

- Mifepristone: 200 mg 24–48 hours before induction.
- Misoprostol: 50–100 mcg pv 6 hourly for 24 hours.

Vaginal use of misoprostol is associated with fewer side effects of pyrexia and shivering than oral use [B].

In gestations of 34 weeks or more, doses of 50–100 mg of misoprostol appear to be effective but require breaking the tablets in half or dissolving in water.

Oxytocin augmentation will be required for some women.

Mechanical methods are rarely required now that misoprostol is widely available.

Where possible, membranes should be left intact for as long as possible, as ascending infection can rapidly develop.

For women who have IUFD and who have had a previous CS, the risk of uterine rupture is increased in IOL. After a single CS, induction is reasonable, but consent must be taken by a senior person (RCOG recommend a consultant), and the risk of uterine rupture discussed. Mifepristone alone (200 mg tds for 2 days) has been shown to lead to labour in two thirds of women.

Vaginal prostaglandin E2 can be used with the caveats on safety that increased rates of uterine rupture are seen in labour with a live baby (0.7–1.25%) [C]. If misoprostol is used a reduced dose is recommended, but the exact dose profile of greatest safety is not yet known. Smaller doses need to be specially prepared as tablets cannot be accurately cut into quarters.

Women with more than one previous CS or a previous non standard uterine incision require individualised management. After one previous CS there are still slightly increased risks of rupture and so careful surveillance must be undertaken during induction, but vaginal birth should be considered as the primary option.

Mechanical methods have been used for women with previous CS. There are no large trials and safety data are limited. It is recommended that these are used in the context of clinical trials only.

Immediate postnatal care

PPH is not uncommon, especially where there is pre-eclampsia, abruption, prolonged fetal death or infection. Prolonged chorioamnionitis and repeated small abruptions predispose to retained placenta. When this occurs it should be dealt with quickly and antibiotic prophylaxis given.

An assessment of thrombosis risk should be made for each woman using standard tools. IUFD does not itself constitute an increased risk, but associated factors (pre-eclampsia, infection, immobility) will do. LMWH should be prescribed along normal guidelines [D].

INVESTIGATIONS

It is important not to make assumptions about the cause of the IUFD that may deny parents full investigations. This is particularly so when a true knot or placental abruption is seen. Parents may wish to have a clear cause quickly identified, but it is the role of the medical and midwifery team to explain that only complete information can provide real answers.

The fetus should be carefully examined after birth. The birthweight and length should be recorded and the placenta weighed. If possible the birthweight centile should be calculated using customised centile charts as this will give a better idea of unidentified growth restriction.

Any dysmorphic signs should be noted and if there is a suspected abnormality at this stage, an examination by a clinical geneticist or interested paediatrician can be helpful (this is particularly important if PM is declined) [E].

Sexing the baby is important for identity and naming, but may be very difficult in early fetal deaths and hydropic babies. Also, where there are dysmorphic features, there may be ambiguity. There must be no attempt to guess the sex by obstetricians or midwives, as this may prove very damaging if the assessment is wrong. If necessary, it may be better to await the result of the initial PM findings or karyotype which can often be determined using rapid methods such as PCR, and available within a day or two. If the sex is not determined and parents do not wish any investigation, it is possible to register the baby as indeterminate sex. Alternatively a consensus can be reached by two experienced practitioners (a senior midwife, obstetrician or neonatologist) and if appropriate the parents can be invited to examine the baby and give their own assessment.

Investigation needs to be tailored to the individual case and thought should be given to include only those tests that are going to help inform or manage.

Investigation of the mother

See Table 47.1

Table 47.1 Investigation of the mother

Investigation of the mother	Aim
Kleihauer	Fetal-maternal haemorrhage/determine dose anti-D
FBC with platelets	
Clotting studies/fibrinogen	Baseline in case of bleeding; abnormalities may suggest pre-eclampsia or DIC
Blood group, antibody screen	Isoimmunisation
Anticardiolipin antibodies (IgG, IgM), lupus anticoagulant screen	Antiphospholipid syndrome
Thrombophilia screen	This is debatable: consider if IUGR or placental pathology; care in counselling as association may be weak. (recommended in RCOG guideline)
Protein S measurement should be deferred until at least 6 weeks postnatally	
Haemoglobin A1c	Diabetes
Urea and creatinine	Renal disease/pre-eclampsia

Investigation of the mother	Aim
Liver function tests	Pre-eclampsia/obstetric cholestasis/acute fatty liver
Bile acids	Obstetric cholestasis
Maternal serology for: syphilis, parvovirus B19, CMV, herpes simplex, rubella (if not immune), toxoplasmosis	
(Consider others if history of travel or symptoms e.g. influenza, malaria)	Transplacental transmission of infection
High vaginal/cervical swabs	Transcervical ascending infection (only relevant if confirmed histology of chorioamnionitis)
Blood cultures	If signs/symptoms suggest maternal sepsis
Parental platelet typing	If USS or PM shows intracranial haemorrhage
Thyroid function	Occult maternal thyroid disease
Anti-Ro/La	If hydrops or PM evidence AV node calcification
Red cell antibodies	If fetal hydrops
Urine screen for cocaine metabolites	If consent given and high index of suspicion
Parental karyotype	If fetal karyotype fails and there is a high index of suspicion of chromosomal disease

Investigation of the fetus

Postmortem examination

Investigation of the fetus and placenta is outlined in table 47.2. Fetal investigation is likely to help with diagnosis and future pregnancy management. Parents should be provided with written and verbal information that covers the aim of PM examination, the extent of the examination, how samples of tissue are dealt with afterwards and whether samples are kept for research or audit. They also need to know how long the process will take and whether there will be any delay in releasing the baby for burial or cremation. Perinatal pathology services should offer a rapid service where there is a cultural need to release a baby for burial quickly, but parents do need to know that some information may not be obtained accurately if the process is speedy (for instance careful examination of the fetal brain usually requires fixation which takes some days). Written consent must be obtained for each part of the process, including the fetal tissues sent for karyotyping.

Parents should have time to consider whether they wish a PM to be done and once they have signed the form there should be at least 12, and in the view of the Human Tissue Authority (HTA), 24 hours until the start of the PM.

Parents should always know that, even after they have signed the consent form, they can change their minds about anything they have agreed to.

What is postmortem examination and how it is performed?

Parents need to know that the person performing the examination is a dedicated perinatal pathologist. Some regions perform their perinatal pathology in a main centre. When this is the case, parents should be told that the baby will need to be transferred and will be rapidly and safely returned. Babies classified as stillborn under UK law must be transferred by the undertaker.

Postmortem examinations may take up to 5–7 working days to complete when the brain needs to be fixed for proper examination. Examinations should be completed within 3 days after receipt of the body if no special examination is required. There will then be additional time for histopathological analysis, microbiology, metabolic studies, etc., which can add significant delays to the final report. It is recommended that at least 60 per cent of reports are issued within 42 days and 90 per cent within 56 days.

The baby is always treated with dignity and respect. The incisions are closed and do not involve the face or limbs. In most cases the baby when dressed will look no different from the way it did before the PM. The exception may be the very small macerated fetus whose skin is so thin that suturing is not possible. In these cases, the baby is wrapped.

Fetal and placental investigation
What tissues are kept?

In general, the pathologist will not need to keep any organs. Samples for histology may be retained, but even these can be returned should the parents wish. Where a postmortem is performed in the first trimester, organs are so small that occasionally whole organs need to be retained to make microscope slides. Again, these can be returned if wished.

Where there is a suspected CNS abnormality, the brain needs to be fixed before examination ideally. This can take 5–7 days, especially in a large term fetus. If this is an important

Table 47.2 Fetal investigation

If potential for fetal abnormality take fetal and placental genetic material for karyotype. Discuss consideration of microarray analysis or single gene testing with pathologist and genetics team (fetal blood, skin, chrondrocytes, placenta)	Use more than one site and use more than one method. Solid tissue better for array analysis
Fetal and placental swabs	Bacterial infection
Fetal blood for bacteriology and virology	Culture, serology for viral infection if suspected; if no cord sample available, cardiac blood should be taken; parental consent required
Placental pathology	Infection, infarction, abruption, trophoblast invasion failure, maternal or fetal vessel thrombosis
PM examination of fetus Limited investigation if PM declined: examination/X-rays/MRI	Structural fetal abnormalities, growth restriction, infection, metabolic syndromes

aspect of the postmortem (usually if there has been antenatal suspicion of abnormality), parents have three options:

1   to forgo this extra information;
2   to delay funeral arrangements until this process is complete;
3   to allow the pathologist to retain the fetal brain and to proceed with funeral arrangements without the brain being returned.

Most parents who have given consent for postmortem will want to wait, and to delay arrangements until the baby can be returned intact.

What other investigations might be needed?

Other information may become available later, which may require further investigations. These would include parental karyotype if a fetal translocation were found or if the fetal karyotype failed but a chromosomal cause were suspected, or antiplatelet antibodies if intracranial haemorrhage is seen.

Karyotype analysis often fails. Where there are specific concerns, the genetic laboratory may be able to help with specific diagnoses by utilising other techniques such as FISH or PCR. Fetal chondrocytes provide the most prolonged cell viability, and a small sample from the iliac crest or patella can sometimes provide a diagnosis. Some have recommended performing a fetal karyotype by transabdominal CVS or amniocentesis to avoid problems associated with delay and infection of the placenta during delivery. Whereas this may be ideal, it may be unacceptable to many mothers at this time. Fetal deaths where there are known abnormalities and no previous karyotype has been taken are the group most likely to benefit from this; however, as alternative techniques increase in the number and type of chromosome problems detectable, the need for this will diminish. A search for single gene problems and consideration to whole genome array analysis will be directed to fetuses where a structural abnormality is seen that may point in the direction of a chromosome or genetic issue, undetected

by karyotype analysis. Array analysis is a science in its early stages. Where copy number variants are seen these will be categorised as varying degrees of likelihood as causative, depending on the findings, parental testing and the current body of knowledge. Array analysis is progressing quickly, but is not yet widely used in the management of stillbirth.

The Kleihauer test will become negative very quickly if there is ABO incompatibility. This test must therefore be performed as soon after confirmation of fetal death as possible and should not be delayed until after delivery. Mothers who have experienced huge fetomaternal transfusion may describe an episode of shivering, feeling unwell or rigors that may pinpoint the event; transfusion reactions have been described in this context.

Maternal glucose metabolism returns to normal almost as soon as the fetus dies. Blood sugar estimation is therefore generally unhelpful. Also, as the derangement is generally mild, HbA1c measurements are usually normal. A suspicion of disordered glucose metabolism may arise if the fetal weight is excessive and islet cell hyperplasia is confirmed (though other diagnoses such as Beckwith syndrome can also present in this manner). Women with unexplained stillbirth have a four-fold increase in glucose abnormalities in subsequent pregnancies. Therefore, if this diagnosis is suspected, formal glucose testing should be undertaken in the next pregnancy [C]. It is established that APS can lead to IUFD, and there is evidence that low-dose aspirin and LMWH improve pregnancy outcome amongst those women who present with recurrent miscarriage (see Chapter 89). Thrombophilia may be associated with stillbirth in growth-restricted fetuses and there may be placental features that point to an underlying thrombophilia. It must be recognised that there are no studies to guide management in the subsequent pregnancy.

Obstetric cholestasis carries at most a marginal increase in the rate of stillbirth, but as it is a recurrent condition, screening for bile salts is worthwhile [E].

It is possible to screen maternal urine for the presence of illegal drugs. This should only be done with the consent of the mother and, in this author's experience, is unhelpful. Most mothers feel guilty enough if they think they have contributed to the death of their baby without needing concrete evidence. Those who divulge information about illicit drug use do not need the additional burden of proof. Those who do not provide this information are unlikely to consent to urine testing.

Can anything else be offered to parents who do not want a PM?

Placental pathology should be offered regardless of whether a full PM is to be performed. However, it is important to be realistic about what information this can yield. Up to 48 hours after fetal death placental morphology does not change very much, but after this time placental morphology changes such that it can be difficult to differentiate pre-existing from PM changes. After 14 days from fetal death placental pathology is unlikely to yield any useful information. It is important that the placental pathology is undertaken by an experienced perinatal pathologist, as ascribing causation based on placental changes is not a straightforward task.

Fetal MRI can provide some information, but cannot replace a full PM yet as a specific skill set is required to ensure accurate diagnoses. However, up to 87 per cent concordance has been seen when used to determine major structural abnormalities, compared with PM examination [C].[5]

Parents need careful counselling by someone who is experienced in dealing with this situation and who understands the processes involved. It is important that obstetricians are trained to seek consent in these cases and understand fully the issues involved. An excellent leaflet explaining PM to parents is produced by the HTA at http://www.hta.gov.uk/policiesandcodesofpractice/modelconsentforms.cfm.

The final facet of obtaining good information at PM is to give the pathologist all the relevant information. Where there are specific suspicions, the pathologist should be informed of these. It is usually helpful to speak directly with the pathologist about the case. This will also enable the doctor responsible for the case to attend the PM if possible.

AFTER DELIVERY

After delivery there are many processes that need to be completed before discharge. The first and most important is to allow the parents as much (or as little) time with the baby as they need. Parents should be allowed to express their own wishes with regard to seeing and holding the baby. Some parents will want to come back to the hospital on a few occasions before they feel able to finally part from their lost baby.

Evidence on whether psychological outcomes are better or worse in women who have close contact with their stillborn infant is conflicting and so it is imperative to be guided by what the parents feel is best for them.

Depression, which can become post-traumatic stress disorder (PTSD), is common and women, their partners and children may need considerable support, access to good-quality counselling and in some cases the support of the perinatal mental health team and GP.

Parents should be offered the opportunity to have photographs taken and, if these are not wanted at the time, they can be kept, as many parents request them later (sometimes a long time later). The parents may want footprints or handprints of the baby to be taken.

Importantly, having a funeral and keeping mementoes is not associated with additional adverse outcomes. Photographs should only be taken after seeking the parents' wishes, as in some cultures taking photographs of the dead is unacceptable.[6]

All units should have a bereavement team to take on the care of parents. These teams are usually acutely aware of cultural requirements and may provide an important liaison between the family and the pathologist, especially where there is a need for funeral arrangements to proceed without delay. Unfortunately, it is often those who have the most to gain from PM who feel the most cultural pressure not to delay burial. Sympathetic discussion can often provide a way forward, and many pathologists will provide an out-of-hours service so that delays can be minimised.

Parents should be provided with the telephone numbers of organisations that may also offer support, such as SANDS, as they sometimes need to talk to people unconnected with the hospital. The bereavement team will also provide a contact number.

LEGAL ISSUES

The law in the UK states that a stillborn baby is one delivered after the 24th week of pregnancy, showing no signs of life.

Further guidance issued by the Department of Health and accepted in Scotland and Northern Ireland states that a baby delivered after 24 weeks, but known or able to be proved by examination to have died before 24 weeks, does not need to be registered. Most often this applies to a co-twin, retained for some time after death; however, occasionally a woman will present with a singleton loss, where it is clear that the death was many weeks earlier. In these cases it must be provable by examination of the development of the fetus that the baby was less mature at the time of birth. In some cases this will require PM examination. In others it may be very obvious, by external examination by an experienced person. Where a PM is needed to establish the potential maturity but this is not wished, the baby should be registered in the normal way.

The parents need the stillbirth certificate in order to register the baby. The attending doctor or midwife can issue the certificate.

When the certificate is completed, it is important not to use abbreviations, or attempt to guess the cause of death. It is extremely difficult to have death certificates changed and parents can be deeply upset to find that a baby has a registered cause of death that is not accurate. The Registrar's office may need to contact the doctor or midwife signing the death certificate, so it is always important to sign and print the name, and important information such as recognised GMC qualifications must not be omitted. The less well the form is completed, the more time the bereaved parents will have to spend at the Registrar's office while he or she tries to contact the doctor or midwife involved.

The mother, or father if the couple were married at the time of the loss, can register the stillbirth. This has to be done within 42 days (21 days in Scotland) and only in exceptional circumstances will this be extended to 3 months. Registration can be delegated to the delivering doctor, midwife or bereavement officer if they have the appropriate supporting information and documentation (most Registrars' websites will have the requirements).

Responsibility for funeral arrangements lies with parents, but can be delegated to the hospital.

The sex of the baby can be added later after PM, but changing the name can be more difficult and will not be permitted in many cases.

The law does not recognise fetal deaths before 24 weeks. The lack of legal recognition means that parents will not have a death certificate for these early fetal losses. It does not mean that they cannot arrange a funeral or cremation if they wish.

Mothers who have delivered a stillborn baby are entitled to normal maternity benefits and payments. Mothers delivering before this time will not be so entitled.

The Coroner has the discretion to be involved where there has been a criminal act, such as assault, and can request a PM. Cases of unattended fresh stillbirth should also be discussed with the coroner.

If there is a suspicion of a criminal act to cause a stillbirth, the police should be informed.

SUPPRESSION OF LACTATION

The onset of lactation often catches women by surprise and is a source of considerable distress when it starts in earnest at about 48 hours. Although not all women need or want lactation suppression, discussion should take place so that advice can be given about how to cope. For some women, simply a good supportive bra, NSAIDs if there is discomfort, and time will be enough. However, about a third of women experience distressing breast pain and so pharmacological measures should be offered to all suitable women. A single dose (1 mg) of cabergoline, a long-acting dopamine agonist, is highly effective. Dopamine agonists for the inhibition of lactation should not be used in women with pre-eclampsia or hypertension [B].[7]

CONTRACEPTION

This subject is best covered by the GP or consultant later, but women do need to know that they can conceive before their first period. A pregnancy conceived quickly may delay the grieving process and, before women go home, it does no harm to include a leaflet on contraception that will meet their needs.

GOING HOME

Although every effort is made to ensure women go home quickly, premature discharge must be avoided. It is undoubtedly more painful for women to have to return with problems, and safety is paramount. Many units have a bereavement suite or family room so that other family members can stay for support until discharge can safely be achieved.

Contact telephone numbers should be given to the woman or a companion, and there should be a contact who knows what has happened and who is easily available should problems occur. The community team will play a central role in the care of the family, and detailed communication with the GP and community midwife is of paramount importance. They must be informed by telephone on the day of the woman's return to the community, and all antenatal appointments must be cancelled. There is a notification process so that mailing regarding baby products which may have been signed up to antenatally can be supressed.

BEREAVEMENT CARE

As perinatal death becomes less common, couples can feel increasingly isolated in their grief. The bereavement team and the community midwife and GP need to be aware of the situation and to react quickly when problems appear to be mounting. It is particularly those couples with high expectations and little family or social support who can be most vulnerable at this time. It is helpful to ensure before discharge that provision is made for the partner to have some time off work, as he will often be forgotten at this time. Also, if the fetal loss has occurred early (20–24 weeks), the patient will need a statement of fitness to work (previously termed a sick note), as maternity leave will not be applicable.

Parents who have other children often wish to receive guidance about explaining the death of the baby to them. Children's books about stillbirth are available. Self-help groups (such as SANDS) also offer support that may sometimes be lacking from professionals. The couple's response to bereavement cannot be predicted by whether they already have children, or the gestation of the fetal loss. Couples respond in different ways and take different amounts of time to heal. The loss of a baby with a severe malformation should not be interpreted as a blessing; it may leave parents with significant fears for the future.

The death of one twin with the survival of the other is especially distressing for parents, who are faced with contradictory psychological processes. It is very difficult to celebrate the birth of one healthy baby and to grieve the death of the other. In this situation, mourning may get postponed or give rise to symptoms of failed grieving, which include the inability to care for and relate to the surviving child appropriately and may contribute to postnatal depression. The Twins and Multiple Births Association (TAMBA) has an excellent parents' leaflet on dealing with the loss of one baby in a multiple pregnancy.

FOLLOW-UP

The obstetrician involved in the antenatal care is the usual choice to conduct the follow-up. However, there may be occasions when the woman requests follow-up by a different practitioner, and when this occurs it should not be questioned. It has traditionally been arranged for follow-up to take place at around the time of the usual postnatal visit. In general it is reasonable to try to schedule a visit once all information is available. Reporting times for PM vary and so it is important to know these before attempting to set a date for review.

Women often experience extreme anxiety coming back to the hospital where they have had such a devastating experience. If possible, a neutral venue should be chosen. In every case, there should be enough time to discuss events.

Ideally, the name of the baby should be ascertained before the interview. The bereavement team should be able to supply this. Not all parents will have named the baby.

Generally, parents need to have time to go through events as they recall them, to ask questions that are important to them, and to receive and understand the results of any tests that have been performed.

Often the issues that are most troubling parents are not those that the medical team see as important, so it is vital to keep an open mind, to encourage parents to talk spontaneously and to be honest in replies. Parents may want to apportion blame to individuals or actions. When this occurs, it is important to be honest and to offer apology where this is deemed necessary. Where there has been a failure of care, parents need to receive sincere apologies and reassurance that action to prevent a similar occurrence will take place. Being half-truthful or dishonest will not prevent or reduce litigation. However, where there has been no failure of care, it is important to support other colleagues' management in discussion with parents.

When an underlying cause for the fetal death has been identified, this must be clearly explained. There may be the need to involve other professionals, such as clinical geneticists, at a later date.

When no cause has been found, parents are often very frustrated. This is always difficult for professionals, as the wish to provide answers is one of our most ingrained rationales. It is important not to try to provide unfounded reassurance, but in all cases a clear plan of management for the next pregnancy should be outlined.

Parents often ask when they can try for another pregnancy. It must not be assumed that all couples will wish to do so, and this issue must be covered sensitively.

Early conception may be associated with very marginally higher risks of preterm birth and SGA babies, but these risk increases are not great enough to recommended delayed conception [C].[8] However, it is important that the grieving process is complete (as much as can ever be so) before the next child. Mothers who conceive quickly may have more problems with anxiety during pregnancy, depression, PTSD and disordered bonding after the next birth. Interestingly, fathers experience greater depression if conception is delayed. Postpartum depression following the birth of the next baby is common and professionals should be alert to this.

It is helpful for parents if the issues discussed can be provided for them in a letter. Many women will not wish to book their next pregnancy at the same hospital, and a clear letter will help the future team to understand events. It is also helpful for parents as an *aide memoire*, as they may not clearly remember some of the points covered. Finally, parents must be given the opportunity to come back if they are unclear about certain aspects and, for some, a pre-conceptual visit is helpful.

Where possible lifestyle adjustments should be recommended prior to conception. These may include weight loss, smoking cessation and drug and alcohol interventions. Stillbirth is commoner in relationships where there is domestic violence. Whilst there is still no clear recommendation regarding effective intervention during pregnancy, if possible the opportunity to enquire and offer help should not be missed. This information must be appropriately shared to help to protect the woman and any existing children, and to protect any baby born in the future.[9]

MANAGEMENT OF THE NEXT PREGNANCY

Management in the next pregnancy will depend on the circumstances of the loss and the results of the investigations.

Some aspects are common to all women who have lost babies in these circumstances. A means of identifying that a baby was lost so that professionals are all aware quickly that there has been a previous loss is important. This may include stickers on notes and icons on computer records.

It is beyond the remit of this chapter to discuss the potential management plans after fetal loss as the causes are very diverse and management must be individualised. The most important facet of management is to try to adhere to the plans that were formulated after the loss of the baby. It is unusual for professionals to disagree to such an extent that a previously agreed plan has to be changed. There may be minor differences of opinion, but it is better to put these aside in the interests of maintaining the faith of the patient in their care when at all possible. When the plan needs to be changed (such as may occur when new information comes to light), it is important to explain clearly why the changes need to be made and how this will improve the prospects of a healthy pregnancy.

After the birth of the next child, parents may require much reassurance that the baby is healthy. An examination by a senior paediatrician can do much to allay fears.

Postnatal depression is common and both families and professionals need to be aware of this.

KEY POINTS

- Confirm fetal death quickly by ultrasound.
- Offer parents choice wherever possible.
- Do not make assumptions regarding the cause of death.
- Offer a full range of investigations tailored to the circumstances of the death.
- The support of a bereavement team is an integral part of care.
- Do not discharge the mother home until it is safe to do so.
- Do not forget lactation suppression and thromboprophylaxis.
- Information should be provided at all stages in a form that parents can understand.
- Management of the next pregnancy should try to follow previously set plans.

Key References

1. Schytte J. Stillbirth, an Executive Summary for the Lancet Series. thelancet.com. April 14, 2011.
2. Gardosi J, Giddings S, Clifford S *et al.* Association between reduced stillbirth rates in England and regional uptake of accreditation training in customised fetal growth assessment. *BMJ* Open 2013;3:e003942.
3. Green-top guideline 55. *Late Intrauterine Fetal Death and Stillbirth.* RCOG, October 2010.
4. NICE. *Diabetes in pregnancy.* NICE Clinical Guideline 63, July 2008.
5. Thayyil S, Sebire N, Chitty L *et al.* for the MARIAS collaborative group. Post-mortem MRI versus conventional autopsy in fetuses and children: a prospective validation study. *Lancet* 2013;382:223–33.
6. Gatrad AR, Sheikh A. Muslim birth customs. *Arch Dis Child Fetal Neonatal Ed* 2001;84:F6–8.
7. National Collaborating Centre for Women's and Children's Health. Single dose cabergoline versus bromocriptine in inhibition of puerperal lactation: randomised, double blind, multicentre study. European Multicentre Study Group for Cabergoline in Lactation Inhibition. Commissioned by NICE, March 2008 (revised reprint July 2008). *BMJ* 1991;302(6789):1367–71.
8. Conde-Agudelo A, Rosas-Bermúdez A, Kafury-Goeta AC. Birth spacing and risk of adverse perinatal outcomes: a meta-analysis. *JAMA* 2006;295:1809–23.
9. NICE. *Domestic violence and abuse: how health services, social care and the organisations they work with can respond effectively.* February 2014. NICE public health guidance 50. guidance.nice.org.uk/ph5.

SECTION FIVE

First Stage of Labour

Chapter 48 Induction of labour

Nina Johns

INTRODUCTION

Induction of labour is the process by which labour is started prior to its spontaneous onset by artificial stimulation of uterine contractions and/or progressive cervical effacement and dilatation, leading to active labour and birth. The clinical need for IOL occurs when it is perceived that the outcome of the pregnancy will be improved if it is interrupted by induction, labour and birth.

IOL has considerable impact on women's experience of labour and birth, as it may be less efficient, more painful and more likely to require epidural analgesia and assisted birth.[1,2] Therefore a well-defined clinical indication is needed, with careful consideration of the benefits and risks, together with a clear explanation to the woman prior to the decision being made.

The indications for IOL need to take into account the level of urgency for birth and suitability of vaginal birth. If the clinical situation necessitates urgent birth prior to the likely completion of an IOL process or vaginal birth is contraindicated, then an emergency caesarean birth may be required. If a woman declines the offer of IOL, a plan for monitoring maternal and fetal wellbeing needs to be made and an opportunity provided for her to discuss the risks and benefits again during her continuing care.

The management of IOL is subject to clear national and international guidance with NICE clinical guidelines (CG070)[1,2] and WHO recommendations.[3] Local pathways of care and clinical decisions should therefore reflect this guidance and be based on the evidence available.

INCIDENCE

IOL is a common obstetric intervention, occurring in approximately 20 per cent of all births in the UK. The rates of IOL vary but have been rising over the last 30 years in most developed countries. The RCOG *Patterns of Maternity Care* report found the mean induction rate for primiparous women was 27.5 per cent and 21.4 per cent for multiparous women in the UK (Fig. 48.1). The report highlights that the wide variation in induction rates is not explained by demographic or clinical risk factors.[4]

Increasing rates of IOL also have an impact on the workflow in maternity departments. The increasing elective workload has to be balanced with the emergency care required for women in spontaneous labour or with pregnancy-related complications. At times of peak activity, this workload can exceed capacity and lead to delays and increase the risk to these women and their babies.

INDICATIONS FOR IOL

The primary indication for IOL is when the outcome for mother and baby will be improved by interrupting pregnancy rather than awaiting spontaneous onset of labour. The decision to proceed with IOL must also take into account the attitude and wishes of the woman, provided her understanding of the risks of induction and the risks of continuing the pregnancy are established.

There are many recognised indications for IOL and for most there is a potential risk of perinatal mortality. The following indications are discussed in further detail where

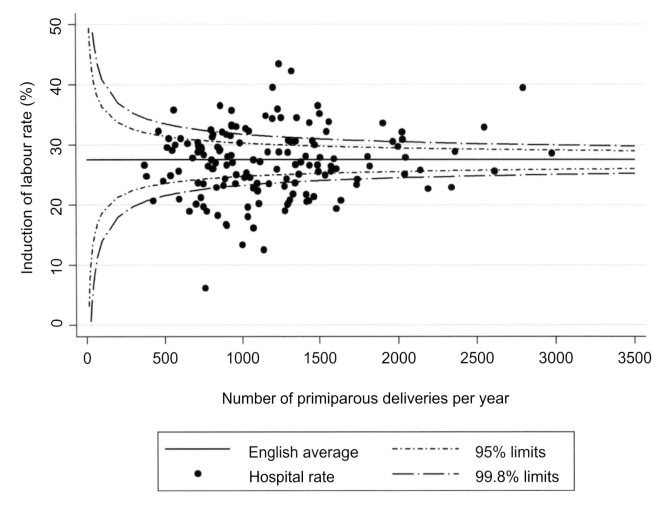

Fig. 48.1 Funnel plot showing rates of induction of labour among primiparous women. RCOG *Patterns of Maternity Care in English NHS Hospitals 2011/12.*

evidence is available to inform decision making or for which recent national guidance has changed.

Prolonged pregnancy

There is established evidence that the risk of perinatal mortality increases with gestational age beyond 40 weeks (Fig. 48.2). Systematic review of RCTs shows that expectant management compared to IOL after 41 weeks' gestation is associated with higher rates of perinatal death, despite the overall incidence being low (2–3/1000 pregnancies). Further, births after 42 weeks' gestation are associated with increased risk of intrapartum and neonatal deaths.[1,2] It is recommended that IOL is offered from 40+7 weeks onwards to avoid prolonged pregnancy. As approximately 20 per cent of women will still be pregnant at 40+7 weeks, local pathways may delay IOL until 40+12 weeks, to facilitate more women to attend in spontaneous labour.

Women who choose not to have IOL should be offered additional antenatal monitoring, which should include as a minimum EFM and ultrasound examination for liquor volume measurement twice weekly.[1]

Pre-labour rupture of membranes at term

Approximately 8–10 per cent of women present with spontaneous rupture of membranes at or beyond 37 weeks' gestation; of these 60 per cent will labour spontaneously within 24 hours. Women should be offered the choice of expectant management following spontaneous rupture of membranes, with the offer of IOL after 24 hours to reduce the risk of serious neonatal infection. (Incidence is 1 per cent with PROM compared to 0.5 per cent in women with intact membranes.) During the period of expectant management women should be advised to check their temperature, report any change in vaginal loss and have fetal movements and heart rate assessed every 24 hours.

Premature pre-labour rupture of membranes

PPROM prior to 37 weeks' gestation occurs in approximately 3 per cent of pregnancies. The resulting risk of preterm birth, maternal and neonatal infection is associated with significant morbidity and mortality. Evidence from RCTs shows

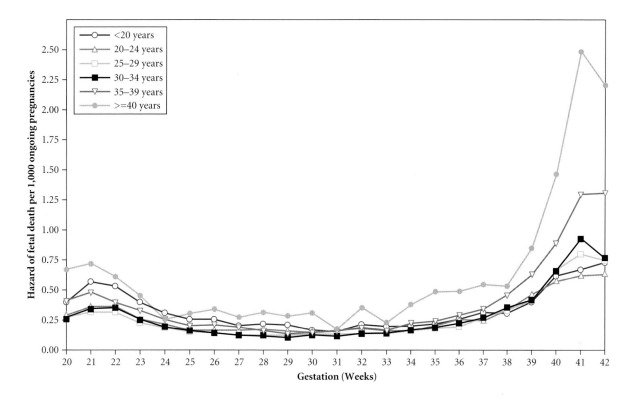

Fig. 48.2 Risk of stillbirth for singleton births without congenital anomalies by gestational age, 2001–2002. U. Reddy *et al. American Journal of Obstetrics and Gynecology* 2006;195:764–70.

that immediate IOL is associated with reduced incidence of chorioamnionitis. However, the increased risk of neonatal morbidity due to prematurity prior to 34 weeks' gestation has led to the recommendation that induction is inappropriate unless there are clinical indicators of sepsis or fetal compromise.[1,2]

Maternal conditions

Diabetes
Confidential Enquiry data have confirmed the higher stillbirth rate for women with diabetes, which is approximately 5 times greater than the national rate. Evidence from RCT and cohort studies shows that IOL between 38–39 weeks' gestation results in reduction in late stillbirth and the intrapartum complications of macrosomia, such as shoulder dystocia. Therefore, IOL is recommended after 38 weeks.[5]

Hypertension
Pre-existing and gestational hypertension are both associated with increased risk of placental abruption, developing pre-eclampsia and increased perinatal mortality. In order to reduce this risk, recent NICE guidance recommends that for women with chronic hypertension whose blood pressure is lower than 160/110 mmHg after 37 weeks, with or without antihypertensive treatment, timing of birth, and maternal

and fetal indications for birth should be agreed between the woman and the senior obstetrician. Further, women with pre-eclampsia after 37 weeks' gestation should be offered IOL.[6]

Obstetric cholestasis
OC is associated with an unpredictable increased risk of stillbirth at all gestations. Systematic review suggests that the uncertain risk to the fetus and the risks of the intervention of IOL should be balanced and discussed with the woman after 37 weeks' gestation. There is additional evidence suggesting that the decision to intervene should also be influenced by the severity of the biochemical abnormalities.[7]

Advanced maternal age
Epidemiological studies show that the average age of women having their first baby is increasing, particularly in women aged over 35 years. Women over 40 have increased rates of intrapartum CS and operative vaginal delivery rates. Their risk of stillbirth at 39 weeks' gestation is similar to that of a 25–29 year old at 41 weeks' gestation and is greater in nulliparous women. IOL is often offered at 39–40 weeks' gestation, particularly in a first pregnancy, after these risks have been discussed with the women, but there is currently no trial evidence that early induction reduces intrapartum complications or perinatal mortality.[8]

Maternal request

Maternal request for IOL is currently not supported by NICE guidance. However, it adds that this may be considered in exceptional circumstances and after discussion of the risks with the women. In practice, these women will often face frustrating delays in the process as their indication for induction will not be prioritised when there are issues of capacity.

Fetal conditions

Small for gestational age

The SGA fetus is defined as having an abdominal circumference or estimated fetal weight below the 10th centile on ultrasound examination and is at greater risk of perinatal mortality and morbidity, particularly if growth restricted.[10] At present the only intervention for IUGR is birth. RCT evidence shows increased risk of adverse perinatal outcome in women offered expectant management versus IOL when SGA was detected beyond 36 weeks' gestation. Therefore it is recommended that IOL can be offered at 37 weeks' gestation. However, rates of emergency CS are increased in this group undergoing IOL and continuous FHR monitoring is recommended once regular uterine contractions commence.[9]

Reduced fetal movements

Women who present on two or more occasions with reduced fetal movements are at increased risk of a poor perinatal outcome compared with those who attend on only one occasion. There are currently no studies to determine whether intervention such as IOL alters perinatal morbidity or mortality in these women. NICE recommends that the decision to induce labour at term in a woman who presents recurrently with reduced fetal movements, when the growth, liquor volume and CTG appear normal, must be made after careful consultant-led counselling of induction on an individualised basis.[10]

Multiple pregnancies

Twin and triplet pregnancies more often present in preterm labour, with nearly 60 per cent of women with twin pregnancies giving birth spontaneously before 37 weeks' gestation. Evidence from studies reporting on all multiple pregnancies together (uncomplicated, spontaneous onset of labour or otherwise) showed an increase in the risk of fetal death per week at term gestations, with significant rise from 37 weeks' gestation. The risk of term perinatal mortality was greater in MC twin pregnancies. It is recommended that women with DC twins should be offered elective birth at 37 weeks, and MC twins at 36 weeks. For triplets there is an increased risk of spontaneous preterm labour and a significantly higher risk of fetal death after 34 weeks 6 days. It is recommended that women with triplet pregnancies should be offered birth at 35 weeks.[11]

Suspected fetal macrosomia

Suspected fetal macrosomia is defined as a birthweight above 4000 g and occurs in approximately 2–10 per cent of births in the UK. Evidence from two systematic reviews comparing IOL versus expectant management showed no difference in maternal or fetal outcomes, such as CS rates or episodes of shoulder dystocia, with suspected fetal macrosomia.[1]

METHODS OF IOL

Spontaneous labour is defined as the onset of regular painful contractions, leading to progressive dilatation of the cervix. The precise steps for the initiation of labour are unknown and methods for IOL aim to bring about dilatation of the cervix and start uterine contractions. Reviews of the available evidence for methods of IOL are summarised in Table 48.1 and discussed below.

Membrane sweeping

Membrane sweeping appears to result in increased local production of prostaglandins. Systematic review shows that membrane sweeping is associated with an increased rate of spontaneous labour and a reduction in need for formal induction, particularly in multiparous women.[1,2] It is associated with an increased incidence of uncomplicated bleeding and pain at the time of examination, but similar maternal (CS rates, maternal infection) and fetal outcomes (compared to no membrane sweep) and appears acceptable to women. Review of the NNT show that to avoid 1 formal IOL, sweeping of membranes would need to be performed in 8 women in pregnancies of 38–42 weeks' gestation. Women should be offered membrane sweeping prior to formal IOL and at the 40- and 41-week antenatal visits.[1,2]

Vaginal prostaglandins

Prostaglandins (PGs) are established in the role of stimulating uterine contractions and cervical change. Vaginal PGs can be administered via a number of preparations: controlled release pessaries, vaginal tablets or gel.

Evidence from systematic review and RCTs shows that, in women with an unfavourable cervix, all preparations of vaginal PGE2 improve cervical status and reduce the need for oxytocin augmentation. In addition, in women with a favourable cervix, vaginal PGs are associated with high rates of achieving vaginal birth within 24 hours compared to placebo and reduced risk of PPH compared to amniotomy plus intravenous oxytocin.

It appears that maternal and fetal outcomes are comparable for all preparations of vaginal PGs and vaginal PGs should be the preferred method of IOL irrespective of cervical status. However, in women with an unfavourable cervix the use of controlled-release pessaries may be preferable because the induction time may be longer and repeated doses of tablet or gel would be required.[1,2]

Table 48.1 Summary of methods of induction of labour

Method of IOL	Level of evidence	Benefit	Potential harm
Membrane sweeping	Systematic review & RCT	Increased spontaneous labour; reduction in IOL; same maternal and fetal outcomes	Increase in uncomplicated bleeding; pain
Vaginal prostaglandins	Systematic review & RCTs	Improved cervical status (unfavourable cervix); higher rates of birth by 24 hours (favourable cervix); less PPH	Uterine hyperstimulation; increased risk of scar rupture in previous CS
Oral PGE2	Systematic review	Similar maternal and fetal outcomes compared to other PGE2 preparations & ARM +/− oxytocin	Significant gastrointestinal side effects
Intravenous PGE2; extra-amniotic PGE2; intracervical PGE2	Systematic review	Similar maternal and fetal outcomes compared to vaginal PGE2 preparations	Increased uterine hyperstimulation with IV PGE2 and significant maternal side effects
Intravenous oxytocin alone	Systematic review	When compared to vaginal PGE2, less likely to achieve cervical change or birth within 24 hours	Increased rate of caesarean birth with intact membranes and unfavourable cervix
Amniotomy with intravenous oxytocin	Systematic review	Comparable to vaginal PGE2 to achieve birth within 24 hours and rates of caesarean birth	Increased PPH (favourable cervix); more invasive for women and requires CEFM
Misoprostol	Systematic review & RCTs	Comparable to vaginal PGE2 at low dose, increased rates of success at higher doses	Significantly higher rates of uterine hyperstimulation; maternal gastrointestinal side effects; not licensed for use in pregnancy in UK
Amniotomy (ARM)	Systematic review (1 RCT)	Similar maternal and fetal outcomes compared to vaginal PGE2 but increased need for oxytocin; no uterine hyperstimulation	Significantly increased need for oxytocin augmentation; risk of infection
Mechanical methods (balloon catheters)	Systematic review & RCTs	Comparable to vaginal PGE2 to achieve birth within 24 hours; less uterine hyperstimulation	Risk of infection; maternal satisfaction unclear
Castor oil	Systematic review & RCT	Small RCT shows improvement of Bishop's score; systematic review shows no difference	All women experienced nausea after ingesting castor oil
Homeopathy	Systematic review	Insufficient data to show benefit	Insufficient data to show harm
Acupuncture	Systematic review but poor quality studies & RCT	Insufficient data to show benefit	Insufficient data to show harm
Herbal supplements	No evidence	No evidence of benefit	Potential harmful effects due to active ingredients

Amniotomy and oxytocin

Amniotomy describes the artificial rupture of the membranes (ARM) and is only possible if the cervical os is open and the membranes are accessible. Systematic review of the RCT evidence for ARM only compared to vaginal PGs showed a significant increased need for oxytocin use but with similar maternal and fetal outcomes at birth.[1] ARM alone is not recommended as a primary method of IOL, but may be considered if vaginal PGs are contraindicated or there is a history of uterine hyperstimulation.

Intravenous oxytocin has been used alone, in combination with ARM, or following cervical preparation with other agents. Systematic review has evaluated the effects of intravenous oxytocin alone compared to vaginal PGs and in combination with ARM. It shows that intravenous oxytocin alone was associated with an unchanged cervical status after 12–24 hours and an increased caesarean birth rate, in women with an unfavourable cervix and intact membranes. Women with ruptured membranes or with a favourable cervix given intravenous oxytocin alone were significantly less likely to give birth vaginally within 24 hours when compared with vaginal PGs.[1]

Systematic review comparing ARM with intravenous oxytocin and vaginal PGs showed no significant differences in not achieving vaginal birth within 24 hours or in caesarean birth rate, but numbers of cases were small. However one RCT, with women with a favourable cervix, showed significant increases in PPH rates in those receiving ARM and intravenous oxytocin compared to those with vaginal PGs. It is recommended that ARM with intravenous oxytocin should not be used as a primary method of IOL, but may be considered if vaginal PGs are contraindicated or there is a history of uterine hyperstimulation. ARM with intravenous oxytocin continues to be the secondary process for IOL if vaginal PGs have not been successful.[1]

Misoprostol

Misoprostol is a synthetic PG producing uterine contractions and can be given orally, vaginally or sublingually. It is not licensed for use in pregnancy in the UK.

Systematic review has compared different doses of oral and vaginal misoprostol with vaginal and intracervical PGs and shown that vaginal misoprostol at low doses is comparable with vaginal PGs, but at higher doses is associated with higher rates of successful IOL but also with greater risk of uterine hyperstimulation. However, the only available preparations of misoprostol are higher-dose tablets and the product is not licensed in the UK, therefore misprostol should not be used for IOL except in cases of IUFD.[1]

Mechanical methods

Mechanical methods studied for use in IOL include balloon catheters or laminaria tents, which are inserted into the cervical canal or into the extra-amniotic space. Balloon catheters appear to be the most commonly used method in the UK. Systematic review has compared mechanical methods with placebo, vaginal or cervical prostaglandin, and with misoprostol and intravenous oxytocin; unfortunately the studies are small, with many different comparisons. It appears that, when compared with all PG preparations, mechanical methods do not change the rate of vaginal birth within 24 hours or the caesarean birth rate.[1] Mechanical methods may be associated with reduced rates of uterine hyperstimulation and may reduce the risk of uterine rupture in the presence of a previous CS scar, but require further evaluation.

CLINICAL PATHWAY AND PROCESS FOR INDUCTION OF LABOUR

The NICE guidance on the IOL care pathway can be found within the guidance and website link: http://pathways.nice.org.uk/pathways/induction-of-labour#path=view%3A/pathways/induction-of-labour/performing-induction.xml&content=view-node%3Anodes-formal-induction.

Monitoring during IOL

How close a woman is to the onset of spontaneous labour will influence the likelihood that IOL will be successful. This is assessed by vaginal examination and cervical status measured using the Bishop's score (Table 48.2). Prior to formal induction, this should be assessed and recorded and maternal and fetal wellbeing established with a normal FHR pattern with EFM and routine maternal observations.

Prior to IOL it is necessary to confirm that the indication for offering induction remains, confirm the fetal lie and presentation, confirm that placental site is not low-lying and inform the woman of the pathway and the risk of complications, including uterine hyperstimulation/tachysystole.

After administration of vaginal PGs, when contractions begin, fetal wellbeing should be assessed with continuous EFM.

Table 48.2 Cervical scoring using modified Bishop's score

Cervical scoring				
Score	0	1	2	3
Dilatation (cm)	<1	1–2	2–4	>4
Length (cm)	>4	2–4	1–2	<1
Consistency	Firm	Average	Soft	
Position	Post	Mid/Anterior		

Once this is confirmed as normal, intermittent auscultation should be used unless there are clear indications for continuous EFM. Bishop's scores should be reassessed 6 hours after vaginal PGE2 tablet or gel insertion, or 24 hours after vaginal PGE2 controlled-release pessary insertion, to monitor progress.[1]

Place of IOL

Facilities should be available for continuous electronic fetal heart rate and contraction monitoring wherever IOL is carried out.

Cohort studies found that woman being induced in the morning were less likely to require intravenous oxytocin and had lower rates of operative vaginal birth and greater maternal satisfaction.[1]

A recent Cochrane review of four studies of outpatient IOL showed no difference in success of induction or birth outcomes, and greater maternal satisfaction during outpatient IOL, but that total hospital stay was the same for inpatient and outpatient pathways.[12] NICE recommends that outpatient induction should be continuously audited and only carried out if safety and support procedures are in place.

SPECIAL CIRCUMSTANCES

Previous caesarean birth

A proportion of women who have had a previous caesarean birth will also have an indication for IOL in a future pregnancy. In addition to the risks of IOL, these women also have the increased risk of uterine rupture. Multiple systematic reviews have compared different methods of induction in women with previous caesarean births and UKOSS have reviewed rates of uterine rupture.[1,13] Systematic review showed inadequate evidence for the preferred method for induction in these cases, though a small RCT showed that vaginal PGs followed by ARM was more effective that ARM alone.[1] However, UKOSS data show a higher risk of uterine rupture with labour induction and that the rate with vaginal PGs was greater than with ARM and intravenous oxytocin. Uterine rupture is more likely to be associated with IOL in women with no previous vaginal birth. It is recommended that women who have had a previous CS may be offered IOL with vaginal PG, CS or expectant management on an individual basis. Women should be informed of the increased risks with IOL, increased risk of need for emergency CS and increased risk of uterine rupture.[1]

IUFD

IUFD after 24 weeks of gestation is estimated to occur in 1 per cent of all pregnancies. Though 90 per cent of women will spontaneously deliver within 3 weeks of the intrauterine death, expectant management is associated with risks of intrauterine infection if the membranes are ruptured, and of DIC. Multiple RCT and observational studies have compared induction methods and shown that misoprostol is most effective and that the use of oral mifepristone reduced the dosage of prostaglandins required to induce labour.[1]

COMPLICATIONS OF IOL

IOL has considerable impact on women's experience of labour and birth, as it may be less efficient, more painful and more likely to require epidural analgesia and assisted birth.[1] In addition to the impact on women's experience, there are additional specific complications.

Failed IOL

Failed induction is defined as failure to establish labour after one cycle of treatment, consisting of the insertion of two vaginal PGE2 tablets (3 mg) or gel (1–2 mg) at 6-hourly intervals, or one PGE2 controlled-release pessary (10 mg) over 24 hours, and is estimated to occur in 15 per cent of cases.[1]

There is little evidence relating to management of failed induction and NICE recommends that each case is reviewed individually to consider whether a further attempt to induce labour can be considered or a caesarean birth is required.

Uterine hyperstimulation

Uterine hyperstimulation can appear as tachysystole (increased uterine contractions) or hypertonus (increased uterine activity with fetal distress), which leads to fetal heart rate changes and occurs in 1–5 per cent of cases depending on the methods of induction used. Systematic review shows low-dose PG preparations carry the lowest risk and that tocolytics can be used to reduce the uterine activity and reversible hyperstimulation. Terbutaline is recommended as first-line treatment; however, if FHR changes remain, emergency caesarean birth may be considered necessary.

Cord prolapse

Cord prolapse is a potential risk when the membranes rupture, especially when the membranes are ruptured artificially. To reduce this risk it is recommended that engagement of the presenting part should be assessed, umbilical cord presentation should be excluded during vaginal examination and ARM should be avoided if the baby's head is high.[1]

Emergency caesarean birth

Patterns of maternity care in English NHS Hospitals 2011/12 show that among primiparous women with induced labours, the mean rate of emergency caesarean was 30.2 per cent.

Among multiparous women whose labours were induced, the mean rate of emergency caesarean was 13.2%.[4] However recent meta-analysis to evaluate whether or not IOL increases the risk of CS in women with intact membranes showed that a policy of induction was associated with a reduction in the risk of CS compared with expectant management in women at term. The authors concluded that this effect may arise from non-treatment effects, and that additional trials are needed.[14]

Delays in care

Whilst there is qualitative evidence regarding the impact of IOL on a woman's experience, there are no data reviewing the impact of the increasing elective workload in maternity departments or the effect of delays in the induction pathway on a woman's experience.[1] It is difficult to justify delays in the elective induction pathway when the indication for induction is the increased risk of continuing the pregnancy. However, balancing the demands of ongoing emergency work with the additional demands of an increasing IOL rate and unpredictable individual response to the intervention continues to challenge maternity services. This also has an unknown impact on the emotional and psychological wellbeing of the mother and her family.

KEY POINTS

- The national and worldwide rates of induction of labour continue to rise occurring in approximately 28% of births in primiparous women in UK in 2011/12.
- Robust indications for the intervention are required which are evidence based and show that IOL will avoid potential harm.
- Pregnancy outcomes, incidence of complications and maternal experience of IOL should be monitored through research, audit and maternity dashboards.
- NICE recommends the method of choice to be two vaginal PGE2 tablets (3 mg) or gel (1–2 mg) at 6-hourly intervals, or one PGE2 controlled-release pessary (10 mg) over 24 hours.

SUMMARY

Induction of labour is one of the most common obstetric interventions. A clear clinical indication is needed to interrupt a pregnancy, with careful consideration of the benefits and risks, together with a full explanation to the woman and her family prior to the decision being made.

References

1. National Collaborating Centre for Women's and Children's Health. *Induction of labour.* Clinical Guideline CG070. 2008, RCOG Press.
2. Induction of labour: Evidence Update July 2013 A summary of selected new evidence relevant to NICE clinical guideline 70 'Induction of labour' (2008) Evidence Update 4.
3. WHO. *WHO recommendations for induction of labour.* ISBN 978 92 4 150115 6 (NLM classification: WQ 440) WHO 2011. http://whqlibdoc.who.int/hq/2011/WHO_RHR_11.10_eng.pdf
4. RCOG. *Patterns of Maternity Care in English NHS Hospitals 2011/12.* NHS Information Centre. *NHS Maternity Statistics 2011–12 Summary Report*, www.hscic.gov.uk/catalogue/PUB09202.
5. National Collaborating Centre for Women's and Children's Health. *Diabetes in pregnancy: management of diabetes and its complications from preconception to the postnatal period.* Clinical Guideline. March 2008, RCOG Press.
6. NICE. *Hypertension in pregnancy.* The management of hypertensive disorders during pregnancy. NICE clinical guideline 107. August 2010 last modified: January 2011. guidance.nice.org.uk/cg107.
7. RCOG. Obstetric Cholestasis. Green-top Guideline No. 43. London: RCOG. April 2011. https://www.rcog.org.uk/globalassets/documents/guidelines/gtg_43.pdf
8. RCOG. *Induction of Labour at Term in Older Mothers.* Scientific Impact Paper No.34. London: RCOG. February 2013.
9. RCOG. *The Investigation and Management of the Small-for-Gestational-Age Fetus.* Green-top Guideline No. 31. London: RCOG. February 2013. Minor revisions, January 2014.
10. RCOG. *Reduced Fetal Movements.* Green-top Guideline 57. London: RCOG. February 2011.
11. National Collaborating Centre for Women's and Children's Health. *Multiple pregnancy: the management of twin and triplet pregnancies in the antenatal period.* Commissioned by NICE. September 2011.
12. Kelly AJ, Alfirevic Z, Ghosh A. Outpatient versus inpatient induction of labour for improving birth outcomes *Cochrane Database Syst Rev.* 2013;11:CD007372.
13. Fitzpatrick KE, Kurinczuk JJ, Alfirevic Z, Spark P, Brocklehurst P, Knight M. Uterine rupture by intended mode of delivery in the UK: a national case-control study. http://www.plosmedicine.org/article/info%3Adoi%2F10.1371%2Fjournal.pmed.1001184
14. Wood S, Cooper S, Rossa S. Does induction of labour increase the risk of caesarean section? A systematic review and meta-analysis of trials in women with intact membranes. *BJOG* 2014;121:674–85.

Chapter 49 Management after previous caesarean section

Lucy Kean

INTRODUCTION

Delivery by caesarean section accounted for 25.5 per cent of deliveries in England in 2012–2013, with rates ranging from 17–40 per cent. In many units, emergency CS rates for primigravidae of 24 per cent are seen. Consequently, the problem of management of women with a scarred uterus in subsequent pregnancies is one of the most common reasons for hospital referral in multigravida. It is a vital part of antenatal care that women are given a clear understanding of the plan of management from early in pregnancy, with the caveat that this may need to be adapted if the pregnancy presents unexpected problems.

UNDERSTANDING THE RISKS

Relative maternal morbidity and mortality

It is almost impossible to assess the relative mortality from CS, as the indication for the CS will undoubtedly have an impact on the outcome. There are no trials to instruct us in this, and adapting information from published reports such as the CEMD is fraught with difficulty. In the most recent CEMD 116 women died after CS, but in only one case was the CS performed for maternal request. In all of the other cases there were compelling maternal or fetal indications for the procedure. Three women died following uterine rupture, though one of these women had a placenta praevia accreta.[3]

Chapter 53 discusses the risks of CS in detail.

A good understanding of the risks of CS is vital in counselling women with regard to subsequent delivery. The risks of both placenta praevia and placenta accreta increase exponentially with each repeat CS, from a baseline risk of 0.26 per cent and 0.01 per cent respectively in an unscarred uterus to 10 per cent and 6.7 per cent after a fourth CS.

In comparing elective repeat caesarean section (ERCS) with vaginal birth after caesarean section (VBAC) it is clear that the main maternal morbidity is encountered by women who need an emergency CS for a failed VBAC. It is therefore vital that when discussing management with a patient, the individual risks and benefits must be considered.

The aim of this chapter is to attempt to quantify these risks in order that, for each individual, appropriate counselling can be undertaken in planning the next delivery.

It is important to realise that women make decisions for a variety of reasons and that their choices may not always be those that we would make ourselves. The recent change in guidance produced by NICE has provided extended choice for all women to chose delivery by CS if they wish.[2]

There is remarkably little evidence to inform practice with regard to the management of previous CS. There are only two small randomised trials comparing trial of labour with elective CS, and most of the available data relate to observational studies.[4]

Candidates should be conversant with the RCOG Green-top guideline *Birth after previous caesarean birth*,[1] the NICE guideline *Caesarean section 2011*[2] and research that has been published since the guidelines were produced.

Repeat elective CS: risks and benefits

Maternal benefits

Caesarean section avoids labour with its risks of:

- Perineal trauma (urinary and faecal problems);
- 5% risk of anal sphincter trauma and 39% risk instrumental delivery;
- The need for emergency CS;
- Scar dehiscence or rupture with subsequent morbidity and mortality.
  It also has the advantage of allowing a planned delivery.

Maternal risks

- Prolonged recovery;
- Future pregnancies would probably require CS for delivery;
- Increased risks of placenta praevia and accreta in subsequent pregnancies;
- Wound infection risk of 10–20 per cent;
- Risk of death 13/100,000.

Fetal benefit

- No risk from intrapartum scar rupture.

Fetal risk

- Increased risk of transient tachypnoea/respiratory distress syndrome (1–3 per cent at 39 weeks, 6 per cent at 38 weeks).

Planned VBAC: risks and benefits

Maternal benefits

- Shorter hospital stay and convalescence (if a vaginal birth achieved);
- Potentially easier future deliveries.

Maternal risks

- Increased risk of transfusion (relative risk 1.7 due to increased need in women with failed VBAC);
- Increased risk of endometritis (relative risk 1.6 due to increased risk in women with failed VBAC);
- Risk of uterine rupture (0.22–1.0 per cent which is stratified by need for intervention i.e. highest risk with prostaglandin IOL, lowest risk for spontaneous delivery) [D];
- Risk of death 4/100,000.

Fetal benefit

- Reduced risk of transient respiratory morbidity.

Fetal risks

- 0.08 per cent risk of hypoxic ischaemic encephalopathy (similar to risk for nulliparous women);
- 0.04 per cent risk of delivery-related death.

A large observational study from Scotland suggested that women with a previous CS were at increased risk of stillbirth at term compared to women with an unscarred uterus. This study showed an absolute risk of 1.1/1000 women at or after 39 weeks for women previously delivered by CS compared to a risk of 0.05 per cent for women with an unscarred uterus. The absolute risk of stillbirth after CS is the same as that for the nulliparous population.[5] A subsequent large Canadian study of similar size showed no significant differences in antepartum stillbirth between the previous CS and previous vaginal delivery groups.[6] The latter paper attempted to control for obesity, a risk factor for both CS and stillbirth. It may be that obesity is the factor that increases the risk, rather than caesarean section [C].

Uterine rupture rate for women undergoing labour after a single prior CS

Uterine rupture is accurately defined as a disruption of the uterine muscle extending to and involving the uterine serosa or disruption of the uterine muscle with extension into the bladder or broad ligament. A uterine dehiscence is defined as disruption of the uterine muscle with intact uterine serosa.[1]

Studies looking at rates of scar rupture are all observational. The most helpful study for informing UK practice reported 35,854 women with a single previous CS, giving birth by means other than elective CS at 37 or more weeks.[7] Multiple births were excluded. This study showed that across the whole group the success rate for VBAC was 74.2 per cent. The uterine rupture rate was higher in women induced using prostaglandins, but not in women induced by other methods. The rupture rate was higher in women who had not previously also delivered vaginally. The overall risk of uterine rupture was 0.35 per cent. Women who had not previously delivered vaginally had a rupture risk of 1 in 210 if they did not undergo IOL with prostaglandins, and 1 in 71 if they were induced with prostaglandins. For women who had previously delivered vaginally the risks were 1 in 514 and 1 in 175 respectively.[7]

The National Institute of Child Health and Human Development (NICHD) has produced a large multicentre prospective cohort study encompassing around 16,000 women undergoing ERCS compared to 18,000 women undergoing planned VBAC, mostly women delivering in tertiary centres. This study gave an overall risk of uterine rupture in the VBAC group of 0.74 per cent. Unsuccessful VBAC had the highest rupture rates of 2.3 per cent [D].[8]

The RCOG Green-top guideline suggests that women know that the risk of rupture is 22–74/10,000 compared to almost no risk for ERCS and a composite risk of 0.5% should be discussed with women.[1]

ADVISING WOMEN ABOUT INDIVIDUAL RISKS

When advising women on subsequent delivery, as much information about the previous CS as possible should be sought.

It is good practice to ask for a copy of the case notes of the previous surgery before making a final decision, as occasionally features may be seen that will alter management, such as extensions of the uterine incision that the woman may be unaware of. It is also important to gain any available information about the circumstances leading to the CS.

Good antenatal planning should individualise the risks and benefits for each woman for each type of delivery, allowing the woman to make the best choice for herself. Research suggests that most women do not have clear ideas about the best choice for delivery and want accurate information and advice individualised for their own set of circumstances. The composite success rate should be quoted at 72–75%.[1]

Type of scar, method of closure and previous operative morbidity

It is recognised that vertical upper-segment uterine scars have a high risk of rupture, often with catastrophic results. Therefore, it is usual to recommend repeat pre-labour CS for women who are known to have undergone previous classical CS. However, despite this, some women will arrive in labour. A scar rupture rate of 12 per cent has been seen in this group.[9] Lower-segment vertical scars are associated with lower rates of uterine rupture of 2 per cent, but it is often very difficult to be sure that the scar did not encroach into the upper segment. With a full discussion of the risks and necessary precautions, women with a low uterine scar should be considered for VBAC.[1] It should not be assumed that a vertical abdominal incision means that the uterine incision will also be vertical; indeed, in most cases a vertical abdominal incision is associated with a transverse uterine incision. Given the extremely high rates of uterine rupture with vertical upper-segment incisions, it is best to err on the side of caution whenever there is doubt. J-shaped and inverted-T-shaped incisions are associated with similar rupture rates to low vertical incisions of 1.9 per cent [D].

In the USA a single-layer uterine closure was the norm for some years. In the UK this trend was not universally adopted and most women continued to undergo a traditional two-layer closure. The evidence on whether a single-layer closure is associated with higher rates of subsequent rupture is conflicting. Because the only studies of rupture are either small or observational the real risks are difficult to quantify. The largest study suggested an increase in risk, with an OR 3.95 (95% CI 1.35–11.9).[12]

One study addressed the issue of rupture related to intrapartum or postpartum pyrexia in the previous caesarean delivery. This study suggested an OR of 4.02 in women experiencing both intrapartum and postpartum pyrexia. However, the study was small and the confidence intervals very wide (1.04–15.5) [D].

Indication for previous CS

The extent to which the reason for previous CS impacts on subsequent successful trial of labour has been evaluated in a meta-analysis of observational studies [D].[13] The results are shown in Table 49.1.

Table 49.1 Successful vaginal delivery in subsequent labour by reason for previous caesarean section (CS)

Indication for previous CS	Success rate (%)
Malpresentation	85
Any reason one previous vaginal delivery	84
Fetal distress	75
Dystocia	67
Oxytocin in this labour	63

Table 49.2 Successful vaginal delivery related to dilatation at arrest of the previous labour

Dilatation at arrest (cm)	Vaginal delivery (%)
0–5	61
6–9	80
10	69

DOES CERVICAL DILATATION AT TIME OF PREVIOUS CS HAVE AN IMPACT ON DELIVERY?

This question has been addressed through observational studies. Only women whose prior CS was for 'failure to progress' were included (Table 49.2).[12]

These data accord with an overall rate of vaginal delivery for dystocia in the previous labour of 69 per cent, which compares well with the data from Rosen et al.,[12] and shows that dilatation at arrest does not signify who will achieve successful delivery next time, though CS for dystocia at any stage reduces the chance of successful VBAC[D].

TRIAL OF LABOUR IN WOMEN WITH MORE THAN ONE PRIOR CS

The NICHD study[8] used a multivariate approach to assess the rupture risk for women who have undergone two or more previous sections. The rupture rate was not higher for these women compared to women with a single previous CS, but they did experience higher rates of transfusion and hysterectomy. Many other smaller observational studies have suggested an increase in risk of 2–3 in women with more than one previous CS. Many of these studies were uncontrolled. One relatively large observational study showed the risk of uterine rupture was increased 2-fold compared with women with only one uterine scar (rupture risk 1.8% vs 0.9%; adjusted OR 2.3, 95% CI, 1.37–3.85).[11] The most recent meta-analysis showed a 1.3 per cent rupture risk for women with two or more CS.[12] It is interesting to note that the VBAC rates between studies vary hugely and it is very likely that there are differing criteria for selection for VBAC in the different participating centres, which may account for the different rupture rates seen.

Success rates vary but should be quoted as 62–75 per cent. Because of small numbers the real risk for rupture in women with three or more sections is difficult to quantify. Small observational studies suggest that the rupture risk may be increased by a factor of 2 or 3.[1]

Women should therefore be counselled that a VBAC is an alternative after two prior lower-segment sections and an individualised risk given where possible based on all the available information.

TRIAL OF LABOUR IN WOMEN WITH OBESITY

In the case of women with a scarred uterus and obesity, decision-making is often difficult. It is recognised that fetal birthweight is usually larger than average, and the prior CS will often have been performed for poor progress in labour, as obesity appears to increase the risks of inefficient uterine activity. The wish to avoid a further abdominal delivery must be balanced against the increased morbidity that occurs if an emergency CS is required. Observational data suggest that for women weighing in excess of 135 kg, the chance of vaginal delivery is very low (13 per cent) and elective CS may be a better option in this very obese group.[15]

The rates of unsuccessful VBAC increase incrementally as BMI increases. Women with a BMI above 30 have an OR for failed VBAC of 2 (95% CI 1.2–3.3).

OTHER RISK FACTORS FOR UNSUCCESSFUL VBAC AND UTERINE RUPTURE

Other risk factors have been evaluated.

Interdelivery interval

The interdelivery interval has been the subject of three studies. All of the studies are retrospective and in all the analysis was limited to women with singleton pregnancies, at term, who had one prior caesarean birth and no prior vaginal births. This will therefore skew the data towards slightly higher rupture rates, as women with a previous vaginal birth form the lowest risk group for rupture. It is noted from these studies that high rupture rates are reported, varying from 0.9 per cent in the lowest rupture groups to 4.8 per cent in the highest rupture rate groups. These studies are all from the USA and all small. At most the OR increase in risk is 2–3 and likely to be most pronounced in the intervals of less than a year.

Maternal age

The success of vaginal birth in all women decreases as age increases, regardless of whether the woman has previously undergone CS. Studies have shown lower rates of successful VBAC in women over 35 but these studies have not controlled for confounding variables. Unsuccessful VBAC carries the highest rate of uterine rupture. It is not surprising therefore that a study has suggested a link between uterine rupture and maternal age.

Other risk factors

Almost every factor known to be associated with lower chances of successful vaginal birth in any setting has been examined in relationship to VBAC and unsurprisingly those factors associated with overall lower rates of vaginal delivery are also associated with lower rates of successful VBAC. These include fetal macrosomia, delivery after 41 weeks, cervical dilatation of <4 cm at admission, non-white ethnicity, male infant and short maternal stature. When discussing choices with women these can be borne in mind. Decision making may therefore vary depending on the circumstances at the time, as some of these factors are dynamic.

ANTENATAL MANAGEMENT

Counselling and documentation

Wherever possible, the records of the delivery leading to CS should be reviewed [E]. Occasionally, facts that the patient may be unaware of may come to light. It is especially important to review records where there is any doubt about the type of uterine scar used. Counselling the patient with regard to the likelihood of success is also important, and review of the previous labour is a necessary part of this counselling.

It is very important to document carefully the discussion of the risks and benefits of both vaginal delivery and CS with the patient. Women should be provided with as accurate information as possible pertinent to their particular set of circumstances. The role of the doctor is to advise and guide where requested. The final choice rests with the woman. Women should be advised that the safest place to labour, should she wish to labour, is in hospital. It is better to support a woman to labour in hospital, even if the clinician feels this is injudicious, than for her to feel unsupported and to choose to labour at home.

If a woman is able to make her choice early in the pregnancy her antenatal care can be tailored around this. If her choice is for VBAC and there are no other factors which place the pregnancy at risk then a scheduled visit at 40 weeks to discuss a strategy should she pass 41 weeks is reasonable. Women can be offered an open appointment to return should they have further questions, but the provision of antenatal care can rest with the community midwife. For women with no identifiable pregnancy-related problems who choose ERCS a date can be provided for CS at 39 weeks so that the woman can prepare. This can be amended if circumstances change.

It is important to establish what choices women who choose ERCS would make should they labour before the date of planned CS. Many but not all women would consider VBAC if spontaneous labour ensues before the planned date.

Planning the delivery

Value of pelvimetry

Pelvimetry performed either clinically or radiographically does not provide any useful information [A]. Four trials of more than 1000 women were included in the most recent Cochrane Review. The trials were generally not of good quality. Women undergoing pelvimetry were more likely to be delivered by CS (OR 2.17, 95% CI 1.63–2.88). No impact on perinatal outcome was detected.[12]

Value of ultrasound for scar thickness

Ultrasound evaluation of the scar antenatally has been investigated as a method of determining women at higher risk of scar rupture during labour. Unfortunately, results do not give a high enough sensitivity for this modality to be used in everyday clinical practice.[1]

Documenting the plan and setting limits

Women are generally keen to avoid a repeat of the previous labour, and so it may be reasonable to avoid the circumstances that led to problems in the previous labour, such as avoiding induction if the CS was for failed induction. Women who underwent CS for poor progress usually need reassurance that limits will be placed on their next labour so that they do not undergo a prolonged labour. Women are significantly more likely to request a repeat CS if they had their initial surgery because of failure to progress in labour than if their initial CS was because of suspected fetal compromise.

It is important when discussing delivery in the antenatal period to agree a clear plan of management with the patient and for this to be carefully documented and easily available to carers in labour. If the agreed plan is for delivery by elective CS, it is good practice to give the patient a date for this, assuming an uncomplicated pregnancy. This can be made with the proviso that if circumstances change, it can be amended, but it does allow women to plan in advance and minimises requests for early delivery later in pregnancy that can compromise neonatal wellbeing. In general, an elective CS should be performed in the 39th week of pregnancy. It is possible to apply a little common sense where women have persistently laboured at 38 weeks before, but it must be remembered that if women have a tendency to go well past their dates, even 39 weeks may be early for some babies.

Assessment of the risk of placenta accreta

This is particularly pertinent in the management of women undergoing delivery after repeated caesarean sections. The risk is highest in women with a coexistent placenta praevia.

Findings suggestive, but not diagnostic, of a placenta accreta on antenatal ultrasound include:

- loss of the normal hypoechoic rim of myometrial tissue beneath the placenta;
- loss of the normal hyperechoic uterine serosa–bladder wall interface;
- presence of tissue of placental echotexture extending beyond the uterine serosa, sometimes seen within the lumen of the bladder;
- sometimes multiple or large placental venous lakes are seen giving the placenta a 'moth-eaten' appearance.

MRI has been suggested as an adjunct to ultrasound. Much depends on the experience of the person performing the scans. False negatives and positives occur with both modalities. Currently, in experienced hands, ultrasound alone is as good as MRI. If an accreta is suspected then it is prudent to take precautions for major haemorrhage. Full consent and discussion of the potential outcomes should be undertaken.

Management of placenta accreta is discussed in Chapter 46, Antepartum haemorrhage.

MANAGEMENT OF LABOUR

All carers on labour wards must be trained in the identification of the signs and symptoms of scar rupture.

Signs and symptoms of scar rupture

The cardinal signs of imminent uterine rupture are:

- worsening CTG changes (especially prolonged variable or late decelerations);
- haematuria;
- secondary arrest;
- small amounts of vaginal bleeding;
- pain over the scar which persists between contractions.

Signs of uterine rupture are:

- fetal bradycardia;
- upward displacement of the presenting part;
- sudden loss of contractions;
- maternal hypotension;
- heavy vaginal bleeding;
- abdominal or shoulder pain.

If the fetus or placenta is extruded into the abdomen, there is very little time to salvage the fetus. Delivery needs to be accomplished within 10 minutes. Most fetuses in this situation are profoundly acidotic at the time of delivery.

The literature is conflicting with regard to signs of impending uterine rupture. Clearly the sign most commonly associated with uterine rupture is a fetal bradycardia. Studies that have examined the CTGs in cases of confirmed rupture have shown bradycardia in almost 100 per cent of cases.

This is however, unhelpful to the clinician on the labour ward as our aim is to intervene before the uterus ruptures.

Ridgeway *et al.* undertook a case–control comparison of the CTGs of women who had a confirmed uterine rupture with those women undergoing VBAC who had a successful vaginal birth. This study differs from others because it compares only women having VBAC. Comparing cases with uterine rupture in the 4 hours preceding the second stage and during the second stage there were no differences in the appearance of any type of deceleration.[17]

Sheiner *et al.*[18] examined CTGs in the period before uterine rupture but compared them to the CTGs of women who did not have a scarred uterus. They demonstrated higher rates of severe fetal bradycardia (4.0% vs 1.0%, p = .064), fetal tachycardia (8.0% vs. 2.3%, p = .042), reduced baseline variability (24.0% vs. 12.5%, p = .021), uterine tachysystole (10.0% vs. 0.8%, P <.001) and disappearance of contractions (6.0% vs. 0, p <.001) in women with uterine rupture as compared to the controls.

Ayres *et al.*[19] examined the CTGs of women who had a uterine rupture and showed that 100 per cent of CTGs showed late decelerations prior to the bradycardia seen with the rupture. They did not compare these to controls.[6]

Therefore, although an abnormal CTG is the most consistent finding in uterine rupture and is present in 55–87 per cent of cases, deciding who is at risk of rupture from who is not is not an easy undertaking, as it appears that CTG changes are commoner in women undergoing VBAC than in the population of women with an unscarred uterus.

Conduct of the labour

General management

Some general steps can be taken on admission in labour to minimise the risks to the mother and fetus. These include:

- Read the plan for labour in the notes and note any discussion points;
- Site intravenous access (though this can be capped and flushed);
- Group and save blood;
- Discuss active management of the third stage;
- Advise continuous EFM once labour is established.

The use of EFM

There are no trials assessing the various modalities of monitoring of the fetus in labour during VBAC. Because bradycardia is seen in uterine rupture, the consensus opinion of the Expert Committee recommends continuous fetal monitoring in labour for women with a uterine scar [E].

The use of oxytocin to augment labour

The use of oxytocin in labour in women with previous CS is contentious. There are no randomised studies to help and only observational data are available [D].

The potential for oxytocin to correct abnormal patterns of labour is the same in women with a previous CS as it is in women without. However, given evidence that in nulliparous women oxytocin use does not reduce the rate of CS its use in the context of previous CS might be questioned.

The studies are all observational. One study attempted to control for dose and duration of oxytocin use and found a doubling in the rate of rupture which was most marked at doses of greater than 20 mu/min. Oxytocin augmentation appears to be associated with an increase in the risk of scar rupture of 2–3.[8,11]

It is vital that, before considering syntocinon, all steps are taken to optimise labour progress. With the advent of small fetal monitors and more mobility with epidural analgesia, it should be possible to allow women the opportunity to mobilise without compromising fetal surveillance. Forty per cent of women will respond to simple measures such as rehydration (see Chapter 50). A more flexible approach should be adopted in women with a uterine scar, and consideration should be given for lower rates of progress before resorting to syntocinon. When syntocinon is thought to be necessary, the decision should be made at consultant level and the risks and benefits should be discussed with the mother [E]. Assessment of progress in labour should ideally be made by the same person and the frequency of vaginal examination may need to be increased as there is some evidence that early intervention for static progress over 2 hours after augmentation can be used to prevent uterine rupture.

INDUCTION OF LABOUR

There have been many concerns voiced about IOL in women with a scarred uterus. Only four small randomised trials assessing the method of induction have been performed. These trials are too small to provide any meaningful data. Several observational studies have been performed, but all of these have limitations.

Clearly success rates for VBAC are lower if IOL is needed. The NICHD study showed a 33 per cent CS rate in induced labours.[8] Other studies have suggested successful vaginal birth in 50–70 per cent of women with a previous vaginal birth undergoing IOL compared to 44–61 per cent of women who have not delivered vaginally previously.

Membrane sweeping

Membrane sweeping is recommended for women where IOL is considered after 40 weeks. There are no trials assessing this approach in women with a previous CS, but it seems a reasonable option and may reduce the need for intervention.

Non-prostaglandin IOL

The NICHD study gave a risk for uterine rupture amongst women induced by non-prostaglandin methods of 89/10,000. This was almost exactly the same as the risk for women augmented in labour (87/10,000).[8] The data from Scotland did not show a significant increase in uterine rupture in women induced with ARM and oxytocin, with rates of 29/10,000.[7] Mechanical methods also include use of hygroscopic dilators, foley catheters and specifically designed catheters when the cervix is not yet suitable for artificial rupture of membranes. These methods are associated with a lower risk for induction than prostaglandins (0.29%).

Prostaglandin IOL

The NICHD study did not show a significantly higher risk of uterine rupture with prostaglandin IOL compared to non-prostaglandin methods of induction (140 vs 89/10,000).[8] The Scottish data showed a higher risk with prostaglandin IOL of 87 vs 29/10,000.[7] Interestingly the figure for prostaglandin IOL in the Scottish study is identical to the risk for non-prostaglandin IOL in the NICHD study, and lower than the risk for prostaglandin IOL in the NICHD study.

Clearly, when deciding on the best strategy the reason for induction must be considered and weighed against the risks of the procedure. Induction at 41 weeks is recommended to prevent the risk of stillbirth after this time. The risk of stillbirth at 41 weeks from epidemiological studies is 2–3/1000 [B]. The risks of perinatal death following IOL in women with a previous CS is 1.1/1000 [D]. Given the possibility that stillbirth may be more common in women with previous CS the marginal benefit of induction past 41 weeks is still probably justified, but the benefits are not as clear cut as they are for women with an unscarred uterus.

An unfavourable cervix at the onset of induction is associated with higher rates of CS but not with any other adverse outcome [D].

Despite the potential increased risk of scar rupture with prostaglandin the guideline development group who produced the most recent NICE guideline on IOL recommend that intravaginal PGE2 be used as the preferred option in women with a previous CS [E]. There are no preparations of prostaglandin that are licensed for use in IOL. The data sheets for the commonly used preparations (PGE2 tablets, gel and slow-release pessaries) all state that use in induction is contraindicated. The NICE guideline (Induction of labour) states that informed consent should be sought and documented.

Documentation:

- Involve a consultant obstetrician in decisions regarding mode of delivery, the need for induction and any decision to augment labour.
- Management plans should be fully documented.
- EFM should be used once labour is established.
- Local guidelines should be developed.
- There should be adequate education of all staff, ensuring awareness of signs and symptoms of uterine rupture.

MANAGEMENT OF THE THIRD STAGE

PPH is commoner in women who have a scarred uterus, probably because of the inability of the scar tissue to contract and increased placental adherence. Therefore, a low threshold for very active management of the third stage should be implemented. This should include:

- oxytocics at delivery of the shoulders;
- prompt delivery of the placenta after separation;
- consideration of continued syntocinon infusion for 4 hours after delivery or a long-acting syntocinon analogue.

If the placenta is retained, the possibility of a placenta accreta must be borne in mind. Therefore, before proceeding to a manual removal, important steps must be taken.

1 Establish the probable placental site from the previous scan reports. Accreta is much more likely if the placenta was noted to be anterior.
2 Cross-match 4 units of blood.
3 Obtain the patient's consent and note that the possibility of accreta has been discussed, with its potential problems and management options.
4 Ensure that senior staff are aware and, if you are inexperienced, ask for help *before* you go to theatre.

If at the time of manual removal a clear plane of cleavage cannot be defined, placenta accreta is likely.

Different treatment options for morbidly adherent placenta have been tried with variable success. These are fully discussed in Chapter 46.

CONCLUSIONS

The current rates of CS of 24 per cent in primiparae will inevitably lead to large numbers of women needing to choose the best method for delivery next time. Vaginal delivery after CS is a safe option if precautions are taken. IOL and augmentation lead to increased rates of scar rupture and must only be undertaken with caution. However, the risks of repeated CS must also be considered, as it is recognised that placenta accreta increases in incidence exponentially with each repeat CS (see Chapter 46). Keeping primary CS rates to a minimum will help to prevent the morbidity associated with both VBAC and repeated CS.

Key points

- A thorough history and examination of the notes should be made when booking a patient who has undergone a previous caesarean section.
- Where information is lacking, it should be sought.
- Vaginal delivery is a valid option after almost any prior lower-segment caesarean section.
- After classical caesarean section, vaginal delivery should be avoided.
- Repeated caesarean sections carry exponentially increasing risks of placenta praevia and accreta, with significant maternal morbidity.

FIRST STAGE OF LABOUR

- The risk of scar rupture in labour after a single caesarean section is approximately 22–74/10,000.
- Oxytocin use in labour probably increases this risk by two to three times.
- Induction of labour may lead to at least a doubling in risk of scar problems but it is possible that the magnitude of increase is higher if prostaglandins are needed.
- The risk of scar rupture may be 2–3 times higher after more than one caesarean section.
- Vigilance for scar rupture in labour is of paramount importance.
- Active management of the third stage should be standard.
- Placenta accreta must be considered if an anteriorly placed placenta is retained.

Key References

1. RCOG. *Birth after previous caesarean birth.* Green-top Guideline 45, February 2007. Revised October 2015. RCOG, London.
2. NICE. *Caesarean section* Clinical guideline 132, November 2011. www.nice.org.uk/cg132
3. Confidential Enquiry into Maternal and Child Health. Saving Mothers' Lives: Reviewing maternal deaths to make motherhood safer: 2006–2008. The Eighth Report of the CEMD in the UK, 2011. London CMACE. *BJOG* 2011;118:1–203.
4. Dodd JM, Crowther CA, Huertas E, Guise JM, Horey D. Planned elective repeat caesarean section versus planned vaginal birth for women with a previous caesarean birth. *Cochrane Database of Systematic Reviews* 2013;12: CD004224.
5. Smith GC, Pell JP, Dobbie R. Caesarean section and risk of unexplained stillbirth in subsequent pregnancy. *Lancet* 2003;362:1779–84.
6. Wood SL, Chen S, Ross S, Sauve R. The risk of unexplained antepartum stillbirth in second pregnancies following caesarean section in the first pregnancy. *BJOG* 2008;115:726–31.
7. Smith GC, Pell JP, Cameron AD, Dobbie R. Risk of perinatal death associated with labor after previous cesarean delivery in uncomplicated term pregnancies. *JAMA* 2002;287:2684–90.
8. Landon MB, Hauth JC, Leveno KJ *et al.* Maternal and perinatal outcomes associated with a trial of labor after prior cesarean delivery. *N Engl J Med* 2004;351:2581–9.
9. Macones GA, Cahill A, Pare E *et al.* Obstetric outcomes in women with two prior cesarean deliveries: is vaginal birth after cesarean delivery a viable option? *Am J Obstet Gynecol* 2005;192(4):1223–8.
10. Tahseen S, Griffiths M. Vaginal birth after two caesarean sections (VBAC-2): a systematic review with meta-analysis of success rate and adverse outcomes of VBAC-2 versus VBAC-1 and repeat (third) caesarean sections. *BJOG* 2010;117(1):5–19.
11. Rosen MG, Dickinson JC, Westhoff CL. Vaginal birth after caesarean: a meta-analysis of morbidity and mortality. *Obstet Gynecol* 1991;77:465–70.
12. Bujold E, Bujold C, Gauthier R. Uterine rupture during a trial of labour after a one-versus-two-layer closure of a low transverse caesarean. *Am J Obstet Gynecol* 2001;184:S18.
13. Rosen MG, Dickinson JC. Vaginal birth after caesarean: a meta-analysis of indicators for success. *Obstet Gynecol* 1994;84:255–8.
14. Ollendorff D, Goldberg JM, Minogue JP, Socol ML. Vaginal birth after Caesarean section for arrest of labour: is success determined by maximum cervical dilatation during the prior labour? *Am J Obstet Gynecol* 1988; 159:636–9.
15. Chauhan SP, Magann EF, Carroll CS, Barrilleaux PS, Scardo JA, Martin JN. Mode of delivery for the morbidly obese with prior Caesarean delivery: vaginal versus repeat Caesarean. *Am J Obstet Gynecol* 2001;185:349–54.
16. Pattinson RC, Farrell E-ME. Pelvimetry for fetal cephalic presentations at or near term. *Cochrane Database of Systematic Reviews* 2007, Issue 2.
17. Ridgeway J, Weyrich D, Benedetti T. Fetal heart rate changes associated with uterine rupture. *Obstet Gynecol* 2004;103:506–512.
18. Sheiner E, Levy A, Ofir K *et al.* Changes in fetal heart rate and uterine patterns associated with uterine rupture. *J Reprod Med* 2004;49(5):373–8.
19. Ayres AW, Johnson T, Hayashi R. Characteristics of fetal heart rate tracings prior to uterine rupture. *Int J Gynaecol Obstet* 2001;74:235–40.

Chapter 50 Poor progress in labour

Graham Tydeman and Alexandra Rice

INTRODUCTION

There is a shortage of randomised evidence regarding poor progress in labour. This applies both in terms of diagnosis and management. As such, much of what is held to be normal is based on lower-quality evidence. The phrase 'failure to progress' (FTP) is used in the literature, which can be taken to mean the end stage of poor progression, although in reality in many situations where FTP is declared, there has actually only been a slowing of progression rather than no progression at all. The CS rate has been steadily increasing with FTP increasing in proportion. In 1985 the WHO declared there was 'no justification for any region to have caesarean section rates higher than 10–15 per cent'. At that time, 15 per cent was an unusually high rate. [1] In a Scottish audit from 1995, the CS rate was 16 per cent and FTP was the sole indication in 50 per cent of emergency cases.[2] In 2012 the Scottish CS rate was 28 per cent.[3] During the same time period, the perinatal mortality rate has remained largely unchanged.[4]

The question is whether there has simply been a greater tendency to diagnose FTP, or has the population changed with more fetuses becoming stuck and if so, why?

If FTP is considered as abnormal labour, then it is worth reviewing the evidence for what constitutes normal labour. Labour is typically separated into latent and active phases. Women are not in 'established labour' until the active phase. Only in the active phase is FTP relevant as there is no imperative to intervene before labour has become 'established'. There is a general consensus that the latent phase carries no inherent risk of harm if it fails to progress. As will become apparent in considering this subject these are generally descriptive terms based on observational studies. Conceptually speaking, labour has become established when the process of delivery has no chance of stopping and will inevitably result in either delivery or fetal impaction. Finally, FTP is a description and whether it is also a diagnosis is debatable. Once FTP has been declared there are many factors influencing management and, particularly in the absence of other clear imperatives such as risk of fetal hypoxia, this should include the woman's choice.

NORMAL LABOUR

Cervical dilatation

Much of what we consider normal labour was established in the 1950s by Friedman.[5] His ground-breaking study published in 1955 involved 500 nulliparous women, at term, who arrived in early labour. As admitted in the paper, it was biased as it excluded those who presented already in advanced labour. Unlike previous studies that had focused on the total length of labour, Friedman plotted progress as a function of cervical dilatation. This work became the gold standard and it started the process by which an individual woman's labour could be compared with normal. A 2003 review stated 'What Friedman did was define labor in a way that lent itself to quantitation and thus to standardization.'[6] He also introduced the idea of the two main phases of labour: latent (from labour onset to the point at which the rate of dilatation begins to change) and active (from that point until complete dilatation) and provided the opportunity to assess variations from normal objectively. On the other hand, Friedman's work only involved women in their first labour and the mean age was only 20 years. In addition, over 50 per cent were instrumental deliveries; the occipito-posterior rate was unusually high at nearly 20 per cent but the caesarean section rate was 1.8 per cent. Cervical dilatation was assessed by both vaginal and rectal examination. Small numbers of women with breech, twins and stillbirth were also included (4 per cent of the total). Heavy sedation, which at the time usually involved a potent mix of opiates, was common. Variations of normal were defined as up to 2 standard deviations from the mean with latent phase having a mean of 8.6 hours +/- 6 hours and the active phase a mean of 4.9 +/-3.4 hours. The active phase was when the rate of dilatation began to accelerate – at just under 3cm dilatation reaching a peak rate of 3 cm/h (+/- 2 cm/h) from about 4 cm. In the final stages, there was a slowing in rate of progress from 9 cm but once full dilatation was achieved, the average length of the second stage was 1 hour (+/- 0.8 hours). The high rate of instrumental deliveries probably explains the short second stage as routine practice in the unit was not to allow the second stage to extend beyond 2 hours. Following the publication of this work, any individual woman's labour could then be compared with 'The Friedman Curve' (Fig. 50.1), an asymmetrical sigmoid curve that was an amalgamation of all labours studied. The introduction of the partogram and the active management of labour were direct consequences of the publication of the Friedman curve.

In the 1990s there were reviews of the Friedman curve from two perspectives – was it still relevant 40 years later and was the initial analysis valid? The original data were not normally distributed and were an amalgamation of 500 different curves but, perhaps most importantly, were never intended to be prescriptive – they were not intended to dictate care in labour. Between 1992 and 1996 and involving nearly four times as many nulliparous women as Friedman, a similar study was organised,[7] but analysed with better statistical tools. This produced some of the first data suggesting Friedman's curve might either be inaccurate or no longer relevant. As a result but also largely in response to the rising CS rate, the US National Institute of Child Health and Human Development organised a very large study to describe contemporary labour. A retrospective review of the case notes of over 200,000 women between 2002 and 2008 was undertaken. This resulted in several important publications including a re-evaluation of the Friedman curve. Focusing on over 60,000 nulliparous women, one publication resulting from this study[8] reported that labours took much longer than as predicted by the Friedman curve with many women not entering the accelerative phase until 6 cm (rather than 4 cm) and the normal rate of progress being up to 6 hours between just 4 and 5 cm and up to 3 hours between 5 and 6 cm. For the second stage, even without an epidural, second-stage 95th centiles were between 3.6 and 2.8 hours for nulliparous and parous women respectively: 3 times longer than from the Friedman data. For both nulliparous and parous women, progress to about 6 cm was similar but thereafter progress was much faster in parous women for the remaining first stage and the second stage. New graphs were produced to provide the basis for a new partogram for nulliparous and parous women (Fig. 50.2). Despite these data, many places still rely on the '1 cm/h after 4 cm' diktat from the accelerative phase of the original Friedman curve. New guidance from the UK acknowledges the uncertainty that 'Essentially there is huge normal variation in the length of time an individual women will be in labour. All we can advise is that first labours will last on average 7 hours and are unlikely to last more than 18 and that in subsequent pregnancies the average duration is 5 hours and unlikely to last more than 14.'[9,10]

Descent of the head

Partograms not only include cervical dilatation but also plot the descent of the head during labour. The Royal College of Midwives describes the need to assess the descent of the head during each vaginal examination[9] and it is commonly taught in midwifery and obstetrics; however, there is much less evidence of what is normal than there is for cervical dilatation. One study from India[11] looked at 100 cases of normal labour

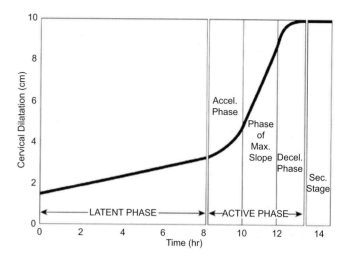

Fig. 50.1 The Friedman curve

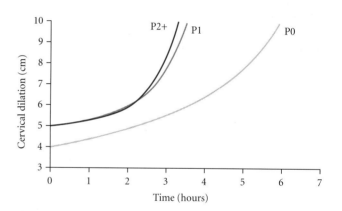

Fig. 50.2 Curves from 2002 to 2008 US data

and concluded that the course of labour was uninfluenced by the degree of engagement. Using a simulator that precisely defined the actual station of the head and using the classification of station from ACOG, another study found reliability poor between observers.[12]

Partograms

Finally, despite their widespread use in almost all labour wards, there is room for debate about the value of partograms in improving outcomes. RCOG promotes their use as 'they result in fewer operative births and less use of oxytocin';[13] however, a Cochrane systematic review[14] from 2008 that included six studies involving nearly 8000 women (two of which were randomised to partogram or no partogram) found no difference in CS or instrumental delivery rates unless the partogram included a latent phase, in which case CS rates were higher with the use of a partogram. The conclusion was: 'We cannot recommend routine use of partogram as part of standard management and care' although the authors did acknowledge that it was such an established part of normal practice that its use could be 'locally determined'.

ABNORMAL LABOUR – FAILURE TO PROGRESS?

First stage – problems with diagnosis

FTP inherently implies an abnormal labour. Its 'diagnosis' is on the increase in relative and absolute terms as the CS rate has risen. Evidence from the UK in 2000[15] showed that with a CS rate of 20 per cent, FTP was the indication in 20 per cent of CS whereas a US study of nearly 40,000 women in 2013[16] with a 30 per cent CS rate showed 35 per cent of CS being performed due to FTP. Of those having a CS for FTP, 40 per cent of nulliparous women and 33 per cent of parous women were at less than 5 cm cervical dilatation at the time of delivery, which begs the question, were they even in established labour?

As we have seen, there has been a strong focus on cervical dilatation as the single measure of progress in labour. For an individual woman being compared to population data, it needs to be considered whether she is a normal representative of that population. Partograms with an action line are commonly in use to aid these comparisons – if the rate of progress falls behind the action line, FTP can be considered to be occurring. Given the body of evidence that normal progress in labour is a sigmoid curve, it perhaps seems odd that action lines are of uniform slope. We have previously considered the evidence as to whether a partogram is of value but there appear to be no studies comparing a partogram with or without an action line. There are several RCTs comparing the effects of action lines of different fixed slopes[17,18,19] and NICE[10] concludes that a 4-hour action line should be used as the use of shorter intervals 'increases interventions without any benefit to mother or baby'. Using a definition of up to 4 cm as the end of the latent phase, NICE goes on to define the diagnosis of delay as 'cervical dilatation of less than 2 cm in 4 hours for first labours or cervical dilatation of less than 2 cm in 4 hours or a slowing in the progress of labour for second or subsequent labours'.

In addition to being nulliparous, a variety of factors have been identified that might make any individual woman's progress differ from the norm. Perhaps it should be questioned whether the use of general population curves should apply to all women. In a manner akin to customised growth charts[20] perhaps there should be customised progress in labour charts. Factors that tend toward slower labour include: induction of labour, premature rupture of membranes, age, epidural, obesity and having been raped.[21,22,23,24] Factors which shorten labour, other than being parous, include oxytocin use[25] and staying upright in the first stage.[26]

Cervical assessment – is full dilatation 10 cm?

As we have seen, measuring the dilatation of the cervix is the standard way that labour is compared with normal but it should be no surprise that there are errors in the assessment of cervical dilatation, particularly between different examiners. For an individual woman, error could be very significant if the conclusion is that she is failing to progress. There is some research evidence from simulators demonstrating significant inter-observer error.[27,28] It makes sense (and is recommended) to minimise error with examinations performed by the same observer where possible[9] but in situations where this good practice occurs, it is also common for a doctor to perform a single final examination prior to intervention. This also makes sense: that person may be taking responsibility for the decision whether to intervene, but they should be aware of the potential for error inherent in their single examination.

The technique of examination is another potential source of error: whether it is performed vaginally or rectally is not unified in the early research and even for vaginal examination there is no unified opinion as to the best way to perform the assessment. Where 10 cm comes from is also difficult to determine and there appears to be a lack of evidence as to the range of normal. The teaching from early obstetric and midwifery textbooks, 1903 to 1953,[29-33] was to avoid unnecessary vaginal examinations – the recommendation was simply one examination at rupture of membranes (to confirm no cord prolapse) and only one more in the second stage, only if there was delay. A normal second stage, of 2–3 hours was quoted for nulliparous and 1 hour for parous. These figures are interestingly more similar to research from the 21st century[8] than from Friedman in 1955.[5] Earlier textbooks also focused on how much cervix was left before full dilatation was achieved rather than how dilated it had become. Not until 1953 is the idea introduced that 3¾ inches (9.5 cm) is the normal aperture for full dilatation[33] but in the same book it was also noted that full dilatation was different for different-sized babies: 3¾ inches for a 7 pound baby but 2½ inches was suggested as full dilatation for a 3 pound baby.

There is almost certainly biological variation with some women never achieving 10 cm despite full dilatation and others having several centimetres of cervix left at 10 cm. There appears to be no evidence as to what dilatation is the range of normal. There is an attraction in focusing attention on how much cervix is left before full dilatation is achieved, rather than how dilated it has become. Full dilatation is a clear end point: there is no cervix left and it has all become incorporated into the lower segment.

Midwives are often still taught using pocketbook cards with various-diameter holes in to learn what 10 cm feels like.[34] Anecdotally some observers simply try to determine how far apart their fingers are at all stages but others do this until there is not much cervix remaining, and then subtract what is left from 10. This is inherently illogical as if there are 3 cm left on one side, then there is likely to be another 3 cm on the other side, which should mean, by simple subtraction, that the dilatation is actually only 4 cm and not 7 cm. However the cervix is rarely perpendicular to the vagina (Fig. 50.3) so it may work in practice and, more importantly, focuses on what remains, which is arguably a more important end point.

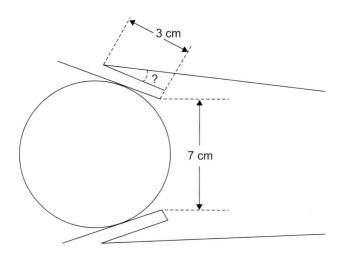

Fig. 50.3 Cervical dilatation

The reality of vaginal examination is likely to be that during training we learn a consensus of what each dilatation 'feels like' in comparison with experienced teachers, rather than attempt to measure a precise reality at each examination. This adds a considerable element of judgement and error.

Second stage

The second stage is typically divided into the passive phase from full dilatation to the start of active pushing. If a normal second stage is up to 3.6 hours[10] it needs to be considered what adverse effects there are of being at one end of the normal range. NICE recommends that it should be no more than 3 hours (1 hour passive and 2 hours pushing) for nulliparous women and 2 hours (1 hour passive, 1 hour pushing) for parous women.[10] In a Canadian study[35] of over 150,000 uncomplicated women there was an increase in a combination of maternal and neonatal adverse outcomes, including PPH/ sepsis and lower Apgar scores/increased admissions to neonatal units, with second stages longer than 2 and 3 hours for parous and nulliparous women respectively.

Causes

Traditional teaching talks in terms of the three P's – power, passage and passenger. In other words are contractions ineffective (power); is the pelvis (passage) insufficient to cope with the presenting part of the fetus (passenger); or is the presenting part too large, possibly as a result of position, to fit through an otherwise normal pelvis? There is a simple attraction to thinking in these terms but unfortunately there is also a lack of evidence that an understanding of the cause leads to any intervention that will alter management – except perhaps in extreme cases such as severe hydrocephalus, massive lower-segment fibroids or pelvic abnormalities when elective CS might prevent 'inevitable' FTP if labour were to commence. There is evidence of prolonged labour and higher

instrumental delivery rates in certain fetal positions such as occipito-posterior[36] but a lack of evidence as to what to do about it that might make a difference. This makes evaluation of these factors in any greater detail of debatable value. Investigations such as pelvimetry or estimation of fetal weight are insufficiently reliable to be of use in practice.[37] Cephalopelvic disproportion (CPD) is the description of a failure of two of the three Ps (passenger and passage). If CPD truly does occur then FTP is the inevitable consequence. The difficulty is that there are no precise ways of determining when CPD has occurred other than by allowing labour to continue long after a suspicion of FTP has been raised, such as occurs in situations where access to intervention is very limited. If the delivery then proceeds by CS then signs such as ballooning of the lower segment, free fluid in the abdomen and a deeply impacted head may confirm the diagnosis of FTP.[10] As such, estimates as to its true incidence are difficult to establish but are reported to only be a few per cent.[38] On the other hand, if a CS for FTP is being performed where there is no absolute evidence of CPD, what is it being done for?

In addition to poor rates of cervical dilatation and failure of descent there are other signs that the head is becoming 'stuck'. Increasing moulding and caput are traditional features along with a feeling of impaction – difficulty in getting a finger around the head due to a lack of room between it and the maternal pelvis. The more marked these features are, particularly if permanent saggital suture overlapping occurs, the higher the chance of true CPD occurring,[39] but again there is lack of evidence to support use of these features to guide management. Perhaps there should at least be an awareness that if these features are not present, it should prompt the person doing the examination to question whether there really is true FTP or whether one of the many sources of error highlighted above might be at play.

Prediction

A variety of parameters have been identified that appear to be associated with an increased chance of FTP, including maternal shoe size, maternal height, maternal pelvimetry and estimations of fetal weight. Unfortunately none of these has yet been found to be sufficiently robust to be useful in practice and NICE recommend they should not be used to guide management.[10]

Population change

Increasing age and obesity have been linked to an increased chance of CS for FTP. In the mid-1970s, 6 per cent of US pregnant women were over 35 years old compared to 20 per cent in 2012.[40] The incidence of obesity in women of childbearing age has doubled in the same time,[41] with studies on adolescents showing relative risk of 1.6 for FTP, even for the mildly overweight (BMI of over 25 kg/m²).[42] A recent study from Scotland showed relative risks of up to 14 times higher for emergency caesarean in the most obese women.[43]

MANAGEMENT

Having excluded all forms of error and having been robust in making the diagnosis, if the conclusion is reached that there has been significant FTP, management in the first stage is CS and in the second stage is either CS or instrumental delivery. Obviously it's not quite that simple and interventions can be tried to accelerate the rate of progress in an attempt to return it to normal but unfortunately none of these interventions has conclusively been shown to improve outcome.

First stage

The use of oxytocin is encouraged by NICE for nulliparous women and has been shown to shorten labour but not to reduce first-stage caesarean sections: 'Oxytocin will bring forward the time of birth but will not influence the mode of delivery or outcomes.'[10] For parous women in particular, there is the concern that if the labour really is obstructed then forcing the uterus to contract more can result in rupture, massive haemorrhage and death. Again to quote NICE, 'Oxytocin should only be started in multiparous women once there has been a full assessment by the obstetrician. Continuous fetal monitoring is required with the use of oxytocin irrespective of the parity. Once oxytocin has been commenced vaginal examinations should occur at 4-hourly intervals; if there has been less than 2 cm of progress the decision should be made as to whether a CS is required.' And furthermore: 'Early use was associated with hyperstimulation as well as increased fetal heart trace concerns but no change in neonatal or maternal outcomes. Current guidelines do not recommend the use of syntocinon in the second stage whether or not regional anaesthesia is in place or not. The only exception to this would be subjectively poor contractions at the start of the second stage in nulliparous patients with regional anaesthesia.'[10]

The package known as the 'active management of labour' that includes early amniotomy and 2-hourly examinations also does not appear to make any difference.[18] One-to-one care from a health professional has benefits in terms of length of labour and other markers such as postnatal depression rates but other than encouraging trends in the original observational studies from the 1970s[44] there remains little evidence that it affects CS rates.

Immobility in the first stage has been associated with longer labours and NICE[10] discourages women from staying supine although encouraging women to mobilise doesn't seem to improve outcomes.

Second stage

Not lying supine and not being in the lithotomy position has been shown to be associated with a shorter second stage and lower rates of instrumental delivery.[45] In the second stage, oxytocin can be used but again without robust evidence that it alters outcome.

CONCLUSIONS

Failure to progress accounts for about a third of all emergency caesarean sections. CS rates are rising with minimal evidence of benefit. Despite much more powerful data from large studies in the 21st century, management of labour continues to rely on practices that emerged following publication of a small study in the 1950s. The key points from later research are that the active phase may not start until 6 cm and that slow progress before then may not be intrinsically harmful. The use of oxytocin may speed things up but not alter outcome. On the plus side there is plenty of room for research: we rely on assessing progress largely by cervical dilatation alone which has untested errors and not even a standardised technique. Research into establishing these errors, standardising technique and perhaps focusing on the amount of cervix until full dilatation is achieved may be interesting. There is evidence that the population is changing and as such it may be wrong to try to reverse the trend in rising caesarean sections for FTP.

A fresh look with new ideas and robust research as to how to tackle rising intervention rates is needed. Sixty years after Friedman, it will be interesting to see where we'll be in another 60.

References

1. Lauer JA, Betrán AP, Merialdi M, Wojdyla D. Determinants of caesarean section rates in developed countries: supply, demand and opportunities for control. *World Health Report* 2010; Background Paper, 29.
2. Scottish Programme for Cinical Effectiveness and Reproductive Health. *Caesarean section in Scotland 1994/5: a National Audit.*
3. National Services Scotland Information Services Division. *Births in Scottish Hospitals.* 2012.
4. National Services Scotland. *Trends in Perinatal Mortality in Scotland – a review over 30 years.* National Services Scotland, 2009.
5. Friedman EA, Primigravid labor; a graphicostatistical analysis. *Obstet Gynecol* 1955 Dec;6(6):567–89.
6. Pitkin R. Review of Friedman. *Obstet Gynecol* 2003;101(2):216.
7. Zhang J *et al.* Reassessing the labor curve in nulliparous women. *Am J Obstet Gynecol* 2002;187:824–8.
8. Zhang J, Landy HJ, Branch DW *et al.* Consortium on Safe Labor. Contemporary patterns of spontaneous labor with normal neonatal outcomes. *Obstet Gynecol* 2010 Dec;116(6):1281–7.
9. NICE/Royal College of Midwives. *Assessing Progress in Labour.* NICE, 2008.
10. Intrapartum care: care of healthy women and their babies during childbirth. NICE. Clinical Guideline 190. December 2014.

11. Kushtagi P. Pattern of descent of foetal head in normal labour. *Journal of the Indian Medical Association* 1995;93(9):336–9.

12. Dupuis O, Silveira R, Zentner A *et al*. Birth simulator: reliability of transvaginal assessment of fetal head station as defined by the American College of Obstetricians and Gynecologists classification. *Am J Obstet Gynecol* 2005 Mar;192(3):868–74.

13. RCOG online teaching: StratOG. http://www.rcog.org.uk/stratog/page/partogram-0

14. Lavender T, Hart A, Smyth RM. Effect of partogram use on outcomes for women in spontaneous labour at term. *Cochrane Database Syst Rev* 2008; Oct 8;4:CD005461.

15. The National Sentinel Caesarean Section Audit. *BJOG* 2000;107(5):579–80.

16. Boyle A, Reddy UM, Landy HJ *et al*. Primary cesarean delivery in the United States. *Obstet Gynecol* 2013 Jul;122(1):33–40.

17. Lavender T, Alfirevic Z, Walkinshaw S. Partogram action line study: a randomised trial. *BJOG* 1998;105(9):976–80.

18. Pattinson RC, Howarth GR, Mdluli W *et al*. Aggressive or expectant management of labour: a randomised clinical trial. *BJOG* 2003;110(5):457–8.

19. Lavender T, Alfirevic Z, Walkinshaw S. Effect of different partogram action lines on birth outcomes: A randomized controlled trial. *Obstet Gynecol* 2006;108(2):295–302.

20. Gardosi J, Chang A, Kalyan B, Sahota D, Symonds EM. Customised antenatal growth charts. *Lancet* 1992;339:283–7.

21. Sheiner E, Levy A, Feinstein U, Hallak M, Mazor M. Risk factors and outcome of failure to progress during the first stage of labor: a population-based study. *Acta Obstet Gynecol Scand* 2002 Mar;81(3):222–6.

22. Epidural versus non-epidural or no analgesia in labour. *Cochrane Database Syst Rev* 2011;12:CD000331.

23. Kominiarek MA, Zhang J, Vanveldhuisen P, Troendle J, Beaver J, Hibbard JU. Contemporary labor patterns: the impact of maternal body mass index. *Am J Obstet Gynecol* 2011 Sep;205(3):244.e1–8.

24. Nerum H, Halvorsen L, Oian P, Sørlie T, Straume B, Blix E. Birth outcomes in primiparous women who were raped as adults: a matched controlled study. *BJOG* 2010 Feb;117(3):288–94.

25. Bugg GJ1, Siddiqui F, Thornton JG. Oxytocin versus no treatment or delayed treatment for slow progress in the first stage of spontaneous labour. *Cochrane Database Syst Rev* 2013 Jun 23;6:CD007123.

26. Lawrence A1, Lewis L, Hofmeyr GJ, Styles C. Maternal positions and mobility during first stage labour. *Cochrane Database Syst Rev* 2013 Aug 20;8:CD003934.

27. Robson S. Variation of cervical dilatation estimation by midwives, doctors, student midwives and medical students in 1985 – a small study using cervical simulation models. Research and the Midwife Conference Proceedings Manchester: University of Manchester, 1991.

28. Tufnell D, Bryce F, Johnson N, Lilford R. Simulation of cervical changes in labour: reproducibility of expert assessment. *Lancet* 1989;8671:1089–90.

29. Jellet. *Short practice of midwifery.* Churchill, 1903.

30. Fairbairn. *A textbook for midwives.* Oxford Medical, 1914.

31. Schuman. *Text book of Obstetrics.* Saunders and Co, 1936.

32. Comyns. *Handbook of midwifery.* Berkeley Cassell and Co., 1943.

33. Myles. *Textbook for midwives.* Livingstone Ltd, 1953.

34. Aspin J. *Vaginal examination – a unique pocket guide.* www.in-practice.co.uk.

35. Allen VM, Baskett TF, O'Connell CM, McKeen D, Allen AC. Maternal and perinatal outcomes with increasing duration of the second stage of labor. *Obstet Gynecol* 2009;113(6):1248–58.

36. Gardberg M, Tuppurainen M. Persistent occiput posterior presentation: a clinical problem. *Acta Obstet Gynecol Scand* 1994 Jan;73(1):45–7.

37. RCOG. *Pelvimetry.* Guideline No. 14. London: RCOG, 2001.

38. Tsvieli O, Sergienko R, Sheiner E. Risk factors and perinatal outcome of pregnancies complicated with cephalopelvic disproportion: a population-based study. *Arch Gynecol Obstet* 2012;285(4):931–6.

39. Buchmann EJ, Libhaber E. Sagittal suture overlap in cephalopelvic disproportion: blinded and non-participant assessment. *Acta Obstet Gynecol Scand* 2008; 87(7):731–7.

40. Ecker JL, Chen KT, Cohen AP, Riley LE, Lieberman ES. Increased risk of cesarean delivery with advancing maternal age: indications and associated factors in nulliparous women. *Am J Obstet Gynecol* 2001 Oct;185(4):883–7.

41. Kim SY, Dietz PM, England L, Morrow B, Callaghan WM. Trends in pre-pregnancy obesity in nine states, 1993–2003. *Obesity* (Silver Spring) 2007;15(4):986–93.

42. Sukalich S, Mingione MJ, Glantz JC. Obstetric outcomes in overweight and obese adolescents. Ovid MEDLINE(R) 1946 to Present with Daily Update. *Am J Obstet Gynecol* 2006;195(3):851–5.

43. Denison FC, Norwood P, Bhattacharya S *et al*. Association between maternal body mass index during pregnancy, short-term morbidity, and increased health service costs: a population-based study. *BJOG* 2014;121(1):72–81; discussion 82.

44. O'Driscoll K, Jackson RJ, Gallagher JT. Active management of labour and cephalopelvic disproportion. *J Obstet Gynaecol Br Commonw* 1970;77:385–9.

45. National Collaborating Centre for Woman's and Children's Health. *Caesarean Section.* National Collaborating Centre for Woman's and Children's Health, 2004.

Chapter 51 Fetal compromise in the first stage of labour

Jenny Blackman and Myles Taylor

MRCOG standards

- The ability to recognise, classify and act appropriately on CTG patterns.
- The ability to perform fetal blood sampling and to be able to interpret the results.

In addition, we would suggest the following.

Theoretical skills

- Know the risk factors for fetal compromise and how they can be recognised either antenatally or in early labour.
- Understand the alterations in placental blood flow during contractions.
- Know the acute intrapartum complications that can lead to fetal compromise.
- Be aware of the different techniques available for assessing fetal wellbeing in labour as well as their individual indications and limitations.
- Be able to quote the risk of serious neonatal morbidity and mortality.

Practical skills

- Be confident in your ability to interpret a CTG, particularly with regard to recognising those babies requiring immediate delivery.
- Be able to perform and interpret additional tests of fetal wellbeing for non-reassuring CTGs that do not necessitate immediate delivery.
- Be able to apply a scalp electrode or perform a real-time ultrasound scan when it is not possible to obtain an adequate fetal heart rate trace using conventional Doppler techniques.

INTRODUCTION

Members of the public, and indeed the legal profession, commonly relate childhood disability to a 'difficult' labour and delivery. However, the Consensus Statement of the International Cerebral Palsy Task Force reported that intrapartum hypoxia could at most be responsible for only one in ten cases of cerebral palsy.[1] Nevertheless, as labour represents about 0.4 per cent (1/280) of the total duration of pregnancy, a 10 per cent contribution to sub-optimal neonatal outcomes reminds us that it is a relatively 'high-risk' period. The fact that uterine perfusion is dramatically reduced during each contraction emphasises the additional stress that labour places on the fetus.

AIMS

The aim of monitoring fetal wellbeing during labour is to prevent birth asphyxia and so reduce perinatal mortality, morbidity and long-term disability. Although all three of these outcomes are uncommon, the use of operative delivery for 'non-reassuring fetal status' remains an everyday occurrence on delivery suites in the UK. This is in part because of a wish to deliver on the downwards slope towards a poor outcome, before it actually occurs. The key question is, what are the poor outcomes that we are trying to prevent? Currently, efforts are focused on reducing intermediate adverse outcomes in the hope that long-term permanent adverse outcomes (death and disability) can be avoided. Such intermediate outcomes include NICU admissions at term, umbilical cord acidosis and base deficit, low Apgar scores and neonatal hypoxic ischaemic encephalopathy at term.

ABSOLUTE OUTCOMES

Perinatal mortality

This remains a widely accepted measure of maternity care, but such crude figures provide little help in assessing intrapartum monitoring. First, they are heavily distorted by very preterm births, in which fetal condition at birth is only one of many factors influencing outcome. Second, perinatal mortality rates also include stillbirths. It is self-evident that fetal monitoring can only be of use when the baby is alive at the onset of labour.

Intrapartum term stillbirths may be a more appropriate mortality figure, as they are often related to events occurring during parturition. The intrapartum stillbirth rate in term singleton pregnancies is reported as only 0.3 per 1000.[2] The influence of fetal monitoring on such a rare event will remain difficult to study.

Long-term morbidity

The achievement of normal long-term neurodevelopment is another major aim of intrapartum fetal assessment. The incidence of cerebral palsy is widely quoted as 2 per 1000. However, as mentioned previously, only in 10 per cent of cases (or 1 in 5000 births) are intrapartum events thought to have been of influence. Once again, the ability of fetal monitoring to impact on such a rarity is difficult to prove or disprove.

All obstetricians should therefore appreciate that intrapartum operative interventions carried out at term because of 'non-reassuring fetal status' are trying to prevent sub-optimal outcomes seen in approximately 1 in 2000 births. It is necessary not only for obstetricians to react appropriately but also to avoid over-reaction.

INTERMEDIATE OUTCOMES

Apgar scores

To improve the recognition of intrapartum factors contributing to the absolute outcomes referred to above, markers of potential long-term morbidity have been used.

The influence of the condition of the baby at birth using Apgar scores taken at 1 and 5 minutes has been widely investigated, particularly in the earliest studies. All now agree that the 1-minute Apgar score purely reflects the need for neonatal resuscitation, regardless of aetiology. Unfortunately, the 5-minute Apgar score also appears to provide little predictive ability for long-term complications unless very low (<4) or moderately low (<7) and remaining so beyond 10 minutes of age.

There is not yet enough evidence to support the use of other similar markers, such as the need for intubation or ventilation.

Arterial or capillary pH

Hypoxaemia will result when gas exchange across the placenta is impaired, with a gradual fetal accumulation of CO_2. This eventually leads to fetal acidaemia, which can be detected by analysing fetal capillary or neonatal arterial pH. The widely accepted lower limit of normal for fetal or neonatal pH is 7.20. This represents two standard deviations below the mean fetal pH seen from intrapartum studies. It must be stressed that this

value was chosen for statistical reasons, not primarily because of an association with neonatal morbidity. Clinical studies suggest that an umbilical arterial pH below 7.00 may be a more reliable marker of potential long-term problems, but the figure of 7.20 remains in everyday use to provide a wide margin of safety. The type of acidosis is also important. In a respiratory acidosis, the PCO_2 is elevated but the base excess is normal, a condition that will be easily resolved with the onset of neonatal respiration and gas exchange. Metabolic acidosis is associated with a transition to anaerobic metabolism and an accumulation of acids such as lactate. It is defined by a base deficit >12 mmol/L and is a marker of moderate to severe neonatal compromise in its own right.

Neonatal encephalopathy

Neonatal behaviour and early-onset medical complications also provide some prognostic information. Neonatal encephalopathy refers to disturbed neurological function in the first week of life. Signs include difficulty maintaining respiration, depressed tone and reflexes, altered level of consciousness and seizures. Moderate to severe neonatal encephalopathy will be seen in most cases of brain damage secondary to intrapartum complications. However, neonatal encephalopathy has poor sensitivity with 75 per cent of cases having no clinical signs of intrapartum hypoxia.

Criteria for intrapartum hypoxic events

No individual intermediate measure can precisely link intrapartum complications to absolute outcomes. Several groups have proposed pathways by which combinations of intermediate measures can help to define a causal intrapartum hypoxic event. The International Cerebral Palsy Task Force has listed criteria essential to link brain injury to an earlier intrapartum hypoxic event.[1] They include:

- evidence of a metabolic acidosis at birth (pH <7.00 and base deficit >12 mmol/L);
- early-onset moderate or severe encephalopathy;
- cerebral palsy of the spastic quadriplegic or dyskinetic type.

Other features that support an intrapartum hypoxic event include:

- a sentinel hypoxic event around the time of labour;
- a deterioration in the fetal heart rate pattern around the time of the sentinel event after a previously normal pattern;
- Apgar scores of <7 for longer than 5 minutes;
- early-onset multi-organ dysfunction
- early imaging evidence of an acute cerebral abnormality.

WHAT TYPE OF FETAL MONITORING IS BEST?

The Dublin Trial of Intermittent versus Continuous Monitoring remains the classic study in this field.[3] Despite subsequent studies, the conclusions have been largely unchallenged. In low-risk pregnancies, electronic continuous monitoring was better at detecting fetal acidosis and led to a reduced incidence of neonatal seizures. However, it did not appear to have any influence on the absolute outcomes of mortality and long-term disability. Meta-analysis seems to support these conclusions, although it is recognised that the data are insufficient to detect a true difference in the rare absolute outcomes of death and disability [Ia]. Most authorities agree that continuous monitoring leads to an increase in operative intervention, although this can be at least partially mitigated by the use of secondary tests of fetal wellbeing.

WHAT IS A HIGH-RISK PREGNANCY?

The presence of any of the following risk factors at the onset of labour would label a fetus as being at 'high risk' of intrapartum hypoxia, for which the consensus is that continuous fetal monitoring should be offered:

- Hypertension/pre-eclampsia;
- Diabetes;
- APH;
- Significant maternal medical disease;
- IUGR;
- Preterm gestation;
- Isoimmunisation;
- Multiple pregnancy;
- Breech presentation;
- Previous caesarean section;
- Significant meconium staining of the amniotic fluid;
- Pre-labour rupture of membranes for >24 hours;
- Oligohydramnios;
- Abnormal umbilical artery Dopplers;
- Post-term pregnancy;
- Epidural analgesia;
- Induced or augmented labour.

Meconium staining of the amniotic fluid remains a marker of risk. In the Dublin trial, ARM was performed on admission, and the 5 per cent of women with either no fluid or significant meconium were excluded from the trial. Despite continuous monitoring and fetal blood sampling, the perinatal mortality rate in this group was 11 per 1000, compared to 2.1 per 1000 in the remaining trial participants. However, in the absence of fetal heart rate abnormalities, the presence of meconium is not an indication for fetal blood sampling.[4]

It is attractive to base intrapartum monitoring plans on a pre-labour assessment of risk. However, risk can change as labour progresses, for example with:

- the onset of vaginal bleeding;
- development of meconium staining of the amniotic fluid;
- maternal pyrexia (>38 degrees or 2 readings of >37.5 degrees 2 hours apart);
- slow progress in labour.

Ongoing risk appraisal can assist the clinician in deciding how long to tolerate a suspicious (but not pathological) CTG before employing secondary tests. It must be remembered that at least 40 per cent of cases of moderate to severe birth asphyxia in term pregnancies will occur to women in whom no antepartum risk factors were identified.[5]

ADMISSION TESTS

Equally attractive to the pre-labour assignment of risk is an early labour reassessment in low-risk pregnancies. In this situation, a screening test is applied to try to identify those fetuses that are more likely to develop intrapartum complications. Tools that have been used in this situation include CTGs, ultrasound assessment of AFV and umbilical artery Doppler. Research suggests that an abnormal admission test is associated with increased levels of obstetric intervention but no significant reduction in adverse perinatal outcomes [Ib].[6,7] The NICE Guideline on Intrapartum Care does not recommend an admission test in women with uncomplicated pregnancies labouring at term.

INTERMITTENT AUSCULTATION

In the low-risk situation, intermittent auscultation, either by Pinard stethoscope or by handheld Doppler, is often advocated. Current guidelines suggest auscultating the FHR every 15 minutes in the active phase of the first stage of labour. This should be for 60 seconds following a contraction, in order to detect significant decelerations. Maternal pulse should also be recorded by palpation to avoid confusion, particularly when an FHR abnormality is suspected.

The main criticisms of intermittent monitoring are that:

- the above standards are often not achievable on busy delivery suites;
- gradual changes such as an increasing baseline or falling variability will be missed;
- there is no certification process for practitioners using intermittent monitoring;
- no hard record from the monitoring is generated and therefore it is impossible to audit any guidelines related to performing the technique.

CONTINUOUS ELECTRONIC FETAL MONITORING

The mainstay of 'high-risk' fetal assessment, EFM relies on several assumptions:

- that abnormal patterns in the FHR will be seen in the presence of compromise;
- that sufficient warning will be given to allow potentially beneficial interventions to be undertaken;
- that caregivers will recognise the abnormality and take appropriate action.

Many events, such as cord prolapse or abruption, may be so acute as to have no preceding period of deterioration in fetal wellbeing. Fetal monitoring may allow recognition of the problem but no advance warning. A similar rapid deterioration may be seen in fetuses with diminished reserves at the onset of labour, such as those babies with IUGR. Alternatively, it has been suggested that a chronically compromised baby may not exhibit the same type of FHR changes when acute compromise is superimposed. CTG abnormalities in this situation may be subtle or even atypical. Low *et al.* found that only 80 per cent of term births with metabolic acidosis exhibited a predictive fetal heart rate pattern.[5] In other words, in one fifth of cases, the obstetrician would have found the CTG acceptable. The pathophysiology behind other causes of neonatal harm, such as infection, may not be associated with severe or typical 'non-reassuring' FHR abnormalities until almost pre-terminal. Finally, events related to the actual delivery (trauma, shoulder dystocia, problems during resuscitation) contribute to morbidity and mortality but cannot be predicted by intra-partum monitoring.

Some cases of abnormal intrapartum monitoring may have their roots in fetal development. Fetal cardiac anomalies are frequently undiagnosed antenatally and carry considerable morbidity and mortality. It is logical to assume that an abnormal heart will respond to the haemodynamic changes of labour atypically. Similarly, it can be difficult to disentangle prenatal neurological damage, occurring before the onset of labour, from that arising during labour. As the control of FHR involves higher centres, damage to these structures will lead to abnormal cardiovascular responses in labour. Thus, although it is tempting to assume that a poor neurological outcome is necessarily due to a stressful labour as reflected by an abnormal CTG, an alternative possibility needs to be considered, namely that pre-existing neurological damage led to an abnormal cardiovascular response to labour.

WHAT IS A NORMAL CTG?[8]

A useful approach that helps to avoid over-reaction is initially to extract those features of a CTG that are normal by systematically reviewing baseline rate, heart rate variability and accelerations.

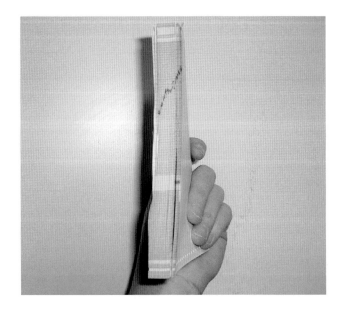

Fig. 51.1 Rising baseline. It is sometimes difficult to see if a baseline is rising or is stable on a short piece of CTG but when a long episode of monitoring is folded and looked at in this manner then the rising baseline is obvious

- *Baseline.* The normal fetal baseline heart rate is 110–160 bpm. There is a small fall in baseline rate as gestation advances. A stable baseline over time is also important (Fig. 51.1). Many women will also have had recent admissions, generating earlier CTGs for comparison.
- *Variability.* FHR variability appears to result from a balance between sympathetic and parasympathetic influences. Therefore, a well-oxygenated nervous system is required for its full expression. Normal variability is >5 bpm. Short periods of reduced variability (particularly when associated with an inactive baby) can be entirely physiological, but in most cases variability will have recovered within 45 minutes.
- *Accelerations.* FHR accelerations represent a response to many minor stresses. Commonly, this is fetal movement, but it also includes palpation or noise. It implies a fetus responsive to external stimuli and, therefore, intact neurocardiac pathways. Most authorities agree that accelerations are the hallmark of fetal wellbeing.

WHAT IS AN ABNORMAL CTG?

- *Baseline.* A continuous and progressive fetal bradycardia indicates fetal hypoxaemia. Fetal bradycardia can arise with any acute reduction in fetal oxygenation, such as cord compression, abruption or uterine hyperstimulation. If the bradycardia is moderate to severe or associated with other CTG abnormalities and the cause cannot be corrected promptly, abdominal delivery will be necessary.

- An isolated tachycardia is rarely, if ever, associated with fetal compromise. Such a tachycardia may be appropriate in some situations. If the baby is very active, the mother will know and the variability will usually be excellent. A fetal tachycardia may arise secondary to a maternal tachycardia, often in response to pain or maternal pyrexia. Clinicians must always be wary of an underlying diagnosis of chorioamnionitis as the fetus is in a hazardous environment that will not be reflected by scalp pH.

- *Variability*. A prolonged period of reduced variability, lasting >90 minutes, is clearly abnormal. The most concerning cause of decreased variability is fetal hypoxaemia, usually chronic, that has globally depressed CNS function. Other aetiologies include pre-existing neurological problems, maternal drugs and congenital heart block.
- *Accelerations*. These will rarely be seen in the presence of a compromised fetus.
- *Decelerations*. Decelerations arouse instant concern in many observers, particularly the less experienced. However, they should never be viewed in isolation, only as a part of the whole clinical picture. Decelerations are usually divided into one of three types, but this can only be determined after observing a pattern repeating over time.
  - *Early decelerations*. These decelerations begin with the onset of a contraction and mirror the shape of the contraction trace. They are usually thought to arise from vagal nerve stimulation secondary to cord compression. They are seen in approximately 1 in 20 first-stage CTGs and, in isolation, are rarely associated with fetal compromise (Fig. 51.2).
  - *Variable decelerations*. Variable decelerations are just that – variable. Each deceleration has a different shape and their timing with regard to contractions is unpredictable. They are the most common type of deceleration and are seen in up to 1 in 8 first-stage traces (Fig. 51.3). They are classically thought to arise from chemoreceptor stimulation secondary to cord compression. They may also result from head compression.
  - *Late decelerations*. Late decelerations begin after the contraction, with the onset, nadir and recovery occurring after the onset, peak and end of a contraction (Fig. 51.4). Only 1–2 per cent of labours demonstrate

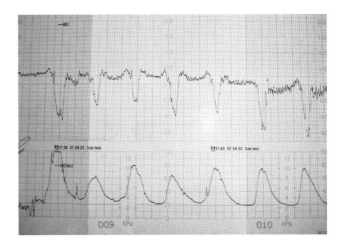

Fig. 51.3 Variable decelerations

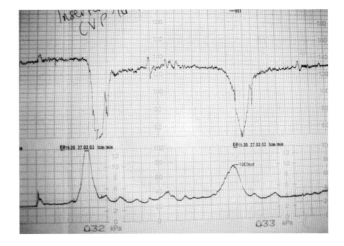

Fig. 51.4 Late decelerations

late decelerations in the first stage of labour. Late decelerations have been postulated to result from direct fetal myocardial depression secondary to hypoxaemia. There may be an additional contribution from chemoreceptor stimulation. Although isolated late decelerations with no other fetal heart rate abnormality are rarely associated with fetal compromise, the presence of any other coexisting abnormalities justifies secondary testing.

CTG INTERPRETATION AND DOCUMENTATION

RCOG and ACOG both recommend a three-tier system of interpretation of the CTG. In the UK, each CTG recording is interpreted as being either normal, suspicious or pathological (Tables 51.1, 51.2) and an appropriate management plan instigated in response. To assist this systematic approach, the use of a structured CTG *pro forma* has been advocated.

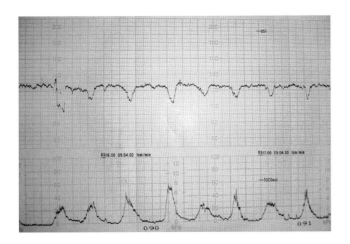

Fig. 51.2 Early decelerations

Table 51.1 Catergorisation of fetal heart rate pattern (NICE Intrapartum Care Guideline 2007)

Category	Definition
Normal	A FHR* trace in which all four features are classified as reassuring
Suspicious	A FHR trace with one feature classified as non-reassuring and the remaining features classified as reassuring
Pathological	A FHR trace with two or more features classified as non-reassuring or one or more classified as abnormal

*Fetal Heart Rate

This encourages a thorough analysis of the CTG in the clinical context, documentation of CTG findings and proposed management plan.

No one element of the CTG should be interpreted in isolation. Regardless of how much intellectual activity is put into the interpretation of the CTG, it remains a screening test only. Even the most worrying pattern (late decelerations with reduced variability) is only associated with acidosis in 50 per cent of cases. Diagnostic or secondary tests are necessary to avoid unnecessary obstetric intervention.

SECONDARY TESTS OF FETAL WELLBEING

Vibro-acoustic stimulation

The use of VAS applied to the maternal abdomen in the presence of a non-reactive antenatal CTG is well documented.[9] The healthy fetus responds with an acceleration in fetal heart rate. The same technique has been applied in the intrapartum period. An acceleration evoked by VAS immediately prior to scalp sampling was never associated with a pH of <7.25. VAS cannot completely eliminate the need for scalp sampling, as only 30 per cent of non-responders will be found to be acidotic. However, it can reduce the need for scalp sampling by up to 50 per cent [B].

Fetal blood sampling

Fetal scalp pH studies remain the principal secondary test of intrapartum fetal wellbeing. It is recommended that all units offering continuous EFM have facilities for FBS. Fetal scalp pH lies between arterial and venous pH but it cannot be determined to which it is closer in advance. As mentioned previously, the lower limit of normal is accepted as a pH of 7.20 in order to allow a wide margin of error. The recommended classification of fetal scalp pH is shown in Table 51.3.

- After a normal result, FBS should be repeated no more than 60 minutes later if the CTG remains pathological, or sooner if there are further abnormalities.
- After a borderline result, FBS should be repeated no more than 30 minutes later.
- An abnormal result should prompt urgent delivery.

Ideally, the base excess should also be measured to distinguish metabolic from respiratory acidosis. There is interest in simply measuring the capillary lactate levels, which provide similar information.[10] Testing systems have now been developed that require smaller volumes of fetal blood than conventional pH studies. This, in conjunction with the ability to sample at lesser dilatations, has led to a lower 'failure-to-sample' rate.

FBS should be performed with the woman in a left lateral position.

Contraindications to FBS include maternal infection with HIV, hepatitis and HSV, suspected fetal haemophilia and prematurity (less than 34 weeks of gestation).

Table 51.2 Classification of fetal heart rate trace features

Feature	Baseline (bpm)	Variability (bpm)	Decelerations	Accelerations
Reassuring	110–160	≥5	None	Present
Non-reassuring	100–109 161–180	40–90 minutes	Typical variable decelerations with over 50% of contractions, occurring for over 90 minutes Single prolonged deceleration for up to 3 minutes	The absence of accelerations with otherwise normal trace is of uncertain significance
Abnormal	<100 >180 Sinusoidal pattern ≥10 minutes	<5 for 90 minutes	Either atypical variable decelerations with over 50% of contractions or late decelerations, both for over 30 minutes Single prolonged deceleration for more than 3 minutes	

Table 51.3 Classification of fetal blood sample results (NICE Intrapartum Care Guideline 2007)

Fetal blood sample result (pH)	Interpretation
≥7.25	Normal
7.21–7.24	Borderline
≤7.20	Abnormal

Scalp stimulation

Most clinicians will have noted that fetuses that respond to scalp sampling with an acceleration almost always have a normal pH. This has been confirmed in formal studies, which showed that 93 per cent of fetuses with a scalp pH >7.20 respond with an acceleration, compared to none of those that are acidotic.[11] This can be useful information when technical difficulties preclude sample collection. However, clinicians should always be wary of scalps that do not bleed, as this may reflect peripheral vasoconstriction in a compromised fetus.

FETAL ECG

The knowledge that changes occur in both the fetal PR interval and ST segment of the fetal ECG in response to hypoxaemia has prompted the use of computerised fetal ECG analysis in combination with conventional CTG to monitor the fetus in labour.

A Cochrane review[12] and a recent meta-analysis[13] compared the effectiveness of EFM with additional ST analysis in vertex term singleton pregnancies with conventional EFM. The combined use of ST analysis (STAN™) and CTG monitoring was associated with a reduction in the number of fetal blood samplings and fewer operative vaginal deliveries. However, there was no difference in the number of babies born with significant metabolic acidosis at birth (defined by pH <7.05 or base deficit >12 mmol/L) or neonatal encephalopathy. There was no difference in the numbers of births by CS or Apgar score <7 at 5 minutes. Monitoring with PR interval analysis did not appear to confer clinical benefit.

There are few data currently regarding the long-term development of infants who participated in these studies.

ST analysis in labour shows promise but there are a number of disadvantages. The technique requires additional equipment and training in interpretation for all caregivers. The use of a spiral fetal scalp electrode is necessary and, if ST analysis is to be commenced where FHR abnormalities are present, it may be necessary to obtain the results of a fetal blood sample before commencing such monitoring.

Non-invasive fECG acquisition using abdominally sited electrodes is now technically possible[14] and in the future may become feasible in clinical practice. This technique avoids the use of a scalp electrode and also allows earlier fECG monitoring in labour.

Computerised CTG analysis

It is well known that there is significant intra-observer and inter-observer variation in the assessment of FHR recordings.

Although the CTG has been the mainstay of monitoring high-risk pregnancies and has remained largely unchanged for more than 40 years, the poor reproducibility and reliability of clinicians to predict fetal compromise using this tool remains a problem and challenge in modern obstetric practice.

Computerised analysis of intrapartum fetal signals has recently been developed but there is no published evidence yet that this technology results in improved perinatal outcomes. Results from prospective randomised trials, comparing intrapartum conventional CTG and computerised analysis of fetal monitoring signals with real-time alerts, are eagerly awaited.

Fetal pulse oximetry

There is no evidence that fetal pulse oximetry is of benefit in labour. The largest RCT to date failed to show any benefit in terms of CS rate or neonatal condition.[15] Fetal pulse oximetry is not in use in the UK and it has not received the support of the ACOG in the USA.

THE MANAGEMENT OF SUSPECTED FETAL COMPROMISE

Improve placental blood supply.

1   Correct maternal hypovolaemia and/or hypotension.
    – Maternal positioning to avoid aorto-caval compression.
    – Intravenous fluids when appropriate.
    – Vasoconstrictors such as ephedrine for lower limb vasodilatation secondary to epidural analgesia.
2   Diminish uterine activity, particularly if excessive.
    – Decrease or stop any oxytocin infusion.
    – Remove vaginal prostaglandins if given recently. This may require vaginal lavage if gels have been used.
    – Use bolus tocolytics (e.g. terbutaline 0.25 mg)

Improve maternal oxygenation.

Maternal oxygen therapy should not be used for more than a short period of time unless there is documented low maternal oxygen saturation. There is no evidence of benefit and a suggestion of possible detrimental effect when applied for more than a few minutes [Ia].

Improve umbilical blood flow.

Increase amniotic fluid volume. Transcervical amnioinfusion may reduce cord compression and frequently leads to an improvement in the FHR. One randomised trial showed a significant reduction in operative intervention and an improvement in cord pH at delivery.[16] Common protocols include infusing 500 mL of Hartmann's solution over 20–30 minutes followed by up to 250 mL/hour. To minimise the risk of amniotic fluid embolus and over-distension, the infusion should be gravity fed.

Decide if delivery is indicated, based upon:

1 the CTG and secondary tests of fetal wellbeing including fetal blood sampling;
2 the whole picture – including obstetric risk factors and progress in labour;
3 other complications, such as abruption, cord prolapse, chorioamnionitis, suspected scar dehiscence.

A CLINICAL APPROACH TO REVIEWING INTRAPARTUM CTGS IN THE FIRST STAGE OF LABOUR

Does the abnormality require immediate delivery if it continues?

Yes (Think little, do lots):

1 Is there a possible precipitant?
   - Cord prolapse/recent epidural/excessive uterine activity/bleeding/scar dehiscence etc.
   - If possible, rapidly take steps to correct any precipitants identified.
   - If no corrective steps are possible or there is no response, deliver by caesarean section.

No (Do little, think lots):

1 For comparison, has there been a 'normal' CTG:
   - earlier in labour?
   - within a few weeks of admission?
2 On the current CTG, what normal features are present?
   - Stable baseline with normal rate;
   - Good variability;
   - Accelerations.
3 On the current CTG, what abnormal features are present?
   Compare 1 and 2 with 3 to decide on the severity of any CTG abnormality and classify as *normal, suspicious* or *pathological.* (See Table 51.1)
4 Is there a possible precipitant?
   - Cord prolapse/cord compression/recent epidural/ excessive uterine activity/bleeding/scar dehiscence etc.
   If possible, take steps to correct any precipitants identified in 4.
5 What risk factors were present in the antenatal period?
6 Were there any recent changes immediately prior to labour?
   - Maternal illness/reduced fetal activity etc.

7 Have any risk factors developed during labour?
   - Meconium/bleeding/poor progress/fever etc.
   - **Then use 5, 6 and 7 to decide:**
   - if and for how long this abnormality can be tolerated before delivering or employing secondary tests of fetal wellbeing (eg. FBS), *and*
   - when to next review the CTG – a deliberate plan is the best approach.

Always try to answer 'What is causing this CTG abnormality?'

Do not forget 'benign' causes, such as recent narcotic analgesia or a rapidly progressing labour.

KEY POINTS

- Intrapartum events rarely lead to perinatal mortality or neurodevelopmental disability after uncomplicated term pregnancies.
- Electronic fetal monitoring is a crude screening test with a poor predictive value for acidosis.
- Always review EFM in the context of the whole pregnancy and labour.
- Secondary tests of fetal wellbeing after non-reassuring CTGs are necessary to avoid over-intervention.
- Intrauterine therapy can improve non-reassuring CTGs and reduce operative delivery.

Published Guidelines

National Institute for Health and Clinical Excellence: *Intrapartum care - care of healthy women and their babies during childbirth.* September 2007.

Key References

1. MacLennan A. A template for defining a causal relation between acute intrapartum events and cerebral palsy: international consensus statement. *BMJ* 1999;319(7216):1054–9.
2. Smith GC. Life-table analysis of the risk of perinatal death at term and post term in singleton pregnancies. *Am J Obstet Gynecol* 2001;184(3):489–96.
3. MacDonald D, Grant A, Sheridan-Pereira M, Boylan P, Chalmers I. The Dublin randomized controlled trial of intrapartum fetal heart rate monitoring. *Am J Obstet Gynecol* 1985;152(5):524–39.
4. Baker PN, Kilby MD, Murray H. An assessment of the use of meconium alone as an indication for fetal blood sampling. *Obstet Gynecol* 1992;80(5):792–6.
5. Low JA, Pickersgill H, Killen H, Derrick EJ. The prediction and prevention of intrapartum fetal asphyxia in term pregnancies. *Am J Obstet Gynecol* 2001;184(4):724–30.

6. Chauhan SP, Washburne JF, Magann EF, Perry KG, Jr., Martin JN, Jr., Morrison JC. A randomized study to assess the efficacy of the amniotic fluid index as a fetal admission test. *Obstet Gynecol* 1995;86(1):9–13.

7. Blix E, Reinar LM, Klovning A, Oian P. Prognostic value of the labour admission test and its effectiveness compared with auscultation only: a systematic review. *BJOG* 2005;112(12):1595–604.

8. Macones GA, Hankins GD, Spong CY, Hauth J, Moore T. The 2008 National Institute of Child Health and Human Development workshop report on electronic fetal monitoring: update on definitions, interpretation, and research guidelines. *Obstet Gynecol* 2008;112(3):661–6.

9. Polzin GB, Blakemore KJ, Petrie RH, Amon E. Fetal vibro-acoustic stimulation: magnitude and duration of fetal heart rate accelerations as a marker of fetal health. *Obstet Gynecol* 1988;72(4):621–6.

10. Wiberg-Itzel E, Lipponer C, Norman M *et al.* Determination of pH or lactate in fetal scalp blood in management of intrapartum fetal distress: randomised controlled multicentre trial. *BMJ* 2008;336(7656):1284–7.

11. Clark SL, Gimovsky ML, Miller FC. Fetal heart rate response to scalp blood sampling. *Am J Obstet Gynecol* 1982;144(6):706–8.

12. Neilson JP. Fetal electrocardiogram (ECG) for fetal monitoring during labour. *Cochrane Database Syst Rev* 2013 May 31;5:CD000116.

13. Schuit E, Amer-Wahlin I, Ojala K *et al.* Effectiveness of electronic fetal monitoring with additional ST analysis in vertex singleton pregnancies at >36 weeks of gestation: an individual participant data meta-analysis. *Am J Obstet Gynecol* 2013 Mar;208(3):187.e1–187

14. Taylor MJ, Thomas MJ, Smith MJ *et al.* Non-invasive intrapartum fetal ECG: preliminary report. *BJOG* 2005;112(8):1016–21.

15. Bloom SL, Spong CY, Thom E *et al.* Fetal pulse oximetry and cesarean delivery. *N Engl J Med* 2006;355(21):2195–202.

16. Schrimmer DB, Macri CJ, Paul RH. Prophylactic amnioinfusion as a treatment for oligohydramnios in laboring patients: a prospective, randomized trial. *Am J Obstet Gynecol* 1991;165(4 Pt 1):972–5.

Chapter 52 Obstetric anaesthesia and analgesia

David M Levy and Duncan S Cochran

MRCOG standards

Candidates are expected to:

- understand and be able to counsel women about the options for pain relief in labour, and their respective risks;
- understand the influence of various complications of pregnancy and labour (e.g. pre-eclampsia, coagulopathy and major haemorrhage) on the choice of anaesthetic.

INTRODUCTION

Obstetric *analgesia* is pain relief in labour; *anaesthesia* is the abolition of sufficient sensation to allow operative delivery.

Provision of analgesia is a key element of the modern management of labour. Women receive education antenatally about the options for analgesia in labour and often have very high expectations on admission to the delivery suite.

Regional (spinal, epidural or combined spinal–epidural) anaesthesia is now used for the vast majority of caesarean sections.

ANALGESIA FOR LABOUR

Modes of analgesia include:

- relaxation therapy;
- immersion in warm water;
- aromatherapy;
- transcutaneous electrical nerve stimulation (TENS);
- inhalation of nitrous oxide – and other inhalational anaesthetics – in oxygen;
- parenteral opioids;
- regional analgesia.

The requirement for pharmacological pain relief in labour is reduced when a known practitioner provides continuous support throughout labour [A].[1] Immersion in water during the first stage of labour reduces analgesic requirements.[2] The evidence underpinning nonpharmacological methods of pain relief in labour (including continuous support, bathing, upright position and massage) has been systematically reviewed.[3]

Transcutaneous electrical nerve stimulation

Electrical impulses are applied to the skin via flexible carbon electrodes from a battery-powered stimulator. Stimulation of A-fibre transmission and local release of β-endorphins modulate pain, closing a postulated 'gate' in the dorsal horn of the spinal cord. The effect is similar to massage of the lower back by a birthing partner.

- Electrodes are placed over the T10–L1 dermatomes on either side of the spinous processes to provide analgesia for the first stage of labour. A second set of electrodes is placed over the S2–S4 dermatomes for second-stage pain relief. Women can control the level of current delivered.
- There is no evidence that TENS provides better analgesia than placebo ('sham' TENS). However, TENS can diminish the need for other analgesic interventions, and is completely free from adverse effects.[4] TENS 'analgesia' seems to be rated more highly in retrospect than contemporaneously.

Opioid analgesia

The analgesic efficacy of opioids in labour is limited, although sedation is almost invariable.[5]

- All opioids can cause decreased Apgar and neurobehavioural scores and neonatal respiratory depression, even when administered many hours before birth.
- Neonatal respiratory depression is readily reversible with naloxone, a specific opioid antagonist. The neonatal dose is 10 mcg/kg IM, repeated if necessary.
- Maternal gastric emptying is inhibited and the incidence of nausea and vomiting increased. An anti-emetic (e.g. cyclizine 50 mg or prochlorperazine 12.5 mg) should be given IM with the chosen opioid.

- Midwives can prescribe and administer controlled drugs in accordance with Nursing and Midwifery Council (Midwives) Rules and locally agreed policies and procedures. In the UK, pethidine is the most widely used IM opioid, although the use of diamorphine is increasing in the UK without evidence of greater efficacy.[6] Comparisons of pethidine 100 mg with diamorphine 5 mg, meptazinol 100 mg and tramadol 100 mg have failed to demonstrate superior analgesic efficacy or a more favourable side-effect profile associated with any one agent.
- Because of the additive risk of maternal respiratory depression, IM opioids should never be given in the event of inadequate regional analgesia without prior reassessment of the woman by an anaesthetist.
- A reduction in baseline CTG variability can make interpretation difficult.

Patient-controlled analgesia

Intravenous opioid by PCA system is useful in women with thrombocytopenia or other haematological reasons for avoiding regional analgesia or IM injections. The potency and rapidity of action of remifentanil can predispose to sudden respiratory depression – as labour pain is episodic as opposed to continuous, the therapeutic window is particularly narrow. There appears to be wide variation in the dose required for effective labour analgesia.

Despite a slower onset of action and less rapid clearance, fentanyl is perhaps the drug of choice, by 20–30 mcg bolus and 5-minute lockout period [E].

Analgesia by inhalation

Sixty to 70 per cent of labouring women in the UK seek analgesia by inhalation of a 50:50 mixture of nitrous oxide and oxygen (N_2O/O_2). Marketed as Entonox® and Equanox®, the gas mixture is supplied in cylinders with a blue body and blue/white shoulders and is piped to labour rooms in many hospitals. The future availability of nitrous oxide is not assured. Protracted inhalation of N_2O can inactivate vitamin B_{12} and inhibit DNA synthesis. Isoflurane and sevoflurane, two fluorinated, potent inhalational anaesthetics, have been studied in labour at low doses, but not yet widely adopted.[5]

- N_2O/O_2 is self-administered by inspiration through a facemask or mouthpiece, which opens a demand valve. Diffusion from alveoli to pulmonary capillaries and delivery to the brain by the cardiac output are not instantaneous. Inhalation should therefore start as soon as a contraction begins, to allow maximum drug effect at the peak.
- The drug is non-cumulative and does not affect the fetus. N_2O/O_2 causes highly variable maternal sedation. Some women appear to be dreaming or drunk; others become somnolent or even briefly unrousable.

- Hyperventilation with N_2O/O_2 can be followed by a short period of apnoea; therefore, the woman should always hold the mouthpiece or mask herself. If she loses consciousness, she will let go. A few breaths of air eliminate the N_2O and consciousness is invariably soon regained.
- A number of studies have questioned the analgesic effect of N_2O/O_2. Pain is often still perceived under the influence of the drug – it is merely rendered more bearable by the intoxicated state. Thirty to 40 per cent of women in labour derive no benefit.
- The risk of cross-contamination between patients sharing breathing systems dictates that mouthpieces and masks should be disposable, or sterilised between patients. Either a new disposable breathing system should be used for each patient, or a disposable breathing system filter interposed between the tubing and mouthpiece/mask.

Regional analgesia for labour

Regional analgesia is the provision of pain relief by blockade of sensory nerves as they enter the spinal cord. Local anaesthetic and/or opioid can be introduced into epidural and/or subarachnoid (intrathecal) spaces.

Comparisons of regional analgesia regimens require careful scrutiny of which drugs have been introduced into which space(s) and their mode of administration (bolus or infusion).

Compared with other analgesic modalities, pain relief from regional blockade is undoubtedly superior.[7] Ninety per cent of consultant obstetric units in the UK provide a 24-hour regional analgesia service. The UK Obstetric Anaesthetists' Association (OAA) captured data in 2011 from 558,256 mothers in 148 units. The regional analgesia rate was 22.7 per cent. In the USA, the rate is 60 per cent.

Contraindications to regional blockade are outlined in Table 52.1. Subcutaneous LMWH within the previous 10–12 hours is a relative contraindication. Scar tissue from previous spinal surgery can make identification of the epidural space difficult, and impede spread of local anaesthetic solution. However, catheterisation of the subarachnoid space might nevertheless be feasible – early referral (ideally with the post-operative radiographs) should be made to an obstetric anaesthetist. Untreated pyrexia in labour raises the possibility of bacteraemia and seeding a vertebral canal abscess in the event of bleeding from an epidural vein. However, the likelihood of such a complication has to be weighed against the probably greater risks of general anaesthesia (e.g. anaphylaxis to succinylcholine) that might otherwise be avoided. Regional analgesia has been shown to cause pyrexia in labour in around 15 per cent of women. Suggested mechanisms include abolition of hyperventilation and sweating (from the lower half of the body) and promotion of shivering. The potential importance is that maternal fever, particularly in association with fetal acidosis, greatly increases the risk of neonatal encephalopathy. Acetaminophen (paracetamol) and active

Table 52.1 Contraindications to regional analgesia, with associated risks

Contraindication	Risk
Uncorrected anticoagulation or coagulopathy	Vertebral canal haematoma
Local or systemic sepsis (pyrexia >38°C not treated with antibiotics)	Vertebral canal abscess
Hypovolaemia or active haemorrhage	Cardiovascular collapse secondary to sympathetic blockade
Patient refusal	Legal action
Lack of sufficient trained midwives for continuous care and monitoring of mother and fetus for the duration of epidural blockade	Delayed recognition and treatment of maternal collapse/convulsion/respiratory arrest or fetal compromise

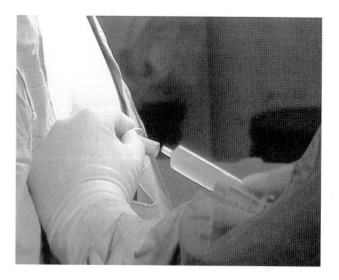

Fig. 52.1 Tuohy needle with loss-of-resistance syringe

cooling are indicated. The link between epidural analgesia and backache has been thoroughly investigated and no evidence of causation found.[7] The risk of permanent neurological injury is probably less than 1:100,000. Obstetric palsies (e.g. compression of the lumbosacral trunk) are far more common.

Regional analgesia does not impair the initiation of breast feeding.

Epidurals and spinals

The epidural space is identified by the loss of resistance to depression of a syringe plunger as a Tuohy needle is advanced (Fig. 52.1) through the ligamentum flavum. A catheter is then threaded through the Tuohy needle (Fig. 52.2) to facilitate bolus top-ups or a continuous infusion. The subarachnoid space, which contains CSF, is a few millimetres deeper, inside the meninges. Needles used for deliberate spinal injection are much finer than Tuohy needles (Fig. 52.3). Unlike local anaesthetics, which prevent the conduction of nerve impulses, opioids act on specific receptors in the spinal cord. Synergistic mixtures of local anaesthetic and opioids (usually fentanyl) have permitted significant reductions in the amount of local anaesthetic used. Side effects specific to opioids are respiratory depression (in the most unlikely event of cephalad spread of opioid to the brainstem) and pruritus.

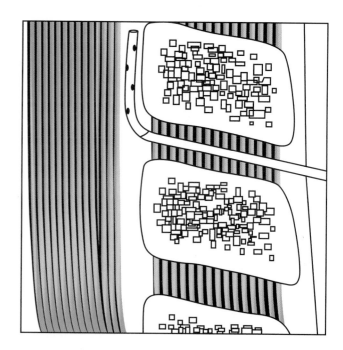

Fig. 52.2 Tuohy needle advanced through the ligamentum flavum, with the catheter in the epidural space

Dural tap

Accidental meningeal puncture with a Tuohy needle is called a 'dural tap'. Eighty-five per cent of women who have a dural tap will develop a severe, characteristically postural headache, caused by leakage of CSF. Only the presence of headache during labour is an indication for elective forceps or vacuum extraction at full dilatation. The definitive treatment is epidural injection of autologous blood (up to 20 mL) – a 'blood patch', best undertaken at 24–48 hours post-delivery. Occasionally, the patch has to be repeated. Women with persistent headache must be followed up until symptom-free. Intracranial

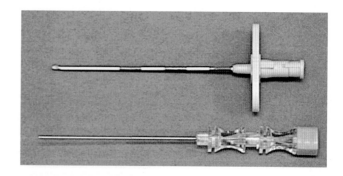

Fig. 52.3 Epidural Tuohy (above) and spinal needles

hypotension (low CSF pressure) can be complicated (albeit very rarely) by cranial subdural haematoma secondary to tearing of a dural bridging vein.

Total spinal

Five to ten times the dose of local anaesthetic is required for an equivalent effect after epidural as opposed to subarachnoid injection. Any communication between epidural and subarachnoid spaces introduces the risk of a large dose of local anaesthetic, intended for the epidural space, reaching the subarachnoid space. A block high enough to impair diaphragmatic innervation and cause respiratory arrest is known as a 'total spinal'. A total spinal should be a survivable event for mother and fetus. The mother will require emergency tracheal intubation and treatment of hypotension. The urgency of CS will be dictated by the FHR pattern. Tracheal extubation should be feasible within 2–3 hours, once the high block has regressed.

Local anaesthetic toxicity

If local anaesthetic is injected inadvertently into an epidural vein, symptoms and signs of local anaesthetic toxicity (Table 52.2) can arise from the effect of high concentrations of local anaesthetic in the CNS. Initial treatment follows the 'ABC' principle: airway, breathing and circulation (with relief of aorto-caval compression). A new, specific and effective treatment has been introduced for local anaesthetic-induced cardiac arrest: intravenous Intralipid™ 20 per cent. The dose for a 70 kg adult is 100 mL. All delivery suites should have a readily available emergency LipidRescue™ box, containing a 500 mL bag of Intralipid 20 per cent, 50 mL syringes and giving set. Details of evolving guidelines for this novel treatment are available at www.lipidrescue.org. One of the deaths in the most recent Report on Confidential Enquiries into Maternal Deaths[8] (accidental IV administration of bupivacaine from an infusion bag intended for epidural use) might have been averted had this therapy been available.

Combined spinal–epidural analgesia

Combined spinal–epidural (CSE) analgesia entails an initial subarachnoid injection of fentanyl (in the UK) mixed with a small amount of local anaesthetic. The spinal injection makes the onset of analgesia considerably faster (5 minutes, as opposed to at least 20 minutes with an epidural). The resulting motor block is sufficiently minimal for women to retain sufficient muscle power to walk in labour. However, depending

on the drug regimen, proprioception (information from joint receptors to maintain balance) might be impaired. The Comparative Obstetric Mobile Epidural Trial (COMET)[9] found that both low-dose infusion epidurals and CSE analgesia resulted in a lower incidence of instrumental vaginal deliveries compared to traditional intermittent (midwife-administered) bolus epidurals (Table 52.3) [B]. It is presumed that this is attributable to the preservation of motor tone and the bearing-down reflex, as mode of delivery was not influenced by whether or not women walked during the first stage of labour. The effect of mobility after full cervical dilatation remains equivocal.[10] A Cochrane review failed to find a difference in overall maternal satisfaction with CSE compared to epidural analgesia, despite the faster onset. CSEs were associated with more pruritus.[11]

Patient-controlled epidural analgesia

Increasing numbers of units (25 per cent in 2011) favour self-administration of epidural opioid and local anaesthetic: patient-controlled epidural analgesia (PCEA).[12] Compared with continuous infusion techniques, PCEA reduces the total administered dose of local anaesthetic, the degree of motor block and the number of anaesthetists' interventions. Some studies suggest that analgesia is improved by a continuous background infusion.

Regional analgesia and progress of labour

Regional analgesia can improve uteroplacental blood flow in labour. However, a fall in blood pressure after a bolus dose of local anaesthetic can precipitate a fetal bradycardia. Adoption of full left-lateral position and treatment of hypotension by i.v. fluid bolus and/or vasopressor should resolve the FHR abnormality.

Despite better pain relief than other methods of analgesia, regional analgesia has been associated with longer first and second stages of labour, an increased incidence of fetal malposition, greater use of syntocinon®, and an increased risk of instrumental vaginal birth. No direct effect on the CS rate has been demonstrated.[7]

A recent large RCT compared neuraxial (subarachnoid) fentanyl (at the initiation of CSE) with parenteral opioid

Table 52.2 Symptoms and signs of local anaesthetic toxicity

Symptoms	Signs
Numbness of tongue or lips	Slurring of speech
Tinnitus	Drowsiness
Light-headedness	Convulsions
Anxiety	Cardiorespiratory arrest

Table 52.3 COMET: analgesic regimen and mode of delivery

Delivery	'Traditional' epidural (n = 353)	Combined spinal epidural (n = 351)	Low-dose infusion epidural
Normal vaginal	124 (35%)	150 (43%)	150 (43%)
Instrumental vaginal	131 (37%)	102 (29%)	98 (28%)
Caesarean section	98 (28%)	99 (28%)	102 (29%)

- $p = 0.04$, 1 DF (degree of freedom) for normal versus other deliveries

(hydromorphone) at the first request for pain relief in labour, with deferral of regional analgesia.[13] Women who received early CSE experienced superior analgesia and a shorter duration of labour. The rates of CS and instrumental delivery were similar (the study had 90 per cent power to detect a 50 per cent difference in CS rate [B].

There is no high-level evidence upon which to withhold modern regional analgesia because an arbitrary degree of cervical dilatation has not yet been achieved.

Instrumental delivery

When epidural analgesia is topped up for instrumental delivery, the block height and density should be adequate for CS, in case the need arises to proceed swiftly to operative delivery if the instrument application fails.

ANAESTHESIA FOR CAESAREAN SECTION

The OAA 2011 data collection identified a CS rate of 24.8 per cent. Fifty-nine per cent were performed under single-shot spinal anaesthesia. Epidural anaesthesia was used in 19.8 per cent of cases (most were topped-up labour epidurals and CSEs). The GA rate was 8.2 per cent (Fig. 52.4). The NICE caesarean section guideline (www.nice.org.uk/Guidance/CG132) includes anaesthesia recommendations.

Categorisation of urgency

Good communication among obstetric, anaesthetic, midwifery and theatre staff is vital for a well-organised caesarean section. A four-point classification (1–4) of urgency of CS

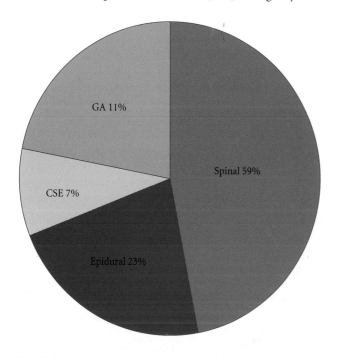

Fig. 52.4 UK caesarean sections, 2011 (NOAD)[21]

(Table 52.4), similar to that used by the National Confidential Enquiry into Patient Outcome and Death (NCEPOD), has been validated by close agreement between anaesthetists' and obstetricians' gradings of more than 400 cases, and recently reassessed.[14] It has replaced the more traditional 'emergency', 'urgent', 'elective' terminology. A decision-to-delivery interval of 30 minutes has become widely adopted as an audit standard, despite lack of any evidence that 30 minutes is a critical threshold in the development of intrapartum hypoxia. Spinal anaesthesia is often appropriate for urgent (Table 52.4) CS, although a CESDI deemed repeated attempts at regional anaesthesia to be inadvisable in the absence of significant risk factors for general anaesthesia.[15] Auditable standards published by the Royal College of Anaesthetists (www.rcoa.ac.uk/docs/ARB-section8.pdf) are listed in Table 52.5.

In-utero fetal resuscitation

Anaesthetists are increasingly attuned to contributing to the multidisciplinary management of in-utero fetal compromise. The Bristol 'SPOILT' acronym is a useful aide memoire:

- Syntocinon® off;
- Position: full left lateral;
- Oxygen;
- Intravenous infusion of crystalloid;
- Low blood pressure: IV vasopressor;
- Tocolysis: SC terbutaline 250 mcg.

Mortality

Maternal mortality attributed to anaesthesia has fallen considerably over the last 50 years (Fig. 52.5). Capnography is arguably the most valuable component of physiological monitoring. Tracheal or oesophageal intubation can be confirmed immediately, with complete accuracy.

Antacid prophylaxis

Fasting intervals of 6 hours for food and 2 hours for fluids (tea/coffee with semi-skimmed milk, or fruit squash) are appropriate for women scheduled for elective caesarean section. Ranitidine diminishes gastric acid secretion; sodium citrate neutralises acid already in the stomach. Ranitidine

Table 52.4 Classification of urgency for caesarean section

Category	Definition
1	Immediate threat to life of woman or fetus
2	Maternal or fetal compromise that is not immediately life threatening
3	Needing early delivery but no maternal or fetal compromise
4	At a time to suit the woman and maternity team

Table 52.5 Audit recommendations: Royal College of Anaesthetists

Proposed standard or target for best practice	>95% RA for category 4 CS
	>85% RA for categories 1 to 3 CS
	<1% RA to GA conversion rate in category 4 CS
	<3% RA to GA conversion rate in categories 1 to 3 CS (this figure of 3% includes regional anaesthetics for labour converted to GA for CS)
Suggested data to be collected	Number of CS, category of CS, type of anaesthetic and reason for its use
	Name and grade of anaesthetist and surgeon
	Conversion rate to GA and reason (e.g. technical difficulty, poor block, maternal request, fetal or surgical reasons)
	In particular, data collected should allow units to identify reasons for a low RA rate (or high)

- CS, caesarean section; GA, general anaesthesia; RA, regional anaesthesia.

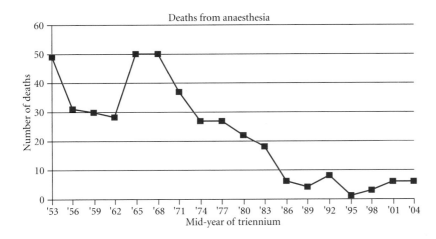

Fig. 52.5 Maternal mortality (number of deaths) from anaesthesia 1952–2005

150 mg should be prescribed for 2 hours before an elective operation and administered 8-hourly to all women in labour with risk factors for CS. Administration of a measure (30 mL) of sodium citrate 0.3M immediately before caesarean section under general anaesthetic should be done. The risk of aspiration of gastric contents is not confined to general anaesthesia: protective laryngeal reflexes may be obtunded in the event of an excessively high regional block, though sodium citrate is not usually given prior to regional anaesthesia.

Regional anaesthesia

Single-shot spinal anaesthesia

Single-shot spinal anaesthesia has become the most popular anaesthetic technique for caesarean section (Fig. 52.4), largely as a consequence of the widespread adoption of pencil-point tip needles (Fig. 52.6). Compared to standard cutting bevel (or Quincke) needle tips, there is less leakage of CSF and a lower incidence of headache requiring epidural blood patch.

Preload – or coload?

A crystalloid fluid preload has become recognised as an ineffective means of preventing hypotension after spinal injection. Its short intravascular half-life prevents a sustained increase in cardiac output before sympathetic blockade develops. Rather than infuse crystalloid before spinal blockade, fluid is best given (from pressurised infusion bag) as the block develops – hence 'coload'. Colloids, such as hydroxyethyl starch, are no longer recommended.

Hypotension is best managed by:

- strict avoidance of aorto-caval compression;
- rapid infusion of crystalloid immediately after intrathecal injection;
- prompt boluses or infusion of vasopressor.

Level of injection

MRI has shown that the conus medullaris of the spinal cord extends below the level of the body of L1 in 20 per cent of patients. Moreover, anaesthetists commonly underestimate the height of their approach. A series of case reports describing

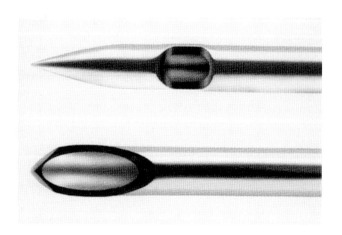

Fig. 52.6 Pencil-point (top) and cutting bevel-tip spinal needles

damage to the conus medullaris has led to an authoritative recommendation that spinal needles should not be inserted higher than the L3/4 interspinous space – practically, the space at or immediately above a line joining the highest points of the iliac crests. Anaesthetists are increasingly using ultrasound probes to identify the space to be used.

Dose of local anaesthetic

Most UK obstetric anaesthetists use hyperbaric bupivacaine 0.5 per cent. Gestation is important when deciding upon the dose for a single-shot spinal. In one study, loss of cold sensation to T4 was achieved with 2.25 mL in all of a group of women at term, but only 16 per cent of women at 28–35 weeks' gestation. The progressively gravid uterus causes increasing vena caval compression, epidural venous engorgement and consequent displacement of the dura and reduced subarachnoid space volume. Postural manoeuvres after intrathecal injection, such as moving from right to left lateral or flexing the knees and thighs, promote cephalad spread of the injectate by influencing vertebral canal blood volume.

Loss of light touch sensation to T5 is a better predictor of pain-free CS under (opioid-free) spinal anaesthesia than loss of cold sensation. Light touch sensation is ascertained by asking if the woman has any appreciation of ethyl chloride dripped on to skin. The extent of the block and modality of testing should be recorded in case a subsequent claim of intra-operative pain has to be defended. The obstetrician must clarify with the anaesthetist that it is appropriate to start surgery.

Spinal anaesthesia can cause, within 5 minutes, a high block with precipitous fall in blood pressure – even despite IV coload and vasopressor. Relief of aortocaval compression by swift delivery of the baby will be required urgently. Obstetricians should not, therefore, leave the theatre suite during induction of spinal anaesthesia.

Opioids

The addition of intrathecal fentanyl, diamorphine or morphine can reduce the incidence of intra-operative visceral pain, although fentanyl does not contribute significantly to postoperative analgesia. Reports of respiratory depression after intrathecal doses of opioids in obstetric practice are conspicuous by their absence. NICE recommends the use of 0.3 mg diamorphine for category 4 CS. Intra-operative pain should be treated promptly by IV alfentanil (0.5 mg increments) or inhaled isoflurane or sevoflurane in an N_2O/O_2 50:50 mixture, IV ketamine (20 mg increments) or conversion to general anaesthesia.

Vasopressors

Ephedrine (alpha and beta sympathomimetic) was regarded as the vasopressor of choice in obstetrics for decades. Persisting reservations about the effects of alpha-agonists on uteroplacental blood flow were founded on studies of Columbian ewes, which did not undergo regional anaesthesia. Randomised comparisons of IV boluses of ephedrine and phenylephrine in women undergoing CS found similar changes in maternal systolic pressure and cardiac output, but significantly lower UA pH in neonates whose mothers had received ephedrine. Increased fetal metabolic rate secondary to ephedrine-induced beta-adrenergic stimulation may be the explanation. Infusions of phenylephrine, compared with ephedrine, are associated with improved maternal haemodynamic control and less nausea and vomiting [B].[16] Phenylephrine is now widely regarded as the vasopressor of choice at CS and should mitigate the slight fetal acidosis that was observed in a meta-analysis of spinals compared with epidurals or general anaesthetics.

Spinal anaesthesia and pre-eclampsia

Over the last few years, it has become accepted by many that pre-eclampsia is not necessarily a contraindication to single-shot spinal anaesthesia; if the abnormal systemic vasoconstriction is of humoral rather than neural aetiology, sympathetic blockade should not, logically, cause precipitous hypotension. Prior vasodilatation by effective antihypertensive treatment (e.g. oral methyldopa or IV hydralazine) with limited intravascular volume expansion seems to avert problematic hypotension. Judicious fluid boluses and small increments of phenylephrine will correct hypotension.

Postoperative analgesia

Supplementation of intrathecal diamorphine or morphine by regular oral, rectal or IV paracetamol (1 g 6-hourly) and diclofenac (50 mg 8-hourly, 12 hours after an initial 100 mg postoperative dose), makes patient-controlled IV morphine unnecessary for most women. NSAIDs are contraindicated in the initial postoperative period if CS has been complicated by excessive bleeding or there is concern about the adequacy of haemostasis (e.g. uterine atony). In pre-eclampsia, prescription of NSAIDs should be deferred until 24 hours postpartum and confirmation of normal renal function. In 2013, the Medicines and Healthcare products Regulatory Agency (MHRA) contraindicated the use of codeine in mothers who are breastfeeding, due to fears of a small risk of respiratory depression in infants in mothers who are 'fast acetylators'.[22]

Transversus abdominis plane (TAP) blocks (Fig. 52.7) have emerged as highly effective adjuncts to other analgesic modalities after general anaesthesia, though have limited use after regional anaesthesia if a long-acting intrathecal opioid has been administered.[17]

Epidural anaesthesia

Few elective caesarean sections are now performed under epidural anaesthesia, because the quality of anaesthesia is generally poorer than that afforded by subarachnoid block. The rate of conversion to general anaesthesia for epidurals is consistently greater than that for spinals. *De novo* epidural anaesthesia is still favoured by some when gradual establishment of block is desired to minimise hypotension e.g in patients with cardiac disease. In severe pre-eclampsia, postoperative infusion of epidural bupivacaine/fentanyl in a high-dependency area will confer optimal analgesia and contribute to blood pressure control. A South African study demonstrated that women who were fully conscious and cooperative after an eclamptic seizure could safely undergo caesarean section under epidural anaesthesia. All women had platelet counts >100 × 10⁹/L and had been treated with magnesium sulphate.[18]

Conversion of labour analgesia

In women in labour deemed high risk for CS – and those with potentially difficult airways – consideration should be given to instituting epidural analgesia early. It should be established that the block is working well, without missed segments. If analgesia in labour has been poor, it is unlikely that anaesthesia for CS will be satisfactory. Conversion of analgesia for labour to surgical anaesthesia for CS takes around 20 minutes. In contrast to single-shot spinal anaesthesia, abrupt changes in blood pressure are unusual. Good communication among midwives, obstetricians and anaesthetists should make general anaesthesia for the woman with a working epidural a rarity.

Even in the event of cord prolapse, traditionally managed without question by general anaesthesia, there might be time for an epidural top-up, provided upward displacement of the presenting part is effective in avoiding cord compression.

Combined spinal–epidural anaesthesia

Some units have adopted CSE anaesthesia as their standard technique for CS, despite lack of evidence of overall superiority compared with single-shot spinals. CSE anaesthesia is useful when there is a possibility that surgery might outlast a single-shot spinal block – a standard intrathecal dose of local anaesthetic lasts typically around 90 minutes. In the event of protracted surgery (e.g. caesarean hysterectomy in a woman with placenta praevia), an epidural catheter will allow extension of the block. However, the initial spinal anaesthetic block precludes ascertainment of correct positioning of the epidural catheter.

Continuous spinal anaesthesia

Threading a fine gauge catheter into the subarachnoid space can permit repeated fractionated bolus doses directly into the CSF compartment, allowing high-quality anaesthesia which can be extended if surgery is protracted. The technique has been reserved for women with cardiovascular risk factors (e.g. complex cardiac disease) for whom abrupt sympathetic blockade might be deleterious.

The US FDA banned microspinal catheters (27 g or smaller) in 1992, in response to a cluster of cases of cauda equina syndrome. The cause was, in all likelihood, pooling of hyperbaric 5 per cent lidocaine (not available in the UK) in the sacral area, as opposed to morbidity associated with the catheter *per se*. A multicentre comparison of continuous intrathecal labour analgesia versus continuous epidural labour analgesia was published in 2008, powered to detect a >1 per cent incidence of neurological complications related to use of the intrathecal

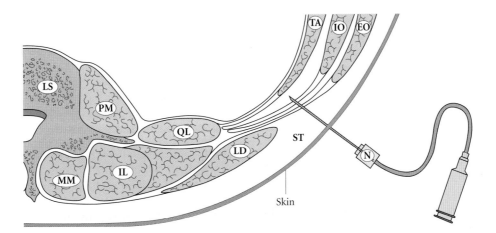

Fig. 52.7 Transversus abdominis plane block. Line drawing of a transverse section through the abdominal wall at the level of the lumbar triangle of Petit (TOP). The floor of the triangle is composed, from superficial to deep, of the fascial extensions of external oblique, internal oblique, and transversus abdominis, respectively, and the peritoneum. The needle is inserted through the triangle, using the loss-of-resistance technique. The needle is shown in the transversus abdominis plane, and the fascial layers have separated as a result of the injection of local anesthetic.

LS, lumbar spine; LD, latissimus dorsi; PM, psoas major; QL, quadratus lumborum; MM, multifidus; IL, iliocostalis; TA, transverse abdominis; IO, internal oblique; EO, external oblique; N, 50 mm blunt-tipped needle; ST, subcutaneous tissue.

catheter [B].[19] There were no permanent neurological deficits in either group.

Placenta praevia and APH

Regional anaesthesia has been associated with reduced estimated blood loss and transfusion requirements at CS with placenta praevia. Although the evidence is not high level, the commonly held obstetric view that placenta praevia mandates general anaesthesia is not supported. Individual risk factors must be considered in every case. Anterior placenta praevia in a woman over 35 who has undergone previous CS suggests a particularly high risk of placenta accreta and massive haemorrhage. General anaesthesia with intra-operative red cell salvage and provision for postoperative ICU admission might be considered prudent.

An important distinction must be made between women with the potential for major intra-operative haemorrhage (as in placenta praevia) but who are normovolaemic (i.e. have not bled), and those who present with antepartum haemorrhage. Pregnant women can compensate for significant blood loss by vasoconstriction, which will be abolished by regional anaesthesia. *Any woman who has bled and is pale and tachycardic is not suitable for regional anaesthesia, regardless of the blood pressure.*

Regional anaesthesia might be ideal for advanced placement of uterine artery balloons immediately before caesarean section, but totally inappropriate for interventional radiological management of haemorrhage.

General anaesthesia

General anaesthesia may be indicated for 'emergency' caesarean sections (Table 52.4) and for other cases for which a regional block is absolutely contraindicated (e.g. uncorrected coagulopathy) or has failed.

Good communication between the anaesthetist and obstetrician is vital in these cases, and the safety of the mother must always remain of paramount importance.

If the history or evaluation of the airway suggests that tracheal intubation might be difficult, awake fibre-optic intubation should be considered. The principal risks of general anaesthesia are:

- airway problems (e.g. failed tracheal intubation);
- aspiration of gastric contents;
- anaphylaxis (principally to succinylcholine).

In the event of anaphylaxis, adrenaline (epinephrine) is likely to improve rather than reduce uteroplacental blood flow. Rapid operative delivery while the anaesthetist administers pharmacological treatment will aid maternal resuscitation.

Depth of anaesthesia

The regimen of thiopental, succinylcholine and intubation has remained standard and largely unchanged since it superseded ether by facemask 50 years ago, and has permitted a lighter plane of inhalational general anaesthesia. General anaesthesia

is 'innocuous and reversible' for the baby, provided maternal oxygenation and normocarbia are maintained, aorto-caval compression is avoided and a paediatrician is present to support neonatal ventilation. If uterine hyperstimulation has been contributory to fetal compromise, uterine relaxation conferred by a volatile agent might be therapeutic. In contrast, a maternal stress response to excessively light general anaesthesia will be to the detriment of uteroplacental blood flow. With inhalational agent monitoring now universally available, the risk of awareness in obstetric anaesthesia should have been consigned to history. Cases of explicit awareness are attributable to failures of basic anaesthetic practice (e.g. inadequate anaesthesia during neuromuscular blockade).[20]

The introduction of sugammadex, a specific antagonist for rocuronium, has offered the possibility of discontinuing the use of succinylcholine (the muscle relaxant with worst side-effect profile), 50 years after its introduction.

Special considerations in pre-eclampsia

Any dubious notion of light general anaesthesia for the baby's benefit should be overridden by efforts to protect the mother's cerebral circulation. A death in the 2005–2009 Confidential Enquiries was attributable to intracerebral haemorrhage sustained in the course of a predictable pressor response to difficult tracheal intubation. A generous bolus dose of opioid or magnesium should be given to supplement the IV induction. Prior communication with a paediatrician is essential in order for preparation to be made for antagonism of opioid and provision of ventilatory support for the neonate.

The onset and duration of succinylcholine are unaffected by therapeutic serum magnesium concentrations. However, the durations of action of all non-depolarising drugs are potentiated, and the use of a peripheral nerve stimulator is essential to ensure adequate reversal at the end of surgery. There should be a low threshold for blood pressure monitoring by radial arterial line, both in theatre and post-operatively in the high-dependency unit.

Any patient whose larynx was noted to be swollen at laryngoscopy, or in whom intubation was traumatic, is at particular risk of laryngeal oedema. Post-operative care must be undertaken in an ICU or high-dependency area with an anaesthetist immediately available. The ominous significance of stridor (impending airway obstruction) must be understood, and vigilance maintained. Should stridor develop, an anaesthetist must be called immediately.

Special considerations for maternal cardiac disease

In labour, the sympathetic blockade consequent upon high-dose, intermittent bolus doses of epidural local anaesthetic must be avoided. Low-dose regimens can be embraced and topped up slowly and carefully if required for operative delivery [E].

Compared to regional anaesthesia, opioid-based general anaesthesia affords greater preservation of systemic vascular resistance. Regional anaesthesia avoids myocardial depression but can lead to unpredictable decreases in preload and/or afterload. General anaesthesia might therefore be preferable for CS in women with fixed cardiac output states. If acute peri-operative deterioration is potentially amenable to surgical remedy (e.g. emergency valve replacement), caesarean section might best be undertaken in a cardiac theatre, with extracorporeal circulatory support immediately available.

Pre-assessment and the role of the anaesthetist

All units should have a referral system between obstetricians and obstetric anaesthetists. Trainees and non-consultant anaesthetists providing out-of-hours cover should never be presented with complex cases 'out of the blue'. Obstetric referrals to a specialist physician's clinic (e.g. cardiology) should be brought to the attention of a consultant obstetric anaesthetist.

Anaesthetists' principal concerns are:

- the feasibility of regional block – which depends on flexion of the lumbar spine and normal coagulation;
- whether tracheal intubation at emergency caesarean section might be hazardous, e.g. because of limited neck flexion/mouth opening;
- the influence of medical conditions and their treatment on the safe conduct of regional or general anaesthesia.

The presence of morbidly obese women admitted in labour or to the antenatal ward should be brought to the attention of the duty obstetric anaesthetist. Morbid obesity should ring as many alarm bells as does severe pre-eclampsia. Regional blockade will almost certainly be a challenge, and general anaesthesia hazardous. A summary care plan with '6 Rs' mnemonic has been introduced at the Royal Berkshire NHS Foundation Trust:

1 Early review by anaesthetist on arrival on labour ward or once established labour has started;
2 Ranitidine throughout labour;
3 Early venous cannulation;
4 Regional block – consider early;
5 Heparin thromboprophylaxis – strongly consider for all but straightforward vaginal births;
6 Senior help will be needed for GA.

Criteria for referral are listed in Box 52.1.

EBM

- The need for analgesia in labour is reduced by the continuous support of a known practitioner.
- Regional blockade is superior to other modalities of analgesia.
- Regional analgesia entails an extremely low risk of neurological complication, and does not increase the incidence of postnatal backache.
- Regional analgesia has been associated with an increased requirement for instrumental vaginal delivery, but not caesarean section.
- Continuous low-dose epidural infusions and CSEs are associated with a lower risk of instrumental vaginal delivery than conventional bolus epidural analgesia.

Box 52.1 Criteria for antenatal anaesthetic referral

Cardiovascular problems

Congenital heart disease

Valvular heart disease

Arrhythmias

Cardiomyopathy

Poorly controlled hypertension

Respiratory problems

Severe asthma (requiring steroids or hospital admission)

Breathlessness which limits daily activity

Cystic fibrosis, or any other chronic pulmonary disease

Neurological/musculoskeletal problems

Any spinal surgery e.g. laminectomy, scoliosis correction

Congenital conditions e.g. spina bifida

Muscular dystrophy, myotonia

Myasthenia gravis

Demyelinating disease (multiple sclerosis)

Spinal cord injury

Rheumatoid arthritis or any condition affecting neck/jaw

Cerebrovascular disease e.g. aneurysm, arteriovenous malformation

Haematological problems

Anticoagulation

Coagulation/platelet disorders, hepatic disease

Patients who have been treated for malignancy e.g. lymphoma, leukaemia (cardiorespiratory legacy of radiotherapy/chemotherapy)

Airway problems

Previous difficult tracheal intubation

Inability to open mouth or move jaw or head normally

Drug-related problems

Cholinesterase abnormalities - succinylcholine (Scoline) apnoea

Allergy or adverse reaction to anaesthetic drugs

Malignant hyperthermia

Drug misusers - with no peripheral venous access

Other

Morbid obesity - BMI >40 kg/m^2

Needle phobia

Panic attacks

Any obscure eponymous syndrome that no one seems to have heard of ... which may pose problems if emergency anaesthesia is needed

Any women with concerns regarding analgesia or anaesthesia e.g. previous problems with inadequate epidural for labour, or pain/awareness during caesarean section

Jehovah's Witnesses

KEY POINTS

- Opioids confer more sedation than analgesia; no one agent is superior.
- Compared to intermittent bolus epidurals, low-dose epidural infusions and combined spinal–epidural analgesia result in a lower incidence of instrumental vaginal deliveries.
- Intravenous Intralipid™ can reverse local anaesthetic-induced cardiac arrest.
- Almost 90 per cent of caesarean sections in the UK are performed under regional anaesthesia.
- Single-shot spinals are the most common regional technique for caesarean section. The addition of opioid to the local anaesthetic can reduce the incidence of intra-operative pain and provide post-operative analgesia.
- Epidural anaesthesia is generally of poorer quality than spinal anaesthesia. A combined spinal–epidural technique is useful when it is anticipated that surgery might be protracted.
- General anaesthesia is indicated for the majority of caesarean sections where there is immediate threat to the life of the mother or fetus and a regional technique is absolutely contraindicated or has failed.
- The principal risks of general anaesthesia are airway problems, aspiration of gastric contents and anaphylaxis.
- Ranitidine should be prescribed for women in labour with risk factors for caesarean section.
- General anaesthesia for caesarean section in placenta praevia is usually unnecessary. Regional anaesthesia is inappropriate for women with signs of significant haemorrhage.
- All units should have a referral system between obstetricians and anaesthetists.
- Sepsis is now the leading direct cause of maternal death, and prompt use of a sepsis bundle should be undertaken if sepsis suspected.

Key References

1. Hodnett ED, Gates S, Hofmeyr GJ, Sakala C. Continuous support for women during childbirth. *Cochrane Database Syst Rev* 2007;3:CD003766.
2. Cluett ER, Burns E. Immersion in water in labour and birth. *Cochrane Database Syst Rev* 2009;2:CD000111.
3. Simkin PP, O'Hara MA. Nonpharmacologic relief of pain during labor: systematic review of five methods. *Am J Obstet Gynecol* 2002;186:S131–59.
4. Dowswell T, Bedwell C, Lavender T, Neilson JP. Transcutaneous electrical nerve stimulation (TENS) for pain relief in labour. *Cochrane Database Syst Rev* 2009;2:CD007214.
5. Wee M. Analgesia in labour: inhalational and parenteral. *Anaesth Int Care Med* 2007;8:276–8.
6. Tuckey JP, Prout RE, Wee MYK. Prescribing intramuscular opioids for labour analgesia in consultant-led maternity units: a survey of UK practice. *Int J Obs Anesth* 2008; 17: 3–8.
7. Anim-Somuah M, Smyth RMD, Howell CJ. Epidural versus non-epidural or no analgesia in labour. *Cochrane Database Syst Rev* 2005;4:CD000331.
8. Lewis, G (ed.) *The Confidential Enquiry into Maternal and Child Health (CEMACH). Saving Mothers' Lives: reviewing maternal deaths to make motherhood safer – 2003–2005.* The Seventh Report on Confidential Enquiries into Maternal Deaths in the United Kingdom. London: CEMACH, 2007: www.cemach.org.uk.
9. Comparative Obstetric Mobile Epidural Trial (COMET) Study Group UK. Effect of low-dose versus traditional epidural techniques on mode of delivery: a randomised controlled trial. *Lancet* 2001;358:19–23.
10. Wilson MJA, MacArthur C, Cooper GM *et al.* Ambulation in labour and delivery mode: a randomised controlled trial of high-dose vs mobile epidural analgesia. *Anaesthesia* 2009;64:266–72.
11. Simmons SW, Cyna AM, Dennis AT, Hughes D. Combined spinal-epidural versus epidural analgesia in labour. *Cochrane Database Syst Rev* 2007;3: CD003401.
12. Halpern S, Carvalho B. Patient-controlled epidural analgesia for labor. *Anesth Analg* 2009;108:921–8.
13. Wong CA, Scavone BM, Peaceman AM *et al.* The risk of caesarean delivery with neuraxial analgesia given early versus late in labor. *N Engl J Med* 2005;352:655–65.
14. Kinsella SM, Scrutton MJL. Assessment of a modified four-category classification of urgency of caesarean section. *J Obstet Gyanaecol* 2009;29:110–13.
15. Focus Group. Obstetric anaesthesia delays and complications. *In: Confidential Enquiry into Stillbirths and Deaths in Infancy, 7th Annual Report.* London: Maternal and Child Health Research Consortium, 2000:41–52.
16. Ngan Kee WD, Lee A, Khaw KS *et al.* A randomised double-blinded comparison of phenylephrine and ephedrine infusion combinations to maintain blood pressure during spinal anesthesia for caesarean delivery: the effects on fetal acid-base status and hemodynamic control. *Anesth Analg* 2008;107:1295–302.
17. McDonnell JG, Curley G, Carney J *et al.* The analgesic efficacy of transversus abdominis plane block after caesarean delivery: a randomised controlled trial. *Anesth Analg* 2008;106:186–91.
18. Moodley J, Jjuuko G, Rout C. Epidural compared with general anaesthesia for caesarean delivery in conscious women with eclampsia. *Br J Obstet Gynaecol* 2001;108:378–82.
19. Arkoosh VA, Palmer CM, Yun EM *et al.* A randomized, double-masked, multicenter comparison of the safety of continous intrathecal labor analgesia using a 28-gauge

catheter versus continuous epidural labor analgesia. *Anesthesiology* 2008;108:286–98.

20. Paech MJ, Scott KL, Clavisi OM *et al.*, the ANZCA Trials Group. A prospective study of awareness and recall associated with general anaesthesia for caesarean section. *Int J Obst Anesth* 2008;17:298–303.

21. M PURVA. NOAD subcommittee National Obstetric Anaesthesia Data for 2011: A report: www.oaa-anaes. ac.uk

22. Codeine: restricted use as analgesic in children and adolescents after European safety review www.mhra.gov. uk/safetyinformation/DrugSafetyUpdate/CON287006

Chapter 53 Caesarean section

Tracey A Johnston

INTRODUCTION

Caesarean section is a routine part of modern obstetric practice, with the aim of reducing maternal and perinatal morbidity and mortality. There is significant geographical variation in CS rates throughout the world, ranging from 0.4 per cent in Chad to 45.9 per cent in Brazil,[1] with significantly higher rates seen in developed countries. The reasons for higher CS rates in developed countries are not all clear, but include socio-demographic factors, clinical practices and, importantly, the attitudes of healthcare professionals and women towards the procedure. The 'right' CS rate is unknown, but in 1985 WHO recommended a CS rate of no higher than 15 per cent.[1] This figure is based on the increased mortality rates in countries with CS rates <10 per cent (i.e. deaths could be avoided if more CS were performed) and the fact that mortality rates are not reduced further where CS rates are >15 per cent, suggesting that many 'unnecessary' CS are performed. More recent evidence supports this figure and suggests that CS rates >15 per cent may actually result in poorer outcomes.[2,3] The CS rate in the UK is currently around 25 per cent, and there are many drivers to try to reduce this. Figures from 2012–13[4] show that the overall CS rate in England was 25.5 per cent, split into 10.7 per cent for elective CS and 14.8 per cent for emergency CS. Elective CS rates showed little variation across England, but there are significant differences in emergency CS rates between organisations.[5]

INDICATIONS FOR CS

Women undergoing CS fall into three main groups:

- women who have a clinical indication for CS;
- women with a previous CS (see Chapter 49), who may opt for either vaginal birth after CS (VBAC) or elective repeat CS (ERCS);
- women who are considering CS with no clinical indication (maternal request CS – MRCS).

There are many clinical indications for CS, both planned and unplanned, but the majority (>70 per cent) are performed for failure to progress in labour, presumed fetal compromise, breech presentation and ERCS.

PLANNED CS

Timing

CS before the onset of labour is associated with increased respiratory morbidity in the neonate, the risk of which decreases after 39 weeks' gestation.[6] For this reason, planned CS should be performed after 39 weeks unless there are maternal or fetal reasons for earlier delivery [B].

Indications

Planned CS should be offered in the following circumstances:

- Breech presentation (see Chapters 41, 57). Following publication of the Term Breech Trial, women should be counselled that vaginal breech birth is associated with an increase in perinatal morbidity and mortality compared to elective CS.[7] Women should therefore be offered elective CS if external cephalic version (ECV) is contraindicated or has failed [A].
- Twin pregnancy where the leading twin is not cephalic, and higher-order multiples (see Chapter 35). Although robust evidence of benefit does not exist, this is currently standard practice in the UK.
- Placenta praevia. Placenta praevia exists where the placenta is implanted either wholly or in part into the lower segment of the uterus. In modern obstetric practice with the routine use of ultrasound, this should always have been identified before delivery. It accounts for approximately 3 per cent of CS, and is associated with an increased risk of major haemorrhage, hysterectomy and maternal mortality. CS for placenta praevia should therefore be carried out by an experienced operator with a consultant immediately available, in a unit with on-site blood transfusion services,[8] following appropriate counselling and consent. In uncomplicated placenta praevia, delivery should be planned between 38 and 39 weeks' gestation [D].

In cases of placenta praevia with a previous CS, the risk of morbidly adherent placenta (MAP – placenta accreta, percreta or increta) is related to the number of previous CS[9] – see Table 53.1. Where placenta praevia is confirmed at 32–34 weeks' gestation in cases of previous CS, colour flow Doppler should be performed to identify MAP. Magnetic resonance (MR) scanning may improve diagnostic accuracy, but the best results are obtained with gadolinium enhancement, which is not used in the UK, and although thought to be without risk, long-term safety for the fetus has not yet been established. When MR scanning is considered, careful discussion regarding the potential risks and benefits should take place and MR scanning used only if acceptable to the woman.[10] Due to the diagnostic accuracy of both imaging modalities, it is best to be prepared for MAP in all cases of placenta praevia with previous CS. When planning and performing CS for potential MAP, the NPSA Intrapartum Toolkit's Placenta Praevia after Caesarean Section Care Bundle[11] should be used to minimise the risk of morbidity. This consists of six elements:

- Consultant obstetrician planned and directly supervising delivery;
- Consultant obstetric anaesthetist planned and directly supervising anaesthesia at delivery;
- Blood and blood products available on site;
- Multidisciplinary involvement in pre-operative planning;
- Discussion and consent includes possible interventions (such as hysterectomy, leaving placenta in situ, cell salvage and interventional radiology);
- Local availability of level 2 critical care bed.

In suspected MAP, in the absence of complications delivery should be planned no earlier than 36–37 weeks' gestation [D]. For both placenta praevia and suspected MAP, the use of cell salvage at the time of surgery is recommended and presently its use is being critically appraised as part of an HTA study (SALVO)[D].

- Maternal HIV infection either not on ART, where the viral load >/= 400 copies/mL despite ART, or if HIV and hepatitis C infection are both present.[10]
- History of primary genital HSV infection occurring in the third trimester.[10]

ERCS

In a small number of cases, ERCS is recommended after the first CS e.g. if there is an upper-segment scar on the uterus (previous classical CS, previous J or T incision), but in most cases the main factor is maternal choice. When counselling a

Table 53.1 Risk of placenta praevia and morbidly adherent placenta with number of previous CS[9]

No. of previous CS	Risk of placenta praevia (%)	Risk of MAP (%)
1	0.6–1.3	11–14
2	1.1–2.3	23–40
3 or more	1.8–3.7	35–67

woman regarding the risks and benefits of ERCS vs VBAC (see Chapter 49), the following should be discussed:[12]

- The VBAC success rate is around 75 per cent [B]. Higher success rates of around 90 per cent are seen in those who have previously had a vaginal birth also.
- The risk of scar rupture during VBAC is low (approximately 1:200) [B].
- With VBAC, the risk of brain damage or death to the baby is low (approximately 1:200), but is higher than the risk if delivery is by ERCS (approximately 1:1000) [B].
- VBAC reduces the risk of respiratory problems in the baby [B].
- The risk of fetal laceration at CS is 1–2 per cent.
- VBAC carries a 1 per cent additional risk of infection and the need for blood transfusion compared to ERCS [B].
- ERCS increases the risk of damage to bowel and bladder, hysterectomy, future placenta praevia/MAP (Table 53.1) [B].

The woman's views should be taken into consideration and if after discussion she wishes ERCS, this should be performed.

MRCS

The number of requests for CS in the absence of a previous CS or an obstetric indication is increasing, with tocophobia (excessive fear of childbirth) and safety for the baby cited as the commonest reasons. In these cases, it is important to explore carefully and document the reasons for such a request, and fully counsel the woman to ensure she is fully informed of the risks and benefits for both the mother (Table 53.2) and the baby (Table 53.3). In cases of tocophobia, referral to an appropriate perinatal mental health professional who has access to the planned place of birth in the antenatal period is indicated. If after all this vaginal birth is still not an acceptable option, then CS should be offered or the woman referred to another obstetrician willing to carry out the procedure.[10]

Table 53.2 Effects on women's health of planned CS compared with planned vaginal birth for women with an uncomplicated pregnancy and no previous CS[10]

Effects around the time of birth	Planned CS	Planned vaginal birth	Relative effect (95% CI)
Reduced after planned CS			
Perineal and abdominal pain during birth	Median score 1.0	Median score 7.3	Not calculable
Perineal and abdominal pain 3 days postpartum	Median score 4.5	Median score 5.2	Not calculable
Vaginal injury	0%	0.56%	Not calculable
Early postpartum haemorrhage	1.1%	6.0%	OR 0.23 (0.06–0.94)
	3.9%	6.2%	RR 0.6 (0.4–0.9)
Obstetric shock	0.006%	0.018%	RR 0.33 (0.11–0.99)
Reduced after planned vaginal birth			
Length of stay	3.2 days	2.6 days	Not calculable
	3.96 days	2.56 days	Not calculable
Hysterectomy for PPH	0.03%	0.01%	RR 2.31 (1.30–4.09)
Cardiac arrest	0.19%	0.03%	RR 4.91 (3.95–6.11)
No difference between CS and vaginal birth			
Perineal and abdominal pain 4 months postpartum	Median score 0.0	Median score 0.17	Not calculable
Injury to bladder/ureter	0%	0.14%	Not calculable
Injury to cervix	0%	0.28%	Not calculable
Iatrogenic surgical injury	0%	0.07%	Not calculable
Pulmonary embolism	0%	0.003%	Not calculable
Wound infection	0.01%	0%	Not calculable
	1.5%	0.9%	RR 1.7 (0.9–3.2)

Effects around the time of birth	Planned CS	Planned vaginal birth	Relative effect (95% CI)
Intra-operative trauma	0.1%	0.3%	RR 0.5 (0.1–3.5)
Uterine rupture	0.02%	0.03%	RR 0.51 (0.25–1.07)
Assisted ventilation/intubation	0.01%	0.005%	RR 2.21 (0.99–4.90)
Acute renal failure	0.004%	0.001%	RR 2.17 (0.58–8.14)
Conflicting findings from studies			
Maternal death	9/737 (cases/controls)	49/9133 (cases/controls)	OR 2.28 (1.11–4.65)
	0%	0%	
	0%	0.002%	
DVT	0%	0.03%	
	0.06%	0.03%	RR 2.2 (1.51–3.20)
Blood transfusion	1.7%	1.9%	OR 0.87 (0.27–2.78)
	0.3%	0.3%	RR 0.89 (0.20–3.99)
	0.3%	0.4%	RR 0.7 (0.2–2.7)
	0.02%	0.07%	RR 0.20 (0.20–0.64)
Infection: wound and postpartum	1.1%	0.8%	RR 1.36 (0.75–2.4)
	0.6%	0.21%	RR 2.85 (2.52–3.21)
Hysterectomy	0.6%	0.1%	P = 0.13
	0.1%	0.01%	RR 9.09 (1.36–60.33)
	0.06%	0.02%	RR 3.60 (2.44–5.31)
Anaesthetic complications	0.4%	0.3%	RR 1.24 (0.34–4.59)
	0.53%	0.21%	RR 2.5 (2.22–2.86)

Table 53.3 Effects on babies' health of planned CS compared with planned vaginal birth for women with an uncomplicated pregnancy and no previous CS[10]

Effects around the time of birth	Planned CS	Planned vaginal birth	Relative effect (95% CI)
Reduced after planned vaginal birth			
NICU admission	13.9%	6.3%	RR 2.20 (1.4–3.18)
No difference between CS and vaginal birth			
Hypoxic ischaemic encephalopathy	0.2%	0.2%	RR 0.81 (0.22–3.00)
Intracranial haemorrhage	0%	0.01%	
Neonatal respiratory morbidity	12%	11.5%	RR 1.04 (0.88–1.23)
Conflicting findings from studies			
Neonatal mortality	0%	0.1%	
	0.17%	0.07%	RR 2.4 (2.20–2.65)
5-minute Apgar	0%	0.5%	
<7	0.6%	1.2%	RR 0.44 (0.07–2.51)

UNPLANNED CS

The commonest reasons for unplanned CS are failure to progress in labour and suspected fetal compromise. For the management of delay in the first stage of labour, see Chapter 50, and for the management of suspected fetal compromise see Chapters 51 and 54. It should be noted that the maternal risks of haemorrhage, infection, bowel injury, bladder damage, hysterectomy and death, although still very low, are higher in unplanned when compared to planned CS, but that the risks of respiratory compromise in the neonate are lower in unplanned compared to planned CS. Second-stage CS merits particular mention, as the rates of both maternal (infection, haemorrhage secondary to both uterine atony and trauma, surgical damage) and perinatal (secondary to difficulties with delivery) morbidity are higher compared to first-stage CS, and it should therefore be undertaken by an experienced operator.

CATEGORISATION OF CS

Historically, CS were classified as either elective or emergency, but this is not specific enough to allow adequate communication regarding the urgency of CS. In 2000, a new system of categorisation was introduced which has been adopted throughout the UK with the purpose of improving communication within the team and auditing process[13] – see Table 53.4.

PRIOR TO CS

- Information: because approximately 1 in 4 women will have a CS, all women should be provided with evidence-based information about CS in the antenatal period. This should include common indications for CS (FTP in labour, suspected fetal compromise and breech presentation account for >70 per cent).
- Consent: informed consent should be obtained, including risks and benefits of the procedure for that specific situation. The operator should be aware of any specific risk factors and include these in the counselling and consent process.
- Blood tests and investigations: a recent Hb should be available to identify those women with significant anaemia, and if there are concerns regarding the need for blood transfusion, blood should be sent for grouping and saving of serum.
- Anaesthesia: mode of anaesthesia to be employed is an anaesthetic decision, and good communication between teams is essential (see Chapter 52).
- Thromboprophylaxis: all women should have a VTE risk assessment performed and thromboprophylaxis given to reduce the increased risk of thromboembolism that is associated with CS. Hydration and early mobilisation are important in all cases, with the addition of graduated anti-embolic stockings and/or LMWH depending on the risk assessment [D].
- The bladder must be emptied prior to the start of surgery. If regional anaesthesia is employed, an indwelling catheter should be used to avoid post-operative urinary retention and re-catheterisation [A].
- Prophylactic antibiotics should be given prior to the skin incision to reduce the risk of post-operative infection, in particular endometritis, wound infection and urinary tract infection [A]. Because of the association between co-amoxiclav and necrotising enterocolitis demonstrated in preterm babies, it is advised to avoid this specific antibiotic as there are acceptable alternatives available. In cases of major haemorrhage or where the procedure lasts longer than 4 hours, a second dose of prophylactic antibiotics should be considered.
- As with any surgical procedure, the WHO surgical safety checklist should be used.

PROCEDURE

In some cases where difficulties are anticipated (e.g. placenta praevia, large fibroids, abnormal lie), ultrasound immediately before surgery can help the operator decide on the best skin incision and site of uterine incision.

Table 53.4 Categorisation of CS[13]

Category	Definition	Examples	Decision to delivery interval
1	Immediate threat to life of mother or fetus	Cord prolapse, prolonged bradycardia, pH <7.20, uterine rupture,	As soon as possible; within 30 minutes
2	Maternal or fetal compromise which is not immediately life threatening	Failure to progress in labour	As soon as possible; within 75 minutes
3	No maternal or fetal compromise but needs early delivery	Failed induction, booked category 4 CS with ruptured membranes not in labour	
4	At a time to suit the woman and her maternity service	'Elective' CS	

Skin incision

There are three different skin incisions that are used in CS:

1 Pfannenstiel – a low transverse, curved, suprapubic inci-sion that uses sharp dissection to open the rectus sheath; the rectus muscles are then separated from the sheath and the peritoneum is then picked up and opened with sharp dissection.

2 Joel Cohen – a slightly higher straight transverse incision that employs blunt dissection to open the rectus sheath and peritoneum after a small transverse incision has been made in the rectus sheath in the midline. This approach is associated with shorter operating times, lower blood loss, less fever and less pain when compared to the Pfannenstiel incision [A].

3 Vertical – usually a midline sub-umbilical incison. Allows access to the abdomen as well as the pelvis and therefore is often employed if access to the upper segment of the uterus is required (some cases of placenta praevia or sus-pected MAP, or large fibroids) or other surgical proce-dures are anticipated. It is associated with increased pain and a higher incidence of wound dehiscence, and more concerns regarding the cosmetic appearance when com-pared to transverse incisions [B].

Uterus

Before incising the uterus, dextrorotation should be corrected, the visceral peritoneum above the bladder should be picked up to identify the upper margin of the lower segment, and the peritoneum should be incised transversely and the blad-der gently pushed down to avoid injury. Following this, inci-sion of the lower segment is the standard approach as the lower segment is thinner and less vascular than the upper seg-ment making the procedure easier. It is also associated with fewer post-operative complications, such as ileus, peritonitis, obstruction and adhesions, as well as a significantly lower risk of scar dehiscence or rupture in a future pregnancy. The uterus is then opened using sharp dissection transversely in the mid-line, and extended using blunt dissection, which is associated with less blood loss, lower incidence of PPH and less need for transfusion when compared with sharp dissection [A]. In cases of second-stage CS, the upper margin of the lower seg-ment (identified by the peritoneal reflection) is higher than usual, and it is therefore important to identify the upper mar-gin carefully then incise the uterus higher than usual to ensure the correct part of the lower segment is opened. Opening the uterus too low will increase the risks of extension and difficulty in delivery.

The second commonest approach is the classical incision. This is a vertical incision in the midline of the upper segment, and indications include:

• preterm delivery where the lower segment is poorly formed;
• ruptured membranes with a transverse lie and the back presenting;

• placenta praevia, to minimise blood loss and/or consider conservative management in cases of MAP, by avoiding incising the placenta;
• lower-segment or cervical fibroids;
• fetal abnormality (e.g. conjoint twins, massive hydroceph-aly, large sacrococcygeal teratomas).

Delivery

In a cephalic presentation, once the uterus is opened the oper-ator's hand is inserted below the head, ensuring flexion and rotation into the occipito-transverse position. Once the head is lifted out of the pelvis into the incision, the assistant applies fundal pressure in a stepwise manner to effect delivery of the head. If the head is high, traditionally short curved forceps have been used to aid delivery, but disposable hand-held vacuum devices are also effective with perhaps a lower risk of trauma.

One of the most frightening situations for a trainee is that of the stuck head at CS. This is commoner in second-stage CS, particularly after failed instrumental delivery. It is essential not to panic and not to fight the uterine activity. Tocolysis using terbutaline, atosiban or GTN can be used to aid uterine relax-ation. When the operator's hand is inserted into the uterus, very often a contraction is provoked and this may prevent the hand getting below the fetal head. It is essential to stop moving and wait for the uterus to relax before trying to advance the hand further. Constant movement of the hand will prolong or provoke a contraction. Once the uterus relaxes the hand can be advanced below the head. If another contraction happens, again stop moving and wait for it to pass. While the uterus is relaxed, the head can be flexed and lifted into the incision, and delivery completed. Occasionally, using the opposite hand is helpful. Failing this, consider delivering by the breech (a high, generous uterine incision as described above for second-stage CS facilitates this). To achieve this, the operator's hand should be run up the fetal back to the breech, flexing it down into the incision. Alternatively, gentle steady traction on one or both legs will bring the breech down into the incision. If the inci-sion is not large enough, this should be extended. A J-shaped extension on one or both sides will generally give more room than a central inverted T-incision. In the vast majority of cases, delivery will be safely achieved with these methods. In general, however, a common response is to push the fetal head up from below, often by a member of staff with little experience in this manoeuvre. This action again provokes a contraction, thus the upward pressure being applied to the fetal head is work-ing against the downward pressure of the contraction. This approach is associated with fracture of the fetal skull and thus should only be used as a last resort. Different devices that are inserted into the vagina to elevate the fetal head are available, but are still undergoing evaluation to prove their effectiveness.

Once delivery of the head is achieved, the shoulders should be released by lateral flexion, with delivery being completed by gentle traction. In cases of breech presentation, either the breech can be flexed and lifted into the incision in a similar manner to the head, or one or both feet/legs can be delivered first with delivery of the breech being achieved by gentle traction. Once the breech is delivered, gentle traction will achieve delivery of the trunk, with the arms being delivered by hooking out or rotation in a similar manner to vaginal breech delivery (breech CS is an ideal opportunity to practise the mechanisms and manoeuvres of vaginal breech delivery). The head can be delivered either by flexion or by the Burns Marshall technique of extension. With a transverse lie, it is better to try to achieve a longitudinal lie before opening the uterus. If this is not possible, once the uterus is open insert a hand and bring either pole into the incision, or find a leg and apply gentle traction to bring the breech round.

Once the baby is delivered, consider delayed cord clamping and cord gases (paired cord gases/umbilical artery pH should be performed after all CS for suspected fetal compromise, to allow review of fetal wellbeing and guide ongoing care of the baby [B]).

Placenta

Following delivery of the baby, 5 IU of oxytocin should be given by slow intravenous injection to facilitate contraction of the uterus and placental separation, and this is associated with reduced blood loss [C]. The placenta should then be delivered by controlled cord traction and the uterine cavity checked to ensure it is empty.

Placenta praevia

In cases of placenta praevia, there may be large sinuses in the lower segment, which continue to bleed and may require suturing. Full-thickness figure-of-eight sutures are effective with less risk of tearing out. Inserting a balloon into the uterus is also effective in controlling bleeding from the lower segment by tamponade.

MAP

If after administration of the oxytocin the placenta fails to separate, different options exist which should have been considered and discussed with the woman before surgery. These include:

- manual/piecemeal removal of the placenta – this is associated with an increased risk of blood loss, and may not be successful in removing all the placental tissue;
- hysterectomy with the placenta *in situ* – this is associated with less blood loss and may be the option of choice if fertility preservation is not an issue;
- conservative management leaving the placenta *in situ* – this can be considered if the woman is keen to preserve her fertility, there has been no antenatal bleeding and the placenta has not been breached at the time of CS. In such cases, the cord should be drained and ligated close to the placental insertion. The membranes should be trimmed close to the placental margins, and the uterus closed in the usual manner. Postnatal follow-up is essential to observe for haemorrhage, infection and to confirm placental resorption [D].[7]

Closure

The uterus should be repaired *in situ*, as exteriorisation is associated with increased pain and no decrease in haemorrhage or infection [A]. Occasionally, however, exteriorisation will allow better visualisation if there are extensions, making repair easier. In such cases, both the anaesthetist and the woman should be warned before the uterus is exteriorised. Both angles of the uterine incision should be identified, then the incision closed in two layers using a continuous absorbable suture. Occasionally, extra haemostatic sutures are required if bleeding persists after application of pressure. Single- versus double-layer closures have been compared in the CAESAR trial[14] and no differences were found in any of the short-term outcomes studied, but there are concerns regarding an increased risk of scar rupture in future pregnancies[15] and it is therefore recommended that until further information is available from the CAESAR follow-up study, two-layer closure should be used [B]. Classical incisions usually require a three-layer closure because of the increased thickness and vascularity. Following closure of the uterus, the adnexae should be inspected, and any adnexal surgery e.g. sterilisation conducted at this point.

With regards to the peritoneum, neither the visceral nor the parietal peritoneum should be sutured at CS, as this reduces operating time and the need for post-operative analgesia, and improves maternal satisfaction [A], but there are no follow-up studies addressing potential long-term complications such as adhesion formation and bowel obstruction. Closure of the anterior abdominal wall depends on the type of incision. In cases of a midline skin incision, mass closure of the rectus sheath and subcutaneous tissues should be employed using a slowly absorbable continuous suture as this is associated with reduced wound pain, sinus formation, incisional hernias and wound dehiscence [B]. In transverse skin incisions, the rectus sheath is closed using a non-locking, continuous, absorbable suture. If there is more than 2 cm of subcutaneous fat this layer should be closed with an absorbable suture, as this decreases the incidence of wound infection [A]. There are different methods of skin closure, including subcuticular sutures (either absorbable which do not require removal, or of material such as prolene which does require removal), interrupted sutures (which require removal) or staples. In women with an increased risk of haematoma or infection, an interrupted method has the advantage of removal of one or two to allow drainage if required. Staples, although quicker to insert, are associated with more pain [A]. Subcuticular absorbable sutures have the benefit of less pain, a good cosmetic effect and no need for removal.

Drains

There is no evidence to support the routine use of drains at CS. Intraperitoneal drains should only be used if there are concerns regarding the risk of ongoing bleeding, and should be of the wide-bore, non-suction variety. The CAESAR study[14] showed no benefit to the routine use of subrectus drains, and these should only be used if clinically indicated, in which case the abdominal peritoneum must be closed. Superficial wound drains do not reduce the incidence of infection or haematoma, and should therefore not be used [A].

Dressings

Following CS, an interactive dressing should be applied and remain in place for 48 hours.[16] As the abdominal cavity is a large potential space it is not possible to apply effective pressure, rendering pressure dressings ineffective at stopping or preventing bleeding, but effective at hiding it. Any wound bleeding should be dealt with by applying effective pressure by pinching the area between the fingers, diathermy, or inserting another suture. The interactive dressing allows the wound to be observed for further bleeding. In other surgical specialities, vacuum dressings are being used in some cases at high risk of infection e.g. morbid obesity, and their use is beginning to be introduced into obstetrics.

POST-OPERATIVE MANAGEMENT

Following CS, women should be cared for on a one-to-one basis by an appropriately trained individual in an appropriate environment until they have regained airway control, are cardiovascularly stable and are able to communicate. Skin-to-skin contact and early breastfeeding should be facilitated as soon as possible. Maternal observations including heart rate, blood pressure, respiratory rate and pulse oximetry should be performed every 5 minutes for the first 30 minutes, then every 30 minutes for the first 2 hours. Thereafter, if stable, the frequency of observations can be reduced dependent on the maternal condition. Women should be encouraged to eat and drink as soon as they feel hungry/thirsty. The catheter is usually removed after 12–24 hours in cases of regional anaesthesia, and early mobilisation is encouraged. In all cases, a discussion regarding the reason for CS and the implications for future pregnancies should take place prior to discharge, including any recommendations regarding mode of birth in the future.

COMPLICATIONS

As with any surgical procedure, there are associated complications of CS. Intra-operative complications include:

- difficulty in gaining access to the uterus, usually secondary to previous surgery;
- difficulty in delivering the baby;
- difficulty in delivering the placenta;
- uterine extensions including into the vagina and broad ligament;
- haemorrhage;
- damage to bowel/bladder/ureter;
- fetal laceration (1–2 per cent).

Anticipation can lead to avoidance, and also allows appropriate help to be summoned in advance. Where such complications arise unexpectedly, appropriate help should be called for e.g. senior obstetric help, urologist, general surgeon. In cases of obstetric haemorrhage at CS, the majority are still secondary to atony, and this should be managed as usual with the use of uterotonic drugs in a stepwise manner, followed by mechanical methods (see Chapter 64). For bleeding secondary to trauma, lacerations should be repaired promptly.

Peripartum hysterectomy

If hysterectomy is being considered, senior help is essential to assist in making the decision as well as performing the surgery. It is wise to remember not to leave the decision too late, as this is associated with increased morbidity. In the UKOSS study of peripartum hysterectomy[17] the vast majority were performed for haemorrhage, with most being for atony and/or MAP, although in many there was more than one cause. Subtotal hysterectomy is a reasonable option in cases of uterine atony, and may be associated with less morbidity, but in cases of MAP, total hysterectomy is more common to ensure the lower pole of the uterus, which is mainly where the haemorrhage is arising from, is removed. When comparing total with subtotal hysterectomy, there were no statistical differences in the rate of bladder or ureteric damage, ovary removal, further surgery and blood transfusion, although it is acknowledged that the numbers were small.[17] In women undergoing peripartum hysterectomy it must be remembered that around 20 per cent will need to go back to theatre, often to control further bleeding, 20 per cent will sustain damage to other organs, and around 20 per cent will suffer from other severe morbidity [B].

Post-operative complications

The major post-operative complications include infection (see Chapter 65) and thromboembolic disease (Chapter 12). CS is associated with a significantly increased risk of both postnatal infection [D] and thromboembolic disease (TED), and the role of prophylactic antibiotics and thromboprophylaxis has been discussed above. There has been a significant reduction in the incidence of TED following the introduction and implementation of the RCOG Green-top Guidelines for both antenatal and postnatal thromboprophylaxis.

FUTURE PREGNANCIES

Prior to discharge, all women should be debriefed regarding the indication for their CS and any complications at the time of surgery. They should be informed whether VBAC is appropriate in the future or whether subsequent deliveries should be by ERCS. In cases of previous CS for a non-recurrent cause, maternal choice should be taken into account in planning future mode of birth.

CONCLUSION

Caesarean section is an integral part of obstetric practice, with around a quarter of babies in the UK being born by this method. There are many drivers to reduce the number of 'unnecessary' caesarean sections. In some cases of planned CS, maternal choice should be considered in the decision-making process, including cases with no previous CS and no medical indication. The implications of CS for future pregnancies, including increased risk of stillbirth, placenta praevia and MAP, must be considered when making the decision to perform a CS. National evidence-based guidance exists for CS.

KEY POINTS

- There are significant geographical variations in CS rates, and the 'correct' CS rate is unknown.
- Maternal choice should be taken into consideration in some cases of elective CS.
- Thromboprophylaxis and prophylactic antibiotics significantly reduce the incidence of post-operative complications.
- Preparation and anticipation are essential to minimise the risks of intra-operative difficulty.
- Two of the most difficult situations are CS at full dilatation, especially following failed instrumental delivery, and placenta praevia in the presence of a previous CS, and in both situations the operator must have strategies in place to minimise the risk of complications.

References

1. WHO. Appropriate technology for birth. *Lancet* 1985;2(8452):436–7.
2. Althabe F, Sosa C, Belizán JM, Gibbons L, Jacquerioz F, Bergel E. Cesarean section rates and maternal and neonatal mortality in low-, medium- and high-income countries: an ecological study. *Birth* 2006;33(4):270–7.
3. Villar J, Valladares E, Wojdyla D *et al*. Caesarean delivery rates and pregnancy outcomes: the 2005 WHO global survey on maternal and perinatal health in Latin America. *Lancet* 2006;367(9525):1819–29.
4. NHS Maternity Statistics – England, 2012-13; Health and Social Care Information Centre, Dec 2013.
5. Bragg F, Cromwell D, Edozian L *et al*. Variation in rates of caesarean section among English NHS trusts after accounting for maternal and clinical risk: cross sectional study. *BMJ* 2010;341:c5065.
6. Morrison JJ, Rennie JM, Milton PJ. Neonatal respiratory morbidity and mode of delivery at term: influence of timing of elective caesarean section. *Br J Obstet Gynaecol* 1995;102:101–6.
7. Hofmeyr GJ, Hannah ME. Planned caesarean section for term breech delivery. *Cochrane Database Syst Rev* 2000;2.
8. RCOG Green-top Guideline No. 27. *Placenta praevia, placenta praevia accreta and vasa praevia; diagnosis and management*. RCOG Press, January 2011.
9. Guise JM, Eden K, Emeis C *et al*. Vaginal birth after cesarean: new insights. *Evidence Report/Technology Assessment* 2010;191:1–397.
10. National Collaborating Centre for Women's and Children's Health. NICE Clinical Guideline *Caesarean Section*. RCOG Press, 2011.
11. RCOG, RCM, NPSA. Placenta praevia after caesarean section care bundle. [http://www.nrls.npsa.nhs.uk/intrapartumtoolkit].
12. RCOG Green-top Guideline No. 45. *Birth after Previous Caesarean Section*. RCOG Press, February 2007.
13. Lucas DN, Yentis SM, Kinsella SM *et al*. Urgency of caesarean section: a new classification. *J R Soc Med* 2000;93:346–50.
14. CAESAR study collaborative group. Caesarean section surgical techniques: a randomised factorial trial (CAESAR). *BJOG* 2010 Oct; 117(11):1366–76.
15. Chapman SJ, Owen J. One- versus two-layer closure of a low transverse cesarean: The next pregnancy. *Obstet Gynecol* 1997; 89:16–18.
16. National Collaborating Centre for Women's and Children's Health. NICE Clinical Guideline *Surgical Site Infection: prevention and treatment of surgical site infection*. RCOG Press, 2008.
17. M Knight, UKOSS. Peripartum hysterectomy in the UK: management and outcomes of the associated haemorrhage. *BJOG* 2007; 114: 1380–7.

SECTION SIX

Second Stage of Labour

Chapter 54 Fetal compromise in the second stage of labour

Myles Taylor

MRCOG standards

Candidates are expected to have:

- the ability to recognise, classify and respond appropriately to CTG patterns;
- the ability to perform fetal blood sampling and to be able to interpret the results.

In addition, we would suggest the following.

Theoretical skills

- Review theoretical knowledge for fetal compromise in the first stage of labour.
- Know the additional physiological stresses placed on the fetus during the second stage of labour.
- Appreciate the physiological (as opposed to pathological) changes seen in a second-stage CTG.

Practical skills

- Be able to recognise a potentially difficult assisted delivery, in order to:
  - decide when to use secondary tests of fetal wellbeing;
  - avoid a traumatic birth in the presence of pre-existing compromise.

INTRODUCTION

The management of suspected fetal compromise in the second stage of labour demands considerable skill, in terms of both decision making and practical ability. Uterine contractions have peaked in terms of strength and frequency, and the resulting intrauterine and uterine wall pressures are further increased by maternal pushing. These pressures will frequently be greater than maternal arterial blood pressure, temporarily abolishing placental perfusion. Compression of the fetal head and umbilical cord is at its greatest, as the amniotic fluid volume has reached a nadir and passage through the rigid bony pelvis has begun. After many hours of stressful labour, fetal reserves may also be reduced or depleted. All these factors combine to make fetal heart rate abnormalities particularly common, although many of these abnormalities will be entirely benign. Having reached full dilatation, there is also an expectation that vaginal birth will be achieved.

Despite the factors detailed above, clinicians must remain wary of undertaking difficult assisted vaginal deliveries in the presence of fetal compromise. For this reason, secondary tests of fetal wellbeing still have a place in the second stage of labour. Such tests can give reassurance that further time for head descent and/or rotation can be allowed, converting a difficult delivery into an easier one or even a spontaneous birth.

DEFINITIONS

See Chapter 51.

WHAT TYPE OF FETAL MONITORING IS BEST IN THE SECOND STAGE?

The debate over the advantages and disadvantages of intermittent auscultation versus continuous electronic monitoring in the first stage of labour also arises when considering fetal monitoring in the second stage. Unfortunately, there is little evidence to inform this discussion. However, an obvious practical disadvantage of intermittent monitoring in the second stage is that it is difficult for an obstetrician called to undertake an assisted delivery to confirm fetal wellbeing. Instead, any concern regarding a difficult delivery should be met with either a short period of EFM or fetal scalp blood sampling.

Intermittent auscultation

In the low-risk situation, intermittent auscultation, either by Pinard stethoscope or by handheld Doppler, remains popular. Conventional guidelines, such as those issued by

RCOG (2007), suggest auscultating the FHR for at least 1 minute at least every 5 minutes in the second stage and the maternal pulse should also be recorded.

WHAT IS A NORMAL SECOND-STAGE CTG?

In an early large study of 1755 second-stage heart rate traces, 75 per cent maintained a normal baseline rate, with about 5 per cent becoming tachycardic.[1] The remaining 20 per cent of traces developed a baseline bradycardia that was transient in one third, persistent in one third and progressive in the remaining third.

Overall, a normal baseline in combination with an absence of decelerations was seen in only one quarter of second-stage heart rate tracings. However, 60 per cent of these 'normal' traces either exhibited no accelerations or poor variability, resulting in 90 per cent of all second-stage CTGs showing some degree of abnormality.

Therefore, the definition of a normal second-stage CTG is difficult. Using standards applied for antenatal or even first-stage CTGs, a normal CTG would appear to be rare in the second stage of labour.

Early studies of second-stage CTG abnormalities related neonatal outcome to Apgar scores rather than cord pH. Provided the baseline heart rate remained normal, only 2 per cent of neonates ended up with a 5-minute Apgar score <7.[1] Later studies found a similar risk of metabolic acidosis in this situation.[2-5]

WHAT IS AN ABNORMAL SECOND-STAGE CTG?

Baseline. Apart from late decelerations, the only FHR pattern that is strongly suggestive of fetal hypoxaemia is a continuous or progressive bradycardia.

Approximately 10 per cent of persistent or progressive bradycardias in the second stage will lead to 5-minute Apgar scores <7.[1] Neither superimposed early nor variable decelerations influence these figures. In later studies, fetal bradycardia was linked with neonatal acidosis.[3-5] Both Piquard *et al.*[6] and *Cordoso et al.*[5] found the mean umbilical artery pH to be lower in the presence of a fetal bradycardia. The severity of the bradycardia also correlates with perinatal risk. Acidosis was found in 30–40 per cent of moderately to severely bradycardic fetuses;[3,4] in more than half of the cases there was a metabolic acidosis. One study found that an FHR of <70 bpm increased the risk of acidosis 26-fold and the risk of metabolic acidosis 5-fold.[2]

A baseline tachycardia is reportedly associated with low 5-minute Apgar scores in 6 per cent of cases[1] and with neonatal acidaemia in up to 20 per cent.[3,4] However, it is rarely linked with a base excess >12 mmol/l.[4]

Variability. The work of Gilstrap *et al.*[3] suggested that absent variability dramatically increased the risk of neonatal acidosis, even in the presence of an otherwise normal CTG. A cord pH <7.20 was seen in 24 per cent of cases with isolated absent variability, compared to 3 per cent of completely normal second-stage traces. Gull *et al.*[7] investigated the inter-relationship between baseline bradycardias and variability. In the presence of a baseline heart rate <100 bpm, the risk of neonatal metabolic acidaemia increased as the interval before loss of variability shortened and as the duration of loss of variability increased. This suggests that loss of variability corresponds to fetal decompensation.

Accelerations. These are not commonly present in the second stage.

Decelerations. Decelerations are remarkably common, and are seen in more than 70 per cent of second-stage heart rate traces.

- *Early decelerations* occur in 14 per cent of second-stage traces. They do not appear to increase the risk of a low 5-minute Apgar score,[1] and should be viewed as benign – regardless of baseline rate.
- *Variable decelerations* are much commoner, being seen in approximately half of second-stage CTGs. After taking into account the baseline heart rate, mild variable decelerations have little influence on the incidence of low Apgar scores.[1] However, deep variable decelerations, with a drop in FHR of <70 bpm, are associated with a 10-fold increase in the risk of metabolic acidosis.[2]
- *Late decelerations* are relatively uncommon in the second stage, being seen in only 5 per cent of traces. However, their presence dramatically increases the chances of a low 5-minute Apgar score, regardless of baseline rate.[1] If the baseline rate is normal, a 5-minute Apgar score <7 is seen in 10 per cent of cases. This increases to 20–25 per cent when superimposed on a persistent or progressive baseline bradycardia. The combination of a baseline tachycardia and late decelerations is associated with a 14 per cent risk of low Apgar scores. The presence of late decelerations increases the risk of metabolic acidosis 17-fold.[2]

ACTIVE VERSUS PASSIVE SECOND STAGE

Many clinicians now divide the second stage of labour into a passive and an active phase. During the former, continued descent of the fetal head occurs with neither maternal effort nor urge to push. The risks of acidosis in this passive phase are probably similar to those of the active first stage. Certainly, Nordstrom *et al.* showed fetal scalp lactate to increase in parallel with the length of *active* pushing in the second stage.[8]

SECONDARY TESTS OF FETAL WELLBEING

Fetal blood sampling

Fetal scalp pH studies remain the principal secondary test of fetal wellbeing in the second stage of labour. There is no evidence that their accuracy falls, and they are usually technically very easy.

Other secondary tests

There has been little investigation into the prognostic ability of other secondary tests of fetal wellbeing, such as vibro-acoustic stimulation, scalp stimulation, fetal ECG or pulse oximetry in the second stage of labour. Combining ST analysis (STAN™) with CTG monitoring has the advantage of reducing operative vaginal delivery rates by 10 per cent.[9] However, guidelines on the use of STAN have emphasised that ST monitoring should not be commenced in the second stage as this risks missing ST changes which have already occurred in cases of pre-existing fetal hypoxia.[10]

THE MANAGEMENT OF SUSPECTED FETAL COMPROMISE IN THE SECOND STAGE OF LABOUR

- **Improve placental blood supply**.
  - Maternal positioning to avoid aorto-caval compression.
  - Intravenous fluids when appropriate.
  - Vasoconstrictors such as ephedrine for lower limb vasodilatation secondary to epidural analgesia.
- **Improve maternal oxygenation**.
  - Maternal oxygen therapy may be helpful if used for a short period while other measures are instituted. However, the routine use of oxygen therapy in the second stage was found to lead to an increase in newborn acidosis.[11]
- **Diminish uterine activity if excessive**.
  - Decrease or stop any oxytocin infusion. In the second stage, bolus intravenous tocolytics have been associated with an increase in instrumental delivery but no improvement in fetal outcome.[12] Their use in this situation should be restricted to cases where a short delay is expected before operative delivery can be undertaken.
- **Decide if delivery is indicated, based upon:**
  - the severity of the CTG abnormality and results of any secondary tests of fetal wellbeing;
  - response to the above interventions to improve the situation;
  - the whole clinical picture, including obstetric risk factors, progress in labour and potential assisted delivery;

- untreatable fetal complications such as abruption, cord prolapse and chorioamnionitis, and scar dehiscence.

There is little evidence to support the use of amnioinfusion in the second stage of labour to reduce cord compression and improve umbilical blood flow.

A CLINICAL APPROACH TO REVIEWING ABNORMAL SECOND-STAGE CTGS

Always ask yourself:

What factors are present that increase the neonatal risk of instrumental delivery?

For example, meconium/macrosomia/malposition/mid-cavity arrest/diabetes/previous shoulder dystocia.

Does the abnormality require immediate delivery?
Yes

Is an assisted delivery likely to be easy?

- Yes – occiput anterior (OA)/low station/little caput or moulding.
  - Deliver in room.
- No – malposition/mid-cavity arrest/major moulding or caput.
  - Undertake delivery in theatre either as trial or directly by caesarean section.
  - Strongly consider FBS before trial of instrumental delivery.

No

Is an assisted delivery likely to be easy?

- Yes – OA/low station/little caput or moulding.
- Has progress been steady in active second stage?
- Yes: offer mother choice of continued pushing for set time before recommending assisted delivery.
- No: consider oxytocin (consider FBS beforehand) if mother wishes to avoid assisted delivery.
  - If no intervention possible to improve situation, recommend assisted delivery in room.
- No – malposition/mid-cavity arrest/major moulding or caput).
  - Has progress been steady in active second stage?
    Yes: consider FBS to allow more time and convert to an easier delivery.
    No: consider FBS and then oxytocin.
  - If inappropriate to intervene to improve progress, recommend delivery.
  - In theatre either as a trial or directly by CS, strongly consider FBS before trial of instrumental delivery.

Published Guidelines

NICE: *Intrapartum care – care of healthy women and their babies during childbirth.* September 2007.

KEY POINTS

- CTG abnormalities are very common in the second stage but many are benign.
- Particular attention should be paid to marked bradycardias, any bradycardia with reduced variability and late or severe variable decelerations.
- Use fetal scalp sampling to avoid potentially difficult instrumental deliveries in the presence of pre-existing fetal compromise.

Key References

1. Krebs HB, Petres RE, Dunn LJ. Intrapartum fetal heart rate monitoring V Fetal heart rate patterns in the second stage of labor. *Am J Obstet Gynecol* 1981;140(4):435–9.

2. Sheiner E, Hadar A, Hallak M, Katz M, Mazor M, Shoham-Vardi I. Clinical significance of fetal heart rate tracings during the second stage of labor. *Obstet Gynecol* 2001;97(5 Pt 1):747–52.

3. Gilstrap LC, 3rd, Hauth JC, Toussaint S. Second-stage fetal heart rate abnormalities and neonatal acidosis. *Obstet Gynecol* 1984;63(2):209–13.

4. Gilstrap LC, 3rd, Hauth JC, Hankins GD, Beck AW. Second-stage fetal heart rate abnormalities and type of neonatal acidemia. *Obstet Gynecol* 1987;70(2):191–5.

5. Cardoso CG, Graca LM, Clode N. A study on second-stage cardiotocographic patterns and umbilical acid-base balance in cases with first stage normal fetal heart rates. *J Matern Fetal Invest* 1995;5:144–9.

6. Piquard F, Hsiung R, Mettauer M, Schaefer A, Haberey P, Dellenbach P. The validity of fetal heart rate monitoring during the second stage of labor. *Obstet Gynecol* 1988;72(5):746–51.

7. Gull I, Jaffa AJ, Oren M, Grisaru D, Peyser MR, Lessing JB. Acid accumulation during end-stage bradycardia in term fetuses: how long is too long? *Br J Obstet Gynaecol* 1996;103(11):1096–101.

8. Nordstrom L, Achanna S, Naka K, Arulkumaran S. Fetal and maternal lactate increase during active second stage of labour. *BJOG* 2001;108(3):263–8.

9. Neilson JP. Fetal electrocardiogram (ECG) for fetal monitoring during labour. *Cochrane Database Syst Rev* 2006;3:CD000116.

10. Amer-Wahlin I, Arulkumaran S, Hagberg H, Marsal K, Visser GH. Fetal electrocardiogram: ST waveform analysis in intrapartum surveillance. *BJOG* 2007;114(10):1191–3.

11. Thorp JA, Trobough T, Evans R, Hedrick J, Yeast JD. The effect of maternal oxygen administration during the second stage of labor on umbilical cord blood gas values: a randomized controlled prospective trial. *Am J Obstet Gynecol* 1995;172(2 Pt 1):465–74.

12. Campbell J, Anderson I, Chang A, Wood C. The use of ritodrine in the management of the fetus during the second stage of labour. *Aust N Z J Obstet Gynaecol* 1978;18:100–113.

Chapter 55 Shoulder dystocia

Jenny Blackman and Myles Taylor

INTRODUCTION

Shoulder dystocia is an acute obstetric emergency requiring rapid intervention to prevent neonatal morbidity and mortality. The relative infrequency of shoulder dystocia means that few obstetricians are truly experienced in its management. However, the high perinatal mortality and morbidity associated with this condition means that all labour ward practitioners must possess a detailed knowledge of the condition and how to overcome it.

DEFINITION

Classically, shoulder dystocia is recognised when the fetal chin retracts firmly back onto the perineum immediately after delivery of the head, the so-called 'turtle-neck' sign. A widely used but not universally accepted definition of shoulder dystocia is a delivery that requires additional obstetric manoeuvres to release the shoulders after gentle downward traction has failed.[1]

A logical approach to the assessment of severity of an earlier shoulder dystocia is essential. Events surrounding the delivery should be considered under three headings.

1 Additional manoeuvres.
   - What steps were required to effect delivery? See 'first-line', 'second-line' and 'third-line' under 'management' below.
2 Fetal complications:
   - Apgar scores and degree of resuscitation required;
   - neonatal unit admission;
   - direct fetal trauma (brachial plexus injury, fractures);
   - long-term disability (neurodevelopmental, palsy).
3 Maternal complications:
   - perineal trauma (extended episiotomy or tear, third-degree tear);
   - postpartum haemorrhage;
   - psychological trauma.

INCIDENCE

The lack of a universally agreed definition for shoulder dystocia hampers any estimate of incidence. As a rough guide less than 1 per cent of deliveries are complicated by shoulder dystocia.

COMPLICATIONS

Fetal

Short-term complications such as fractures of the humerus or clavicle are not uncommon. However, these heal well and have an excellent prognosis. Transient brachial plexus injury, such as Erb's palsy, is also relatively common. Fortunately, with early recognition, prompt physiotherapy and even neurosurgical treatment, most improve over time, leaving only 1–2 per cent of shoulder dystocia cases with long-term dysfunction. Hypoxic–ischaemic encephalopathy may develop after severe cases and carries a risk of later neurodevelopmental disability. Perinatal mortality secondary to shoulder dystocia was reported in 56 cases in the UK in 1994–95, an incidence of approximately 1 in 25,000 births.[2]

Maternal

Possible complications include excessive blood loss from extensive perineal, vaginal and cervical lacerations and extension of perineal trauma into third- or fourth-degree tears.

AETIOLOGY

The mechanics underlying shoulder dystocia have been reviewed by Johnstone and Myerscough.[3] Although the bisacromial diameter is larger than the biparietal diameter, the shoulders have the advantage of inherent mobility. As the fetal head passes through the pelvic outlet, the shoulders simultaneously enter the pelvic inlet. Ideally, the shoulders should enter the pelvis transversely, although they are usually oblique, with the posterior shoulder moving towards the sacrosciatic notch. As restitution of the fetal head occurs, the shoulders rotate through the pelvis and the anterior shoulder presents under the symphysis pubis.

In cases of true shoulder dystocia, either the anterior shoulder or, in severe forms, both the anterior and posterior shoulders are arrested at the pelvic inlet. It is a common misconception that the pelvic outlet and perineum contribute to shoulder dystocia.

PREDISPOSING FACTORS

There are well-recognised antenatal factors associated with shoulder dystocia such as a history of previous shoulder dystocia, macrosomia >4.5 kg, maternal diabetes, maternal obesity and induction of labour.

Excessive fetal size

The incidence of shoulder dystocia is known to increase in line with birthweight. Below 3.5 kg, the reported incidence is 0.2–0.8 per cent, rising to 5–23 per cent with birthweights above 4.5 kg.[4,5]

Despite this relationship, half of all shoulder dystocia cases occur with babies of normal birthweight. This may be because some babies that fail to meet an absolute criterion for macrosomia (such as a birthweight >4.0 kg) are actually relatively 'large for gestation' for that particular woman. Unfortunately, it is difficult to know in advance the 'intended' birthweight for any individual woman's offspring. However, customised fetal growth charts are increasingly available; these use maternal ethnic origin, build and parity to individualise predicted fetal weight at any gestation.

Clinicians must remain wary of any clinical situation or condition that is likely to increase fetal weight abnormally. Maternal diabetes, long known to be associated with a risk of excessive fetal growth, is a major risk factor [B].[6] Other causes of fetal macrosomia, either relative or absolute, include maternal obesity, multiparity and post-dates pregnancies.

Diabetes

Babies born to diabetic mothers have a 2- to 4-fold increase in the incidence of shoulder dystocia compared with babies of non-diabetic mothers of the same birthweight.

Previous history of shoulder dystocia

Overall recurrence risks for shoulder dystocia are approximately 10–15 per cent.[7,8] These may underestimate the risks, since CS may have been advised for those pregnancies in which a poor outcome occurred after shoulder dystocia.

Intrapartum events

Relative disproportion is often suggested by poor progress in labour, but this is a poor predictor of subsequent shoulder dystocia.[6,9] Shoulder dystocia has been associated with secondary arrest and mid-cavity instrumental deliveries,[9] but since this reflects a significant failure of descent, it is again highlighting poor progress in labour.

Parturition has long been linked with the three Ps – the passages, the passenger and the powers. It may be that inefficient uterine contractile activity underlies some cases of shoulder dystocia. It has been suggested that the endogenous powers pushing the shoulders through the birth canal in cases of shoulder dystocia are actually more important than the traction forces generated by the obstetrician.[10] An aetiological role for the 'powers' is also suggested by the increased incidence of shoulder dystocia found in induced labours, associated with an increased risk of dysfunctional labour and operative delivery.[5,9,11]

PREDICTION OF SHOULDER DYSTOCIA

Despite evidence for antenatal and intrapartum factors associated with shoulder dystocia, models for prediction of this emergent obstetric event are highly unreliable even when a combination of predisposing factors are present.

Review of previous delivery

A careful review of the events surrounding an earlier delivery is essential, using the system outlined under 'Incidence'. This must include a review of the previous maternity notes, which may necessitate correspondence with other units.

Screening for gestation diabetes

If there is any suspicion of excessive fetal growth in a previous pregnancy (regardless of birthweight), a glucose tolerance test should be arranged for 28 weeks' gestation. If impaired glucose tolerance is found, measures should be implemented to minimise any fetal effects [C].

Pelvimetry

There is no evidence to support the routine use of pelvimetry in this situation. Its use should be highly selective. Examples of situations in which it might be considered include marked shoulder dystocia with a small baby or a predisposing factor for pelvic contraction, such as a previous significant fracture.

Identification of fetal macrosomia

The prediction of fetal weight, either clinically or by ultrasound, is inaccurate in the third trimester where the margin of error in predicting birthweight exceeds 10 per cent. Thus information gained from prenatal assessment of size can only be used as one risk factor in the overall clinical picture. It facilitates advance planning and preparation but, in isolation, should not dictate any particular management. The recognition of significant macrosomia in association with other risk factors, particularly diabetes or a previous birth with shoulder dystocia, requires careful assessment.

SHOULDER DYSTOCIA PREVENTION

Early induction

Evidence from observational and randomised trials does not support the use of induction to prevent shoulder dystocia in suspected fetal macrosomia in a non-diabetic woman.[11,12,13]

As mentioned previously, induced labours are reported to have a higher incidence of shoulder dystocia. However, there is evidence that in the presence of maternal diabetes, the incidence of shoulder dystocia is reduced with early IOL. The current NICE recommendation for diabetic women, irrespective of macrosomia, is to offer elective delivery from 38 weeks' gestation.

A meta-analysis of 5 RCTs of specific treatment for gestational diabetes including offering early IOL compared with usual care concluded that the incidence of shoulder dystocia was significantly reduced in those specifically treated.[14]

Elective caesarean section

The ACOG Practice Bulletin 22 Guideline recommends considering elective caesarean section when the birthweight is predicted to be greater than 5 kg in non-diabetics or 4.5 kg in diabetics [D].[15] Despite this, it acknowledges that such a policy would result in 443 caesarean sections in diabetic women to prevent a single permanent newborn injury.

Extremely macrosomic babies (>5 kg) may have a 26-fold increase in shoulder dystocia and, in this group, a much higher incidence of brachial plexus injury. However, the difficulty in accurately predicting birthweight means that choosing the appropriate timing and mode of delivery it is not straightforward.[16]

At present, there are few grounds on which to recommend elective caesarean section on the basis of fetal size alone. Decisions should be individualised, based on an appreciation of all risk factors present.

Diabetic control

It is logical to suppose that tight diabetic control may reduce the incidence of fetal macrosomia. At present, there is a small body of evidence to support this assumption [C].

Intrapartum management

Advance planning

Antenatal risk factors for shoulder dystocia should be noted.

- Reassessment of risk should be carried out if there is poor progress in labour. In women believed to be at significant risk, advance preparation is essential.
- Midwifery and medical staff should establish a contingency plan involving:
  - who needs to be aware of the potential problem;
  - who will be present at the delivery;
  - what steps will be taken should difficulties arise.

In mothers who have failure of descent in the second stage, the presence of other risk factors for shoulder dystocia will influence not only if but also where and by whom an instrumental delivery is attempted. Although a trial of instrumental delivery in theatre does not reduce the risk of shoulder dystocia, it ensures the presence of adequate staffing to deal with it efficiently.

An epidural should always be considered in situations in which there is judged to be a considerable risk of shoulder dystocia, particularly if it is felt that maternal distress may interfere with cooperation.

Prophylactic use of the McRoberts manoeuvre is not recommended prior to delivery of the head in view of the absence of evidence for its benefit.

Early diagnosis allows prompt intervention. If there is difficulty delivering the face and chin or the head remains tightly applied to the vulva, retracts or there is failure of restitution then shoulder dystocia may be anticipated. Examination to define the location of the anterior shoulder (above or below the symphysis) can be helpful.

SHOULDER DYSTOCIA MANAGEMENT

There are no randomised trials to provide guidance for the management of this obstetric emergency.

Manoevres to overcome shoulder dystocia cannot solely be learnt from a book. Practical training in obstetric emergencies is strongly recommended, as offered on an ALSO© Course, PROMPT course or similar.

High-fidelity simulations should be used.[17]

Recent evidence has shown that sustained practical staff training improved the management of shoulder dystocia with extremely low morbidity and no cases of permanent obstetric brachial plexus injury in over 17,000 vaginal births.[18]

Help should always be summoned as soon as a problem is recognised. Clearly stating the nature of the emergency "Shoulder dystocia!" to the arriving team has been shown to prompt a coordinated response.[19]

As well as additional midwives, neonatology and anaesthetic staff should be called.

Identify a 'scribe' to note times of staff attendance and manoeuvres performed using a designated *pro forma*.

Fundal pressure is not recommended as this can cause uterine rupture. Maternal pushing should be discouraged as this may lead to further impaction of the shoulders.

An episiotomy should be considered but it is not mandatory. An episiotomy or extension of an episiotomy serves to create increased vaginal access to perform internal manoeuvres but may cause considerable maternal trauma.

The steps for approach to management of shoulder dystocia are described in the RCOG guideline on shoulder dystocia.

Manoeuvres for shoulder dystocia are aimed at addressing one or a combination of the following:

- increasing the size of the pelvis (McRoberts and all-fours position);
- decreasing the bisacromial diameter of the fetal shoulders (externally by suprapubic pressure or internally by delivery of the posterior arm);
- changing the relationship of the bisacromial diameter in the mother's bony pelvis (internal rotational manoevres).

SIMPLE FIRST-LINE MEASURES

The first step should always be the McRoberts manoeuvre which is successful in up to 90 per cent of cases. Remember to maintain the head in a neutral position (axial and in line with the fetal spine), avoiding excessive lateral traction.

- The McRoberts manoeuvre involves hyperflexion of the maternal thighs onto the maternal abdomen, either by the mother herself or by a pair of assistants. It has been shown radiographically to flatten the lumbosacral curve and lessen any obstruction from the sacral promontory.

- Suprapubic pressure is often used simultaneously. Using a stance similar to that of CPR, pressure is exerted obliquely on the posterior aspect of the anterior shoulder. The aim is to move the shoulders into the wider oblique diameter of the pelvis and force the anterior shoulder under the symphysis pubis.

SECOND-LINE MEASURES: INTERNAL MANIPULATIONS

Failing correction of the problem with simple measures further manipulations will be required either by internal rotational manoeuvres or by delivery of the posterior arm. These may involve considerable discomfort to the mother (and distress to her partner) and warning should be given.

The aim of these manoeuvres is to rotate the fetal trunk into an oblique position to allow delivery of the shoulders.

The most spacious part for access is the sacral hollow and the hand should be introduced into the posterior vagina. A generous episiotomy may be required.

Internal rotational manoeuvres

- *Rubin's manoeuvre.* By approaching the anterior shoulder from behind attempts should be made to rotate the shoulders into the oblique diameter of the pelvis, using a finger hooked into one axilla. Ideally, one should attempt to move the fetus in a direction that allows the shoulder to move inwards towards the chest, which will decrease the dimensions of the shoulders. Once disimpacted, traction can again be tried.
- *Wood's screw manoeuvre.* If simple rotation fails and the posterior shoulder is below the sacral promontory, Wood's screw manoeuvre should be attempted. Approach the posterior fetal shoulder from the front and rotate the posterior shoulder through 180° so that it becomes the anterior shoulder. By simultaneously combining this with a degree of downward traction, the rotated shoulder remains within the pelvis and appears under the symphysis.
- *Reverse Woods screw manoeuvre.* Approach the posterior shoulder from behind and rotate the fetus in the opposite direction from Rubin or Woods screw manoeuvres – this may be successful when previous manoeuvres have failed.

Delivery of the posterior arm

By advancing a hand into the uterus posteriorly and finding the fetal hand, delivery of the posterior fetal arm can be achieved by sweeping it across the fetal chest.

The 'All-fours' technique

The decision to move the mother into this position will depend on the setting, feasability and accoucheur. It may be tried (and is reported with high success[20]) if simple measures fail either before or after attempting internal manoeuvres.

If delivery still has not been achieved then repeating the above stepwise approach of manoeuvres is recommended.

THIRD-LINE MEASURES

If all the above measures have been tried and retried and the baby is still alive, third-line measures could be considered. However, the likelihood of any individual obstetrician gaining experience of these techniques within the UK is remote. Furthermore, publication bias means that clinicians often only report their successes. It is likely that heroic measures have, on many occasions, been followed by stillbirth, neonatal death or profound disability, at a cost of considerable maternal morbidity.

- *Cleidotomy* or deliberately fracturing the fetal clavicle(s) can be used to shorten the biacromial diameter. However, this can be difficult to perform and can lead to injury of underlying vascular and pulmonary structures.
- *Zavenelli manoeuvre.* The fetal head is replaced into the uterus by reversing the steps of parturition. This may require additional uterine relaxation, using either bolus tocolytics or general anaesthesia. Abdominal rescue describes intrauterine manipulation through a transabdominal hysterotomy to facilitate vaginal delivery.
- *Symphysiotomy* can lead to a 2–3 cm increase in the bony pelvic diameters. However, there is a significant risk of long-term maternal morbidity. Special skills and equipment are required, including a solid-bladed scalpel. The urethra must be catheterised and displaced laterally. In the absence of an epidural, local anaesthesia is needed. It is likely that the fetus will have been severely compromised by the time a symphysiotomy could be safely performed on most UK labour wards.

AFTER DELIVERY

- Postpartum haemorrhage and significant maternal trauma are associated with shoulder dystocia.
- The baby should always be carefully examined by the neonatologist.
- Explanation of events is essential for the mother and her partner. Mothers must understand what went wrong, both to minimise inappropriate blame of themselves or others and so that they may alert their caregivers in the next pregnancy.

DOCUMENTATION

After a delivery complicated by shoulder dystocia, it is important that the details surrounding the delivery are accurately recorded. A designated *pro forma* is ideal for this purpose. (see http://www.rcog.org.uk/files/rcog-corp/ GTG42_25112013.pdf). This is important for medico-legal reasons. For example, brachial plexus injury is the most common reason for litigation and where Erb's palsy is present, it is important to determine whether the affected shoulder was anterior or posterior, since trauma to the posterior shoulder plexus is unlikely to be due to action by the accoucheur (RCOG Guideline No.42).

Not only should the individual document their part in the management of the shoulder dystocia with care and detail, but the medical records should be reviewed contemporaneously, checking for completeness and consistency between healthcare professionals.

Good documentation is also useful for helping form a plan in any subsequent pregnancy.

It is important to record the following:

- time of the delivery of the head;
- the direction the head is facing after restitution;
- the manoeuvres performed, their timings and order;
- time of the delivery of the body;
- the staff in attendance;
- the condition of the baby, Apgar scores, and cord pH blood levels;
- estimated maternal blood loss.

KEY POINTS

- Neither fetal macrosomia nor shoulder dystocia can be reliably predicted.
- The presence of known risk factors, particularly two or more, should trigger advance preparations to deal with or avoid the situation, before it actually arises.
- Since shoulder dystocia will often occur without warning, obstetricians must have well-rehearsed strategies to overcome it.

Published Guidelines

American College of Obstetricians and Gynecologists. ACOG Practice Bulletin Number 22. *Fetal Macrosomia* Clinical Management Guidelines for Obstetricians/ Gynecologists. November 2000.

Focus Group – Shoulder dystocia. *In: Confidential Enquiry into Stillbirths and Deaths in Infancy,* 5th Annual Report, Section 8, Focus Group – Shoulder Dystocia. London: HMSO, 1996.

Royal College of Obsetricians and Gynaecologists. RCOG Guideline No. 42 Shoulder Dystocia (2nd edn March 2012).

Key References

1. Resnik R. Management of shoulder girdle dystocia. *Clin Obstet Gynecol* 1980;23(2):559–64.
2. Hope P, Breslin S, Lamont L *et al.* Fatal shoulder dystocia: a review of 56 cases reported to the Confidential

Enquiry into Stillbirths and Deaths in Infancy. *Br J Obstet Gynaecol* 1998;105(12):1256–61.

3. Johnstone FD, Myerscough PR. Shoulder dystocia. *BJOG* 1998;105(8):811–5.

4. Mocanu EV, Greene RA, Byrne BM, Turner MJ. Obstetric and neonatal outcome of babies weighing more than 4.5 kg: an analysis by parity. *Eur J Obstet Gynecol Reprod Biol* 2000;92(2):229–33.

5. Acker DB, Sachs BP, Friedman EA. Risk factors for shoulder dystocia in the average-weight infant. *Obstet Gynecol* 1986;67(5):614–18.

6. Acker DB, Sachs BP, Friedman EA. Risk factors for shoulder dystocia. *Obstet Gynecol* 1985;66(6):762–8.

7. Smith RB, Lane C, Pearson JF. Shoulder dystocia: what happens at the next delivery? *BJOG* 1994;101(8):713–5.

8. Lewis DF, Raymond RC, Perkins MB, Brooks GG, Heymann AR. Recurrence rate of shoulder dystocia. *Am J Obstet Gynecol* 1995;172(5):1369–71.

9. McFarland M, Hod M, Piper JM, Xenakis EM, Langer O. Are labor abnormalities more common in shoulder dystocia? *Am J Obstet Gynecol* 1995;173(4):1211–4.

10. Gonik B, Walker A, Grimm M. Mathematic modeling of forces associated with shoulder dystocia: a comparison of endogenous and exogenous sources. *Am J Obstet Gynecol* 2000;182(3):689–91.

11. Dublin S, Lydon-Rochelle M, Kaplan RC, Watts DH, Critchlow CW. Maternal and neonatal outcomes after induction of labor without an identified indication. *Am J Obstet Gynecol* 2000;183(4):986–94.

12. Combs CA, Singh NB, Khoury JC. Elective induction versus spontaneous labor after sonographic diagnosis of fetal macrosomia. *Obstet Gynecol* 1993;81(4):492–6.

13. Gonen O, Rosen DJ, Dolfin Z, Tepper R, Markov S, Fejgin MD. Induction of labor versus expectant management in macrosomia: a randomized study. *Obstet Gynecol* 1997;89(6):913–7.

14. Horvarth K, Koch K, Jeitler K *et al.* Effects of treatment in women with gestational diabetes mellitus; systemic review and meta-analysis. *BMJ* 2010;340:c1395.

15. Sokol RJ, Blackwell SC. ACOG practice bulletin: Shoulder dystocia. Number 40, November 2002. *Int J Gynaecol Obstet* 2003;80(1):87–92.

16. Vidarsdottir H, Geirsson RT, Hardardottir H, Valdimarsdottir U, Dagbjartsson A. Obstetric and neonatal risks among extremely macrosomic babies and their mothers. *Am J Obstet Gynecol* 2011 May;204(5):423.e1–6.

17. Crofts JF, Bartlett C, Ellis D, Hunt LP, Fox R, Draycott TJ. Training for shoulder dystocia: a trial of simulation using low-fidelity and high-fidelity mannequins. *Obstet Gynecol* 2006;108:1477–85.

18. Crofts JF, Bartlett C, Ellis D, Hunt LP, Fox R, Draycott TJ. Prevention of brachial plexus injury - 12 years of shoulder dystocia training: an interrupted time-series study. *BJOG* 2015;Feb 17.Epub ahead of print.

19. Siassakos D, Bristowe K, Draycott TJ *et al.* Clinical efficiency in a simulated emergency and relationship to team behaviours; a multisite cross-sectional study. *BJOG* 2011;118:596–607.

20. Bruner JP, Drummond SB, Meenan AL, Gaskin IM. All-fours maneuver for reducing shoulder dystocia during labor. *J Reprod Med* 1998;43(5):439–43.

Chapter 56 Instrumental vaginal delivery

Tracey A Johnston

INTRODUCTION

Instrumental vaginal delivery (IVD) is an essential part of the obstetrician's armamentarium, and s/he must be competent and confident in both forceps and vacuum for non-rotational delivery, and at least one technique for rotational delivery. Second-stage caesarean section (see Chapter 53) is associated with increased maternal and neonatal morbidity,[1] and therefore should be avoided if safely possible. The risks are higher for CS following failed instrumental delivery, and neonatal morbidity is increased with sequential use of instruments.[2] Thorough assessment and selection of the most appropriate mode of birth are therefore essential to minimise morbidity, as is skill in performing the procedure. National guidance exists[3] which addresses the indications and contraindications for intervention, the relative merits of forceps and vacuum, classification of operative delivery and prerequisites for operative delivery, as well as place of delivery and aftercare. As with CS there are geographical variations in the incidence of IVD, but the rate has remained relatively constant in the UK for the past few years, with the most recent figures for England showing a rate of 12.8 per cent, with 6.8 per cent being forceps and 6 per cent being vacuum.[4] This is despite an increase in the CS rate, which has not been associated with a concomitant reduction in operative vaginal birth.

REDUCING THE NEED FOR IVD

There are several evidence-based strategies that should be routine practice on the labour ward to reduce the need for operative intervention. It has been established for some time that one-to-one care in labour reduces intervention and improves maternal satisfaction, especially when the continuous carer is not a member of staff [A].[5] This raises the question regarding the use of doulas as a cost-effective mechanism for increasing the normal birth rate. The mother being supine or in lithotomy in second stage increases the rate of IVD [A].[6] Epidural analgesia is associated with an increased operative vaginal delivery rate,[7] but the COMET trial demonstrated that more modern methods of regional analgesia such as combined spinal epidural and 'mobile' epidurals improved the normal delivery rate mainly by reducing the IVD rate [B].[8] In nulliparous women with an epidural, delayed pushing by extending the passive second stage of labour is associated with a reduction in IVD [B],[9] as is the judicious use of oxytocin in the second stage [B].[10] The BUMPES trial has recently finished recruitment and seeks to determine whether maternal position in second stage with an epidural influences mode of birth.[11]

CLASSIFICATION

Standardised terminology should be used when defining and classifying IVD. Table 56.1 sets out the preferred classification, adapted from ACOG.[12]

Table 56.1 Classification for instrumental vaginal birth (adapted from ACOG, 2000)

Outlet Vertex visible
Fetal skull has reached pelvic floor
Saggital suture is in the anterior–posterior position with no more than 45° of rotation
Fetal head at or on the perineum
Low cavity Vertex 2 cm or more below the ischial spines but not on the pelvic floor
* Rotation of 45 degrees or less from the occipito-anterior position
* Rotation of more than 45 degrees including the occipito-posterior position
* Rotation of more than 45 degrees including the occipito-posterior position
Mid cavity Head no more than 1/5 palpable abdominally
Vertex between ischial spines and spines +2 cm
* Rotation of 45 degrees or less from the occipito-anterior position
* Rotation of more than 45 degrees including the occipito-posterior position
High cavity Head >2/5 palpable abdominally
Presenting part above ischial spines
Instrumental birth is not recommended in this situation

INDICATIONS

IVD is used to expedite delivery by shortening the second stage of labour. There are both maternal and fetal indications for IVD (Table 56.2) but it must be remembered that no indication is absolute, and each case must be assessed individually and the risks and benefits of continued pushing balanced against those of intervention. The commonest indications for IVD are confirmed fetal acidaemia (following FBS) or suspected fetal compromise (abnormal CTG), and delay in second stage. Chapter 54 covers fetal compromise in the second stage and will therefore not be discussed further here.

Table 56.2 Indications for instrumental vaginal birth

Maternal	Prolonged second stage
	Maternal fatigue
	Poor maternal effort (e.g. dense epidural block)
	Certain maternal medical disorders
Fetal	Confirmed fetal acidaemia
	Presumed fetal compromise

Delay in second stage

The NICE guideline for Intrapartum Care[9] sets out a definition and recommended limits for the length of the second stage

of labour for nulliparous and multiparous women. These recommended limits are based on the increased risks of mainly maternal compromise, such as chorioamnionitis, operative birth, PPH and perineal trauma. With appropriate fetal monitoring and intervention if indicated, prolonged second stage does not appear to be associated with significantly increased neonatal morbidity.[9] Passive second stage of labour is defined as the finding of full dilatation of the cervix before or in the absence of involuntary expulsive contractions. The onset of the active second stage of labour is defined by the baby being visible, expulsive contractions with a finding of full dilatation of the cervix or other signs of full dilatation of the cervix, or active maternal effort following confirmation of full dilatation of the cervix in the absence of expulsive contractions. With regard to the normal length of the active second stage, it varies depending on parity and whether the woman has an epidural. The range and upper limit of normal for the active second stage in women giving birth to their first baby is about 0.5–2.5 hours without an epidural, and 1–3 hours with an epidural, and for women giving birth to second or subsequent babies, up to about 1 hour without an epidural, and 2 hours with an epidural. Delay should be diagnosed in nulliparous women when the active second stage has lasted 2 hours and birth is not imminent, and when the active second stage has lasted 1 hour and birth is not imminent in multiparous women.[9] When an epidural is *in situ*, birth should be achieved within 4 hours of the diagnosis of second stage, irrespective of parity,[9] and this must be borne in mind when implementing delayed pushing (i.e. prolonging the passive second stage), which is associated with a significant reduction in the incidence of mid-cavity and rotational IVD.[13] When delay in second stage is diagnosed, operative intervention should be considered to achieve birth. In most cases this will be by IVD, but in some cases second-stage CS is appropriate (Chapter 54).

Other maternal indications

With respect to maternal fatigue and poor maternal effort, supportive measures should be employed including appropriate analgesia, but if these measures are not successful, operative intervention can be offered.

Maternal medical disorders which merit shortening of the active second stage should usually be identified in the antenatal period and appropriate discussion and planning put in place. Such conditions include New York Heart Association class III and IV maternal cardiac disease, severe hypertension (crisis), proliferative retinopathy and myasthenia gravis. Accidental dural puncture is not an indication for IVD [C].

CONTRAINDICATIONS

There are few absolute contraindications to IVD, the main one being lack of appropriate skill in performing the procedure.

Vacuum should not be used below 34 weeks' gestation because of the increased susceptibility of the preterm infant to cephalohaematoma, intracranial haemorrhage, subgaleal haemorrhage and neonatal jaundice [D]. The safety of vacuum is not clear between 34 and 36 weeks' gestation [D]. Vacuum is also contraindicated in face presentation, although forceps can be used if mento-anterior. Fetal bleeding disorders (e.g. thrombocytopenia, haemophilia) and bone disorders associated with fractures (e.g. osteogenesis imperfecta) are relative contraindications, but a non-rotational low cavity IVD is associated with less trauma than CS if the head is deep in the pelvis. Careful assessment and a skilled operator are required in these cases, as is appropriate instrument selection taking into account that forceps reduce the haemorrhagic risk compared to vacuum and vacuum reduces the risk of fracture compared to forceps.

Blood-borne viral infection is not a contraindication to IVD [D] (although fetal scalp electrodes and FBS should be avoided), although difficult IVD with an increased risk of fetal laceration is probably best avoided. FBS and fetal scalp electrodes again are not contraindications to IVD, as the risk of significant scalp haemorrhage with vacuum is minimal [C].

PREREQUISITES

To minimise risk to both mother and baby, careful case and instrument selection are vital. Before embarking on an instrumental delivery, specific prerequisites must be fulfilled.

- An operator with the required skills and a willingness to abandon the procedure if indicated.
- Cephalic presentation not more than ⅕ palpable per abdomen (in certain circumstances skilled operators may perform a vacuum extraction with a higher presenting part e.g. second twin). The presenting part should be the vertex, although forceps can be used in mento-anterior face presentations, and in brow presentations where the pelvis is adequate and the fetus small (e.g. late preterm). In these circumstances, the operator must have the appropriate level of expertise to conduct these more complicated instrumental vaginal deliveries.
- Cervix fully dilated with ruptured membranes (again, skilled operators may perform vacuum extraction prior to full dilatation in specific circumstances e.g. acute bradycardia in a parous woman approaching full dilatation).
- Adequate pelvis – beware significant moulding.
- Position of the presenting part *must* be known to ensure correct application of both forceps and vacuum.
- Informed consent of the mother – this is usually verbal consent, but if there is time written consent should be obtained if possible. In cases of trial of instrumental birth, written consent for the trial and possible caesarean section should be obtained.[14]
- Adequate analgesia – often regional analgesia although a pudendal block can be used, particularly if regional

anaesthesia is declined or there are concerns regarding fetal wellbeing.
- Bladder empty and catheter removed or balloon deflated.
- There is no prerequisite for episiotomy, as it is not clear from the evidence whether routine episiotomy protects against anal sphincter injury in either forceps or vacuum, and restrictive use using the operator's clinical judgement is reasonable [B].

PLACE OF DELIVERY

IVD can be conducted in the labour room or in theatre. In cases where a higher failure rate may be anticipated, delivery should be performed as a trial in theatre to facilitate immediate recourse to CS if IVD is unsuccessful [C]. Such cases include malposition, mid-cavity/head palpable abdominally (no more than ⅕), big baby and raised maternal BMI.[1] Increased perinatal morbidity is seen where there is a delay between failed IVD and CS, whereas there is no difference in neonatal outcome when failed IVD followed by immediate CS is compared to immediate CS without an attempt at IVD.[15] In cases where there is a concern over fetal wellbeing, timescales must be taken into account. On average, IVD undertaken in the delivery room takes around 15 minutes, whereas IVD following transfer to theatre takes around 30 minutes,[16] thus the risks of delaying delivery by transferring to theatre must be balanced against the risks of a failed IVD in the room.

CHOICE OF INSTRUMENT

There are many different types of forceps and vacuum devices available. For forceps, the easiest way to categorise them is secondary to their physical characteristics. Forceps are either curved or straight, depending on whether they have a pelvic curve or not, and either have a long or a short shank. In the UK, the only short forceps available are short curved forceps, or Wrigley's forceps. These are generally used for 'lift-out' deliveries, when the vertex is at the introitus. The only straight forceps available are long straight forceps, or Kielland forceps, which are used for rotational deliveries (see later). The most commonly used forceps are long curved forceps of which there are around 700 varieties, with very little to choose between them (e.g. Neville-Barnes, Haig-Ferguson, Andersons and so on).

There are also different types of vacuum extractors and cups, again with different pros and cons. In current practice, the disposable hand-held vacuum device (Kiwi™ Omnicup, Clinical Innovations Europe Ltd, Abingdon UK) seems to be the most commonly available vacuum in many units, and indeed may be the only device available. Unfortunately, higher failure rates have been reported in RCTs comparing Kiwi with conventional vacuum [B][17,18] although the failure rate decreases in skilled hands.[19]

With conventional vacuum, there are a variety of cups. Metal cups come in different sizes and are generally either OA or OP cups, with OP cups having the tubing insertion point on the side to allow placement over the flexion point on a deflexed, OP position. Large, soft silastic cups gained popularity for their ease of application and lower incidence of scalp trauma, but have been shown to have a higher failure rate when compared to rigid cups [A].[20]

With any vacuum delivery, poor cup placement is associated with an increased failure rate, which is why it is essential to determine where the flexion point is to enable correct cup placement over the flexion point. If the cup is placed correctly over the flexion point (a flexing median application), the failure rate for vacuum extraction should be in the region of 4 per cent. A flexing paramedian application increases the failure rate to around 17 per cent, a deflexing median application with the cup placed too far anteriorly is associated with a failure rate of 29 per cent and a deflexing paramedian application has a failure rate of up to 35 per cent. These figures confirm the importance of correct cup placement and firmly refute the 'suck it and see' approach which unfortunately does still exist. Unless the flexion point is clearly identified and the cup placed correctly, any attempt at vacuum delivery should not proceed.

When using vacuum, there is no evidence of benefit in a slow, incremental increase in pressure compared to a rapid increase.[21]

When selecting which instrument to use, the operator must take into account their personal skill set and the particular clinical scenario in each case, as the objective must always be to achieve delivery safely with the first instrument of choice. For non-rotational deliveries, the options are either non-rotational forceps or vacuum, and there are pros and cons to both [A] (Table 56.3). Operators should be skilled in the use of both instruments, and fully understand the impact of different clinical situations on likely outcome. In cases of outlet deliveries, there may be little to choose between the two in terms of success rates, but overall forceps are associated with a significantly increased success rate compared to vacuum [A], and achieve delivery more quickly,[9] which is an important feature to consider in cases where delivery needs to be achieved quickly. Factors which should warn the operator of an increased risk of failure with vacuum include: excessive caput or moulding (may be an indicator of relative cephalo-pelvic disproportion, less likely to achieve adequate seal), malposition, and poor maternal effort (particularly following epidural top-up or spinal for a trial in theatre). Most trainees become comfortable with vacuum before forceps, but when looking at the pros and cons listed in Table 56.3, with fully informed counselling it may be that, given that there is no difference in long-term outcomes, most women would be prepared to accept more pain and discomfort, and increased rates of perineal trauma, to optimise the chance of success with the first instrument of choice and ensure less trauma to and concerns about their baby.

In cases where rotation is required to achieve delivery, there are three options:

- manual rotation and either forceps or vacuum to complete delivery;

Table 56.3 Outcomes when vacuum compared to forceps

Vacuum compared to forceps	OR	95% CI
Procedure:		
More likely to fail with selected instrument	1.69	1.31–2.19
No difference in CS rates	0.56	0.31–1.02
Reduction in the use of anaesthesia	0.59	0.51–0.68
Takes longer to achieve delivery[9]		
Maternal:		
Reduction in maternal genital tract injury	0.41	0.33–0.50
Reduced pain during birth	1.5	0.5–4.2
Reduction in severe perineal pain at 24 hours	0.54	0.31–0.93
Increase in maternal anxieties about the baby	2.17	1.19–3.94
No difference in incontinence at 5 years	1.47	0.44–4.92
Neonatal:		
Increased risk of cephalohaematoma	2.38	1.68–3.37
Increased risk of retinal haemorrhage	1.99	1.35–2.96
No difference in Apgar score <7 at 1 minute	1.13	0.76–1.68
No difference in scalp and facial injuries (excluding cephalohaematoma)	0.89	0.7–1.13
No difference in need for phototherapy	1.08	0.66–1.77
No difference in perinatal death	0.8	0.18–3.52

- rotational vacuum;
- rotational forceps.

Many such deliveries are conducted as trials in theatre with regional anaesthesia, which limits maternal effort, and clinicians must be skilled in at least one of the above techniques. Rotational vacuum is most commonly used, but the higher failure rates must be taken into account. Using a conventional vacuum device with a rigid OP cup will maximise the chances of success. Manual rotation can indeed avoid IVD, as following rotation maternal effort may be successful in achieving birth without further assistance. The fetal head is flexed and then rotated into the occipito-anterior position, and held there until either the mother pushes and the head descends, or either vacuum or forceps are applied to achieve delivery. The most effective instrument in achieving rotational delivery is Kielland forceps, but in many units the skill in using them has disappeared, mainly because of concerns over increased maternal and perinatal morbidity. There are reports in the literature regarding poor outcomes with Kielland forceps, but many of these are old and from uncontrolled observational studies and in many cases the fault lies with poor case selection and an unwillingness to abandon the procedure at the appropriate time. A recent review of almost 900 cases shows that neonatal admission rates following rotational forceps delivery are no higher when compared to normal birth and vacuum delivery, and are lower than emergency CS. In terms of maternal morbidity, rotational forceps delivery was associated with lower rates of PPH than emergency CS [B].[22] This demonstrates that in skilled hands rotational forceps still have a valuable place in modern obstetrics in terms of safely achieving vaginal birth and avoiding second-stage CS.

WHEN TO ABANDON

It is essential before embarking on an instrumental delivery that the operator has the appropriate skills, and in particular knows when to abandon the procedure. Both maternal and neonatal morbidity are increased with prolonged, repeated or excessive traction in the absence of progress. If there is no descent after the first pull, the situation should be reassessed and requesting senior help should be considered, as this may be indicative of an increased risk of failure. Possible explanations to exclude are incorrect determination of position or station (OP instead of OA), incorrect cup placement (not over the flexion point), poor maternal effort (particularly with vacuum, and with spinal or dense epidural blockade), cephalo-pelvic disproportion and, rarely, equipment failure (leak in the vacuum system). If delivery is not imminent after three pulls, if the vacuum cup detaches three times, or delivery is not completed within 30 minutes of the decision to deliver, then the procedure should be abandoned [B], with recourse, in the majority of cases, to CS. As the success rate with forceps is higher than with vacuum, there is a temptation to try forceps if vacuum fails. This practice is associated with an increased risk of perinatal trauma [B], especially intracranial haemorrhage, retinal haemorrhage and feeding difficulties,[2] and the risk of this must be balanced against the risks of CS following failed IVD (see Chapter 53). In cases where the head is in the low cavity or on the perineum, forceps may be the safer option, but caution must be exercised and this should be a senior decision.

POST-DELIVERY CARE

Paired cord gases should be obtained in cases where fetal compromise is suspected, and a careful examination of the neonate conducted, assessing for any signs of trauma secondary to the instrument used. Any injuries should be explained to the parents and documented, and if there are concerns the baby should be seen by an appropriately qualified practitioner. It is good practice for the operator to note any marks on the neonate to confirm where the instrument used was placed e.g. is the chignon over the flexion point? Are any forceps marks in the correct place? This gives immediate feedback regarding appropriate application and placement, and will inform skill development. Maternal aftercare should include appropriate analgesia (paracetamol and diclofenac if no contraindications), a venous thromboembolism risk assessment and thromboprophylaxis if indicated [D][23] and good bladder care. The timing and volume of the first void should be monitored and documented [C], and assessment of post-void residual carried out if retention is suspected, to avoid over-distension injury. If regional anaesthesia has been used, an indwelling catheter should be left *in situ* for 12 hours after delivery. There is no evidence to support the use of antibiotic prophylaxis in cases of IVD [A]. The women should be given a full explanation of the indication for IVD, preferably by the operator, to ensure she has full understanding as well as the opportunity to ask questions. She should also be informed of the high chance of a successful vaginal birth in future pregnancies [B].[24]

TRAINING

Inexperience and inadequate training are associated with adverse outcomes,[25] and training is a key component of patient safety initiatives.[26] The RCOG curriculum specifies the training requirements for IVD (Core Module 11), and trainees should have both formative and summative objective structured assessments of technical skill (OSATs) performed to ensure achievement and maintenance of competencies. Hands-on experience cannot be replaced in total by other learning modalities. More experienced operators are more likely to achieve successful IVD[27] and formal postgraduate training is associated with a reduction in both neonatal and maternal morbidity.[28] This requires appropriate supervision by clinicians who have achieved the appropriate competencies, and increased consultant presence on the labour ward will facilitate this.

SECOND STAGE OF LABOUR

KEY POINTS

- One-to-one care in labour, non-supine position in second stage, delayed pushing in the presence of epidural analgesia and the judicious use of oxytocin all reduce the need for IVD.
- The main indications for IVD are fetal compromise and delay in second stage.
- Successful delivery is more likely to be achieved with forceps, and more quickly, than with vacuum.
- Sequential use of instruments is associated with increased neonatal morbidity.
- Correct case selection, correct instrument selection and appropriate skills are all essential to optimise success rates.
- Know your limitations and ask for help!

References

1. Murphy DJ, Leibling RE, Verity L et al. Early maternal and neonatal morbidity associated with operative delivery in second stage of labour: a cohort study. Lancet 2001;358:1203–7.
2. Gardella C, Taylor M, Benedetti T et al. The effect of sequential use of vacuum and forceps for assisted vaginal delivery on neonatal and maternal outcomes. Am J Obstet Gynecol 2001;185:896–902.
3. RCOG Green-top Guideline No. 26: Operative Vaginal Delivery. RCOG Press, January 2011.
4. NHS Maternity Statistics – England, 2012–13; Health and Social Care Information Centre, Dec 2013.
5. Hodnett ED, Gates S, Hofmeyr GJ, Sakala C. Continuous support for women during childbirth. Cochrane Database Syst Rev 2007;3:CD003766.
6. Gupta JK, Hofmeyr GJ, Smyth RMD. Position in the second stage of labour for women without epidural analgesia. Cochrane Database Syst Rev 2000;1:CD002006.
7. Anim-Somuah M, Smyth R, Howell C. Epidural versus non-epidural or no analgesia in labour. Cochrane Database Syst Rev 2005;4:CD000331.
8. Comparative Obstetric Mobile Epidural Trial (COMET) Study Group UK. Effect of low-dose mobile versus traditional epidural techniques on mode of delivery: a randomised controlled trial. Lancet 2001;358(7):19–23.
9. National Collaborating Centre for Women's and Children's Health. Clinical Guideline No. 55: Intrapartum care: care of healthy women and their babies during childbirth. London: RCOG Press, 2007.
10. Saunders NJ, Spiby H, Gilbert L et al. Oxytocin infusion during second stage of labour in primiparous women using epidural analgesia: a randomised double-blind placebo-controlled trial. BMJ 1989;299:1423–6.
11. A study of position during the late stages of labour in women with an epidural - BUMPES: a randomised controlled trial. ISRCTN35706297.
12. ACOG. Practice Bulletin No. 17: Operative vaginal delivery. Washington DC, USA: ACOG, 2000.
13. Roberts CL, Torvaldsen S, Cameron CA et al. Delayed versus early pushing in women with epidural analgesia: a systematic review and meta-analysis. BJOG 2004;111(12):1333–40.
14. RCOG. Consent Advice No. 11: Operative vaginal delivery. London: RCOG, 2010.
15. Revah A, Ezra Y, Farine D, Ritchie K. Failed trial of vacuum or forceps – maternal and fetal outcome. Am J Obstet Gynecol 1997:176;200–4.
16. Murphy DJ, Koh DK. Cohort study of the decision to delivery interval and neonatal outcome for emergency operative vaginal delivery. Am J Obstet Gynecol 2007;196:145.e1–7.
17. Attilakos G, Sibanda T, Winter C et al. A randomised controlled trial of a new handheld vacuum extraction device. BJOG 2005;112:1510–15.
18. Groom KM, Jones BA, Miller N, Peterson-Brown SA. A prospective randomized controlled trial of the Kiwi Omnicup versus conventional ventouse cups for vacuum-assisted vaginal delivery. BJOG 2006;113:183–9.
19. Baskett TF, Fanning CA, Young DC. A prospective observational study of 1000 vacuum assisted deliveries with the Omnicup device. J Obstet Gynecol Can 2008;30:573–80.
20. Johanson R, Menon V. Soft versus rigid vacuum extractor cups for assisted vaginal delivery. Cochrane Database Syst Rev 1999;4:CD000446.
21. Suwannachat B, Lumbiganon P, Laopaiboon M. Rapid versus stepwise negative pressure application for vacuum extraction assisted vaginal delivery. Cochrane Database Syst Rev 2008;3:CD006636.
22. Stock SJ, Josephs K, Farquharson S et al. Maternal and neonatal outcomes of successful Kielland's rotational forceps delivery. Obstet Gynecol 2013;121(5):1032–9.
23. RCOG Green-top Guideline No. 37a. Thrombosis and Embolism during Pregnancy and the Puerperium, Reducing the Risk. RCOG Press, November 2009.
24. Bahl R, Strachan B, Murphy DJ. Outcome of subsequent pregnancy three years after previous operative delivery in the second stage of labour: cohort study. BMJ 2004;328:311–14.
25. Johnstone T. Minimizing risk: obstetric skills training. Clin Risk 2003;9:99–102.
26. Murphy DJ, Leibling RE, Patel R et al. Cohort study of operative delivery in the second stage of labour and standard of obstetric care. BJOG 2003;110:610–15.
27. Olah KS. Reversal of the decision for CS in the 2nd stage of labour on the basis of a consultant VE. J Obstet Gynaecol 2005;25(2):115–16.
28. Cheong YC, Abdullahi H, Lashen H, Fairlie FM. Can formal education and training improve the outcome of instrumental delivery? Eur J Obstet Gynecol Reprod Biol 2004;113:139–44.

Chapter 57 Breech presentation

Alexander M Pirie

Alexander M Pirie

MRCOG Standards

Module 1: Clinical skills
- Communicate effectively.
- Take notes concisely and accurately.

Module 3: Information technology, clinical governance and research
- Understand how to perform, interpret and use clinical audit cycles.
- Understand the production and application of clinical standards, guidelines and care pathways and protocols.
- Understand the skill necessary to critically appraise scientific trials and literature.
- Understand the principles and legal issues surrounding informed consent.

Module 5: Core surgical skills
- Demonstrate an understanding of the issues surrounding informed consent, including knowledge of complication rates, risks and likely success rates of different operations.

Module 8: Antenatal care
- Demonstrate skill in listening and conveying complex information (e.g. concerning risk).
- External cephalic version.

Modules 10 and 11: Management of labour and management of delivery
- The exam may test certain aspects of practical skill relating to normal and abnormal delivery.
- Vaginal breech delivery including second twin.

INTRODUCTION

Seasoned obstetricians are vexed long in our wakeful nights by the memories of a sick child born by vaginal breech birth. Tragic outcomes for breech are well recognised, yet they happen even after caesarean sections as well as technically flawless vaginal breech births. The cause of an unhappy outcome is often not the mode of birth. Every experienced midwife and obstetrician recalls happy memories of mothers who birth their breech so smoothly and naturally, that we worry wakefully that our modern tilt towards caesarean section may be costly and invasive, introducing morbid and mortal risk whilst taxing young mothers with prolonged recovery times.

As we lean towards CS (based on better short-term neonatal outcomes), we fear a future where the rising CS rate multiplies the risks of haemorrhage, transfusion, sepsis, visceral injury and 'returns to theatre' as well as the psycho-social and parenting implications of longer recovery times. Caesarean for breech increases the likelihood of more complex caesarean in subsequent pregnancies, with an escalation in the challenging realities of placenta accreta with catastrophic haemorrhage, obstetric hysterectomy, uterine scar rupture, cerebral palsy and maternal death. Caesarean sections carry resource implications for facilities and finance as well as the learning of new skills for complex repeat obstetric surgery, as well as the loss of obstetric skills in vaginal breech birth. And we need to consider both resource-rich and resource-poor settings, as well as the increasing plight of women who may move from rich country to poor (e.g. after failed asylum application) with dire consequences for their next pregnancy if they have a scarred uterus.

Research to help us guide a mother's choice between caesarean and vaginal birth has evolved from the primordial soup of expert opinion, up through the jungles of retrospective and prospective cohort studies, to the shining Grade A quality of randomised trials, meta-analysis and systematic review. The dawn of a regularly revised RCOG guideline systematically produced by a multidisciplinary expert group is a shining beacon for modern practice, yet still we are left with shadowy uncertainties. The spectres of controversy and critique still haunt labour suites and courtrooms as we weigh the risks in the longer term. The hired guns of obstetric litigation duel their heavy arguments for cause and effect before the civil courts. It has been said that some expert obstetricians may be more comfortable discoursing in a lawyer's chambers than using head, hand and heart in a busy labour suite. Unlike the high scientific standard of proof which all doctors assume for research trials (95% probability; $p < 0.05$), or the high standard of proof ('beyond reasonable doubt') in criminal trials, a civil court trial for medical negligence applies the lowest standard of proof ('balance of probabilities') which means the judge awards success to the side whose argument appears to be more probable than not (in other words, at least 51%

probability of being true). Yet the history of science is punctuated by seemingly probable arguments that turn out to be wrong. The Earth can look fairly flat, despite being round.

Critical appraisal of both research and litigation, and qualitative research on which outcomes are important to women, must blend in the crucible of our understanding if we are to transform care into a gold standard for breech babies and supporting their mothers' informed choices.

Eight questions faced by hands-on obstetricians are worth meditation by the MRCOG candidate:

1   How would you counsel a woman in antenatal clinic at 37 weeks' gestation whose baby is found to be a breech presentation, and ensure she had 'informed choice'?
2   What if a woman were first found to be breech at 7 cm dilatation in labour at term?
3   What if the gestation were 24 weeks, 28 weeks or 32 weeks in a labouring woman?
4   What about twins where either the first or second twin is breech?
5   What would you do if she politely refused your recommendations?
6   Could you write a guideline and set audit standards for performing ECV?
7   Can you overview and critically appraise the evidence for the options of vaginal breech versus caesarean birth?
8   Can you demonstrate using a model the recognised manoeuvres for assisted vaginal breech birth and its complications, and discuss the minimisation of the common neonatal injuries?

This chapter aims to inspire you, the reader, to answer these questions, to breed excellence in your future clinical practice, to strengthen your ability to contribute to service, research and quality improvement, and for you to flourish in the MRCOG examination.

PREVALENCE

The frequency of breech presentation at term is around 3 per cent of pregnancies at 37 weeks.[1-4] This figure has been very constant over the last century. It is much commoner with preterm babies, perhaps due to the mobile, smaller baby and immature brain, such that the prevalence at 28 weeks' gestation is around 20–30 per cent.

TYPES OF BREECH

Extended breech is commonest (70 per cent) and easiest of all breeches to deliver vaginally with the buttocks fitting roundly into the cervix. The legs are extended at the knees and flexed at the hips, with the feet up near the face. It is sometimes confusingly called 'frank' breech.

Flexed breech has the knees flexed and the feet at or below the breech. This is sometimes called a 'complete' breech.

Footling breech has one or both legs extended at the hip and knee, so the foot may prolapse down the birth canal with a high risk of cord prolapse.[5,6]

CAUSES

Ultrasound has become an essential tool for discerning any underlying cause, where management of the underlying condition is an important facet of management of breech. Many breeches are idiopathic, and an old hypothesis was that neural immaturity prevents flexion of the legs, leaving them in extension which then splints the trunk, preventing the flexion necessary for the natural forward roll to cephalic presentation.[1-6]

There are fetal, placental and maternal factors that increase the prevalence of breech:

- polyhydramnios (e.g. maternal diabetes, fetal anomaly such as oesophageal or duodenal atresia);
- oligohydramnios (associated with fetal growth restriction, amniorrhexis, renal tract dysgenesis);
- fetal anomaly (e.g. hydrocephalus, myelomeningocele, aneuploidy);
- placenta praevia;
- uterine anomaly (e.g. bicornuate uterus);
- pelvic mass (e.g. uterine fibroids, ovarian cyst);
- prematurity;
- multiple pregnancy;
- multiparity.

DIAGNOSIS

A woman with a breech presentation may complain of a hard lump or discomfort under her ribs. The firm round 'cricket ball' feeling of the baby's head may be felt in the upper abdomen, and the presenting part will be soft without the usual hard 'ballotable' head. For those with experience of auscultation of the fetal heart, it will be loudest above the maternal umbilicus rather than below.

On vaginal examination the presenting part is soft, although a tightly moulding breech deep in the pelvis can occasionally be mistaken for a head with the natal cleft and anus simulating the sagittal fissure and fontanelle, and so a high degree of vigilance should be maintained. It used to be said to beware the deeply engaged head for the head may not be there at all, if it were actually a breech. Palpation of the hard ischial tuberosities and sacrum helps differentiate the breech from a face presentation where the malar bones, hard chin and mouth can be felt.[5,6]

Screening for breech is an important function of the late antenatal check, and this satisfies Wilson's WHO Criteria for a screening test.[7] Clinical suspicion of breech after 36 weeks should be confirmed by ultrasound. Even in experienced hands, palpation in the absence of ultrasound still misses the diagnosis of breech, particularly in women with high BMI.[1,5,6]

Detection of breech with 100 per cent sensitivity is an argument for routine ultrasound late in antenatal care.

The first recognition of breech presentation is sometimes at vaginal examination in labour, which is less than ideal for enabling informed choice and planned CS. Women in threatened preterm labour are at higher risk of breech presentation and so need particular suspicion for breech with a documented discussion of the risks and benefits of the options for birth.

COMPLICATIONS

The risks of vaginal breech birth are well known but must be balanced against the significant risks of CS for this and future pregnancies. The harms of vaginal breech are:[1-6]

- cord prolapse, particularly with footling or flexed breech, where the presenting part does not seal the birth canal at membrane rupture;
- visceral injury, particularly perinephric haematoma: where the fetal abdomen has been grasped during delivery instead of the buttocks;
- fractures of femur and humerus: where limbs are manipulated particularly with the nuchal arm, or much rarer bilateral nuchal arms;
- brachial plexus injury with subsequent Erb's or Klumpke's palsy;
- dislocation of hips: common with the shallow acetabulum characteristic of breech, but more so if legs released using non-standard manoeuvres;
- cord compression: once the head has entered the pelvis, the cord can undergo compression released only by delivery, especially if the cord is round the neck. This can cause relative hypovolaemia and asphyxia and is often blamed for hypoxic brain injury in vaginal breech;
- arrest of the after-coming head: the obstetrician's nightmare where the head gets stuck but the cord and body have delivered;
- tentorial tear and intracranial haemorrhage: thought to result from the unmoulded breech head being delivered too rapidly, and the base of the skull is pulled apart from the bones of the cranial vault exerting force on the tentorium and veins of Galen.

MANAGEMENT

Decision models and the 'Inner Consultation'

The main management decision is between the three options of external cephalic version, vaginal breech birth or caesarean section, and the specifics will vary with antenatal or intrapartum diagnosis, term or preterm, causes, parity and choice. I would like to reflect on how we enable informed choice and support women in their decision making. This is highly relevant to performing well in the structured clinical examination in the MRCOG, as well as becoming the best doctors that we can be.

In the past, obstetricians in the UK have used a highly directive model of counselling, often described as 'paternalistic'. This is where the 'expert' paternal figure issues 'doctor's orders' as to what the patient should do, and the paternal figure is framed as protecting the patient from risk. This is still the expected model in some subcultures where the doctor is not expected to give the patient a choice, and the idea of supporting the patient's legal right to bear their own personal risks of harm seems cavalier. It is vital that the doctor recognises the potential for such 'framing error' in communication within sub-cultures, as the offering of choice can be perceived as the options being equally devoid of risk. Such patients say afterwards that they were offered a choice therefore assumed the risks were negligible, otherwise they believe the protective paternal figure would have forbidden choice. I know of legal cases for damaged babies where women have come from cultures where doctors were expected to give orders rather than choices, and the women have refused medical advice to have intervention because it was presented as a choice.

Nowadays, the shared-decision model of care involves partnership with patients and enables informed choice.[8,9] The post-modern western society is suspicious and critical of expert authority, and women place high value on personal autonomy and the right to choose and bear calculated personal risk. Adults make risk decisions every day when they smoke, drink and drive cars and so we value making our own decisions about our own medical care. Where women's autonomy and choice are not respected, women can exert their legal right to have a home birth, and this probably carries higher risks for a vaginal breech than labour in hospital. The NHS Constitution[9] and the NICE guideline for Intrapartum Care[10] specifically instruct that 'patients should have the opportunity to make informed decisions about their care and treatment, in partnership with their healthcare professionals'. Patients are, after all, experts in their own lives.

A skilled consultation requires good counselling and listening skills. The following 'three-domain decision model' imposes useful structure on the consultation and allows rapid shared analysis of the issues for each woman.

1 The first domain is the woman's perception of the risks associated with each option. There is good evidence that risk is notoriously over- or under-perceived by doctors and patients, and creating perspective to show the true size of each risk is crucial. Also, care has to be taken in applying population risks to individuals. The population risk for an adverse event may be e.g. 1 per cent, but the adverse event will either happen (100% risk) or not happen (0% risk) to that individual, irrespective of the population risk.
2 The next domain is the woman's values. Some women place very high value on vaginal birth; they may view labour as a transformative 'rite of passage' and feel deeply traumatised if they are persuaded to have a CS. Other

women place high value on the perceived convenience and control of planned CS. It needs to be established what is important to each woman, rather than the doctor make paternalistic value judgements as to what they imagine should be important.

3   The final domain is intuition or gut instinct. Sometimes we are confused by too much information and over-thinking, creating cognitive dissonance with our subliminal intuitive intelligence. There is a significant literature on intuitive knowledge, and it is probably unwise to go against a woman's gut feeling about how she should have her baby, after a full discussion of the other domains.

The concept of the 'inner consultation' is useful in providing non-directive counselling, because doctors bring their own conscious and unconscious bias to polarise their counselling. Inner consultation involves the doctor reflecting deeply upon their own feelings after the 'outer consultation' with the patient, and being open to the idea that unconscious processes drive our actions, which are often irrational and not always helpful to our patients. Such reflection brings the unconscious bias to light, and allows us to serve our patients more skilfully. In the Inner Consultation, there are no irritating patients, only irritable doctors! [10]

For example, we may see ourselves as risk averse for compassionate reasons, protecting our patients from harm. The unconscious driver may be our narcissistic urge not to look bad if things go wrong, or to be the powerful 'saviour' who fixes people. In becoming conscious of this, we can move from 'narcissistic conscientiousness' to 'compassionate conscientiousness' and better support our patients in their decisions by removing our own selfish drivers from the consultation.

Sometimes we are driven by a memory or fear of a single tragic outcome from the past, which is as irrational as generalising outcomes from an 'n=1' research trial. Or we are driven by the internalisation of a role model such as a persuasive teacher, who themselves were driven by irrational processes or outdated evidence. We could then harm large numbers of patients in trying to prevent a single unlikely complication on the basis of our single bad experience. GPs are now selected for their ability to 'bear uncertainty' so as to protect their patients from over-investigation and overly interventional approaches, where harms can exceed benefits. The price of bearing this uncertainty is sometimes being wrong, but that is seen as worthwhile in the face of the benefit of protecting the majority from harm.

And sometimes we have delusions of power over circumstances. For example, we may be rationally aware of an association of a bad outcome with a certain condition (e.g. fetal growth restriction and stillbirth, breech babies and neonatal morbidity) but be in denial that our interventions are ineffective, or come at high cost in terms of service provision or introducing new risks. We are then treating ourselves rather than our patients.

If the obstetrician recognises their own psychological tendencies in relation to clinical risk and their understanding of probabilities, we become less directive in our counselling and skilful enablers of truly informed choice, in line with each woman's legal right.[9]

UNDERSTANDING THE CONTROVERSY BETWEEN CAESAREAN SECTION AND VAGINAL BREECH

Most people interpret their world by seeing patterns, forming hypotheses around those patterns, and then continuing to see the world through this frame or hypothesis even though new facts may refute their hypothesis. If we see our beliefs as hypotheses, we are perhaps more able to let them go in the face of contesting evidence. But if we see our hypotheses as truth, or part of our identity, we can become emotional rather than rational, and we project our shadows onto our challengers unconsciously minimising our psychological distress. The history of the debate between vaginal breech and CS is often clouded by such 'believers' or 'enthusiasts' on each side clinging to their prior viewpoints, and each interpreting new findings in ways that support their prior belief. Much emotion is attached to obstetricians' beliefs about caesarean versus vaginal birth for myriad reasons. A single tragic experience of vaginal breech, or a single tragic experience of a CS, can bias in either direction and the various unconscious drivers listed under the 'inner consultation' conspire to leave us with beliefs which are less rational than we would often like to believe. Expert opinion may fly in the face of contrary factual evidence, because experts are tainted by the cognitive bias which comes from their own status as expert.

Obstetric policies around issues like CS have huge impact on society, financially, physically, socially and psychologically. We need vocal, thinking obstetricians engaging in dialectical discourse where opposing views are comfortably argued, and dangerous 'group think' avoided by accommodating a contrarian 'devil's advocate' to challenge conditioned group norms. This will help us cultivate self-awareness around our psychological tendencies if we are to discover the best way to deliver breech babies. We also need to support qualitative research to identify the vital 'patient-reported outcomes' which are the true objective of good medicine. And we should remain conscious that what seems obvious at first often turns out to be wrong.

So let us try to understand the obstetric dialectic around published evidence and the RCOG guidelines on breech.[1]

The Term Breech Trial

This extraordinary trial was published in 2000 and involved 121 centres in 26 countries, including the UK, to recruit 2088 women.[11] Their babies were extended or flexed breech, and they were randomised to either CS or vaginal breech birth. The analysis was performed on an 'intention to treat' basis which is important, because the trial was designed to inform us how to advise (or 'treat') women in antenatal clinic with breech presentation, rather than analyse the results on how the baby ended up being born. Almost 10 per cent of the women randomised to CS actually had a vaginal breech birth, and only 57 per cent of those randomised to vaginal birth actually had a vaginal birth. This tells us that the conversion to CS rate in women assigned to vaginal birth is around 43 per cent. It is important for you to make women aware of that when choosing vaginal birth when counselling for informed choice.

The trial was stopped early when the data monitoring committee noted the event rate (mortality and morbidity) was higher than expected, so the trial never reached its full statistical power. However, perinatal mortality, neonatal mortality or serious neonatal morbidity was significantly lower for the women randomised to planned CS by two thirds (RR 0.33, 95% CI 0.19–0.56). There were 17 morbid or mortal 'events' in the 1041 women in the planned CS group compared with 52 'events' out of the 1039 women in the planned vaginal birth group. There were no significant differences in terms of maternal mortality or serious maternal morbidity.

The authors concluded that 'planned caesarean section is better than planned vaginal birth for the term fetus in the breech presentation; serious maternal complications are similar between the groups'. When the trial was published, there was a massive change in worldwide obstetric practice towards CS for breech. However, the controversy, criticisms and follow-up studies which ensued are a fascinating social study in themselves. The controversy created a vital dialectic in the search for the truth of how we should organise obstetric services.

Cochrane systematic reviews 2003 and 2011

The Cochrane trial register contains three randomised trials in this area. The meta-analysis[12] contains 2396 patients and given that most of the data were from the Term Breech Trial, the results showed the same two-thirds reduction in perinatal and neonatal mortality and serious morbidity in the planned CS group. Interestingly, the highest reduction in mortality was in countries with already low mortalities, such as the UK.

However, the meta-analysis did show that planned CS was associated with increased short-term maternal morbidity (RR 1.29, 95% CI 1.03–1.61) although three months after delivery, the women allocated to CS reported less urinary incontinence (RR 0.62, 95% CI 0.41–0.93) and less perineal pain although more abdominal pain.

Vitally, at two years there were no differences in the combined outcome 'death or neurodevelopmental delay' and maternal outcomes at two years were also similar.[13] This important fact is discussed later under 'Controversy'.

In subgroup analysis, the perinatal mortality, neonatal mortality/serious neonatal morbidity was still halved (RR 0.49, 95% CI 0.26–0.91) even after the exclusion of women with prolonged labours, inductions or augmentations, footlings or the protocol violation of no experienced obstetrician being present.[12] Another subgroup analysis based on actual mode of delivery found that adverse perinatal outcomes were least with

CS before labour, then increased progressively with CS in early labour, later labour and vaginal birth.[14] Subgroup analysis has well-known methodological limitations (as trials are not designed to answer the questions fished out in later retrospective analyses) and care should be taken in drawing confident conclusions from this type of secondary analysis.[15]

Cost effectiveness

A policy of planned CS was associated with lower healthcare costs in countries with low perinatal mortalities (mean difference of $877 Canadian). Vitally, however, this did not include the future costs which may be associated with a scarred uterus e.g. likelihood of repeat CS, risk of uterine rupture and its consequences, which limits the value of the cost analysis.[12]

This has been a presented as a powerful set of arguments to support a policy of recommending planned CS for a woman found to be breech in the antenatal setting. It is harder to know how this can be extrapolated to other settings, such as initial diagnosis of breech in labour, preterm breech and twins.

The controversy: obstetric dialectics

Enormous controversy followed these publications in the obstetric world. The two-year follow-up showing no difference in the combined outcome 'death or neurodevelopmental delay' was entirely unexpected, and suggested there was no real long-term benefit of CS over vaginal birth.[3,13] The higher number of deaths in the vaginal birth group was balanced by the higher number of delayed infants in the CS group. Those neurologically delayed infants in the CS group had appeared healthy in the perinatal morbidity figures. This confirms the long-known fact that early neonatal morbidity is not a good predictor of long-term disability.

Also, although the combined outcome was a primary outcome determined prior to starting the trial, one must be careful of making a value judgement and equating a developmentally delayed infant with a baby which has died.

Likewise the apparent cost effectiveness of planned CS did not include the forward costs of the scarred uterus (e.g. increased likelihood of repeat CS, placenta accreta, uterine rupture, etc.), leading RCOG to advise the uncertainty to be communicated to women when supporting them in making their birth choices by the time the 2006 guideline was published.[1,12]

The trial was heavily criticised for its protocol violations (e.g. experienced obstetricians were not always in attendance, some breeches were footling which should have been excluded, many women were recruited in active labour and there was large institutional variation in the standards of care), although the subgroup analyses (which have methodological limitations) refuted this to some extent.[3,16-18]

The trial was also criticised for not requiring ultrasound assessment of the baby, to exclude fetal growth restriction and macrosomia, to assess the attitude for exclusion of stargazers (see below) or to confirm breech type. Three per cent of the babies in the trial were actually cephalic. Seven out of 16 perinatal deaths were due to undiagnosed fetal growth restriction. Continuous EFM was not required by the trial protocol and only one third of the babies had it. Of the 18 babies with serious early neonatal morbidity that were followed up, 17 of them were neurologically normal at 2 years and one died of congenital subglottic stenosis, a complication not obviously related to the mode of delivery.

In fact, at 2 years of age, the only significant difference in infant outcome was fewer 'medical problems in the past several months' in the vaginal birth group (15% vs 21%, p = 0.02). The neonatal immune system is stimulated by labour, and there may be causal relations between absence of labour and later allergic and auto-immune disease.[19,20] In the trial, women had a 97 per cent chance of having a neurologically normal 2-year-old, regardless of planned mode of birth. Those randomised to a trial of labour had a 6 per cent absolute lower chance (or 30 per cent relative risk reduction) of having a 2-year-old child with fewer 'medical problems in the last few months', consistent with the idea that labour confers benefits on the child's immune system.

There were calls for the authors to publish formal withdrawal of their conclusions, on the basis of the methodological critique. Others criticised the fact that the *Lancet* had fast-tracked the paper through its peer review process, thus invalidating the 'sanctity' of the peer-review process.[17] The fast track was justified by the *Lancet* on the basis of the mortal significance of the authors' conclusions, but they were accused of doing so against the advice of some of their own peer reviewers.

By 2012, some Australian obstetricians were calling for the early criticisms of the trial to be revisited as the first maternal deaths were now being reported from the complications of the original CS for the subsequent pregnancies.[18]

There is a strong argument that in units where vaginal breech is common practice, and where strict criteria are rigorously applied antenatally and during labour, vaginal breech birth is a safe option. A prospective cohort study tested this, recruiting 2526 women with planned vaginal deliveries where 71 per cent successfully had a vaginal birth and the neonatal morbidity and mortality was only 1.60 per cent (95% CI 1.14–2.17), much lower than the 5 per cent in the Term Breech Trial and not significantly different to the planned section group.[21]

THE SHORT- AND LONG-TERM RISKS OF CAESAREAN SECTION

In popular belief (as well as doctors who are not obstetricians) CS is a safe, simple operation, almost like going to the hairdressers. However, women must be made aware of the risks of haemorrhage, transfusion, sepsis, visceral injury and 'returns to theatre' in the short term as well as the psychosocial and parenting implications of longer recovery times. CS for breech increases the likelihood of having another CS in subsequent pregnancies, and repeat sections are surgically more complex with risks of placenta accreta with catastrophic haemorrhage,

obstetric hysterectomy, uterine scar rupture, cerebral palsy and maternal death.[22–26]

THE WOMAN ALREADY IN LABOUR

EBM

The RCOG guideline conclusions:
- Women should be informed that planned CS carries a reduced perinatal mortality and early neonatal morbidity for babies with a breech presentation at term compared with planned vaginal birth.
- Women should be informed that there is no evidence that the long-term health of babies with breech presentation at term is influenced by how they are born.
- Women should be advised that planned CS for breech carries a small increase in serious immediate complications for them compared with planned vaginal birth.
- Women should be advised that the long-term effects of planned CS for term breech on future pregnancy outcomes for them and their babies are uncertain.

Enabling informed choice is more challenging where a woman is diagnosed with breech for the first time whilst she is in labour. Pain, analgesia and the labour process itself produce cognitive distraction such that choices may not be made that would have been made in the cold seat of an antenatal clinic. Advice as to mode of delivery will be based on an assessment of her wishes (using the three-domain decision model described above where possible), her gestation, parity, previous labour performance, fetal wellbeing and any underlying cause for breech. The rate of progress of labour will also be a factor.

Care needs to be taken in extrapolating the recommendations to a woman with a breech in antenatal clinic, to a woman with a breech already progressing in labour. The risks of CS in labour are higher than the risks of a planned CS. Subgroup analysis from the Term Breech Trial based on actual mode of delivery found that adverse perinatal outcomes were least with CS before labour, then increased progressively with CS in early labour, later labour and vaginal birth.[14] Furthermore, the risks of a CS at or near full dilatation (second-stage CS) are particularly higher than at other times, and this needs to be weighed against the risk of vaginal breech birth and the skills available.[23–25]

THE PRETERM BREECH

The current research evidence on the term breech baby does not readily extrapolate to the preterm breech, where the baby is smaller, the risks are different and caesarean may need to be by the more complex classical method rather than lower segment (especially before 28 weeks). With a higher mortality for preterm babies, CS may also needlessly compromise a woman's future pregnancies.

The current RCOG guidelines advise that the mode of delivery for preterm labour should be discussed with the woman and her partner but that routine CS is not advised unless there are other factors.[1] While there are retrospective cohort study data showing better outcomes after CS, even the authors themselves are reluctant to attribute this to the mode of delivery as there are other sources of bias in this type of study. Poor neonatal outcomes relate more to the complications of prematurity than to vaginal birth.

On current evidence, the proven benefits to the preterm baby are with use of antenatal steroids, consideration of maternal magnesium sulphate infusion for fetal neuroprotection and delayed cord clamping, rather than mode of delivery.

On the other hand, if the woman is not in labour but there is a strong indication for delivery of the preterm baby, CS would then become appropriate.

Head entrapment is uncommon, but is a significant fear for the obstetrician assisting a woman with preterm vaginal breech birth. The smaller baby can deliver while the cervix is not completely dilated and the head can get stuck above the cervix. Gentle insertion of a finger into the cervix can frequently flex the head to bring a smaller diameter through the cervix. Alternatively, Durer's incisions on the cervix can be performed to release the head. With appropriate analgesia, the fingers of the left hand can gently grasp the cervix whilst the right hand inserts scissors to make cuts at the 4 and 8 o'clock positions, and these can be sutured postpartum if they continue to bleed.

Management points for preterm breech in labour

- What has caused labour? (e.g. abruption, amniorrhexis, sepsis, cervical weakness, polyhydramnios);
- Documentation and discussion of options;
- Neonatal counselling in anticipation of outcomes;
- Tocolysis to allow maternal steroid benefits;
- Antenatal steroids;
- Magnesium sulphate for fetal neuroprotection;
- Analgesia (e.g. epidural may allow obstetric manoeuvres such as Durer incisions, and the softened pelvic floor may be protective to the immature skull as well as preventing maternal pushing before full dilatation);
- Gentle handling during delivery to minimise bruising, visceral and intracranial injury;
- There may be a benefit to the baby of being delivered within the membranes (*en caulle*);
- If CS is required, for smaller babies before 28 weeks, the lower segment may be empty or unformed, and consideration should be given to the low classical section, or J- or T-shaped uterine incisions. This minimises the traction and trauma to the fragile preterm baby. The abdominal incision (as opposed to the uterine incision) however is usually still low transverse;

- Cord clamping should be delayed by a timed 30 seconds, with the baby held dependent in a birth bag to prevent evaporation and heat loss;
- Senior paediatrician present at delivery.

FIRST TWIN IS BREECH

In assisting the woman to make an informed choice, it seems reasonable to extrapolate the research findings from singleton breech to twins where the first twin is breech.[1] This would be to advise the woman of the reduced perinatal complications for the first baby, but the increase in short-term complications for her, and less certain longer-term issues for future pregnancy.

There is a traditional anxiety about breech/cephalic twin pairs 'interlocking' where the after-coming head gets stuck above the second twin's head. This is rare (around 1 in 817 where twin I is breech) and is signalled by slow descent of the trunk. It is treated either by external displacement of twin II head upwards, or by immediate CS. It is an argument for performing breech/cephalic twin deliveries in an operating theatre rather than a labour suite.

SECOND TWIN IS BREECH

For the 40 per cent of twins where the first twin is a cephalic presentation but the second twin is non-vertex, current guidelines do not support routine CS.[1] Various cohort studies and small randomised trials have shown no benefit to CS, although these are statistically under-powered to show small but significant differences.

Where the second twin begins as non-vertex, once the first baby has delivered, the second twin often turns to cephalic spontaneously. Alternatively, the obstetrician can perform ECV in uterine diastole, followed by amniotomy at the height of a contraction. Many practitioners prefer to perform internal podalic version, by grasping the feet through the membranes then performing amniotomy at the height of contraction (to minimise the risk of cord prolapse) followed by breech extraction. This is probably the only agreed indication for active breech extraction in UK practice.

PRACTICAL SKILLS

External cephalic version

The RCOG guidelines advise that women with a breech baby should be offered ECV as it lowers their chances of having a CS.[27] For every six women attempting ECV, it will prevent one of them having a CS. About 50 per cent of ECV attempts are successful in turning the baby, but the baby can turn back again. Also women following successful ECV have a higher rate of obstetric intervention than women who have not had ECV.

ECV should be offered from 36 weeks' gestation in nulliparous women and from 37 weeks in multiparous women.

Conduct of external cephalic version

- Informed consent to include discussion of 50 per cent likelihood of success and small risk of placental abruption or cord entanglement (of the order of 0.5 per cent). They should also be advised that it can be uncomfortable but that they can stop any time they wish. Ideally, this information would be provided in a written form.
- Ultrasound to confirm breech, type of breech and position of spine as well as to exclude placenta praevia, fibroids or fetal anomaly.
- It is common practice to obtain 30 minutes of CTG to assess fetal wellbeing.
- Lay patient with head slightly below feet to allow breech to disengage. Left lateral tilt or a wedge can be used to prevent aorto-caval compression.
- Terbutaline can be given to aid uterine relaxation as this improves the chances of success. The woman should be warned that it can cause tachycardia and feelings of anxiety.
- A mixture of nitrous oxide and air can be used to aid relaxation.
- The obstetrician should elevate the breech from the pelvis and attempt to flex the baby by gently pushing the head forwards towards the breech.
- Then a forward roll should be attempted. Sometimes the baby just has to be flexed and held for a kick to cause it to turn itself.
- If this fails, a backward flip can be attempted.
- If this fails, the fetal heart should be checked followed by a 30-minute CTG. The mother should be advised to attend if there is bleeding or amniorrhexis.
- A discussion needs to follow as to the alternatives of vaginal breech birth or CS, and full documentation is essential.
- Anti-D prophylaxis if appropriate.

Absolute contraindications to ECV

- Where caesarean is necessary for other reasons;
- Antepartum haemorrhage within 7 days;
- Abnormal CTG;
- Major uterine anomaly;
- Ruptured membranes;
- Multiple pregnancy (except after delivery of first twin).

Conditions such as fetal growth restriction, pre-eclampsia and previous CS are not absolute contraindications, but many obstetricians would not perform ECV in these situations.

Conduct of assisted vaginal breech birth

Breech extraction vs assisted vaginal breech

Firstly, don't make the common error of confusing *assisted vaginal breech delivery* with *vaginal breech extraction*,[5,6] as these are very different techniques.

Vaginal breech extraction is when you apply traction on the baby to pull it down, either by fingers in the flexed groin, or pulling on a foot or feet. In the UK this is not recommended for a vaginal breech except for a second twin, usually after podalic version. The worry is that traction can cause the trunk and neck to de-flex (by the Moro reflex), making the baby look upwards ('stargazing') which would draw the highest cephalic diameter (mento-vertical) down and make delivery difficult.

Assisted vaginal breech delivery is when the natural process of labour including maternal effort causes flexion and descent of the baby, and the obstetric manoeuvres are only used to free the head and limbs. Traction is avoided almost completely, at least until after birth of the umbilicus.

Assessment criteria for assisted vaginal breech

Prior to assisting a vaginal breech birth, it is vital to consider the following criteria:[1]

- Woman's choice based on accurate understanding of risks and benefits to herself and baby.
- Factors excluded which are likely to exacerbate mechanical difficulties e.g. placenta praevia, fibroids, hydrocephalus or myelomeningocele, pelvic disruption (e.g. childhood rickets).
- Fetal growth restriction is often associated with breech presentation. The associated placental insufficiency means the baby will be less likely to tolerate the cord compression associated with the later stages of breech delivery.
- Large babies may be more likely to benefit from CS e.g. estimated weight above 3800 g; diabetic macrosomia may also be associated with higher susceptibility to hypoxia.
- Extended ('frank') breech is easiest to deliver vaginally, followed by flexed ('complete') breech. Footling breech at term where hip and knee are both extended is probably best delivered by CS.
- Clinical pelvimetry should confirm adequacy of pelvis and help exclude feto-pelvic disproportion.
- Previous obstetric history such as previous CS would usually preclude vaginal breech birth (although there are small cohort studies with largely successful outcomes).

Ultrasound prior to vaginal breech

The obstetrician assisting a vaginal breech birth should be appropriately trained in the use of ultrasound[1] for the following:

- Exclude placenta praevia and fibroids;
- Exclude macrosomia and fetal growth restriction;
- Identify type of breech;
- 'Stargazers' with hyperextended necks may have poorer outcomes (thought to be due either to nuchal cord, uterine anomalies or congenital iniencephaly);
- Estimated fetal weight can be calculated. Although there is no good evidence to support its use, and there is at least 15 per cent error in the estimate, many practitioners recommend CS if the estimate is above 3800 g, as per the RCOG guidelines.

Clinical pelvimetry

Many practitioners recommend clinical pelvimetry prior to vaginal breech to help exclude feto-pelvic disproportion, but the evidence base is weak and the assessments are highly subjective.[1–4] X-ray and MRI pelvimetry have been extensively used in the past but studies have failed to show their usefulness in predicting vaginal birth or improving neonatal outcomes. A method of clinical pelvimetry is as follows.

- Ensure the woman understands the purpose, process and discomfort of pelvic assessment and freely gives consent.
- Remember to document the name and presence of the chaperone.
- Gently insert a finger in the vagina and palpate posteriorly up to the sacral promontory. The distance from the promontory to the lower surface of the pubic symphysis is the 'obstetric conjugate diameter'. It serves as a clinical approximation of the pelvic inlet (which cannot be directly measured clinically as it's the distance from the promontory to the upper surface of the pubic symphysis).
- It is held that the obstetric conjugate diameter should be more than 11.5 cm for successful vaginal breech. The obstetrician should know the length of his/her own forefinger to each knuckle and to the pollex–metacarpal angle. My own is 17.5 cm with 11.5 cm forefinger length, so if I can't reach the promontory, that is a good sign.
- From the promontory, the finger should turn towards the sacrum, and then palpate the depth of the sacral curve. Ideally the curve is deep and capacious rather than flat. (Take greater care if the rectum is full.)
- Turn the fingers towards the front and gently open them to palpate the ischial spines in the mid-pelvis, which should not be too prominent. If analgesia is appropriate (e.g. epidural), the intertuberous distance should accommodate a closed fist.
- Fingers facing the front, gently palpate the angle under the pubic symphysis. The ideal sub-pubic arch allows space for two fingers to be side by side unlike the android pelvis where the fingers are crushed into overlap.

Continuous EFM

The commonest avoidable cause of perinatal morbidity and mortality in breech has been identified as sub-optimal care in labour.[1,3] For this reason, continuous EFM is recommended. Although FBS can be performed from fetal buttocks, the higher background risk for breech babies means that CS may be the better response to CTG abnormalities in breech labour.

Induction or augmentation of labour

Although there is no high-quality evidence to inform practice in the area of induction or augmentation, many experienced obstetricians worry that slow progress in labour may represent feto-pelvic disproportion and the RCOG guideline advises against augmentation. IOL is supported by the RCOG guidelines 'where individual circumstances are favourable'. ACOG currently do not support the use of oxytocin either for induction or augmentation, whereas the Canadian College supports oxytocin only for augmentation where there is uterine inertia.[1–4]

Analgesia

There were arguments in the past in favour of epidural analgesia because it allowed obstetric manoeuvres to be performed with ease, such as Durer's incisions, forceps to the after-coming head, etc. It was also argued that the softer pelvic floor with the dense motor block common with older-style epidurals (which used more local anaesthetic than opioid) offered protection to the vulnerable fetal skull, particularly with preterm breech. Epidural may also prevent maternal pushing before full dilatation. In the absence of strong evidence to the contrary, the current RCOG guidelines recommend individualised discussion with each woman, offering the full range of analgesic options including spinal, epidural or pudendal block.

Timing of first and second stages of breech labour

Active labour is diagnosed when there are strong regular uterine contractions and the cervix is 4 cm or more dilated. Uterine contractions before this dilatation are part of the latent phase of the first stage of labour. The Term Breech Trial protocol allowed for normal progress to be anything more than 0.5 cm per hour. However, there are more recent data suggesting that progress from 5 cm to 10 cm should not be more than 7 hours.[3,10,11]

Full dilatation is more difficult to diagnose with a breech presentation than cephalic, because the softer presenting part starts to descend through the cervix before full dilatation, and so an experienced practitioner should confirm full dilatation, trying to assess around the sides of the presenting part and above in case a rim of cervix is hiding there. Correct diagnosis is essential because timing the length of the second stage is an important criterion for good outcome. The Term Breech Trial allowed for a second stage of 3.5 hours. Based on this and later data, it seems reasonable to allow 90 minutes of passive second stage for the breech to descend and up to 60 minutes of active second stage, giving a maximum full second stage of 2.5 hours.[3,10,11] If strict safety criteria are being applied, it would seem prudent to recommend CS if the baby has not delivered by this time, even if the breech is on the perineum (assuming accurate diagnosis of the onset of full dilatation).

Neonatology

Because breech babies frequently have low Apgar scores, a neonatologist of sufficient experience should be present at the birth.

Technique of assisted vaginal breech[1,3,5,6,27]

1 Ensure again that the woman has made an informed choice which has been documented.
2 Perform ultrasound and clinical pelvimetry as above and discuss analgesia, continuous fetal monitoring and the indications for changing to CS (slow progress or CTG

abnormality). Discuss birth positions (most experience is with the lithotomy position) and what will happen at delivery in terms of waiting, pushing and assisting, and who will be present (anaesthetist, neonatologist, midwife, etc.).

3 The active first stage of labour should progress at 0.5–1 cm per hour with supportive coaching. Slow progress or CTG abnormalities should give strong consideration to CS given the higher background risk for breech babies.

4 At full dilatation, the traditional advice is patience and 'Keep your hands off the breech until it's climbing the perineum.' Significant delay in descent in the second stage or significant CTG abnormalities should give strong consideration for CS as feto-pelvic disproportion and cord compression are risks. Otherwise, the appearance of the fetal anus at the perineum should be patiently awaited with uterine contractions and maternal effort alone.

5 Once the fetal breech is at the perineum, with her agreement, the woman is placed in the lithotomy position with some lateral tilt or a wedge to minimise aorto-caval compression. If there is no epidural, a pudendal block or perineal block can be inserted as appropriate.

6 If the perineum is being distended, an episiotomy can be performed with consent around now, taking care to avoid the fetal genitalia. There is an old argument to avoid episiotomy as the firm perineum encourages flexion of the baby, but selective episiotomy is supported by the RCOG guideline if thought to be appropriate.

7 The breech usually enters the pelvis with the inter-trochanteric diameter in the pelvic transverse (sacro-posterior) then rotates through 90° so the breech appears at the perineum in the sacro-lateral position. As descent occurs by uterine contraction and maternal effort, the breech usually rotates to the sacro-posterior position again as the shoulders enter the pelvis with the bisacromial diameter in the pelvic transverse. Although advice at this stage is 'Keep your hands off the breech', and no traction should be applied, it is acceptable to perform small rotational movements to help 'get the back up' to sacro-posterior.

8 Visceral injury is a real risk to breech babies, as are deep haematomas in thighs, calves and arms. Gentleness in handling the baby is essential, and the rotational movement should be applied by grasping the buttocks with the thumbs against the bony sacrum. With larger hands it is tempting to grasp round the abdomen and kidneys but this can cause perinephric haematomas and adrenal trauma (Fig. 57.1).

9 Spontaneous delivery of the buttocks and trunk should continue to the level of the umbilicus when many practitioners advise gently pulling down a loop of cord to protect against compressive cord injury. Others advise against handling cord as it may cause vasospasm. Each situation must be judged on its own merits.

10 For the extended breech climbing the perineum (once the umbilicus has delivered), two fingers can be slid along

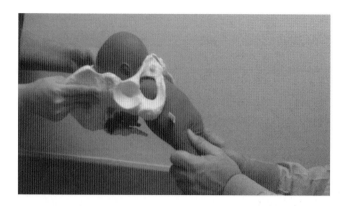

Fig. 57.1 Fingers grasp sacrum not kidneys (with the assistance of Ruth Cavey-Wilcox and Sami Saba)

the posterior surface of the fetal thigh towards the popliteal fossa. Gentle pressure along the thigh causes slight abduction of the hips along with gentle pressure on each popliteal fossa to allow flexion of the knee in its natural plane of movement which brings the foot down, expediting delivery (Pinard's manoeuvre). Gentleness and natural planes of movement will help avoid femoral fracture and hip dislocation.

11 Now the legs and trunk have delivered, the breech is allowed to hang on the perineum until the lower border of the fetal scapula is seen under the pubic arch.

12 This is a critical stage because the cord is now delivered and at risk of compression as the head enters the pelvis. Ideally, delivery from now should occur within 3 minutes. This is more time than it may seem, and sufficient for allowing calm progression through the appropriate delivery manoeuvres. The obstetrician should be aware of the risk of panic at this stage, because traction and firm grasping of the abdomen or limbs should be avoided. Traction can cause the head to de-flex or the arms to extend, making the delivery all the more fraught. Remind yourself that the baby will deliver, once all the practised moves are made, and it's important to portray calm to the patient and delivery team so that everyone cooperates and the mother feels safe and does not tense up and lose control.

13 When the scapula is seen and the baby's back is up, slide two fingers up the baby's spine, then laterally over the fetal shoulder and down the arm to splint the humerus and gently push the fetal arm over the chest and down in a 'windscreen wiper' movement for delivery of the hands. Gentleness and natural planes of joint movement will minimise the risk of humeral fracture and shoulder dislocation. The baby can be rotated 90° to either side to make this easier, but the abdomen should not be grasped, only the buttocks with thumbs pressing on the hard sacrum. If the baby is slippery and hard to rotate, a drape can be used to wrap the baby which also helps keep it warm (Fig. 57.2).

SECOND STAGE OF LABOUR

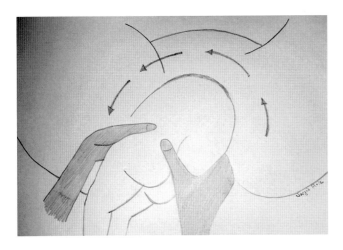

Fig. 57.2 Rotating the baby (Lovset manoeuvre) (by courtesy of Dr Nargis Pirie)

14 The main issues around delivery of the fetal head are promoting and maintaining flexion to minimise arrest of the after-coming head and gentle, slow delivery to minimise the risk of reverberation injury from sudden compression–decompression of an unmoulded head. With the head in flexion, the smallest diameter of the fetal head is brought down (the sub-occipito-bregmatic diameter, same as in occipito-anterior vertex births). De-flexion will increase the diameter to the sub-fronto-occipital diameter (same as in occipito-posterior cephalic births) and extension will bring the widest diameter into play, the mento-vertical.

15 The trunk, arms and legs have been delivered and can be supported by the obstetrician while the trunk is allowed to hang on the perineum, allowing flexion of the head. When the nape of the neck (hairline) is seen under the pubic arch, the head can be delivered by one of three methods, all of which should be gentle and slow. The RCOG guideline states there is no evidence to favour one over another although concerns have been expressed about the Burns-Marshall method where hyperextension of the neck can be dangerous. The three methods are:

- *Mauriceau-Smellie-Veit (MSV) manoeuvre*: the baby's trunk is supported along the forearm of the obstetrician who pushes the fingers of the supporting arm against the fetal malar bones to pull the head into flexion. The other hand can be applied to the nape of the neck to increase the flexion. Traditionally, a finger was placed in the fetal mouth to cause flexion, but this can result in jaw dislocation unless it is done very gently. This two-handed flexion manoeuvre splints and protects the cervical spine, and the head is moved towards the mother's back rather than her feet to allow a controlled delivery of the head (Fig. 57.3).

- *Forceps to the after-coming head*: some obstetricians favour this method because they believe the cradling effect of the forceps protects the head against compression–decompression injury as well as allowing flexion and controlled descent. A scrubbed assistant is

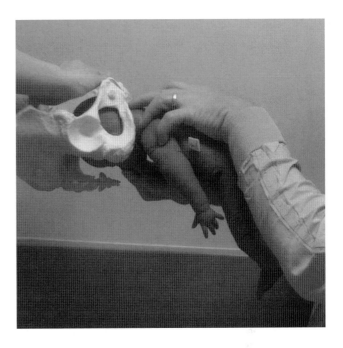

Fig. 57.3 Flexing the head in MSV manoeuvre (with the assistance of Ruth Cavey-Wilcox and Sami Saba)

required to hold the baby's trunk and legs just above the horizontal plane, taking care not to over-extend the neck. The forceps are applied by wandering them over the head in the 4 and 8 o'clock positions with the other hand guiding the tips and protecting the maternal tissues. Any long-handled forceps can be used (including Kiellands), although Piper's forceps were specifically developed for this purpose if they are available (I have never seen them in the UK). Gentle traction is applied during a contraction with maternal effort. The direction of traction is towards the floor until the chin and mouth are seen, then the forceps and trunk are raised upwards for the head to be delivered.

- *The Burns-Marshall method*: a scrubbed assistant wraps a drape round the baby's trunk and legs to improve grip and keep baby warm. The legs and trunk are gently swept upwards, extending the neck. Great care is required not to hyperextend the neck as such concerns have been voiced about this method. This allows the head to flex within the pelvis and effect delivery. I personally have very little experience of the method.

Managing the complications of assisted vaginal breech

The following manoeuvres should be practised on models until deeply internalised for their instinctive use in emergency.

1 *Delay in head entering the pelvis*: if the trunk and legs have delivered but the head does not engage, the RCOG guideline recommends suprapubic pressure by an assistant to assist flexion of the head (Bracht's manoeuvre) (Fig. 57.4). The buttocks can be grasped and used to

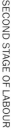

SECOND STAGE OF LABOUR

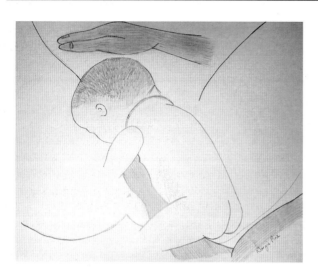

Fig. 57.4 Suprapubic pressure in Bracht manoeuvre (by courtesy of Dr Nargis Pirie)

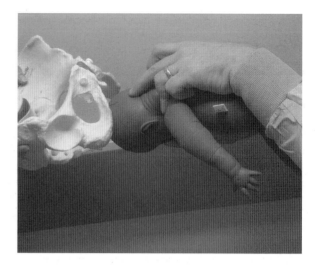

Fig. 57.5 Flexion and descent with MSV manoeuvre (with the assistance of Ruth Cavey-Wilcox and Sami Saba)

rotate the baby sideways at the same time, to allow the long axis of the head to enter the pelvis in the transverse or oblique diameter. Failing this the MSV manoeuvre can be used as described above, but this time with the hand inside the birth canal (Fig. 57.5).

2 *Arrest of the after-coming head*: if the trunk, legs and arms have delivered but the head has arrested despite the manoeuvres already described, the RCOG guideline recommends consideration of Durer's cervical incisions if the cervix is not completely dilated, or consideration of symphysiotomy or even replacing the trunk and performing CS, all of which have been successfully described.

3 *Nuchal arm or arms*: if the arms are not in their usual position of being flexed across the fetal chest or face, they may be trapped behind the neck. It is rare for this to be both arms. The buttocks should be grasped (a drape helps with this) and the baby rotated in the direction of the trapped hand. This 'unwinds' the arm from the neck and allows delivery as above. The manoeuvre can be reversed to 'unwind' the other arm.

4 *Extended arms*: Lovset's manoeuvre[28] involves grasping the buttocks, exerting gentle downwards traction and rotation with the back in the anterior oblique position, then flexing the baby laterally by lifting the trunk upwards to bring the posterior shoulder into the pelvis. The baby is then gently rotated to bring that posterior shoulder anteriorly under the symphysis where the arm can then be delivered. This is then reversed to deliver the other arm.

5 *Posterior rotation of the trunk*: occasionally, the baby has not been kept with the back upwards, perhaps because of rapid delivery. The head is then in an occipito-posterior position. It can sometimes be rotated to occipito-anterior (taking great care not to place rotational strain on the cervical spine) where delivery can be completed as normal. If it cannot be rotated, a reverse Prague

manoeuvre can be used where the right hand lifts the baby's feet upwards and forwards to flex the baby, and the left hand cradles beneath the shoulders pulling gently downwards to flex the head and effect delivery.

Developing and maintaining assisted breech delivery skills

With the increasing use of CS, most practice for assisted breech will come from use of a model pelvis and doll. I personally prefer a bony or plastic pelvis to the covered mannequins as it lets you see the diameters correctly. The manoeuvres should be practised over and over again by every MRCOG candidate until they are second nature. When delivering a breech at CS, it is also possible to use similar manoeuvres (although it's more akin to a breech extraction), and this is an ideal way to rehearse the motor skills in safe handling of a vaginal breech (but remember no traction in the latter). Labour suites should organise regular 'skills drills' where the whole team manage an unexpected breech birth together. Courses widely available in the UK such as ALSO, MOET and PROMPT also include breech delivery skills.

KEY POINTS

- Breech affects 3 per cent of babies at term and 20 per cent at 28 weeks, and can be a siren for later development problems.
- Ultrasound can be used to assess the cause of breech which may direct subsequent management e.g. placenta praevia, fetal anomaly.
- Caesarean section has become the favoured recommendation in most circumstances, on the basis of research evidence and guidelines based on better early neonatal outcomes, but these are still subject to debate and

further analysis as longer-term infant outcomes seem no different yet the risks to mothers are higher.

- Routine CS is not currently advised for preterm breech babies in labour.
- Twins in labour may benefit from CS where the first twin is breech as for singleton pregnancies, but not so where only the second twin is breech.
- Vaginal breech delivery skills should be practised until they are intuitive on birth simulators, and standard manoeuvres for minimisation of risks, for the situations where vaginal breech is still inevitable.
- Evidence and RCOG guidelines around breech should be critically appraised and form a vital part of MRCOG preparation and subsequent Continuing Professional Development.

CONCLUSION

The research on vaginal breech has borne fruit which remains ripe for debate around evidence quality, the ethics of choice and service provision, and most of all the apprenticed skill of the obstetrician in counselling, enabling informed choice and safely conducting external cephalic version or an assisted vaginal breech birth and minimising the chance of complications. This is a rich seam of gold for the aspiring MRCOG candidate to explore and demonstrate their excellence in the Membership exam, and beyond into a lifetime of practicing the craft.

References

1. RCOG. *The Management of Breech Presentation*, Guideline No. 20b. London: RCOG Press, 2006, reviewed 2010.
2. The Royal Australian and New Zealand College of Obstetricians and Gynaecologists College Statement: C-Obs 11. *Management of Breech Presentation at Term*. RANZCOG, 2013.
3. Society of Obstetricians and Gynaecologists of Canada. *Vaginal Delivery of Breech Presentation (Guideline 226) 2009*. Canada: Society of Obstetricians and Gynaecologists of Canada.
4. ACOG. Committee Opinion No. 340, Mode of term singleton breech delivery. *Obstet Gynecol* 2006;108:235–7.
5. Donald I. *Practical Obstetric Problems*. London: Lloyd-Luke Ltd, 1974.
6. Chassar Moir J, Myerscough PR. *Munro Kerr's Operative Obstetrics*. 8th edn. London: Balliere, Tindall and Cassell, 1971.
7. Wilson JMG, Jungner G. *Principles and practice of screening for disease*. Geneva: WHO, 1968.
8. Neighbour R. *The Inner Consultation: how to develop an effective and intuitive consulting style*. 2nd edn. Oxford: Radcliffe Publishing Ltd, 2004.
9. Department of Health. *The NHS Constitution*. London: Crown Office, 2013.
10. NICE. *Intrapartum care: care of healthy women and their babies during labour (CG190)*. London: NICE, 2014.
11. Hannah ME, Hannah WJ, Hewson SA, Hodnett ED, Saigal S. Planned caesarean section versus planned vaginal birth for breech presentation at term: a randomised multicentre trial. Term Breech Trial Collaborative Group. *Lancet* 2000; 356:1375–83.
12. Hofmeyer GJ, Hannah M, Lawrie TA. Planned caesarean section for term breech delivery. *Cochrane Database Syst Rev* 2011.
13. Whyte H *et al.* Outcomes of children at 2 years after planned caesarean birth versus planned vaginal birth for breech presentation at term: The international randomised term breech trial. *Am J Obstet Gynecol* 2004;191:864.
14. Su ML, McLeod L, Ross S *et al.*; Term Breech Trial Collaborative Group. Factors associated with adverse perinatal outcome in the Term Breech Trial. *Am J Obstet Gynecol* 2003;189:740–5.
15. Kotaska A. Inappropriate use of randomised trials to evaluate complex phenomena: Case study of vaginal breech delivery. *BMJ* 2004;329:1029.
16. Glezerman M. Five years to the term breech trial: the rise and fall of a randomized controlled trial. *Am J Obstet Gynecol* 2006;194(1):20–5.
17. Bewley S, Shennan A. Peer review and the Term Breech Trial. *Lancet* 2007;369(9565):906.
18. Lawson GW. The term breech trial ten years on: primum non nocere? *Birth* 2012;39(1):3–9.
19. Negele K, Heinrich J, Borte M *et al*. Mode of delivery and development of atopic disease during the first 2 years of life. *Pediatr Allergy Immunol* 2004;15:48–54.
20. Laubereau B, Filipiak-Pittroff B, von Berg A *et al*. Caesarean section and gastrointestinal symptoms, atopic dermatitis, and sensitisation during the first year of life. *Arch Dis Child* 2004;89:993–7.
21. Goffinet F, Carayol M, Foidart J-M *et al*. For the PREMODA Study Group. Is planned vaginal delivery for breech presentation at term still an option? Results of an observational prospective survey in France and Belgium. *Am J Obstet Gynecol* 2006;194:1002–11.
22. Armstrong CA, Harding S, Matthews T, Dickinson JE. Is placenta accreta catching up with us? *Aust N Z J Obstet Gynaecol* 2004;44: 210–3.
23. McKelvey A, Ashe R, McKenna D, Roberts RJ. Caesarean section in the second stage of labour: a retrospective review of obstetric setting and morbidity. *Obstet Gynaecol* 2010;30(3):264–7.

SECOND STAGE OF LABOUR

24. Bahl R, Strachan B, Murphy DJ. Outcome of subsequent pregnancy three years after previous operative delivery in the second stage of labour: cohort study. *BMJ* 2004;328:311.

25. Murphy DJ, Liebling RE, Verity L, Swingler R, Patel R. Early maternal and neonatal morbidity associated with operative delivery in second stage of labour: a cohort study. *Lancet* 2001;358 (9289):1203–7.

26. Van Roosmalen J, Meguid T. The dilemma of vaginal breech delivery worldwide. *Lancet* 2014; 383(9932):1863–4.

27. RCOG. *External Cephalic Version and Reducing the Incidence of Breech Presentation*, Guideline No 20a. London: RCOG Press, 2006, reviewed 2010.

28. Løvset J. Shoulder delivery by breech presentation. *J Obset Gynaecol Brit Emp* 1937;44:696–704.

Chapter 58 Perineal trauma

Lucy Kean

MRCOG standards

Theoretical skills

- Have a clear understanding of the impact of severe vaginal trauma and be able to counsel women about vaginal delivery following third-degree or fourth-degree tears.
- Have completed the programme of FGM e-modules developed by Health Education England.
- Be able to identify and refer women in antenatal clinic who have undergone female genital mutilation.
- Have attended a course on repair of third- and fourth-degree perineal trauma.

Practical skills

- Be able to recognise and grade the degree of perineal trauma, including recognition of the degree of anal sphincter damage.
- Be able to repair second- and third-degree perineal trauma.
- Be able to repair fourth-degree trauma under supervision.
- Have attended skills drills on obstetric collapse.
- Be able to recognise and manage paravaginal haematomas.

In addition, we suggest the following.

Theoretical skills

- Revise your knowledge of pelvic anatomy.

INTRODUCTION

Perineal trauma is a common event in first labours, affecting up to 90 per cent of first-time mothers. It is a cause for concern for many women and in some countries has led to a large increase in the numbers of women requesting elective caesarean section. Considerable postnatal morbidity and occasionally mortality can be attributed to this, and therefore a clear understanding of the best management of perineal trauma is mandatory for every clinician working in obstetrics.

ANATOMY OF THE PELVIC FLOOR AND DEFINITIONS OF TRAUMA

In order to understand the pathophysiology of perineal trauma, an understanding of the anatomy of the pelvic floor is required.

First-degree trauma is defined as injury to the perineal skin alone. Second-degree trauma involves injury to the perineum including the perineal muscles but not involving the anal sphincter. Figure 58.1 shows the muscles of the perineum and the usual extensions of mediolateral and midline episiotomy.

Third-degree extensions involve any part of the anal sphincter complex (external and internal sphincters) and fourth-degree encompasses extension into the rectal mucosa.

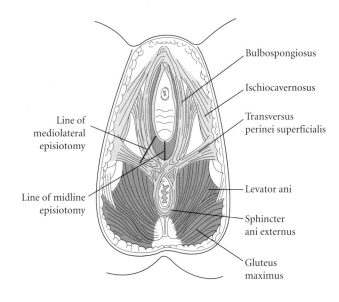

Fig. 58.1 Muscles of the perineum

RCOG recommends classifying anal sphincter damage as follows:[1]

- 3a: less than 50 per cent of the external anal sphincter (EAS) is torn;
- 3b: more than 50 per cent of the external anal sphincter is torn;
- 3c: tear involving the internal anal sphincter (almost always involves complete disruption of the external sphincter);
- 4th degree: injury to the both the external and internal anal sphincter complex and anal epithelium.

FIRST- AND SECOND-DEGREE PERINEAL TRAUMA

In a first pregnancy, perineal trauma affects up to 90 per cent of women, with episiotomy rates of 40–60 per cent being common in many countries. Following delivery the perineum is often the source of much discomfort and pain for many women. Morbidity to the perineum may persist for weeks to years post-delivery. This can result in a cascade of events such as dyspareunia, psychosexual dysfunction, maladjustment to motherhood and relationship breakdown. Minimising the risk of perineal trauma should therefore be at the forefront of care during labour.

RISK FACTORS FOR PERINEAL TRAUMA

It is recognised that perineal trauma is associated with:

- larger infants;
- prolonged labour;
- instrumental delivery.

Instrumental delivery and forceps delivery in particular increase the risk of extended trauma, with as many as 60 per cent of women experiencing ultrasonographically visible anal sphincter defects in research studies.[2] Long second stage also appears to contribute to perineal damage. Malposition of the fetal head in labour is a risk factor for long labour and instrumental delivery and thus perineal trauma.

REDUCING THE RISK OF PERINEAL TRAUMA

Perineal massage

Perineal massage antenatally appears to slightly reduce the need for episiotomy in first-time mothers and reduce pain at three months in women who have had a baby before. Fifteen women need to undertake this to avoid one case of trauma, but this is a simple technique that women can be taught in parent education classes and has no harm [A].[3] Also the application

of warm compresses during the second stage has been shown to reduce the incidence of third- and fourth-degree tears. The physiology behind this is very unclear, but as women find this acceptable, there is no reason not to use this [A].[4]

The role of episiotomy

Liberal use of mediolateral episiotomy does not appear to reduce the incidence of third-degree tears. In the most recent Cochrane evaluation, eight studies involving 5541 women were examined. In the routine episiotomy group, 75 per cent of women had episiotomies; in the restrictive episiotomy group 28 per cent did.

Combining trials of restrictive policy for episiotomy compared with standard care gives the following results:

- less severe perineal trauma (RR 0.67, 95% CI 0.49–0.91);
- more anterior perineal trauma (RR 1.84, 95% CI 1.61–2.10);
- less suturing (RR 0.71, 95% CI 0.61–0.81);
- fewer healing complications (RR 0.69, 95% CI 0.56–0.85);
- no difference in:
  - severe vaginal/perineal trauma (RR 0.92, 95% CI 0.72–1.18);
  - dyspareunia (RR 1.02, 95% CI 0.90–1.16);
  - urinary incontinence (RR 0.98, 95% CI 0.79–1.20);
  - pain scores.

Midline episiotomy certainly increases the risk of extended trauma, with a reported OR of 4.5–6 for third-degree or fourth-degree tears [A].[5]

NICE has recommended that:

- There is considerable high-level evidence that the routine use of episiotomy (trial mean 71.6%, range 44.9–93.7%) is not of benefit to women either in the short or longer term, compared with restricted use (trial mean 29.1%, range 7.6–53.0%) [A].
- Where an episiotomy is performed, the recommended technique is a mediolateral episiotomy originating at the vaginal fourchette and usually directed to the right side. The angle to the vertical axis should be between 45 and 60 degrees at the time of the episiotomy [A].[6]

This final point is an important practice point, as a common error made by inexperienced practitioners is to angle the episiotomy too vertically. Perineal stretching at crowning makes the perineum appear broader and therefore a much more horizontal angle of incision is required than would be expected. In a prospective case–control study there was a 50 per cent relative reduction in risk of sustaining third-degree tear observed for every 6 degrees away from the perineal midline that an episiotomy was cut. Recent data from Scandinavia have shown that education of practitioners regarding the mechanism of birth and the correct angle of episiotomy (and also using a hands-on approach) led to a reduction in extended trauma of 50 per cent. These data are not randomised and so we must be careful in using this in practice, but good education regarding birth and how to perform episiotomy is vital.

Conduct of normal birth

The conduct of delivery has also been examined in three studies. Changing established practice is obviously difficult, in one study there was only 73 per cent compliance in the 'hands poised' group (vs 95 per cent in 'hands on').[7] Across the three relevant studies the rates of perineal trauma were similar in both groups: 29 per cent first-degree trauma and 37 per cent second-degree trauma. Thus, conduct of the delivery in terms of a hands-on or -off approach showed no advantage of one method over the other.

The use of Lidocaine spray has been evaluated and shown to have no effect on pain, but possibly a small reduction in trauma rates [B].[6]

Birth position in women without an epidural does not influence perineal trauma rates (increased spontaneous trauma but reduced episiotomy rates in women who were not supine). Non-supine positions were also associated with higher rates of bleeding but fewer fetal heart rate abnormalities, a marginally shorter second stage (by 4.28 mins) and less pain [A]).[6]

Mode of delivery

Mode of delivery has a large impact on rates of perineal trauma. Of course, elective CS prevents damage to the perineum from labour-related events, and reducing the rates of instrumental vaginal delivery will reduce the incidence of perineal trauma.

Ventouse delivery appears to be associated with less perineal trauma (see Chapter **). Ventouse delivery (risk difference 0.06, 95% CI 0.10, 0.02) and spontaneous birth (0.11, 95% CI 0.18, 0.04) causes less anal sphincter trauma than forceps delivery. However, at 5-year follow-up there is no difference in reported symptoms in women delivered by either ventouse or forceps. Therefore, given that the highest rates of severe perineal damage occur in women for whom two instruments are needed to achieve delivery, the first choice must be the instrument most likely to deliver the baby safely and with which the obstetrician is experienced.

Episiotomy has been recommended when instrumental vaginal delivery is performed. This is not based on any randomised evidence.[8] Ventouse delivery in a multiparous woman may not require any episiotomy, and an intact perineum may result. However, a forceps delivery in a nulliparous woman is likely to require episiotomy and a good technique with a correct angle of cut will minimise the risk of extended trauma [C].[9]

Prolonged second stage and epidural analgesia

The issue of epidural analgesia and instrumental delivery are closely linked and trials that attempt to divide the two are difficult to perform. Epidural analgesia has been shown to be associated with an increased risk of instrumental vaginal delivery, with the attendant perineal morbidity [A]. There is an association between long second stage and perineal trauma, with increased risk of severe trauma in women experiencing long second stages. However, it has been shown that allowing a passive second stage in nulliparae with continuous epidural analgesia reduces the incidence of difficult instrumental delivery (RR 0.79, 95% CI 0.66–0.95). Spontaneous delivery is also slightly more likely among women who delay pushing (RR 1.09, 95% CI 1.00–1.18).[10] NICE recommends that consideration should be given to the use of oxytocin, with the offer of regional analgesia, for nulliparous women if contractions are inadequate at the onset of the second stage. NICE guidance is clear that for nulliparous women:

- Birth would be expected to take place within 3 hours of the start of the active second stage in most women.
- A diagnosis of delay in the active second stage should be made when it has lasted 2 hours and women should be referred to a healthcare professional trained to undertake an operative vaginal birth if birth is not imminent.

And for multiparous women:

- Birth would be expected to take place within 2 hours of the start of the active second stage in most women.
- A diagnosis of delay in the active second stage should be made when it has lasted 1 hour and women should be referred to a healthcare professional trained to undertake an operative vaginal birth if birth is not imminent.[6]

This has involved a culture change for many units where recourse to instrumental delivery if birth is not imminent after an hour of pushing has been normal practice.

REPAIR TECHNIQUES FOR FIRST-DEGREE AND SECOND-DEGREE TRAUMA

Adequate lighting, analgesia and any necessary assistance are mandatory before attempting to repair a tear or episiotomy. It is unacceptable to perform a perineal repair with inadequate anaesthesia just as performing a CS without adequate anaesthesia would be considered unacceptable.

Before commencing a repair, a full examination should take place. The vaginal apex must be identified and the anal sphincter inspected. If the practitioner is inexperienced in the examination of the anal sphincter, someone with experience should be called at this stage. One study has shown that when the practitioner is uncertain, re-examination by a trained person identifies significantly more anal sphincter ruptures.

Minor first-degree trauma that is not bleeding and where the skin edges are opposed does not need closure; however, a careful examination should be undertaken to ensure no damage to the perineal muscles has occured.

Women should be advised that second-degree trauma should be sutured, as this leads to faster healing and less gaping of the perineum.

It is vital to ensure that the apex of the vaginal component is secured, as paravaginal haematoma formation can occur if the apex is missed. When individual bleeding arteries are identified, they should be ligated separately. Once the repair is complete, it is important to perform the following.

1   Remove any vaginal tampon placed to aid visualisation.
2   Count swabs and ensure none is retained.
3   Count and dispose carefully of any needles.
4   Inspect the repair to ensure vascular haemostasis.
5   Perform a rectal examination to ensure no sutures have breached the rectal mucosa and to palpate the anal sphincter to ensure it is intact.
6   Prescribe analgesia.
7   Document the repair, using a diagram if necessary.
8   Document that the swab and needle count is correct.

Retained swab is now seen as a 'never event' by the national patient safety agency (NPSA) and all units must have procedures in place for the counting of swabs and the recording of any that are placed within the vagina to aid visualisation. A particular area of danger is when a swab is placed into the vagina and then the patient moved to the operating theatre.

Evidence for suture technique

The Cochrane Review showed that continuous suture techniques compared with interrupted sutures for perineal closure (all layers or perineal skin only) are associated with:

- reduction in analgesia use associated with the continuous subcutaneous technique vs interrupted stitches for repair of perineal skin (RR 0.70, 95% CI 0.59–0.84);
- reduction in suture removal in the continuous suturing groups vs interrupted (RR 0.56, 95% CI 0.32–0.98);
- no difference in long-term pain.

Using a two-stage method where the skin is left unsutured but approximated is associated with very slightly less pain at 14 days (RR 0.86, 95% CI 0.76–0.98), and interestingly a slight reduction in the need for re-suturing, despite more reported gaping at 7–10 days [A].[10]

Evidence for suture material

In modern practice synthetic sutures are used. Comparisons between rapidly absorbable and medium absorbable sutures show there is little difference, but a slight increase in the need for suture removal if medium absorbable sutures are used.

Braided sutures have not been compared with monofilament sutures.

Follow-up

In general, most first-degree and second-degree perineal repairs will heal without problems. Important issues relate to the failure to identify anal sphincter damage, which may only become apparent later. Women who have experienced difficult vaginal deliveries may value the opportunity to discuss their delivery at a later date.

The ideal setting for follow-up for women experiencing persistent problems after delivery is a dedicated clinic. Where this is not available a team approach involving obstetricians and physiotherapists, with access to appropriate investigative techniques such as endo-anal ultrasound and manometry, is important. Urinary problems are amenable to biofeedback techniques, and physiotherapy input is vital to ensure that these are appropriately taught and reinforced.

The incidence of childbirth-related perineal wound dehiscence is unknown; figures of 0.1 per cent to 4.6 per cent have been reported, dependent on the degree of the initial trauma. Wound breakdown, when it occurs, happens remarkably quickly, with most women presenting at 4–5 days. It is devastating and can lead to depression and impaired breastfeeding.

Because of the association of breakdown with infection, many units have advocated allowing healing by secondary intention. This can take many weeks and women often request primary re-closure. There are only a few small trials examining this, of which only two are randomised. Women in the early suturing arm resumed sexual intercourse more quickly, but no other differences were seen. These trials did not include satisfaction or depression in their outcomes. All women received antibiotics [B].[11]

Clearly this is an area in which further research is urgently needed. In the meantime an open-minded approach is probably best, and the adoption of the view that healing by secondary intention is best should be re-evaluated.

THIRD-DEGREE AND FOURTH-DEGREE TRAUMA

Incidence

Internal anal sphincter incompetence results in insensible faecal incontinence, whereas external anal sphincter incompetence is associated with faecal urgency. Third-degree tears are reported in approximately 2.8 per cent of primigravidae and 0.4 per cent of multigravidae. The reported rates will vary amongst units with different rates of instrumental delivery. New-onset symptoms of faecal incontinence are reported in 10 per cent of primigravidae undergoing instrumental vaginal delivery at 10 months, and in 3 per cent of primigravidae undergoing spontaneous vaginal delivery. Some of these new symptoms are attributable to pudendal neuropathy, as 5 per cent of women report new symptoms after emergency CS, whereas new-onset bowel symptoms are very uncommon after elective CS. Some degree of faecal urgency probably related to occult anal sphincter damage is much more common, with 44 per cent of women reporting this at 5 years following instrumental delivery of their first baby.

Ultrasonographically visible anal sphincter defects are apparent in 82 per cent of women undergoing forceps delivery and in 48 per cent of ventouse deliveries. However, most women report infrequent problems, and there is no difference in long-term follow-up between forceps and ventouse delivery.[12]

Research studies investigating anal sphincter damage have demonstrated sphincter defects visible on ultrasound in 36 per cent of women after vaginal delivery of their first baby, though two thirds of these will be asymptomatic. The much higher incidence of problems demonstrated in research studies underlines two important facts:

1   women are embarrassed about faecal problems after childbirth;
2   ultrasonographically demonstrated lesions do not translate into confirmed problems of faecal continence.

Anal sphincter damage is mainly limited to first deliveries, whereas pudendal nerve damage can be cumulative. Pudendal nerve damage occurs during labour as the nerve becomes compressed and stretched. Delivery late in first stage or second stage by CS does not prevent this. It has also been shown that ultrasonographically visible anal sphincter defects can be demonstrated in women who were demonstrated to have an intact anal sphincter at the time of delivery. The mechanism for this late disruption is unclear. It may be related to infection or haematoma formation, or possibly to partial unrecognised sphincter ruptures.

Women who have undergone a primary repair of a third- or fourth-degree tear have a 10 per cent risk of wound breakdown and a 0.3–0.4 per cent risk for fistula formation.

Risk factors for third-degree and fourth-degree tears

The risk factors for third-degree and fourth-degree tears are shown in Table 58.1.

Risk factors are cumulative, and in some cases the risks may be greater than the sum of two individual risks; for instance

Table 58.1 Factors associated with increased risk of third-degree tears

Factor	Odds ratio
Primigravida	2–7
Second stage of labour of .60 minutes (including passive second stage)	2
Instrumental vaginal delivery	1.7–7
Midline episiotomy	5–11
Macrosomia (>4 kg)	2.9
Persistent occipito-posterior position	1.7
Epidural analgesia	1.5
Prior third-degree tear	4
Induction of labour	2
Shoulder dystocia	4

the risk of severe trauma when two instruments are needed is much greater than the summed risks for each individual instrument.

Repair

Identification of extent of damage

All women sustaining perineal trauma should be carefully examined to assess the severity of damage to the perineum, vagina and rectum. All staff performing perineal repair must be confident in their ability to diagnose anal sphincter injury. It is imperative to examine carefully for rectal extension, as **small buttonhole tears** can be overlooked and lead to fistula formation.

When disrupted, the anal sphincter retracts, forming a dimple on either side of the anal canal. Rupture of the rectal mucosa will almost always involve damage to both the internal and external anal sphincters.

A good repair of the sphincter is imperative, as this is the factor most strongly associated with future faecal continence.

Conduct of the repair

The most recent Cochrane review of techniques used to repair the EAS included six eligible trials, of variable quality, involving 588 women. There was considerable heterogeneity in the outcome measures, time points and reported results. In one of the six trials all of the repairs were carried out by one of two practitioners only. In the others experienced practitioners within the department undertook the repairs.

Comparing the overlap technique with an end-to-end repair the results showed:

No statistically significant difference in:

- perineal pain (RR 0.08, 95% CI 0.00–1.45, one trial, 52 women);
- dyspareunia (average RR 0.77, 95% CI 0.48–1.24, two trials, 151 women);
- flatus incontinence (average RR 1.14, 95% CI 0.58–2.23, three trials, 256 women) between the two repair techniques at 12 months;
- quality of life;
- flatus incontinence at 36 months follow-up (average RR 1.12, 95% CI 0.63–1.99, one trial, 68 women);
- faecal incontinence at 36 months (average RR 1.01, 95% CI 0.34–2.98, one trial, 68 women).

Lower incidence of:

- faecal urgency (RR 0.12, 95% CI 0.02–0.86, one trial, 52 women);
- lower anal incontinence score (standardised mean difference [SMD] 0.70, 95% CI 1.26 to −0.14 [author check], one trial, 52 women) in the overlap group;
- deterioration of anal incontinence symptoms over 12 months (RR 0.26, 95% CI 0.09–0.79, one trial, 41 women) [A].[13]

For partial thickness EAS tears the new RCOG guidance recommends an end to end technique, avoiding figure of eight sutures. If the EAS tear is full thickness, either an overlap or end to end technique is acceptable with equal outcomes.

Whichever method is used it is important to ensure that the muscle is correctly approximated with long-acting sutures so that it is given adequate time to heal. In the case of 3b tears some practitioners advocate cutting the remaining fibres to perform an overlap repair.

The repair must be performed or directly supervised by a practitioner trained in the repair of third-degree and fourth-degree trauma. There must be adequate analgesia. In practice, this means either a regional or general anaesthetic, as local infiltration does not allow enough relaxation of the sphincter to allow a satisfactory repair. The lighting must be adequate and an assistant is usually needed. This means in practice that repair should usually be undertaken in the operating theatre, though if the prerequistes are met, repair in the room, after senior discussion is also reasonable.

Repair of the rectal mucosa should be performed first. 2:0 polyglycolic acid interrupted sutures with the knots placed on the mucosal side are commonly used and are less irritant than PDS sutures. Next, the layers of the internal sphincter should be replicated across the defect with interrupted sutures of 2:0 or 3:0 Vicryl or PDS. The torn external sphincter is then repaired. This should be re-approximated with either three or four figure-of-eight sutures, or an overlap technique.

A 2.0 or 3.0 polydioxanone suture (PDS) is ideal. Polyglycolic acid is also used. A single study comparing the two showed no difference in outcomes at 12 months [B]. However, the longer tensile retention of PDS and its monofilament characteristics make it especially suitable. Short half-life treated polyglactin sutures (Vicryl Rapide™) are not acceptable as they do not have a long enough half-life to ensure muscle healing. Also, non-absorbable sutures should not be used in the acute setting as these can form a focus for infection, requiring removal. The knots should be buried beneath the superficial perineal muscles, to minimise knot migration.

The remainder of the perineal repair is undertaken as for second-degree trauma. It is imperative to ensure that a good repair of the perineal muscles is performed, as a short or deficient perineum makes injury in future deliveries more likely.

Retention of urine secondary to the anaesthesia or repair is common and a urinary catheter should be inserted until spontaneous voiding is achieved.

Postoperative precautions

It is common practice after delayed anal sphincter repair to use a constipating regimen to allow the repair to heal before stools are passed. This is difficult in recently delivered women who have very different needs from those of the surgical patient. Constipative regimens have been compared with stool-softening regimens. It is concluded that constipative management leads to more pain and a longer postoperative stay compared to stool-softening regimens, but with no difference in repair success. Lactulose and a bulk agent such as Fybogel are recommended for 5–10 days.

It is common sense to give a broad-spectrum antibiotic. There is only one randomised trial on this which showed a large reduction in wound breakdown. It is important to include an antibiotic that will cover possible anaerobic contamination, such as metronidazole. This should be prescribed orally rather than per rectum [C].

Adequate oral analgesia should be prescribed. Paracetamol, NSAIDs and opioid analgesia are acceptable. However, opioids used alone can exacerbate constipation, and thus the former should be used first. A laxative should be prescribed, but bulking agents avoided as they can exacerbate urgency.

Re-evaluate the thrombosis risk and provide appropriate thromboprophylaxis.

Before the mother goes home:

- ensure that she has had a chance to discuss the delivery with a senior member of the team;
- prescribe necessary analgesia and stool softeners;
- advise on perineal hygiene;
- counsel that 60–80 per cent of women will be asymptomatic following healing of the repair;
- provide a contact number in case problems occur;
- make an initial plan for short-term management with a physiotherapist;
- counsel that sutures occasionally migrate and fragments may be passed per vaginum or, occasionally, per rectum; help should be sought if there are concerns;
- give an appointment for follow-up at 6–12 weeks.

DOCUMENTATION

Clear written or electronic notes in black ink must be made following any perineal trauma. These must include:

- clear record of the extent of trauma (measurements are helpful);
- type of analgesia/anaesthesia;
- comprehensive notes of the procedure undertaken and suture material used (including evidence of anal sphincter examination);
- documentation of a swab and needle count before and after the procedure with the name of the second checker;
- estimated blood loss (measured ideally);
- post-operative instructions covering all aspects (fluid replacement, extra monitoring, antibiotics, thromboprophylaxis, stool softeners);
- pre-discharge instructions as necessary;
- follow-up needs.

The notes must be signed, with the date and time. The operator's name should be printed and a contact or pager number given if possible.

SECOND STAGE OF LABOUR

FOLLOW-UP

All women who have sustained a third-degree or fourth-degree tear should be offered follow-up by someone interested in this field. A team approach as outlined earlier is best. Physiotherapy should include augmented biofeedback, as this has been shown to improve continence.

At 6–12 weeks, a full evaluation of the degree of symptoms should take place. This must include careful questioning with regard to faecal and urinary symptoms. A standard questionnaire for women to complete before attending is helpful in precisely delineating the degree of symptoms. Symptomatic women should be offered investigation, including endo-anal ultrasound and manometry [C].

Asymptomatic women with low squeeze pressures and a demonstrable sphincter defect of more than a quadrant should be counselled regarding the pros and cons of future deliveries. Women with ongoing severe symptoms should be considered for secondary surgery. As pudendal neuropathy can take at least 6 months to improve, any further surgical intervention is best deferred until at least this time; however, in exceptional cases in which sphincter disruption is demonstrated and faecal incontinence is debilitating, surgery may be required earlier.

Women with mild symptoms should be advised to avoid gas-producing foods and bulking agents, and constipating agents and biofeedback offered.

Counselling about subsequent delivery

Women can be divided into one of three or four groups with regard to their next delivery.

Previous third-/fourth-degree tear, no ongoing symptoms

These women should be counselled that there is approximately a 5–7 per cent risk of further anal sphincter damage in a subsequent vaginal delivery. This recurrence is not predictable antenatally. Women who were transiently incontinent after their first delivery are particularly at risk of worsening of symptoms, and 17–24 per cent may develop worsening symptoms after subsequent delivery.[14]

When women opt for subsequent vaginal delivery, every effort should be made to avoid instrumental vaginal delivery. There is no evidence that episiotomy prevents muscle damage, and most women appreciate an intact perineum if that can be achieved. The second stage should not be prolonged. Women need careful counselling about epidural analgesia with reference to both the type of delivery and length of second stage. Where anal sphincter damage does not occur, new-onset symptoms are usually attributable to pudendal neuropathy, which usually improves with time. Transient flatus incontinence is reported by 10 per cent of women delivered without further sphincter damage.

Women who continue to be symptomatic

The majority of these women will have a demonstrable defect on ultrasound. There is a risk of worsening of symptoms, which may then make life much more difficult. Women should be carefully counselled with regard to the additional effects of worsening pudendal damage and the small risk of further muscle damage. The majority of women in this group may opt for CS, but for those choosing vaginal delivery, every effort should be made to avoid operative vaginal delivery and lengthy second stage.

Women who have undergone a secondary anal sphincter repair

The consensus is that these women should be delivered by CS [E]. However, there are no data to advise women who wish to try for a vaginal delivery. Again, instrumental delivery and long second stage should be avoided where possible.

Women who are asymptomatic but have demonstrable anal sphincter defects or abnormal manometry on testing

This is a difficult group to manage, as there are few data to advise management. These women are at risk of new symptoms following subsequent delivery. Those at most risk appear to be women with a full quadrant defect, and these women may wish to choose CS next time [C].[14]

The plan for delivery must be clearly documented in the case notes.

PERINEAL TRAUMA AND FEMALE GENITAL MUTILATION

Female genital mutilation (FGM) is defined as all procedures involving partial or total removal of the external female genitalia or other injury to the female genital organs, whether for cultural or other non-therapeutic reasons. The practice of FGM is very common in parts of the Middle East and Africa but also to some extent in India and Indonesia. Somalia, Egypt and Sudan are the countries with the highest rates of FGM. It is important to note that the practice is not limited to particular cultural or religious groups and all women from areas of risk must be sensitively questioned and examined.

For most women, the procedure will have been undertaken when they were children. Some women may not have any recollection of the procedure, and for some women it will be seen by them as a normal thing to have happened. Many women experience physical and psychological damage for many years following FGM.

It is vital that questioning is undertaken with sensitivity. It is usually easier to refer to the practice as 'cutting' as most women understand what is meant by this.

The practice involves removal of parts of the female genital organs, including the labia minora, infundibulum, clitoris and, in some cases, the labia majora. It is important to ascertain the extent of the FGM as complications are more likely with type III FGM.

Classification of types of FGM procedures (WHO) is as follows:

- Type I. Partial or total removal of the clitoris and/or the prepuce (clitoridectomy);
- Type II. Partial or total removal of the clitoris and the labia minora, with or without excision of the labia majora (excision);
- Type III. Narrowing of the vaginal orifice with creation of a covering seal by cutting and appositioning the labia minora and/or the labia majora, with or without excision of the clitoris (infibulation).
- Type IV. All other harmful procedures to the female genitalia for non-medical purposes e.g. pricking, piercing, incising, scraping and cauterising.

Piercing is part of this WHO classification and is classed at type 4 FGM. This is reportable to HSCIC (see below).

Ninety per cent of women who have undergone FGM will have types I, II or IV.

Under the 1985 and 2003 Acts in England and the Prohibition of Female Genital Mutilation (Scotland) Act 2005 it is illegal to perform FGM for traditional or ritual reasons, and is punishable by imprisonment for up to 14 years. It is also illegal to remove an individual to another country for the purposes of FGM. Interestingly, responsibility for decisions regarding surgical reduction of the labia for cosmetic/comfort reasons has been derogated to doctors. It is advised that where a doctor is unsure of the legal position of any request an ethical committee and a legal opinion should be sought and compliance with the FGM acts ensured.

If the unborn child, or any other child in the family, is considered to be at risk of FGM then reporting to social services or the police must occur.

FGM in a woman under 18 must be reported to the police within a month of detection, and if there is a family history of FGM, this must be recorded in the personal child health record (Red book) of the baby.

In the main, the issues seen with FGM are those related to the sequelae of the procedure. Type III is most often associated with physical problems, but all women are at risk of the psychological problems related to FGM.

Physical problems include:

- UTI;
- chronic inflammation and scarring;
- epidermoid and sebaceous cysts (which can become infected);
- fistulae;
- risk of blood born viruses (HIV, Hep B and C).

Psychological problems are common with one third to one half of women displaying symptoms of PTSD, depression, fear of childbirth and other anxiety states.

Obstetric complications are more likely with the more severe types of FGM. An increase in the rates of CS, PPH,

neonatal resuscitation and stillbirth are seen with types II and III FGM, with type III posing the highest risk.

In settings where high-quality intrapartum care is available FGM does not appear to lead to a longer second stage, but perineal tears and the need for episiotomy are much more common.

Additional screening for hepatitis C should be offered in early pregnancy.

De-infibulation pre-conceptually is the best option where this is likely to be needed.[15]

When women who are likely to have undergone FGM are seen in antenatal clinic it is vital that they are sensitively questioned and examined and that a careful plan of management is made for delivery. Psychological support should be offered. A discussion regarding whether de-infibulation is advised antenatally or intrapartum should be undertaken by a senior professional with experience in this area, and all women should be referred to the local specialist team.

Examination in clinic can determine whether de-infibulation is indicated. If the introitus is sufficiently open to permit vaginal examination and if the urethral meatus is visible, then de-infibulation is unlikely to be necessary. Usually a midline anterior episiotomy (division of the labia) is required. A catheter may need to be passed to identify the urethra when the anterior episiotomy is performed. A carefully placed posterior mediolateral episiotomy will be needed if there is rigid scar tissue. Great care must be taken when performing the posterior mediolateral episiotomy, as the presence of the scar tissue can lead to extensive tears if not appropriately managed.

Women should be informed that re-infibulation will not be undertaken under any circumstances. Perineal repair should be undertaken as for a woman without FGM.

Postnatal care should include regular inspection of the perineum to ensure healing, as poor or delayed healing is common.

Women who have had defibulation performed during pregnancy or delivery should be re-examined in any future pregnancy, as reinfibulation between pregnancies is not uncommon.

In response to the paucity of prosecutions since the law was enshrined, there has been a recent intercollegiate document produced to improve the awareness and understanding of responsibilities regarding women and children who have undergone, or who are at risk of, FGM.[16] The nine recommendations are:

1 Treat it as child abuse. FGM is a severe form of violence against women and girls. It is child abuse and must be integrated into all UK child safeguarding procedures in a systematic way.
2 Document and collect information. The NHS should document and collect information on FGM and its associated complications in a consistent and rigorous way.
3 Share that information systematically. The NHS should develop protocols for sharing information about girls at risk of – or girls who have already undergone – FGM with other health and social care agencies, the Department for Education and the police.

4 Empower frontline professionals. Develop the competence, knowledge and awareness of frontline health professionals to ensure prevention and protection of girls at risk of FGM. Also ensure that health professionals know how to provide quality care for girls and women who suffer complications of FGM.

5 Identify girls at risk and refer them as part of child safeguarding obligation. Health professionals should identify girls at risk of FGM as early as possible. All suspected cases should be referred as part of existing child safeguarding obligations. Sustained information and support should be given to families to protect girls at risk.

6 Report cases of FGM. All girls and women presenting with FGM within the NHS must be considered as potential victims of crime, and should be referred to the police and support services.

7 Hold frontline professionals accountable. The NHS and local authorities should systematically measure the performance of frontline health professionals against agreed standards for addressing FGM and publish outcomes to monitor the progress of implementing these recommendations.

8 Empower and support affected girls and young women (both those at risk and survivors). This should be a priority public health consideration; health and education professionals should work together to integrate FGM into prevention messages (especially those focused on avoiding harm e.g. NSPCC 'Pants' Campaign, Personal, Social and Health Education, extracurricular activities for young people).

9 Implement awareness campaign. The government should implement a national public health and legal awareness publicity campaign on FGM, similar to previous domestic abuse and HIV campaigns.

Following this document there is now a legal requirement to report every case of FGM to the Health and Social Care information Centre via the enhanced dataset. This requires notifying of the patient in an identifiable form and must be discussed with the woman. There is also a legal requirement to inform the police and social care of FGM in any minor (under 18).

ACUTE HAEMATOMA

Incidence

The reported incidence of puerperal haematomas varies widely, ranging from 1 in 309 to 1 in 1500. However, large and clinically significant haematomas complicate between 1 in 1000 and 1 in 4000 deliveries.

Aetiological factors

Aetiological factors include:

- Episiotomy (85–90 per cent of cases);
- Instrumental vaginal delivery;
- Primiparity;
- Hypertensive disorders;
- Older mothers.

Multiple pregnancy, vulval varicosities, macrosomic infants and prolonged second stage have all been implicated, but their contribution is probably small.

In two thirds of haematomas, failure to achieve perfect haemostasis at the time of repair, particularly at the upper end of the incision, has been implicated. However, haematomas can occur without any perineal laceration, due to stretching and avulsion of vessels during delivery.

The anatomy of the perineum and vagina plays an important part in the limitation or extension of haematoma formation. Infralevator haematomas, most commonly associated with vaginal delivery, are limited superiorly by the levator ani, medially by the perineal body and from extension onto the thigh by Colles fascia and the fascia lata. These may extend into the ischiorectal fossa. They usually arise from small vulvar or labial vessels, branches of the inferior rectal, inferior vesical or vaginal branch of the uterine arteries. They usually present as vulval pain out of proportion to that expected from an episiotomy, with an ischiorectal mass and discoloration. Continued bleeding or urinary retention may also occur.

In contrast, supralevator haematomas have no fibrous boundaries. They may be paravaginal or supravaginal. They arise from branches of the uterine artery, the inferior vesical and pudendal artery. Bleeding can track into the broad ligament, the retroperitoneal and presacral spaces. Thus they present as rectal pain and pressure, an enlarging rectal or vaginal mass or with hypovolaemic shock.

Broad ligament haematomas will cause upward and lateral displacement of the uterus. The uterus feels well contracted and there may be little revealed vaginal bleeding. As these haematomas are above the pelvic diaphragm; they are more rarely associated with vaginal delivery, although they can occur if genital trauma extends into the fornices or if a cervical tear is sustained. They may also occur in cases of uterine rupture or scar dehiscence.

Following delivery, the vulvar and paravaginal tissues are loose and oedematous. They can accommodate large amounts of blood before a haematoma becomes obvious and gives rise to symptoms (500–1500 mL). Blood loss estimation is therefore extremely difficult and it is usually grossly underestimated.

Presenting symptoms

Infralevator haematomas

- Vaginal swelling;
- Continued vaginal bleeding;
- Severe rectal/vaginal pain;
- Urinary retention.

If postpartum blood loss was moderate, bleeding into the haematoma may produce signs of shock.

Supralevator haematomas

- Cardiovascular collapse;
- Uterine displacement;
- Abdominal or rectal pain;
- Continued vaginal bleeding.

Urgent MRI or CT scanning may help in the identification of supravaginal haematomas.

Management

Small, non-expanding haematomas of less than 3 cm can be managed conservatively. Larger or expanding haematomas require surgical management to prevent pressure necrosis, septicaemia, haemorrhage and death. Full maternal resuscitation in conjunction with anaesthetic colleagues is vital. Blood loss is likely to be significantly underestimated and early recourse to transfusion is necessary. As for repair of genital trauma, adequate analgesia, assistance and lighting are needed.

If the haematoma lies beneath a repair, this should be taken down. If no repair was made, an incision in the inferior portion of the mass near the introitus should be made. Clot is evacuated and the area involved is irrigated with saline. Individual bleeding points should be ligated, although it is more common to find diffuse ooze from very friable haemorrhagic paravaginal tissue. If the tissues allow, a layered closure or primary closure should be undertaken; however, the tissues are generally very difficult to place sutures into, as they are extremely friable. If sutures appear to be tearing out, closing the defect over a soft suction drain such as a Jackson–Pratt drain with a tight pack in the vagina for 12–24 hours may achieve the necessary reduction of dead space and control of bleeding. A urethral catheter will be needed, both to allow effective bladder emptying and to monitor urinary output. Prophylactic broad-spectrum antibiotics should be given, as the risk of subsequent infection is reasonably high and late problems are often attributable to infection. There must be a high index of suspicion if repeated symptoms occur, as the risk of recurrence in the first 12–48 hours is high (approximately 10 per cent). Special vigilance after pack removal is particularly important.

Large paravaginal and supravaginal haematomas can be much more complicated. Extension into the retroperitoneal space or broad ligament can be life threatening. The cervix should be carefully examined to assess cervical lacerations. This is best accomplished by grasping the cervix with a sponge holder, starting at 12 o'clock. A second sponge holder is placed at 2 o'clock and the cervix examined between the two. If intact, the first holder is moved to 4 o'clock. By working around the cervix in this way the whole circumference can be examined and tears identified. Tears must be repaired with full-thickness interrupted sutures, ensuring that the apex is identified. A combined vaginal and abdominal approach may be needed to evacuate clot, identify bleeding and secure haemostasis. An abdominal approach is always needed for tears of the cervix or upper vagina where the apex cannot be identified and

bleeding is occurring. **Ureteric injury can result from blindly placed deep sutures in the fornix.**

Internal iliac artery ligation, hysterectomy and radiological embolisation techniques have all been described to control intractable bleeding.

Careful observation in a high-dependency area is required for 12–24 hours, as recurrence of the haematoma may occur in up to 10 per cent of cases. These women are likely to have lost very large amounts of blood and the strategy for major obstetric haemorrhage should be followed. Early recourse to surgery, antibiotics and transfusion has improved maternal mortality in this life-threatening situation.

It is important that measures to reduce thromboembolism are not ignored in these women, as they have a high risk of thrombosis. Whilst many surgeons may wish to defer heparins until the risk of recurrence is lessened, other measures such as full-length thromboembolic stockings, compression boots and leg exercises can all be safely implemented without increasing the risk of recurrence.

KEY POINTS

- Episiotomy does not prevent third-degree and fourth-degree tears. Midline episiotomy increases the risk of such trauma.
- Perineal massage antepartum reduces the risk of third-degree and fourth-degree trauma in primiparae by a small amount.
- There are higher rates of ultrasonographically visible anal sphincter defects after forceps compared with ventouse, but no difference in maternal symptoms at 5 years.
- Leaving the perineal skin approximated but not closed is associated with less perineal dysaesthesia. If the skin is sutured, a subcuticular suture causes less short-term pain.
- A loose continuous repair without locking the vaginal component is associated with less short-term pain.
- Overlap is probably marginally superior to end-to-end approximation of the anal sphincter in repair of third-degree tears.
- FGM is illegal and the national guidance is that all cases should be reported. Local guidelines will exist as to how this is done.

Key references

1. RCOG. *Management of Third- and Fourth-Degree Perineal Tears.* Clinical Green-top Guideline No. 29. London: RCOG Press, 2015.
2. Sultan AH, Johanson RB, Carter JE. Occult anal sphincter trauma following randomized forceps and vacuum delivery. *Int J Obstet Gynecol* 1998;61:113–19.
3. Beckmann MM, Stock OM. Antenatal perineal massage for reducing perineal trauma. *Cochrane Database of Systematic Reviews* 2013,4:CD005123. DOI: 10.1002/14651858.CD005123.pub3.

4. Aasheim V, Nilsen ABV, Lukasse M, Reinar LM. Perineal techniques during the second stage of labour for reducing perineal trauma. *Cochrane Database of Systematic Reviews* 2011,12:CD006672. DOI: 10.1002/14651858. CD006672.pub2.

5. Carroli G, Mignini L. Episiotomy for vaginal birth. *Cochrane Database of Systematic Reviews* 2009,1: CD000081. DOI: 10.1002/14651858.CD000081.pub2.

6. NICE. *Intrapartum Care. Care of healthy women and their babies.* Clinical guideline 55. London: NICE, 2007.

7. McCandlish R, Bowler U, Van Asten H *et al.* A randomised controlled trial of care of the perineum during second stage of normal labour. *BJOG* 1998;105:1262–72.

8. RCOG. *Operative Vaginal Delivery.* Clinical Green-top Guideline No. 26. London: RCOG Press, 2011.

9. To come

10. Kettle C, Dowswell T, Ismail KMK. Continuous and interrupted suturing techniques for repair of episiotomy or second-degree tears. *Cochrane Database of Systematic Reviews* 2012,11:CD000947. DOI: 10.1002/14651858. CD000947.pub3.

11. Dudley LM, Kettle C, Ismail KMK. Secondary suturing compared to non-suturing for broken-down perineal wounds following childbirth. *Cochrane Database of Systematic Reviews* 2013,9: CD008977. DOI: 10.1002/14651858.CD008977.pub2.

12. Johanson RB, Heycock E, Carter J, Sultan AH, Walklate K, Jones PW. Maternal and child health after assisted vaginal delivery: five-year follow-up of a randomised controlled study comparing forceps and ventouse. *BJOG* 1999;106:544–9.

13. Fernando RJ, Sultan AH, Kettle C, Thakar R. Methods of repair for obstetric anal sphincter injury. *Cochrane Database of Systematic Reviews* 2013,12: CD002866. DOI: 10.1002/14651858.CD002866.pub3

14. Fynes M, Donnelly V, Behan M, O'Connell PR, O'Herlihy C. Effect of second vaginal delivery on ano-rectal physiology and fecal continence. *Lancet* 1999;354:983–6.

15. RCOG. *Female genital mutilation and its management.* Clinical Green-top Guideline No. 53. London: RCOG Press, 2009.

16. Royal College of Midwives. *Tackling FGM in the UK: Intercollegiate recommendations for identifying, recording and reporting.* RCM, July 2015.

SECTION SEVEN

Postpartum Complications

Chapter 59 Perinatal asphyxia

Andrew Currie

INTRODUCTION

Perinatal asphyxia is an important cause of death and disability in the term neonate. Although the pathophysiology of the asphyxial process is understood, there are currently few interventions available that preserve brain function and few treatment modalities have been subject to RCTs. Mild therapeutic hypothermia has recently shown positive results and is discussed later in the chapter.

A number of clinical, biochemical and radiological markers of hypoxic–ischaemic damage are available, but their use in predicting outcome requires caution.

Perinatal asphyxia can lead to the neonatal condition called 'hypoxic–ischaemic encephalopathy' (HIE). Neonatal encephalopathies are a heterogeneous group of disorders clinically defined by a disturbance in the neurological function of the neonate in the early days of life. They are the result of a number of causes including hypoxic–ischaemic insults, metabolic disorders, sepsis, drug exposure, intracranial bleeds, neurological malformations, etc. Neonatal encephalopathies are usually grouped into mild, moderate or severe (or alternatively stage I, II and III) depending on the severity of symptoms and signs. These range from mild hyperalertness in very mild cases through to stupor, severe hypotonia, seizures and respiratory embarrassment in severe cases.

The most common single cause for neonatal encephalopathy is HIE, secondary to some perinatal asphyxial process. However, it is important to understand both from a clinical point of view and a medico-legal perspective that not all neonatal encephalopathies are the result of hypoxia or asphyxia and other causes should be ruled out, especially when the clinical history is ambiguous. Thus, it is more appropriate to use the term 'neonatal encephalopathy' without ascribing a particular cause until appropriate investigations have been undertaken.

DEFINITION

The terms 'birth asphyxia' and 'perinatal asphyxia' are widely used to describe an intrapartum hypoxic–ischaemic insult in a term infant. However, the precise clinical definition varies, making interpretation of data on incidence, clinical manifestations and outcome difficult.

It is unclear if premature infants, with their immature CNS, exhibit the same responses to hypoxic–ischaemic insults as term infants. Preterm infants are of course at higher risk of cerebral insults outside the intrapartum period.

INCIDENCE OF HYPOXIC–ISCHAEMIC INJURY

The incidence varies depending on the definition used and whether preterm infants are included. The incidence appears to be higher in developing countries, although preterm infants are often included in published data. With improvements in antenatal and intrapartum monitoring, the incidence appears to have fallen in some published UK studies, from 6.0 per 1000 live births in the early 1980s[1] to 1.0 per 1000 live births in the mid-1990s. Subsequently, population surveys in the UK show the rates appear to have stabilised over recent years at around 1.2 per 1000 live births [C].[2]

PREVENTION

In order to prevent brain injury caused by hypoxia–ischaemia, there needs to be awareness as to when and under what conditions the injury might occur. Most available information relates to the detection of problems during the intrapartum period. However, it is clear that not all hypoxic–ischaemic insults occur intrapartum and that many occur prior to labour and delivery [C].[3] In recent years, major advances in antenatal assessment have been made and a number of tools for the antenatal assessment of fetal wellbeing are now widely used, including monitoring fetal movements, fetal heart rate, biophysical profiles, fetal growth and blood flow velocity in umbilical and fetal blood vessels (see Chapter 37, Tests of fetal wellbeing).

One group at particular risk of hypoxic–ischaemic brain injury is the preterm fetus. As well as the traditional methods of improving outcome delivered in the peripartum period (i.e. the administration of maternal betamethasone), there is increasing evidence that the maternal administration of a loading dose of intravenous magnesium sulphate (followed by a maintenance dose) significantly reduces long-term neurodevelopmental morbidity (RCOG Scientific Opinion Paper, No. 29, 2011).

The aim of intrapartum monitoring is to detect 'fetal compromise'; this is often used as a marker for hypoxia–ischaemia. Detection of fetal compromise does not help in timing the hypoxic insult, as it may reflect the infant's inability to mount a normal physiological response to an earlier hypoxic event. Intrapartum assessments of fetal wellbeing/fetal compromise include:

- monitoring of fetal heart rate, either intermittently or continuously;
- assessment of fetal acid–base status;
- passage of meconium *in utero*.

It should be noted that the detection of fetal compromise is a poor predictor of HIE or later cerebral palsy.

Once concerns have been raised regarding the wellbeing of the infant, in order to ensure optimum resuscitation, it is vital that communication is made to neonatal staff prior to delivery. It is essential that staff attending the delivery are appropriately trained in neonatal resuscitation and are given any relevant details in the maternal history that may affect resuscitation; for example, placental abruption, for which the infant may require blood during the resuscitation.

PATHOPHYSIOLOGY OF BRAIN INJURY

Perinatal asphyxia occurs when a lack of oxygen and acidosis cause organ impairment. Deprivation of oxygen to the brain can occur in two ways:

1 **hypoxaemia** – a reduction in the amount of oxygen in the blood;
2 **ischaemia** – a reduction in the amount of blood perfusing the brain.

Although brain injury occurs at the time of the hypoxic–ischaemic insult, it is now well established that neuronal damage is an ongoing process which starts at the time of the primary injury and following a 'latent' period continues, despite resuscitation, into the recovery phase (secondary injury).

This is supported clinically by the delay of up to 24–48 hours before typical signs of encephalopathy are observed, with further delays before radiological changes are seen on either ultrasound or MRI [C].[4]

Following a hypoxic–ischaemic insult, cell death occurs in two phases. The mechanisms involved are different and are influenced by the severity and nature of the original insult. The neuronal injury resulting from hypoxic–ischaemic insult in a term infant is 'selective neuronal necrosis'. It is unaffected by resuscitation and occurs 5–30 minutes after the onset of ischaemia. Primary neuronal death predominantly affects the watershed areas of the cerebral cortex, is bilateral and usually symmetrical. Many neurons do not die during this primary phase; they do, however, appear vulnerable to further injury and death as a result of severe cerebrovascular dysfunction. This appears to trigger a series of biochemical events resulting in secondary neuronal death as a result of apoptosis. Evidence from animal and early clinical studies indicates that a therapeutic window exists between the primary and secondary phases when intervention may prevent secondary neuronal death and subsequently improve neurological outcome.[5]

AETIOLOGY

Perinatal asphyxia may be the result of an acute event or may occur as a result of chronic hypoxia (Box 59.1). It is important to note that in many cases no single factor is identified and that asphyxia may be caused by several antenatal factors or antenatal and intrapartum factors coexisting. It is difficult accurately to quantify the timing of hypoxic–ischaemic insults, as reported studies differ widely in their definitions, methodologies and inclusion criteria. It has been estimated that approximately 20 per cent of insults occur antenatally, 35 per cent occur intrapartum and, in a further 35 per cent, there are both antenatal and intrapartum factors involved.[3] In the remaining cases, the timing is difficult to define. It is clear that despite differences in definition, intrapartum events contribute to a significant proportion of cases.

Box 59.1 Causes of and associations with perinatal asphyxia

Impaired maternal oxygenation
Maternal cardiovascular disease
Impaired uterine blood flow
Vascular disturbance, pre-eclampsia, diabetes
Maternal hypotension/hypovolaemia
Impaired placental function
Placental infarction
Abruption
Post-maturity
Infection

Impaired blood flow to cord, e.g. cord compression/prolapse

Abnormal fetal haemoglobin

Rhesus haemolytic disease

Twin–twin transfusion

Feto-maternal transfusion

Maternal drugs

Cocaine

Failure to establish adequate cardiopulmonary circulation after birth

Meconium aspiration

Congenital cardiorespiratory disease

CLINICAL FEATURES AND MANAGEMENT OF HIE

Despite the subjective nature of the scoring system, the universal method employed to assess an infant's wellbeing at birth is the Apgar score. Infants who have been exposed to a hypoxic insult will invariably have low Apgar scores beyond 1 minute; however, other factors not associated with asphyxia can also lower the Apgar score e.g. anaesthetic agents and prematurity. Despite this, there is good evidence that prolonged depression of the Apgar score is associated with death or major neurological disability [C].[6]

It is essential that personnel trained in neonatal resuscitation are present prior to the delivery of an asphyxiated infant. Resuscitation should establish a secure airway, ensure adequate oxygenation and restore circulation. Some severely affected infants will require endotracheal intubation and ventilation in the delivery room; however, others will require little in the way of initial resuscitation, but will deteriorate after the first 24 hours. Intravenous fluids, and in particular colloid, should be used with caution in restoring the circulation in severe asphyxia, the exception being where there is a clear history of antepartum haemorrhage or placental abruption; in such cases, O-negative blood should be administered in the delivery room.

If, despite appropriate resuscitation, there is no spontaneous cardiac output by 10 minutes or respiratory activity by 30 minutes, the outlook for both term and preterm infants is poor.

Post-resuscitation management

Infants who have experienced an asphyxial insult develop the clinical syndrome known as HIE. After resuscitation, the infant may be flaccid and unresponsive. The clinical signs progress over the first 24–48 hours before gradual improvement is seen. The severity of HIE can be graded clinically as mild, moderate or severe, as shown in Table 59.1.[1] The management after hypoxia–ischaemia is crucial, as the affected infant is still at risk of reperfusion injury.[5] Transfer to a neonatal intensive care unit with facilities for cerebral and systemic monitoring is of the utmost importance. Full supportive care is required, with great attention to detail. As well as general intensive care, specific neurological monitoring and care should also be given.

General management

During episodes of hypoxia, blood flow is distributed in order to preserve blood supplies to vital organs, namely the brain, heart and adrenals. This leaves other organs, particularly the kidney, liver and gut, prone to ischaemic damage. With this in mind, blood pressure should be continuously monitored and hypotension avoided in order to ensure cerebral perfusion and to prevent further underperfusion of other organs. Hypotension is common and usually due to myocardial dysfunction rather than hypovolaemia. It should be treated promptly with volume expansion and/or inotropes as clinically indicated. Care should be taken not to overload infants with fluid, as acute tubular necrosis and inappropriate antidiuretic hormone release are common sequelae. Maintenance fluids should be restricted by 25 per cent for the first 48 hours or so, based on regular clinical assessment of hydration, serum and urinary electrolytes, urine output and specific gravity and the infant's weight.

Asphyxiated infants are at risk of developing necrotising enterocolitis and therefore oral feeds should be introduced with caution. Prevention of tissue catabolism is important and thus nutritional support should be provided by parenteral nutrition until feeds are established.

Respiratory support with endotracheal intubation should only be undertaken if hypercapnia develops, if the infant has prolonged or frequent convulsions, or if there is coexisting respiratory disease. Hyperventilation is not recommended, as hypocapnia reduces cerebral perfusion and may compound the ischaemic insult. Respiratory support is guided by regular

Table 59.1 Clinical grading for HIE[7]

Grade I (mild)	Grade II (moderate)	Grade III (severe)
Irritability	Lethargy	Comatose
Mild hypotonia	Marked abnormalities in tone	Severe hypotonia
Poor suck	Requires tube feeds	Failure to maintain spontaneous respiration
Hyperalert	Seizures	Prolonged seizures

arterial blood gas analysis. Hypoxia should be avoided and the PaO_2 kept between 8 and 12 kPa (60–90 mmHg).

Neonatal meningitis may present in a similar way to HIE and therefore if there is any doubt, a lumbar puncture should be performed and treatment commenced. Routine antibiotics have no part to play in the treatment of HIE.

Disseminated intravascular coagulation is not uncommon in severe cases of HIE, and therefore regular assessments of clotting status should be made. Treatment includes additional vitamin K, platelets, cryoprecipitate and/or fresh frozen plasma infusions.

Neurological management

Much of the management after hypoxic–ischaemic insults has not been subject to RCTs. Probably the one major exception to this is the series of recent multicentre studies investigating mild hypothermia as a neuroprotective measure (see below under Therapeutic hypothermia for treatment of HIE).

In severe HIE, cerebral oedema and raised intracranial pressure (ICP) are commonly observed. Management strategies to lower ICP have included the administration of hyperosmolar agents and lowering $PaCO_2$. There is no evidence that hyperventilation and the ensuing hypocarbia are beneficial in reducing ICP, and therefore accepted practice is to maintain the $PaCO_2$ within the normal range [E].

The use of hypertonic saline has been shown to be beneficial in lowering ICP in animal models and in adults. Its use has not been evaluated in the neonate and it cannot be recommended. There is no evidence for the use of mannitol, furosemide or steroids in the treatment of cerebral oedema in neonates.[7]

Seizures are a salient feature of HIE. Frequent and prolonged clinically evident seizures should be treated promptly with anticonvulsant(s). Phenobarbital is the drug of choice, as recent evidence suggests that the use of phenytoin, diazepam or chloral hydrate confers no benefit [A].[7] Anticonvulsants can be stopped once seizures are controlled. The use of early prophylactic phenobarbital as a 'neuroprotector' in HIE has been subject to a meta-analysis, which concluded that routine use is not recommended in perinatal asphyxia [A].[8]

Glucose metabolism in HIE has been extensively studied and yet is still not fully understood. Normoglycaemia should be maintained, as there is evidence that both hypoglycaemia and hyperglycaemia may worsen brain injury.

New neuroprotective strategies

A number of new neuroprotective strategies have evolved in recent years.[5,7] Most have been used in animal models, with only a few trials in the human neonate. The rationale behind these interventions is in the prevention of reperfusion injury. Interventions have included magnesium sulphate, calcium channel blockers, allopurinol as a free radical scavenger, the Chinese herb *Salvia miltiorrhizae*, naloxone and hypothermia. Of these alternatives, selective hypothermia is the only strategy that has shown positive results.

Therapeutic hypothermia for treatment of HIE

As mentioned earlier, neuronal cell death is the result of a combination of primary and secondary cellular energy failure. There is little that can be done to prevent primary neuronal cell death; however, between these two phases there is a latent period of several hours which may serve as a therapeutic window to prevent the secondary energy failure.

There is clear evidence that fever on top of HIE results in a worse outcome.[9] In addition, a number of animal studies have shown that cooling ameliorated the delayed energy failure and inhibited neuronal cell apoptosis. As a result, over recent years, a number of large clinical trials have taken place studying the effects of therapeutic hypothermia in HIE. A recent meta-analysis of these studies has concluded that induced mild hypothermia to a core temperature of 33.5°C resulted in a reduction in the combined outcome of mortality and neurodevelopmental disability at 18 months in term infants with moderate or severe HIE. As a result of this and a more recent multicentre clinical study confirming these results, it is generally agreed that therapeutic hypothermia should be offered in cases of moderate and severe HIE.

The treatment is primarily a preventative strategy treatment, so it is important that cooling is commenced as soon as HIE is suspected, and ideally within 6 hours of birth before clinical evidence of secondary neuronal cell death (such as seizures) appears.

INVESTIGATIONS

Continuous integrated single-channel EEG monitoring is now in widespread use and is very useful both from a clinical treatment point of view and prognostically.

The value of neuroimaging is limited in the first 24–48 hours of life. Ultrasound evidence of lesions in the thalami and basal ganglia, focal infarctions and changes in periventricular white matter are usually seen after the first 48 hours of life. Their presence before this suggests an antenatal insult.

MRI is useful in asphyxiated infants. Early scans characteristically show brain swelling and abnormal signal intensity within the basal ganglia, periventricular white matter, subcortical white matter and cortex. Late MRI findings associated with poor outcome include delayed myelination as a marker for neuronal loss and extensive white matter changes.

OUTCOME

Determining the outcome after perinatal asphyxia is difficult for a number of reasons:

- the definition of asphyxia varies;
- there is variation in the outcomes assessed – mortality, motor, behavioural, etc.;
- there is varied inclusion/exclusion of preterm infants;
- the age at time of assessment varies.

POSTPARTUM COMPLICATIONS

What is clear, however, is that the neurological outcome depends on the severity of the insult. It is well recognised that term infants with grade I HIE (mild) have no long-term developmental problems, whereas severe HIE is associated with a poor outcome. It is more difficult to predict the outcome of moderate HIE as there are few readily available reliable markers of long-term impairment. One early predictor of adverse outcome is the severity of the neurological abnormalities found on clinical examination, particularly in association with discontinuous activity on EEG. Severe acidosis associated with poor Apgar scores, multi-organ failure and encephalopathy immediately after birth are also markers of poor outcome [C].[10]

The major neurological sequelae in surviving infants are motor deficits and, in particular, spastic quadriplegia and dyskinetic cerebral palsy. There may also be associated visual or intellectual impairment or epilepsy. It is important to note that not all cerebral palsy is the result of perinatal asphyxia and not all asphyxiated infants develop cerebral palsy [C].[11]

SUMMARY

- Phenobarbital is the drug of choice for convulsions secondary to HIE.
- There is as yet no evidence to support routine seizure prophylaxis in infants with HIE.
- Most infants with severe HIE will develop neurological sequelae. Most infants with mild HIE will have no long-term sequelae. Infants in the moderate category remain the most difficult in whom to predict outcome.
- Therapeutic hypothermia has been proven to improve outcomes in HIE and should be offered as early as possible as part of these infants' intensive care.

KEY POINTS

- Most cases of HIE have an intrapartum element.
- However, not all infants with HIE develop cerebral palsy, and not all children with cerebral palsy demonstrate HIE.
- Damage due to HIE occurs in two phases: the initial insult and then further reperfusion injury (primary and secondary cellular energy failure).
- Damage is usually symmetrical and affects watershed areas.
- A persistently depressed Apgar score is generally associated with poor outcomes.
- Mild therapeutic hypothermia is now recognised as an important part of the management of moderate to severe HIE.

ACKNOWLEDGEMENT

This chapter has been revised and updated. The author and editors acknowledge the contribution of Sandie Bohin to the chapter on this topic in the previous edition of the book.

Key References

1. Levene MI, Kornberg J, Williams THC. The incidence and severity of post-asphyxial encephalopathy in full term infants. *Early Hum Dev* 1985;11:21–6.
2. Trent Neonatal Survey Report 2007. Trent Infant Mortality and Morbidity Studies. Leicester University, 2005–2007.
3. Volpe JJ. Hypoxic–ischaemic encephalopathy: clinical aspects. *In: Neurology of the Newborn*, 3rd edn. Philadelphia: WB Saunders, 1995.
4. Sie LT, Van der Knapp MS, Van Wezel-Meyler G *et al.* Early MR features of hypoxic–ischaemic brain injury in neonates with periventricular densities on sonogram. *Am J Neuroradiol* 2000;21:852–61.
5. Cornette L, Levene MI. Post-resuscitative management of the asphyxiated term infant. *Semin Neonatol* 2001;6:271–82.
6. Nelson KB, Ellenberg JH. Apgar scores as predictors of chronic neurological disability. *Pediatrics* 1981;68:36–44.
7. Whitelaw A. Systematic review of therapy after hypoxic–ischaemic brain injury in the perinatal period. *Semin Neonatol* 2000;5:33–44.
8. Evans DJ, Levene MI. Anticonvulsants for preventing mortality and morbidity in full-term newborns with perinatal asphyxia. *Cochrane Database Syst Rev* 2007;3:CD001240.
9. Lieberman E, Eichenwald E, Mathur G *et al.* Intrapartum fever and unexplained seizures in term infants. *Pediatrics* 2000;106:983–8.
10. Yudkin PL, Johnson A, Clover LM, Murphy KW. Clustering of perinatal markers of birth asphyxia and outcome at age five years. *BJOG* 1994;101:774–81.
11. Blair F, Stanley FJ. Intrapartum asphyxia: a rare cause of cerebral palsy. *J Pediatrics* 1988;112:515–19.
12. RCOG Scientific Opinion Paper, No:29, 2011. https://www.rcog.org.uk/globalassets/documents/guidelines/sip29.

POSTPARTUM COMPLICATIONS

Chapter 60 Neonatal resuscitation

Andrew Currie

INTRODUCTION

Health professionals involved with childbirth should be capable of providing life support to the newly born when the need arises.

To facilitate this, various professional bodies have been developed, including the UK Resuscitation Council, the European Resuscitation Council and the International Liaison Committee on Resuscitation (ILCOR).[1-3] Each professional body has produced guidelines and training programmes to improve resuscitation practices.

Much of resuscitation procedure is based on 'best practice', with very little evidence-based medicine to support it. This is hardly surprising given the ethical dilemmas that would be created by trying to perform RCTs of resuscitation techniques.

This chapter concentrates on the essential steps required to provide safe and appropriate resuscitation to the newborn. It draws on recommendations from the above resuscitation bodies and, where possible, the evidence is reviewed.

INCIDENCE

Most studies show that approximately 90–95 per cent of all births require no resuscitation. The other 5–10 per cent need some form of respiratory support, with possibly up to 1–2 per cent requiring full cardiopulmonary resuscitation.[4]

PHYSIOLOGICAL CHANGES

Many physiological adaptations occur to the infant at birth.[5] The most important involve the cardiovascular system, respiratory system and thermoregulatory mechanisms.

Respiratory

In utero, the lungs are full of fluid (30–35 mL/kg in term infants). Pulmonary pressures are suprasystemic, thus reducing blood flow to the fetal lung. To adapt to extrauterine life, lung fluid production reduces near term. In addition, the mechanics of birth include the birth canal exerting an immense extrathoracic pressure on the infant during its descent, squeezing lung fluid from the trachea and upper airways. With delivery, a natural 'recoil' of the airways (along with the infant's first respiratory efforts) helps to inflate the lungs. Subsequent breaths become progressively easier, due to development of a functional residual capacity and improving lung compliance. Dispersal of surfactant to form a monolayer within the alveolar system further improves lung mechanics by lowering surface tension and ensuring alveoli remain open, even in expiration.

Cardiovascular

Major features of the fetal cardiovascular system include high pulmonary pressures and a series of three anatomical right-to-left shunts.

1   The ductus venosus carries blood from the placenta back to the fetus (effectively connecting the umbilical vein to the inferior vena cava).
2   The foramen ovale is important in diverting blood from the right atrium to the left, thus bypassing the lungs.
3   The ductus arteriosus diverts blood from the pulmonary artery to the aorta.

Following birth, the pulmonary pressures fall. This is as much to do with changes at a cellular level (including the effects of cytokines, prostaglandins and the influence of endogenous nitric oxide) as with the mechanics of lung inflation.

The ductus venosus closes soon after clamping of the umbilical cord, with establishment of the normal venous circulation. The fall in pulmonary pressures allows greater blood flow into the pulmonary circulation. This increases the blood volume returning to the left atrium, with consequent closure of the foramen ovale and increased systemic pressures; these in turn reverse the shunting across the ductus arteriosus. The ductus arteriosus subsequently closes under the influence of increasing oxygen concentrations and prostaglandins. As a result, the normal neonatal circulation is established. The conversion of the fetal to the neonatal circulation may take several days to complete.

Thermoregulation

The infant is born naked and wet into a hostile environment. Immature thermoregulatory mechanisms can lead to cold stress with serious morbidity, such as acidosis, hypoglycaemia and respiratory distress. Equally, pyrexia may be as dangerous, studies showing that it worsens cerebral hypoxic injury.[6] Hence an essential part of neonatal resuscitation is maintenance of a normal body temperature.

AETIOLOGY

Many causes have been associated with a potentially compromised infant at birth. These can be divided into maternal, fetal and intrapartum. A list of the more common is shown in Box 60.1.

Box 60.1 Common causes for a compromised newborn infant

Maternal
Chronic ill-health
Drug ingestion (legal and illegal)
Hypertension
Diabetes mellitus
Anatomical abnormalities
Placenta praevia
Fetal
Multiple pregnancies
Prematurity
Post-term (>42/52)
IUGR
Congenital abnormalities
Liquor disturbances (oligohydramnios/polyhydramnios)
Hydrops
Isoimmunisation
Intrauterine infection

Intrapartum
Fetal distress
Abnormal presentation
Prolapsed cord
Antepartum haemorrhage
Prolonged rupture of membranes
Thick meconium
Instrumental deliveries

MANAGEMENT OF THE RESUSCITATION

Basic principles (fundamental to optimise patient outcome)

- As with any resuscitation, the ABC (airway, breathing, circulation) approach is the most appropriate. The vast majority of neonatal 'arrests' are primarily due to respiratory problems. Hence, heavy emphasis is placed on ensuring an adequate airway and efficient ventilation delivery to the child.
- Good preparation is essential to optimise clinical management.
- Resuscitation of the newborn is a team approach. Clear communication is essential.
- The ability to assess a situation and act accordingly on a regular basis is crucial. The ability to use basic knowledge in a safe, logical and adaptive manner makes resuscitation of the patient a more rewarding process.

Preparation

Good preparation is as important to a successful outcome as the actual resuscitation itself. Preparation involves more than getting equipment ready.

Medical history

Accurate medical information is invaluable. Although a detailed medical history is ideal, time is often against this. It is vital to establish key facts quickly.

Useful questions that may influence the actual resuscitation process include the following:

- How many infants should we expect? This will dictate numbers of personnel and amount of equipment, as well as help inform likelihood of complications.
- What is the gestation? While the basics of resuscitation remain the same, priorities and expectations will differ and may influence the approach taken.
- Are there any congenital anomalies (e.g. congenital diaphragmatic hernia)? Specific conditions do influence the approach taken to resuscitation.

- Has the mother had any relevant medication in the last few hours (e.g. opiates)? This may affect the infant's response to resuscitation.
- Has there been any meconium prior to delivery? Again, this will influence the approach taken to the resuscitation procedure (see below under Meconium).

Personnel

All workers involved in birth should be able to provide basic neonatal life support, and regular updates of skills should be undertaken. Ideally, somebody trained in advanced neonatal life support should also be readily available.

Resuscitation is a team event. Individuals should understand their roles. Ideally, two to three people make an effective team: one to look after the airway, one to look after the cardiovascular circulation and the third to assist with drugs, fluids and additional equipment. One person should take the role of leader; this ensures clarity of the roles and efficient team working.

Other important tasks that may be delegated in the acute situation include informing neonatal unit staff who will be looking after the infant following resuscitation and communicating with the parents, who need to be informed of events as early and fully as possible.

Communication and documentation

Often, the source of mishaps and complaints is poor communication. In addition, poor documentation makes post-hoc reviews very difficult. The importance of accurate information gathering, documentation and communication cannot be emphasised enough. Accurate timing must be recorded and all records (midwifery, obstetric and neonatal) should be consistent. In the acute situation, if sufficient staff are available, one team member should be asked to keep a record of times and procedures.

Environment

A brightly lit, warm and draft-free room is ideal. As well as reducing morbidity due to heat loss, an appropriate environment ensures that attendants can see and assess the infant.

The infant's temperature should be kept in the normothermic range. Hyperthermia is associated with increased neuronal damage in cases of perinatal hypoxia. In the normal situation hypothermia is equally associated with increased morbidity, particularly in the premature infant. However, multicentre trials in recent years have shown that induced mild hypothermia in the early hours after birth is neuroprotective in term infants with moderate or severe perinatal asphyxial hypoxia.[7] These studies managed infants with core temperatures at 33.5°C for up to 72 hours.

It is speculative to relate these studies to the acute resuscitation when often the clinical picture is unclear; however, it has become accepted practice to turn off the radiant heater on the resuscitaire as a means of passively cooling a term infant in the presence of possible perinatal hypoxia. Despite this it should be the case that for most situations the recommendation remains that during the acute resuscitation of the newborn maintenance of normothermia, and certainly prevention of hyperthermia, should be the rule [E].[7]

Equipment

Having the right equipment, which is reliable, is paramount to a successful resuscitation. Box 60.2 shows a list of essential equipment.

Within the hospital setting, all essential equipment is found on a resuscitaire – best described as a mobile, open cot. The heat and warmth sources are located above a firm, flat surface. A clock is attached. There are usually two sources of oxygen (piped and cylinders), with two outlets. Air supplies should also be available on resuscitaires. Studies have indicated that resuscitation with air is as effective as oxygen[8] in term infants [A]. There is also increasing concern about the detrimental effects of hyperoxia to the lungs and eyes in the preterm infant. Thus, it is now felt that the initial approach to resuscitation of the newborn should be with the use of air and only if there is a poor response to this should introduction of oxygen be considered. The availability of an air/oxygen blender to better manage the concentration of oxygen used is considered to be a better approach.

Box 60.2 Essential equipment for neonatal resuscitation

Equipment
Light source
Source of warmth (heater and/or warmed linen)
Flat surface (±firm mattress)
Clock
Suction apparatus (able to deliver suction up to 100 mmHg)
Suction catheters
Oxygen supply
Ventilation system (either 'bag-valve-mask' or 'facemask and T-piece', or both)
Oxygen saturation monitor
Endotracheal tubes (various sizes from 2.5 to 4.0 mm internal diameter)
Introductory stylet
Fixation kit for endotracheal tube
Laryngoscopes (with straight blades and spare bulbs)
Oropharyngeal airways
Nasogastric tubes
Umbilical venous catheters
Scalpel
Intravenous cannulae
Intraosseous cannula
Syringes and needles
Fluids and medications

Suction apparatus is intrinsic in the resuscitaire. The rest of the equipment should be readily available, stored in various drawers mounted on the resuscitaire.

The resuscitaire should be situated in the delivery room. Fluids and medications may or may not be stored with the resuscitaire. If not, they should be in a readily accessible place for emergency use.

It is the responsibility of the individuals using equipment for resuscitation to ensure that they are competent with its use and that it is working properly. All resuscitation equipment should be checked daily, as well as before and after each use.

THE RESUSCITATION PROCESS

This section assumes birth is taking place in a maternity suite with a resuscitaire; however, the principles can be applied to any setting.

Fig. 60.1 shows a step-by-step approach. Each step is explained in more detail below.

Step 1

With the birth of the whole baby, the clock is started and the infant is transferred to the resuscitaire. The infant is placed with the head in the 'neutral position', towards the resuscitator. The neutral position involves the head being placed so that the eyes are looking directly upward. This position helps maintain airway patency.

The infant should be kept warm. For the term infant and larger preterm infant, this may be achieved by drying with a warm towel. A vigorous, not aggressive, rub with the towel serves the dual purpose of drying the infant and stimulating breathing. The infant is then wrapped in a second warm towel. Evidence indicates that for the premature infant in the delivery suite (less than 30 weeks' gestation) heat loss is best managed

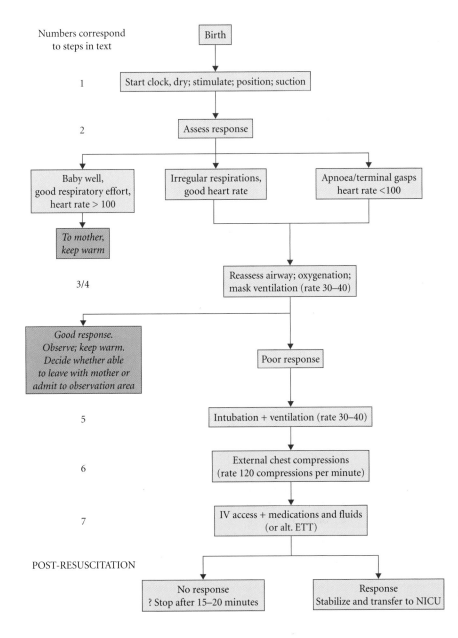

Fig. 60.1 Neonatal resuscitation in the delivery room. ETT, endotracheal tube.

by placing it directly into a plastic bag, without drying, under a radiant heat source.

The airway must be correctly positioned and also needs to be clear. Babies have secretions in their oropharynx at birth. Assuming these are not copious and the infant is vigorous, the infant will clear them independently. Routine oropharyngeal suctioning is to be avoided [E].

Infants with excessive secretions, or those with thick meconium (see below under Special situations) and/or blood, need suctioning. A suction catheter can be placed in the oropharynx; care must be taken not to push the catheter too far back, and some authorities advocate not inserting it further than 5 cm. A suction pressure of 100 mmHg is appropriate. Excessive toileting of the oropharynx causes reflex bardycardia and laryngospasm.

These initial steps should take no more than 20–30 seconds.

Step 2

The infant is then assessed. Initial assessment should include heart rate, respiratory effort and colour. This should have occurred by 30 seconds of age.

Assessment (and reassessment) is vital to a successful outcome. Many workers use the Apgar score (Table 60.1) to aid them. This was originally described by Virginia Apgar, an anaesthesiologist, in 1953. Whilst this is a useful tool, it has its limitations. Apgar scores are carried out at 1 minute and 5 minutes of life. Further scores may be done at 5-minute intervals depending on subsequent progress. It is an internationally recognised assessment tool, giving an indication of the neonate's condition after birth. However, it would be inappropriate to delay resuscitating an apnoeic infant with a profound bradycardia at birth, while waiting for a low 1-minute Apgar score.

From the initial assessment, the infant will fall into one of three groups.

1   Well, healthy and vigorous. The child has a good respiratory effort, is pink centrally, and the heart rate is >100 bpm. This infant can be wrapped up and given to the parents.

Table 60.1 Apgar scoring system

Parameter	Score		
	0	1	2
Heart rate	0	<100	>100
Breathing	Apnoeic	Irregular	Good
Colour	White	Blue	Pink
Muscle tone	Floppy	Some movement	Active
Reflex response	None	Grimace	Cough, cry, sneeze

2   Cyanosed, poor respiratory effort, with or without a heart rate <100 bpm. This infant needs further intervention.
3   White, apnoeic or terminal gasps, with absent heartbeat or profound bradycardia (<60 bpm). This infant needs full intensive resuscitation.

If the child's condition is still a cause for concern, the previous interventions should be checked.

- Is the airway clear and positioned correctly?
- Has the child responded to stimulation?

Step 3

The person resuscitating the infant must ensure the airway is patent before proceeding, as without this any further resuscitation steps will be futile. Manoeuvres which are useful to learn include the one-person or two-person jaw thrust. Both of these are used to lift the tongue up and help open the oropharynx by lifting the lower jaw forward (with the infant lying supine) so it juts just above the upper jaw. Remember the most common cause for an obstructed airway in the newborn is loss of muscle tone and the tongue falling backward.

Another useful technique is the use of a Guedel airway. The easiest way of selecting the right size airway is by measuring the Guedel from the angle of the jaw to the middle of the jaw. This is then placed in the mouth using a laryngoscope blade to lift the lower jaw and tongue and passing the Guedel airway over the blade.

Once the operator is happy the infant's airway is patent, the infant's response should be reassessed. If there is still concern with their breathing, ventilation should be commenced.

Indications for ventilation are:

- an apnoeic infant, or one with gasping respirations despite the above interventions;
- an infant that remains cyanosed despite adequate oxygen delivery.

At this stage in the resuscitation, the infant should be no more than 1 minute of age. This is time enough to know if simple interventions are going to work, without causing further insult by undue delay.

Ventilation is performed either with a bag–valve–mask (bvm) apparatus or a facemask plus T-piece connector.

- The bvm is attached to a gas supply (air plus oxygen) and should have a reservoir bag attached. This helps to increase the concentration of oxygen to near 100 per cent if needed. (In practice it is probably nearer 60–80 per cent with a refill bag, as opposed to 30–40 per cent without; 100 per cent oxygen concentration is difficult to achieve with bvm devices due to leakage at various points.) It is recommended that 500 mL bags be used to aid efficient delivery of ventilatory breaths. These devices have a 'pop-off' valve, which is set to between 20 and 30 cmH$_2$O. (The 'pop-off' valve reduces the risk of excessive peak pressures, which could cause overinflation.) The facemask is applied over the nose and mouth. For neonates, a circular facemask forms the best seal. Positive pressure is applied by squeezing the bag fully, then allowing it to reinflate before the next breath.

- The facemask plus T-piece is also attached to an appropriate air and oxygen supply. Again the facemask is applied over the nose and mouth to form a seal. Above the facemask is a hole over which the resuscitator's thumb is applied to create a positive pressure. The peak pressure can be set using a pressure gauge.

Both techniques are easily learnt, although the T-piece plus facemask probably results in more reliable delivery of a set positive pressure compared to the bvm technique. Certain types of T-piece plus facemask apparatus can also deliver positive end-expiratory pressure (PEEP), which is advantageous in helping to create and maintain a functional residual capacity.

When starting ventilation, five 'rescue' breaths should be administered. These are more sustained breaths, designed to overcome the high airways resistance present in the lungs of the infant who has not breathed. This is much easier to achieve using the T-piece plus facemask technique, in which the thumb can be applied for 1–2 seconds at a set pressure. With the bvm technique, prolonged breaths are difficult to achieve, but higher pressures can be applied by locking the 'pop-off' valve (NB: this should only be done by an experienced operator).

Following these initial rescue breaths, the infant's response should be assessed. If there is still concern regarding respiration, regular ventilation should be commenced. This is delivered at a rate of 30–40 breaths per minute, with each breath lasting approximately 0.5 seconds. The peak pressure should be set to achieve adequate lung expansion without overdistension. Clinically, this can be assessed by chest movement, breath sounds, colour and heart rate, as well as improving spontaneous respiratory effort. Ventilation should be stopped once good, spontaneous, respiratory effort is achieved.

Step 4

Next, use of supplementary oxygen may be considered.

Studies in recent years looking at use of air vs oxygen for resuscitation have questioned the previously long-accepted 'best practice' of using 100 per cent oxygen for resuscitation. Animal and clinical trials indicate that resuscitation with air in the term infant is as effective as 100 per cent oxygen and may even be advantageous [C].[9] Concerns exist relating to the effects of oxygen on the respiratory centres, as well as its direct effects on lungs by means of free radical production. Such effects are even more contentious in the preterm infant. As a result it has become accepted practice to commence resuscitation using air and then add oxygen if there is a poor response. It is important to ensure the airway is patent and good ventilation technique is being applied before using oxygen.

To help with this step, application of an oxygen saturation monitor to the right hand in the newborn can be very helpful.

Remember the oxygen saturations in the well newborn term infant will gradually rise from approximately 60 per cent at birth to over 90 per cent by 10 minutes of age without the use of supplemental oxygen.

Recent guidelines from ILCOR and the UK Resuscitation Council have emphasised the importance of adequate airway and ventilation, leaving the decision to use oxygen to be considered depending on the clinical situation [E].[3]

Step 5

After another 30–60 seconds of facemask ventilation, if there is still inadequate response, endotracheal intubation for more efficient ventilation should be considered.

Indications for intubation include:

- poor respiratory effort despite appropriate interventions as above;
- thick meconium at delivery;
- anticipated need for long-term ventilatory support.

Intubation is achieved using a straight-bladed laryngoscope held in the left hand and an endotracheal tube held in the right hand. The laryngoscope blade size can be chosen to suit the infant. Thus a size 1 blade is suitable for term infants, whereas a size 0 is better suited to preterm infants. A size 00 is available for extremely premature infants with small mouths.

The blade is inserted into the mouth in the midline and the laryngoscope is pulled forward and upward, thus bringing the lower jaw and tongue up and forward until the uvula is visible. At this point it may be necessary to suction the oropharynx using a suction catheter in the right hand. The blade is then advanced over the back of the tongue into the venecular and pulled forward. This elevates the epiglottis, revealing the glottis and vocal cords. It should be remembered that the larynx in the newborn is more 'floppy' than in adults, hence to aid vision, external downward pressure over the cricoid cartilage may be needed to help bring the vocal cords into view. An alternative technique is to place the laryngoscope in the oropharynx as far as it will go, pull the lower jaw and tongue forward and upward to maximise vision and then gradually withdraw the laryngoscope until the epiglottis slips into view, with the vocal cords visible below. This is quicker, but can be more traumatic if not performed carefully.

Once the vocal cords are visualised, the endotracheal tube can be inserted. There is a choice between a straight-sided and a shouldered endotracheal tube (Coles tube). The shouldered tube is stiffer, to help intubation. An introductory stylet can be used to help stiffen whichever endotracheal tube is used.

For resuscitation purposes, oropharyngeal intubation is best practised [E], as this is simpler and quicker than nasopharyngeal intubation – a technically more demanding skill.

Once the endotracheal tube has been positioned, the ventilatory circuit can be attached and ventilatory breaths delivered. Adequate air entry should be confirmed (equal chest movement, breath sounds, appropriate colour and heart rate). If there is any doubt about whether the tube is in the correct position, it should be removed and the infant ventilated with a facemask system whilst the situation is reassessed.

The act of intubation should take no longer than 20–30 seconds from the time of inserting the laryngoscope blade in the mouth until the endotracheal tube is attached to the ventilatory circuit. While performing this action, the infant is effectively being asphyxiated, thus undue delay is unacceptable.

Endotracheal intubation should not be attempted by inexperienced practitioners without appropriate supervision.

Ventilation breaths are delivered at a rate of 30–40/minute, the same as for mask ventilation. Slightly higher rates (up to 60 breaths/minute) may be used for premature infants.

Once intubation has been established, the practitioner must be alert to potential complications, such as a blocked or displaced endotracheal tube, equipment failure and pneumothorax.

Step 6

Once the airway and breathing have been addressed, the next step is to assess the circulation. The heart rate and pulses should be checked. Useful sites include the base of the umbilical cord or brachial pulse, as other pulses can be difficult to elicit. Infants with a heart rate of <60 bpm which have not responded to appropriate ventilation require external chest compressions. This is performed by depressing the lower half of the sternum by one third of the antero-posterior diameter of the chest. In practice, for most infants this equates to 1–2 cm.

Chest compressions can be performed either using both thumbs over the lower sternum, with the hands wrapped around the chest, or by placing the index and middle fingers over the lower sternum. It is more important that appropriate sternal compressions are performed, regardless of which technique is preferred. A rate of 120 chest compressions per minute (two per second) should be attained. If ventilation is being undertaken at the same time, a ratio of three chest compressions to one breath is appropriate. Chest compressions should be stopped once the cardiac rate is >60–80 bpm.

Step 7

This step involves vascular access, use of medication and volume expansion.

- Vascular access may be needed for advanced resuscitation.
  Use of the umbilical vein is the quickest and most effective means of achieving access. An umbilical catheter, primed with 0.9 per cent saline, should be inserted to a depth of approximately 5 cm. Alternative forms of access include the use of peripheral intravenous cannulae (but only if a peripheral vein is readily accessible) or an intraosseous needle. The endotracheal tube can also be used for quick access for certain medications (e.g. adrenaline).
- Medication:

  – Adrenaline (epinephrine) is probably the most important medication available. It can be given via any route, most commonly intravenous or endotracheal. The recommended dose is 0.1–0.3 mL/kg of 1:10,000 solution (or 10–30 µg/kg). Following administration, 1–2 minutes of ventilation and chest compressions are performed. This dose may be repeated every 1–2 minutes. Higher doses (i.e. 100–300 µg/kg or 0.1–0.3 mL/kg of 1:1000 solution) are no longer recommended as there is no evidence that this is beneficial and, indeed, some studies suggest higher doses of adrenaline may be detrimental to the infant [B].[3]
  – Sodium bicarbonate remains controversial. It may be useful in prolonged resuscitations when sustained cellular acidosis may affect myocardial contractility. If used, administration should be limited to a 4.2 per cent solution in aliquots of 1.0–2.0 mL/kg intravenously. The aim is to improve acidic conditions in the heart and thus improve myocardial contractility, as well as facilitating the beneficial effects of adrenaline.
  – Naloxone may be used in the infant with respiratory depression as a result of maternal intrapartum opiate analgesia. The dose is 200 µg intramuscularly. Naloxone is not a substitute for appropriate resuscitation, which should always take precedence. Also, it is best avoided in infants of drug-dependent mothers, as it can result in a severe withdrawal state in these infants. Finally, the caregiver should note that naloxone has a shorter half-life than most opiates and doses may need to be repeated.
  – Dextrose. Hypoglycaemia is a major problem in prolonged resuscitations. Hence, small aliquots of dextrose may be required. A dose of 2–3 mL/kg of 10 per cent dextrose should be adequate.
  – Use of volume replacement.
  – Blood. If there is any suggestion of haemorrhage, O-negative blood should be used: 10–20 mL/kg can be given as a bolus and the response assessed.
  – For other causes of circulatory disturbance, volume replacement with a crystalloid or colloid can be useful in the resuscitation scenario. The dose is again 10–20 mL/kg. Following a Cochrane review[10] that found the use of albumin to be detrimental, most authorities recommend crystalloids, such as 0.9 per cent saline [A].

Glucose solutions must not be used for volume replacement.

POST-RESUSCITATION

Continuing care

Once the infant has been successfully resuscitated, it is essential that provision for ongoing care be provided. This may simply involve handing a well infant to the mother to keep warm and feed, with attendants available to ensure there is no deterioration, or transfer of the sick infant to a NICU for ongoing intensive care.

Before any transfer, the infant should be reassessed clinically. All lines, including endotracheal tubes, intravenous cannulae, nasogastric tubes and monitoring leads, should be secured. The need for ongoing medication and fluids should be considered.

Comprehensive documentation, including interventions, responses and subsequent management plans, should be completed and signed legibly. The family should be fully informed of events.

Discontinuing care

Unfortunately, not all resuscitation attempts are successful and the decision to stop resuscitative attempts can be extremely difficult. As a guide, it is appropriate to consider discontinuing attempts if there is no spontaneous circulation by 15 minutes [E].

Non-initiation of resuscitation

This can also be a contentious issue and it is important that units develop guidance in this area. Most practitioners would accept that it is inappropriate to routinely attempt resuscitation in infants less than 23 weeks' gestation or 400 g birthweight. Equally, it is ethically acceptable not to resuscitate infants with lethal anomalies, such as anencephaly or trisomy 13 and 18.

In cases of uncertainty, an alternative approach is to commence resuscitation, and withdraw intensive care only once more information is available. However, it should be remembered that both withdrawal and withholding of intensive care are ethically equivalent.

With such decisions, the family should be fully informed and involved, as they will have to live with the consequences.

SPECIAL SITUATIONS

Extreme prematurity

These infants have much greater difficulties due to their immature physiology. Their lungs are poorly developed, lack surfactant and have poor lung compliance. They thus experience greater degrees of respiratory distress. Many infants less than 30 weeks' gestation require early ventilation, with administration of surfactant. Indeed, some practitioners advocate 'elective' intubation of all infants less than 28 weeks. This has become contentious with greater awareness of the damage caused by barotrauma and oxygen toxicity.

Premature infants have a much greater surface area to body mass ratio, and thus lose heat much more quickly than term infants. Their cardiovascular systems are also immature, with

poor autoregulation of the cerebral circulation. Care should be exercised when administering volume expanders.

The major practical differences in the approach to resuscitation of a premature infant include: use of a sterile plastic bag and a radiant heat source instead of drying with warm towels; consideration of elective early intubation and administration of surfactant to minimise lung injury; and special attention to avoid excessively high oxygen concentrations. Oxygen saturation monitors can help with the aim of keeping oxygen saturations below a maximum of 95 per cent.

Meconium

Whereas it was previously taught that all infants with meconium present prior to delivery should have their airway viewed and suctioned under direct vision, it is now accepted that this approach can be detrimental in the majority of cases [A].[11] As a rule, infants born in good condition with good respiratory effort do not require airway visualisation or oropharyngeal suctioning. Infants with depressed respiratory effort at birth should have their airway inspected and cleared prior to any other resuscitative efforts. The aim of this is to prevent inhalation of any meconium into the lungs of the compromised infant, as this can cause mechanical problems with breathing, as well as a chemical pneumonitis.

Hydrops

The main problem at birth, regardless of the cause, is the presence of large effusions (pleural, pericardial and peritoneal). These often need draining as a matter of urgency at delivery. Probably the quickest method is the use of an 18 or 20 FG cannula attached to a syringe. This can be advanced into the effusion to be drained, while maintaining gentle negative pressure on the syringe. As soon as fluid is aspirated, the cannula should be advanced over the needle, which is removed. In this way, the cannula can act as a temporary drain until a more permanent one can be inserted.

Congenital diaphragmatic hernia

At birth, the major concerns relate to the degree of lung hypoplasia and amount of bowel and other abdominal content in the chest. Early control of the infant's ventilation in addition to preventing the infant swallowing air and thus inflating the stomach in the chest is generally felt to be best practice. To this end, the infant may be best managed with early intubation and muscle relaxation soon after birth. A large-bore nasogastric tube is inserted to keep the bowel empty.

Owing to lung hypoplasia, caution with positive pressure ventilation must be exercised to prevent pneumothorax.

Nitric oxide ventilation and extracorporeal membrane oxygenation can be used for intensive care and should be considered early in management, depending on the infant's response.

Congenital cardiac disease

Management depends on the lesion. There are too many to discuss in this chapter, except to say that infants with duct-dependent lesions should be commenced on a low-dose prostaglandin infusion early after birth. Otherwise, for the purposes of early neonatal resuscitation, there is no need for other special measures.

Polyhydramnios

The main difference over the usual resuscitation process in this circumstance is to exclude a possible oesophageal atresia by inserting a large-bore nasogastric tube.

SUMMARY

This chapter briefly discusses the process of resuscitating the newborn infant. It emphasizes the ABC approach, with a need for continual appraisal of a situation. It should be stressed that the vast majority of infants require no, or minimal, intervention. Equally, for those who do need help, most problems are related to the respiratory system, and attention to detail with regard to the airway and ventilation will be all that is required.

- Resuscitation should initially start with managing temperature control and ensuring a patent airway [E].
- In the term baby, air is as good as 100 per cent oxygen for resuscitation and may have additional benefits [B].
- High doses of adrenaline are no longer recommended as they confer no additional advantage and may be detrimental [C].

KEY POINTS

- The vast majority of infants need nothing more active than keeping warm at birth.
- Nearly all neonatal resuscitations involve respiratory failure as the primary event.
- Optimizing airway patency is the most important part of neonatal resuscitation.
- Always remember the ABC approach.
- Do not forget to keep the infant warm.

ACKNOWLEDGEMENT

This chapter has been revised and updated. The author and editors acknowledge the contribution of Sandie Bohin to the chapter on this topic in a previous edition of the book.

Key References

1. Royal College of Paediatrics and Child Health and RCOG. *Resuscitation of Babies at Birth*. London: BMJ Publishing Group, 1997.
2. Phillips B, Zideman D, Wyllie J *et al*. European Resuscitation Council Guidelines 2000 for Newly Born Life Support. A statement from the Paediatric Life Support Working Group and approved by the Executive Committee of the European Resuscitation Council. *Resuscitation* 2001;48:235–9.
3. International Consensus Conference on Cardiopulmonary Resuscitation and Emergency Cardiovascular Care Science with Treatment Recommendations. *Circulation* 2005;112:111–99.
4. Kattwinkel J, Niermeyer S, Nadkarni V *et al*. Resuscitation of the newly born infant. *Circulation* 1999; 99:1927–38.
5. Bhutani VK. Extrauterine adaptations in the newborn. *Semin Neonatol* 1997;2:1–12.
6. Gunn AJ, Bennet L. Is temperature important in delivery room resuscitation? *Semin Neonatol* 2001;6:241–9.
7. Jacobs SE, Hunt R, Tarnow-Mordi WO *et al*. Cooling for newborns with hypoxic ischaemic encephalopathy. *Cochrane Database Syst Rev* 2007;4:CD003311.
8. Rabi Y, Rabi D, Yee W. Room air resuscitation of the depressed newborn: A systematic review and meta-analysis. *Resuscitation* 2007;72:353–63.
9. Saugstad OD. Resuscitation of newborn infants with room air or oxygen. *Semin Neonatol* 2001;6:233–9.
10. Alderson P, Schierhout G, Roberts I, Bunn F. Colloids versus crystalloids for fluid resuscitation in critically ill patients. *Cochrane Database Syst Rev* 2000;2:CD000567.
11. Halliday HL, Sweet DG. Endotracheal intubation at birth in vigorous term meconium-stained babies. *Cochrane Database Syst Rev* 2002;4:CD000500.

Chapter 61 Common neonatal problems

Andrew Currie

Andrew Currie

INTRODUCTION

Most babies are born healthy and remain so throughout their lives. However, they can develop a number of common problems which, while not necessarily life threatening, may nonetheless cause significant morbidity and parental anxiety.

This chapter introduces the reader to the most common problems encountered at or shortly after birth, concentrating in the main on those relating to the term fetus/neonate.

At the end of this chapter, there is a brief summary of the more complicated problems associated with prematurity.

INCIDENCE

There are no reliable figures relating to how often paediatricians are asked to review infants for anything other than a newborn check.

Infants requiring paediatric input fall into two main groups. The first group comprises those that require acute care. These infants are primarily seen within the delivery suite shortly after birth. Paediatricians are called either to the resuscitation or for acute problems such as 'the grunting infant'.

The other group comprises infants seen on the postnatal wards. They are usually several hours of age, and any concern is less acute. Table 61.1 summarises an audit of common, non-life-threatening problems seen within one unit during a one-year period, and gives an indication of the concerns paediatricians are asked to respond to on the postnatal wards. The birth population was approximately 5500 births per year. Routine newborn examinations and acutely ill infants have been excluded.

It can be seen from this table that many common problems in the newborn period are not serious health issues, but nonetheless can cause considerable morbidity and anxiety.

Table 61.1 Numbers of infants presenting with common problems on the postnatal wards over a 12-month period, in a birth population of 5500 per year

Clinical condition(s)	Total number
Hips	213
Jaundice	99
Cardiac murmurs	33
Antenatal anomalies	25
Birth trauma	16
Surgical	23
Hypothermia	2
Hypoglycaemia	5
Vomiting	2
Infection	23
Maternal infection	34
Other maternal conditions	23
Family history	64
Genetic	15
Skin lesions	31

COMMON NEONATAL COMPLICATIONS PRESENTING IN THE FIRST 24 HOURS

Respiratory/grunting (transient tachypnoea of the newborn)

One of the most common problems that paediatricians review is acute respiratory embarrassment. Tachypnoea and 'grunting' are the most common concerns. 'Grunting' is the descriptive term given to the noise made by forced expiration against a closed glottis. It is essentially a sign of alveolar disease: the alveoli do not open adequately, hence the infant tries to open them by increasing his or her intrathoracic pressure. Most commonly, 'grunting' and tachypnoea are caused by excess lung fluid, which has not fully cleared following birth. These signs usually appear within the first few hours after birth and settle within 24–48 hours. The infant is otherwise well and observation is usually all that is required. This condition is often referred to as transient tachypnoea of the newborn (TTN). It must be remembered that this is a diagnosis of exclusion. More serious conditions, such as sepsis, aspiration, pneumothorax or respiratory distress syndrome, should be excluded. The signs of acute respiratory embarrassment are the same for many aetiologies;[1] thus, such infants should be seen by a paediatrician. If the signs are not settling quickly (i.e. within a few hours), if they worsen or if there are other risk factors in the history, the infant should be admitted to a neonatal unit for further investigation and management. This complication is common among babies delivered by elective caesarian section (CS), with as many as 15 per cent of neonates being affected [B].[1]

Hypoglycaemia

This subject causes much anxiety and continues to generate much controversy.[2] It is now accepted that many newborn infants go through a period of relatively low blood glucose levels shortly after birth. Assuming they are otherwise well, they can utilise alternative fuel sources, such as ketones and lactate, in the short term. This means that for term infants of average birthweight, it is unnecessary to monitor blood glucose and start invasive treatments. They should be left alone to establish breast- or bottlefeeding normally. The importance of hypoglycaemia is to identify and treat the 'at-risk' infant. Examples include:

- preterm infants (<36 weeks);
- growth-restricted babies;
- the infants of diabetics;
- infants with perinatal asphyxia;
- septic infants;
- infants with inborn errors of metabolism.

In these groups, a blood glucose <2.6 mmol/L is generally accepted to indicate hypoglycaemia [E]. Any infant presenting with low blood glucose must be carefully examined for the underlying cause and treated accordingly. The treatment of hypoglycaemia involves the administration of glucose. In the well infant, feeding with milk should be the first-line treatment. If this is not successful, or if there are indicators to suggest the infant is unwell, intravenous dextrose may be needed (a 10 per cent solution should be used initially). It may be necessary to give intravenous bolus doses (small boluses of 2–3 mL/kg of 10 per cent dextrose, followed by an infusion). All infants requiring additional glucose should be admitted to a neonatal unit.

Hypothermia

This can be defined as a rectal temperature <36°C. It is most commonly seen in growth-restricted and preterm small infants, or as part of the clinical picture in the sick infant. Newborn infants are born exposed and wet, and can lose heat very quickly if not dried and covered adequately. Hypothermia can cause significant morbidity; infants are lethargic and feed poorly. More seriously, hypothermia is associated with hypoglycaemia, metabolic acidosis and respiratory distress.

The septic infant may also present with hypothermia rather than pyrexia. Hence, when dealing with the cold newborn, the first concern is to look for the underlying cause. Once this has been dealt with, specific measures to warm the child include a warm environment (this may seem obvious, but it is often found that delivery rooms are environmentally unfriendly for the newborn infant), drying the infant adequately and dressing him or her in warm clothes (including skin-to-skin contact with the mother and warm towels and covers), and the use of a radiant heater or warming mattresses. For extreme hypothermia, more invasive measures, such as reheating with warmed plasma expanders or exchange transfusions with warmed blood, have been used. However, it is debatable whether these convey any benefit over the use of a radiant heater and warming mattress.

Fractures

These are not common. Fracture of the clavicle is the most frequently seen, followed by the humerus, femur and skull bones. Fractures usually result from traumatic deliveries, for example in association with shoulder dystocia and difficult instrumental deliveries [D].[3] However, this is not inevitably the case and certainly the medical literature gives examples of apparently unexplained fractures.

Clavicular fractures are best treated conservatively and have an excellent prognosis. Mild analgesia may be helpful.

Fractures of long bones may require some form of simple splinting to immobilise the limb and thus reduce pain.

Skull fractures are more serious, and the possibility of underlying haemorrhage must be considered.

The majority of neonatal fractures will heal uneventfully with conservative treatment.

Cephalohaematomas

These result from bleeding between the periosteum and skull bones, and take the shape of the underlying skull bone. As they resolve, they may exacerbate jaundice, and the possibility of associated injury (such as skull fracture or intracranial bleeding) should be ruled out. Most cephalohaematomas are benign and resolve without problems. During resolution, the swelling may increase in size; this is usually due to fluid shift into the haemorrhage by osmosis as the clot breaks down. The carers should be warned of this, as it can cause concern.

Nerve palsies

Erb's palsy and facial palsy are the most common nerve palsies. Erb's palsy is due to damage to the brachial plexus (cervical roots C5, 6 and 7), and is commonly associated with traction on the neck and shoulders during difficult deliveries,[3] although cases occurring in infants delivered by CS have been reported. The result is usually a flaccid arm held in a pronated and internally rotated position. Recovery rates vary according to different studies. Between 49 and 94 per cent make a full recovery, with most improving by 12 months of age.[4] Early physiotherapy can help, and surgical treatment techniques to repair damaged nerves are now available for those cases that do not resolve spontaneously. Such cases should be referred early.

Facial palsies are commonly ascribed to obstetric manoeuvres, such as the use of forceps causing pressure damage; however, facial palsies also occur in infants delivered normally.[3] Most are probably the result of external pressure causing a lower motor neuron injury, and the prognosis is excellent. If an upper motor neuron lesion is suspected, the infant should be investigated for possible cerebral injury or congenital disorders. There is no specific treatment required.

Sternomastoid tumours

These are the result of bleeding into the sternomastoid muscle. They are not normally recognised at birth, and do not become obvious until a few weeks of age. Physiotherapy is required to prevent contracture of the muscle. The prognosis is good.

Traumatic cyanosis

This is a petechial rash present over the face and head, and may extend to the upper body, although the rest of the child is usually spared. It is probably the result of venous congestion, resolves spontaneously and is only of importance because it has been mistaken for true cyanosis. Simple reassurance is all that is required.

Lacerations

Occasionally, the infant may suffer skin lacerations during delivery, usually during CS. They are usually superficial and heal without problems. Suturing or use of steristrips may be needed for deeper wounds.

THE NEWBORN EXAMINATION

This is included in this chapter because it plays a major role in the care of the newborn. It entails a clinical examination of the infant, carried out in the first week of life. It is meant as a screening health check, although there has been much controversy concerning its usefulness. At least 80 per cent of mothers find it a useful and reassuring process.[5]

It is probably not worth performing this examination within the first 24 hours of life, as there is a high chance of both false-negative and false-positive findings. Equally, assuming the infant is well, a 24-hour interval provides a chance for the infant to recover from the stresses of birth, and allows bonding to occur.

The newborn examination should be performed in a well-lit, warm room to prevent the exposed infant getting cold.

As with all medical examinations, it helps to have a routine system. By convention, the neonatal check is performed from the head and working down. Auscultation of the heart is opportunistic, as the infant needs to be quiet. A full explanation of the examination process would be lengthy, and the reader is referred to any of the standard textbooks of neonatology for this. A few points to remember include the need for proper hand hygiene when examining infants, and that the infant should not be left exposed for prolonged periods of time. It is often best to leave the nappy area until last. As part of the newborn check, parents should be asked about the passage of urine and stool, as well as any feeding concerns. In addition, a check should be made of the weight and head circumference. Increasingly, early neonatal pulse oximetry is used as part of the examination to screen babies for both undiagnosed cardiac (i.e. congenital heart disease) and non-cardiac (i.e. occult infection) anomalies. This test has very good sensitivity and specificity of diagnosis.[6]

COMMON NEONATAL PROBLEMS PRESENTING ON THE POSTNATAL WARD

Feeding

This is a huge subject and is one of the most common causes of anxiety in mothers.

There are two methods of feeding infants: breastfeeding and the use of formula milk feeds. Breastfeeding is clearly the best choice for a number of reasons, including the following:

- it adapts to the infant's nutritional needs;
- it has anti-infective properties;
- it helps with bonding;
- it helps the mother lose weight;
- it aids contraception;
- it is convenient and free.

However, there are a few problems associated with breastfeeding. Contrary to many mothers' preconceptions, breastfeeding is not always established readily. This can lead to a sense of failure and to the abandonment of breastfeeding if no support is available. Ill and preterm infants do not readily feed. In this situation, facilities should be available to help with the expression of breast milk until such time as the child is ready to suckle. There are often concerns about milk volumes; these are usually helped by support and reassurance. Test weighing has previously been used to try to quantify the amount of milk an infant is getting; however, this is not only unhelpful, but indeed can be positively detrimental to breastfeeding as it often instils a further sense of failure in the mother.

Other problems include concern about inverted nipples, cracked nipples, engorged breasts, overfeeding and weaning. These concerns should be easily addressed with the right support and information. Mastitis can also cause problems, but is not a reason to stop breastfeeding. Antibiotics or non-steroidal anti-inflammatory drugs (NSAIDs) may be indicated. There are very few contraindications to breastfeeding. Probably the most common are chronic ill-health in the mother (such as cystic fibrosis), potential infective risk (e.g. HIV in developed countries), acute ill-health in both the mother and infant, and certain metabolic disorders in the infant (such as phenylketonuria and galactosaemia).

Artificial feeding with formula milk is the alternative. Problems specific to this include:

- poor preparation of feeds;
- inadequate sterilisation;
- cost.

Other problems common to both methods include problems with sucking and swallowing coordination. These may be due to anatomical factors, such as cleft palates or large tongues, as well as physiological factors, such as immaturity of the sucking reflexes.

Vomiting can be a major problem, and is most commonly due to gastro-oesophageal reflux. Assuming that the infant is well and growing, reassurance is usually all that is needed. Examination to exclude other causes of vomiting, such as pyloric stenosis and sepsis, should be performed. Failure to thrive is often due to feeding problems, but usually presents later in life. Bilious vomiting is pathological until proven otherwise, and should always prompt the search for a cause.

Urine/stools

It is not uncommon for neonatologists to be asked to review an infant who has either not passed urine or not opened his/her bowels. Either situation is usually benign. A detailed history, including review of the antenatal progress and birth, is important. The external genitalia and anus should be examined as part of the assessment.

Most infants pass urine within the first 24 hours. This is often missed if it occurs at the time of birth. If there is any doubt but the infant otherwise appears well, it is worth placing cotton wool ball(s) in the nappy. An infant who has not passed urine within the first couple of days or in whom there is any other concern may need further investigation to exclude either obstruction (such as posterior urethral valves in males) or renal disease.

An infant who has not opened his or her bowels within the first 2–3 days should also be reviewed. Obstruction due to anal atresia should be obvious shortly after birth; however, conditions such as anal stenosis and Hirschprung's disease are easily missed if not considered. Investigation in such situations may involve gentle rectal examination, radiological tests and possibly rectal biopsy. Advice should be sought from a neonatologist and/or paediatric surgeon.

Weight loss

It is normal for infants to lose weight in the first week of life. This is predominantly due to water loss. Breastfed infants tend to lose slightly more weight than bottlefed infants. By 1 week of age, infants should start putting weight on. The average weight gain is 20–30 g/day in term infants. Weight loss in excess of 10 per cent is unusual and needs further investigation. There is a long list of causes of excess weight loss, ranging from inadequate intake, through inadequate nutritional content, to feed intolerance and ill-health.

Skin lesions

Skin lesions are a common cause of concern in the otherwise well newborn. They include the following:

- *Birthmarks* such as the flammeus naevus (or 'stork mark') and port wine stains. It should be noted that strawberry birthmarks do not appear until a few weeks of age. Another birthmark is the Mongolian blue spot (very common in Asian and Afro-Caribbean babies), which consists of blue macules found over the back and is caused by melanocytes in the deep dermal layers.
- *Skin defects*, such as the aplasia cutis lesion. This is a congenital absence of the skin over the scalp. It usually has a punched-out appearance, with a healed edge, and it is important to distinguish it from trauma. These lesions usually heal spontaneously, by granulation. Plastic surgery, when the child is older, is required for larger lesions.

- *Rashes.* Common rashes include erythema toxicum neonatorum, a red maculopapular rash, which comes and goes in the first few days and is of no clinical significance. Miliaria may also cause concern; this rash is caused by obstruction of sweat glands. Pustular rashes are common; most are sterile, but possible infection needs to be excluded. Nappy rashes include napkin dermatitis and candidiasis, both of which are very common and cause considerable anxiety.
- *Skin tags.* These can occur anywhere on the body; common sites are around the ears, anus and vagina. Pre-auricular skin tags have classically been associated with renal disorders, although the evidence is tenuous.

Facial problems

- *Clefts of the lip* are usually obvious at birth. With better antenatal screening, many are now diagnosed on antenatal ultrasonography. The possibility of an associated chromosomal disorder should be considered, although most are independent of any other disorder. Although cosmetically they may look very abnormal, the surgical results are excellent. Parents need careful counselling from an early stage, including the use of 'before and after surgery' photographs for reassurance. During the neonatal period, the main concern is one of feeding, and referral for specialist advice at an early stage is paramount.
- Isolated *clefts of the palate* are almost never detected antenatally. They may be detected at a newborn check or can present in the early neonatal period as difficulty in feeding, apnoeas, choking episodes, poor feeding and chest infection. They are often associated with syndromes, and a meticulous neonatal examination should be performed. Referral to a geneticist may be indicated if there are other dysmorphic features. The specialist cleft lip and palate centre should be involved at an early stage.
- *Soft palate defects* can be particularly difficult to diagnose and may not be detected until late in childhood. They can result in feeding problems, as well as speech difficulties, and it is thus important that the palate is visualised to the back of the mouth, as well as palpated as part of the newborn examination.

Orthopaedic

- *Talipes* ('club foot') is a common referral for paediatric assessment. It is important to differentiate between fixed talipes and positional talipes. The former needs referral to orthopaedic surgeons and physiotherapy, whereas the latter is of no consequence and the parents can be reassured.
- Examination of the *hips* is performed to detect dislocation. The hip should be held in a flexed, slightly internally rotated position, between index finger and thumb, while the knee is stabilised within the palm of the hand. The hip is then downwardly displaced to see if it can be dislocated. It is then externally rotated and upward pressure is exerted on to the outer trochanter of the hip with a view to reducing a dislocated hip. These are essentially the Ortolani and Barlow manoeuvres and are designed to diagnose a dislocatable or dislocated hip (in which case a 'clunk' should be felt). This is to be distinguished from a clicky hip, which is usually either due to poor examination technique or lax ligaments around the joint. Dislocated and dislocatable hips need referral to the orthopaedic team. Ultrasonography is useful to discriminate where there is uncertainty. It is also indicated in babies at greater risk of dislocated hips (breech deliveries, positive family histories). The use of double nappies is no longer recommended.

Accessory digits

It is not uncommon for infants to be born with accessory fingers and toes. Most of these are pre-axial and not associated with any other problems. The infant should be thoroughly examined for other anomalies. Most accessory digits are attached by a thread of skin, and are easily dealt with by tying off with a suture. Those with thicker bases should be referred to a plastic surgeon.

Surgical

- *Hernias.* Common hernial sites include the umbilicus and inguinal canal. Umbilical hernias are easily reducible and usually resolve spontaneously. They are more common in Afro-Caribbean and Asian infants. Inguinal hernias are more serious. They are up to six times more common in males than females and there is an increased incidence of complications in the newborn. Early referral to a paediatric surgeon for operative correction is advised. Premature infants more commonly develop inguinal hernias than term infants.
- *Bilious vomiting* always needs investigating; although it may be innocent, the risk of intestinal obstruction or other serious pathology must be considered.
- *Hydrocoeles* are due to fluid accumulation in the scrotum as a result of incomplete closure of the processus vaginalis. They can be differentiated from inguinal hernias because it is possible to get above them and they transilluminate. Most hydrocoeles resolve spontaneously.
- *Hypospadias* occurs in approximately 1:300 male infants. It is characterised by a congenitally short urethra that opens on to the ventral surface of the penis, an abnormally formed foreskin, and chordee of the penis. Referral to a paediatric urologist is required. The parents should be advised not to have the child circumcised, as the foreskin is vital in any reconstructive surgery. The possibility of

chromosomal abnormalities (especially sex chromosome problems) needs to be considered in severe cases.

- *Undescended testes* are common in the newborn male. Most are unilateral, and reassurance that descent will occur is all that is required. If the testicle has not descended by one year of age, referral to a paediatric surgeon is warranted. Bilaterally undescended testicles are much more unusual and require further investigation to exclude underlying disorders, such as intersex or hormonal disorders of the pituitary–adrenal–testicular axis.

Genetic

Paediatricians are commonly asked to review an infant whose appearance has given cause for concern. Most of the time, simple reassurance is all that is required. However, in all cases the child should be carefully and thoroughly examined. There are many dysmorphic features – too numerous to list here. In cases where doubt exists, further advice should be sought from a clinical geneticist. Chromosomal tests, as well as other investigations (dictated by the presenting condition), may be needed. It is important that the parents are carefully counselled. If doubt exists, this should be explained, to avoid erroneous conclusions being made.

Eyes

- The vast majority of *sticky eyes* are due to blocked tear ducts; simple toileting with lukewarm sterile water and cotton wool or gauze is all that is required. If the discharge persists, or is particularly copious, infections should be considered, and a swab sent for microbiological culture and sensitivity. The eyes should then be treated with topical antibiotics. Staphylococcal infections are the most common and are usually successfully treated with either topical gentamicin or neomycin. Chloramphenicol eye drops are also available and popular, but can mask chlamydial infection. Chlamydial infection should be considered if the discharge is copious or persistent. *Chlamydia* requires special culture mediums to grow, and is treated with chlortetracycline eye ointment plus systemic erythromycin.
- Congenital *cataracts* are rare. The newborn check is designed to detect them by looking for the normal red reflex with an ophthalmoscope. If a cataract is present, the red reflex will be absent, or partially obscured, depending on the size of the cataract. In this situation, urgent referral to an ophthalmologist is required. With early intervention, it is possible to improve subsequent vision.

Cardiac murmurs

Heart murmurs are a common finding in newborn infants; however, most cardiac murmurs in the newborn are innocent flow murmurs – these are especially audible in the first days of life. As a general rule, identification of a cardiac murmur should lead to a careful clinical examination, an ECG and measurement of limb oxygen saturations in the right arm and lower limbs (i.e. pre-ductal and post-ductal oxygen saturations). The majority of infants will be found to have a soft systolic murmur (i.e. with a grading of 1–2/6), a normal cardio-vascular examination, no significant change in pre-ductal and post-ductal oxygen saturations, and a normal ECG. These infants can be reviewed in 4–6 weeks, as the chance of a significant cardiac lesion is very small. Parents should be warned of the small risk of a cardiac defect; if they have any concerns, such as the child getting breathless, tired, not feeding or going blue, they should seek medical advice urgently.

Infants who do not meet these criteria should be referred to a paediatric cardiologist for further investigation.

Maternal group B streptococcal infection

It is generally accepted that infants of group B *Streptococcus* (GBS) carriers are at greater risk of infection. However, quantifying that risk is difficult. Equally, given the high carriage rate amongst the normal population (estimated between 30 and 50 per cent), it is difficult to ascertain the best treatment approach.

GBS disease is divided into early and late onset.

Early-onset GBS disease is caused by passage of the infant through the genital tract in a carrier mother (many women are carriers and few babies are affected). It may present as:

- a clinical picture which mimics severe perinatal asphyxia;
- severe respiratory failure at birth;
- signs of early neonatal sepsis, such as temperature instability, lethargy, irritability, respiratory signs and tachycardia.

It is a neonatal emergency with potentially life-threatening consequences.

Universal pregnancy screening programmes and the use of prophylactic antibiotics are not recommended in the UK (see Chapter 44).

In an attempt to identify at-risk babies, it is recommended that infants born to mothers who are GBS carriers and have one or more of the following features deserve special attention:

- previous infant born with GBS disease;
- spontaneous onset of premature labour;
- prolonged rupture of membranes;
- evidence of invasive GBS disease in the mother.

If mothers are given sufficient antibiotics early enough in the labour, the infant should be adequately covered [A].[7]

If this does not occur, or the infant is in any way unwell, he or she should be screened and treated with intravenous antibiotics. Subsequent management will depend on the clinical course and the results of cultures.

Late-onset GBS disease is probably related to infection after birth from a carrier mother. It can be present days or weeks later, most commonly with pneumonia or meningitis.

Renal

In addition to determining whether or not a baby has passed urine (see above under Urine/stools), other renal problems usually relate to infants who have been found to have renal anomalies during antenatal ultrasound screening. Assuming the infant is well, repeated scanning can be performed within the first few weeks of life; many anomalies will have resolved. If there are continuing abnormalities, further investigation is required to delineate the nature of the anomaly.

Infants with significant bilateral renal anomalies on antenatal ultrasound (e.g. bilateral dysplastic, cystic kidneys or bilaterally dilated ureters) need more urgent investigation. They should also be monitored for failing renal function.

Metabolic

The Guthrie test is a screening test performed on all newborn infants within the first week of life. It involves the collection of blood drops from a heel prick, and screens for:

- hypothyroidism;
- phenylketonuria;
- cystic fibrosis (in certain parts of the UK, immunoreactive trypsin levels are measured).

In addition, a few parts of the UK are also using the test to screen for sickle cell disease and medium-chain acyl-coenzyme A dehydrogenase deficiency (MCAD). The test should be performed once the infant has been established on feeds for a few days.

Sacral dimples

Sacral dimples are a common finding, usually at the base of the spinal column. It is also important to ask about bowel actions and urine excretion and to check the lower limbs for normal movements and power. Assuming the base is easily seen and there are no other abnormalities, simple reassurance is all that is required. If the base is not visualised, or if the sacral dimples are larger than 0.5 cm diameter or associated with other features, such as tufts of hair, ultrasound investigation and paediatric review are indicated.

The most commonly associated problem is tethering of the spinal cord, which usually presents later in life.

Umbilical cord

The umbilical cord is a common source of concern. The cord stump usually falls off within a few days.

- The most serious problem is one of *infection*. It is common for the cord stump itself to become colonised with commensal organisms, resulting in a 'sticky' or 'smelly' cord stump. Assuming the infant is otherwise well, with no signs of ascending infection, simple toileting with sterile saline or water is all that is needed [A].[8]

- Should there be any signs of spreading infection or systemic illness, the infant must be treated immediately. Ascending infection from the cord stump is usually due to *Escherichia coli*, other Gram-negative organisms or *Staphylococcus aureus*, and is a neonatal emergency requiring intravenous antibiotics.

- Umbilical stump *granulomas* do not present until after the cord stump has separated. Most resolve, although some practitioners treat them with application of a silver nitrate stick. Great care should be exercised so as not to cause chemical burns to the surrounding skin. They must be differentiated from a patent urachus, which is an embryological remnant connecting the bladder to the base of the umbilical cord and can result in passage of urine. It requires surgical correction.

Jaundice

Jaundice is a common and potentially serious problem with numerous causes:

- physiological jaundice, due to overloading of the immature hepatic system as a result of excessive red blood cell breakdown: the infant develops an unconjugated hyperbilirubinaemia between the second and fifth days, settling by a week of age;
- sepsis;
- haemolysis due to rhesus or ABO incompatibility.

Acute haemolytic disease usually presents within the first 24–48 hours of life, thus any baby appearing jaundiced within this time must be investigated.

Treatment may not be necessary. The most important reason for treating jaundice is to prevent kernicterus, which is associated with severe unconjugated hyperbilirubinaemia and may result in death or major neurological sequelae. Most infants can be treated with simple phototherapy, although for more serious cases exchange transfusions are needed.

Prolonged jaundice is also of concern in the neonate. As a general rule, any term infant with evidence of jaundice beyond 10–14 days of age, or a preterm infant after 3 weeks of age, should be considered as having prolonged jaundice. There are numerous causes, of which the most common is 'breast milk jaundice' (a diagnosis of exclusion). All infants with prolonged jaundice should be investigated. It is particularly important to exclude an obstruction (e.g. biliary atresia), which can be treated successfully with surgical intervention if diagnosed early.[9]

PROBLEMS ASSOCIATED WITH PREMATURITY

Respiratory distress syndrome (also known as hyaline membrane disease) is due to a lack of surfactant in the lungs, leading to acute respiratory failure. The severity varies from mild respiratory symptoms, requiring minimal input, to severe respiratory failure, requiring full intensive care and complex ventilator strategies.

Respiratory distress syndrome can either recover or develop into chronic lung disease (bronchopulmonary dysplasia). Other complications include pulmonary interstitial emphysema and other airleak syndromes.

Effectively, every system in the premature infant is at greater risk of problems. Premature infants are at risk of cardiovascular instability and hypotension requiring treatment. They are susceptible to cerebral insults, especially intraventricular haemorrhage and periventricular leukomalacia (the development of cysts in the periventricular areas at a few weeks of age) due to ischaemic injury. Their immature immune systems put them at higher risk of sepsis. They easily become anaemic, due to marrow immaturity, as well as the need for frequent phlebotomy. Their gastrointestinal system is vulnerable. They often show feed intolerance initially, and there is a high risk of necrotising enterocolitis. (Necrotising enterocolitis is a serious condition which affects the lining of the bowel; it probably results from infection superimposed on bowel that has suffered an ischaemic insult.)

Premature infants also have a higher risk of long-term sequelae, including poor growth, neurodevelopmental disabilities and chronic lung disease.

CONCLUSION

This chapter highlights some of the more common problems facing the newborn infant. It concentrates on acute problems occurring in the delivery suite shortly after birth and on concerns that subsequently present on the postnatal wards. Most of the common problems occurring after the first hours following birth are not life threatening, but do cause significant anxiety and morbidity.

ACKNOWLEDGEMENT

This chapter has been revised and updated. The author and editors acknowledge the contribution of Sandie Bohin to the chapter on this topic in the previous edition of the book.

KEY POINTS

- Most common neonatal problems are not life threatening.
- Recognising the sick infant from the well infant is vital to avoid disaster.
- The newborn examination is a clinical screening test, and as such its limitations should be borne in mind.

Key References

1. Dani C, Reali MF, Bertini G *et al.* Risk factors for the development of respiratory distress syndrome and transient tachypnoea in newborn infants. Italian Group of Neonatal Pneumology. *Eur Respir J* 1999;14:155–9.
2. Cornblath M, Hawdon JM, Williams AF *et al.* Controversies regarding definition of neonatal hypoglycemia: suggested operational thresholds. *Pediatrics* 2000;105:1141–5.
3. Perlow JH, Wigton T, Hart J *et al.* Birth trauma. A five- year review of incidence and associated perinatal factors. *J Reprod Med* 1996;41:754–60.
4. Pollack RN, Buchman AS, Yaffe H, Divon MY. Obstetrical brachial palsy: pathogenesis, risk factors, and prevention. *Clin Obstet Gynecol* 2000;43:236–46.
5. Wolke D, Dave S, Hayes J *et al.* Routine examination of the newborn and maternal satisfaction: a randomised controlled trial. *Arch Dis Child Fetal Neonatal Ed* 2002;86:F155–60.
6. Ewer AK, Middleton LJ, Furmston AT *et al.* PulseOx Study Group. Pulse oximetry screening for congenital heart defects in newborn infants (PulseOx): a test accuracy study. *Lancet* 2011;378(9793):785–94.
7. Smaill F. Intrapartum antibiotics for Group B streptococcal colonisation. *Cochrane Database Syst Rev* 2002;(3):CD000115.
8. Zupan J, Garner P. Topical umbilical cord care at birth. *Cochrane Database Syst Rev* 2002;3: CD001057.
9. Johnson LH, Bhutani VK, Brown AK. System-based approach to management of neonatal jaundice and prevention of kernicterus. *J Pediatr* 2002;140:396–403.

Chapter 62 Perinatal mortality

James Drife

MRCOG standards

Theoretical skills

- Know the definitions of the perinatal mortality rate and its subdivisions.
- Have knowledge of the way in which perinatal deaths are classified, and the leading causes.
- Know how perinatal mortality rates can be kept low or reduced further.

Practical skills

- Recognise that reducing perinatal mortality requires practical obstetric skills.
- Recognise the need for attention to detail in both antenatal and intrapartum care.
- Recognise that skills in risk management are highly relevant.

INTRODUCTION

Although babies may die at any time during pregnancy, and obstetric complications such as preterm labour may result in death of the infant several weeks after delivery, perinatal mortality is strictly defined as stillbirths and deaths of babies in the first week of life. In all countries the perinatal mortality rate (PMR), even with this relatively limited definition, is much higher than the maternal mortality rate. In the UK in 2009 the PMR (7.6 per 1000 live and stillbirths)[1] was 66 times higher than the maternal mortality rate (11.4 per 100,000 maternities), though exact comparison is difficult because of the different denominators (see Chapter 28).

The PMR is widely used as an indicator of the quality of obstetric care and enables comparisons to be made among nations, regions and indeed individual hospitals. The causes of perinatal mortality, however, include a wide range of conditions, such as antepartum haemorrhage, congenital anomalies and preterm labour. For useful clinical lessons to be learned, perinatal mortality must be subdivided by the stage at which death occurred and by the causes.

The two components of the PMR, the stillbirth rate and the neonatal death rate, reflect different aspects of care and tend to be reported separately. Indeed, in England and Wales the most recent report from the Office for National Statistics (ONS)[2] did not include the overall PMR. Instead it reported that the neonatal mortality rate had fallen steadily in the previous decade (from 3.8 per 1000 in 2000 to 2.9 in 2011) while the stillbirth rate had remained virtually unchanged (5.3 per 1000 in 2000 and 5.2 per 1000 in 2011). Interestingly, the static stillbirth rate was not one of the ONS report's 'key findings', although it is the subject of increasing concern and research.[3]

DEFINITIONS

The following definitions are those used in the UK and published in the annual reports of the Centre for Maternal and Child Enquiries (CMACE) which, with its predecessor the Confidential Enquiry in Maternal and Child Health (CEMACH), conducted perinatal surveillance from 2003 to 2009 and produced UK-wide perinatal statistics for the first time.

- *Stillbirth.* The legal definition in England and Wales is 'A child which has issued forth from its mother after the 24th week of pregnancy and which did not at any time after being completely expelled from its mother breathe or show any other signs of life'.
- *Early neonatal death.* Death of a liveborn infant occurring less than 7 completed days (168 hours) from the time of birth.
- *Perinatal mortality rate.* The number of stillbirths and early neonatal deaths (those occurring in the first week of life) per 1000 live and stillbirths.

CMACE also gathered data on deaths that fall outside the strict definition of perinatal mortality. In some regions, for example, late fetal deaths were notified. Other categories and definitions are as follows:

- *Late fetal loss.* Death occurring between 20 weeks + 0 days and 23 weeks + 6 days. If gestation is not known or not sure, all births of at least 300 g are reported.
- *Neonatal death.* Death before the age of 28 completed days following live birth.
- *Late neonatal death.* Death from age 7 days to 27 completed days of life.
- *Post-neonatal death.* Death at age 28 days and over, but under 1 year.
- *Infant death.* Death in the first year following live birth, on or before the 365th day of life (366th in a leap year). Infant deaths therefore include early and late neonatal deaths and post-neonatal deaths.

When infant and neonatal death rates are calculated, the denominator is 'per 1000 live births'. This is slightly different from the denominator 'per 1000 live and stillbirths' which is used to calculate the late fetal loss rate, the stillbirth rate and the PMR.

Definitions of 'stillbirth'

Miscarriages are not included in the PMR. In the UK miscarriages do not have to be registered but it is legally necessary to register stillbirths – i.e. babies born dead after 24 weeks. The dividing line between miscarriage and stillbirth, however, is arbitrary and may vary from country to country. In the United States, for example, there is no single definition used in all states.

In the UK the dividing line was 28 weeks until 1992. When it was lowered to 24 weeks, the official stillbirth rate rose by nearly 30 per cent. The change was made because, with neonatal care, many fetuses born alive at under 28 weeks can now survive. Indeed, survival is possible even below 24 weeks, but this was retained as the dividing line in the UK partly because, under British law, therapeutic abortion for social reasons is allowed up to 24 weeks' gestation.

Internationally, the definition and terminology are inconsistent and this has contributed to confusion about stillbirths.[4] The official definition of the World Health Organization (WHO) is:

> *The death of a fetus weighing at least 500 g (or when birthweight is unavailable, after 22 completed weeks of gestation or with a crown–heel length of 25 cm or more), before the complete expulsion or extraction from its mother.*

In many parts of the world it may be difficult to define gestation exactly, which is why the WHO definition includes fetal weight or measurement. For international comparisons, however, a definition which includes 'early fetal stage' (22–28 weeks) losses is unhelpful, and WHO has agreed that when countries are being compared stillbirth should be defined as fetal death in the third trimester (≥1000 g birthweight or ≥28 completed weeks of gestation).[5]

In all countries, if a baby is born alive and dies soon after delivery, this is classified as a neonatal death irrespective of the gestation. This may lead to some anomalies. For example, in the UK a baby born at 23 weeks' gestation will be included in the national statistics if death occurs after delivery but not if death occurs before delivery.

CONFIDENTIAL ENQUIRIES INTO PERINATAL DEATHS

History

In England and Wales the Confidential Enquiry into Maternal Deaths (CEMD) has been running continuously since 1952, and this method was extended to the deaths of babies in 1992, when the Confidential Enquiry into Stillbirths and Deaths in Infancy (CESDI) was set up. Its aim was to improve understanding of the risks of death from 20 weeks of pregnancy to 1 year after birth, and of how these might be reduced. From 1996, CESDI was managed by a consortium of four Royal Colleges – those of Midwives, Obstetricians and Gynaecologists, Paediatrics and Child Health, and Pathology. In 2002, CEMD and CESDI joined to form the CEMACH, which was part of NICE.

In 2009, CEMACH became CMACE, an independent charity funded mainly by the National Patient Safety Agency (NPSA). In 2011 CMACE was closed down and the only data available for 2010–12 are those collected by ONS. In 2012 the Healthcare Quality Improvement Partnership (HQIP) passed the responsibility for the enquiry to the National Perinatal Epidemiology Unit (NPEU) and from 1 January 2013 data have been collected electronically by MBRRACE-UK (which stands for Mothers and Babies – Reducing Risk through Audits and Confidential Enquiries across the UK).[6]

Although this short history produced a bewildering proliferation of acronyms, the aims of MBRRACE-UK are the same as those of its predecessors. Obstetricians should be pleased that the 'confidential enquiry' method of improving care is now being more widely used, after being pioneered 60 years ago by the RCOG and the (then) Ministry of Health when they set up the CEMD. Enquiries into perinatal deaths, however, require a larger infrastructure than the CEMD. Every year in the UK there are around 6000 perinatal deaths (Table 62.1), compared with about 100 maternal deaths.

Table 62.1 Numbers of perinatal deaths in the UK in 2009[1]

Total births	794,906
Stillbirths	4125
Early neonatal deaths	1945
Late neonatal deaths	566
Total number of perinatal deaths	6070
Perinatal mortality rate (per 1000 total births)	7.6
Stillbirth rate (per 1000 total births)	5.2
Neonatal mortality rate (per 1000 live births)	3.2

Methods

Between 2009 and 2011, every maternity unit in England, Wales and Northern Ireland had a CMACE coordinator who notified the regional office of each death using a 'Perinatal Death Notification Form'. That form contained details of the mother's background, previous pregnancies and medical history, the current pregnancy and delivery, and the outcome including the cause of death. Autopsy data were not required. In addition, deaths were reported to CMACE by pathologists, coroners, child health systems and local congenital anomaly registers, leading to a very high level of ascertainment. Collaboration with the equivalent organisation in Scotland (NHS Quality Improvement Scotland) provided UK-wide statistics and the National Perinatal Mortality Surveillance programme published a report every year.[1]

In June 2012 MBRRACE-UK started work on a secure, web-based electronic data collection system.[6] Data are now collected on 'late pregnancy losses' (i.e. from 22 weeks' gestation), stillbirths, early and late neonatal deaths and post-neonatal deaths (up to 1 year from delivery). Details are requested of the woman's demographic information, health and previous pregnancies, as well as about the current pregnancy and its outcome. Lead users from each maternity unit in the UK have been recruited to facilitate the accuracy and completeness of the data, which are cross-checked with registration data from the ONS.[7] A guideline has been produced to help with data entry, and care is taken to ensure that the system is secure and the anonymity of cases is maintained.

The work programmes of MBRRACE-UK

CESDI, CEMACH and CMACE reported on specific subjects, such as intrapartum-related deaths, sudden unexpected deaths in infancy and deaths around the limits of fetal viability. MBRRACE-UK is undertaking similar focused enquiries. As well as its surveillance of perinatal deaths and the CEMD (see Chapter 28) there are confidential enquiries into a rolling programme of selected maternal morbidity topics and selected stillbirth and infant morbidity and mortality topics. The first maternal morbidity topic was sepsis, and the first perinatal topics were congenital diaphragmatic hernia and, for 2014, unexplained stillbirth at term. Analysis of perinatal cases is done by panels from each English region, Scotland, Northern Ireland and Wales.

Perinatal postmortem examination

Autopsy data are not necessarily required by MBRRACE-UK, but postmortem examination after stillbirth can provide additional information in up to 65 per cent of cases of intrauterine deaths at >20 weeks' gestation. Worldwide, however, rates of perinatal autopsy began to decline in the 1990s, and CMACE reported a reduced uptake of postmortems between 2000 and 2009.[1] These falls were partly due to 'organ retention' controversies in the UK and elsewhere, when it came to light

that organs had been retained after postmortem without the permission of parents having been specifically sought. Several official bodies produced guidelines to ensure that parents are better informed, and that clinicians who discuss postmortems with parents understand the process so that consent is full and informed. Policies to promote the uptake of perinatal postmortem include the availability of specialist perinatal pathologists, education (of both staff and the general public) in the value of postmortem, and senior staff involvement in counselling regarding the procedure. The consent process is crucial and is best carried out by a specialist bereavement midwife or a consultant involved with the care of the woman.[8]

INCIDENCE

Worldwide

Of the 140 million babies born every year, at least 2.65 million are stillborn,[4] and two estimates for 2000 put the figure at around 3.2 million.[5] A similar number die in the first 4 weeks of life. Three quarters of all neonatal deaths happen in the first week and the risk is highest on the first day. Low- and middle-income countries account for 98 per cent of the world's stillbirths, with global rates ranging from 2/1000 total births in Finland to 40/1000 total births in Pakistan and Nigeria. Over 40 per cent of all stillbirths (an estimated 1.19 million) are intrapartum, mostly associated with obstetric emergencies, while the others are antepartum stillbirths associated mainly with maternal infection and intrauterine growth retardation (IUGR).[4]

These figures are estimates because accurate data are often lacking. Some years ago the Director-General of WHO summed up the problem in developing countries as follows:

There are between 7 and 8 million perinatal deaths, but we do not know exactly how many are stillbirths and how many are early neonatal deaths. In many cases, births of infants who die soon after birth are neither recorded nor counted … Although the exact medical causes in countries may differ, the problem is simple: the common denominator for these deaths is the lack of appropriate and quality services, confounded by poverty.

In Europe, PMRs are relatively low but still show marked variations. The Euro-Peristat project began in 1999, coordinated from Paris and supported by the European Commission, and now gathers data from almost all European countries – which is no easy task. In the most recent Peristat report the stillbirth rate after 28 weeks of gestation ranged from 1.5 per 1000 total births in the Czech Republic to 4.3 in France, while the overall stillbirth rate (>22 weeks) ranged from under 4 per 1000 to over 8. Neonatal mortality rates (up to 28 days from delivery) ranged from 1.2 per 1000 live births in Iceland to 5.5 per 1000 in Romania.[9]

These results can be affected by differences between countries in the way that data are collected, which is one reason why data collection is difficult. The Peristat report acknowledges that under-reporting of maternal deaths is widespread in Europe but does not comment on whether this may also be a problem with perinatal deaths. International comparisons are an incentive to countries to improve care but may also discourage them from developing the systems needed to identify all eligible cases and thus push up their figures.

The UK

In the UK every effort is made to ensure that all maternal and perinatal deaths are identified. Data on perinatal mortality have been collected for the last 60 years, during which time there has been a dramatic reduction in perinatal deaths. In 1963 in England and Wales the stillbirth rate was >17 per 1000 total births and the neonatal death rate was >14 per 1000 live births. By 1999 these rates had fallen to 5.0 and 3.9 respectively. It is hard to know how much of this improvement was due to better health of the population and how much to better healthcare, but it is clear that improvements in neonatal intensive care, for example, played a major role in improving the survival rates of babies after preterm delivery.

In 2009, however, the UK stillbirth rate remained at 5.2 per 1000, although the neonatal mortality rate had fallen to 3.2 (Table 62.1). Indeed the UK stillbirth rate has remained largely unaltered since 1992, when the 24-week definition was introduced. The CEMACH report for 2005 commented that 'This lack of progress in reducing the stillbirth rate is a matter of public concern.' The 2009 CMACE report was less outspoken, simply pointing to a non-significant decrease (from 5.4 to 5.2) over the previous decade, but MBRRACE-UK has announced that stillbirth will be a priority for further investigation.[7]

The UK is far from unique, however, in having a static stillbirth rate. A recent review and meta-analysis pointed out that: 'Stillbirth rates in high-income countries have shown little or no improvement over the past two decades.'[10]

AETIOLOGY

General risk factors

The review of high-income countries mentioned above[10] identified several modifiable risk factors, of which the highest-ranking was maternal overweight and obesity (BMI >25 kg/m^2). Other risk factors included advanced maternal age, smoking and primiparity. Among disadvantaged populations, maternal smoking may contribute to as many as 20 per cent of stillbirths. Pregnancy disorders are also risk factors, as are pre-existing diabetes and hypertension. Abruption and small for gestational age (SGA) demonstrate the role of placental pathology in stillbirth.

In the UK, CMACE identified these and other risk factors for perinatal mortality.[1] In 2009, of the women who had a stillbirth or neonatal death, 10 per cent had a BMI of over 35 kg/m^2 – twice the background UK prevalence rate. Other risk factors include the extremes of maternal age, with the

risk of stillbirth increased by a factor of 1.4 among teenage mothers and 1.7 among women over 40. Social deprivation was associated with a 1.6-fold increase in the risk of both stillbirth and neonatal death. Mothers from ethnic minorities were at increased risk. Those of black ethnic origin were 2.1 times more likely to have a stillbirth and 2.4 times more likely to have a neonatal death, compared to mothers of white ethnic origin. Among mothers of Asian ethnic origin, the risks of both these outcomes were increased 1.6-fold. The effects of ethnicity and social class on perinatal mortality are less marked than their effects on maternal mortality but the same groups are at risk.

Classification of perinatal deaths

For many years analysis of perinatal deaths relied mainly on three systems, the Extended Wigglesworth classification (which was based on pathophysiology), and the Obstetric (Aberdeen) and the Fetal and Neonatal Factor classifications. Deficiencies in these systems became increasingly obvious, however. The main problem was that a majority of stillbirths were classified as 'unexplained'. To address this, other systems were developed, such as the ReCoDe (Relevant Condition at Death) system, which focused on the clinical conditions associated with the death rather than why the death occurred.[11] This system reduced 'unexplained' stillbirths from 66 per cent to 15 per cent, and identified 57 per cent of previously 'unexplained' stillbirths as 'growth restricted'.

CMACE developed a new classification of its own, also aimed at providing more insight into why babies die and identifying better intervention strategies. This is the classification that was used in the final CMACE report,[1] and it is discussed in the next section.

Table 62.2 CODAC Level I categories: primary causes of death

0 Infection	Infectious causes of death
1 Neonatal	Conditions, diseases and events specific to neonatal life
2 Intrapartum	Mechanics and events of parturition or its consequences
3 Congenital anomaly	Congenital anomalies, chromosomal anomalies and structural malformations
4 Fetal	Fetal conditions, diseases and events
5 Cord	Cord conditions, diseases and events
6 Placenta	Conditions, diseases and events of the placenta and membranes
7 Maternal	Maternal conditions, diseases and events
8 Unknown	Unknown, unexplained and unclassifiable causes of death
9 Termination	Terminations of pregnancy

EMBRRACE-UK has adopted another classification, the cause of death and associated conditions (CODAC) system,[12] which can record more detail about the influences on any particular death. It has been widely used around the world, in both developed and developing countries, and should allow better international comparisons. The system has ten main categories, as shown in Table 62.2.

The system has three levels. Each of these ten Level I categories is subdivided at Level II (giving a total of 94 subcategories) and again at Level III. The aim is to report not only the main cause of death but also the associated relevant conditions so that scenarios of combined events and conditions are captured. Examples of how to use the system are provided in the EMBRRACE-UK guideline.[7]

Causes of perinatal mortality

Table 62.1 shows that stillbirths account for more than two thirds of all perinatal deaths. This may surprise some professionals. We tend to 'blank' antenatal stillbirths, feeling that little can be done to prevent them. Compared to cot deaths (which are much less common), professional and public awareness of stillbirth is low. Mothers who experience stillbirth say they did not know the problem still existed, and in 2009 a campaign was launched by the Stillbirth and Neonatal Death Society (SANDS) to raise awareness and promote research. The name of the campaign, 'Why17?' drew attention to the fact that on average there are 17 perinatal deaths each day in the UK – ten times the number of cot deaths.

The 2009 CMACE report (the most recent report on perinatal mortality in the UK at the time of writing) classified the causes according to the CMACE system.[1] Table 62.3 shows that the proportion with 'no antecedent factors' was still the largest category but had fallen to 27.5 per cent. This was a major improvement on older reports in which almost 75 per cent of

stillbirths were 'unexplained' according to the Wigglesworth criteria. The second leading cause, 'Specific placental conditions', is a pathological diagnosis – CMACE encouraged examination of the placenta when consent for postmortem was withheld – and the question for clinicians is whether the condition causing the placental pathology can be recognised during pregnancy.

At number 5 in Table 62.3, 'Mechanical' causes of death are mainly cord problems (cord around the neck, prolapsed cord and other entanglements). Much less common in this category are malpresentations and uterine rupture. Number 10, 'Associated obstetric factors', includes spontaneous premature labour, premature rupture of the membranes, and deaths categorised as due to birth asphyxia.

Obstetricians and paediatricians want different information from the analysis of neonatal deaths, and CMACE had a specific classification system for each of the two specialties. Table 62.4 shows the obstetric causes, with the leading category being 'Associated obstetric factors'. Within this category the largest subgroups were spontaneous premature labour

Table 62.4 Causes of neonatal deaths in the UK* in 2009[1] (maternal and fetal classification) (n = 2115)

Cause	Percentage
1. Associated obstetric factors	26.6
2. Major congenital anomaly	23.6
3. No antecedent obstetric factors	12.4
4. Infection	10.1
5. Antepartum or intrapartum haemorrhage	9.4
6. Specific fetal conditions	4.4
7. Hypertensive disorders of pregnancy	3.1
8. Mechanical	2.8
9. Unclassified	2.5
10. Maternal disorder	2.1
11. IUGR	1.8
12. Specific placental conditions	1.2

- *Excluding Scotland

Table 62.5 Causes of neonatal deaths in the UK* in 2009[1] (neonatal classification) (n = 2115)

Cause	Percentage
1. Respiratory disorders	34.4
2. Major congenital anomaly	23.7
3. Neurological disorders	12.4
4. Extreme prematurity (<22 weeks)	8.5
5. Infection	7.9
6. Gastrointestinal disease	4.1

Table 62.3 Causes of stillbirths in the UK* in 2009[1] (n = 3373)

Cause	Percentage
1. No antecedent factors	27.8
2. Specific placental conditions	11.5
3. Antepartum or intrapartum haemorrhage	11.4
4. Major congenital anomaly	9.1
5. Mechanical	8.1
6. IUGR	6.6
7. Hypertensive disorders of pregnancy	5.9
8. Infection	5.1
9. Maternal disorder	5.0
10. Associated obstetric factors	4.0
11. Specific fetal conditions	3.8
12. Unclassified	1.7

- *Excluding Scotland

(continued)

Table 62.5 Causes of neonatal deaths in the UK* in 20091 (neonatal classification) (n = 2115) (*continued*)

Cause	Percentage
7. Other specific causes	3.5
8. Unclassified	3.4
9. Sudden unexpected deaths	2.0
10. Injury / trauma	0.1

and premature rupture of the membranes, which together accounted for 20 per cent of neonatal deaths. Also included in this category was 'intrapartum anoxia', which accounted for 3.3 per cent.

In the neonatal classification of neonatal deaths (Table 62.5) the leading cause is 'respiratory disorder'. Almost 90 per cent of these deaths were in babies born before 32 weeks' gestation. It is not immediately obvious from this table that the main underlying cause of neonatal death is preterm delivery.

Under the previous classification systems, 'intrapartum anoxia' accounted for 8 per cent of perinatal deaths – a proportion which did not change between 1999 and 2007, despite intensive intrapartum fetal surveillance. This was highlighted by the Chief Medical Officer in 2006 as a major cause for concern. In the 2009 CMACE report 'intrapartum-related' deaths still accounted for 8.6 per cent of all perinatal deaths. It is to be hoped that the new and more detailed analysis of these cases will be the first step in reducing this total.

PREVENTION

Worldwide

At the Millennium Summit in New York in 2000, world heads of state named reducing child mortality and improving maternal health among the global Millennium Development Goals. The targets for 2015 were to reduce the under-5 mortality ratio by two thirds and the maternal mortality ratio by three quarters from their 1990 levels. Neither perinatal mortality nor stillbirth was specifically mentioned but strategies for reducing perinatal mortality overlap with those for reducing maternal mortality. A shared theme is the need for functioning health systems which can provide emergency obstetric care.

In developed countries like the UK, the reduction in intrapartum stillbirths during the last 50 years means that most stillbirths occur in the antepartum period. In low-resource countries, however, there is a preponderance of term and intrapartum stillbirths which could be prevented by known risk assessment methods and by prompt delivery, often by caesarian section (CS). The fact that stillbirth is not formally included in any of the major global disease campaigns underlines current fears that 'inappropriate fatalism regarding stillbirths among care givers and policymakers will virtually guarantee that no progress occurs'.[13]

In 2011 the *Lancet* ran an informative series of articles on stillbirth in both developing and developed countries. The final article of this series, entitled 'The vision for 2020',[13] discussed research themes, and the highest priority theme for low and middle-income countries was how to 'adapt and scale up the most effective components of intrapartum care, particularly the appropriate use of caesarean section.' Other priorities were the improvement of antenatal care and effective mortality audit.

Efforts to reduce stillbirths will also help to reduce early neonatal mortality. For reduction of late neonatal and infant mortality, promotion of breastfeeding is particularly important in developing countries. Not only does it provide appropriate nourishment for the newborn, but it also reduces the risk of infection from artificial feeding, provides passive immunity through maternal antibodies, and acts as a natural contraceptive to ensure adequate pregnancy spacing.

The UK

Perinatal mortality can be reduced only if there is a will to do so, and for many years this seemed to be lacking, at least as far as stillbirth was concerned. The mood is now changing, with the prospect of more research into the causes of fetal death. In the following paragraphs the potential for further reducing the PMR will be discussed under the main themes which emerged from the 2009 CMACE report.[1]

Congenital malformation

Congenital abnormalities accounted for 23 per cent of perinatal deaths in 2009 (Tables 62.4 and 62.5). Current screening for congenital abnormalities includes universal fetal anatomy scanning in mid-pregnancy, and screening for chromosomal abnormalities through ultrasound and/or biochemical tests in the public and private sectors. Down's syndrome, the commonest chromosomal abnormality, does not usually cause neonatal death, and therefore the biochemical screening programme has little effect on perinatal mortality.

Around 18 per cent of lethal congenital anomalies at birth are cardiovascular and these constitute the leading cause of death in this category. The cardiovascular system, however, is difficult to visualise adequately at routine ultrasound screening. Specialist cardiac screening is carried out for fetuses at high risk but is too expensive in terms of personnel and equipment to be offered routinely.

The fetal spine is easier to visualise, and most neural tube defects (NTDs) are identified at a gestation at which the woman can be offered termination of pregnancy. This has resulted in a decrease in perinatal mortality from this condition but an increase in therapeutic termination. Ideally, congenital malformations would be prevented rather than being diagnosed early enough for termination, but this is difficult to achieve. The government has advised that all women should take periconceptual folic acid to reduce the incidence of NTDs, but only a minority do so. Sixty countries including the USA have introduced mandatory fortification of flour with folic acid, but Britain is not one of them.

Intrauterine growth restriction

The 2009 CMACE report confirmed what previously had been strongly suspected – that IUGR is a factor in many of the stillbirths previously classified simply as 'antepartum fetal death'. In 6.6 per cent of cases IUGR was given as the primary cause but when all cases were counted it was associated with 19 per cent of all stillbirths. Risk factors identified among this group were maternal smoking and obesity, extremes of maternal age, and black ethnicity. Previous studies have found that many of the mothers had noticed a change in fetal movements.

Past recommendations have included better screening for IUGR and better communication with mothers so that those with concerns about reduced fetal movements can be seen promptly for checks on fetal wellbeing. Women at risk need particular attention. A Scandinavian study showed that the increased perinatal mortality among ethnic minority women is due to delay in seeking antenatal care, inadequate management of IUGR, misinterpretation of cardiotocographs (CTGs) and poor communication.[14] A study in New Zealand showed that women who miss antenatal visits are at increased risk, and that SGA fetuses who are not identified as such in the antenatal period are more at risk of being stillborn.[15]

For all women, routine antenatal care too often fails to identify IUGR. Current UK guidelines recommend screening by fundal height measurement, despite a Cochrane review showing no evidence of benefit. Its sensitivity may be improved by using customised growth charts. Another approach would be routine ultrasound scanning in the third trimester, which is normal practice in France. More evidence is needed, however, on how best to replace the outdated and inadequate technique of fundal height measurement, and how to identify the malfunctioning placenta at an earlier stage.[3]

Intrapartum-related deaths

In the UK in 2009 there were 288 intrapartum stillbirths and 232 intrapartum-related neonatal deaths. Together they represent 8.6 per cent of perinatal deaths, and in relation to the total number of births (794,906) a risk of 1 in 1529. This risk is almost exactly the same as it was in 1994–5, when a detailed CESDI study of intrapartum-related deaths found sub-optimal care in over 78 per cent of the cases, in which alternative management 'might' (25 per cent) or 'would reasonably be expected to' (52 per cent) have made a difference to the outcome. The main findings of that report were failure to recognise risk factors before labour, and inadequate assessment of the fetus during labour by heart rate monitoring and blood sampling. There has been no similar confidential enquiry into intrapartum-related deaths since then. The decision of MBBRACE-UK to investigate unexplained stillbirths is therefore very welcome.

There have, however, been new guidelines on standards of care in labour[16] and national evidence-based guidelines on the use and interpretation of electronic fetal monitoring (EFM). These had a gratifying response at local level and the 2002 CESDI report noted that 'Intrapartum-related mortality has now decreased significantly from 0.95 (1994) to 0.62 (1999) per 1000 live births and stillbirths.' Since 1999, unfortunately, the figure has been static, at 0.56 per 1000 in 2007 and 0.66 in 2009.

The emphasis now is on identifying 'low-risk' women and promoting normal birth. This requires adequate numbers of midwives but there are persistent concerns about the levels of staffing in UK labour wards. Pressure has come not only from the 17 per cent increase in the number of deliveries between 2000 and 2009 but also from the high proportion of deliveries to women born outside the UK – now almost 25 per cent nationally and over 70 per cent in some parts of London. These women are at higher risk and require extra care.

Immaturity

In the 2009 CMACE report 'extreme prematurity' accounted for 8.5 per cent of neonatal deaths but this category included only infants born before 22 weeks' gestation. The contribution of premature delivery after this stage is harder to discern as it is spread among the other categories of the neonatal classification. For example, infants born before 32 weeks' gestation accounted for all but one of the deaths from intraventricular haemorrhage, as well as the 90 per cent of neonatal deaths from respiratory disorders mentioned previously.

Advances in neonatal care have improved the survival of premature infants to a remarkable degree in the last three decades. Survival rates for babies born at 27–28 weeks' gestation are now around 90 per cent, although about 20 per cent of these infants survive with some degree of impairment. It is now well recognised that antenatal steroids given to the mother will reduce the risk of perinatal mortality from respiratory distress syndrome, but they must be given at least 24 hours before delivery and sometimes it is impossible to delay delivery long enough for them to work.

Prevention of preterm birth is now the major challenge for obstetrics. Some reduction can be achieved by measures including smoking cessation, avoidance of multiple embryo transfers, cervical cerclage, progesterone supplementation and avoidance of unnecessary iatrogenic preterm delivery, but these have a relatively small effect on the overall preterm birth rate. More research is needed on disease mechanisms and on biomarkers to predict preterm birth, and there is a need for more engagement with pharmaceutical companies to convert knowledge into available therapies.[17]

Clinical risk management

For many years it has been standard practice for maternity hospitals to hold perinatal mortality meetings to review cases of perinatal death. The clinical history and pathological findings are examined and the implications for the management of similar cases are discussed. Many hospitals have extended this method to include 'near-miss' incidents. It is essential that such discussions take place in a blame-free atmosphere, so that constructive suggestions can be made for improving care.

These meetings have tended to focus on the 'person approach', recognising the importance of individuals, but there is increasing emphasis on the 'systems approach' to risk management. This recognises and indeed expects staff to make errors. It concentrates on improving the system to reduce the chance of errors occurring, to recognise them when they do occur and to prevent adverse consequences. The emphasis is on support for staff rather than blame. This is the most constructive approach to reducing perinatal mortality and morbidity and the associated burden of obstetric litigation.

SUMMARY

Worldwide, there are around 6 million perinatal deaths annually, of which about half are stillbirths. All but 2 per cent of these deaths occur in developing countries, where the main causes are poverty, malnutrition and, importantly, lack of access to healthcare. Improvements could be made by basic hygiene, access to trained healthcare workers and promotion of breastfeeding, but reduction in perinatal mortality requires functioning healthcare systems delivering emergency obstetric care.

In the UK, perinatal mortality is comparatively low but could be reduced still further. Intrapartum management has been improved by training in the interpretation of electronic monitoring and more involvement of senior staff, but regular updating is needed and pressures on midwives need to be recognised. Congenital malformations can be detected during pregnancy, but more can be done to prevent them. Neonatal care continues to improve survival rates after preterm delivery but prevention of preterm labour is a considerable obstetric challenge and needs further research. Recognition of at-risk pregnancies requires meticulous antenatal care, and more research is needed to improve the diagnosis and management of IUGR. In this regard, particular attention must be paid to high-risk groups such as obese women and those from ethnic minorities.

EBM

- Maternal steroid administration before preterm delivery reduces perinatal mortality [Ia].
- The evidence does not support the routine use of EFM in low-risk labours.
- Dietary supplementation in chronically malnourished women reduces perinatal mortality [Ib].

KEY POINTS

- The perinatal mortality rate is the number of stillbirths and deaths in the first week of life per 1000 live and stillbirths.
- Globally the perinatal mortality rate is around 50–60.
- Worldwide, perinatal mortality is due to poverty, malnutrition and infection and lack of emergency obstetric care. It could be reduced by better access to healthcare.
- In the UK the perinatal mortality rate is currently 7.6.
- More than two thirds of perinatal deaths in the UK are stillbirths. Over the last 15 years the neonatal death rate has fallen but the stillbirth rate has not changed.
- Congenital malformations account for 23 per cent of perinatal deaths.
- Antepartum stillbirths could be reduced by more focused antenatal care, concentrating on the detection of IUGR and on better communication with at-risk women.
- The main underlying cause of neonatal death is preterm delivery. There is a need for more research on prevention of preterm birth.
- Perinatal postmortems require fully informed consent from parents, and sensitive counselling is very important.

Key References

1. CMACE. *Perinatal mortality 2009*. United Kingdom: CMACE, 2011.
2. ONS. *Statistical Bulletin. Infant and perinatal mortality in England and Wales by social and biological factors, 2011*. Newport: ONS, 2012.
3. Smith GCS. A bonfire of the tape measures. *Lancet* 2011;377:1307.
4. Lawn JE, Blencowe H, Pattinson R. Stillbirths: When? Where? Why? How to make the data count? *Lancet* 2011;377:1448–63.
5. Cousens S, Blencowe H, Stanton C *et al*. National, regional, and worldwide estimates of stillbirth rates with trends since 1995: a systematic analysis. *Lancet* 2011;377:1319–30.
6. Knight M. How will the new Confidential Enquiries into Maternal and Infant Death in the UK operate? The work of MBRRACE-UK. *The Obstetrician and Gynaecologist* 2012;15:65.
7. MBRRACE-UK Newsletters 02 and 04, and Guidelines for Perinatal and Infant Death data entry. Available at: www.npeu.ox.ac.uk/mbrrace-uk.
8. Stock SJ, Goldsmith L, Evans MJ, Laing IA. Interventions to improve rates of postmortem examination after stillbirth. *Eur J Obstet Gynecol Reprod Biol* 2010;153:148–50.
9. Zeitlin J, Mohangoo A, Delnord M (eds). *European Perinatal health report: health and care of pregnant women and babies in Europe 2010*. Paris: Euro-Peristat, 2013.

10. Flenady V, Koopmans L, Middleton P. Major risk factors for stillbirth in high-income countries: a systematic review and meta-analysis. *Lancet* 2011;377:1331–40.

11. Gardosi J, Kady SM, McGeown P, Francis A, Tonks A. Classification of stillbirth by relevant condition at death (ReCoDe): population based cohort study. *BMJ* 2005;331:1113–7.

12. Froen JF, Pinar H, Flenady V *et al.* Causes of death and associated conditions (Codac) – a utilitarian approach to the classification of perinatal deaths. *BMC Pregnancy and Childbirth* 2009;9:22.

13. Goldenberg RL, McClure EM, Bhutta ZA. Stillbirths: the vision for 2020. *Lancet* 2011;377:1798–805.

14. Saastad E, Vangen S, Froen JF. Suboptimal care in stillbirths – a retrospective audit study. *Acta Obstet Gynecol Scand* 2007;86:444–50.

15. Stacey T, Thompson JM, Mitchell EA, Zuccollo JM, Ekeroma AJ, McCowan LM. Antenatal care, identification of suboptimal fetal growth and risk of late stillbirth: findings from the Auckland Stillbirth Study. *Aust N Z J Obstet Obstet Gynaecol* 2012;52:242–7.

16. Royal College of Obstetricians and Gynaecologists; Royal College of Midwives; Royal College of Anaesthetists; Royal College of Paediatrics and Child Health. *Safer childbirth: minimum standards for the organisation and delivery of care in labour.* London: RCOG Press, 2007.

17. Norman JE, Shennan AH. Prevention of preterm birth: why can't we do any better? *Lancet* 2013;381:184–5.

Chapter 63 Postpartum collapse

Peter J Thompson

INTRODUCTION

Postpartum collapse is a major cause of maternal mortality and morbidity in both the developed and developing worlds. Although the most common causes of postpartum collapse are not confined to the immediate postpartum period, because of the rapid haemodynamic, hormonal and anatomical changes occurring at this time, there is an increased prevalence of these conditions.

Although many of these conditions require specific management plans, the generic treatment of a shocked patient, i.e. airway protection, administration of oxygen and gaining intravenous access, is common to all.

DEFINITION

Postpartum collapse is the onset of shock in the immediate period following delivery of the fetus.

PREVALENCE

There are no good denominator data available to accurately determine the incidence of this condition, though from recent observational studies of severe maternal morbidity at any stage in pregnancy, not all of which result in collapse, the incidence is thought to be between 0.14 and 6 per 1000 [D].[1]

AETIOLOGY

There are many causes of postpartum collapse, with the most common and most important being listed in Table 63.1. Many of these aetiologies have common pathways via hypovolaemia, whether it be absolute hypovolaemia, as in haemorrhage, or relative hypovolaemia secondary to changes in the autonomic nervous system, as in uterine inversion. It is noteworthy that with the exception of psychiatric cases all the main conditions that contribute to both direct and indirect maternal mortality in the UK are represented in this list.

In addition many women who collapse are known to show deterioration in their basic observations, temperature, pulse rate, blood pressure, respiratory rate and urine output. It is for this reason that organisations such as NICE have recommended the introduction of early warning systems, though these have not as yet been shown to improve outcome [E]. In obstetrics a specific early warning system has been developed and implemented in most units in the UK, the Modified Early Obstetric Warning System, MEOWS.

The management of many of these conditions has been described elsewhere in this book, and will therefore not be addressed here. This chapter concentrates on the causes of postpartum collapse marked with an asterisk in Table 63.1.

Table 63.1 Aetiology of postpartum collapse

Pulmonary emboli	Vasovagal attacks*	Uterine inversion*
Septic shock	Epileptic convulsions	Cardiac arrest*
Haemorrhage	Cerebrovascular accidents	Cardiac arrhythmia
Amniotic fluid embolus*	Eclampsia	Iatrogenic*

* See text for explanation.

Vasovagal attacks

Vasovagal attacks are relatively common occurrences and are induced by many external stimuli, which result in extreme emotions, such as fright, anxiety or phobias. They are frequently preceded by a prodromal state consisting of dizziness, nausea, sweating, tinnitus and yawning. The aetiology is one of vasodilatation, leading to a pooling of blood and therefore a relative hypovolaemia. As a result, the heart begins to empty, stimulating mechanoreceptors in the wall of its left ventricle. This, in turn, acts centrally to initiate further vasodilatation and a bradycardia. These attacks usually resolve spontaneously, although it is advisable to position the patient flat and then elevate her legs to encourage central venous return and hence adequate filling of the heart [E]. Similar syncopal episodes may also be present in patients with cardiac disease, specifically those women who have arrhythmias or obstructive heart disease.

Cardiac arrest

Cardiac arrest during the postnatal period is usually associated with hypovolaemia, obstructive heart disease or complex congenital heart disease. However, with increasing maternal age at the time of delivery, ischaemic heart disease is now seen more commonly. Indeed, in the Confidential Enquiry into Maternal Deaths (CEMD) 2006–08,[2] six women died following myocardial infarction (three of these cases were secondary to ischaemic heart disease) and a further five women died of ischaemic heart disease where no evidence of myocardial infarction was found at autopsy. The rate of myocardial infarction is usually quoted as one in 10,000 births. The interim publications from UK Obstetric Surveillance Service (UKOSS) have only found 2.4 cases per 100,000 maternities, with further efforts being made to ascertain if this is a true incidence or if it represents under-reporting.[3] Reversible causes of cardiac arrest are listed in Table 63.2.

Table 63.2 Reversible causes of cardiac arrest

Four Hs	Four Ts
Hypovolaemia	Tension pneumothorax
Hypoxia	Cardiac tamponade
Hyper/hypokalaemia, hypocalcaemia, acidaemia	Thromboembolic or mechanical obstruction
Hypothermia	Toxic or therapeutic substance in overdose

Resuscitation of women who have had a cardiac arrest in pregnancy is usually complicated by the fact that, when supine, a gravid uterus will compress the inferior vena cava, decreasing venous return. Emptying the uterus by delivering the fetus will improve stroke volume by 60 per cent and is therefore mandatory if resuscitation is not rapidly successful

and delivery should occur within 5 minutes [D]. Although this latter problem is not present in the immediate postpartum period, the uterus may still be of sufficient size to cause significant aortocaval compression, and therefore resuscitation should be conducted with the uterus displaced to the left [D]. Previously it was recommended that this be achieved by placing the woman on a tilt, with a reported increased cardiac output of 25 per cent when compared to a supine patient.[4,5] However recent recommendations suggest that the preferred option is displacing the uterus as described above.

Management consists of diagnosing and treating any reversible cause of the arrest, while simultaneously following the European Resuscitation Council Guidelines 2010 for Adult Advanced Life Support.[6] These are summarised in Fig. 63.1. Once a cardiac arrest has been diagnosed it is essential that resuscitation begins promptly, as survival is related to early CPR and, if appropriate, defibrillation. It is therefore a prerequisite that staff are trained on a regular basis so that they are able to both provide this level of basic life support and to use an automated electronic defibrillator. The previously recommended precordial thump is thought to have a very low success rate, and then only when administered within the first few seconds of the onset of the cardiac arrest. It is therefore no longer recommended outside a critical care environment as it may delay calling for help [D]. Basic life support should begin once the airway is opened and it is confirmed that the unconscious patient is either not breathing or is performing only occasional gasps. The initial part of the resuscitation is to perform chest compression at a rate of 100 per minute and a compression to ventilation ratio of 30:2. The most recent guidelines suggest that chest compression begins before rescue breaths are given as in these initial moments of a non-asphyxial cardiac arrest oxygenation of the blood is high, but delivery of oxygen to the myocardium and brain is poor. Chest compression is often performed sub-optimally and the person leading the resuscitation needs to rotate the person performing chest compressions regularly, approximately every 2 minutes. There is also significant emphasis in the new guideline regarding performing uninterrupted chest wall compression.

Post-resuscitation care should include transfer of the patient to a critical care unit or coronary care unit [D]. Patients who are hypothermic should not be warmed and those who are pyrexial should receive antipyretics [C].

Amniotic fluid embolus

Amniotic fluid embolism is rare, with estimates of the incidence varying between 1.3 and 12.5 per 100,000.[7] Good denominator data are at present being collected by UKOSS and these preliminary results show an incidence of 1.9 per 100,000 (CI 1.6–2.3) with a mortality rate of 24 per cent, lower than previously thought.[3] Due to its high mortality rate, there were 13 direct maternal deaths attributable to amniotic fluid embolism in the years 2006–08.[2] The aetiology is still debated, but appears to be an anaphylactic reaction to the passage of amniotic fluid and particulate matter into the

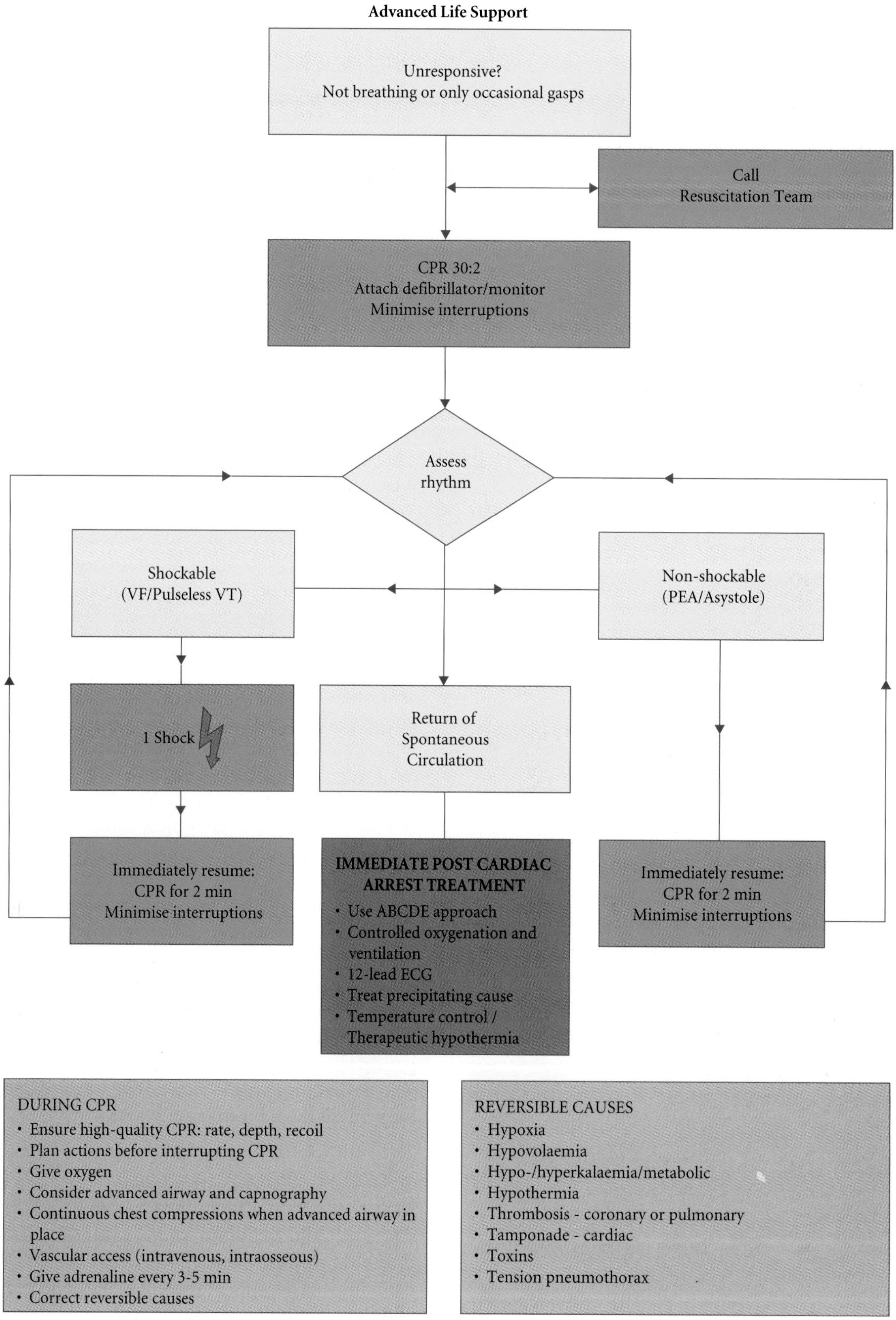

Advanced Life Support

Unresponsive?
Not breathing or only occasional gasps

Call
Resuscitation Team

CPR 30:2
Attach defibrillator/monitor
Minimise interruptions

Assess
rhythm

Shockable
(VF/Pulseless VT)

Non-shockable
(PEA/Asystole)

1 Shock

Return of
Spontaneous
Circulation

Immediately resume:
CPR for 2 min
Minimise interruptions

**IMMEDIATE POST CARDIAC
ARREST TREATMENT**

- Use ABCDE approach
- Controlled oxygenation and
  ventilation
- 12-lead ECG
- Treat precipitating cause
- Temperature control /
  Therapeutic hypothermia

Immediately resume:
CPR for 2 min
Minimise interruptions

DURING CPR
- Ensure high-quality CPR: rate, depth, recoil
- Plan actions before interrupting CPR
- Give oxygen
- Consider advanced airway and capnography
- Continuous chest compressions when advanced airway in
  place
- Vascular access (intravenous, intraosseous)
- Give adrenaline every 3-5 min
- Correct reversible causes

REVERSIBLE CAUSES
- Hypoxia
- Hypovolaemia
- Hypo-/hyperkalaemia/metabolic
- Hypothermia
- Thrombosis - coronary or pulmonary
- Tamponade - cardiac
- Toxins
- Tension pneumothorax

Fig. 63.1 European resuscitation guidelines for advanced life support (copyright European Resuscitation Council – www.erc.edu – 2014/017, reproduced with permission). PEA pulseless electrical activity; VF ventricular fibrillation; VT ventricular tachycardia

lungs. This results in a biphasic model where initially patients develop pulmonary hypertension and hypoxia presenting as respiratory distress, central cyanosis and circulatory collapse, with survivors undergoing a resolution of the pulmonary hypertension and subsequent development of left ventricular failure.[8] Approximately half of the patients who survive the initial insult develop disseminated intravascular coagulopathy (DIC). Diagnosis of the condition is suspected when patients collapse in labour or shortly after delivery with signs of central cyanosis, although confirmation of the diagnosis can be made on examination of lung tissue at postmortem, or on examination of blood films for the presence of squames or fetal hair. If however the mother dies, diagnosis should be confirmed by immunochemistry. Management of these patients revolves around the generic treatment of shock and coagulopathies, with the former often requiring the information provided by pulmonary artery wedge pressures to guide inotropic interventions [D]. Although high-dose hydrocortisone has been suggested as an appropriate treatment, no studies have examined this.

Uterine inversion

Uterine inversion is a rare condition, occurring with an incidence of one in 10,000 pregnancies. Although maternal death secondary to uterine inversion is well recognised, in the CEMD 2006–08[1] there was only one such case, and in the previous triennial report covering 2003–05, no such deaths were documented. In the recent case uterine replacement was not attempted.

The degree to which the fundus of the uterus inverts is variable, with the mildest form being dimpling of the fundus and the most severe being complete inversion, where the fundus of the uterus passes through the cervix. There is no agreement on the aetiology of this condition, although several factors appear to be associated with its occurrence. These include:

- mismanagement of the third stage of labour, either by inappropriate traction during controlled cord traction or too-rapid removal of the placenta during manual removal;
- maternal age >25 years;
- a sudden rise in intra-abdominal pressure in the presence of a relaxed uterus;
- a fundally placed placenta with a short umbilical cord.

Patients present with a picture of shock in the absence of visible blood loss. This shock appears to be of neurogenic origin secondary to traction on structures adjacent to the uterus. The fundus of the uterus may be visible at the introitus; however, if not, it will be detected on vaginal examination. This latter examination is mandatory in all patients who appear to be shocked in the immediate postpartum period in the absence of visible blood loss [E]. Not only can this lead to the exclusion of a diagnosis of an inverted uterus, but a diagnosis of a supralevator haematoma will also be excluded.

Treatment is based on the principles of managing a shocked patient and then replacing the uterus as soon as possible. If the diagnosis is made immediately, the uterus can often be replaced manually prior to the onset of shock. However, once the uterus has been inverted for only a few minutes, the tissues surrounding it constrict, preventing its replacement. In this circumstance, manual replacement may be possible using general anaesthesia [D]. If this fails, O'Sullivan's hydrostatic technique may be attempted: the vagina is filled with warm saline while being blocked at the introitus with the attendant's fist. The hydrostatic pressure resulting from the instillation of 4–5 L of saline may be sufficient to balloon the vagina and reverse the inversion [D].

Should neither of these techniques result in replacement of the uterus, a laparotomy and Haultain's procedure should be performed before the uterus becomes ischaemic from obstruction of its blood supply. At laparotomy, traction is placed on the round ligaments and an incision is made through the muscular ring in the posterior uterine wall. Continued manual pressure on the fundus from the vagina and traction of the round ligaments will allow replacement of the uterus, and the incision is closed [D]. In all these treatment options, it needs to be remembered that if the placenta is still attached it should not be removed until the uterus has been replaced, as the uterus will be unable to contract and constrict the placental bed blood vessels and therefore major haemorrhage may ensue [E].

In all the previously described management options, once the uterus is correctly sited, a Syntocinon infusion should be commenced to encourage contraction of the uterus [E]. It should be noted that a recurrence rate of approximately 30 per cent has been quoted in the literature, although recent figures are unavailable.

Iatrogenic causes

Iatrogenic causes of loss of consciousness in the postnatal period include inappropriate advice on positioning the woman, with a resultant syncopal episode, and reactions to the administration of drugs. Although any drugs may be administered at this time, those that are most frequently used include syntocinon, ergometrine and local anaesthetics.

Syntocinon may cause sudden hypotension and, in women who are supine and have recently haemorrhaged, can be sufficient to result in loss of consciousness. This situation should be managed as for any shocked patient, with the appropriate positioning of the woman, protection of the airway and the administration of oxygen and intravenous fluids. In the previous CEMD, it has been reiterated that syntocinon should be used with care in such situations. Ergometrine, which is usually administered along with syntocinon, is a powerful smooth-muscle constrictor and is contraindicated in women with severe hypertension, as it may precipitate a hypertensive crisis and haemorrhagic cerebrovascular accident.

In women with inadequate analgesia, infiltration of the perineum with a local anaesthetic is mandatory prior to surgical repair of the perineum. Lidocaine, the most widely used local anaesthetic for this purpose, is ideally suited, with an onset and duration of action after infiltration of 5 minutes and 1 hour, respectively (maximum plasma concentrations occur at 25 minutes). Overdosage usually presents as light-headedness, sedation, paraesthesia, twitching and convulsions. However, if the drug is administered intravenously, it may result in the precipitation of cardiac arrhythmias and cardiac arrest. This is one of the reversible causes of cardiac arrest and should be managed according to the guidelines described by the European Resuscitation Council [E].[6] In addition, in the event of local anaesthetic-induced cardiac arrest, if there is no rapid response to normal CPR then a lipid emulsion should be administered as per the regimen in the British National Formulary.

It is therefore imperative for all healthcare professionals who infiltrate with lidocaine to ensure that injections are not intravenous and to be aware of the maximum dose of lidocaine that can be administered safely. This will depend, among other things, upon the patient's size and the degree of vascularity of the area being infiltrated. This latter variable can be altered by the administration of a vasoconstrictors to the local anaesthetic. The recommended maximum dose of lidocaine is 200 mg (500 mg if administered with adrenaline). However, this situation is complicated by the fact that most local anaesthetics are labelled in percentage solutions and hence professionals need to understand how much lidocaine there is in a specified percentage solution. This equation is shown below.

One litre of a 100 per cent solution contains 1 kg of the active ingredient. Therefore, 10 mL of 0.5 per cent lidocaine contains:

$$\frac{1000\,g \times 10\,mL \times 0.5}{1000\,mL \times 100} = 0.05\,g = 50\,mg$$

EBM

- There are few randomised controlled trials of the management of acute postpartum collapse.
- There are, however, internationally accepted evidence-based guidelines for adult resuscitation.

KEY POINTS

- All healthcare practitioners should be aware of the local guidelines to treat the shocked patient.
- European guidelines are available for resuscitation following cardiac arrest.
- Pregnant women who have had a cardiac arrest need to have their uterus displaced to the left.
- Prompt replacement of an inverted uterus may be life saving.
- Local anaesthetic solutions are labelled in per cent and can easily be converted into milligrams.
- Local and national guidelines are essential for the management of these conditions.
- Good denominator data for many of the conditions that cause postpartum collapse are being collected by UKOSS.

References

1. RCOG. *Maternal collapse in pregnancy and the puerperium*. RCOG Green-top guideline No 56. London: RCOG, January 2011.
2. Saving Mothers' Lives: Reviewing maternal deaths to make motherhood safer: 2006–2008. The Eighth Report of the CEMD in the United Kingdom. *BJOG* 2011;118 supplement 1–203.
3. Knight M, Workman M, Fitzpatrick K *et al. UKOSS Annual Report 2013*. Oxford: National Perinatal Epidemiology Unit, 2013.
4. Lee RV, Rodgers LD, White LM, Harvey AC. Cardiopulmonary resuscitation of the pregnant woman. *Am J Med* 1986;81:311–18.
5. Uckland K, Novy MJ, Peterson EN. Maternal cardiopulmonary dynamics IV. The influence of gestational age on the maternal cardiovascular response to posture and exercise. *Am J Obstet Gynecol* 1969;104:856–64.
6. Nolan JP, Soar J, Zideman DA *et al.* On behalf of the ERC Guidelines Writing Group. *Resuscitation* 2010;81:1219–76.
7. Gilbert WM, Danielsen B. Amniotic fluid embolism: decreased mortality in a population-based study. *Obstet Gynecol* 1999;93:973–7.
8. Clark SL. New concepts of amniotic fluid embolism: a review. *Obstet Gynecol Surv* 1990;45:360–8.

Chapter 64 Postpartum haemorrhage

Peter J Thompson

MRCOG standards

Theoretical skills

- Understand the definitions and differing aetiologies of primary and secondary postpartum haemorrhage.
- The techniques for control of postpartum haemorrhage.
- Retained placenta.
- Appropriate use of blood products.

Practical skills

- Demonstrate skills in acute resuscitation.
- Recognise a postpartum haemorrhage and be able to both initiate and coordinate a multidisciplinary-based plan of management.
- Complete objective structured assessment of technical skill in perineal repair and manual removal of placenta.

INTRODUCTION

Haemorrhage is still one of the leading causes of maternal mortality in the United Kingdom with postpartum haemorrhage (PPH) playing a significant role in the deaths of nine women in the last triennial report.[1] Any discussion of PPH must cover both the primary and secondary conditions, although the majority of this chapter is aimed at the management of primary PPH.

DEFINITIONS

The differentiation between primary and secondary PPH is more than an academic discussion, as the aetiology, clinical presentation, treatment and prognosis of the two conditions are very different.

PPH is subclassified as follows:

- Primary PPH is defined as the loss of 500 mL of blood from the genital tract following, but within the first 24 hours of, the delivery of the baby. A caveat is added in that if the blood loss is <500 mL, but is sufficient to cause hypovolaemic shock in the patient, this is also classified as a primary PPH. A new definition of massive PPH has been introduced, being the loss of greater than 1000, 1500 or 2500 mL of blood. Owing to the relatively low risks of blood loss below these levels, this is thought to be of greater clinical relevance. The incidence of this complication is being used in some units as an indicator of the standard of maternity care and is being promoted by RCOG as one of their clinical indicators on the maternity scorecard.[2,3]
- Secondary PPH is more of a subjective diagnosis, as its definition is blood loss from the genital tract of a volume greater than expected after the first 24 hours, but within the first 12 weeks of delivery.

INCIDENCE

The incidence of primary PPH in the developed world is approximately 5 per cent of all deliveries.[4] The incidence of massive PPH in the United Kingdom has been reported as 6.7 per 1000. This figure was obtained by analysis of a cohort of 48,865 women who delivered in a one-year period. Although significant morbidity will be associated with this condition, other data concerning its incidence are limited. However in the last triennial report on maternal mortalities in the UK there were five deaths secondary to PPH, half the number in the previous report. Despite this decrease in prevalence in three of these cases there was a lack of routine observations performed in the postnatal period.[1]

AETIOLOGY

The most common aetiology of primary PPH is uterine atony, followed by genital tract trauma.

Uterine atony may have many causes, including retained placental fragments, and is associated with prolonged labour, multiple pregnancies, polyhydramnios, instrumental deliveries and grand multiparity. Other somewhat rarer causes include coagulopathies, pathological placentation (e.g. placenta accreta) and uterine inversion. These rarer causes retain a significant level of importance because of their relative over-representation among severe cases of haemorrhage.

The major aetiological factors associated with secondary PPH are retained placental fragments and endometritis.

MANAGEMENT

It is important to discuss the options for the prevention of PPH with women antenatally. It has been well established that active management of the third stage of labour, with the administration of syntometrine at the time of delivery of the infant's anterior shoulder followed by controlled cord traction, is associated with a relative risk of PPH of greater than 1l of 0.34 (95% CI 0.14–0.87) [A].[5] However, there is a substantial increase in the risk of maternal side effects, such as nausea with active management of the third stage of labour when compared to physiological management.[5] Whilst most episodes of PPH occur in women with no known risk factors, those with recognised risk factors should be encouraged to deliver in a consultant-led unit with consideration given to siting of an intravenous cannula and blood being taken for estimation of the haemoglobin concentration, and serum should be grouped and saved [E]. Such women include those in the risk categories mentioned above, as well as women who have had a previous PPH, who have a risk of recurrence of approximately 25 per cent. Examination of the placenta post-delivery should identify a proportion of women who have retained placental fragments and who will require manual removal of the placenta. Relative risks for the development of PPH that are present in the antenatal and intrapartum period are listed in the RCOG guideline on this topic.[6]

Significant PPH is an obstetric emergency that requires a multidisciplinary team for optimum management [E]. Initial management is dependent upon rapid diagnosis. This is difficult, as it is well recognised that both obstetricians and midwives are poor at accurately estimating blood loss at the time of delivery. This can be further confounded by the ability of fit young women to maintain their blood pressure, either with or without a tachycardia, until they have lost approximately 15 per cent of their blood volume.

Resuscitation

Immediate management needs to revolve around the principles of ABC: airway, breathing and circulation. In this case this is likely to involve resuscitation of the hypovolaemic patient with the application of facial oxygen, siting of two large-bore (14/16 G) intravenous cannulae, fluid administration and examination to determine the aetiology of the haemorrhage, often performing uterine massage [E]. At this time blood should also be taken for diagnostic tests, including full blood count, coagulation screen, urea and electrolytes and cross

match (4 units). Although for many years clinical teaching has been that fluid replacement by colloid is superior to the use of a crystalloid, examination of randomised controlled trials (RCTs) in patients with hypovolaemia has failed to show any benefit with the preferential use of colloids [A].[7] Although these studies are in the non-pregnant population, it is reasonable to extrapolate this conclusion to fit pregnant women. In this early stage of resuscitation, it is important to obtain blood for a full blood count, clotting studies and group- and cross-matching. If the haemorrhage is thought to be 'massive' then the local massive haemorrhage protocol should be formally initiated at this time.

Disseminated intravascular coagulation

DIC is a life-threatening complication of massive haemorrhage. Regardless of the aetiology, the management should revolve around maintaining an adequate intravascular volume and treating the underlying cause, in this case stopping the haemorrhage. This condition is discussed in more detail in Chapter 46, Antepartum haemorrhage. However, one should aim to follow four basic principles:

1 to maintain the intravascular volume;
2 to administer fresh frozen plasma (FFP) at a rate to keep the activated partial thromboplastin:control ratio <1.5;
3 to administer packed platelets to maintain a platelet count $>75 \times 10^9$/L;
4 to administer cryoprecipitate to keep the fibrinogen level >1 g/L.

Although administration of blood components should be guided by haematological results in conjunction with a senior haematologist, as described above, this should not be delayed until the patient is moribund, as successive Confidential Enquiries into Maternal Deaths (CEMDs) have identified delay in transfusion as a significant contributor to maternal mortality [D]. In addition if blood is required but fully cross-matched units are not available then O rhesus-negative blood can be administered, though in most cases group specific uncross-matched blood can be available within 10–15 minutes.

Specific management strategies

Uterine atony can be managed pharmacologically or by a combination of pharmacological and surgical interventions. If the placenta is thought to be complete, the uterus is clinically atonic and there are no significant signs of genital tract trauma, an examination in theatre may be avoided by the administration of ergometrine followed by a syntocinon infusion. Although the former has significant side effects, including nausea, vomiting and hypertension, its tonic action on the uterine muscle is a valuable adjunct to therapy with syntocinon alone. However, caution is necessary in patients with pre-eclampsia, who may suffer episodes of severe hypertension following the administration of ergometrine.

Should these efforts fail to control the bleeding, examination of the genital tract needs to be performed with adequate lighting and patient analgesia. This usually means examination in an operating theatre with the patient having a regional or general anaesthetic. If the bleeding is significant, this examination should not be delayed in order to obtain blood results; if the anaesthetist is concerned about the risks of siting a regional anaesthetic in the presence of a possible coagulopathy or hypotension, then immediate resuscitation should be followed by the administration of a general anaesthetic [E].

Examination under anaesthesia should include examination of the vagina, cervix and, in the case of continued bleeding, exploration of the uterine cavity digitally to identify and remove any retained fragments of the placenta. If the uterine cavity is explored digitally, this should be covered by the administration of a broad-spectrum antibiotic. At this time, if no other cause for the haemorrhage has been identified, administration of prostaglandin analogues, either intramuscularly (if carboprost is available) or rectally (if only misoprostol or gemeprost is available), is advisable. The success of carboprost administration was as high as 88 per cent in one study. Misoprostol administration has also been thought to be effective in decreasing blood loss in cases of primary PPH, although there are limited data on optimal dosage, route and efficacy.[8] Suggested dosages of these uterotonics can be seen in Table 64.1. Bimanual compression of the uterus may also need to be performed at this stage; this decreases blood loss partly because of the fact that it puts the uterine arteries under tension. In addition to uterotonics, drugs that promote coagulation can be administered, such as tranexamic acid and recombinant factor VIIa. These drugs are not, however, without risk, with recombinant factor VIIa in particular having a recognised risk of thrombotic cerebrovascular accidents and myocardial infarction.

Table 64.1 Suggested dosages for uterotonics

Uterotonic	Route of administration	Dosage
Syntocinon	IV	Bolus dose of 5 IU, followed if necessary by an infusion of 40 IU in 40 mL of saline run at 10 mL/hour
Syntometrine	IM	1 mL
Ergometrine	IV/IM	250–500 µg
Carboprost	IM	250 µg every 15–90 minutes, to a maximum of 2 mg (eight doses)
Misoprostol	PR	800 µg
Gemeprost	Intrauterine	1–2 mg

If these pharmacological and basic surgical steps have not achieved haemostasis, the uterus can be packed by either a traditional technique using gauze[9] or, as has more recently been described, balloon insufflation.[10,11] This technique can be employed regardless of whether the abdomen is open or closed, and may therefore avoid the need for open laparotomy [D]. Indeed, the provisional data on the use of balloon insufflation using a Rusch urological balloon appear very encouraging, although there are problems related to when and by how much the balloon should be deflated.

Should these steps fail, the patient will require a laparotomy. At that time, either unilateral or bilateral uterine artery ligation can be performed, with success rates reported of more than 90 per cent [D].[12]

This technique involves placement of a suture through the broad ligament to include 2–3 cm of myometrium. The suture should be placed approximately 2 cm above the point where an incision for a lower-segment caesarean section (CS) would be, thus ligating the ascending branch of the uterine artery and avoiding inclusion of the ureter in the suture.

Arterial ligation has been modified into a series of stepwise procedures producing uterine devascularisation. This technique, described in Egypt, involves five steps: unilateral ligation of the uterine artery at the level of the lower segment; bilateral ligation of the uterine artery at the level of the lower segment; low ligation of the uterine artery after mobilisation of the bladder; unilateral ovarian vessel ligation; and bilateral ovarian vessel ligation [D].[13] The first two of these steps resulted in haemostasis in more than 80 per cent of cases in the original report. Although ligation of the internal iliac arteries has been well described in the literature, it requires a high level of surgical skill and is reported as avoiding hysterectomy in only 50 per cent of cases.[14] The surgical time and complication rate in this series were also higher than when a hysterectomy was performed. After all these levels of uterine devascularisation, subsequent menstruation and successful pregnancies have been reported.

The use of compression sutures of the uterus has been reported from Switzerland and the UK,[15,16] although their exact role in the treatment of PPH has yet to be established. Compression sutures are only of possible benefit if bimanual compression of the uterus results in significant decrease in blood loss. Initially, the operation described by B-Lynch involves inserting a compression suture through a lower uterine segment incision, either the CS incision or making a new incision. The suture is placed 3 cm below the incision and 3 cm in from its lateral border, through the uterine wall and cavity, exiting through a similar position on the superior aspect of the incision 3 cm above and 4 cm in from the lateral border. It then passes over the uterine fundus 3–4 cm from the right cornu and passes posteriorly down the uterus to enter the posterior uterine wall at the same level as the upper anterior entry point. The suture is then placed under moderate tension, while an assistant compresses the uterus. It is then placed back through the posterior wall on the left at a similar point as on the right. The suture is passed back over the fundus and then inserted through the upper and lower incisions on the left in a similar fashion as on the right. It is then tied. Initially, this technique was described using a 2-catgut suture on a 70 mm round-bodied hand needle. However, since the withdrawal of catgut, an alternative suture would be 1-monocryl.

A modification of the technique without opening a previously intact uterus has also been described.

Other options, such as arterial embolisation and the use of recombinant factor VIIa, have been successfully described; however, good denominator data on the success rates of these are not available at this time.[17,18]

The importance of good denominator data is demonstrated by the UK Obstetric Surveillance System (UKOSS), where rare conditions are identified and registered with a central coordinating body. One such study into the prevalence of peripartum hysterectomy showed that 50 women who subsequently went on to have a hysterectomy had had a B-Lynch suture inserted, which compares to the nine cases in the world literature where this procedure failed.

Data on all three of these procedures are now being collected by UKOSS.

Hysterectomy with ovarian conservation may be required as a life-saving procedure. In the UK, it has a reported incidence of approximately 4.1 per 10,000 deliveries.[19] Experienced obstetricians need to be involved in the decision-making process during this cascade of events and, where possible, the patient and her relatives should be kept fully informed.

Selective arterial embolisation has been described both prior to hysterectomy and for persistent bleeding following hysterectomy. However, as mentioned above, its efficacy is still unknown and at the present time its use is limited by its availability.

The post-operative management of these patients may include the use of critical care units, with careful monitoring of central venous pressure being a recommendation from consecutive maternal mortality reports [D]. In the long term, these patients may also need professional counselling, especially if they have undergone a hysterectomy, and a debriefing with the lead clinician in charge of the patient's care is likely to improve patient understanding and satisfaction [E].

The management of secondary PPH may, if severe, follow similar lines to the above. However, if milder, the management will depend upon the aetiology of the condition, with patients with suspected endometritis being treated with broad-spectrum antibiotics and those with suspected retained fragments of the placenta by uterine exploration. Because of the high incidence of infection, it is important that any uterine instrumentation is covered by administration of a broad-spectrum antibiotic [E]. In this situation, the role of ultrasound in the detection of retained products of conception is limited, because of the difficulty in distinguishing between placental tissue and an organised blood clot on ultrasonographic examination [E].

EBM

- A systematic review of RCTs shows that active management of the third stage of labour decreases the incidence of PPH.
- A systematic review of the optimal choice of fluid for resuscitation shows no advantage in choosing a colloid before a crystalloid.
- No high-order avoidance exists to support one form of surgical management of PPH over any other.
- There are few RCTs of the management of PPH.
- A series of retrospective and prospective studies has shown that even with severe haemorrhage, a combination of medical and surgical treatment should avoid the need for hysterectomy in the vast majority of cases.
- The efficacy of different therapies for peripartum haemorrhage is being assessed by UKOSS.

KEY POINTS

- PPH is still a cause of maternal mortality in the United Kingdom.
- Active management of the third stage of labour decreases the risk of PPH.
- Early identification of PPH with accurate estimation of blood loss is essential.
- Acute management requires a multidisciplinary approach with the involvement of senior clinicians.
- It is important to monitor central venous pressure in severe cases.
- Early transfusion and correction of coagulopathy is fundamental.
- All units need their own detailed protocols for the management of massive PPH.

Key References

1. Cantwell R, Clutton-Brock T, Cooper G *et al.* Saving mothers' lives. Reviewing maternal deaths to make motherhood safer: The eighth edition of the CEMD in the UK. *BJOG* 2011;118:1–203.
2. Waterstone M, Bewley S, Charles Wolfe C. Incidence and predictors of severe obstetric morbidity: case–control study. *BMJ* 2001;322:1089–94.
3. Arulkumaran S, Chandraharan E, Mahmood T *et al. Maternity dashboard clinical performance and governance score card.* Good Practice No 7. London: RCOG, 2008.
4. Anonymous. The management of postpartum haemorrhage. *Drug Ther Bull* 1992;30:89–92.
5. Begley CM, Gyte GML, Devane D, McGuire W, Weeks A. Active versus expectant management for women in the

third stage of labour. *Cochrane Database of Systematic Reviews* 2011,11: CD007412.

6. RCOG Prevention and management of postpartum haemorrhage. Green-top guideline No. 52. London: RCOG, April 2011

7. Perel P, Roberts I, Ker K. Colloids versus crystalloids for fluid resuscitation in critically ill patients. *Cochrane Database of Systematic Reviews* 2013,2: CD000567.

8. Mousa HA, Blum J, Abou El Senoun G, Shakur H, Alfirevic Z. Treatment for primary postpartum haemorrhage. *Cochrane Database of Systematic Reviews* 2014,2: CD003249.

9. Maier RC. Control of postpartum hemorrhage with uterine packing. *Am J Obstet Gynecol* 1993;169:317–23.

10. Katesmark M, Brown R, Raju K. Successful use of a Sengstaken–Blakemore tube to control massive postpartum haemorrhage. *Br J Obstet Gynaecol* 1994;101:259–60.

11. Johanson R, Kumar M, Obhrai M, Young P. Management of massive postpartum haemorrhage: use of a hydrostatic balloon catheter to avoid laparotomy. *Br J Obstet Gynaecol* 2001;108:420–2.

12. O'Leary JA. Uterine artery ligation in the control of post cesarean hemorrhage. *J Reprod Med* 1995;40:189–93.

13. Abd Rabbo SA. Stepwise uterine devascularization: a novel technique for management of uncontrolled postpartum hemorrhage with preservation of the uterus. *Am J Obstet Gynecol* 1994;171:694–700.

14. Annonymous. Postpartum haemorrhage. *Clin Obstet Gynecol* 1994;37:824–30.

15. Schnarwller B, Passweg D, von Castleberg B. Erfolgreiche Behandlung einr medikamentos refraktaren Uterusatonie durch Funduskompressionsnahte. (Successful treatment of drug refractory uterine atony by fundus compression sutures.) *Geburtshilfe Frauenheilkd* 1996;56:151–3.

16. B-Lynch C, Coker A, Lawal AH, Abu J, Cowen MJ. The B-Lynch surgical technique for the control of massive postpartum haemorrhage: an alternative to hysterectomy? Five cases reported. *Br J Obstet Gynaecol* 1997;104:372–5.

17. Ahonen J, Jokela R. Recombinant factor VIIa for life-threatening post-partum haemorrhage. *Br J Anaesth* 2005;94:592–5.

18. Badawy SZ, Etman A, Singh M et al. Uterine artery embolization: the role in obstetrics and gynecology. *Clin Imaging* 2001;25:288-95.

19. Knight M on behalf of UKOSS. Peripartum hysterectomy in the UK: management and outcomes of the associated haemorrhage. *BJOG* 2007;114: 1380-7.

Chapter 65 Postpartum pyrexia

Peter J Thompson

INTRODUCTION

Historically, postpartum sepsis was most commonly secondary to infection with group A *Streptococcus*, and the prognosis was poor. Although the advent of antimicrobial therapy has significantly improved the prognosis, the last triennial Confidential Enquiry into Maternal Deaths (CEMD) report demonstrates that puerperal sepsis is not a disease of the past as although this report noted a fall in maternal mortality, the opposite was true for deaths secondary to sepsis. Indeed, one of the 10 recommendations from the report concerns the management of genital tract sepsis as this was identified as the leading cause of direct maternal death. The increase from previous reports shows that in 26 cases a woman's maternal death was due to sepsis, with 13 of these deaths being due to group A streptococcal infection.[1]

DEFINITIONS

Normal core body temperature is 37–37.5°C, with a diurnal variation of body temperature resulting in evening temperatures being 0.5–1°C higher than those in the morning. Oral and axillary temperatures are usually 0.4 and 1°C lower than core temperature, respectively. Persistent elevation of body temperature above those normal levels is termed 'pyrexia' or fever. The standard definition for puerperal fever used for reporting rates of puerperal morbidity is an oral temperature of 38.0°C or more on any two of the first 10 days postpartum, or 38.7°C or higher during the first 24 hours postpartum. For definitions of sepsis and severe sepsis see the relevant chapter, though it is worth reiterating here that septic shock is defined as the persistence of hypoperfusion of organs causing organ dysfunction that is not corrected by adequate fluid replacement.

PREVALENCE

Following delivery, pyrexia is common, with fever secondary to disorders of the breast occurring in approximately 18 per cent of healthy mothers.[2,3] Benign fever with resolution in the first 24 hours occurs with an incidence of 3 per cent.[4] Fever associated with infection is also common, with urinary tract infection (UTI) occurring in 2–4 per cent of women following delivery and endometritis in 1.6 per cent. Infections of the lower genital tract are uncommon and account for only approximately 1 per cent of cases of puerperal infection.[5]

AETIOLOGY

The aetiology of pyrexia following delivery can be separated into four broad categories:

1. benign fever;
2. breast engorgement;
3. infections of the urogenital tract;
4. distant infections.

The most common infections of the urogenital tract are endometritis, UTIs and infections of perineal repairs. Although not all pyrexias are of an infective origin, infection is the most important diagnosis and a detailed history should be taken and thorough examination performed to identify possible sites of infection. Rare causes of infection should be borne in mind in those patients who have recently been in tropical countries. Specific infections in the puerperium are caused by the same organisms that cause these infections at other times; however in addition one should consider the possibility of Lancefield group A streptococcal infection and the possibility of influenza, both of which are known to carry a significant mortality risk in pregnancy and the puerperium. In 2009 the risks of community-acquired group A streptococcal infection were circulated by the Inspector of Microbiology and Infection Control, where he quoted a 20–50 per cent mortality rate.

The development of endometritis is secondary to contamination of the uterine cavity with vaginal organisms during labour and delivery, with subsequent invasion of the myometrium. Endometritis is usually a polymicrobial infection associated with mixed aerobic and anaerobic flora. Bacteraemia may be present in 10–20 per cent of cases. The organisms that contribute to this condition include groups A and B beta-haemolytic streptococci, aerobic Gram-negative rods, *Neisseria gonorrhoeae* and certain anaerobic bacteria.

Regardless of the aetiology of the pyrexia, the common pathway appears to be the production of endogenous pyrogens released by leukocytes in response to an antigenic stimulus. These then act on the hypothalamus, which in turn acts on the vasomotor centre, resulting in an increased production of heat and a decrease in heat loss.

MANAGEMENT

Prophylaxis

Prophylaxis against infections in the puerperium is particularly important in the case of delivery by caesarean section [A],[6] although there is no good evidence supporting the use of antibiotics at the time of instrumental delivery [A][7] and recent publications from NICE suggest that women with congenital heart disease do not require antibiotic prophylaxis against infective endocarditis.[8] If, however, women with congenital heart disease develop pyrexia, then this must be excluded and close liaison with local cardiologists should be maintained [E], as in previous triennial reports into maternal mortality there were indirect deaths attributable to infectious endocarditis. In the most recent report there were three such deaths: two late coincidental deaths in drug users and one from secondary acute endocarditis.[1]

In cases where puerperal women have been exposed to H1N1 infection or been in contact with people with invasive group A streptococcal infection prophylaxis may be indicated and liaison with infectious disease units is indicated [E].

In addition all postnatal women should have their observations taken and recorded on a modified obstetric early warning system chart, MEOWS. Most importantly, abnormal observations need to be documented and acted upon.

General management

Management will depend upon the origin of the pyrexia; however a general philosophy of following a sepsis care bundle will both help to identify patients and then lead to the initiation of a general treatment package. One such example of a treatment package is the Sepsis Six (Box 65.1). Instigation of such sepsis care bundles have seen the rates of mortality from septic shock decrease from 46.5 per cent in 2001 to 18 per cent in the recently published PRoCESS trial; this was the mortality rate in the usual care arm of the trial where 70 per cent of hospitals were using protocolised management of septic shock [B].

Because of the diverse nature of aetiologies mentioned above, a thorough history and examination need to be per-

Box 65.1 Sepsis Six

1. Administer high-flow oxygen
2. Take blood cultures
3. Give broad-spectrum intravenous antibiotics
4. Give intravenous fluids
5. Measure serum lactate and haemoglobin
6. Accurately measure the urine output

formed, paying particular attention to examination of the breasts, chest and any wound sites. This includes an abdominal examination of the uterus for tenderness, a sign of endometritis. The endometrial cavity should be thought of as a wound site in this situation [E]. Features that are more typical of a benign fever are the presence of early low-grade pyrexia in the absence of any other symptomatology.

Appropriate cultures should be taken and, depending on the clinical features present, these may include wound and vaginal swabs, midstream specimens of urine, sputum samples and blood cultures. Management should consist of supportive therapy to ensure hydration and, where necessary, the administration of regular paracetamol, which acts as an antipyretic and will improve patient comfort, while not altering the course of the disease process [B].[9] In cases of severe septicaemia, transfer to a critical care unit may be required so that inotropic support can be initiated; however it is essential that administration of broad-spectrum antibiotics occurs within one hour of diagnosing a septic state. This is known to improve survival rates.

Specific management

This should be aimed at the administration of an appropriate antibiotic, which may need to be given intravenously in the first instance. In line with controls assurance standards, all hospitals should have an antibiotic policy determined by examination of the antibiotic sensitivities of organisms that have been detected within that unit. These policies need to be regularly reviewed, easily accessible and well promoted throughout the hospital. Once the relevant culture results are available, it is essential that any empirical antibiotic therapy commenced is reviewed in light of the known antibiotic sensitivities.

The management of proven endometritis has been shown to be optimal if antibiotics that cover *Bacteroides fragilis* and other penicillin-resistant anaerobic bacteria are used. When uncomplicated endometritis is clinically improving on intravenous therapy, there appears to be no advantage in continuing oral therapy [A].[10] As no single antibiotic regimen has yet been shown to be superior to others in the treatment of UTIs, therapy should be determined by policies based on the antibiotic sensitivities of bacteria isolated locally [A].[11]

As already mentioned, the Health Protection Agency in England has noted an estimated 62 per cent increase in the incidence of invasive group A streptococcal infections, with a reported increased mortality rate of 25 per cent. While not all these cases were in postpartum women, some fatalities were. A high index of suspicion should be maintained when patients present with symptoms suggestive of invasive group A streptococcal sepsis, such as general malaise, high fever, severe muscle aches, dizziness, hypotension, confusion, unexplained diarrhoea and vomiting, localised muscle tenderness, pain out of proportion to external signs and a flat red rash over large areas of the body.

Red-flag signs that are suggestive of influenza or group A streptococcal infection can be seen in Table 65.1. Where either of these conditions is suspected appropriate cultures including throat swabs should be taken and antibiotics or antiviral therapy commenced without awaiting the results of these cultures as in the sepsis bundle above.

Where group A streptococcal sepsis is suspected, immediate liaison with a consultant microbiologist is required, the Health Protection Unit must be informed and any contacts who show signs or symptoms of non-invasive group A

streptococcal infection should be treated with penicillin V or, if allergic, azithromycin, and their appropriate contacts traced and treated.[12]

Women thought to have H1N1 infection should be treated with oseltamivir and infection control regimens put in place, including wearing personal protective equipment; in addition in the case of aerosol-generating procedures such as intubation, FFP3 masks should be worn. Although a recent Cochrane review has questioned whether the use of oseltamivir results in a clinically significant benefit in healthy young adults, this review did not consider the benefits in a pregnant population, believing them to already be proven.[13]

Wound infections and endometritis may both be complicated by abscess formation. In these circumstances, antibiotic therapy alone is insufficient, and surgical drainage will be required [E]. The long-term complications of endometritis include subfertility [D].

The management of fever associated with breast problems is detailed elsewhere (see Chapter 67, Problems with breastfeeding).

Table 65.1 Red-flag symptoms for H1N1 infection and invasive group A streptococcal infection

H1N1 infection	Invasive group A *Streptococcus*
Temperature of 38°C	Temperature of 38°C
Cough	Hypotension
Rhinorrhoea or other upper respiratory symptoms	General malaise
Headache	Severe myalgia
Chills	Localised muscle tenderness
Myalgia, which can be severe	Pain out of proportion to the external signs
Vomiting and/or diarrhoea	Flat red rash over parts of the body
	Vomiting and/or diarrhoea

EBM

- Systematic reviews of randomised controlled trials (RCTs) show:
  - a decrease in infective morbidity following caesarean section if prophylactic antibiotics are used;
  - in cases of endometritis, antibiotics that cover *Bacteroides fragilis* and other penicillin-resistant anaerobic bacteria should be used;
  - if the endometritis is uncomplicated, oral therapy following intravenous therapy is unnecessary.
- RCTs show that the administration of paracetamol to pyrexial patients increases their comfort and does not affect the progress of the disease.
- Expert opinion regarding controls assurance suggests that all hospitals should have their own antibiotic policy.
- In cases of proven sepsis expert opinion is that broad-spectrum intravenous antibiotics should be administered within 1 hour of diagnosis and a sepsis bundle be initiated.

KEY POINTS

- Puerperal sepsis is still a significant and increasing cause of maternal mortality.
- A thorough examination and acquisition of appropriate cultures are mandatory.
- The NHS Executive has produced guidelines regarding controls assurance which suggest that all hospitals should have their own antibiotic policy.
- Paracetamol administration is safe and improves patient comfort.
- Implementation of sepsis bundles has decreased the mortality from sepsis in the general population.

Key References

1. Saving Mothers' Lives: Reviewing maternal deaths to make motherhood safer: 2006–2008. The Eighth Report of the CEMD in the UK. *BJOG* 2011;118 supplement 1–203.

2. Almeida OD Jr, Kitay DZ. Lactation suppression and puerperal fever. *Am J Obstet Gynecol* 1986;154:940–1.

3. Marshall BR, Hepper JK, Zirbel CC. Sporadic puerperal mastitis. An infection that need not interrupt lactation. *J Am Med Assoc* 1975; 233:1377–9.

4. Ely JW, Dawson JD, Townsend AS *et al*. Benign fever following vaginal delivery. *J Fam Pract* 1996;43:146–51.

5. Sweet RL, Ledger WJ. Puerperal infectious morbidity: a two-year review. *Am J Obstet Gynecol* 1973;117:1093–100.

6. Hofmeyr GJ, Smaill FM. Antibiotic prophylaxis for cesarean section. *Cochrane Database Syst Rev* 2002;(3):CD000933.

7. Liabsuetrakul T, Choobun T, Peeyananjarassri K, Islam QM. Antibiotic prophylaxis for operative vaginal delivery. *Cochrane Database Syst Rev* 2004;(3): CD004455.

8. NICE. *Prophylaxis against infectious endocarditis.* Guideline 64. NICE, 2008.

9. Prescott LF. Paracetamol: past, present, and future (review). *Am J Ther* 2000;7:143–7.

10. French L, Smaill FM. Antibiotic regimens for endometritis after delivery. *Cochrane Database Syst Rev* 2004;(4):CD001067.

11. Vazquez JC, Villar J. Treatments for symptomatic urinary tract infections during pregnancy. *Cochrane Database Syst Rev* 2001;(4):CD002256.

12. Duerden BI. *Increase in invasive group A streptococcal infections in England.* Department of Health, Central Alerting System April 2009, gateway reference 11632.

13. Jefferson T, Jones MA, Doshi P *et al*. Neuraminidase inhibitors for preventing and treating influenza in healthy adults and children. *Cochrane Database of Systematic Reviews* 2014, Issue 4. Art. No.: CD008965. DOI: 10.1002/14651858.CD008965.pub4.

Chapter 66 Disturbed mood

Peter J Thompson

MRCOG standards

Theoretical skills
Understand the epidemiology, aetiology, pathophysiology, clinical characteristics, prognostic features and management of:
- manic depression, psychoneurosis, puerperal disorders (baby blues, depression), mood disorders, schizophrenia, reaction to pregnancy loss.

Practical skills
- Observation of the above.

INTRODUCTION

There is significant morbidity and mortality associated with mood disorders in pregnancy, with the morbidity being in both social and physical terms. In the past, it was felt that pregnancy had a protective affect with fewer women committing suicide than would be expected;[1] however, this has been contradicted by reports into maternal mortality in the UK and evidence suggests that the prevalence of psychiatric disorders at conception is the same as in the female non-pregnant population. In the last Confidential Enquiry into Maternal Deaths (CEMD) triennial report there were 13 indirect deaths caused by suicide, with another 16 late maternal deaths. Of the 13 indirect deaths four were during the antenatal period. When all 29 women are considered, most of these deaths were violent (87 per cent) with over half secondary to hanging or multiple injuries from jumping from a height. Of these women, 19 had a past history of psychiatric illness, but in the nine cases where this was identified it was considered to have been appropriately managed in only four cases.[2]

Antenatal disorders of mood tend to involve the management of pre-existing psychiatric conditions. However, while any psychiatric condition can arise in the postnatal period, either as a recurrence or *de novo*, there are specific postnatal disorders of mood. These fall into three broad categories: 'baby blues', postnatal depression and puerperal psychosis. This section aims to cover all four of the areas above.

DEFINITIONS

'Baby blues' (or postpartum blues) is the term used to describe the transient experience of tearfulness, anxiety and irritability that frequently occurs in the first few days following delivery.

In comparison, postpartum psychosis is defined as a severe mental disorder usually occurring in the first 4 weeks after delivery, characterised by the presence of irrational ideas and unusual reactions to the baby. In addition, these patients also suffer fewer specific symptoms, such as restlessness, irritability, insomnia and lability of mood.

The symptoms of postnatal depression do not differ from the symptoms of depression at other times of life, but a temporal association with childbirth distinguishes it from other forms of depression. There does, however, seem to be little agreement on what the limits of this temporal relationship are, which makes assessment of the literature more difficult. Most studies are limited to depression with onset within 3 months of delivery, although some studies extend this limit to 6 months.

INCIDENCE

As antenatal disorders of mood disturbance are usually due to pre-existing psychiatric conditions, the incidence is approximately the same as amongst non-gravid women of a similar age.

More than 50 per cent of women suffer from postpartum blues, usually commencing on the fourth or fifth postnatal day.[3] The incidence of postnatal depression is approximately 10–15 per cent,[4] whereas postnatal psychosis is rare, occurring in 0.1 per cent of cases.[5]

AETIOLOGY

Antenatal conditions

As already mentioned, although antenatal mood disorders are usually secondary to pre-existing conditions, they can be precipitated for the first time by a significant life event – the pregnancy. Pregnancy can place an additional strain on many relationships, not to mention the worries of future financial burdens, which may be sufficient to destabilise a susceptible individual. Therefore, these conditions may be secondary to the social implications of pregnancy rather than the pregnancy itself.

Baby blues

As the immediate postnatal period is a time of significant physiological and social change, it is not surprising that a significant number of mothers suffer from disorders of mood. Baby blues is a self-limiting condition that has not been associated with any specific metabolic or endocrinological disturbance. It is more common in women following their first delivery, and some authors believe that sufferers are not more likely to have a past psychiatric history than non-sufferers. Other factors such as lack of sleep, hospitalisation and pain have been implicated in the aetiology of this condition.

Postnatal depression

The social and physiological changes seen at this time are also relevant to postnatal depression and puerperal psychosis. Although it is still true that no specific endocrinological change has been associated with the onset of postnatal depression, it has previously been hypothesised that the fall in both progesterone and oestrogen concentrations is implicated, as these hormones are known to have psychoactive properties. Unlike baby blues, postnatal depression is associated with a past history of psychiatric illness. One of the problems with determining the aetiology of this condition is that not all experts even recognise it as a separate disease entity.

Puerperal psychosis

Whether puerperal psychosis is a discrete disease entity or a rapidly evolving affective psychosis is a matter of much debate. The aetiology of puerperal psychosis is poorly understood; however, it does appear to be more common following the first delivery and in patients with previous bipolar disorders, and is recognised as having a 25 per cent risk of recurrence in subsequent pregnancies. Many patients also suffer from recurrent relapsing affective disorders for the remainder of their lives.[6]

MANAGEMENT

Antenatal conditions

Management of psychiatric illnesses during pregnancy is similar to that outside pregnancy and should include both pharmacological and non-pharmacological therapies. The main concerns for both women and their physicians are the effects that psychotropic drugs may have on the fetus, due to

their high transplacental transfer rates. Indeed, although these drugs are not licensed for use in pregnancy, it is well established that if medication is withdrawn for mood disorders, anxiety disorders and schizophrenia, there are high rates of relapse during pregnancy. In view of this, several reviews have been published examining the possible teratogenic effects of these drugs (see Chapter 27, Medication in pregnancy). However, as new data are established daily on the adverse effect of drugs, readers are encouraged to search for the latest systematic reviews and teratology databases for themselves, e.g. http://toxbase.u5e.com/.

Overall, antidepressants as a group have not been associated with an increase in major malformations, although in the case of paroxetine, and more recently fluoxetine, both the relevant drug company and the FDA in the US issued a warning regarding cardiac malformations following paroxetine usage in the first trimester [D].[7]

Following treatment in the first trimester of pregnancy, benzodiazepines, antipsychotic medications and lithium have all been associated with small but significantly increased risks of teratogenicity in the offspring. Therefore, women with a psychiatric disorder who are pregnant or who are trying to conceive should be counselled regarding the relative risks of disease relapse and fetal exposure to medication, and where appropriate an alternative, safer drug may be prescribed [C].

Women with a past history of psychiatric problems are at an increased risk of developing postnatal depression, and should therefore be identified and offered increased professional support following delivery [E]. Screening for mood disorders is a routine part of antenatal care in the UK, and should occur both antenatally and postnatally. Early diagnosis and treatment can help reduce the negative impact of mental illness on the whole family unit.

In addition to the above it is usually recommended that women with significant disorders of mood will require a written care plan, which is formulated by a multidisciplinary team, and may include liaison with the social service sector to implement a safeguarding plan for the unborn child.

Baby blues

Research into the management of this condition is limited, with the only significant research being focused on an attempt to identify women who are at increased risk of developing either postnatal depression or puerperal psychosis. Management consists of providing a supportive environment for the new mother, with both professionals (particularly midwives) and the family working together [E]. Drug therapy is not indicated, as the condition is usually self-limiting. Those women in whom the condition persists beyond 10–14 days[9] and those who have marital difficulties appear to have an increased risk of developing puerperal psychosis.

NICE has recommended in its guideline on postnatal care of women that resolution of these symptoms should be confirmed between 10 and 14 days post-delivery, and if they have not resolved, assessment for postnatal depression performed and where appropriate further referral instigated [E].[10]

Postnatal depression

Whether or not postnatal depression is a separate disease entity from depression, there is no doubt that it can have significant long-term effects on the mother–infant relationship and the development of the infant. Therefore, early detection and appropriate treatment are essential. The Edinburgh Postnatal Depression Score is a self-report scale that has ten items relating to symptoms of depression. The detection rates of postnatal depression in the community can be improved by implementation of the Edinburgh Postnatal Depression Score at a 6-weeks postnatal check [C].[11]

The treatment of postnatal depression in the past has mainly revolved around social support and supportive therapy, the administration of sex hormones (oestrogen and progesterone) and the prescription of antidepressants. In the case of sex hormone therapy, a systematic review of studies that used oestrogen or progesterone to treat women with postnatal depression showed discouraging results. Treatment with high doses of oestrogen did appear to reduce the depression scores of women with severe postnatal depression, but the potential side effects of thromboembolic disease, endometrial hyperplasia and inhibition of lactation make this an unattractive therapy for women to take. Progesterone therapy was associated with a higher incidence of postnatal depression than placebo. This could be because the mood elevation seen with natural progesterone is not an effect of synthetic progestogens.[12] Therefore, these medications cannot be recommended for women with postnatal depression [A]. Modern therapy, therefore, revolves around supportive therapy and pharmacological treatments.

Early involvement of a psychiatrist with experience in this condition is essential [E] and if the patient requires hospitalisation, it is preferable to avoid separation from the baby, which will necessitate admission to a specialised mother-and-baby unit [D]. Ten trials have been included in a systematic review of the treatment of postnatal depression with psychosocial and psychological interventions as compared with the usual postpartum care.[13] This review showed a risk ratio of 0.44 (CI 0.24–0.88) for the evidence of depression at 1 year in favour of the interventions [A].

There are sparse data where the role of antidepressants for the treatment of this condition has been investigated in the context of an randomised controlled trial (RCT), though a recent review in the Cochrane database has shown an increased response and remission rate when comparing selective serotonin re-uptake inhibitors (SSRIs) to treatment with placebo. This analysis does however point out the limitations of the review, including the small numbers of patients involved [A].[14] NICE has recommended that for women with a new onset of mild to moderate depression in the postnatal period, self-help strategies, non-directive counselling and brief courses of cognitive–behavioural therapy or interpersonal psychotherapy should be offered first, with antidepressant medication

reserved for those who are resistant to the above, those with a history of severe depression and those who decline psychological treatment. For those with moderate depression with a history of a depressive episode or those with severe depression during the postnatal period, treatment should be with structured psychological treatment or, if the patient has a preference for them, with antidepressants. If antidepressants are to be used then NICE recommends that the drugs of first choice are SSRIs (with the exclusion of paroxetine). If these treatments fail separately, a combination of the two treatments should be considered [E].[8]

Puerperal psychosis

This is a psychiatric emergency and its treatment requires hospitalisation. As it is preferable to avoid separation of the mother from her infant, admission to a specialized mother and baby unit should be arranged, where antidepressant and neuroleptic medication can be initiated and supervised by psychiatrists [C]. Failure to treat the condition aggressively is associated with rates of infanticide as high as 4 per cent [C].[15] This aggressive treatment may include electro-convulsive therapy [D].

EBM

- Systematic review of two RCTs shows progesterone therapy to be of no benefit, although oestrogen therapy may decrease the severity of depression when used as adjunctive therapy.
- An RCT has shown that fluoxetine is as effective as cognitive–behavioural therapy for the treatment of postnatal depression.
- Cohort studies show that the Edinburgh Postnatal Depression Score is effective in detecting women at risk of postnatal mood disorders.
- Retrospective cohort studies show that most drugs used to treat psychiatric conditions are relatively safe to use in pregnancy.

KEY POINTS

- Most drugs used to treat psychiatric disorders are relatively safe to use in pregnancy.
- Postnatal screening for postnatal depression using the Edinburgh Postnatal Depression Score is effective.
- The best treatment for postnatal depression appears to be cognitive–behavioural therapy, with the administration of antidepressants where necessary. The antidepressants of choice are SSRIs.
- Puerperal psychosis is a psychiatric emergency.
- Most women who commit suicide following or during pregnancy have a significant history of mental health disorders.

References

1. Appleby L. Suicidal behaviour in childbearing women. *Int Rev Psychiatry* 1996;8:107–15.

2. Saving Mothers' Lives: Reviewing maternal deaths to make motherhood safer: 2006–2008. The Eighth Report of the CEMD in the UK. *BJOG* 2011;118 supplement 1–2033.

3. Kendell RE, McGuire RJ, Connor Y, Cox JL. Mood changes in the first three weeks after childbirth. *J Affect Disord* 1981;3:317–26.

4. Cox JL, Murray D, Chapman G. A controlled study of the onset, duration and prevalence of postnatal depression. *Br J Psychiatry* 1993;163:27–31.

5. Kumar R, Robson KM. A prospective study of emotional disorders in childbearing women. *Br J Psychiatry* 1984;144:35–47.

6. Davidson J, Robertson E. A follow-up study of postpartum illness, 1946–1978. *Acta Psychiatr Scand* 1985; 71:451–7.

7. National Teratology Information Service (NTIS). *Use of Paroxetine in Pregnancy*. Newcastle upon Tyne: NTIS, Regional Drug and Therapeutics Centre, 2005.

8. NICE. *Antenatal and postnatal mental health. Clinical Management and Service Guidance*. NICE Clinical Guideline 45. London: NICE, 2007. Available from ‹www.nice.org.uk/guidance/CG45/niceguidance/pdf/English›.

9. Robinson GE, Stewart DE. Postpartum psychiatric disorders. *CMAJ* 1986;134:31–7.

10. Demott K, Bick D, Norman R *et al. Clinical guidelines and evidence review for postnatal care: routine postnatal care of recently delivered women and their babies.* London: National Collaborating Centre for Primary Care and Royal College of General Practitioners, 2006.

11. Georgiopoulos AM, Bryan TL, Wollan P, Yawn BP. Routine screening for postpartum depression. *J Fam Pract* 2001;50:117–22.

12. Dennis CL, Ross LE, Herxheimer A. Oestrogens and progestins for preventing and treating postpartum depression. *Cochrane Database Syst Rev* 2008; 4:CD001690.

13. Dennis CL, Hodnett ED. Psychosocial and psychological interventions for treating postpartum depression. *Cochrane Database Syst Rev* 2007;4:CD006116.

14. Essali A, Alabed S, Guul A, Essali N. Preventive interventions for postnatal psychosis. *Cochrane Database of Systematic Reviews* 2013;6:CD009991. DOI: 10.1002/14651858.CD009991.pub2.

15. D'Orban PT. Women who kill their children. *Br J Psychiatry* 1979;134: 560–71.

Chapter 67 Problems with breastfeeding

Peter J Thompson

INTRODUCTION

Although a physiological process, breastfeeding is an action that women perform for only a small part of their lives. For it to be successful, not only do the correct physiological processes have to occur, but both the mother and neonate need to adapt to this situation, and whereas some mothers and babies seem to be able to establish it without any problems, others do not. Increasingly, the proportion of women breastfeeding has been identified as a high priority for the government in their White Paper 'Our Healthier Nation'.[1] Indeed, the WHO recommends exclusive breastfeeding until the age of 6 months.[2] For these targets to be reached, interventions of proven benefit need to be employed throughout the health service. To this aim, UNICEF has developed a programme whereby maternity services that employ their Ten Steps to Successful Breastfeeding and seven-point plan for sustaining breastfeeding can apply for Baby Friendly status. These are evidence-based standards designed to promote, protect and support breastfeeding, with new standards produced in 2012. They cover topics including the establishment of local policies, training of staff, antenatal and postnatal education of women and the establishment of support groups. As an incentive to maternity services, many clinical commissioning groups in England are insisting on their acute trusts achieving Baby Friendly status. Other initiatives to encourage breastfeeding have included trials concerning supplying breastfeeding mothers with monetary incentives.

DEFINITIONS

There are extensive data in the literature supporting the concept that the optimum food for babies is breast milk. The benefits bestowed upon the infant are pertinent in both the short and long term. Included in these benefits is reduced morbidity from respiratory, gastrointestinal, urinary tract and middle ear infections, as well as a decreased tendency towards atopy and obesity. For the mother, there are both health benefits, such as a decrease in the incidence of epithelial ovarian cancer and premenopausal breast cancer, as well as financial benefits. Therefore, conditions that interfere with breastfeeding constitute important epidemiological health issues.

INCIDENCE

The last national audit in 2010 showed that following delivery approximately 81 per cent of women in the UK commence breastfeeding, a 5 per cent rise from the survey performed in 2005. Breastfeeding is much more common among women from least-deprived areas, those educated over the age of 18, those in ethnic minorities, those aged over 30 and women in England rather than other parts of the United Kingdom.[3] However, in the UK, these rates fall to approximately 69 per cent after 1 week, 55 per cent at 6 weeks and 34 per cent at 6 months. All of these are significant rises on the figures found in the 2005 survey. Despite these increases the number of women exclusively breastfeeding at 6 months of age is still less than 1 per cent.

AETIOLOGY

The establishment of lactation is dependent upon a variety of influences, including the production of prolactin from the anterior pituitary gland and oxytocin from the posterior pituitary gland. These hormones stimulate milk production and ejection, respectively. However, problems with lactation are rarely due to pituitary–hypothalamic-axis dysfunction. Indeed, the main reasons why women neither initiate breastfeeding nor continue it as long as in other European countries appear to relate to social and cultural issues. This section does not attempt to discuss these, but concentrates on the management of mastitis, breast abscess formation, enforced separation of mother and baby, and poor infant feeding. Many of these problems are interrelated and it has been suggested that the majority can be avoided by using a technique of feeding on demand and attaching the baby to the nipple in the correct position from the first feed onwards.[4]

MANAGEMENT

Mastitis

Mastalgia is defined as painful breasts. The prevalence of this condition varies with the duration of breastfeeding, though of women who fed for 6 months 46 per cent complained of breast engorgement, blocked milk ducts or mastitis.[3] The aetiology of this condition revolves around the imbalance between the production of milk and infant consumption that occurs in a small proportion of women. When milk production exceeds the infant's requirements, the alveolar spaces within the breasts become distended, with the breast feeling hot, swollen and tender. This swelling leads to compression of the capillaries, which in turn increases the arterial pressure to the breasts, causing compression of the connective tissues and a decrease in lymphatic drainage. This results in the formation of oedema and engorgement of the breast (obstructive mastitis), which may develop into infective mastitis.

Five factors have been associated with the development of breast engorgement: delayed initiation of feeds, infrequent feeds, time-limited feeds, a late shift from colostrum to milk production, and the habit of administering supplementary feeds.[5] Therefore, avoidance of these will significantly decrease the incidence of this problem.

Many interventions have been proposed for the treatment of breast engorgement, some of which have been the subject of systematic reviews, which have examined both traditional and modern treatments. The most effective treatments tested involved the use of anti-inflammatory agents [B]. The agents tested are not available in the UK, and it is uncertain whether these results are applicable to similar agents. Interventions, such as the topical application of cabbage leaves, the use of gel packs and ultrasound treatment, all showed an improvement in symptoms, though not to a greater extent than placebo. It has been postulated that these improvements are secondary to warming and physically massaging the breast [A].[6]

As previously mentioned, breast engorgement may become complicated by infection, leading to infective mastitis. The most common causative organism is *Staphylococcus aureus*, with others occasionally being implicated, including *Staphylococcus epidermidis*, groups A, B and F beta-haemolytic *Streptococcus*, *Haemophilus influenzae* and *Escherichia coli*. Management consists of the administration of an antibiotic that is effective against beta-lactamase-producing bacteria and encouraging the mother to continue breastfeeding or manually expressing milk [B].

Breast abscess formation

Although uncommon, the exact prevalence of this condition is not well reported, with the better estimates being in the region of 0.4 per cent.[7] It does, however, appear to be more common in women over 30 years of age, primiparous women and particularly following mastitis, with a reported incidence of 5–11 per cent most commonly following inadequate treatment of the mastitis.[8] Not surprisingly, therefore, the prevention of abscess formation is achieved by the avoidance of milk stasis.[9,10] However, unlike for infective mastitis, most authors would recommend that feeding from the affected breast ceases when pus is draining from the nipple [C]. The commonest causative organism is, as with mastitis, *Staphylococcus aureus*. Once formed, abscesses require either surgical drainage, under general anaesthesia,[11] or preferably needle aspiration with or without ultrasound control,[12,13] with concomitant administration of broad-spectrum antibiotics [C]. Ultrasound-guided aspiration is most successful when the abscess is 3 cm or less in diameter, with failure being associated with abscesses greater than 5 cm in diameter [B].[14] Repeat needle aspiration may be required and should continue until the abscess is less than 4 mm in diameter. When surgical drainage is performed, choice of incision for the drainage is controversial; circumferential incisions give optimum cosmetic results, but radial incisions carry a smaller risk of damage to other lactiferous ducts. Therefore, it would seem sensible to perform circumferential incisions to drain superficial abscesses, whereas deep abscesses should be drained via a radial incision [E].

Enforced separation of mother and baby

Separation of mother and baby, usually secondary to the ill-health of one or both parties, may have a significant impact on the establishment of breastfeeding. The successful long-term establishment of breastfeeding is dependent upon frequent feeding,[6] and this is obviously complicated when the parties are physically separated or when one or other party is too ill to feed. Indeed, ensuring that mothers and babies are together 24 hours a day is one of the 'Ten Steps to Successful Breastfeeding' promoted by UNICEF. However, systematic reviews have failed to show improved prevalence of long-term breastfeeding in groups of women who commence feeding early (within 30 minutes) when compared to those who commence feeding their infants between 4 and 8 hours post-delivery, though early skin-to-skin contact does appear to prolong duration of breastfeeding [A].[15,16]

If breastfeeding is to be established in these circumstances, the expression of breast milk, in place of frequent feeds, is essential [D]. This can be done by hand or mechanically, with collection of the milk in a container to feed the infant at a later date.

This problem is seen commonly in babies admitted to a neonatal unit and, because of the previously noted advantages of breastfeeding such children, many units have established milk banks to store this milk. There are occasions when breastfeeding may be contraindicated, for example maternal HIV infection, or relatively contraindicated, for example severe maternal ill-health. In such conditions, it may be appropriate to prescribe a dopamine antagonist, such as cabergoline, which will cause the production of milk to stop.

Poor infant feeding

Poor infant feeding secondary to ill-health has already been considered above. Poor technique of breastfeeding is another cause of poor feeding. A systematic review of increased support for mothers by healthcare professionals has shown a significantly decreased risk of discontinuation of breastfeeding. This effect was larger when there was both professional and lay support and the effect increased further when these supporters were UNICEF trained [A].[17]

EBM

Systematic reviews of randomised controlled trials (RCTs) show that:

- prolonged breastfeeding is not more prevalent in women who perform the first feed within 30 minutes of birth;
- support from a professional person increases the likelihood of a woman exclusively breastfeeding;
- the treatment of choice for breast engorgement is an anti-inflammatory agent.

There are few RCTs on the management of the other breast pathologies mentioned above, with most evidence coming from cohort or retrospective studies.

KEY POINTS

- Breastfeeding is beneficial to both mother and infant.
- A high proportion of women never commence breastfeeding and, of those who do, fewer than half will still be breastfeeding at 6 months.
- Women with obstructive and infective mastitis should continue to breastfeed.
- Women with breast abscesses should discontinue breastfeeding and will require needle aspiration or surgical drainage.

References

1. Department of Health. *Our healthier nation.* London: HMSO, 1998.
2. WHO. *Global strategy for infant and young child feeding.* 2003. Available from: http://apps.who.int/iris/bitstream/10665/42590/1/9241562218.pdf?ua=1
3. The Health and Social Care Information Centre *The infant feeding survey 2010.* 2012. Available from: http://www.hscic.gov.uk/catalogue/PUB08694›.
4. Inch S, Renfrew MJ. Common breastfeeding problems. *In*: Iain Chalmers I, Enkin M, Keirse MJNC (eds). *Effective Care in Pregnancy and Childbirth*, vol. 2. Oxford: Oxford University Press, 1989: 1375–89.
5. Moon JL, Humenick SS. Breast engorgement: contributing variables and variables amenable to nursing intervention. *J Obstet Gynecol Neonatal Nurs* 1989;18:309–15.
6. Mangesi L, Dowswell T. Treatments for breast engorgement during lactation. *Cochrane Database of Systematic Reviews* 2010, Issue 9. Art. No.: CD006946. DOI: 10.1002/14651858.CD006946.pub2.
7. Amir LH, Forster D, McLachlan H, Lumley J. Incidence of breast abscess in lactating women: report from an Australian cohort. *BJOG* 2004;111:1378–81.
8. Berens PD. Prenatal, intrapartum and postpartum support of the lactating mother. *Paediatr Clin North Am* 2001;48:365–75.
9. Thomsen AC, Hansen KB, Moller BR. Leukocyte counts and microbiologic cultivation in the diagnosis of puerperal mastitis. *Am J Obstet Gynecol* 1983;146:938–41.
10. Thomsen AC, Espersen T, Maigaard S. Course and treatment of milk stasis, non-infectious inflammation of the breast, and infectious mastitis in nursing women. *Am J Obstet Gynecol* 1984;149:492–5.
11. Benson EA. Management of breast abscesses. *World J Surg* 1989;13:753–6.
12. Karstrup S, Solvia J, Nolose CP et al. Acute puerperal breast abscesses: US-guided drainage. *Radiology* 1993;188:807–9.
13. Schwarz RJ, Shrestha R. Needle aspiration of breast abscess. *Am J Surg* 2001;182:117–19.
14. Eryilmaz R, Sahin M, Hakan Tekelioglu M, Daldal E. Management of lactational abscesses. *Breast* 2005;14(5):375–9.
15. Renfrew MJ, Lang S, Woolridge MW. Early versus delayed initiation of breastfeeding. *Cochrane Database Syst Rev* 2000;(3):CD000043.
16. Moore ER, Anderson GC, Bergman N, Dowswell T. Early skin-to-skin contact for mothers and their healthy newborn infants. *Cochrane Database of Systematic Reviews* 2012, Issue 5. Art. No.: CD003519. DOI: 10.1002/14651858.CD003519.pub3.
17. Renfrew MJ, McCormick FM, Wade A, Quinn B, Dowswell T. Support for healthy breastfeeding mothers with healthy term babies. *Cochrane Database of Systematic Reviews* 2012, Issue 5. Art. No.: CD001141. DOI: 10.1002/14651858.CD001141.pub4.

SECTION EIGHT

Reproductive Gynaecology

Chapter 68 Normal and abnormal development of the genitalia

Rebecca Deans and Sarah M Creighton

MRCOG standards

Theoretical skills

- Revise your knowledge of the embryological development of the male and female urogenital system.
- Understand the situations in which a disruption in these pathways can lead to disorders of sex development, Müllerian anomalies and Wolffian duct remnants.
- Understand the classification of Müllerian anomalies.
- Know about first-line investigations for disorders of sex development and Müllerian anomalies and treatments available in tertiary referral centres.

Practical skills

- Be able to take an appropriate history.
- Be able to initiate appropriate investigations to enable a diagnosis and/or tertiary referral

INTRODUCTION

Fetal development of the gonads, external genitalia, Müllerian ducts and Wolffian ducts can be disrupted at a variety of points, leading to a wide range of conditions with a large spectrum of clinical presentations. Disorders of sex development (DSD) occur when there is a disruption of either gonadal differentiation or fetal sex steroid production or action. Müllerian anomalies and Wolffian duct remnants occur when there is disruption of the embryological development of these systems. An understanding of embryology, as well as molecular genetics, helps us determine the biological basis of these conditions. Many of these cases present in infancy, with initial investigations and treatment performed by paediatric endocrinologists. Some will present for the first time to the gynaecologist and fertility subspecialist with primary amenorrhoea or infertility. Paediatric and urological surgeons may have initially treated others. Patients with DSDs may have coexisting medical problems and require thorough evaluation. As well as anatomical and fertility concerns for these patients, there are often many psychological issues; therefore management in a multidisciplinary team (MDT) is essential for the management of more complex cases. In some conditions, the optimal operative management is still uncertain, and there is currently debate regarding the optimal timing or need for genital surgery in patients with DSD conditions who present in childhood.

NORMAL EMBRYOLOGICAL DEVELOPMENT OF THE INTERNAL AND EXTERNAL GENITALIA

Genetic sex is determined at the moment of conception by the presence or absence of the Y chromosome, and after week 6 should guide the subsequent development of the fetus down one of two standard pathways – male or female. Until this time, development is the same in all fetuses. Primordial germ cells (the precursors of gametes) can be seen at 3 weeks in the endoderm of the yolk sac wall. During weeks 5 and 6, they migrate by amoeboid movement to the genital ridge (future gonad), an area of mesenchyme medial to the developing mesonephros and Wolffian (or mesonephric) duct. During week 6, primitive sex cords form around the germ cells in the indifferent gonad. The two Müllerian (or paramesonephric) ducts also appear lateral to the Wolffian ducts. At the same time, at the caudal end of the fetus, the cloacal membrane folds and is separated into the anterior urogenital and posterior anal parts. The urogenital section with the genital tubercle will become the future external genitalia, and by week 7 consists of a genital tubercle, urogenital membrane, urogenital folds and, more laterally, labioscrotal swellings. At the end of week 7, the urogenital membrane has degenerated and the urogenital sinus freely communicates with the amniotic fluid.

The first noticeable divergence in male and female fetuses is the differentiation of gonadal structure. The indifferent gonad has the potential for testicular or ovarian development.

The presence of intact germ cells seems necessary for the ovary to develop, but this is not required for testicular development. The gonad remains undifferentiated until around 42 days. After gonadal differentiation has occurred, the presence or absence of gonadal hormone production and other fetal factors then guides the development of the Müllerian ducts, Wolffian ducts and external genitalia. Sertoli cells in the fetal testis secrete anti-Müllerian hormone (AMH – also called Müllerian inhibiting substance, MIS), leading to active regression of the Müllerian ducts. Early Leydig cells commence production of testosterone which acts through the androgen receptor on the Wolffian ducts, leading to the development of the vas deferens, seminal vesicle and epididymis. Testosterone is converted to its active metabolite dihydrotestosterone (DHT). The fetal ovaries do not secrete androgen or AMH, and therefore there is female external genital development, growth of the Müllerian ducts and spontaneous regression of the Wolffian ducts.

STANDARD MALE PATHWAY

In an XY fetus, activation of the SRY (sex-determining region of the Y chromosome) gene at the end of week 6 guides the indifferent gonad to commence development into a testis.[1] Other autosomal genes (e.g. WT1, SOX9, SF1) are also involved in this genetic cascade.[2] The medullary sex cord cells become Sertoli cells, surrounding the primitive germ cells. At puberty, these will become the seminiferous tubules surrounding the spermatozoa. Sertoli cells produce AMH, which acts locally to cause apoptotic regression of the adjacent Müllerian ducts from 7 weeks. The appendix testis and prostatic utricle are usually all that remain of the Müllerian ducts in the male.

At around weeks 8–10, Leydig cells appear in the testis and start to secrete testosterone. The control of testosterone production may be independent initially, then under the control of placental human chorionic gonadotrophin (hCG) through the shared leutinizing hormone/hCG receptor (LHCGR), and subsequently by 20 weeks the hypothalamic pituitary (gonadotrope) axis becomes active and fetal leutinizing hormone (LH) production controls steroidogenesis. Testosterone acts through the androgen receptor and causes development of the Wolffian ducts into the vasa deferentia, and later the seminal vesicles and epididymides. Testosterone is also released into the circulation and undergoes peripheral conversion to its more active metabolite DHT by the enzyme 5α-reductase type 2, and acts on the target tissues of the perineum resulting in development and growth of the genital tubercle, urogenital sinus, urogenital folds and labioscrotal swellings into the glans penis, penile shaft, urethral tube and scrotum, respectively. The penis is similar in size to the clitoris at 14 weeks and, under the influence of DHT, continues growing until birth. Testicular descent is mediated by the Leydig cells under the influence of the hypothalamic pituitary (gonadotrope) axis, commences at 12 weeks, and is usually complete by week 34.

STANDARD FEMALE PATHWAY

Traditionally, ovarian development in an XX fetus has been considered a 'default pathway'; however, emerging research indicates that a distinct set of genes are expressed in the developing ovary and required for maintaining ovarian integrity and actively opposing testicular development (DAX1, WNT4/RSPO1), termed 'anti-testis' genes.[3–5] These genes, in combination with the absence of the SRY gene, cause the indifferent gonad to commence ovarian differentiation at around week 7. The sex cord cells degenerate and secondary sex cords form and surround the primordial germ cells. Between 5 and 24 weeks, rapid mitotic expansion of primordial oogonia occurs, followed by first meiotic division (8–36 weeks), and subsequently meiotic arrest as primordial follicles. The presence of ovaries is not required for regression of the Wolffian ducts, and it is the absence of local testosterone that causes their regression at 10 weeks. The paroophoron, epoophoron and Gartner's cysts are all that may remain of the Wolffian ducts in the female. The absence of circulating testosterone also leads to an absence of peripheral DHT and directs the genital tubercle, urogenital sinus, urogenital folds and labioscrotal swellings to develop into the clitoris, lower vagina, labia minora and labia majora, respectively.

As AMH is not produced by the fetal ovary, the Müllerian ducts continue to develop. These paired mesodermal ducts originate in week 5, lateral to the Wolffian ducts at the third to fifth thoracic segment. They are thought to be associated with the basement membrane of the Wolffian ducts and grow caudally guided by them. The cranial ends of the Müllerian ducts are independent of the Wolffian ducts and remain separate as the Fallopian tubes. At the pelvis, the Müllerian ducts cross the Wolffian ducts anteriorly to lie medially next to each other. At weeks 8–10, the pelvic Müllerian ducts have fused and subsequent breakdown of their medial walls leads to a single tube, which will become the upper vagina, cervix and the uterine epithelium and glands. Surrounding mesenchymal tissue will become the myometrium and stroma. At their caudal end, the fused Müllerian ducts form the Müllerian tubercle, which connects with a thickened area of the urogenital sinus that develops into the paired sinovaginal bulbs. This connection of the endodermal urogenital sinus and mesodermal Müllerian ducts forms the vaginal plate – a column of squamous tissue. It remains unknown how much of each tissue (and possibly some of the Wolffian duct) contributes to this developing vagina. In weeks 10–16, the vaginal plate enlarges and develops a cavity, which is separated from the urogenital sinus by an endodermal membrane.

Gradual change of the lower Müllerian duct epithelium from columnar to stratified squamous epithelium occurs, ending at the future external cervical os. By month 5, the urethra and vagina are separated by a septum, and the endodermal membrane between the vagina and urogenital sinus breaks down to form the hymen. The urogenital sinus forms the vaginal vestibule.

HUMAN SEX DEVELOPMENT

Human sex development can be divided into three main parts:

1 chromosomal sex (presence of X and/or Y chromosome);
2 gonadal sex (development of the gonad into either testis or ovary);
3 phenotypic or anatomic sex (appearance of the internal and external genitalia).

This differs from the concept of gender or 'brain sex', which encompasses gender identity (which is one's self-representation), gender role behaviour and sexual orientation. Occasionally, there is discordance between sex and gender, as well as the elements of gender. It is important to note that no single category dictates someone's sex, and it is important to consider all components of sex when managing the patient with DSD.

KEY POINTS

- The *SRY* gene directs the gonad to become a testis.
- The absence of the *SRY* gene in combination with 'anti-testis' genes differentiates the gonad to the ovary.
- The presence or absence of androgens acting via androgen receptors determines external genital development.
- The presence of gonadal testosterone production leads to Wolffian duct differentiation into vas deferens, epididymis and seminal vesicle.
- The presence of gonadal AMH production leads to Müllerian duct regression.
- The absence of gonadal AMH production allows Müllerian duct differentiation into the upper vagina, cervix, uterine glands and epithelium and Fallopian tubes.
- The absence of gonadal testosterone production allows Wolffian duct regression.
- The genital and urinary systems are closely associated and therefore abnormalities that occur in the Müllerian system commonly affect the renal system.
- Definition of sex encompasses chromosomal sex, gonadal sex, and phenotypic sex. Gender relates to psychosexual development.

ABNORMAL EMBRYOLOGICAL DEVELOPMENT: DISORDERS OF SEX DEVELOPMENT

Definition and classification

Over the last 20 years, there has been a significant increase in the understanding of the underlying aetiology of many forms of abnormal embryological development. Clinicians were becoming increasingly aware that traditional terms,

such as intersex, true hermaphroditism, female pseudohermaphroditism and male pseudohermaphroditism, were confusing, inaccurate and often considered negative by the patients involved. Therefore, a new consensus meeting was held in 2005, and one of the main elements to emerge was a new nomenclature system for this group of disorders, which is more generic, diagnostically accurate and less derogatory.[6–8]

The term 'disorders of sex development' or DSD was established to describe congenital conditions with atypical development of chromosomal, gonadal or anatomical sex. This encompasses a blend of the physically defining features associated with males or females, i.e. karyotype, gonadal structure, internal genitalia and external genitalia, and covers a diverse range of conditions including individuals with standard male or female genitalia who may have a variety of internal genital organs and karyotype, and also those with ambiguous external genitalia. In addition, an updated classification system was proposed (Table 68.1) which divides conditions into:

- sex chromosome DSD;
- 46XY DSD;
- 46XX DSD.

This new classification system also embodies a wider range of disorders, for instance sex chromosome DSD includes Turner's syndrome (45X) and Kleinfelter's syndrome (47XXY), which were not previously considered 'intersex' conditions. Similarly, female patients with congenital adrenal hyperplasia (CAH), who were traditionally considered to have an adrenal disease, are now included as 46XX DSD due to the surgical and reproductive consequences associated with this disorder. Although there are a large number of DSD conditions, only the more common conditions have been considered in this chapter (Table 68.2).

With new knowledge concerning fetal sexual differentiation and development, greater awareness and understanding

Table 68.1 Updated nomenclature for disorders of sex development: adapted from Ref. 6, with permission

Terminology used previously	Proposed new terminology
Intersex	Disorders of sex development (DSD)
Male pseudohermaphrodite	
Undervirilisation XY male	
Undermasculinisation XY male	46XY DSD
Female pseudohermaphrodite	
Overvirilisation of an XX female	
Virilisation of an XX female	46XX DSD
True hermaphrodite	Ovotesticular DSD
XX male or XX sex reversal	46XX testicular DSD
XY sex reversal	46XY complete gonadal dysgenesis

Table 68.2 Key features of DSD conditions

DSD condition	Karyotype	External genitalia	Internal genitalia	Special features
Congenital adrenal hyperplasia (CAH)	XX	Virilised/masculinised	Uterus and ovaries	Coexisting glucocorticoid (and sometimes also mineralocorticoid) deficiency requiring steroid replacement therapy
Complete androgen insensitivity syndrome (CAIS)	XY	Female	Testes	Absent pubic and axillary hair; at risk of osteoporosis; gonadal malignancy risk small until after 50 years of age
Swyer's syndrome	XY	Female	Streak gonads and uterus	High risk of gonadal malignancy; poor breast development; normal axillary and pubic hair
5α-reductase deficiency	XY	Female or ambiguous at birth, virilising/masculinising at puberty	Testes	In those with testes *in situ*, 60–80% undergo change of gender from female to male at some point from late childhood onwards
17β-hydroxysteroid dehydrogenase – type 3 deficiency	XY	Variable; often female or ambiguous at birth, virilising/masculinising at puberty	Testes	In those with testes *in situ*, 60–80% undergo change of gender from female to male at some point from late childhood onwards
46XX/XY ovotesticular DSD	71% XX 20% XX/XY 7% XY 2% other	Often ambiguous	Mix of ovary and/or testis and/or ovotestes; uterus or male ducts	Fertility described as both males fathering a child and females carrying a pregnancy

of female sexual function and a more patient-centred emphasis on condition management, it is hoped that patient care will be improved in this group of individuals. Although there are no RCTs or even adequate long-term data to inform the management of DSD, currently expert opinion and a few small cohort studies and retrospective, uncontrolled trials form the basis of management.[9] Disclosure of important aspects of the patient's condition (karyotype, gonadal status, fertility potential) is essential.[10]

Incidence

The incidence of DSD conditions in the UK is unknown. An estimate for the prevalence is one in 2000.[11] Conditions with autosomal recessive inheritance are more prevalent in communities in which consanguinity is common.

Aetiology

Most DSD conditions occur due to a genetic or environmental disruption to the pathway of fetal sexual development. This disruption can be of gonadal differentiation or development, sex steroid production, sex steroid conversion or tissue utilisation of sex steroids.

Presentation and investigation

Every DSD condition has a spectrum of severity and therefore may present in a variety of ways:

- ambiguous genitalia at birth;
- mismatch of fetal chromosomal results, such as amniocentesis or chorionic villus sample with phenotype at birth;

- salt-losing crisis in neonatal life (CAH);
- sibling history of intersex;
- ambiguity of the genitalia developing in childhood or puberty;
- inguinal hernia with unexpected gonad;
- pelvic mass with gonadal tumour;
- primary amenorrhoea or pubertal delay;
- infertility;
- sexual dysfunction;
- part of a syndrome with other anomalies (e.g. renal anomalies in Denys–Drash syndrome).

Initial investigation will depend on presentation, but should include karyotype, testosterone, LH, follicle-stimulating hormone (FSH), 17-hydroxyprogesterone and pelvic ultrasound scan. Further investigation will depend on initial findings, external genital appearance and clinical presentation, and may include androstenedione, DHT, oestradiol, 24-hour urinary collection for steroid metabolites, hCG stimulation test, synacthen test, renal ultrasound scan, MRI and DNA for genetic testing.

Management

The areas to consider in intersex management are:

- accurate diagnosis;
- need for hormone replacement therapy;
- screening for associated medical conditions;
- providing information on the condition;
- psychological treatments;
- disclosure of diagnosis;
- genetic counselling for other family members;
- sex assignment for children;
- gonadal malignancy risk;
- fertility options;
- genital surgery options for ambiguous genitalia;
- vaginal enlargement options;
- access to peer support.

Accurate diagnosis at presentation is essential, and referral to an appropriate paediatric or adult multidisciplinary DSD service (endocrinology, gynaecology, surgery and psychology expertise), where available, is ideal. Individuals with different DSD conditions may require specific medical and surgical treatments; however, all should have access to experienced clinical psychologists and peer support via the relevant national support organisations. Over the past decade, a major shift in management has been the recognition that all patients have a right to information concerning the details of their condition, and the provision of this information and the options available need sensitive communication in a supported environment. Ideally, this should be with the expertise of a trained clinical psychologist. It is no longer considered good practice to withhold condition details from the patient.[8,10] There is no evidence other than clinical experience and ethical evaluation on which to base this management, as

there have been no studies evaluating long-term psychological outcomes with concealed or revealed diagnosis information; however, it is considered that disclosure should be planned with the opportunity for ongoing dialogue,[12] and in general disclosure is associated with enhanced psychosocial adaptation.[10] Gonadal malignancy and fertility options vary with the different DSD conditions.[8]

Cases presenting at birth or in childhood may be seen by a paediatric gynaecologist as part of a DSD team, but more often will be under the care of a paediatric endocrinologist, paediatric surgeon or paediatric urologist. The majority of these cases will have presented due to ambiguous genitalia. After thorough evaluation and diagnosis, sex of rearing is assigned and cosmetic genital surgery is considered where relevant. Currently, many neonates with ambiguous genitalia are assigned as females. The rationale for early feminising genital surgery for the more severely virilised cases includes relative technical ease of surgery, negating the need to disclose the disorder to the patient, and an assumed 'one stage' procedure, with the theoretical aim of initially aiding parental acceptance of the child's assigned gender, and later improving the psychological outcomes for the child.[13,14] All of the indications for genital surgery are now being re-evaluated, and current management based upon clinical audits and vocal adult patient support groups has led to recommendations to delay unnecessary genital surgery till an age of informed consent, and to individualise care.

At present, it remains unknown whether infant genital surgery has an effect on parental acceptance of assigned gender or on later psychological outcomes for the child. Small cohort studies suggest that the majority of infants undergoing genital surgery will require repeat genital treatment (surgery or vaginal dilatation therapy) at or after puberty, mainly for vaginal introital stenosis but also for cosmesis. Sexual function in subjects with DSD has been noted to be impaired compared to population controls.[15,16] Sexual function following feminising genital surgery also contributes to loss of sensation and subsequent reduced sexual function.[19] Small observational studies of adults who had undergone clitoral reduction surgery in childhood have suggested that orgasm is reduced[14,20,21] and that genital surgery may contribute to adult sexual dysfunction.[22–24] Whether sexual impairment is due to genital surgery or simply the DSD condition is still debated.[16] Certainly the role of vaginoplasty in the child is less clear and therefore deferring this procedure until adolescence where informed consent may be ascertained is generally the recommendation.[16,17]

Gynaecologists are more often involved in the care of the older child developing ambiguous genitalia at puberty, or in follow-up of adults who underwent feminising genital surgery as children. In many subjects born with ambiguous genitalia, there will be vaginal hypoplasia or agenesis, and the gynaecologist will need to discuss the treatment options at the appropriate time. Where childhood surgery has been performed, there is a strong possibility that repeat surgery may be required for vaginal stenosis, hypoplasia or genital cosmesis. This treatment is indicated to improve psychological and sexual outcomes; however, there have been no studies to provide evidence that improvements in these outcomes are achieved.

Enlargement procedures for vaginal hypoplasia include self-dilatation therapy or surgical vaginoplasty. These interventions are offered to improve psychological and sexual outcomes. There is disagreement about both the optimal timing and the choice of intervention; however, it is recommended that these should be performed during or after adolescence.[25] There is a consensus now that vaginal dilatation therapy is the treatment of choice for vaginal hypoplasia due to the absence of surgical risk, including the later risk of malignancy in vaginal graft material. In a retrospective study, the success of dilators was as high as 86 per cent for achieving normal vaginal length, and 81 per cent of patients were able to have intercourse free of pain,[26] but success depends on the motivation of the patient, and the appropriate time to start treatment must be individualised. Concomitant psychological support may improve outcomes. The surgical vaginoplasty method depends on the genital configuration and surgeon's expertise. In some cases, the aim of vaginoplasty is to open up the lower vagina, with the upper vagina being normally developed. A pull-through vaginoplasty with complete separation of the vagina from the urethra may be required where the vagina does not reach the perineum but instead has joined the urethra near to the bladder, forming a single urogenital perineal opening (the high-confluence vagina). In conditions in which the entire vagina is hypoplastic or absent, there are many vaginoplasty techniques: laparoscopic tension via an external traction device, peritoneal grafting, amnion grafting, skin grafting, bowel grafting, muscle flaps, labial expansion flaps, etc. Each method has different risks and benefits. The surgical risks include malignancy (in graft material), contracture leading to introital stenosis or loss of vaginal length, vaginal prolapse, dry vagina or excessive vaginal discharge.

EBM: Genital surgery for ambiguous genitalia

- There is only minimal evidence to inform management.
- There have been few studies of psychological outcomes after childhood clitoral and genital surgery.
- Cohort studies include beneficial effects of surgery and minimising families' concerns and distress.[14,17]
- Cohort studies suggest the cosmetic and anatomical outcomes of vaginal and clitoral childhood surgery may be poor.[15]
- Control-matched cohort studies of adult female sexual function suggest that childhood cosmetic clitoral surgery impairs sexual function but does not prevent orgasm.[14,20,21]

EBM: Vaginal enlargement procedures for vaginal agenesis or hypoplasia

- The treatment of choice is dilator therapy and should be the first line in the absence of previous surgery.
- Vaginal dilator therapy should be reserved for adolescent and adult patients and avoided in children.
- Studies suggest that vaginal enlargement self-dilatation therapy is successful in up to 86 per cent of cases.[26,27]
- Studies show that childhood vaginal enlargement surgery may require revision in up to 90 per cent of cases.[17,18]
- There are no RCTs of the outcomes of different vaginoplasty techniques.
- Retrospective uncontrolled studies have not shown one method of vaginoplasty surgery to have superior results to another method.

46XX DSD – ABNORMAL EMBRYOLOGICAL DEVELOPMENT OF MÜLLERIAN DUCTS AND PERSISTENCE OF WOLFFIAN STRUCTURES

Abnormal development of the Müllerian ducts can lead to a wide range of conditions. Many are subtle variations of normal Müllerian anatomy, and often remain asymptomatic or require no treatment. Others are transverse or longitudinal structural abnormalities or agenesis of parts of the Müllerian ducts, and may present to the gynaecologist in a variety of ways. An understanding of the timing and sequence of embryological development of the entire urogenital system helps in understanding the range of conditions that occur. Occasionally, Müllerian anomalies may be associated with other conditions such as renal or spinal abnormalities or, more rarely, developmental defects of the cloaca such as bladder exstrophy, cloacal anomalies or anorectal anomalies. Ovarian development is independent of Müllerian duct development. Also considered in this section are lower transverse vaginal septae and the imperforate hymen (which derive from the urogenital sinus endoderm) and persistence of Wolffian duct remnants.

Müllerian anomalies

Definitions

There have been many attempts to classify Müllerian abnormalities, and the American Fertility Society classification is historically the most widely used (Fig. 68.1). Congenital Müllerian abnormalities generally fall into one of three groups: normally fused single Müllerian system with agenesis of one or more parts; unicornuate systems (unilateral hypoplasia or agenesis of one Müllerian duct); or lateral fusion failures (including didelphic and bicornuate anomalies).

I. Hypoplasia/ agenesis (a) vaginal (b) cervical (c) fundal (d) tubal (e) combined	II. Unicornuate (a) communicating (b) non- communicating (c) no cavity (d) no horn	III. Didelphus
		IV. Bicornuate (a) complete (b) partial
V. Septate (a) complete (b) partial	V. Arcuate	VII. DES drug related

Fig. 68.1 American Fertility Society classification of Müllerian anomalies. (From The American Fertility Society classifications of adnexal adhesions, distal tubal occlusion, tubal occlusion secondary to tubal ligation, tubal pregnancies, Müllerian anomalies and intrauterine adhesions: *Fertil Steril* 1988; 49: 944-55.) Reproduced with permission of the American Society for Reproductive Medicine: DES, diethylstilbestrol.

Rokitansky syndrome (agenesis of the uterus and vagina) is considered separately later in this section. More recently a new classification system has been developed by ESHRE/ESGE[28] which classifies abnormalities of uterus (U0–6), with two subclasses incorporated, the cervix (C0–4) and vagina (V0–4). This system is complex and as yet is not in widespread clinical use.

Incidence

The prevalence is thought to be 0.5 per cent in the female population.[29] The incidence in women with infertility is substantially higher. The most common are septate and bicornuate anomalies.

Aetiology

The cause of Müllerian anomalies is unknown; they may be due to genetic errors, teratogenic events or a combination of these. Only a minority of cases appear to have a family history. It is assumed that there has been failure of fusion of the two Müllerian ducts, failure of one or both ducts to develop, or failure of resorption of the areas of Müllerian duct fusion. The causes of transverse vaginal septae are unknown.

Presentation and investigation

The spectrum of anomalies is wide and around 75 per cent of these women will remain asymptomatic. The remaining 25 per cent will present in a variety of ways. Secondary sexual development is normal as ovarian development and function are independent of Müllerian duct and urogenital sinus growth.

Presentation of Müllerian anomalies

- primary amenorrhoea;
- cyclical abdominal pain (obstruction to menstruation);

- severe dysmenorrhoea (obstruction to menstrual drainage from one Müllerian duct, e.g. the non-communicating rudimentary horn associated with a unicornuate uterus);
- pelvic mass – haematocolpos (vagina distended with menstrual blood) or haematometra (uterus distended with menstrual blood);
- menorrhagia;
- dyspareunia (transverse or longitudinal vaginal septae);
- infertility and recurrent miscarriage;
- ectopic pregnancy;
- obstetric complications, e.g. preterm birth, abnormal lie and uterine rupture.

Investigation of Müllerian anomalies

This includes an assessment of the internal and external uterine contours. Ultrasound, MRI and a hysterosalpingogram are often used, sometimes in association with laparoscopy or hysteroscopy. Imaging of the renal tract is also indicated.

Management

Management of these anomalies depends on the type of anomaly and the presenting features. Symptomatic uterine and longitudinal vaginal septae can be resected hysteroscopically. The horns of a bicornuate uterus can be joined together into one cavity by an abdominal metroplasty. Any form of obstruction to menstrual flow requires surgery to relieve the obstruction and prevent pain and endometriosis. The didelphic uterus is often associated with vaginal septae that can lead to unilateral obstruction and requires careful vaginal surgery to remove the septum. Transverse vaginal septa can be of varying thicknesses, and complete removal is essential to try to prevent a stenotic ring at the site of surgery. For thick transverse vaginal septa, a combined abdomino-perineal procedure is often required.

The hymen usually opens after the fifth month of fetal life. An imperforate hymen presents either in neonatal life with a mucocolpos or at puberty with haematocolpos. A purple-blue bulge at the introitus associated with primary amenorrhoea is diagnostic. Surgery to create an adequate window for vaginal drainage cures the problem.

Rokitansky syndrome (also called Mayer–Rokitansky–Kuster–Hauser (MRKH) syndrome)

Definition and incidence

This condition is agenesis or hypoplasia of the vagina and uterus. The uterus is either absent or consists of a small central rudimentary uterine bud or bilateral uterine buds on the pelvic side walls. The incidence in the UK is estimated as between one in 4000 and one in 6000 females.

The aetiology remains unknown. The control mechanisms leading to Müllerian duct regression in males and Müllerian duct survival and growth in females are not well defined.

Presentation and management

The usual presentation is primary amenorrhoea with normal secondary sex characteristics. Occasionally, the condition is identified in childhood. Investigation is as standard for primary amenorrhoea, and should exclude intersex conditions and include renal tract imaging due to the 30–40 per cent incidence of associated renal anomalies.

Management needs to encompass both psychological interventions, to help with aspects such as accepting the diagnosis, living with the condition, forming relationships and improving sexual function and quality of life outcomes, and interventions that can be used to enlarge or create the vagina. The aim of vaginal enlargement techniques (both surgical vaginoplasty and self-applied vaginal dilatation therapy) is to improve sexual function; however, there have been no studies to assess the effectiveness of these interventions on this outcome. Vaginoplasty surgery and dilators should not be used in childhood. Uterine transplant is not an option for the foreseeable future, although tissue engineering techniques may eventually provide new treatment options. As ovarian function is normal, fertility is possible via surrogacy.

Incomplete regression of the Wolffian system

Parts of the Wolffian duct may fail to regress completely in females, presenting as cysts lateral to the Müllerian duct. Usually these are incidental findings and most are asymptomatic, although they can grow to be large. The epoophoron and paraoophoron can be found beside the ovary in the mesosalpinx. Gartner's duct (the lower part of the Wolffian duct) cysts can occur anywhere from the broad ligament down to the vagina, and may present as vulval or vaginal masses. Wolffian remnants are also seen in the cervix. Very rarely, the Wolffian system may persist as the primitive mesonephric system draining functioning glomeruli, and an extra ureter can be found emptying into the vagina.

KEY POINTS

- Abnormalities of the Müllerian system are asymptomatic in 75 per cent of women.
- Imaging of the renal tract should be performed whenever abnormalities of the Müllerian system are found.
- This condition should be considered high on the list of differential diagnosis in patients presenting with painless amenorrhoea, and normal secondary sexual development.

46XX DSD – Congenital adrenal hyperplasia

This condition occurs in an XX fetus due to an enzyme deficiency (usually 21-hydroxylase) in the adrenal gland. The XX fetus proceeds down the female development pathway, with ovarian formation and development of the Müllerian ducts into uterus, cervix and upper vagina. Owing to the adrenal enzyme deficiency, cortisone production is deficient, and so the adrenal gland undergoes hyperplasia to try to produce sufficient cortisol. A by-product of this survival mechanism is the production of large quantities of androgens. These high circulating androgen levels lead to masculinising effects at the external genitalia, and ambiguous genitalia or normal-looking male genitalia at birth.

This is one of the most common DSD conditions, with a UK population prevalence estimated at one in 10,000, of whom half are female. It is the only DSD condition that can be life threatening, as unrecognised cortisol deficiency can lead to a salt-wasting crisis in the neonate. Management aims to correct the cortisol deficiency and excess androgen production. Gender assignment at birth is usually female due to the presence of ovaries and uterus with fertility potential. Genital surgery to cosmetically feminise the appearance has been standard practice in the past, although there is now controversy concerning the benefits and risks of this procedure.[8] Adolescents and adults considering surgery to reduce the size of the clitoris, for cosmetic concerns or due to pain during sexual intercourse, are counselled that the actual risk of damage to clitoral orgasm is unknown, but is estimated at 20–25 per cent. At puberty, a review of the vagina is necessary to identify obstruction, stenosis or hypoplasia.

Other causes of XX fetal virilisation

In a manner similar to that of CAH, other exogenous causes of androgens (e.g. maternal androgen-secreting tumours or the use of virilising drugs such as danazol in pregnancy) may rarely lead to masculinising of the external genitalia in an XX fetus.

46XY DSD – Androgen receptor defects: CAIS

Androgen insensitivity syndrome occurs due to the complete inability of the body to respond to androgens. The cause is a disruption of the androgen receptor gene on the long arm of the X chromosome. Previously the condition was called testicular feminisation, due to the erroneous assumption that the testes must be producing a feminising factor. In this condition, an XY fetus proceeds initially down the pathway of male fetal sexual determination. The *SRY* gene leads to normal testicular development, and both AMH and testosterone are normally produced. The AMH ensures regression of the Müllerian duct; however, due to the lack of ability of all body cells to respond to androgen, female external genitalia develop and female CNS organisation occurs. The result is an XY female with absent Müllerian structures, normal female genitalia, variable vaginal hypoplasia, absent or sparse pubic and axillary hair, normal breast development, normal female behaviour and gender identity and intra-abdominal testes that produce high levels of circulating testosterone.

Androgen insensitivity syndrome can also occur as a partial form (partial androgen insensitivity syndrome, PAIS) in which some response to androgens occurs. The aetiology of this condition is less well understood, although some cases have a disruption in the androgen receptor gene allowing some function. Presentation is a spectrum from ambiguous genitalia to a normal male phenotype with infertility. For those cases identified in early infancy, assignment of sex of rearing is difficult, with no data concerning outcome. Future sexual function as male or female is unknown, with physical growth of the genitalia being unpredictable and a lack of scientific knowledge about how sexual orientation and gender identity develop. It is likely that both male- and female-type behaviours and gender identity are at least partly pre-programmed by the fetal sex steroid environment, and in PAIS the fetal sex steroid environment is unknown.

46XY DSD – Gonadal dysgenesis

In this condition (also known as Swyer's syndrome), disruption at the very start of the male sex determination pathway causes an XY fetus to divert to the female development pathway. In 15–30 per cent of cases, the fault lies with the *SRY* gene, and gonadal testicular differentiation does not occur. In the remaining cases, disruption of other testis-determining genes is assumed to be the cause. In the absence of SRY activation, ovarian determination probably occurs, but cannot be sustained due to the lack of a second X chromosome. The result is a dysgenetic (abnormally formed) streak gonad. As this gonad produces neither AMH nor testosterone, the external genital development is female and the Müllerian ducts develop into the vagina, uterus and cervix.

The streak gonad again fails to produce hormones at puberty, leading to the usual clinical presentation of primary amenorrhoea with poor breast development. In contrast to CAIS, these women have normal pubic and axillary hair and the presence of a normal uterus. Investigation will show raised gonadotrophins and low testosterone and oestradiol levels. Menstruation usually commences with hormone replacement therapy (oestrogen and progesterone are necessary), and pregnancy is possible with donor oocytes. Gonadectomy is recommended due to the high malignancy risk of dysgenetic gonads.

Other forms of XY gonadal dysgenesis that can lead to DSD conditions are less well understood. Partial gonadal dysgenesis with some testicular function, and mixed gonadal dysgenesis (a unilateral testis and a contralateral streak gonad) are conditions that usually present with variable degrees of genital masculinisation or ambiguity. Regression of each Müllerian duct depends on the local concentration of AMH produced by the fetal gonad on each side, and unilateral uterine development can occur if one gonad is more dysgenetic and hence produces less AMH than the contralateral gonad (see Chapter 69, Karyotypic abnormalities).

46XY DSD – Androgen biosynthetic defects (5-α-reductase type 2 deficiency and 17-β-hydroxysteroid dehydrogenase type 3 deficiency)

These conditions may present in a similar fashion with genital ambiguity at birth. In the past, most cases were assigned to a female sex of rearing; however, this management is currently under review and now each case is individually considered.[8] Both are autosomal recessive conditions in which an XY fetus initially starts down the male development pathway with normal testis development. However, there is a deficiency of enzymes involved in androgen synthesis, leading to mainly female external genital development. If left untreated in childhood, both conditions will result in increasing masculinisation at puberty, and possibly a change in gender identity from female to male for some individuals. 5-α-Reductase-type 2 is the enzyme responsible for the peripheral conversion of testosterone to the more potent androgen DHT required for fetal genital masculinisation. 17-β-Hydroxysteroid dehydrogenase type 3 is the gonadal enzyme needed for the final step in testosterone production in the fetal testis, i.e. conversion of androstenedione to testosterone. Each of these enzymes has more than one isoenzyme, and it is likely that activation of other isoenzymes is responsible for the virilisation seen at puberty.

Clinical presentation of both these conditions is usually mild ambiguity of the genitalia (clitoromegaly) at birth or in early childhood in an XY female. However, the presentation can be variable, and a number of these patients will present to a gynaecologist with virilisation at puberty. Müllerian structures are absent and Wolffian structures are present. The testes are intra-abdominal in childhood, and often descend to the inguinal canal or labioscrotal folds after puberty. Without childhood intervention, secondary sexual development is usually masculine, with poor breast development and normal pubic and axillary hair. The incidence of these conditions is unknown, but with the new scientific knowledge of these enzymes over the past decade, 17-β-hydroxysteroid dehydrogenase type 3 deficiency is now being diagnosed in some cases previously labelled as CAIS. In cases diagnosed in childhood, the management and assignment of gender are difficult. There have been insufficient cohorts raised as either males or females from childhood to evaluate the outcomes of adult gender identity, sexual function, psychological outcomes and quality of life. Fertility may be possible as a male, although infertility is common. Diagnosis is by DNA serum samples, and urinary steroid profile (either 24 hour or spot sample).

46XX/46XY DSD

This condition is defined by the presence of both ovarian tissue with Graafian follicles and testicular tissue containing distinct tubules in one person. It is said to be the rarest

DSD condition, but has a higher prevalence in some areas, such as Africa. The gonads can be any mix of ovary, testes and ovotestes. The aetiology is unknown.

Most cases present with ambiguous genitalia, although clinical presentation is very variable. The degree of genital masculinisation is thought to be a reflection of the amount of functional testicular tissue. The spectrum of internal genital development is influenced by the composition of the adjacent gonad, with up to 80 per cent having internal female organs and therefore being potentially fertile. The karyotype is 46XX in the majority, with a smaller proportion having a mosaic XX/XY karyotype, and only a minority having a 46XY karyotype. At present, there are insufficient data from cohort studies to advise on optimal management in terms of gender assignment in childhood.

Key References

1. Harley VR, Clarkson MJ, Argentaro A. The molecular action and regulation of the testis-determining factors, SRY (sex-determining region of the Y chromosome) and SOX9 (SRY-related high-mobility group HMG box 9). *Endocr Rev* 2003;24:466–87.

2. Warne GL, Zajac JD. Disorders of sexual differentiation. *Endocrinol Metab Clin North Am* 1998;27:945–67.

3. Nef S, Schaad O, Stallings NR *et al*. Gene expression during sex determination reveals a robust female genetic program at the onset of ovarian development. *Dev Biol* 2005;287:361–7.

4. Beverdam A, Koopman P. Expression profiling of purified mouse gonadal somatic cells during the critical time window of sex determination reveals novel candidate genes for human sexual dysgenesis syndromes. *Hum Mol Genet* 2006;15:417–31.

5. Parma P, Radi O, Vidal V *et al*. R-spondin1 is essential in sex determination, skin differentiation and malignancy. *Nat Genet* 2006;38:1304–9.

6. Hughes IA, Houk C, Ahmed SF, Lee PA. LWPES Consensus Group; ESPE Consensus Group. Consensus statement on management of intersex conditions. *Arch Dis Child* 2006;91:554–63.

7. Lee PA, Houk CP, Ahmed SF, Hughes IA. Writing Group for the International Intersex Consensus Conference. *Pediatrics* 2006;118:753–7.

8. Houk CP, Hughes IA, Ahmed SF, Lee PA. Summary of consensus statement on intersex disorders and their management. *Pediatrics* 2006;118:753–7.

9. Creighton S, Minto C. Managing intersex. *BMJ* 2001;323:1264–5.

10. Liao LM, Green H, Creighton SM, Conway GS. Patient experiences in obtaining and giving information about disorders of sex development. *Br J Obstet Gynaecol* 2010;117:193–9.

11. Blackless M, Charuvastra A, Derryck A *et al*. How sexually dimorphic are we? Review and synthesis. *Am J Hum Biol* 2000;12:151–66.

12. Carmichael P, Ransley P. Telling children about a physical intersex condition. *Dialogues Pediatr Urol* 2002;25:7–8.

13. Warne G, Grover S, Hutson J *et al*. A long-term outcome study of intersex conditions. *J Pediatr Endocrinol Metab* 2005;18:555–67.

14. Crouch NS, Minto CL, Liao LM *et al*. Sexual function and genital sensation after feminizing genitoplasty for congenital adrenal hyperplasia: a pilot study. *BJU Int* 2004;93:135–8.

15. Köhler B, Kleinemeier E, Lux A *et al*. Satisfaction with genital surgery and sexual life of adults with XY disorders of sex development: results from the German clinical evaluation study. *J Clin Endocrinol Metab* 2012;97:577–88.

16. Callens N, van der Zwan YG, Stenvert LS Drop *et al*. Do surgical interventions influence psychosexual and cosmetic outcomes in women with disorders of sex development? *J ISRN Endocrinology* 2012;276742.

17. Creighton SM, Minto CL, Steele SJ. Objective cosmetic and anatomical outcomes at adolescence of feminising surgery for ambiguous genitalia done in childhood. *Lancet* 2001;358:124–5.

18. Alizai NK, Thomas DFM, Lilford RJ *et al*. Feminizing genitoplasty for congenital adrenal hyperplasia: what happens at puberty? *J Urol* 1999;161:1588.

19. Gastraud F, Bouvattier C, Duranteau L *et al*. Impaired sexual and reproductive outcomes in women with classical forms of congenital adrenal hyperplasia. *J Clin End Metab* 2007;92:1391–6.

20. Randolph J, Hung W, Rathlev MC. Clitoroplasty for females born with ambiguous genitalia: a long-term study of 37 patients. *J Pediatr Surg* 1981;16:882–7.

21. Newman K, Randolph J, Parson S. Functional results in young women having clitoral reconstruction as infants. *J Pediatr Surg* 1992;27:180–3.

22. May B, Boyle M, Grant D. A comparative study of sexual experiences. *J Health Psychol* 1996;1:479–92.

23. Dittmann RW, Kappes ME, Kappes MH. Sexual behavior in adolescent and adult females with congenital adrenal hyperplasia. *Psychoneuroendocrinology* 1992;17:153–70.

24. Nordenskold A, Holmdahl G, Frisen L *et al*. Type of mutation and surgical procedure affect long term quality of life for women with congenital adrenal hyperplasia. *J Clin Endocrinol Metab* 2008;93:380–6.

25. Statement of the British Association of Paediatric Surgeons Working Party on the Surgical Management of Children Born with Ambiguous Genitalia, July 2001. Available at ‹http://www.baps.org.uk/›.

26. Ismail-Pratt IS, Bikoo M, Liao LM *et al*. Normalisation of the vagina by dilator treatment alone in complete

androgen insensitivity syndrome and Mayer-Rokitansky-Kuster-Hauser Syndrome. *Hum Reprod* 2007;22: 2020–4.

27. Robson S, Oliver GD. Management of vaginal agenesis: review of 10 years practice at a tertiary referral centre. *Aust NZ J Obstet Gynaecol* 2000;40:430–3.

28. Grimbizis GF, Gordts S, Di Spiezio Sardo A *et al.* The ESHRE/ESGE consensus on the classification of female genital tract congenital anomalies. *Gynecol Surg* 2013;10:199–212.

29. Nahum GG. Uterine anomalies. How common are they and what is their distribution among subtypes? *J Reprod Med* 1998;43:877–87.

Chapter 69 Karyotypic abnormalities

Diana Fothergill

INTRODUCTION

There are a number of karyotypic abnormalities that may present to the gynaecologist with an initial complaint of primary amenorrhoea. Others will have been diagnosed in childhood but are referred on for further management by paediatricians and endocrinologists. Some karyotypic abnormalities have little impact on gynaecological problems, but those affecting the sex chromosomes are covered briefly in this chapter. This is a rapidly changing field of medicine, and more sophisticated tests can lead to refinements in original diagnoses, so it may be appropriate to repeat genetic investigations or to test other cell lines.

TURNER'S SYNDROME (45X AND MOSAICS)

This is probably the commonest abnormality in females involving the sex chromosomes. Although 1 in 2500 live-born girls are affected, most pregnancies with this abnormality miscarry, probably secondary to major cardiac defects. It is estimated that 10 per cent of all miscarriages have a 45X karyotype.[1] The incidence does not rise with increasing maternal age, but screening early pregnancies for increased nuchal thickness has led to more cases being diagnosed antenatally, as cystic hygroma and non-immune hydrops are frequently features of Turner's syndrome. Over half of these girls will have some form of mosaicism. The rate of detection is partly dependent on how hard it is looked for, as the cell lines may vary in different tissues. If Turner's syndrome is clinically suspected but the blood karyotype is normal, it is advisable to check a second tissue such as a skin biopsy.[2]

Over two-thirds of Turner's syndrome cases result from loss of a paternal sex chromosome; in some there are fragments of a sex chromosome still present. If this is a Y chromosome, there is a 12 per cent risk of gonadoblastoma development, and gonadectomy is usually advised.[2]

Physical abnormalities associated with Turner's syndrome

- Growth failure: low birthweight and short stature;
- ovarian failure: no secondary sexual development in most cases, occasionally secondary amenorrhoea in mosaicism;
- inverted, widely spaced nipples, and shield chest;
- webbed neck;
- puffy hands and feet in babies due to lymphoedema;
- low hairline;
- cubitus valgus;
- short fourth metacarpal;
- high, arched palate, micrognathia and defective dental development;
- renal dysgenesis;
- left-sided cardiac malformations, coarctation of the aorta;
- distortion of the Eustachian tube leading to otitis media;
- nail dysplasia;
- eye deformities.

Intelligence is usually normal, but there is an increased risk of impairment of non-verbal skills, e.g. maths and visuospatial.[3] The phenotypic abnormalities result in most cases being diagnosed in infancy and childhood. The girls are then usually referred to a gynaecologist after optimal growth potential has been achieved using growth hormone, for advice about long-term hormone replacement therapy (HRT). However, spontaneous pubertal development can occur, particularly in girls with mosaicism. In most girls, ovarian failure will have occurred early in life; although they have a uterus and vagina, they will not develop any secondary sexual characteristics without hormonal supplements. A low dose of oestrogen is given initially to encourage steady growth of the breasts; this is usually started after the age of 12 years, as the administration of oestrogen promotes epiphyseal fusion, which stops further growth.[4] The dose of oestrogen is gradually increased over 2 years. The transdermal route is preferred as it has better effects on bone density; it can be started at 6.25 μg/24hrs, by cutting patches into quarters, increasing to 12.5 mcg after a year. If the girl presents initially at an older age, the starting dose can be 12.5 μg as these girls are usually very keen to commence their pubertal development and be like their peer group. The uterus will respond to oestrogen therapy, so after 2 years it is necessary to add progestogens cyclically to produce regular endometrial shedding, or in a continuous combined regime to suppress endometrial development. HRT should be continued until at least the age of 50 years. Cryopreservation of ovarian tissue may be an option for future fertility, particularly for girls with mosaicism.[5] Mothers have also preserved their oocytes for their daughters' future use.

There are a number of long-term health issues which affect women with Turner's syndrome:

- hypertension;
- coarctation of the aorta – 11%; bicuspid aortic valve – 16%; dissecting aortic aneurysm;
- diabetes – 25%;
- hypothyroidism – 25–30%;
- coeliac disease – 4–6%;
- sensorineural hearing loss – 50%;
- renal disease;
- eye problems – red–green colour blindness in 8%, and increased risk of amblyopia;
- osteoporosis.

Premature mortality in women with Turner's syndrome is three times higher than in the general population.[6] The gynaecologist may be the only point of regular medical contact and needs to be aware of these issues, particularly when pregnancy is desired. A full cardiological assessment is advisable before referral to an assisted conception unit for counselling about treatment with donor oocytes.[7] Clinical pregnancy rates are reported to be comparable to those of other women with primary ovarian failure but there is an increased risk of complications including diabetes and hypertension in the pregnancy, and delivery by caesarian section (CS) may be required because of the woman's short stature.[8]

Ideally women with Turner's syndrome should have annual checks of blood pressure, thyroid function and liver function tests, lipids and glucose. Every 3–5 years they should have an echocardiogram, bone densitometry and audiogram.[9]

EBM

- There is little published evidence on the effects of long-term HRT in women with Turner's syndrome and on the optimal preparation to be used.
- Oestrogen therapy has been shown to increase bone mineral density.

Patients with Noonan's syndrome have a similar phenotypic appearance to Turner's syndrome. Noonan's syndrome has an autosomal dominant trait with no abnormality of the sex chromosomes and there is no effect on ovarian function.[10]

47XXX

These girls are not often referred to gynaecologists, although 47XXX is the most common female chromosomal abnormality, occurring in about 1 in 1000 live-born females. They may have genitourinary abnormalities but are of normal or tall height, and sexual development occurs normally. Academic performance is usually below average; there may be motor and speech delay, and attention deficit. The ovaries often fail prematurely and women may present with secondary amenorrhoea and require HRT. Somewhat surprisingly, most women give birth to chromosomally normal children, but prenatal diagnosis should be considered.

48XXXX, 49XXXXX

These are very rare disorders. Almost all girls with these karyotypes have developmental delay and learning difficulties. Craniofacial anomalies such as hypertelorism, upslanting palpebral fissures and a flat nasal bridge are commonly found, as is ovarian dysfunction.

46XY

Characteristically, this diagnosis is made when a phenotypically normal girl presents with primary amenorrhoea or delayed puberty. There are a variety of conditions that are associated with this karyotype.

In androgen insensitivity syndrome, the problem lies with the end-organ response to testosterone. It is an X-linked recessive disease due to mutations in the *AR* gene. The testes are functional and Müllerian inhibition factor is produced, so the uterus and vagina do not develop. Dilator therapy is usually indicated to allow intercourse. Breast development usually takes place, as circulating testosterone is peripherally converted to oestrogen, but there is absent pubic hair due to the abnormal androgen receptors.[11]

In Swyer's syndrome, or pure gonadal dysgenesis, there is a lack of functional gonadal tissue and, as a consequence, Müllerian structures persist and a normal uterus and vagina are found. Breast development does not normally occur and typically girls present above average height with delayed puberty. Pubic and axillary hair may be present due to the effect of peripherally produced androgens. Treatment is similar to that for Turner's syndrome, with oestrogen to develop the breasts and the addition of progestogens to cause withdrawal bleeds. Donor egg and embryo pregnancies have been reported.[12]

Streak gonads may be present; as there is a 30 per cent risk of malignant change, gonadectomy is advised.[3]

STRUCTURAL ABNORMALITIES OF THE X CHROMOSOME

There are many abnormalities that can occur in the X chromosome. The commonest is an isochromosome for the long arm, most often found in mosaic form with 45X. Deletions of part of the long or short arm have variable effects depending on the level at which the deletion has occurred. If the short arm is missing, most girls will be of short stature; if the long arm is missing, there is usually gonadal dysgenesis. It is of interest to note that although one X chromosome is inactivated, it is necessary to have two normal X chromosomes to maintain fertility.

KEY POINTS

- Karyotypic abnormalities are a common cause of primary amenorrhoea.
- HRT is required in all patients with ovarian failure.
- Ovum donation may be an option for fertility.
- Turner's syndrome has long-term health implications.

Key References

1. Pinsker JE. Turner syndrome: updating the paradigm of clinical care. *J Clin Endocrinol Metab* 2012;97:E994–1003.
2. Bondy CA. Care of girls and women with Turner syndrome: a guideline of the Turner Syndrome Study Group. *J Clin Endocrinol Metab* 2007;92:10–25.
3. Cools M, Drop SL, Wolffenbuttel KP *et al.* Germ cell tumours in the intersex gonad: old paths, new directions, moving frontiers. *Endocr Rev* 2006;27:468–484.
4. RCOG. Scientific Impact paper no 40. *Sex steroid treatment for pubertal induction and replacement in the adolescent girl 2013.* http://www.rcog.org.uk/womens-health/clinical-guidance/sex-steroid-treatment-pubertal-induction-and-replacement-adolescent-.
5. Borgstrom B, Hreinsson J, Rasmussen C *et al.* Fertility preservation in girls with Turner syndrome: prognostic signs of the presence of ovarian follicles. *J Clin Endocrol Metab* 2009;94:74–80.
6. Schoemaker MJ, Swerdlow AJ, Higgins CD *et al.* Mortality in women with Turner syndrome in Great Britain: a national cohort study. *J Clin Endocrinol Metab* 2008;93:4735–42.
7. Practice Committee of the American Society for Reproductive Medicine. Increased maternal cardiovascular mortality associated with pregnancy in women with Turner syndrome. *Fertil Steri* 2012;97:282–4.
8. Alvaro Mercadal B, Imbert R, Demeestere *et al.* Pregnancy outcome after oocyte donation in patients with Turner's syndrome and partial X monosomy. *Hum Reprod* 2011;26:2061–8.
9. Conway GS, Band M, Doyle J, Davies MC. How do you monitor the patient with Turner's syndrome in adulthood? *Clin Endocrinol* 2010;**73**:696–9.
10. Chacko E, Graber E, Regelmann MO *et al.* Update on Turner and Noonan syndromes. *Endocrinol Metab Clin N Am* 2012;41:713–34.
11. Mendoza N, Motos MA. Androgen insensitivity syndrome. *Gynecol Endocrinol* 2013;29:1–5.
12. Sauer MV, Lobo RA, Paulson RJ. Successful twin pregnancy after embryo donation to a patient with XY gonadal dysgenesis. *Am J Obstet Gynecol* 1989;161:380–1.

Chapter 70 Menarche and adolescent gynaecology

Diana Fothergill

INTRODUCTION

Puberty marks the change from childhood to adolescence, with the development of breasts and secondary sexual hair and the onset of menstruation. At the same time there is a period of accelerated growth. The age at which the changes take place is variable, but it is abnormal for there to be no sign of secondary sexual development at the age of 13 years.

The trigger for the changes to start is an increasing frequency and amplitude of pulses of gonadotrophin release. The ovaries are then stimulated to begin to produce oestrogen, which acts on the breast tissue to promote growth. This usually begins at around the age of 9 and takes about 5 years to be completed. There is evidence to suggest that this is occurring at a younger age, particularly in African-American girls, prompting a reassessment of the age at which precocious puberty should be investigated.[1]

Causes of precocious puberty

- Idiopathic;
- McCune–Albright syndrome (a genetic disorder of the bone with *café au lait* spots, polyostotic fibrous dysplasia and hormone excess);
- tumours of the adrenal or ovary-producing steroids;
- cerebral tumours;
- ingestion of exogenous oestrogens.

Pubic hair growth is stimulated by androgens released by the ovary and the adrenal gland. Breast and pubic hair development is described in five stages following the classification by Marshall and Tanner (Table 70.1).[2] Growth charts indicate the range of normal ages at which these stages are attained.

Table 70.1 Marshall and Tanner staging

Stage	Breast	Pubic hair
I	Pre-adolescent, elevation of papilla only	No pubic hair
II	Breast bud – elevation of breast and papilla as small mound; enlargement of areolar diameter	Sparse growth of long downy hair along the labia
III	Further enlargement but no separation of the contours	Hair coarser, darker and more curled; over mons
IV	Projection of the areola and papilla to form a secondary mound above the level of the breast	Adult-type hair but no spread to thighs
V	Mature; areola recessed to general contour of breast	Adult, with horizontal upper border and spread to thighs

In most girls, breast development starts before the growth of pubic hair.

Even before these changes are obvious, there is acceleration of growth, which is frequently accompanied by a rapid increase in shoe size. The peak height velocity, of approximately 8 cm/year, occurs just before the onset of menses – on average around the age of 12 years. Oestrogen promotes closure of the epiphyses, so final height is usually attained about 2 years after menarche.

Menarche occurs 2.3 ± 1 years after the onset of breast development. The average age of menarche has declined and is now 12.52 years in white girls and 12.06 years in African-Americans.[3] The factors involved include improved nutrition and genetic influences: daughters often undergo menarche at a similar age to their mothers. Initial menstrual cycles are usually anovulatory and often irregular for several years.

DELAYED PUBERTY

Most referrals to gynaecologists are because of concern about delay in the onset of menstruation. In order to determine the likely cause for this it is first important to establish whether puberty itself is delayed. A detailed history should be taken, asking about general health, the age at which breast and pubic hair development started, and if the girl has had a growth spurt or still appears to be growing. Any chronic illness may lead to constitutional delay in puberty. The family history should include the age when mother and siblings went through puberty.[4] Teenage girls may be reluctant to answer questions and the mother frequently gives much of the history, but it is important to address the girl rather than talking directly to the mother. Examination should include accurate measurement of height, together with assessment of the stage of breast and pubic hair development, and these should be plotted on growth charts. The examination should be sensitively performed – ask the girl if she wishes her mother to be present, as some feel more embarrassed with the mother there – and only expose one part of the body at a time. An internal examination should not be performed; inspection of the external genitalia is all that is necessary, as further assessment of the internal organs will be achieved by ultrasound scanning of the pelvis.

Investigations usually include:

- measurement of gonadotrophins – follicle stimulating hormone (FSH) and luteinising hormone (LH) – and oestrogen;
- karyotyping;
- ultrasound scan of the pelvis to confirm the presence of the uterus and ovaries;
- possibly X-ray to determine bone age.

Additional biochemical tests to assess thyroid function, prolactin and 17-α-hydroxyprogesterone may be appropriate.

ABSENT BREAST AND PUBIC HAIR DEVELOPMENT

Hypogonadotrophic hypogonadism

The majority of girls with low gonadotrophins have constitutional delay in puberty; there will often be a family history of delayed puberty. Another possibility is that it may be secondary to chronic illness, for example cystic fibrosis.

Girls with anorexia nervosa have low levels of gonadotrophins and, if the problem starts at a young age, will have absent or poorly developed secondary sexual characteristics. A similar situation is found in many athletic girls, the classic example being gymnasts, who have a low bodyweight and very low body fat. This can lead to the 'female athletic triad', with disordered eating, amenorrhoea and osteopenia, and an increased risk of stress fractures.[5]

Congenital deficiency of gonadotrophins is more rarely encountered; it may be associated with anosmia due to hypoplasia of the olfactory lobes, when it is known as Kallman's syndrome. Brain imaging will be necessary to establish this diagnosis.

Acquired deficiency may follow damage to the hypothalamus or pituitary as a result of trauma, tumour such as a craniopharyngioma, irradiation or infection – frequently secondary to hydrocephalus. Infiltration of these organs can also occur in haemochromatosis, which may be secondary to transfusions for sickle cell disease or thalassaemia and to Wilson's disease.

In all these conditions, ultrasound will confirm the presence of an immature uterus and small, inactive ovaries. The bone age will help to differentiate cases of constitutional delay, as it will be behind chronological and height age.

Treatment may be required if there are no signs of spontaneous onset of puberty, although most girls with constitutional delay will proceed to normal development if left untreated. A study conducted on untreated girls indicated that they experienced considerable distress, which affected their success at school, work or socially; 50 per cent would have preferred to receive treatment.[6] Pulsatile gonadotrophins have been used but are very difficult to sustain, as they require a subcutaneous injection attached to a portable pump for several months. The more widely used approach is to give low doses of ethinyl oestradiol 1–2 mg/day for 3–6 months, or a 25 μg transdermal patch cut into eighths or quarters. Frequently, spontaneous sexual maturation then occurs, but if not, the dose is gradually increased over several years.

Hypergonadotrophic hypogonadism

This occurs when there is failure of gonadal development. The normal release of gonadotrophins occurs, but as there is no response from the gonad, there is no negative feedback to control gonadotrophin levels. The commonest cause is Turner's syndrome (45X), or other genetic problems (see Chapter 69). Other causes include damage to the ovaries by irradiation, surgery, chemotherapy or infection. Galactosaemia is also associated with ovarian failure and its management presents a challenge, as oral preparations of oestrogen and progesterone contain lactose. Autoimmune ovarian failure may be associated with other autoimmune disorders such as Addison's disease, vitiligo and hypothyroidism.

One of the less common causes of congenital adrenal hyperplasia is the deficiency of 17-α-hydroxylase. This enzyme is required to produce both oestrogen and testosterone, so virilisation does not occur at birth, but there is also a failure of development of secondary sexual characteristics.

The treatment consists of gradually increasing levels of oestrogen replacement, combined with progesterone to induce withdrawal bleed once endometrial development has been stimulated.

NORMAL BREAST AND PUBIC HAIR DEVELOPMENT

Anatomical causes

If puberty has progressed normally but the girl has failed to menstruate, the commonest cause is an anatomical abnormality, such as Müllerian agenesis, which is described in detail in Chapter 69. Girls with an imperforate hymen or transverse vaginal septum usually present as an emergency with cyclical abdominal pain, possibly with a palpable abdominal mass. The blockage prevents the flow of menstrual blood and there is usually a tense blue bulge seen at the introitus. Ultrasound scanning may show a distended vagina containing blood, and normal ovaries. Where there is a thin imperforate hymen, treatment is straightforward, as incision will allow the blood to drain and the mass will resolve. Treatment of a thicker and possibly higher septum is more complex and is best dealt with in a tertiary referral centre, as injudicious excision can result in stricture formation which is difficult to treat and will lead to considerable problems with intercourse.

Hyperprolactinaemia

This is more often a cause of secondary amenorrhoea, but can present as primary amenorrhoea and there may not be any galactorrhoea. A high prolactin level should prompt investigation for a pituitary adenoma. Treatment is the same as in the older female, with dopamine agonists such as cabergoline, which will result in the onset of menstruation.

Congenital adrenal hyperplasia

Menarche is often delayed in this condition, and when menstruation starts it may be erratic. Poor control of the condition, often due to poor compliance with treatment, may be the cause. The ovaries also often have a polycystic appearance on scan. Fertility rates in these women are poor for a number of reasons: infrequent ovulation, difficulties in achieving penetrative sex, and failure to form relationships.[7]

NORMAL BREAST BUT SCANTY OR ABSENT PUBIC HAIR DEVELOPMENT

This is the classical presentation of androgen insensitivity syndrome. The karyotype will be XY. Pubic hair fails to grow because of end-organ insensitivity to androgens, but breast development occurs due to peripheral conversion of androgens to oestrogen. No hormonal treatment is required.

MENORRHAGIA AND DYSMENORRHOEA

As initial menstrual cycles are usually anovular, they are normally painless, but bleeding may be prolonged.

Girls are often referred to gynaecologists because of concern about missing school, particularly when studying for state examinations, due to heavy and painful periods. Almost invariably they are accompanied by a mother who will tell you about the problems she had with her periods. It is very important to speak to the girl herself to try to establish if there is a genuine problem, and to make some effort to quantify the loss by the degree of soakage of the pads used. The number of pads used per day may be quite misleading, and as most women do not know what amount of loss is normal, it can be very difficult for a girl to know whether she is actually experiencing an abnormal amount of bleeding.

Excessive menstrual loss will usually result in a fall in the haemoglobin level, and occasionally the loss can be so great that emergency admission and transfusion are required. Many of these girls will have an underlying medical disorder. It is most important to exclude a coagulation disorder, such as von Willebrand's disease, or a platelet dysfunction, which may be present in a third of these cases.[8,9] There may be no previous personal or family history of bleeding symptoms. If such a disorder is found, it may be possible to treat the girl with desmopressin on a cyclical basis.[10]

The oral contraceptive pill is usually prescribed and, where blood loss is recurrently excessive, it can be helpful to prescribe this continuously for three or more cycles to reduce the frequency of withdrawal bleeds. However several studies have reported that the number of days of bleeding is not statistically different from conventional cyclic dosing.[11] The levonorgestrol intrauterine system (Mirena) has also been used successfully. The uterine cavity has to be at least 5–6 cm to enable insertion, and a general anaesthetic is likely to be required.[12]

Occasionally girls present with life-threatening haemorrhage. The options for treatment include medroxyprogesterone acetate 5 mg orally every 1–2 hours for 24 hours and then 20 mg daily for 10 days, or a 50 µg oral contraceptive pill taken 6-hourly for 48 hours, then reduced to once daily over the next 3 days.[13] Intravenous oestrogen has also been used (40 mg 4-hourly for 24 hours) combined with a highly progestational oral contraceptive pill, but is not readily available in many pharmacies. It is rarely necessary to perform a diagnostic curettage.

Dysmenorrhoea usually responds to simple analgesia or oral contraceptives. However, where these measures fail, it is important to bear in mind the possibility of partial obstruction of menstrual flow. There are a number of reported cases of obstructed hemivagina and uterine horn associated with ipsilateral renal agenesis.[14] The usual presentation is severe cyclical pain with an abdominal mass due to a hemihaematometra and haematocolpos. Removal of the occluded vaginal septum allows drainage and relief of symptoms. Endometriosis occurs in many of these patients, presumably secondary to the enforced retrograde menstrual flow.

There are many causes of chronic pelvic pain in young women, including psychosomatic factors. It is important to realise that endometriosis should be excluded in chronic pelvic pain that has not responded to simple measures. Laparoscopy may be indicated. The symptoms are often not those typically encountered in older women.[15]

EBM

All girls with menorrhagia who are found to be anaemic should be investigated for a bleeding disorder, including testing for von Willebrand's disease and platelet function defects.

KEY POINTS

- Secondary sexual characteristics start to develop in most girls by the age of 14 years.
- Menarche normally occurs 2 years after breast development has commenced.
- Ovarian failure is the commonest cause of delayed puberty – karyotyping and gonadotrophins are essential investigations.
- Tests for bleeding disorders should be performed for any girl with moderate to severe menorrhagia.
- Endometriosis can occur in teenagers.

Key References

1. Kaplowitz PB, Oberfield SE. Re-examination of the age limit for defining when puberty is precocious in girls in the United States: implications for evaluation and treatment. The Drug and Therapeutics and Executive Committees of the Lawson Wilkins Pediatric Endocrine Society. *Pediatrics* 1999;104:936–41.

2. Marshall WA, Tanner JM. Variations in pattern of pubertal changes in girls. *Arch Dis Child* 1969;44:291.

3. Anderson SE, Must A. Interpreting the continued decline in the average age at menarche: results from two nationally representative surveys of U.S. girls studied 10 years apart. *J Pediatr* 2005;147:753–60.

4. Palmert MR, Dunkel L. Delayed puberty. *N Engl J Med* 2012;366:443–52.

5. Gordon CM, Nelson LM. Amenorrhoea and bone health in adolescents and young women. *Curr Opin Obstet Gynecol* 2003;15:377–84.

6. Crowne FC, Shalet SM, Wallace WH *et al*. Final height in girls with untreated constitutional delay in growth and puberty. *Eur J Pediatr* 1991;150:708–12.

7. Mulaikal RM, Migeon CJ, Rock JA. Fertility rates in female patients with congenital adrenal hyperplasia due to 21-hydroxylase deficiency. *N Engl J Med* 1987;316:178–82.

8. Smith YR, Quint EH, Hertzberg RB. Menorrhagia in adolescents requiring hospitalization. *J Pediatr Adolesc Gynecol* 1998;11:13–15.

9. Chi CC, Pollard D, Tuddenham EGD, Kadir RA. Menorrhagia in adolescents with inherited bleeding disorders. *J Pediatr Adolesc Gynecol* 2010;23:215–22.

10. Lee CA, Chi C, Pavord SR *et al*. The obstetric and gynaecological management of women with inherited bleeding disorders: review with guidelines produced by a taskforce of UK Haemophilia Centre Doctors' Organisation. *Haemophilia* 2006;12:301–36.

11. Edelmann A, Gallo MF, Nichols MD *et al*. Continuous versus cyclic use of combined oral contraceptives for contraception: systematic Cochrane review of randomized controlled trials. *Hum Reprod* 2006; 21:573–8.

12. Pillai M, O'Brien K, Hill E. The levonorgestrel intrauterine system (Mirena) for the treatment of menstrual problems in adolescents with medical disorders, or physical or learning disabilities. *BJOG* 2010;117: 216–21.

13. Slap GB. Menstrual disorders in adolescence. *Best Pract Res Clin Obstet Gynaecol* 2003;17:75–92.

14. Stassart JP, Nagel TC, Prem KA *et al*. Uterus didelphys, obstructed hemivagina, and ipsilateral renal agenesis: the University of Minnesota experience. *Fertil Steril* 1992;57:756–61.

15. Propst AM, Laufer MR. Endometriosis in adolescents. Incidence, diagnosis and treatment. *J Reprod Med* 1999;44:751–8.

Chapter 71 Ovarian and menstrual cycles

Mohammed Khairy and Rima Dhillon

MRCOG standards

Theoretical skills

- Have a thorough understanding of the physiology of the menstrual cycle.
- Be able to explain dysfunction in the cycle (e.g. anovulation) with reference to ovarian and uterine physiology.
- Understand the mechanism of action of drugs that affect the cycle.

Practical skills

- Be able to interpret the menstrual and gynaecological history.
- Be able to initiate appropriate investigations to enable a diagnosis.

INTRODUCTION

Successful human reproduction depends on optimal spermatogenesis and ejaculatory function in males, and an exquisitely regulated hypothalamic–pituitary–ovarian (HPO) axis and endometrial preparation in females. The HPO axis orchestrates steroidogenesis and folliculogenesis (oogenesis) in the ovary, culminating in monthly ovulation. This is mirrored in cyclic endometrial preparation in the uterus for implantation of a pregnancy or cyclic menstruation in the absence of implantation.

Understanding the regulation of ovarian and menstrual function is therefore crucial to the rational management of many gynaecological disorders. These include delayed puberty, amenorrhoea, anovulatory infertility, abnormal uterine bleeding and also ovarian stimulation in assisted reproduction treatment.

In this chapter we will address the basic facts about the different compartments of the HPO axis controlling the ovarian and menstrual cycles.

THE HPO AXIS

The hypothalamus

The hypothalamus contains neurons secreting gonadotrophin-releasing hormones (GnRH) in the ventro-medial nucleus. These neurones would have migrated in fetal life from the olfactory placode. Failure of migration of these neurons results in congenital absence of GnRH or hypogonadotrophic hypogonadism, usually associated with anosmia (Kallmann's syndrome). The hypothalamic GnRH centre receives afferent neurons from the limbic system, olfactory centre, occipital cortex and other nuclei in the hypothalamus controlling energy metabolism and the stress response.[1]

During intrauterine life and shortly after birth these neurons secrete GnRH in a pulsatile manner into the hypothalamic hypophyseal portal circulation. Here the neurons stimulate the GnRH receptor-bearing gonadotrophs in the anterior pituitary resulting in the synthesis and pulsatile secretion of gonadotrophins (FSH and LH).[2]

The amount of GnRH reaching the systemic circulation is very low and its half-life is very short (2 minutes); therefore GnRH pulses cannot be easily measured. Instead the LH pulses (half-life of 20 minutes) can be measured in the circulation and so are used as indirect measure of GnRH pulses. The pulsatile secretion of GnRH is essential for maintaining gonadotrophin secretion and ovarian activity. Sustained exposure to GnRH (as seen in the use of GnRH analogues) leads to an initial increase of gonadotrophins (flare response) which is followed after 10–14 days by down-regulation and desensitisation of GnRH receptors with subsequent very low levels of gonadotrophins and ovarian steroid hormones.[2]

Shortly after birth the GnRH pulse generator becomes completely suppressed and remains so till puberty. It is believed that attainment of a critical level of fat content leads to leptin hormone signalling from adipose tissue that releases the GnRH pulse generator from the prepubertal inhibition, with initiation of puberty.

During the reproductive years the hypothalamic GnRH pulse centre is under the influence of various endocrine and paracrine regulators. Some of these exert a stimulatory effect, for example leptin, insulin, activin and high levels of oestrogens at ovulation. Others exert an inhibitory effect, for example ghrelin, inhibin, corticotrophin-releasing hormone (CRH), thyrotrophin-releasing hormone (TRH), prolactin, oestrogens, progestins, androgens, opioids and melatonin.

These regulators mediate their actions primarily by neuropeptide and amine transmitters namely kisspeptin (stimulatory), pro-opiomelanocortin (stimulatory), neuropeptide Y (inhibitory), dopamine (inhibitory), GABA, serotonin and norepinephrine.

It follows that reproductive function (as initiated by GnRH pulses) is under the influence of energy levels (leptin, insulin, ghrelin), stress (CRH, TRH, opioids), gonadal signals (oestrogens, progestins, androgens, inhibins, activin) and light/dark signals (melatonin). Various pharmacological agents which affect the neurotransmitters' levels can also affect reproductive function.[2] The GnRH pulse frequency and amplitude is dependent on the balance of these signals as well as on the timing, duration and amplitude. For example, the rapid rise of oestrogens at the time of ovulation triggers the LH surge, and the sustained level of GnRH inhibits gonadotrophins. Other pituitary hormones also have an inhibitory effect on GnRH and gonadotrophin secretions as in hyperprolactinaemia. Pathological lesions disconnecting or damaging the hypothalamic hypophyseal portal circulation lead to disruptions of the GnRH pulses and a state of hypogonadotrophic hypogonadism (as part of hypopituitarism).[1,2]

The pituitary gland

The pituitary gonadotrophins FSH and LH are both glycoprotein hormones. These hormones share a common alpha unit with other glycoprotein hormones, such as thyroid stimulating hormone (TSH) and human chorionic gonadotrophin (hCG), but each has a unique beta subunit. All these hormones act on transmembrane G-protein receptors that cause an increase in cyclic adenosine monophosphate (cAMP). There is cross-responsiveness of these receptors to the various glycoprotein hormones.[3]

The gonadotrophins are secreted from the pituitary gland mainly in response to GnRH pulses from puberty onwards. The GnRH receptors are membrane receptors which are down-regulated by sustained exposure of gonadotrophs to GnRH.[3]

The FSH hormone has a half-life of 4 hours and is under the influence of both GnRH and gonadal hormones; therefore its pulses are not accurately reflective of GnRH pulses. LH pulses, with a short half-life, are a more accurate reflection of GnRH pulses. These LH pulses are of higher frequency (every 60–90 minutes) and lower amplitude in the follicular phase of ovarian cycles, compared with the lower frequency (120–160 min) and higher amplitude signals in the luteal phase.[3]

CLINICAL POINTS

- The down-regulated GnRH receptors, following prolonged administration of a GnRH analogue, are responsible for the pituitary suppression and prevention of natural ovulation in cycles of in-vitro fertilisation (IVF). A similar effect has been achieved, although for a shorter period, using GnRH antagonists, which act by competitive blockade of GnRH receptors rather than down-regulating the GnRH receptors. In GnRH antagonist cycles, the GnRH agonist can be used to initiate a surge of LH, similar to natural cycles, with less risk of inducing ovarian hyperstimulation syndrome.
- An exaggerated positive feedback of leptin in obese women and patients with polycystic ovarian syndrome leads to an increase in GnRH/LH pulse frequency, with an increase in ovarian androgen production leading to chronic anovulation. On the other hand, there is a subset of morbidly obese women in whom there is a congenital leptin deficiency with increased caloric intake and low FSH/LH levels.
- Stress- and/or weight-related amenorrhoea are due to combined inhibitory signals by the neuropeptide Y and stress hormones, leading to suppressed GnRH secretion and functional hypothalamic amenorrhoea.

CLINICAL POINTS

- The similar structural activity of hCG and TSH explains the transient hyperthyroidism seen in states of increased hCG, such as molar pregnancies and hyperemesis gravidarum.
- Spontaneous activating mutations of G-protein linked to receptors of glycoprotein pituitary hormones lead to a condition of precocious puberty called McCune–Albright syndrome (MAS). The classic triad of features in MAS (polyostotic fibrous dysplasia, autonomous endocrine hyperfunction and *café au lait* skin pigmentation) can be explained by activation of the G-protein's alpha subunit and increased intracellular cAMP levels.

The ovary

Embryologically ovarian tissue is formed from three main types of cells:

1   Primordial germ cells derived from endodermal cells of the yolk sac which migrate at 6 weeks of intrauterine life

to the genital ridge. During the 6th to 8th week of development, the primordial germ cells grow and begin to differentiate into oogonia.

2   Coelomic (sex cord) cells which develop into granulosa cells that surround the oogonia to form the primordial follicles.

3   Mesenchymal (sex stromal) cells which later form the theca cells and other ovarian stromal cells.

Until 10 weeks of gestation the germ cells and surrounding sex cord and sex stromal cells are not differentiated, and the gonadal ridges are bi-potential gonads. These gonads develop into ovaries by lack of paracrine factors transcripted by the genes in the sex determining region on the Y chromosome (*SRY*).[3,4]

THE OVARIAN CYCLE

Gonadotrophin-independent phase

By 12 weeks of gestation some germ cells (oogonia) start to enter into meiosis and become primary oocytes surrounded by flattened granulosa cells to form primordial follicles. The primary oocytes are arrested in the prophase stage of the first meiotic division (diploid cell). The remaining oogonia have ongoing cycles of mitosis and reach a peak number of 5–6 million at 20 weeks' gestation.

The few primary oocytes that survive are those that are surrounded by flat, spindle-shaped follicular or pregranulosa cells. This oocyte–pregranulosa cell complex is enclosed by a basement lamina. At this stage of development, the primary oocyte with its surrounding single layer of pregranulosa cells is called a primordial follicle. Primordial follicles are 30–60 μm in diameter. The first primordial follicle usually appears around 6 weeks into intrauterine life, and the generation of primordial follicles is complete by about 6 months after birth.[3,4]

The first step in follicular growth is that a primordial follicle becomes a primary follicle. The primary follicle forms as the spindle cells of the primordial follicle become cuboidal cells. In addition, the oocyte enlarges. Thus, the primary follicle contains a larger primary oocyte that is surrounded by a single layer of cuboidal granulosa cells.

The secondary follicle contains a primary oocyte surrounded by several layers of cuboidal granulosa cells. The granulosa cells of a primary follicle proliferate and give rise to several layers of cells. In addition, stromal cells differentiate, surround the follicle and become the theca cells. These theca cells are on the outside of the follicle's basement membrane. The oocyte increases in size to a diameter of about 120 μm. As the developing follicle increases in size, the number of granulosa cells increases to about 600, and the theca cells show increasing differentiation. The progression to secondary follicles also entails the formation of capillaries and an increase in the vascular supply to developing follicular units.

The increasingly abundant granulosa cells secrete fluid into the centre of the follicle creating a fluid-filled space called the antrum. At this stage, the follicle is now called a tertiary follicle. In tertiary follicles, gap junctions are formed between theca and granulosa cells. In addition, tight junctions and desmosomes exist between adjacent cells. Gap junctions may also exist between the oocyte and the granulosa cells closest to the oocyte and may function as channels to transport nutrients and paracrine signals from the granulosa cells to the oocyte and vice versa. The granulosa cells closest to the oocyte also secrete a layer of mucopolysaccharides (the zona pellucida).

These stages occur independent of gonadotrophin stimulation and under the effect of local autocrine and paracrine factors such as growth differentiation factor (GDF) and anti-Müllerian hormone (AMH). The latter is produced from the granulosa cells and reaches the systemic circulation in levels proportional to the secondary follicle pool. In the absence of further gonadotrophin stimulation the secondary follicles undergo apoptosis and atresia.

This process of gonadotrophin-independent recruitment to secondary follicles and apoptosis in absence of gonadotrophins is continuous during intrauterine, pre-pubertal and reproductive life till depletion of the follicular pool at the age of menopause. Unlike spermatogenesis, the atretic follicles cannot be replenished; therefore the ovarian reserve of follicles is a finite pool. On average the number of primordial follicles is about 1–2 million at birth and decreases to about 400,000 at initiation of puberty and is less than 1000 by the age of menopause, with only about 500 oocytes destined to ovulate during a woman's reproductive lifespan. The rate of loss of the primordial follicle pool is variable among individual females, with variable age of loss of fertility and menopause (40–55 years). It is believed that natural fertility is lost around 10 years earlier than the age of menopause (fixed-interval hypothesis). The duration of the gonadotrophin-independent phase is around 74–80 days.[3,4]

Gonadotrophin-dependent phase

In the absence of pituitary gonadotrophins, the growing follicles in the ovary will be destined to atresia (apoptosis). The rise of pituitary gonadotrophins during the reproductive years, as a result of release of hypothalamic GnRH pulse centre from pre-pubertal inhibitory signals, leads to rescue of the preantral/antral follicles.

The number of rescued and recruited follicles depends on the pool of secondary follicles available at the time of the rise of FSH, which is indirectly related to the total pool of primordial follicles in the ovary (ovarian reserve). It also depends on the level of FSH and duration of rise (**selection window**).

A critical step of this rescue process is the induction of aromatase enzyme activity in the granulosa cells which converts the androgens synthesised in the theca cells into oestrogen under the effect of LH.

Therefore the two gonadotrophins, FSH and LH, act preferentially on the two main steroid-producing cells (granulosa and theca cells) in the ovary. The main effect of FSH is the rescue of granulosa cells (and oocytes) from atresia and induction of aromatase activity. The main role of LH is the stimulation of steroidogenesis by acting on theca cells to synthesise androgenic substrates that are converted into oestrogens in the granulosa cells. This is called **the two cell, two gonadotrophins theory**. The effect of this synchronised action of FSH and LH is conversion of the microenvironment of the secondary pre-antral follicles from one dominated by androgens into one dominated by oestrogens.

The effect of the latter is further proliferation of the granulosa and theca cells with accelerated production of oestrogen and peptide hormones (inhibins, activin, follistatin) and formation of a cavity (antrum) in which the oocyte is surrounded by a few layers of granulosa cells projecting into the cavity.

The follicular cavity fluid contains a myriad of growth factors and signalling molecules involved in bidirectional communication between the oocyte and surrounding granulosa.[3,4]

Inhibins/activin/follistatin and insulin-like growth factors

The granulosa cells of the growing follicles secrete a group of proteins which are important for regulating the HPO axis. In the early follicular phase FSH induces granulosa cells to secrete activin and inhibin A. Activin augments FSH action by increasing its receptors and up-regulates granulosa cell proliferation and aromatase enzyme production. Activin also inhibits the theca cells, androgen production.

Inhibin A exerts a negative feedback effect on the pituitary synthesis and secretion of FSH and stimulates theca cell LH receptors and androgen production. The granulosa cells also secrete follistatin, which combines activin and inhibits its action; it also directly suppresses FSH synthesis and secretion by the pituitary.[5,6]

As the follicular phase progresses (Fig. 71.1) inhibin A activity predominates over activin. This facilitates the selection of the dominant follicle which is able to maintain steroidogenesis in the face of declining FSH levels. Concurrent with these effects the insulin-like growth factor-2 (IGF-2) and its binding protein (IGF2 BP) modulate intra-ovarian activity of FSH and LH so that in androgen-dominant follicles there is a higher concentration of IGF2 BP and lower concentration of bioavailable IGF-2. This leads to decreased FSH action on the granulosa and less steroidogenic activity with less oestradiol production and follicular atresia.[5,6] This could be one of the mechanisms for arrest of follicles and anovulation in polycystic ovary syndrome in the presence of hyperinsulinaemia and hyper-androgenaemia.

In the luteo-follicular transition and early follicular phase, inhibin B is secreted by the granulosa cells, recruited from the secondary follicles pool, to enter the gonadotrophin-dependent phase.[5,6]

The dominant follicle

In the mid-follicular phase (usually on day 7–8 of a 28-day cycle) selection of a dominant follicle (which is usually over 10 mm in diameter at that stage) occurs by the effect of rising oestrogen and inhibin A levels produced by actively growing follicles. This results in a negative feedback effect on the pituitary gonadotrophin (FSH/LH) secretion, and starvation of most of the follicles of the necessary FSH to support granulosa cell proliferation and aromatase activity. The dominant follicle expands in size with an exponential rise of oestradiol levels. This further accentuates the decline in FSH levels and leads to atresia of the rest of the follicles. In natural cycles selection of a single dominant follicle and monofollicular ovulation is the rule, whilst in ovarian stimulation cycles the prolonged exogenous FSH stimulation leads to support and survival of more than one follicle.[3,4]

The dominant follicle (Fig. 71.1) accumulates more fluid in the follicular cavity and its granulosa cells become organised into three compartments: mural granulosa cells surrounding the antrum; cumulus oophorus (which is a stalk of granulosa cells connecting the oocyte to the mural granulosa); and corona radiata (which is a layer of granulosa cells in direct contact with the oocyte). The oocyte with its surrounding corona radiata and cumulus oophorus are bathed within follicular cavity fluid. The latter separates it from the mural granulosa and outer theca cells. The follicle is now is known as the pre-ovulatory or Graafian follicle.[3,4] The Graafian follicle continues to produce oestrogen, independent of FSH stimulation, and has the highest number of granulosa cells and oestradiol levels with the lowest androgen-to-oestrogen ratio. This follicle also develops LH receptors in the granulosa cells, which helps with maturation of the oocyte and prepares the follicle for the ovulatory stimulus of the LH surge. The LH receptors also ensure adequate progesterone production by the luteinised granulosa cells from the corpus luteum after ovulation.[3,4]

Ovulation

When the estradiol (E2) levels peak to 300–400 pg/ml (500–900 pmol/L) (which usually coincides with a follicle size of 18–20 mm), the pituitary gland responds by a surge of LH levels to about 15–30 IU/L. This leads to a cascade of changes in the Graafian follicle and leads to ovulation within 36 hours (34–39 hours) of the onset of the LH surge.

The LH surge initiates the following changes in the Graafian follicle and ovary:

1   Resumption of meiosis in the oocyte with extrusion of the first polar body (the oocyte becomes haploid), and the oocyte becomes arrested into the metaphase of the second meiotic division which is completed at fertilisation with extrusion of second polar body.

2   Induction of angiogenesis and increased vascularity and capillary permeability in the theca cell layers with increased production of follicular fluid and increase in intrafollicular pressure.

3   Synthesis and secretion of various prostaglandins that help increase blood flow in the follicular wall and stimulate smooth muscle cells within the ovarian stroma that help expel the oocyte.

4   Activation of matrix metalloproteinases and other proteolytic enzymes that digest the follicular wall and ovarian capsule at the site of the follicle to facilitate follicular rupture and oocyte release the i.e. ovulation.

5   LH stimulates progesterone synthesis by the granulosa and theca cells shortly before ovulation. This further accentuates the LH surge and ensures adequate luteinisation of the theca and granulosa cells and adequate corpus luteum function later.

The resulting effect of these changes is follicular wall rupture with release of follicular fluid and the oocyte and its surrounding cumulus cells. This is usually picked up by the fimbrial end of the tube, and is transported to the ampullary part of the fallopian tube where fertilisation may occur.

In a regular 28-day cycle the gonadotrophin-dependent phase (follicular phase of the ovarian cycle) lasts about 14 days. However, this is variable amongst individuals and leads to variable lengths of the follicular phase and subsequent variable menstrual cycle lengths as the corpus luteum lifespan is nearly fixed at about 14 days. The timing of ovulation is therefore difficult to predict prospectively; however a fertile period when ovulation is likely to occur can be predicted using the woman's menstrual history and cycle lengths.[3,4]

The luteal phase

After the release of the oocyte–cumulus complex the follicular antrum is filled with blood and new blood vessels forms. The theca–lutein cells become full of cholesterol (luteinised) and the resulting structure is called a corpus luteum. The corpus luteum produces oestrogen, progesterone (P4) and inhibin A in response to LH pulses. These in turn suppress FSH and LH secretion by the pituitary. In the face of declining FSH and LH levels the corpus luteum functions for only about 10 days, with peak activity at about 7 days after ovulation (mid-luteal

peak of progesterone on day 21 of a 28-day cycle). It then enters into an apoptosis and regression phase of about 4 days if pregnancy does not occur. In the absence of pregnancy, the corpus luteum has a fairly predictable life span of 14 days. The falling oestradiol and progesterone levels lead to apoptosis and shedding of the endometrium. The falling ovarian steroid levels release the hypothalamus and pituitary from the negative feedback effect, with a subsequent increase in FSH levels and ensuring a new cycle of recruitment of secondary follicles. The luteo-follicular transition phase is characterised by increasing FSH levels, low oestradiol and progesterone levels and high inhibin B secreted by the granulosa cells of recruited follicles.[3,4]

If pregnancy occurs the hCG produced by the trophoblast of the implanting embryo rescues the corpus luteum from apoptosis and atresia, enabling the corpus luteum to function and produce progesterone till 10–12 weeks' gestation when the placenta takes over this function.[3,4]

THE MENSTRUAL CYCLE

The endometrium undergoes cyclic changes which mirror the effect of the hormones produced by the growing follicles and corpus luteum in the ovary.

In the early follicular phase the endometrium is rebuilt from the basalis layer after its superficial layer has been shed in the menses of the previous cycle. The prevailing oestradiol secreted from the ovary leads to active mitosis and proliferation of the endometrial glands and stroma. This leads to an increase in the thickness of the endometrium from 2–3 mm to about 6–8 mm by the end of this **proliferative phase**.

Following ovulation the prevailing progesterone hormone leads to more functional maturation of the endometrial glands and decidualisation of the endometrial stroma. Histologically these changes are reflected in enlarged tortuous endometrial glands that are full of secretions; hence this phase is called the **secretory phase**. The stroma appears oedematous with an increased number and coiling of the spiral arteries and pericapillary leukocytic and cellular infiltrates, a process called decidualisation. The effect of the epithelial changes is secretion of adhesion molecules, such as integrins and glycodelins, which mediate the attachment of the blastocyst (in the case of successful fertilisation) that initiates the implantation process. The effect of stromal decidualisation is recruitment of immunological cells (natural killer cells, dendritic cells) that help regulate the trophoblastic invasion and effect changes in the spiral arteries that lead to the development of the early placenta. The peak of secretory changes in the endometrium is 7–9 days after ovulation when the endometrium is most receptive to implantation of the blastocyst, the so called **implantation window**.

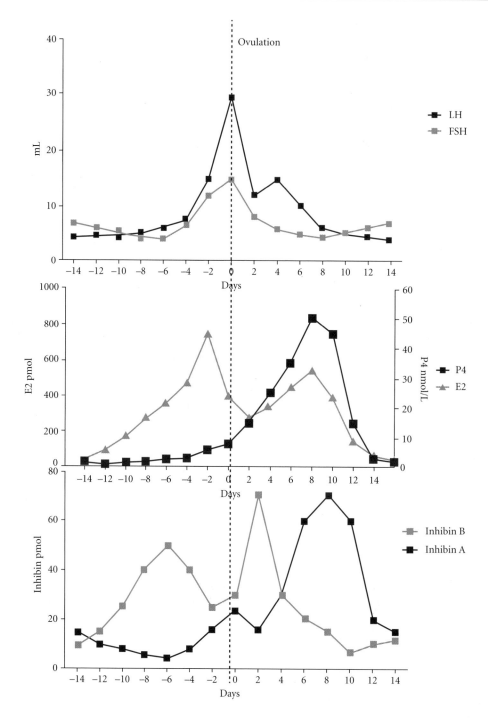

Fig. 71.1 Depiction of the changes of pituitary hormones (FSH/LH), ovarian steroids (E2, P4) and ovarian peptide hormones in a normal ovarian and menstrual cycle

REPRODUCTIVE GYNAECOLOGY

If fertilisation occurs and a blastocyst successfully implants in the endometrium the trophoblast of the implanting embryo secretes hCG which rescues the corpus luteum. This prolongs the lifespan of the corpus luteum and maintains progesterone secretion till about 10 weeks' gestation when the developing placenta takes over the hormonal production (luteo-placental shift). As a result of maintenance of oestrogen and progesterone production and stability of the decidua,

pregnant women will experience the physiological amenorrhoea of pregnancy.

If there was no fertilisation or a blastocyst could not successfully implant then the declining corpus luteum function (starting around day 10–12 after ovulation and almost complete by day 14) is associated with falling oestrogen and progesterone levels. This in turn initiates apoptosis in the endometrium with release of prostaglandins and lysosomal enzymes from the cells, setting waves of vasoconstriction leading to ischaemia. There is further breakdown of blood vessels and cells followed by vasodilatation, with escape of blood cells (erythrocytes, leukocytes, platelets) as well as various proteolytic enzymes (metalloproteinases, enkephalinases, fibrinolysins) into the endometrial stroma. The effect of these waves of vasoconstriction and vasodilatation with apoptosis and proteolysis culminates into endometrial sloughing at the junction of superficial and basal layers forming the menstrual bleeding. In concert with these changes the released prostaglandins from the endometrium, as well as the myometrial cells under the effect of falling progesterone levels, lead to myometrial contractions. This leads to expulsion of the menstrual blood from the uterus.[3,4]

A normal menstrual phase is expected to last 2–6 days and the amount of bleeding is generally 20–80 ml. The rising oestradiol level caused by the recruited follicles leads to rapid repair and rebuilding of the endometrium and the end of the menstrual phase.

Menstrual bleeding in ovulatory cycles (oestrogen/progesterone withdrawal bleeding) is characterised by being synchronised and less prolonged and associated with menstrual cramps due to higher levels of prostaglandins, while in anovulatory dysfunctional menses are usually prolonged, erratic, heavy and painless. Cases of dysfunctional menorrhagia (prolonged and/or heavy menses due to mainly anovulation and/or dysfunctional molecular changes in the endometrium in the absence of significant pathological changes) may benefit from progestins only or sequential oestrogens/progestin treatment to mimic the oestrogen/progesterone withdrawal bleeding in normal cycles. The prostaglandin synthetase inhibitors (such as non-steroidal anti-inflammatory agent mefenamic acid) are also used as a treatment of dysfunctional menorrhagia.

CLINICAL POINTS

- Luteal phase defect is a condition characterised by either a short luteal phase or a subnormal secretion of progesterone in the luteal (secretory) phase leading to defective implantation, with either infertility or miscarriage. In IVF cycles due to prolonged pituitary suppression and lack of hormonal support of the corpus luteum, luteal phase support is given by administering progesterone either vaginally or by intramuscular injection to help implantation and improve pregnancy rate.

- In a healthy pregnancy the hCG level usually shows a long linear rise every 48 hours until it reaches a peak of around 100,000 IU/L around 10 weeks' gestation. The minimum rise of hCG level in viable intrauterine pregnancies is generally around 53–66 per cent of baseline. This level of rise, however, is not observed in most ectopic pregnancies. This serves as the basis of monitoring of early pregnancy complications with serial hCG levels. There is, however, a considerable overlap between viable and non-viable pregnancies and ectopic

gestations in hCG levels, and the interpretations of findings should be in conjunction with transvaginal ultrasound scans and in the context of clinical presentation and risk factors.[8,9]

KEY POINTS

- The ovarian and menstrual cycles are tightly coordinated in order to ensure a receptive endometrium at the time at which the embryo is ready to implant.

- The pituitary hormones LH and FSH are regulated by feedback from the ovarian sex steroids (oestrogens and progestone) and peptides (inhibin).

- Advancements in IVF are underpinned by an understanding of the interplay between the pituitary gonadotrophins and ovarian steroids and glycoproteins. This has allowed for the development of drugs to influence the menstrual cycle, including injectable gonadotrophins to stimulate multiple follicular development for IVF.

- Anovulation should be investigated by using timed measurements of FSH, LH and progesterone, sometimes with additional measurement of prolactin and thyroid function.

- Underlying cause for anovulation needs to be established before considering treatment options.

References

1. Tobet SA, Schwarting GA. Mini review: recent progress in gonadotropin-releasing hormone neuronal migration. *Endocrinology* 2006;147:1159.

2. Kaiser UB, Conn PM, Chin WW. Studies of gonadotropin-releasing hormone (GnRH) action using GnRH receptor-expressing pituitary cell lines. *Endocr Rev* 1997;18:46.

3. Halvorson LM. Reproductive endocrinology. *In*: Hoffmann BL, Schorge J, Schaffer JL, Bradshaw KD, Halvorson LM, Cunningham FG (eds). *Williams Gynaecology*. 2nd edn. New York: McGraw Hill, 2012, 400–439.

4. Carr BR. The ovary and the normal menstrual cycle. *In*: Carr BR, Blackwell RE, Azziz R (eds). *Essential reproductive medicine*. New York, McGraw-Hill, 2005, 79.

5. De Kretser DM, Hedger MP, Loveland KL *et al*. Inhibins, activins, and follistatin in reproduction. *Hum Reprod Update* 2002;8:529.

6. Muttukrishna S, Tannetta D, Groome N *et al*. Activin and follistatin in female reproduction. *Mol Cell Endocrinol* 2004;225:45.

REPRODUCTIVE GYNAECOLOGY

7. Schipper I, Hop WC, Fauser BC. The follicle-stimulating hormone (FSH) threshold/window concept examined by different interventions with exogenous FSH during the follicular phase of the normal menstrual cycle: duration, than magnitude, of FSH increase affects follicle development. *J Clin Endocrinol Metab* 1998;83:1292.

8. Barnhart KT, Sammel MD, Rinaudo PF *et al.* Symptomatic patients with an early viable intrauterine pregnancy: HCG curves redefined. *Obstet Gynecol* 2004;104:50.

9. Kadar N, DeCherney AH, Romero R. Receiver operating characteristic (ROC) curve analysis of the relative efficacy of single and serial chorionic gonadotropin determinations in the early diagnosis of ectopic pregnancy. *Fertil Steril* 1982;37:542.

Chapter 72 Contraception and termination of pregnancy

Kulsum Jaffer

MRCOG standards

Learning outcomes

- To understand and demonstrate appropriate knowledge, skills and attitudes in relation to fertility control – contraception, sterilisation and termination of pregnancy

Theoretical skills

- Thorough understanding of all methods of contraception – reversible, irreversible and emergency contraception.
- Methods, risks and laws relating to termination of pregnancy.

Practical skills

- Candidates should be able to take an appropriate history and counsel patients requesting contraceptive advice, sterilisation and termination of pregnancy.
- DFSRH, LoC IUT and LoC SDI are highly recommended.

Table 72.1 Definition of UKMEC categories (from reference 2, with permission)

UKMEC	Definition of category
1	A condition with **no restriction for the use** of the contraceptive method.
2	A condition where the **advantages of the contraceptive method generally outweigh the theoretical or proven risks**.
3	A condition where the **theoretical or proven risks of the contraceptive method outweigh the advantages**. Expert clinical judgement and/or referral to a specialist contraceptive provider is recommended.
4	A condition which represents an **unacceptable health risk** if the contraceptive method is used.

INTRODUCTION

Many factors determine the method of contraception a person chooses. To be effective, contraception must be used correctly and consistently. Contraceptive effectiveness is usually presented in terms of failure rates rather than success rates and is expressed as failure rates per 100 Woman Years (WY). One WY is equal to 13 cycles. Most contraceptive users are medically fit and can use any contraceptive method safely. However, some medical conditions are associated with increased health risks when certain contraceptives are used, either because the method adversely affects the condition or because the condition, or its treatment, affects the contraceptive. The World Health Organization (WHO) published the WHO Medical Eligibility Criteria (WHOMEC)[1] for contraceptive use which relates to the safety (in terms of direct health risk) of using a contraceptive method by women with certain medical conditions or using certain drugs. The UK Medical Eligibilty Criteria (UKMEC)[2] were adapted from WHOMEC for use by UK clinicians in line with national health policies, needs, priorities and resources (Table 72.1).

FERTILITY AWARENESS METHODS

These are more commonly known as natural family planning (NFP). They have been defined by the WHO as 'the voluntary avoidance of intercourse by a couple during the fertile phase of the menstrual cycle in order to avoid a pregnancy'.[3] Fertility awareness (FA) methods are associated with higher failure rates than other available methods of contraception. They are often perceived as being better for women's health than hormonal and intrauterine methods. Some choose natural methods on moral or religious grounds, others because they have experienced, or have concerns about, the side effects of artificial methods or because they have medical conditions which limit their contraceptive choice.[4] FA methods rely on the fact that there are only certain days during the menstrual cycle when conception can occur. Following ovulation, the ovum is viable within the reproductive tract for a maximum of 24 hours. However, the life span of the sperm is considerably longer, in the region of 3–7 days. These methods require long periods of sexual abstinence. They provide low and varying levels of efficacy and do not provide any protection against sexually transmitted infections (STIs).

Cycle or rhythm method

Cycle length is recorded for a minimum of six cycles. Likely fertile days are then calculated allowing for the survival time of sperm and ova, using the following formula:

First fertile day = shortest cycle minus 20
Last fertile day = longest cycle minus 10

This method requires a significant period of sexual abstinence, e.g. in cases of a regular 28-day cycle, 10 days of sexual abstinence are required during each cycle.

Temperature method

Following ovulation there is a rise in the progesterone levels which produces a rise in the basal body temperature of 0.2–0.4°C that is maintained until the onset of menstruation. The fertile phase ends after 3 consecutive high temperatures are recorded (>0.2°C above the 6 preceding recordings). This is known as the '3 over 6' rule. Intercourse is avoided from the onset of menstruation until the day on which the third higher-level temperature has been recorded. Intercourse is then allowed until the onset of the next menstruation. In case of a 28-day cycle abstinence is required for about 18 days per cycle. Infection, illness and medication can affect the body temperature and interfere with the method. A failure rate of 1.20 per 100 WY has been reported.[5]

Cervical mucus method (Billings method)

During the follicular phase of the cycle the cervical mucus appears like raw egg white (i.e. it is clear, slippery and stretchy: spinnbarkeit phenomenon). The final day of the 'fertile mucus' is considered to be the day when ovulation is most likely to occur. Abstinence must be maintained from the day when fertile mucus is first identified until 3 days after the peak day. The end of the fertile period is characterised by the appearance of 'infertile mucus' which is scanty and viscous. Semen, sexual excitement, spermicides, lubricants, bleeding and vaginal infections can confuse mucus assessment. The actual failure rate for typical use has been reported as 22 per 100 WY.[6]

Cervical palpation method

Daily self-palpation of the cervix helps to detect the changes occurring in the size of the external os and its position relative to the introitus. The cervix rises during the follicular phase of the cycle. At ovulation it reaches peak height from the introitus with maximum softness and the os admits a fingertip. The cervix then descends, becomes closed and firm and is closer to the vulva towards the end of the luteal phase.

Minor clinical indicators of fertility

Ovulation pain (mittelschmerz), mid-cycle show of blood, onset of breast symptoms, skin and mood changes can occur in some women. When present they can be helpful in confirming the major signs.

Various combinations of FA methods can be used to increase the accuracy of identification of the fertile and infertile periods.

Personal fertility monitors

Persona is a small hand-held device that is able to detect urine concentrations of estrone-3-glucuronide (E3G) and luteinising hormone (LH) and thus signifies the start and end of the fertile period. On potentially fertile days, a red light indicates the need for abstinence from intercourse. Safe days are indicated by a green light and a yellow light implies that a urine sample is required. Following the urine test, a red or green light will be displayed depending on the LH and E3G ratio. Persona can be used for cycle lengths between 23 and 35 days. It cannot be used if a woman is experiencing menopausal symptoms, is breastfeeding, has recently given birth, is taking hormones or is on tetracyclines. The failure rate is around 6 per 100 WY.

Lactational amenorrhoea method (LAM)

A woman who is fully breastfeeding and is amenorrhoeic during the first 6 months after childbirth has a 2 per cent chance of getting pregnant [B]. Hence LAM is categorised as one of the NFP methods.[7]

BARRIER METHODS

These provide a physical barrier which stops the sperm from getting into the vagina or upper genital tract. There are many types available including male and female condoms, caps, diaphragms, sponges and spermicides. They provide varying degrees of protection from STIs, including HIV and premalignant and malignant disease of the cervix.

Male condom

The majority of these are made from fine latex rubber. Those who suffer from latex sensitivity can use polyurethane condoms [C]. Oil-based lubricants and vaginal preparations drastically reduce the strength of the condom [C]. Failure rates for condoms range from 2 to 18 per 100 WY.

Female condom (femidom)

This is a polyurethane sheath, 15 cm long and 7.5 cm in diameter with rings at both ends. It is stronger than the male latex condom with less risk of splitting and is not weakened by oil-based lubricants and vaginal preparations. Failure rates are in the region of 5–21 per 100 WY.

Occlusive caps

These comprise the diaphragms, cervical and vault caps and the Vimule. They should be used in combination with spermicides to provide maximum protection [C]. Occlusive devices are available in a range of sizes and initially need to be fitted by trained personnel. They require a high degree of motivation for successful use which is reflected in the varying rates of efficacy.

Diaphragm

A diaphragm is a thin latex rubber or silicone hemisphere, the rim of which is reinforced by a flexible flat or coiled metal spring. The flat spring diaphragm is for the normal vagina, whereas the coil and arcing spring ones are for the tight and lax vaginae respectively. Their external diameters range from 55 to 95 mm, with 5 mm increments. The diaphragm should lie across the cervix extending from the posterior vaginal fornix to behind the symphysis pubis. Urinary tract infections are more common in diaphragm users. Inflammatory reactions, abrasions or even frank ulcers can also be caused by local pressure.

Cervical caps

These are the Dumas, Vimule and Prentif caps made from latex. The FemCap is made from silicone. It snugly fits onto the cervix by suction.

Vaginal sponge

This is made of polyurethane foam and impregnated with spermicide. It is inserted in the vagina to cover the cervix. It acts as a carrier for the spermicide and absorbs the semen. The 'Today' and 'Protectaid' contraceptive sponges have currently been withdrawn from the UK market.

Spermicides

These are chemicals that bring about sperm death by causing osmotic changes in the sperm. The most common spermicide is Nonoxino-9. It can cause vaginal irritation and ulceration and may increase the risk of HIV transmission. The use of condoms lubricated with Nonoxinol-9 is not recommended [B]. Spermicides are used in conjunction with barrier methods.

Coitus interruptus

This is the withdrawal of the penis from the vagina before ejaculation takes place and therefore requires considerable control on the part of the man. Failure rates of about 10 per 100 WY have been quoted.[8]

COMBINED HORMONAL CONTRACEPTION (CHC) (BOXES 72.1, 72.2)

This includes the combined oral contraceptive (COC) pill, the transdermal patch and the vaginal ring. The patch and the

Box 72.1 CHC: UKMEC Category 3 – Risks generally outweigh benefits

CHC: UKMEC Category 3 – Risks generally outweigh benefits
Breastfeeding – between 6 weeks and 6 months postpartum and fully or almost fully breastfeeding
Postpartum – <21 days postpartum
Smoking – aged ≥35 years and smoking <15 cigarettes per day, or stopped smoking <1 year ago
Obesity - BMI >35 kg/m^2
Cardiovascular disease – multiple risk factors for arterial cardiovascular disease
Hypertension - elevated blood pressure >140–159 mmHg systolic or >90–94 mmHg diastolic; also adequately controlled hypertension
Family history of venous thromboembolism (VTE) in a first-degree relative aged <45 years
Immobility (unrelated to surgery) – e.g. wheelchair use, debilitating illness
Known hyperlipidaemias – e.g. familial hypercholesterolaemia
Migraine without aura, at any age – continuation of the method
Past history (>5 years ago) of migraine with aura at any age
Undiagnosed breast mass – initiation of the method
Past history of breast cancer and no evidence of recurrence for 5 years; carriers of known gene mutations associated with breast cancer (e.g. *BRCA1*)
Diabetes – with nephropathy/retinopathy/neuropathy; or other vascular disease
Gallbladder disease – symptomatic medically treated or current
History of cholestasis – past COC-related
Viral hepatitis – acute or flare
HIV – on antiretroviral therapy (drug interactions)
Drugs which induce liver enzymes – e.g. rifampicin, rifabutin, ritonavir, St John's Wort and certain anticonvulsants (i.e. phenytoin, carbamazepine, barbiturates, primidone, topiramate, oxcarbazepine) and lamotrigine

Box 72.2 CHC: UKMEC Category 4 – Unacceptable health risk and should not be used

---

CHC: UKMEC Category 4 – Unacceptable health risk and should not be used

Breastfeeding – <6 weeks postpartum

Smoking – aged ≥35 years and smoking ≥15 cigarettes per day

Cardiovascular disease – multiple risk factors for arterial cardiovascular disease

Hypertension – blood pressure ≥160 mmHg systolic and/or ≥95 mmHg diastolic; or vascular disease

VTE – current (on anticoagulants) or past history

Major surgery with prolonged immobilisation

Known thrombogenic mutations

Current and history of ischaemic heart disease

Stroke

Valvular and congenital heart disease – complicated by pulmonary hypertension, atrial fibrillation, history of subacute bacterial endocarditis

Migraine headaches – with aura at any age

Breast disease – current breast cancer

Diabetes – with nephropathy, retinopathy, neuropathy or other vascular disease

Viral hepatitis – active or flare

Cirrhosis – severe decompensated disease

Liver tumours – benign hepatocellular adenoma and malignant hepatoma

Systemic lupus erythematosus (SLE) – positive or unknown antiphospholipid antibodies

---

ring are no different from the pill in terms of mechanism of action, safety and efficacy. However, there is no data regarding the major side effects of the ring and the patch therefore at present it is advisable that the data for COCs also applies to the NuvaRing and the Evra patch.

Mode of action

All CHCs inhibit ovulation. The vaginal and cervical mucus becomes scanty and viscous and inhibits sperm transport. The endometrium becomes atrophic and is unreceptive for implantation.

Non-contraceptive benefits

CHCs decrease menstrual pain and blood loss. There is a decrease in the incidence of functional ovarian cysts, benign ovarian tumours, benign breast disease, pelvic inflammatory disease (PID) and acne. There is also a 50 per cent reduction in ovarian and endometrial cancers which continues for 15 years after stopping the CHC. There is a possible protective effect against rheumatoid arthritis, thyroid disease and duodenal ulceration.

Major side effects

Venous thromboembolism

The most common serious risk of CHC is VTE. This risk is the most during the first year of CHC use. If a woman is not on any CHC, the risk of VTE is 4–5 per 10,000 WY. The risk of VTE with COCs is double that of the non-users (9–10/10,000 WY). The Danish retrospective study[9] and the MEGA case-controlled study[10] have not only found an increased relative risk (RR) for VTE with desogestrel and gestodene but also with cyproterone acetate and drosperinone compared to levonorgestrel (LNG). Pill users who have a factor V Leiden mutation have up to 20 times the risk of VTE compared to non-pill users.

Myocardial infarction

A meta-analysis of 23 studies showed that there is an overall increased risk of 2.5 of myocardial infarction with current COC use compared with never users.[11] This risk increases with smoking and hypertension.

Stroke

The risk of ischaemic stroke is increased among current users of COCs (RR 2.7) [B]. This risk is further increased with smoking and hypertension and in migraine sufferers.

Migraine

The risk of ischaemic stroke is increased in migraine sufferers and the use of CHC further increases this risk. Migraine with aura at any age is a UKMEC 4 category for CHC use.

Cancer

Breast cancer
A large meta-analysis showed that there is an increased risk of breast cancer with COC use (RR 1.24), which is an increase of 24 per cent above the background risk. This increased risk occurs soon after starting COC and is not duration dependent but disappears after 10 years of discontinuation of the COC.[12]

Cervical cancer
There is a slight increased risk of cervical intra-epithelial neoplasia, cervical cancer and also the morbidity from it with the duration of COC use [B].

COC pill

This is almost 99 per cent effective. COC formulations are either fixed dose or phasic, when the dose of the estrogen and progestogen changes during the cycle. Phasic preparations are designed to mimic the body's cyclical variation in hormone levels. Additional precautions are not needed when using CHCs with antibiotics (non-enzyme-inducing). Zoely and Qlaira are the relatively newer COCs.

Zoely

This contains 1.5 mg of estradiol and 2.5 mg of nomegestrol acetate (NOMAC). It has a 24/4 regimen with no pill-free interval. The 17β-estradiol is identical to the endogenous human 17β-estradiol whereas NOMAC is a progestogen with strong antigonadotrophic and mild antiandrogenic properties. Randomised studies have shown that its efficacy is comparable to other COCs.

The withdrawal bleeding is shorter and lighter and there is a higher incidence of absent withdrawal bleeds. There have been some withdrawals from trials due to weight gain, acne and lack of withdrawal bleeding. The effect on haemostatic and metabolic parameters is less than other COCs but this clinical relevance is yet to be established.

Missed-pill guidelines for Zoely are as follows:

- **Day 1–7:** The missed pill should be taken as soon as possible and extra precautions should be used for the next 7 days.
- **Day 8–17:** The last missed pill should be taken as soon as possible. The rest of the pack is taken in the usual manner.
- **Day 18–24:** Omit the inactive pills and start the next pack straight away or discard the active pills and take the inactive ones before starting the new pack.

Qlaira

Qlaira is a COC containing estradiol valerate (E2V) and dienogest (D) in the doses shown in Table 72.2.

Reducing the pill-free interval has been shown to decrease mood changes, headaches, menstrual loss and pelvic pain. Therefore, it may be suitable for women who complain of estrogen withdrawal symptoms (as above). In situations when extra precautions are needed, 9 days of extra precautions are needed for Qlaira instead of the 7 days for conventional COCs. It delivers 17B estradiol (E2) which is a body identical estrogen. Studies have shown that it has less effect on the haemostatic parameters and lipid profile than Microgynon 30 and Logynon. It may therefore prove useful for women over 35 and those with uncomplicated diabetes.[13] It contains 26 active and two placebo tablets. Hence the pill-free interval is reduced to 2 days. Reducing the pill-free interval has been shown to decrease mood changes, headaches, menstrual loss and pelvic pain. Therefore, it may be suitable for women who complain of estrogen withdrawal symptoms (as above). Pearl index (failure rate) is 0.4 per 100 WY which is similar to those reported for other COCs.

Qlaira has different missed-pill guidelines to the other COCs. The following guidelines should be followed if one pill is missed for more than 12 hours:

Table 72.2 Dosage of E2V and D in Qlaira

Days	2	5	17	2	2
E2V	3 mg	2 mg	2 mg	1 mg	0
D	0	2 mg	3 mg	0	0

- **Days 1–17:** Take the missed pill immediately and the next tablet at the usual time (even if it means taking two on the same day). Continue with the tablet taking in the normal way. Abstain or use an additional contraceptive method for 9 days.
- **Days 18–24:** Discard the rest of the packet. Start taking the day 1 pill from a new packet immediately and continue taking these pills at the correct time. Abstain or use an additional contraceptive method for 9 days.
- **Days 25–26:** Take the missed tablet immediately and the next tablet at the usual time (even if it means taking two tablets on the same day). Additional contraception is not necessary.
- **Days 27–28:** Discard the forgotten tablet and continue tablet taking in the normal way. Additional contraception is not necessary.

Dianette

This contains 35 μg of ethinyl estradiol and 2 mg of cyproterone acetate. It is not licensed as an oral contraceptive but is used as one. It is used for treating moderate to severe acne and hirsutism. There is an increased incidence of VTE in Dianette users more than the second generation COCs. A few cases of severe depression have been reported with Dianette. Therefore it has been advised by the Committee on Safety of Medicines (CSM) that it should be withdrawn 3–4 cycles after the condition for which it was prescribed initially has resolved.

Evra patch

With this patch 20 μg of ethinyl estradiol and 150 μg of norelgestromin are released every 24 hours. It is the first transdermal contraceptive applied once weekly for 3 weeks followed by a patch-free week (3 weeks on, 1 week off). The Pearl index is 1.24 per 100 WY. It has been reported that contraceptive efficacy is reduced in women weighing over 90 kg. It provides a new delivery system and another contraceptive choice for women. Efficacy, cycle control and safety profile are similar to COCs.

NuvaRing

This is a flexible, latex-free ring made of plastic and ethylene vinyl acetate which releases 120 μg of etonogestrel (ENG) and 15 μg of ethinyl estradiol daily. It is 54 mm in diameter and 4 mm thick. It is placed vaginally once every 3 weeks and following a 1-week ring-free interval a new ring is inserted. Efficacy and cycle control are comparable to the COCs. Side-effect profile is also similar to that of COCs. However, women have reported more vaginal symptoms of vaginitis, leukorrhoea, foreign body sensation, coital problems and expulsion.[14] It provides another useful contraceptive for women.

Missed-pill guidelines for COC

See Figure 72.1

| If ONE pill has been missed (more than 24 hours and up to 48 hours late) | If TWO OR MORE pills have been missed (more than 48 hours late) |

Continuing contraceptive cover
- The missed pill should be taken as soon as it is remembered
- The remaining pills should be continued at the usual time

Continuing contraceptive cover

- The most recent missed pill should be taken as soon as possible
- The remaining pills should be continued at the usual time
- Condoms should be used or sex avoided until seven consecutive active pills have been taken. This advice may be overcautious in the second and third weeks, but the advice is a backup in the event that further pills are missed.

Minimizing the risk of pregnancy

Emergency contraception (EC) is not usually required but may need to be considered if pills have been missed earlier in the packet or in the last week of the previous packet.

Minimising the risk of pregnancy

If pills are missed in the first week (Pills 1 - 7)	If pills are missed in the second week (Pills 8 - 14)	If pills are missed in the third week (Pills 15 - 21)
EC should be considered if unprotected sex occurred in the pill-free interval or in the first week of pill-taking	No indication for EC if the pills in the preceding 7 days have been taken consistently and correctly (assuming the pills thereafter are taken correctly and additional contraceptive precautions are used).	OMIT THE PILL-FREE INTERVAL by finishing the pills in the current pack (or discarding any placebo tablets) and starting a new pack the next day.

Fig. 72.1 Advice for women missing combined oral contraceptive pills (except Qlaira and Zoely). (Reproduced from FFPRHC/FSRH guidance - combined oral contraception - missed pills recommendations, CEU Guidance May 2011, with permission.)

Table 72.3 Tailored regimens for use of combined hormonal contraception (CHC). (From FSRH – CHC Guidance October 2011, updated August 2012, with permission)

Type of regimen	Suggested regimen	CHC-free period
Extended use	Tricycling (3 cycles taken continuously back to back i.e. 3 pill packets or 3 rings, or 9 patches)	7 days taken after finishing the 3rd packet, 3rd ring or 9th patch
Shortened pill-free interval	3 weeks of CHC use	4 days taken after each packet of pills, each ring or 3rd patch
Extended use with shortened pill-free interval	Method used continuously (≥21 days; pill-, patch- and ring-free weeks omitted) until breakthrough bleeding occurs for 3–4 days	4-day interval
Extended use with standard pill-free interval	Method used continuously (≥21 days; pill-, patch- and ring-free weeks omitted) until breakthrough bleeding occurs for 3–4 days	7-day interval

Extended prescribing regime for CHCs

Continuous or extended regimens of CHC use are advocated by the Faculty of Sexual and Reproductive Healthcare (FSRH). These are safe but are out of product licence. These regimens are only applicable for monophasic pills (Table 72.3).

PROGESTOGEN-ONLY PILLS (POPs) (BOXES 72.3, 72.4)

Mode of action

POPs alter cervical mucus and prevent sperm penetration. The endometrium is altered so that it is not conducive for implantation. In addition, traditional POPs can inhibit ovulation but this can be variable – up to 60 per cent, whereas in the case of the desogestrel-only pill, Cerazette, 97 per cent of the cycles are anovulatory. Therefore, inhibition of ovulation is the main mode of action of Cerazette [C].

Effectiveness

Failure rates for traditional POPs vary from 0.3 to 8.0 per 100 WY, but are lower for women aged over 40 years (0.3 per 100 WY) compared to younger women. The failure rates of the traditional pills and Cerazette are similar [B]. There is no evidence to suggest that the efficacy of any POP is reduced in women weighing >70 kg and therefore one pill per day is advised as per licence [B].

Side effects

Changes in the bleeding pattern are common. Two in 10 women are amenorrhoeic, whereas 4 in 10 have regular bleeding and another 4 in 10 have irregular bleeding. Mood changes can occur with POP use.

Risks

There is no causal association between POP use and cardiovascular disease (VTE, myocardial infarction and stroke) or breast cancer. Women of any age with a history of migraine (with or without aura) can safely use POPs.

Missed-pill guidelines for POPs

See Figure 72.2.

Box 72.3 POP: UKMEC Category 3 – Risks generally outweigh benefits

> **POP: UKMEC Category 3 – Risks generally outweigh benefits**
>
> Current and history of ischaemic heart disease and stroke – continuation of the method
>
> Past history of breast cancer and no evidence of recurrence for 5 years
>
> HIV – on antiretroviral therapy (drug interactions)
>
> Cirrhosis – severe (decompensated)
>
> Liver tumours – hepatocellular adenoma and malignant hepatoma
>
> SLE – positive or unknown antiphospholipid antibodies

Box 72.4 POP: UKMEC Category 4 – Unacceptable health risk and should not be used

> **POP: UKMEC Category 4 – Unacceptable health risk and should not be used**
>
> Breast disease – current breast cancer

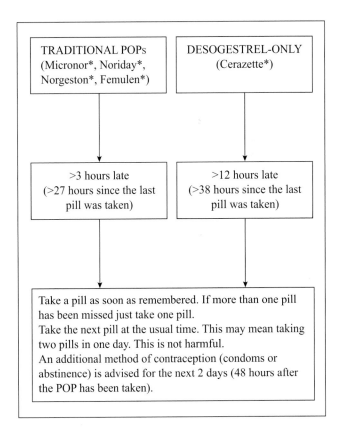

Fig. 72.2 Missed-pill guidelines for POP. (Reproduced from FFPRHC/FSRH – Clinical guidance Progestogen-only Pill, November 2008 with permission.)

LONG-ACTING REVERSIBLE CONTRACEPTION (LARCs) (BOXES 72.5, 72.6, 72.7, 72.8)

- LARC methods require administering less than once per cycle or month.
- They are more cost effective than COCs even at 1 year of use.
- Intrauterine devices, systems and implants are more cost effective than injectables.
- Increased uptake will reduce unintended pregnancies.

The LARC methods are:

- Non-hormonal: Intrauterine device (IUD or Cu-IUD);
- Hormonal: – Intrauterine system (IUS);
  - Progestogen-only injectable contraception (POIC);
  - Progestogen-only implant (POI);

Box 72.5 IUD: UKMEC Category 3 – Risks generally outweigh benefits

IUD: UKMEC Category 3 – Risks generally outweigh benefits
Postpartum – between 48 hours and <4 weeks
VTE – current (on anticoagulants)
Ovarian cancer – initiation of the method
Pelvic tuberculosis – continuation of the method
AIDS – initiation of the method
SLE – initiation of the method in women with severe thrombocytopenia

Box 72.6 IUD: UKMEC Category 4 – Unacceptable health risk and should not be used

IUD: UKMEC Category 4 – Unacceptable health risk and should not be used
Pregnancy, puerperal sepsis and immediate post-septic abortion
Unexplained vaginal bleeding – initiation of the method
Gestational trophoblastic disease (GTD) – persistently elevated beta-human chorionic gonadotrophin (hCG) levels or malignant disease
Cervical cancer – initiation of the method in women awaiting treatment
Endometrial cancer – initiation of the method
Ovarian cancer – initiation of the method
Current PID, symptomatic and asymptomatic chlamydial infection or purulent cervicitis or gonorrhoea – initiation of the method
Pelvic tuberculosis – initiation of the method

Box 72.7 LNG-IUS: UKMEC Category 3 – Risks generally outweigh benefits

LNG-IUS: UKMEC Category 3 – Risks generally outweigh benefits
Postpartum – between 48 hours and <4 weeks
Current and past history of ischaemic heart disease – continuation of the method
Stroke – continuation of the method
Pelvic tuberculosis – continuation of the method
AIDS – initiation of the method
Cirrhosis – severe, decompensated
Liver tumours – hepatocellular adenoma and malignant hepatoma
SLE – positive or unknown antiphospholipid antibodies

Box 72.8 LNG-IUS: UKMEC Category 4 – Unacceptable health risk and should not be used

LNG-IUS: UKMEC Category 4 – Unacceptable health risk and should not be used
Puerperal sepsis
Post-septic abortion
Unexplained vaginal bleeding – initiation of the method
GTD – persistently elevated beta-hCG levels or malignant disease
Cervical cancer – initiation of the method in women awaiting treatment
Endometrial cancer – initiation of the method
Ovarian cancer – initiation of the method
Breast cancer – current
Current PID, symptomatic and asymptomatic chlamydial infection or purulent cervicitis or gonorrhoea – initiation of the method
Pelvic tuberculosis – initiation of the method

Intrauterine contraception – IUD and LNG-IUS

The gold standard IUDs are the T-shaped IUDs with banded copper on the arms and containing at least 380 mm² copper. They last for 10 years whereas other Cu-IUDs and LNG-IUSs are for 3–5 years [C].

Jaydess, a new LNG-IUS Jaydess is licensed for 3 years. It contains 13.5 mgs of LNG which is released at a rate of 6–10 mcg/day. It is slightly smaller than the Mirena and has a silver ring for identification from the Mirena on ultrasound.

It is not recommended for the treatment of heavy menstrual bleeding ((HMB) nor offers protection from endometrial hyperplasia.

Levosert contains 52 mgs of LNG and is licensed for 3 years for contraception and treatment of HMB. It is not licensed for endometrial protection.

A Cu-IUD inserted in a woman at the age of 40 years or over can be retained for 1 year after the last menstrual period if aged over 50 years or 2 years if under 50 years or until contraception is no longer required [C]. The LARC guideline recommends that women who have the LNG-IUS inserted at or after the age of 45 years and are amenorrhoeic may retain the LNG-IUS until the menopause [E].

Effectiveness

Failure rates are less than 2 per cent with TCu380A and TCu380S coils and less than 1 per cent for LNG-IUS [C].

Mode of action

IUDs work by inhibiting fertilisation by direct toxicity [B]. An inflammatory reaction within the endometrium can also have an anti-implantation effect. Copper is toxic to the ovum and the sperm and the copper content of the cervical mucus inhibits sperm penetration as well. LNG-IUS works primarily by its effect on the endometrium, preventing implantation. In addition, its effect on cervical mucus reduces sperm penetration [B].

Insertion and removal prerequisites

A sexual history should be taken from all women attending for IUD/IUS insertions to assess the risk of STIs. Prior to IUD/IUS insertion, women at higher risk of STIs (age <25 years, change in sexual partner, or more than one partner in the last year) should be offered testing for Chlamydia trachomatis, as a minimum [C]. For women assessed as being at higher risk of STIs, and whose test results are not available at the time of the insertion, then the use of prophylactic antibiotics to cover chlamydia should be considered (Good Practice).

Additional protection is never needed at IUD insertion, as the mode of action is by inhibition of fertilisation and implantation and these effects are immediate after insertion. It is however required before IUD removal, as viable ova or sperm may be present in the female genital tract before removal. The woman is therefore advised to abstain, use condoms or start a CHC 7 days before removal [C].

Antibiotic prophylaxis for the prevention of infective endocarditis is NOT recommended in women undergoing intrauterine insertion or removal even in women with conditions where the risk of endocarditis is increased.[15]

Discontinuation

The most common reasons for discontinuation of intrauterine contraception are unacceptable vaginal bleeding and pain.

Another reason is PID/infection. Discontinuation rates for all reasons are similar for different IUDs – framed or frameless – and for LNG-IUS [A].

Risks

Expulsion

Expulsion of intrauterine contraception occurs in approximately 1 in 20 women and is most common in the first 3 months after insertion and often during menstruation [B]. A Cochrane review found a small excess in expulsions with Multiload Cu375 compared to TCu380A in the fourth and subsequent years. The expulsion rate for a frameless Cu-IUD was higher than the TCu380A at 1 year. Early expulsions with a frameless device (GyneFix) are common.[16]

In general there is no difference in the rates of expulsion of the various IUDs and between IUD and IUS [A].

PID

Although there is a six-fold increase in the risk of PID in the 20 days after the insertion of intrauterine contraception the overall risk is low unless there is exposure to STIs [B].

Management

In a woman with an intrauterine contraceptive *in situ* and with signs and symptoms suggestive of pelvic infection then appropriate antibiotics should be commenced. Where possible triple swabs should be taken prior to commencing antibiotic therapy. There is no need to remove the device at this stage. The intrauterine method can be removed if symptoms fail to improve 72 hours after commencement of antibiotics.

The removal should be carried out at an appropriate time (see above in prerequisites for insertion and removal). There may even be a need to give emergency hormonal contraception following the removal. The woman should be followed up to ensure resolution of symptoms, counselling for safer sex and partner notification. The partner also needs to be treated with appropriate antibiotics.

Presence of Actinomyces-like organisms (ALOs)

ALOs can be detected on smears in women who have intrauterine contraception *in situ*.

Management

If there are no signs or symptoms suggestive of pelvic infection then there is no need to remove the device. Neither there is any need for subsequent screening.

If symptoms of infection develop then the woman should be advised to seek medical advice. Other causes of infection, e.g. STIs, should be considered at this stage.

Perforation

The risk of uterine perforation associated with intrauterine contraception is up to 2 per 1000 insertions [B]. It is more common at the time of insertion. Women should be informed about signs and symptoms of uterine perforation and infection. There should be a 6-week interval after an asymptomatic, suspected perforation before an IUD/IUS insertion is attempted again.

Management

If perforation is suspected at the time of insertion the procedure should be stopped and vital signs (blood pressure and pulse rate) and level of discomfort monitored until they are stable. An ultrasound scan and/or plain abdominal X-ray should be organised to locate the device if it has been left *in situ*.

Ectopic pregnancy

The ectopic pregnancy rate for Cu-IUD users is 0.02 per 100 WY (0.3–0.5 per 100 WY for those not using contraception) [A].

Bleeding patterns and pain

Spotting, light bleeding, heavier or longer periods are common in the first 3–6 months following Cu-IUD insertion (C). These bleeding patterns usually decrease with time.

Irregular bleeding and spotting is common during the first 6–8 months of LNG-IUS insertion. By 1 year amenorrhoea or light bleeding ensues [B].

Management

Women who experience problematic bleeding while using an intrauterine contraceptive should have a sexual history taken to establish STI risk and/or be investigated for gynaecological pathology if clinically indicated. When these have been excluded, bleeding problems in cases of LNG-IUS can be treated with mefenamic acid or ethinylestradiol (alone or as an oral contraceptive) provided there are no contraindications to estrogen therapy. Non-steroidal anti-inflammatory drugs or antifibnolytics, e.g. tranexamic acid, can be used to treat abnormal bleeding with Cu-IUDs.

Vasovagal syncope

The incidence of vasovagal syncope at intrauterine contraception insertions is 0.2–2.1 per cent. The signs of syncope are sweating, pallor and bradycardia: a pulse of <60 bpm.

Management

- Abandon procedure, lower head or raise legs;
- Remove instruments and + coil;
- Monitor blood pressure and pulse;
- Administer oxygen (FSRH – essential for intrauterine-contraception-inserting clinics).

Medication

- Atropine IV (0.6 mg/mL) (bradycardia: heart rate <40 bpm or systolic blood pressure <90 mmHg);
- Repeat every few minutes up to a dose of 3 mg.

Lost threads

Management

Women should be advised to use another method until it is confirmed that the device is *in situ*. The cervical canal can be explored with a thread retriever or a Spencer Wells forceps to bring the threads down if they are in the canal. If this is not successful then an ultrasound scan of the pelvis should be organised. If the intrauterine method is not located on ultrasound then a plain X-ray of the abdomen should be arranged to identify an extrauterine location. It is presumed that the intrauterine method has been extruded, if there is failure to visualise the device on X-ray.

Pregnancy

Management

An ectopic pregnancy should be excluded. If the threads of the device are visible then the intrauterine method should be removed up to 12 weeks' gestation. Women who become pregnant with an intrauterine contraception *in situ* should be informed of the increased risks of second-trimester miscarriage, preterm delivery and infection if the intrauterine method is left *in situ*. Removal would reduce adverse outcomes but is associated with a small risk of miscarriage.

Hormonal side effects

Due to the systemic absorption of LNG (though in very small amounts) progestogenic side effects such as headaches, mood changes, acne, breast tenderness or change in libido can occur with LNG-IUS [C].

Ovarian cysts

There has been a slightly increased incidence of functional ovarian cysts in LNG-IUS users compared to IUD users [B].[17]

Non-contraceptive benefits

LNG-IUS reduces menstrual blood loss and decreases pain and is therefore used as first-line therapy for heavy menstrual bleeding. It provides endometrial protection from the stimulatory effects of oestrogens and is used with oestrogen therapy in the management of menopausal symptoms [B]. It can also be used in the management of endometriosis.

PROGESTOGEN-ONLY INJECTABLE CONTRACEPTION (BOXES 72.9, 72.10)

Three POICs are available in the UK. They are:

- Depot medroxyprogesterone acetate (DMPA) 150 mg given as deep intramuscular (IM) every 12 weeks. It is the most commonly used POIC in the UK.

Box 72.9 POIC: UKMEC Category 3 – Risks generally outweigh benefits

UKMEC Category 3 – Risks generally outweigh benefits
Cardiovascular disease – multiple risk factors for arterial cardiovascular disease
Hypertension – vascular disease
Current and history of ischaemic heart disease and stroke
Unexplained vaginal bleeding
Breast cancer – past and no evidence of disease for 5 years
Diabetes – nephropathy, retinopathy, neuropathy and other vascular disease
Cirrhosis – severe (decompensated)
Liver tumours – hepatocellular adenoma and malignant hepatoma
SLE – positive or unknown antiphospholipid antibodies

Box 72.10 POIC: UKMEC Category 4 – Unacceptable health risk and should not be used

POIC: UKMEC Category 4 – Unacceptable health risk and should not be used
Breast cancer - current

- Subcutaneous DMPA (Sayana Press) 104 mg given subcutaneously every 13 weeks. It has been available in the UK since June 2013. It is bioequivalent to IM DMPA. It is administered via Unijet which is a new delivery system and is in a pre-filled injector which needs to be shaken vigorously to ensure a uniform suspension. It can be injected into the upper anterior thigh or anterior abdomen. Rates of bone loss, amenorrhoea, weight gain and return to fertility are the same as for IM DMPA. It will be beneficial for women who are on anticoagulants as there is less likelihood of haematoma formation. Also it may be more advantageous for very obese women when there is concern that the injection may not reach the muscle.
- Norethisterone enanthate (NET-EN) 200 mg, licensed for short-term use. It is also given deep IM but 8-weekly.

Mode of action

The main mode of action is inhibition of ovulation [C]. Thickening of the cervical mucus prevents sperm penetration into the upper reproductive tract. It also brings about changes in the endometrium making the environment unfavourable for implantation.

Effectiveness

The failure rate of DMPA is <4 in 1000 over 2 years [A].

Return of fertility

There is a delay in the return of fertility of up to 1 year with POIC [C]. However there is no evidence to suggest that fertility is reduced in the long term.

Discontinuation

Fifty per cent of POIC users will discontinue the method within 1 year. The main reasons for discontinuation are bleeding problems and weight gain [B].

Side effects

Bleeding problems

Amenorrhoea, spotting, infrequent bleeding or prolonged bleeding can occur with POICs. Amenorrhoea is more likely as duration of use increases. A third of women are amenorrhoeic at 3 months and 70 per cent by 12 months of use [B].[18]

Women who experience problematic bleeding while using a POIC should have a sexual history taken to establish STI risk and/or be investigated for gynaecological pathology if clinically indicated. When these have been excluded bleeding problems can be treated with mefenamic acid or ethinylestradiol (alone or as an oral contraceptive) provided there are no contraindications to estrogen therapy [C]. Sometimes giving the injection 2 weeks earlier helps with the bleeding but this is not evidence based.

Weight gain

The average weight gain among women using DMPA is between 2 and 6 kg. It tends to be more in women with a BMI >30 than in those with a BMI of <25.

Health concerns

Cardiovascular disease

POICs do not appear to be associated with an increased risk of stroke, VTE or myocardial infarction [C]. They are medically safe for women when estrogens are contraindicated.

Bone mineral density (BMD)

Concerns have been raised about the potential detrimental effects of DMPA on BMD. There has been particular concern about use of DMPA in women aged <18 years (who have not yet attained their peak bone mass) and among older women (who are approaching the menopause, when bone loss will occur). DMPA is associated with a small loss of BMD which mostly recovers when DMPA is discontinued [B]. There is no evidence that DMPA increases fracture risk in present or past users [E].

The Department of Health MHRA[19] issued guidance that was endorsed by the FSRH on the use of DMPA as follows:

- In women aged under 18 years DMPA may be used as first-line contraception after all options have been discussed and considered unsuitable or unacceptable [C].
- A re-evaluation of the risks and benefits of treatment for all women should be carried out every 2 years in those who wish to continue use [E].
- For women with significant lifestyle and/or medical risk factors for osteoporosis other methods of contraception should be considered.

Drug interactions

Enzyme-inducing drugs do not reduce the contraceptive efficacy of DMPA. Therefore the injection intervals do not have to be reduced [C].

Non-contraceptive benefits

This improves dysmenorrhoea and the symptoms of endometriosis.

PROGESTOGEN-ONLY IMPLANT (BOXES 72.11, 72.12)

Nexplanon is the only POI available in the UK. It has replaced Implanon. Nexplanon is bioequivalent to Implanon. It is a single rod which contains 68 mg of ENG in a membrane of ethylene vinyl acetate. It is licensed for 3 years [C] just like Implanon. Nexplanon is radio-opaque and has a different introducer and insertion technique to the Implanon.

Other POIs are Norplant, a six-rod LNG implant, and Jadelle, a two-rod LNG implant. These implants are licensed for 5 years' use. They are not available in the UK but UK healthcare professionals may see women who have had them inserted in other countries.

Box 72.11 POI: UKMEC Category 3 – Risks generally outweigh benefits

UKMEC Category 3 – Risks generally outweigh benefits
Current and history of ischaemic heart disease and stroke – continuation of the method
Unexplained vaginal bleeding
Breast cancer – past and no evidence of disease for 5 years
Cirrhosis – severe (decompensated)
Liver tumours – hepatocellular adenoma and malignant hepatoma
SLE – positive or unknown antiphospholipid antibodies

Box 72.12 POI: UKMEC Category 4 – Unacceptable health risk and should not be used

POI: UKMEC Category 4 – Unacceptable health risk and should not be used
Breast cancer - current

Mode of action

The main mode of action is inhibition of ovulation [B]. Thickening of the cervical mucus prevents sperm penetration into the upper reproductive tract. It also brings about changes in the endometrium making the environment unfavourable for implantation.

Effectiveness

The overall pregnancy rate is <1 in 1000 over 3 years' use [B]. The interaction of any enzyme-inducing medication, e.g. certain anticonvulsants, antiretroviral therapy, rifampicin or rifabutin, is not harmful to women but it is likely to reduce the effectiveness of the implant.

Therefore CONSISTENT USE OF CONDOMS IS RECOMMENDED.

Use of other contraceptives should be encouraged for women who are long-term users of any of these drugs.

Side effects

Bleeding problems

Bleeding irregularities are common with POIs. They include prolonged bleeding, irregular bleeding and oligomenorrhoea/amenorrhoea. Up to 20 per cent of women using implants will be amenorrhoeic [C].

Women who experience problematic bleeding while using a POI should have a sexual history taken to establish STI risk and/or be investigated for gynaecological pathology if clinically indicated. When these have been excluded, bleeding problems can be treated with mefenamic acid or ethinylestradiol (alone or as an oral contraceptive) provided there are no contraindications to estrogen therapy [C].

Weight gain

This has been reported in various studies ranging from 3–12 per cent.

Other changes

Mood changes and loss of libido can occur. Acne can improve, occur or worsen whilst using the implant. There is no evidence of a causal association between the use of an implant and headache [C].

Discontinuation

Rates of up to 43 per cent within 3 years have been reported [C]. A third of the women discontinue because of bleeding irregularities. Less than 10 per cent discontinue the method because of other side effects.

Complications with removal

Complications (only in the region of 1 per cent of removals) include deeply sited, non-palpable, broken or migrated implants. As Nexplanon contains barium sulphate it is radio-opaque. Hence it can be identified on X-rays. Ultrasound and MRI can also be used to locate the implants.

Complicated implants should be referred to specialised centres for removal.

Health concerns

VTE

There is little or no increase in the risk of VTE with the use of POIs [C].

BMD

There is no evidence to suggest that POIs have any clinically significant effect on BMD [C].

Endocarditis

Prophylactic antibiotics to prevent endocarditis are not needed for insertion and removal of implants [E].

EMERGENCY CONTRACEPTION

Emergency contraception (EC) prevents a pregnancy following any unprotected sexual intercourse (UPSI). In 2002, a Judicial Review ruled that pregnancy begins at implantation and *not* at fertilisation: thus EC is not considered an abortifacient. Three methods of EC are available in the UK:

Intrauterine device

A copper IUD can be inserted up to 5 days after the first episode of UPSI. If the timing of ovulation can be estimated, insertion can be beyond 5 days of UPSI, as long as it does not occur beyond 5 days after ovulation [C]. It is effective immediately after insertion. IUDs with banded copper on the arms and containing at least 380 mm^2 of copper have the lowest failure rates and should be the first-line choice, particularly if the woman intends to continue the IUD as long-term contraception [A]. The failure rate is 1 per cent.

Prerequisites

Prior to emergency IUD insertion, women at higher risk of STIs (age <25 years, change in sexual partner, or more than one partner in the last year) should be offered testing for *Chlamydia trachomatis* (as a minimum) [C]. For women assessed as being at higher risk of STIs, if results of testing are not available at the time of emergency IUD insertion, the use of prophylactic antibiotics, at least to cover chlamydia, should be considered (Good Practice).

Mode of action

This is the same as for routine IUDs.

Contraindications

The same contraindications apply as for routine IUD insertions.

Hormonal methods

Progestogen-only emergency contraception (POEC)

LNG – Levonelle 1500, Levonelle One Step

Mode of action

Its exact mode of action is not known but it is thought that it works mainly by inhibiting ovulation. It prevents follicular rupture. LNG is given in a single dose of 1.5 mg as soon as possible after UPSI and within 72 hours [A]. However it can also be given up to 96 hours outside product licence, but there is limited evidence of efficacy [E]. It can be used more than once in a cycle. The WHOMEC for contraceptive use advises that there are no medical contraindications to the use of hormonal EC. Women who are on liver enzyme-inducing drugs should be advised to take double the dose, i.e. 3 mg of LNG [C]. This use is outside the product licence.

Ulipristal acetate (UPA)

ellaOne

This is a selective progesterone receptor modulator (SRPM).

Mode of action

Its primary mode of action is thought to be inhibition or delay of ovulation. It can prevent ovulation after the LH surge has started.

How should it be used?

One tablet should be taken orally as soon as possible, but no later than 120 hours after UPSI or contraceptive failure. If vomiting occurs within 3 hours, another tablet should be taken. Ulipristal is not recommended to be used more than once per cycle as the safety of efficacy of repeated exposure has not been assessed. If hormonal contraception is continued after administering UPA, barrier contraception should be used until the next period or withdrawal bleed.

Effectiveness

Individual studies suggest that UPA is as effective as LNG for EC. There have been no studies comparing the efficacy of UPA to the IUD for the purpose of EC. A meta-analysis suggests that regardless of the type of EC drug used, the risk of pregnancy is significantly increased with increasing BMI.[21]

Contraindications

UPA is contraindicated when there is a hypersensitivity to any of its excipients. It is not recommended in those with severe hepatic impairment, or in women with severe asthma. Breastfeeding women are advised not to breastfeed for 1 week after treatment as it is found in breast milk up to 5 days after intake.

Side effects

The most commonly reported side effects are abdominal pain and menstrual disorders, e.g. irregular vaginal bleeding, premenstrual syndrome and uterine cramps.

Does UPA interact with other drugs?

Liver enzyme inducers, e.g. rifampicin, phenytoin, carbamazepine, ritonavir and St John's Wort, may reduce plasma concentrations of UPA and may reduce efficacy. Use of UPA with antacids, proton pump inhibitors and H2 receptor antagonists, or any other drugs that increase gastric pH, may reduce absorption of UPA and decrease efficacy. Therefore it is not advisable to use UPA with liver enzyme-inducing drugs and drugs that increase gastric pH.

UPA binds to progesterone receptors and so may reduce the efficacy of progestogen-containing contraceptives. The CEU (Clinical Effectiveness Unit) therefore advises 14 days of extra precautions if commencing CHC, 16 days with Qlaira and 9 days with POP following UPA administration.

QUICK-STARTING CONTRACEPTION

Quick-starting contraception is contraception, when a woman requests it rather than waiting for the next period.

The clinician has to be reasonably certain that the woman is not pregnant or at risk of pregnancy. If the woman's preferred method is not available then a bridging method, e.g. CHC or POP, can be used till the preferred method is available.

Quick starting can also be initiated immediately after EC administration, but extra precautions need to be observed (Table 72.4). A pregnancy test should be advised 3 weeks after the last episode of UPSI.

STERILISATION

Sterilisation is a permanent and usually an irreversible method of contraception. In the UK about 50 per cent of couples over the age of 40 use this method.

Counselling and written information regarding the procedure, its risks, benefits and failure rates should be provided to the client. Discussion and information should also be given regarding other methods, especially the long-acting reversible methods of contraception.

Both men and women should be informed that reversal operations are rarely provided by the NHS.

Female sterilisation: tubal occlusion

Methods

Female sterilisation usually involves blocking both Fallopian tubes during laparotomy, mini-laparotomy, laparoscopy or via hysteroscopy.

The Pomeroy technique is the most widely used ligation technique. It involves using absorbable sutures to tie the base of a loop of the Fallopian tube near the mid-portion and cutting off the top of the loop. This procedure destroys 3–4 cm of the tube, making reversal more difficult.

Table 72.4 Summary of additional contraceptive requirements when quick-starting contraception. (Adapted from FSRH Quick Starting Contraception, CEU September 2010)

Method	Method of EC	Requirements for additional contraception (condoms/avoidance of sex)
Combined oral contraceptive pills (except Qlaira)	Quick starting after POEC	7 days
	Quick starting after UPA EC	14 days
Qlaira combined oral contraceptive pill	Quick starting after POEC	9 days
	Quick starting after UPA EC	16 days
Combined vaginal ring/transdermal patch	Quick starting after POEC	7 days
	Quick starting after UPA EC	14 days
Progestogen-only pill (traditional/desogestrel)	Quick starting after POEC	2 days
	Quick starting after UPA EC	9 days
Progestogen-only implant	Quick starting after POEC	7 days
	Quick starting after UPA EC	14 days
Progestogen-only injectable	Quick starting after POEC	7 days
	Quick starting after UPA EC	14 days

A modified Pomeroy procedure rather than Filshie clip application may be preferable for postpartum sterilisation performed by mini-laparotomy or at the time of caesarian section (CS), as this leads to lower failure rates [B]. Mechanical occlusion of the tubes by either Filshie clips or rings should be the method of choice for laparoscopic tubal occlusion [A]. Diathermy should not be used as the primary method of tubal occlusion because it increases the risk of subsequent ectopic pregnancy and is less easy to reverse than mechanical occlusive methods [C].

Hysteroscopic sterilisation by tubal cannulation and placement of intrafallopian implants

Micro-inserts made from nickel–titanium and stainless steel are inserted hysteroscopically through the cornual ends of both tubes. This can be performed under local anaesthesia and/or intravenous sedation. These generate fibrosis around the devices and the tubes are occluded by 3 months after the procedure. Additional contraception needs to be used until a hysterosalpingogram is performed at 3 months to confirm full occlusion of the tubes. It is an irreversible procedure and the failure rates quoted are the same as for the other methods of tubal occlusion.

Risks

Efficacy
The failure rate for female sterilisation is 1 in 200. Women should be informed that with tubal occlusion pregnancy can occur several years after the procedure.

Safety
There is no evidence to suggest that there is an increased incidence of bleeding problems and consequently an increased hysterectomy rate after tubal occlusion.

Adverse events for placement of intrafallopian implants include uterine or tubal perforation, infection, device migration or expulsion, pelvic pain and vasovagal reaction.

Male sterilisation: vasectomy

Methods
The technique of vasectomy involves division of the vas with fascial interposition or diathermy. RCOG advises that a no-scalpel technique should be used to identify the vas as there is a lower rate of early complications [A]. The procedure can be carried out under a local anaesthetic and is safer than female sterilisation. Following the procedure, men should be advised to use effective contraception until two consecutive semen samples 4 weeks apart confirm azoospermia. (The first sample should be taken at least 8 weeks after surgery.)

Risks

Failure rate
The failure rate for vasectomy is 1 in 2000. Both early and late failures can occur. Therefore men should be informed that pregnancies can occur several years after vasectomy. Early failures can occur because the wrong structure has been occluded (leaving one or both vasa intact) or because the vas is partially occluded (if ligatures or clips are applied too loosely). There could be congenital duplication of one or both vasa. Although the vasa may have been occluded bilaterally, if there are any more vasa, spermatozoa can still be released. Recanalisation of the vas can occur at an early or late stage. Early recanalisation is recognised by post-vasectomy sperm counts which may at first be azoospermic or reduced but then rapidly increase again. Late recanalisation presents with a pregnancy several months or years after two consecutive azoospermic samples.

Chronic testicular pain
This is probably due to distension and granuloma formation in the epididymis and vas deferens following the operation [B]. Men should be informed of this and reassured that there is no sinister association.

Cancer
There is no increase in testicular or prostatic cancers following the vasectomy operation [B].

Heart disease
There is no increased incidence of heart disease associated with vasectomy.

INDUCED ABORTION

The 1967 Abortion Act came into effect on 27 April 1968. The Human Fertilisation and Embryology Authority (HFEA) made changes to the Abortion Act in 1990 which came into effect on 1 April 1991. Section 4 of the Abortion Act 1967 states that no person is under any obligation to participate in any treatment authorised by the act. This does not apply in an emergency, where the woman's life is in immediate danger or there is immediate risk of grave or permanent injury.

The Abortion Act 1967 states that:

- the abortion must be performed within an NHS hospital or approved clinic;
- the Chief Medical Officer must be informed of the abortion that has taken place;
- two registered medical practitioners must certify in good faith that the operation is being performed for grounds specified within the act.

The 1967 Abortion Act amended by the HFEA in 1990 has five categories. They are:

A   The continuance of the pregnancy would involve risk to the life of the pregnant woman.

B   The termination is necessary to prevent grave permanent injury to the physical or mental health of the pregnant woman.

C   The pregnancy has not exceeded its 24th week and the continuance of the pregnancy would involve risk, greater than if the pregnancy were terminated, or injury to the physical or mental health of the pregnant woman.

D   The pregnancy has not exceeded its 24th week and the continuance of the pregnancy would involve risk, greater than if the pregnancy were terminated, or injury to the physical or mental health of any existing child(ren) of the family of the pregnant woman.

E   There is substantial risk that if the child were born it would suffer from such physical or mental abnormalities as to be seriously handicapped.

Ninety-eight per cent of abortions are carried out under the terms of 'C' of the Abortion Act.

Abortion under clause 'E' of the abortion act is legal beyond 24 weeks. Common reasons are chromosomal abnormalities and congenital malformations. Down's syndrome is the most commonly reported chromosomal abnormality.

Pre-abortion management

Pre-abortion management should include non-directive counselling to address alternatives to abortion, i.e. continuing with the pregnancy, adoption or fostering.

The majority of women will come to a decision quickly but there will be others who will require additional support. Care pathways for additional support, including access to social services, should be available.

A full medical history is taken. An ultrasound scan is usually carried out prior to the procedure to confirm an intrauterine pregnancy and its gestation. Blood tests include haemoglobin measurement, a full blood count and ABO and rhesus grouping [C]. Other tests are carried out if indicated depending on clinical grounds. Chlamydia screening should be offered to all. Details of the abortion methods, the procedures and their risks should be discussed with the woman. In order to prevent repeat terminations, discussion of future contraception is vital at this stage. Antibiotic prophylaxis at the time of surgical abortion reduces infective complications, whereas there is limited evidence of decreasing infections in case of medical abortions.

The following regimens are suitable for periabortion prophylaxis [C]:

- Metronidazole 1 g rectally or 800 mg orally prior to or at the time of abortion
  plus
- Doxycycline 100 mg orally twice daily for 7 days, commencing on the day of abortion
  OR

- Metronidazole 1 g rectally or 800 mg orally prior to or at the time of abortion
  plus
- Azithromycin 1 g orally on the day of abortion.

All chlamydia-positive women should have a full STI screening and contact tracing and treatment of partners.

Methods (Table 72.5, Fig 72.3)

Surgical procedures

Vacuum aspiration should be avoided at gestations below 7 weeks as the failure rate is higher. Conventional vacuum aspiration is an appropriate method at gestations of 7–15 weeks and can be carried out either under local or general anaesthesia [B]. For first-trimester suction termination, either electric or manual aspiration devices may be used, as both are effective and acceptable to women and clinicians. For gestations above 14 weeks, surgical abortion by D&E, preceded by cervical preparation, is safe and effective and should be undertaken by specialist practitioners who have a reasonable caseload to maintain their skills. Cervical preparation should be considered in all cases. The various regimens are:

- Up to 14 weeks: misoprostol 400 mg vaginally or sublingually 3 hours before surgery;
- 14–18 weeks: osmotic dilators.

Medical abortion

Medical abortion using mifepristone plus prostaglandin is the most effective method of abortion at gestations of less than 9 weeks [A].

The following regimen is safe and effective:

- Mifepristone* 200 mg orally followed 36–48 hours later by misoprostol 800 μg vaginally or sublingually. A second dose of 400 mg of misoprostol may have to be given for

  * This regimen is unlicensed.

Table 72.5 Abortion methods at different gestational ages

Gestation	Method
Up to 9 weeks	Early medical termination
Up to 10 to 11 weeks	Manual vacuum aspiration (MVA)
6 to 16 weeks	Vacuum aspiration under local or general anaesthesia
Above 14 weeks	Dilatation and evacuation (D&E) (cervical preparation)
9+ to 24 weeks	Medical method

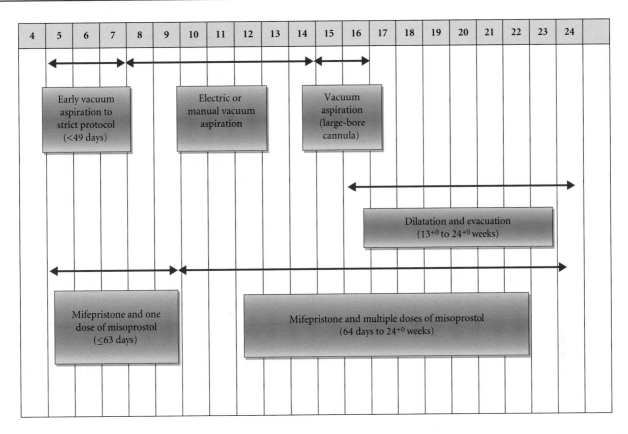

Fig. 72.3 Summary of abortion methods appropriate for use in abortion services in Great Britain by gestational age in weeks. (Reproduced from: FSRH Clinical Effectiveness Unit reports and reviews, 2008–2009, London: RCOG; with the permission of RCOG.)

gestations between 7 and 9 weeks if abortion has not occurred 4 hours after administration of misoprostol.

For gestations between 9 and 24 weeks the regimen is as follows:

- Mifepristone* 200 mg orally followed 36–48 hours later by misoprostol 800 μg vaginally. A maximum of 4 further doses of misoprostol 400 μg may be administered at 3-hourly intervals, vaginally or orally (depending on the amount of bleeding).

  * This regimen is unlicensed.

Complications

Retained products of conception

This is the commonest complication following abortion, more so following a medical abortion. An ultrasound scan is helpful in diagnosing retained products but the decision to intervene and perform a surgical evacuation should be made on clinical grounds.

Haemorrhage

The risk of haemorrhage is 1 in 1000 abortions. The risk is lower for early abortions (occurring in less than 1 in 1000 and rising to 4 in 1000 at more than 20 weeks) [B].

Uterine perforation

The incidence is 1–4 in 1000. The risk is lower for abortions performed early in pregnancy and those performed by experienced clinicians [B].

Uterine rupture

This has been reported in association with mid-trimester medical abortion. However, the risk is under 1 in 1000 [B].

Cervical trauma

The risk of damage to the external cervical os at the time of surgical abortion is moderate (no greater than 1 in 100) [B]. The risk is lower when abortion is performed early in pregnancy and when it is performed by an experienced clinician. Cervical preparation prior to the procedure decreases the risk of cervical trauma.

Failed abortion and continuing pregnancy

All methods of first-trimester abortion carry a small risk of failure to terminate the pregnancy (less than 1 in 100) necessitating another procedure.

Post-abortion infection

Genital tract infection, including PID of varying degrees of severity, can occur. The risk is reduced when prophylactic antibiotics are given or when lower genital tract infection has been excluded by bacteriological screening [B].

Future reproductive outcome

There is no evidence to suggest that induced abortion has any effect on subsequent ectopic pregnancy, placenta praevia or fertility. However, it may be associated with a small increase in the risk of subsequent miscarriage or preterm delivery [B].

Psychological sequelae

There is no evidence to suggest that these are increased following an induced abortion.

Aftercare

Rhesus prophylaxis

Anti-D immunoglobulin G (250 IU before 20 weeks of gestation and 500 IU thereafter) should be given to all non-sensitised Rhesus-negative women within 72 hours following abortion, whether by surgical or medical methods [B].

Contraception

This should have been discussed at the pre-abortion assessment. The chosen method of contraception can be initiated immediately following the abortion. Oral contraceptives can be commenced on the following day of the procedure. Injectables can be administered on the same day, whilst the subdermal implant and intrauterine contraception can be inserted immediately following a first- or second-trimester termination of pregnancy. Sterilisation can also be safely performed at the time of induced abortion. However, this is associated with higher rates of failure and regret on the part of the woman [B].

Follow-up

Women should be given written information about the symptoms they may experience following the abortion. They should be given a 24-hour telephone helpline number to contact in case of any problems. Routine follow-up following a successful abortion is not necessary.

Published guidelines

FFPRHC Guidelines at www.ffprhc.org.uk or www.fsrh.org:

- Barrier Methods for Contraception and STI Prevention, August 2012
- Combined Hormonal Contraception, October 2011
- CEU Guidance: Quick-Starting Contraception, September 2010
- CEU Statement: Hysteroscopic Sterilisation, October 2010
- CEU Statement: Nexplanon,® updated November 2010
- CEU Statement: Update on use of Ulipristal (ellaOne) in breastfeeding women, March 2013
- Emergency Contraception Guidance, updated January 2012
- CEU Statement: Estradiol/Nomegestrol Combined Pill. Zoely,© May 2013
- Intrauterine Contraception, November 2007
- Management of Unscheduled Bleeding in Women Using Hormonal Contraception, May 2009
- Missed-Pill Recommendations, May 2011
- Progestogen-only Pills, updated June 2009
- Progestogen-only Injectable Contraception, updated June 2009
- Progestogen-only Implants, April 2008
- Statement on Drug Interactions between Hormonal Contraception and Ulipristal Products: ellaOne® and Esmya,® November 2012
- CEU statement: Subcutaneous Depot Medroxyprogesterone Acetate (Sayana Press®) New product review, FSRH, June 2013
- UK Medical Eligibility Criteria for Contraceptive Use, 2009
- UK Selected Practice Recommendations for Contraceptive Use, 2002
- Use of UPA in breastfeeding women. FSRH, updated from CEU, March 2013
- Ulipristal Acetate (ellaOne), October 2009

RCOG Guidelines at www.rcog.org.uk:

- Male and Female Sterilisation. Evidence-based Clinical Guideline Number 4, January 2004
- The Care of Women Requesting Induced Abortion. Evidence-based Clinical Guideline Number 7, November 2011

NICE Guidelines at www.nice.org.uk:

- Long-acting Reversible Contraception (C630)
- Hysteroscopic Sterilisation By Tubal Cannulation And Placement Of Intra-Fallopian Implants. NICE Interventional Procedure Guidance 315, September 2009

Key References

1. WHO. *Medical Eligibility Criteria for Contraceptive Use.* 3rd edn. WHO, 2008.
2. FSRH. *UK Medical Eligibility Criteria for Contraceptive Use.* FSRH, 2009.
3. WHO. 9th Annual Report, 1980.
4. Glasier A, Gebbie A. *Handbook of Family Planning and Reproductive Healthcare.* 5th edn. Edinburgh: Churchill Livingstone Elsevier, 2008.
5. Marshall J. A prospective trial of mucothermic method of natural family planning. *Int Rev Nat Fam Plann.* 1985;9:139–43.
6. WHO. A prospective multicentre trial of the ovulation method of natural family planning II. The effectiveness phase. *Fertil Steril* 1981;36:591–8.
7. Kennedy KI, Rivera R, McNeilly AS. Consensus statement on the use of breastfeeding as a family planning method. *Contraception* 1989;39:477–96.

REPRODUCTIVE GYNAECOLOGY

8. Guillebaud J. *Contraception: Your Questions Answered.* 5ᵗʰ edn. Edinburgh: Churchill Livingstone Elsevier, 2009.

9. Lidegaard Ø, Løkkegaard E, Svendsen AL, Agger C. Hormonal contraception and risk of venous thromboembolism: national follow-up study. *BMJ* 2009;339:b2890.

10. Van Hylckama Vlieg A, Helmerhorst FM, Vandenbroucke JP, Doggen CJM, Rosendaal FR. Effects of oestrogen dose and progestogen type on venous thrombotic risk associated with oral contraceptives: results of the MEGA case-control study. *BMJ* 2009;339:b2921.

11. Khader YS, Rice J, John L, Abueita O. Oral contraceptive use and the risk of myocardial infarction: a meta-analysis. *Contraception* 2003;68:11–17.

12. Collaborative Group on Hormonal Factors in Breast Cancer. Breast cancer and hormonal contraceptives: collaborative re-analysis of individual data on 53,297 women with breast cancer and 100,239 women without breast cancer from 54 epidemiological studies. *Lancet* 1996;347:1713–27.

13. Mansour D. Qlaira: A 'natural' change of direction. *Journal of Family Planning and Reproductive Healthcare* 2009;35 (3):139–142.

14. Shimoni N, Westhoff C. Review of the vaginal contraceptive ring (Nuva Ring). *Journal of Family Planning and Reproductive Healthcare* 2008;34(4):247–50.

15. FSRH CEU. *Recommendation: Antibiotic prophylaxis for intrauterine contraceptive use in women at risk of bacterial endocarditis.* FSRH, July 2008.

16. Kulier R, O'Brien P, Helmerhorst F, Usher-Patel M, D'Arcangues C. Copper-containing, framed intrauterine devices for contraception. *Cochrane Database Syst Rev* 2007;(4):CD005347.

17. Robinson GE, Bounds W, Kubba AA, Adams J, Guillebaud J. Functional ovarian cysts associated with the levonorgestrel releasing intrauterine device. *Br J Fam Plann* 1989;14:132.

18. Canto De Cetina TE, Canto P, Ordoñez Luna M. Effect of counseling to improve compliance in Mexican women receiving depot-medroxyprogesterone acetate. *Contraception* 2001;63:143–146.

19. Medicines and Healthcare Products Regulatory Agency. *Updated Guidance on the Use of DepoProveraContraception,* 8 November 2004. Available from: http://www.mhra.gov.uk/Safetyinformation/Safetywarningsalertsandrecalls/Safetywarningsandmessagesformedicines/CON1004262.

20. FSRH. *New Product Review: Ulipristal Acetate (ellaOne).* CEU. October 2009.

21. Ulmann A, Scherrer B, Mathe H, Gainer E, HRA Pharm. Meta-analysis demonstrating superiority of the selective progesterone receptor modulator ulipristal acetate versus levonorgestrel for emergency contraception. Abstract and Poster Presentation presented at the 8th Congress of the European Society of Gynecology, Rome, Italy, 10–13 September 2009.

22. Lohr P, Fjerstad M, DeSilva U, Lyres R. Abortion. *BMJ* 2014;348:29–33.

Chapter 73 Endometrial function

Hilary OD Critchley and Christine P West

MRCOG standards

- Understand the physiology of normal menstruation.

INTRODUCTION

The main function of the endometrium is to receive a fertilised ovum (blastocyst) during implantation. As this occurs relatively infrequently, cyclical breakdown and regeneration of the endometrium during the menstrual cycle are pivotal reproductive events. These changes are under the control of the hypothalamic–pituitary–ovarian axis, with ovarian steroids acting directly within the endometrium via local intracellular receptors. Many other local mediators are involved in the complex and dynamic processes that take place within this metabolically highly active organ.

ENDOCRINE REGULATION OF ENDOMETRIAL FUNCTION

The uterine endometrium is a target organ for sex steroids and is exposed to an orchestrated sequence of circulating oestrogen, progesterone and progesterone withdrawal (result of regression of the corpus luteum in absence of pregnancy). Sequential exposure to oestrogen and progesterone, as a consequence of cyclical ovarian activity, results in repeated episodes of cellular proliferation and differentiation with regular menstrual bleeding.[1,2] The proliferative phase of the endometrial cycle corresponds to the ovarian follicular phase. The secretory phase of endometrial differentiation is under progesterone domination and corresponds to the ovarian luteal phase. In the follicular phase, oestrogen secreted from the dominant follicle promotes regeneration and proliferation of the endometrium with up-regulation of both oestrogen (ERs) and progesterone receptors (PRs). The mid-secretory phase is a period of peak exposure to circulating progesterone and is often referred to as the 'implantation window'.

Endometrial expression of sex steroid receptors permits the endometrium to respond to ovarian oestradiol and progesterone. Exposure of the endometrium to these sex steroids, acting via their cognate receptors (ERs and PRs) results in a cascade of gene expression that is essential for preparation of the endometrium in anticipation of successful implantation. In the absence of a pregnancy, the corpus luteum regresses, progesterone levels fall and progesterone withdrawal is the trigger for the cascade of events that culminate in shedding of the upper zone of the endometrium.

Menstruation is a fundamental reproductive process in women and displays all the hallmarks of an inflammatory event. Equal in importance to the shedding of the endometrium is its regeneration (repair), which commences 36 hours after the onset of bleeding and is normally completed by day 5–6 of the cycle. The processes involved in endometrial repair remain to be defined; however they are likely to share common features with wound-healing processes. Thus endometrial repair will involve overlapping phases of inflammation, its resolution, tissue formation, remodelling and angiogenesis.[3,4] The capacity of the human endometrium to efficiently regenerate each month also supports the presence of adult progenitor cells within the local endometrial environment (for a detailed review of this aspect of endometrial biology see Gargett *et al.* 2012[4]).

MORPHOLOGICAL CHANGES

The three classic phases of the menstrual cycle are the oestrogen-dominated proliferative phase, the post-ovulatory and progesterone-dominated secretory phase, and the menstrual phase.[5]

The endometrium is composed of two layers. The upper functional layer is shed during menstruation. During the follicular phase of the cycle the endometrium proliferates from the basal layer in response to oestradiol. The developing glands are initially straight and tubular within a compact stroma but later become more convoluted. Following ovulation, exposure to rising levels of progesterone from the corpus luteum induces secretory changes in the endometrial glands. Sub-nuclear vacuoles appear initially, followed by evidence of glandular secretory activity. This is accompanied in the late luteal phase by oedema and predecidual changes in the stroma and increased coiling of the spiral arterioles, which supply the endometrium.

Failure of conception results in regression of the corpus luteum and an abrupt decline in circulating levels of oestrogen and progesterone. In the endometrium there is loss of tissue fluid, stromal infiltration of leukocytes and intense vasoconstriction of the spiral arterioles. Distal ischaemia and vasodilatation lead to tissue breakdown and bleeding from the damaged vessels. Thirty-six hours after the onset of bleeding, the process of endometrial regeneration commences in the basal layer.[6]

CELLULAR AND MOLECULAR EVENTS

Progesterone is the endocrine signal that is responsible for the establishment and maintenance of pregnancy. Progesterone withdrawal is the primary initiating event for the cascade of molecular and cellular events that lead to menstruation. Following shedding of the upper functional layer, the endometrium displays remarkable and immediate regenerative capacity.[3]

The precise local mechanisms involved in the control of the highly coordinated cyclical tissue 'injury' and 'repair' that occur in the absence of a pregnancy have still to be fully elucidated. Modern molecular technologies have permitted an expansion of knowledge of gene profiles across the menstrual cycle, including during the 'putative window' of implantation and at the time of progesterone withdrawal.

Valuable insight about progesterone action and endometrial function has come from the observations of pharmacological withdrawal of progesterone from the endometrium. Studies with PR ligands have identified local mechanisms that may be targeted in order to modulate both endometrial receptivity and endometrial bleeding.[7]

The molecular and cellular mechanisms within the uterine endometrium regulating the key reproductive events – implantation and menstruation – involve complex interactions between the endocrine, vascular and immune systems.[3,8] Oestrogen and progesterone, via cognate receptors, regulate the expression of a cascade of local factors within the endometrium that act in a paracrine, autocrine and intracrine manner.

The receptors for sex steroids are members of a large family of nuclear transcription factors that regulate the expression of numerous genes. Members of the nuclear receptor super-family expressed by endometrial cells include progesterone (PR), oestrogen (ERα and ERβ), androgen (AR) and glucocorticoid receptors (GR). The role for these latter two receptors in regulation of endometrial function has thus far received limited attention.[9] The endometrial expression of the PR, ERα and ERβ varies temporally and spatially across the menstrual cycle. Both endometrial ERα and PRs are up-regulated during the proliferative phase by ovarian oestradiol and subsequently down-regulated in the secretory phase by progesterone. The administration of a PR antagonist,

mifepristone (RU486) in the early secretory phase will block the progesterone-induced down-regulation of PR (and ERα) in non-pregnant human endometrium.

The localisation of the PRs in the human endometrium is well documented, with maximal expression in glandular and stromal cells during the mid-late proliferative phase and decreased expression in epithelial cells (maintenance of stromal expression) in the secretory phase.[10] There are two main isoforms, PRA and PRB. Both are nuclear receptors that shuttle between the cytoplasm and nucleus. PRA and PRB are reduced in the glandular epithelium during the secretory phase; however PRA is maintained in the stroma.[11–13] PRs are not present in endometrial endothelial cells or immune cells, indicating that actions of progesterone on these cell types are indirect or paracrine in nature. It is this differential expression of PRs that may explain the early reversibility of induction of menstruation. Early P-withdrawal events occur in PR-positive cells enabling cessation of the inflammatory response with the replacement of progesterone. Subsequent events probably involve PR-negative cells, e.g. immune cells, thereby rendering the cascade of events leading to endometrial breakdown (menses) inevitable.

Oestrogen action is mediated by the two subtypes of oestrogen receptor referred to as ERα and ERβ. These two structurally related subtypes of ER are derived from separate genes. In the upper functional layer, ERα expression increases in both glandular and stromal cells in the proliferative phase and declines in the secretory phase due to suppression by progesterone. In the basal layer, ERα is expressed in glandular and stromal cells throughout the menstrual cycle. In the endometrium, the only sex steroid receptor present in the endothelium and smooth muscle walls of endometrial vessels is ERβ. Thus any direct effects of oestrogen on endometrial vessels, including angiogenesis and permeability, will be mediated by ERβ, and the actions of progestins will be mediated indirectly by perivascular stromal cells. The function of ERβ in the uterus is still to be determined. The physiological role of endometrial AR has also not been established. During the normal cycle stromal cells are the predominant cell type expressing the ARs and thus androgen effects in the endometrium are likely to be mediated by the stroma. A more detailed discussion of the mechanisms of steroid receptor function in the endometrium is outwith the scope of this brief review.

The availability of molecular technologies, including microarray studies and detailed bioinformatics analysis, has contributed to the expanding literature on gene profiles during the progesterone-dominant 'receptive phase' of human endometrium.[14] This knowledge is important for understanding the requirements for a receptive endometrium and successful implantation and how disturbances of endometrial structure and function may play a role in subfertility. Equally important is the insight such knowledge has provided for fertility control (contraception). Valuable insight about progesterone action, progesterone withdrawal and endometrial function has come from the observations of pharmacological withdrawal of progesterone from the endometrium. Studies with ligands for the PR have advanced our understanding of local mechanisms that may be targeted to modulate both endometrial receptivity and endometrial bleeding.

Disturbances of the tightly controlled sequence of injury and repair events within the endometrium contribute to menstrual disorders, such as heavy menstrual bleeding (HMB). A new classification of causes of abnormal uterine bleeding (see Chapter 75) should facilitate future research into endometrial disorders which contribute to such problems.[15,16] Early studies of menstruation identified a role for prostaglandins (PGs). Progesterone withdrawal results in increases in endometrial PG synthesis and decreases in PG metabolism. More recent research has shed light upon the complex molecular and cellular events within the endometrium following withdrawal of progesterone.[1,3,8] Local mediators within the endometrium that have been implicated in the regulation of the menstrual process include: cyclooxygenase-2 (COX-2), the inducible enzyme responsible for synthesis of PGs; chemokines (e.g. CXCL8, neutrophil chemotactic factor, interleukin-8 (IL-8); and CCL-2, monocyte chemotactic peptide-1, MCP-1); and a role for hypoxia.[3] PG synthesis via COX-2 is relevant since non-steroidal anti-inflammatory drugs (NSAIDs) are widely used in the treatment of menstrual complaints including heavy and painful periods. Changes in the structure and viability of the endometrium are due to the release of mediators that degrade the extracellular matrix including matrix metalloproteinases (MMPs).[17] A phenomenon of blood vessel function at menstruation is modest platelet aggregation and fibrin deposition compared to that following vessel damage elsewhere in the body. It is notable that menstrual bleeding extends over 3–5 days and is not accompanied by scarring. The uterus is a rich source of PGs and uterine fluid contains high fibrinolytic activity and fibrin degradation products, suggesting active fibrinolysis occurs. Indeed agents targeting the fibrinolytic system are a first-line management for complaints of HMB. Given limitations with current treatments, novel therapeutic interventions are being explored, including the role(s) for selective progesterone modulators (SPRMs) in the pre-surgical and medical management of uterine fibroids.[18]

Following menstruation the endometrium rapidly repairs with regeneration of all cell types (epithelial, vascular and stromal). The exposed surface is rapidly covered with fibronectin, leukocytes are removed and the epithelium regenerates. Full repair is usually complete by day 6 of the menstrual cycle. A host of local mediators are involved in endometrial repair, including IL-8 endothelins and vascular endothelial growth factor (VEGF). These factors also play a key role in the angiogenic processes necessary for reconstitution of the endometrial vasculature.[3]

ACKNOWLEDGEMENT

We thank Sheila Milne for assistance with manuscript preparation.

References

1. Jabbour HN, Kelly RW, Fraser HM, Critchley HO. Endocrine regulation of menstruation. *Endocr Rev* 2006;27:17–46.

2. Critchley HO, Maybin JA. Molecular and cellular causes of abnormal uterine bleeding of endometrial origin. *Semin Reprod Med* 2011;29:400–9.

3. Maybin JA, Critchley HO. Steroid regulation of menstrual bleeding and endometrial repair. *Rev Endocr Metab Disord* 2012;13:253–63.

4. Gargett CE, Nguyen HP, Ye L. Endometrial regeneration and endometrial stem/progenitor cells. *Rev Endocr Metab Disord* 2012;13:235–51.

5. Noyes RW, Hertig AT, Rock J. Dating the endometrial biopsy. *Fertil Steril* 1950;1:3–25.

6. Garry R, Hart R, Karthigasu KA, Burke C. Structural changes in endometrial basal glands during menstruation. *BJOG* 2010;117:1175–85.

7. Critchley HO, Kelly RW, Baird DT, Brenner RM. Regulation of human endometrial function: mechanisms relevant to uterine bleeding. *Reprod Biol Endocrinol* 2006;4 Suppl 1:S5.

8. Critchley HO, Kelly RW, Brenner RM, Baird DT. The endocrinology of menstruation: a role for the immune system. *Clin Endocrinol (Oxf)* 2001;55:701–10.

9. Critchley HO, Saunders PT. Hormone receptor dynamics in a receptive human endometrium. *Reprod Sci* 2009;16:191–9.

10. Lessey BA, Killam AP, Metzger DA, Haney AF, Greene GL, McCarty KS, Jr. Immunohistochemical analysis of human uterine estrogen and progesterone receptors throughout the menstrual cycle. *J Clin Endocrinol Metab* 1988;67:334–40.

11. Brosens JJ, Hayashi N, White JO. Progesterone receptor regulates decidual prolactin expression in differentiating human endometrial stromal cells. *Endocrinology* 1999;140:4809–20.

12. Wang H, Critchley HO, Kelly RW, Shen D, Baird DT. Progesterone receptor subtype B is differentially regulated in human endometrial stroma. *Mol Hum Reprod* 1998;4:407–12.

13. Mote PA, Johnston JF, Manninen T, Tuohimaa P, Clarke CL. Detection of progesterone receptor forms A and B by immunohistochemical analysis. *J Clin Pathol* 2001;54:624–30.

KEY POINT

Knowledge of basic uterine physiology is necessary to understand the physiological basis of disorders of the menstrual cycle. Future research efforts should aim to delineate cellular and molecular pathways that may be targets for therapeutic intervention when implantation or menstruation is problematic.

REPRODUCTIVE GYNAECOLOGY

14. Giudice LC. Microarray expression profiling reveals candidate genes for human uterine receptivity. *Am J Pharmacogenomics* 2004;4:299–312.

15. Munro MG, Critchley HO, Broder MS, Fraser IS. FIGO classification system (PALM-COEIN) for causes of abnormal uterine bleeding in nongravid women of reproductive age. *Int J Gynaecol Obstet* 2011;113:3–13.

16. Woolcock JG, Critchley HO, Munro MG, Broder MS, Fraser IS. Review of the confusion in current and historical terminology and definitions for disturbances of menstrual bleeding. *Fertil Steril* 2008;90: 2269–80.

17. Salamonsen LA. Tissue injury and repair in the female human reproductive tract. *Reproduction* 2003;125:301–11.

18. Donnez J, Tatarchuk TF, Bouchard P *et al.* Ulipristal acetate versus placebo for fibroid treatment before surgery. *N Engl J Med* 2012; 366:409–20.

Chapter 74 Uterine fibroids

Christine P West

MRCOG standards

Theoretical skills

- Understand the epidemiology, pathophysiology and clinical features of uterine fibroids.
- Understand the principles of investigation by imaging and hysteroscopy.
- Understand the nature, complications and adverse effects of medical, surgical and radiological management of fibroids.

Practical skills

- Be familiar with hysteroscopic assessment of submucosal fibroids.
- Understand the surgical techniques of hysterectomy and myomectomy and be able to recognise and manage their complications.

INTRODUCTION

Uterine fibroids, also known as myomas or leiomyomas, are benign tumours arising from the myometrium. They are composed of round whorls of smooth muscle and connective tissue and may be single or multiple. Their site may be intramural, submucosal or subserosal and their presentation and symptoms vary according to their size and situation within the uterus. While they may present with heavy menstrual bleeding (HMB) or pressure symptoms, they are commonly asymptomatic, found incidentally by ultrasound examination.

Uterine fibroids are a frequent indication for gynaecological intervention, most commonly hysterectomy. In the past many hysterectomies were carried out for asymptomatic fibroids because of concerns about the nature and consequences of a pelvic mass. Advances in imaging have facilitated the diagnosis of fibroids and enabled more women to be managed conservatively. Fibroids may be implicated in the causation of miscarriage and subfertility, but this chapter primarily addresses the evidence base for the management of abnormal uterine bleeding associated with the fibroids.

PREVALENCE

The prevalence of uterine fibroids in women of reproductive age has been estimated at around 25 per cent, based on clinical presentation. With the widespread use of imaging techniques it is now apparent that the actual prevalence may be much higher[1] with the majority of women reporting no symptoms. One community study of 1364 women in the USA[2] reported cumulative incidences of up to 70 per cent by the age of 50 in white women and over 80 per cent in black women, although the corresponding number considered clinically relevant was 35 and 50 per cent respectively. However, another large multistate study of 5023 women screened in early pregnancy reported a prevalence of only 11 per cent.[3]

Increased prevalence of fibroids is reported in women presenting with HMB. In studies in which heavy blood loss has been objectively confirmed by direct measurement,[4] 40 per cent of women with losses above 200 mL were found to have fibroids, compared with only 10 per cent whose losses were below 100 mL. Although a causal relationship with HMB has not been firmly established, it is likely that fibroids contribute to heavy bleeding if present submucosally or where intramural fibroids cause distortion of the endometrial cavity. There is little evidence that subserosal or pedunculated fibroids contribute to heavy blood loss.[4] Similarly the only direct association between uterine fibroids and nulliparity or infertility was found in women with submucosal fibroids.[5]

EPIDEMIOLOGY

It is evident that the incidence of fibroids increases with age and that fibroids subsequently regress in size and undergo degeneration after the menopause.[1] Rates among black women are two to three times greater than among white women and fibroids occur at a younger age.[5] Other risk factors include a younger age at menarche, reduced parity and a family history of fibroids.[5] Child-bearing has a protective effect which increases with the number of live births but decreases as the length of time from the last birth increases.[5] Smoking and the long-term use of the oral contraceptive pill and

Depo-Provera are associated with a reduced risk[6] and users of the levonorgestrel-releasing intrauterine system (LNG-IUS) for contraception have a lower rate of development of fibroids compared with users of copper-containing devices.[6] Other possible risk factors, less consistently reported, include increased BMI, reduced physical exercise and high consumption of red meat, with a protective effect from exercise and consumption of green vegetables.[5]

The majority of fibroids do not increase in size during pregnancy[1] although degenerative changes may occur secondary to altered vascularity, with around 5 per cent of women developing clinical and ultrasound features of red degeneration.

PATHOPHYSIOLOGY

The development of fibroids involves the transformation of normal smooth muscle cells (myocytes) into abnormal myocytes followed by stimulation of growth into clinically apparent tumours. Fibroids contain increased levels of receptors for both oestrogen and progesterone compared with normal myometrium.[7] Within the uterus angiogenesis or new blood vessel formation occurs in response to cyclical fluctuations in steroid hormones. Fibroids are relatively avascular but there is abnormal proliferation of surrounding blood vessels, leading to a hypothesis that abnormal angiogenesis plays a key role in the development of fibroids. Within fibroids there is altered expression of various angiogenic growth factors, including epidermal growth factor (EGF), vascular EDF and transforming growth factor beta. Abnormal responses of these various growth factors to physiological fluctuations of ovarian steroid hormones appear to play a key role in the development of fibroids.[7] It is likely that genetic factors are also involved[1] but currently it remains unclear how fibroids begin to grow and there is no explanation for their heterogeneity in terms of numbers, size, site and behaviour within and between individuals.

Transformation of a benign fibroid to highly malignant leiomyosarcoma was thought to occur in a small minority of cases but genetic studies[1] now indicate that sarcomas have a distinct origin.

MANAGEMENT

This chapter will review the evidence underlying the treatment of women with fibroids who present with symptoms, in particular HMB. In common with all gynaecological disorders, the age and reproductive intentions of the individual woman and her preferences in relation to the various treatments will play a key role in management. Options for women desiring future fertility or those actively seeking a pregnancy will differ from those who have completed childbearing. Psychosocial and cultural factors also influence decision making.

Investigation

Suspicion of fibroids is usually based on a history of HMB together with the presence of a pelvic mass or a palpably enlarged uterus on pelvic or abdominal examination. Pressure symptoms may be present. History, followed by abdominal and pelvic examination, should be supplemented by a full blood count if heavy bleeding is a presenting feature.[8] If the uterine enlargement is no greater than a 10–12 week gestation size, medical management can be initiated within primary care without further investigation, after exclusion of pregnancy.[8] Failure to respond to medical therapy or a uterus that is palpable abdominally is an indication for further assessment [E].[8]

Investigation of abnormal bleeding is covered elsewhere (Chapter 75) but these recommendations also apply to investigation of women with suspected fibroids. Transvaginal ultrasound should be the preliminary investigation [A],[1,6,8] combined with abdominal ultrasound where the uterine enlargement is in excess of 12-week size. It is important to visualise the ovaries and endometrium and, where possible, to document the size, number and position of individual fibroids as well as the overall uterine dimensions [E]. MRI has no advantage over ultrasound for the detection and routine imaging of fibroids[1,8] and is considerably more costly. However it has greater precision and is associated with less inter-observer variation than other techniques, particularly with larger uteri [B]. Where submucosal fibroids are suspected (Table 74.1), MRI, hysteroscopy or transvaginal saline infusion sonography improves diagnostic accuracy [A].[1,8]

The presence of a large pelvic mass will give rise to concerns regarding its nature. A recent large literature review[9] concluded that uterine leiomyosarcoma (LMS) is very rare with an overall incidence of 0.64/100,000 per year. Its estimated prevalence in a presumed fibroid is 0.14% [C]. Risk is positively correlated with age and is extremely low below the age of 40 [C]. Rapid fibroid enlargement is a feature of LMS but in the absence of factors such as pain or abnormal bleeding it is poorly predictive.[1,9] Fibroid growth during ovarian suppressive treatment with a GnRH agonist or after menopause should raise suspicion about its nature. There are no features which can predict an LMS on any imaging technique with certainty [C]. Characteristics which should lead to a suspicion of sarcoma include solitary lesion, oval shape, size >8cm, high vascularity with central necrosis and absence of calcification[9] [D]. Gadolinium-enhanced MRI scanning can be a helpful assessment tool[1,9] [C]. Elevation of serum LDH and LDH isoenzyme 3 has been reported in leiomyosarcoma although its role in diagnosis is currently unclear.

Table 74.1 Classification of submucosal fibroids

Type	Description
0	Pedunculated
1	Less than 50% intramural
2	Greater than 50% intramural

Endometrial biopsy should be carried out if there is prolonged irregular bleeding in women over 45 or those with other risk factors for endometrial cancer or uterine sarcoma [D].[8]

Conservative management

Asymptomatic fibroids do not require active management and there is no consensus regarding the need for on-going surveillance. First-line management of HMB in women with uterine fibroids should follow national guidelines.[8] Iron deficiency anaemia should be treated with oral iron. Some women will wish to avoid further treatment, either medical or surgical, and this preference should be respected [E]. The evidence supporting the use of medical therapies for HMB in women with fibroids is reviewed below.

Medical management

Non-hormonal therapy

Non-steroidal anti-inflammatory drugs (NSAIDs) are not effective in the reduction of heavy bleeding secondary to the presence of fibroids[6] but may be beneficial for management of pain associated with degeneration[10] as well as menstrual pain (see Chapter 76) [C]. There have been no randomised controlled trials (RCTs) evaluating antifibrinolytics in the management of HMB associated with fibroids, but results of a non-random comparative study[11] reported a blood loss reduction of around 50 per cent in women with clinically diagnosed fibroids. On the basis of this information, tranexamic acid should be used in preference to NSAIDs in the first-line management of fibroid-associated HMB [C].

Combined oral contraceptives

There is no evidence that the oral contraceptive pill causes enlargement of fibroids;[6] indeed, long-term use may be protective [C].[5,12] Good-quality data on the use of the combined oral contraceptive pill (COCP) in the treatment of fibroid-associated HMB is lacking. An early comparative study demonstrated a 50 per cent reduction in measured blood loss with a high-dose COCP in women with clinically diagnosed fibroids.[11] A small RCT comparing a COCP (30 μg ethinylestradiol plus 150 μg levonorgestrel) with the LNG-IUS[13] reported a reduction in measured blood loss of only 13 per cent after 12 months of treatment with the COCP, although there was a reduction of 53.5 per cent using pictorial assessment charts [B]. Mean haemoglobin at 12 months was 10.2 g/dL in the group treated with the COCP. There are no data on continuous COCP use in women with fibroid-related HMB or on use of tranexamic acid in conjunction with a COCP although these options may be used in clinical practice [E]. While the use of the combined pill is not contraindicated in women with fibroids who desire contraception [B], available data suggest that it has limited effectiveness in the control of HMB, particularly when this is associated with anaemia [B].

Levonorgestrel-releasing intrauterine system

The role of the LNG-IUS has not been fully evaluated in women with fibroids. The presence of fibroids greater than 3 cm and significant cavity distortion are regarded as contraindications to inclusion in large-scale clinical trials of its use for HMB,[8] thus limiting availability of high-quality information. In the only prospective RCT to date, in which the LNG-IUS was compared with a low-dose COCP in women with fibroids and HMB,[13] blood loss measured by the alkaline haematin method reduced by 91 per cent after 12 months with the LNG-IUS [B]. Recruitment was restricted to fibroids less than 5 cm in diameter and with no cavity distortion. Treatment failure was reported in 6 out of 29 participants (23 per cent) in this group.

A systematic review of 10 small prospective studies of the LNG-IUS in 269 women with HMB and fibroids reported consistent reduction of menstrual loss and improvement in haematological parameters [C].[14] Where stated, uterine size greater than 12 weeks' gestation or significant cavity distortion were exclusion criteria. Rates of amenorrhoea varied between 5 and 50 per cent at 12 months. A prospective cohort study comparing LNG-IUS use in women with and without fibroid-related HMB[15] reported a 27 per cent prevalence of breakthrough bleeding in the fibroid group after 3 years of use compared with 9 per cent in the women without fibroids. The incidence of expulsion may be increased in the presence of fibroids. Using data from the studies cited above,[14,15] the rate of expulsion of the LNG-IUS was 8 per cent among 248 women with fibroids, compared with only 1 per cent of 86 without fibroids.[14,15] Another study reported a greater rate of expulsion with fibroids greater than 3 cm[13] but numbers were small. There is no evidence that use of the LNG-IUS has any significant effect on the growth of fibroids.[14]

On the basis of this information, the use of the LNG-IUS can be beneficial in women with HMB associated with fibroids, including those with anaemia [B] but data is limited to those with uteri below 12 weeks' gestation size and without significant cavity distortion [C]. Even within these limitations, women should be warned of the increased risk of prolonged breakthough bleeding and of expulsion [C].

Progestogens and androgens

Progestogens, even in high doses, do not shrink fibroids:[6] thus use of oral progestogens in women with fibroids should be purely symptomatic and in a regimen that is effective for HMB (Chapter 75) i.e. for 21 days out of 28.[8] The long-term use of depot medroxyprogesterone acetate (DMPA) may protect against the development of fibroids [C][16] but there is no evidence to support its use for fibroid-related symptoms.

Both the androgen danazol[6] and the androgenic antiprogesterone gestrinone[6] (see Chapter 77) reduce fibroid size and blood loss during treatment [B] and may be helpful in the short-term control of fibroid-associated bleeding but their role in relation to other therapies is unclear. Androgenic side effects are fewer with gestrinone compared with danazol.

Antiprogesterones and selective progesterone receptor modulators (SPRMs)

A systematic review of three RCTs of the antiprogesterone mifepristone[17] has highlighted the potential role of antiprogesterones for the treatment of fibroids. At a dose of either 5 mg or 10 mg daily for 3 to 6 months, mifepristone significantly reduced menstrual blood loss, assessed pictorially, compared with placebo. However there was no significant effect on fibroid or uterine volume. In a controlled trial of the SPRM ulipristal acetate, women with fibroid-related excessive menstruation were randomised between 5 mg or 10 mg of the active drug and placebo for a treatment period of 13 weeks.[18] Over 70 per cent of the women in both active treatment groups developed amenorrhoea with a corresponding improvement in haemoglobin and haematocrit. Fibroid volume was reduced by 25 per cent in the women treated with 10 mg and by 12 per cent with 5 mg of ulipristal acetate. A further study by the same group compared both doses of ulipristal acetate with the gonadotrophin-releasing hormone (GnRH) analogue leuprolide acetate 3.75 mg/month, given for 13 weeks.[19] Reduction of menstrual blood loss and rates of amenorrhoea were similar in all three groups but median onset of amenorrhoea was 7 days in the women treated with ulipristal acetate, compared with 21 days for leuprolide acetate. Moderate to severe vasomotor side effects were reported by 10 and 40 per cent of the women respectively, with serum oestradiol remaining in the mid-follicular range in the women treated with ulipristal acetate, compared with postmenopausal levels with the GnRH analogue. However overall uterine volume reduction was significantly greater with the GnRH analogue (47 per cent compared with 20–22 per cent).

Both these studies were carried out in women due to undergo surgery for their fibroids. However approximately half the women in both studies opted not to undergo surgery at the end of the 13-week treatment period. Follow-up of these women showed a slower regrowth of the fibroids after ulipristal acetate, indicating its potential role in the medical management of fibroids.

There have been concerns about antiprogestogenic effects on the endometrium. Endometrial biopsies from the women in the above trials of ulipristal acetate have shown non-physiological changes, including extensive cystic glandular dilatation but with inactive epithelium and no evidence of hyperplasia.[20] These changes are collectively referred to as progesterone receptor modulator-associated endometrial changes and had regressed in the majority of the samples taken 6 months after treatment.

Current evidence is that ulipristal acetate is effective for rapid control of HMB secondary to fibroids [B]. It is licenced in the UK for short-term use at a daily dose of 5 mg for 3 months prior to hysterectomy. This would have particular application for women presenting with severe anaemia. Treatment should be started in the first week of the menstrual cycle. The licence has recently been extended so that 3 month courses of treatment can be repeated intermittently after treatment free intervals of at least one full menstrual cycle. Currently there is limited data on its effect on surgical outcomes or on longer term use beyond four courses of treatment for medical management of fibroid associated symptoms.

GnRH analogues

Treatment with GnRH agonists induces amenorrhoea and shrinkage of fibroids [A].[6,10] However, after cessation, regrowth is rapid. These changes are secondary to temporary ovarian suppression, and long-term treatment with GnRH agonists carries a risk of bone loss. Currently the role of these agents is largely limited to preoperative shrinkage of fibroids, although there is scope for their longer-term use with the addition of hormonal add-back.

Shrinkage of fibroids with a GnRH agonist prior to hysteroscopic or conventional surgery has been advocated on the basis of reduced fibroid size and vascularity. Their use prior to hysterectomy or myomectomy has been the subject of a systematic review[21] that was based on 26 RCTs. When used together with iron therapy for 3 to 4 months prior to surgery, they are effective in the treatment of preoperative anaemia [A]. They significantly reduce intra-operative blood loss, particularly in women with very large uteri, and significantly increase the likelihood of a transverse rather than a midline abdominal incision or a vaginal rather than an abdominal hysterectomy [A]. However, their cost effectiveness for routine use for women who do not fall into these specific categories has been challenged.[22]

There have been no randomised trials of GnRH agonists prior to hysteroscopic myomectomy, although they are widely used in this situation. One non-randomised controlled study[23] reported a significant reduction in operating time, blood loss, volume of distending medium and treatment failure following pre-treatment with a GnRH agonist [C].

In women who have contraindications to surgery or decline surgery and in whom other medical measures have failed, long-term relief of HMB may be achieved with GnRH agonists in combination with low-dose hormone replacement therapy (HRT).[6,10] It has been suggested that the GnRH agonist should be administered alone for 3 months to obtain fibroid shrinkage[6] before addition of the HRT [E]. Add-back therapy with tibolone maintains fibroid shrinkage and symptom relief while reducing vasomotor symptoms and preventing bone loss [B].[24] Low-dose oral oestrogen–progestogen combinations also relieve hypo-oestrogenic side effects and protect bone[6,10] and are less costly than tibolone. Currently there is a lack of evidence relating to the optimum choice of add-back therapy.

HRT in menopausal women with fibroids

Conservative management is often offered to women with symptomatic fibroids who are perimenopausal on the basis that their symptoms will resolve spontaneously when they reach the menopause. It is therefore relevant to consider the effect of HRT on fibroids. Limited information from RCTs suggest that oral combined HRT or tibolone does not promote the growth of fibroids [B][10] although enlargement of fibroids has been reported with transdermal use[C].[6] However HRT may increase the risk of heavy bleeding in women with submucosal fibroids.[10] On the basis of this information, oral continuous combined HRT preparations or tibolone can be used for the relief of vasomotor symptoms in postmenopausal women with fibroids [B] although they may increase bleeding problems related to fibroids or delay their resolution.

SURGICAL TREATMENT

Hysteroscopic surgery

Small submucous fibroids are implicated in heavy and abnormal menstrual bleeding and can be removed hysteroscopically. However, assessment of the effectiveness of hysteroscopic resection has been based on case series from single centres.[6,8] The procedure is normally restricted to Type 0 and Type 1 fibroids (Table 74.1) that are less than 3–5 cm in diameter, although removal of Type 2 fibroids has also been described using a staged approach and pre-treatment with a GnRH analogue[D].[6,10] The complications of hysteroscopic surgery include fluid overload, uterine perforation, haemorrhage and infection (see Chapter 75). Case review and cohort studies[6,8,25] have reported relief of menstrual symptoms in 69–85 per cent of women after up to 15 years of follow-up [C]. Effectiveness can be increased by concurrent endometrial resection in women not desiring future pregnancies.[8,25] For women with asymptomatic submucous fibroids who are trying to conceive naturally or with the aid of IVF, removal by resection is recommended[10] on the basis that it improves the chance of conception[26] [C] but the quality of the evidence is poor[27] and there are no data to support an improvement in pregnancy outcome. For relief of HMB associated with small submucous fibroids, hysteroscopic removal is likely to be cost effective [C].[28]

Abdominal myomectomy

Myomectomy is a well-established alternative to hysterectomy for symptomatic women wishing to preserve their fertility.[6,10,26,28] Reduction of menstrual bleeding in more than 80 per cent of women has been reported in retrospective case series[6] [D] but there is no relevant data from randomised trials. Recurrence of fibroids is common, with a 5-year cumulative recurrence rate of 62 per cent in one case series.[28] Haemorrhage is a potential problem at myomectomy and several interventions to reduce operative blood loss have been tested in small randomised trials.[29] Significant reduction was seen with vasopressin, misoprostol, tranexamic acid, gelatine–thrombin matrix, chemical dissection with mesna and pericervical tourniquet although there is no clear consensus as to which is most effective.[29] Uterine artery embolisation (UAE) can be used prior to myomectomy in selected cases[10] but experience of this is limited. GnRH agonists have been shown to reduce operative blood loss when used for the pretreatment of large uteri [A].[21] Women consenting to myomectomy need to be specifically counselled regarding the potential risk of emergency hysterectomy (less than 1 per cent) in the event of severe operative haemorrhage [E].

Subserosal and intramural fibroids may be removed successfully by laparoscopy in specialist centres but the laparoscopic approach is usually restricted to cases with no more than three fibroids and diameters smaller than 8 cm [C].[10] Larger fibroids require morcellation or removal by opening the upper vagina in order to maintain the benefits of a laparoscopic approach. Larger fibroids require morcellation or removal by opening the upper vagina to maintain the benefit of a laparoscopic approach. Women must be thoroughly counselled about the risks of morcellation[9] (see section below on hysterectomy) and laparoscopic techniques avoided if there are any clinical or imaging features which raise suspicion of a possible uterine sarcoma.

A meta-analysis of six randomised trials comparing laparoscopy with laparotomy for abdominal myomectomy[30] concluded that laparoscopy takes longer but is associated with reduced blood loss, faster recovery and fewer overall complications [A]. Data on menstrual bleeding outcome were not included. However there was no difference in other outcomes, including pregnancy rate or fibroid recurrence. In contrast to earlier studies, the incidence of scar rupture in pregnancy was not increased with the laparoscopic approach, presumably as a consequence of improved suturing techniques. Procedural costs are not significantly different.[28] There is no evidence that removal of subserosal or intramural fibroids enhances fertility[26,27] or improves pregnancy outcome and there remains a lack of evidence relating to the effectiveness of removing fibroids which are not causing endometrial cavity distortion for reduction of HMB.

Uterine artery embolisation

This technique was initially performed for the control of postpartum haemorrhage (PPH) but is now widely used for the treatment of symptomatic fibroids and is approved in the UK by NICE,[8] by RCOG and by the Royal College of Radiologists (RCR).[31] It is performed under radiological screening after selective catheterisation of the uterine arteries via one or both femoral arteries. Particles, most commonly polyvinyl alcohol, are injected to embolise the uterine vascular bed.[31,32] It is carried out under local anaesthesia but usually requires overnight hospitalisation for opiate analgesia because of severe but short-lived post-procedural ischaemic uterine pain. Fibroid shrinkage is gradual and progressive, reaching a mean of around 60 per cent at 6 months[10] with further reduction thereafter. Improvement in pain and pressure symptoms is reported by 80–90 per cent of women[28,31] in prospective cohort studies [C]. Median measured menstrual blood loss reduction following UAE has been reported as 50 per cent after 6–9 months and 80 per cent after 36–48 months [C].[33]

Early side effects of treatment include puncture site bruising, pain and mild febrile reactions (post-embolisation syndrome).[31] The latter is treated with rest and NSAIDs and usually resolves within 10–14 days. Later complications (Table 74.2) include vaginal discharge, delayed passage of infarcted submucosal fibroids and ovarian failure, the latter mainly in women over 45. The most important major

Table 74.2 Complications of uterine artery embolisation[31,34]

Complication	Incidence
Procedure related:	
Groin haematoma	<1%
Arterial complications	<1%
Non-target embolisation	<1%
Early (within 30 days):	
Post-embolisation syndrome	16–18%
Late (usually after 30 days:	
Septicaemia requiring emergency hysterectomy	<1%
Spontaneous fibroid expulsion	7–10%
Fibroid impaction requiring surgical intervention	3–5%
Prolonged vaginal discharge	12–16%
Endometritis	0.5%
Ovarian failure – all ages	1.5–7%
Ovarian failure under age 45	<1%

complication is severe sepsis, which may necessitate emergency hysterectomy.

A systematic review of four RCTs[32] comparing UAE with hysterectomy concluded that UAE is associated with a shorter procedure and duration of hospital stay, reduced risk of blood transfusion and faster return to normal activities compared with surgery [A]. Satisfaction and quality-of-life scores were similarly high in both groups at 2 and 5 years of follow-up although further intervention rates were higher following UAE (see below). The rate of major complications was lower after UAE although the difference was not significant, but minor complications were more frequent and more likely to occur following discharge from hospital (see Table 74.2). The incidence of ovarian failure, measured by serum follicle stimulating hormone (FSH), showed no difference after 5 years of follow-up when compared with hysterectomy and ovarian conservation. Only one RCT compared UAE with myomectomy and again satisfaction rates were high and not significantly different after 2 years of follow-up.[32]

UAE is contraindicated in women with asymptomatic fibroids [E], those with current or recent pelvic infection [A] and in cases where there is serious doubt about the nature of a pelvic mass. In the latter situation, MRI is superior to ultrasound in confirming the diagnosis of fibroids[9] and therefore is recommended for routine use prior to UAE.[31] Bleeding irregularities should be investigated prior to UAE [E]. Although the size or number of fibroids is not known to influence outcome, fibroids in certain sites require special consideration.[31] Pedunculated subserous fibroids may infarct and become detached into the peritoneal cavity, and large submucosal fibroids may detach and cause cervical obstruction following embolisation, requiring surgical intervention. Women consenting to UAE should be warned of the remote risk of emergency hysterectomy (less than 1 per cent) in the event of severe post-procedural sepsis [E].

Long-term outcome of UAE

Up to one third of women in the randomised trials had required a further procedure for fibroids 5 years following UAE,[32] compared with only 4–10 per cent after surgery. These included hysterectomy, repeat embolisation and hysteroscopic or other vaginal procedures. Reinterventions were lower, at 23 per cent after 7 years in a large cohort study,[34] possibly reflecting the influence of patient self-selection. The need for further treatment is age related with only 10 per cent of those over 40 at the time of treatment requiring a further procedure.[31]

In women who have not completed child-bearing, the choice between myomectomy and UAE will be influenced by prospects for future pregnancy. A systemic review of observational studies reported an ongoing pregnancy rate of 63.7 per cent after UAE compared with 77.9 per cent after myomectomy with live-birth rates of 57.8 per cent and 77.4 per cent respectively [C].[35] Further information from randomised trials is awaited.

Information on new fibroid growth after UAE is lacking. One study reported a prevalence of new fibroid growth in only 7 per cent of women 5 years after UAE compared with 60 per cent after myomectomy.[36] Although numbers in the myomectomy group were very small, this figure is consistent with data from a large case series.[28] Further information from longer-term follow-up will be important in counselling women.

Results to date strongly support the use of UAE for symptomatic fibroids [A]. Although the initial costs of UAE are significantly less than those of hysterectomy, this advantage appears to lessen with time so that by 5 years overall costs are similar. A cost–utility analysis comparing UAE, hysterectomy and myomectomy[37] showed that quality-adjusted life years (QALYs) gained over 5 years were high after all three interventions but marginally higher after hysterectomy at a lower total cost because of the avoidance of reinterventions. Myomectomy was more costly than UAE but overall differences were marginal. Further information on predictors of long-term outcome of UAE would enable clinicians to target treatment more effectively. There is also a clear need for more randomised studies and longer-term follow-up of UAE in women actively seeking future pregnancy.

MRI-guided focused ultrasound (MRg-FUS)

This technique uses a high-frequency, high-energy ultrasound beam to destroy fibroid tissue by coagulative necrosis, in conjunction with an MRI thermal mapping system to visualise the anatomy and monitor the temperature of the tissue.[28,38] It is performed as an outpatient procedure under light sedation. The technique remains under development and data is mainly limited to results of small-scale prospective or retrospective cohort studies of women not seeking future fertility.[10,28,38] These studies report significant improvement in fibroid-related symptoms in 50–80 per cent of women and reduction in fibroid volume of 10–25 per cent after 6–12 months [C]. Treatment failed in up to 30 per cent of women by 12 months.

However recovery is rapid and morbidity is low. There is potential for tissue injury such as burns to skin and nerves.

The treatment has limitations as it is time consuming, taking 2–4 hours to treat a single fibroid and due to safety concerns only a small proportion of the fibroid volume may be treated.[10,38] The latter restriction may be relaxed with greater experience of the technique. Most studies have excluded uteri with greater than four fibroids and diameters greater than 10 cm although prior shrinkage with GnRH analogues has been described.[38] The procedure is not suitable for fibroids close to the bowel, bladder or sacrum or for non-enhancing or pedunculated fibroids and the presence of surgical scars may be a contraindication. Due to these factors, up to 40 per cent of women may be technically ineligible for the treatment. This is in contrast to UAE where over 90 per cent are technically eligible.[39]

MRg-FUS has been approved by the FDA in the USA for treatment of women not desiring future fertility[C]. Limited recent experience with women seeking fertility has been reassuring. However, randomised comparisons of its outcome compared with surgery and UAE are required to assess whether it has clear advantages over available alternatives. Theoretically it would seem to be of potential use in women desiring future fertility for treatment of single fibroids encroaching on the endometrium. Until further data are available its role remains unclear.

Other conservative options

Endometrial ablation is not specifically contraindicated for women with fibroids although the presence of fibroids greater than 3 cm or significant cavity distortion have been exclusion criteria for large-scale clinical trials. Most second-generation techniques are not suitable for women with large or distorted cavities although first-generation methods can be used in conjunction with resection of submucosal fibroids in women with HMB not desirous of future pregnancy.[10] The presence of uterine fibroids was found to significantly increase the risk of further surgery following endometrial ablation in an English cohort study of over 100,000 women.[40]

Myolysis or heat destruction of fibroids using various energy sources has been investigated in small-scale trials[10,28] but only focussed ultrasound, described above, has developed to a clinically useful degree. Laparoscopic uterine artery occlusion has been described but evidence is limited[10,28] and it has no obvious advantage over radiological embolisation.

Hysterectomy

Hysterectomy offers a definitive cure for women with heavy bleeding associated with fibroids who have completed childbearing [A][31] and is still the most commonly performed procedure for this indication. Although expensive in the short term and not without risk[6,8,10,28] (see Chapter 75), it may provide a cost-effective option for women who are less likely to benefit from more conservative approaches. Further information based on larger comparative studies is needed to enable clinicians and patients to make an informed choice. The abdominal route has been most commonly used for large

uteri although the vaginal route can be used by experienced operators,[8] usually after GnRH pre-treatment. Laparoscopic techniques are increasingly available in large centres. These involve the use of morcellation which can lead to rare complications such as direct injuries to intestine or blood vessels and seeding of tissue fragments within the peritoneal cavity leading to growth of parasitic fibroids.[9] There has been particular concern about reports of intraperitoneal seeding of unsuspected uterine sarcoma, leading to advice from the FDA discouraging the use of power morcellators.[9] Although the low prevalence and lack of specific diagnostic features makes preoperative diagnosis of LMS difficult, it has been suggested that laparoscopic morcellation should be avoided in women over the age of 40 with clinical or imaging features which raise concerns about the nature of a presumed fibroid.[9] However as yet there are no agreed guidelines, apart from the need for detailed patient information and informed consent [E].

EBM

These recommendations are based on three evidence-based clinical guidelines (two specific to the management of fibroids) and ten systematic reviews or meta-analyses. Some of the recommendations regarding management are based on information from non-randomised trials, case series or prospective cohort studies.

KEY POINTS

- Management of uterine fibroids should be based on the nature of the symptoms and the reproductive wishes of the individual woman [E]. Asymptomatic fibroids, even if very large, do not routinely require active management [E].
- Transvaginal ultrasound, combined with abdominal ultrasound for uteri larger than 12 weeks' gestation size, is the primary investigation for suspected fibroids [A].
- Both hysteroscopy and transvaginal sonohysterography (saline infusion sonography) are of value in the further investigation of suspected submucosal fibroids [A].
- MRI scanning should not be used as a primary investigation but has greater diagnostic accuracy than ultrasound and is indicated if there is doubt about the nature of a uterine mass or for assessment of suitability for UAE [B].
- LMS is very rare with an estimated prevalence of 0.14% in a presumed fibroid and is extremely rare below the age of 40. MRI with contrast enhancement may prove helpful in distinguishing between LMS and fibroid [C].
- Tranexamic acid should be used in preference to NSAIDs in the symptomatic management of HMB associated with fibroids [C].
- COCPs are not contraindicated in the presence of fibroids and may protect against fibroid growth [B] but have limited effectiveness in reduction of HMB, especially when this is associated with anaemia [B].
- Progestogens do not shrink fibroids but may relieve HMB at high doses if used continuously or for 21 days out of 28 [D].

- Progestogen-releasing IUDs are beneficial for fibroid-associated HMB [B] but evidence is based on cases without significant cavity distortion and patients should be warned of an increased risk of expulsion [C].
- Gestrinone or danazol can be used for the short-term management of fibroid-associated HMB [B].
- Selective progesterone receptor modulators have potential as a medical alternative to surgery for management of symptomatic fibroids but current evidence is limited to short and medium term use.
- GnRH agonists shrink fibroids and relieve HMB [A] and may be used in conjunction with add-back low-dose continuous combined HRT or tibolone for longer-term treatment [B].
- Treatment with low-dose oral combined HRT or tibolone is not contraindicated for relief of menopausal symptoms in women with fibroids but may cause a recurrence of bleeding problems related to fibroids or delay their resolution [C].
- GnRH agonists are useful adjuncts to surgery in cases of anaemia, very large fibroids and where uterine shrinkage may result in a transverse abdominal incision or a vaginal rather than an abdominal hysterectomy [A].
- Heavy bleeding associated with the presence of Type 1 or 2 submucous fibroids may be relieved by hysteroscopic resection [C].
- Myomectomy is an alternative surgical treatment for women with HMB and other fibroid-associated symptoms who wish to retain their fertility [C].
- Haemorrhage is a potential problem at myomectomy and interventions are available to reduce operative blood loss [B].
- Laparoscopic myomectomy is associated with shorter hospital stay and faster recovery than laparotomy in selected cases [B] but there is no evidence relating to its role in women with fibroid-associated HMB.
- UAE is an effective alternative to hysterectomy for symptomatic fibroids in women who have completed child-bearing [A] but up to one third of women require further intervention because of lack of symptom control.
- UAE is not contraindicated for women wishing to conserve fertility but the pregnancy outcome is less favourable compared with myomectomy [C].
- MRI-guided focussed ultrasound is of potential use as a uterus-conserving option for selected women with symptomatic fibroids [C] but further information based on larger RCTs is required.
- Hysterectomy is an effective treatment for symptomatic fibroids in women who have completed childbearing [A]. The optimum technique and safety of the laparoscopic approach for removal of large fibroids have yet to be determined.

References

1. Parker WH. Etiology, symptomatology and diagnosis of uterine myomas. *Fertil Steril* 2007;87:725–736.
2. Baird DD, Dunson DB, Hill MC, Cousins D, Schectman JM. High cumulative incidence of uterine leiomyoma in black and white women: ultrasound evidence. *Am J Obstet Gynecol* 2003;188:100–107.
3. Edwards DRV, Baird DD, Hartman KE. Association of age at menarche with increasing number of fibroids in a cohort study of women who underwent standardized ultrasound assessment. *Am J Epidemiol* 2013;178:426–433.
4. Rybo G, Leman J, Tibbin R. Epidemiology of menstrual blood loss. *In*: Baird DT, Michie EA (eds). *Mechanisms of menstrual bleeding*. New York: Raven Press, 1985, 181–93.
5. Schwartz SM. Epidemiology of uterine leiomyomata. *Clin Obstet Gynecol* 2001;44:316–326.
6. Farquhar C, Arroll B, Ekeroma A *et al*. An evidence-based guideline for the management of uterine fibroids. *Aust N Z J Obstet Gynaecol* 2001;41:125–140.
7. Tal RT, Segars JH. The role of angiogenic factors in fibroid pathogenesis: potential implications for future therapy. *Hum Reprod Update* 2014;20:194–216.
8. National Collaborating Centre for Women's and Children's Health. *Heavy menstrual bleeding*. London: RCOG Press, 2007.
9. Brolmann H, Tanos V, Grimbizis G et al. On behalf of the European Society of Gynecological Endoscopy (ESGE) steering committee on fibroid morcellation. Options on fibroid morcellation: a literature review. *Gynecol Surg* 2015;12:3-15.
10. Marret H, Fritel X, Ouldamer L *et al.*; CNGOF (French College of Gynecology and Obstetrics). Therapeutic management of uterine fibroid tumours: updated French Guidelines. *Eur J Obstet Gynecol Reprod Biol* 2012;165:156–164.
11. Nilsson L, Rybo G. Treatment of menorrhagia. *Am J Obstet Gynecol* 1971;10:713–20.
12. Qin J, Yang T, Kong F, Zhou Q. Oral contraceptive use and uterine leiomyoma risk: a meta-analysis based on cohort and case-control studies. *Arch Gynaecol Obstet* 2013:288:139–148.
13. Sayed GH, Zakherah MS, El-Nashar SA, Shaaban MM. A randomized clinical trial of a levonorgestrel-releasing intrauterine system and a low-dose combined oral contraceptive for fibroid-related menorrhagia. *Int J Gynaecol Obstet* 2011;112:126–130.
14. Zapata LB, Whiteman MK, Tepper NK, Jamieson DJ, Marchbanks PA, Curtis KM. Intrauterine device use among women with uterine fibroids: a systematic review. *Contraception* 2010:82;41–55.
15. Magalhaes J, Aldrighi JM, de Lima GR. Uterine volume and menstrual patterns in users of the levonorgestrel-releasing intrauterine system with idiopathic menorrhagia or menorrhagia due to leiomyomas. *Contraception* 2007:75:193–198.
16. Lumbiganon P, Rugpao S, Phandhu-fung S, Laopaiboon M, Vudhikamraksa N, Werawatakul Y. Protective effect of depot-medroxyprogesterone acetate on surgically treated uterine leiomyomas: a multi-centre case-control study. *BJOG* 1995;103:909–914.
17. Tristan M, Orozco LJ, Steed A, Ramirez-Morera A, Stone P. Mifepristone for uterine fibroids. *Cochrane Database*

of Systematic Reviews 2012, Issue 8. Art. No:CD007687. DOI:10.1002/14651858. CD007687.pub2.

18. Donnez J, Tatarchuk TF, Bouchard P *et al.*; PEARL 1 Study Group. Ulipristal acetae versus placebo for fibroid treatment before surgery. *N Engl J Med* 2012; 366:409–420.

19. Donnez J, Tomaszewski J, Vazquez F *et al.*; PEARL II Study Group. Ulipristal acetate versus leuprolide acetate for uterine fibroids. *N Engl J Med* 2012; 366:421–432.

20. Williams AR, Bergeron C, Barlow DH, Ferenczy A. Endometrial morphology after treatment of uterine fibroids with the selective progesterone receptor modulator, ulipristal acetate. *Int J Gynaecol Pathol* 2012;31:556–569.

21. Lethaby A, Vollenhoven B, Sowter M. Pre-operative GnRH analogue therapy before hysterectomy or myomectomy for uterine fibroids. *Cochrane Database of Systematic Reviews* 2001, Issue 2. Art. No.:CD000547. DOI:10.1002/14651858.CD000547.

22. Farquhar C, Brown PM, Furness S. Cost effectiveness of pre-operative gonadotrophin releasing analogues for women with uterine fibroids undergoing hysterectomy or myomectomy. *BJOG* 2002;109:1273–1280.

23. Perino A, Chianchino N, Petronio M, Ciltadini E. The role of leuprolide acetate depot in hysteroscopic surgery: a controlled study. *Fertil Steril* 1993; 59:507–510.

24. Palomba S, Affinito P, Tommaselli GA, Nappi C. A clinical trial of the effects of tibolone administered with gonadotropin-releasing hormone analogues for the treatment of uterine leiomyomata. *Fertil Steril* 1998;70:111–118.

25. Derman SG, Rehnstrom J, Neuwirth RS. The long-term effectiveness of hysteroscopic treatment of menorrhagia and leiomyomas. *Obstet Gynecol* 1991;77:591–594.

26. Pritts EA, Parker WH, Olive DL. Fibroids and infertility: an updated systematic review of the evidence. *Fertil Steril* 2009;91:1215–1223.

27. Metwally M, Cheong YC, Horne AW. Surgical treatment of fibroids for subfertility. *Cochrane Database of Systematic Reviews* 2012, Issue 11. Art.No.:CD003857. DOI:10.1002/14658. CD003857.pub3.

28. Levy BS. Modern management of uterine fibroids. *Acta Obstet Gynaecol Scand* 2008;87:812–823.

29. Kongnyuy EJ, Wiysonge CS. Interventions to reduce haemorrhage during myomectomy for fibroids. *Cochrane Database of Systematic Reviews* 2011, Issue 11. Art. No.:CD005355.DI10.1002/14651858. CD005355.pub4.

30. Jin C, Hu Y, Chen X-c *et al.* Laparoscopic versus open myomectomy – a meta-analysis of randomized controlled

trials. *Eur J Obstet Gynecol Reprod Biol* 2009; 145:14–21.

31. RCOG, RCR. *Clinical recommendations on the use of uterine artery embolisation (UAE) in the management of uterine fibroids.* 3rd edn. London: RCOG and RCR, 2013.

32. Gupta JK, Sinha A, Lumsden MA, Hickey M. Uterine artery embolization for symptomatic uterine fibroids. *Cochrane Database of Systematic Reviews* 2012, Issue 5. Art.No.:CD005073. DOI:10.1002/14651858. CD005073.pub3.

33. Khaund A, Moss JG, McMillan N, Lumsden MA. Evaluation of the effect of uterine artery embolisation on menstrual blood loss and uterine volume. *BJOG* 2004;111:700–705.

34. Dutton D, Hirst A, McPherson K, Nicholson T, Maresh M. A UK multicentre retrospective cohort study comparing hysterectomy and uterine artery embolisation for the treatment of uterine fibroids (HOPEFUL study): main results on medium-term safety and efficacy. *BJOG* 2007;114:1340–1351.

35. Sud S, Maheshwari A, Bhattacharya S. Obstetric outcomes after treatment of fibroids by uterine artery embolization: a systematic review. *Exp Rev of Obstet Gynecol* 2009;4:429–441.

36. Ananthakrishnan G, Murray L, Ritchie M *et al.* Randomized comparison of UAE with surgical treatment in patients with symptomatic uterine fibroids (REST Trial): Subanalysis of 5-year MRI findings. *Cardiovasc Intervent Radiol* 2013;36:676–681.

37. You JHS, Sahota DS, Yuen PM. Uterine artery embolization, hysterectomy or myomectomy for symptomatic uterine fibroids: a cost-utility analysis. *Fertil Steril* 2009;91:580–588.

38. Hesley GK, Gorny KR, Woodrum DA. MR-guided focused ultrasound for the treatment of uterine fibroids. *Cardiovasc Intervent Radiol* 2013:36;5–13.

39. Froling V, Kroncke FV, Schreiter NF *et al.* Technical eligibility for treatment of magnetic resonance-guided focused ultrasound surgery. *Cardiovasc Intervent Radiol* 2014:37;445–50.

40. Bansi-Matharu L, Gurol-Urganci I, Mahmood TA, Templeton A, van der Meulen JH, Cromwell DA. Rates of subsequent surgery following endometrial ablation among English women with menorrhagia: population-based cohort study. *BJOG* 2013;120:1500–1507.

41. McPherson K, Metcalfe MA, Herbert A *et al.* Severe complications of hysterectomy: the VALUE study. *BJOG* 2004;111:688–694.

Chapter 75 Abnormal uterine bleeding

Christine P West

INTRODUCTION

Menstruation is an issue of concern to many women in contemporary society. In the past, large family sizes, prolonged breastfeeding and reduced life expectancy limited the number of menstrual cycles experienced, but currently women may experience more than 400 menstrual periods during reproductive life, and problems related to menstruation are a common cause of referral, both to GPs and to gynaecologists. Abnormal bleeding can be a consequence of pelvic pathology, including malignant disease, but the majority of women who present with menstrual problems have no underlying abnormality. Indeed, a significant proportion of women with symptoms of heavy bleeding are found to have normal menstrual blood loss if the volume is measured objectively. Concern about the widespread use of hysterectomy in this situation has led to a well-developed evidence base for medical management. This evidence base, together with less invasive surgical methods, has increased the range of available options.

DEFINITIONS

The 2007 evidence-based guideline, commissioned by NICE,[1] rejected use of the term menorrhagia in favour of heavy menstrual bleeding (HMB). HMB is defined as 'excessive menstrual blood loss which interferes with the woman's physical, emotional, social and material quality of life, and which can occur alone or in combination with other symptoms'. The former definition of heavy blood loss, based on measured loss of more than 60 to 80 mL per period,[2] is used only as a research tool. Problems that may be associated with heavy bleeding include pain and mood swings (see Chapters 76 and 79). Other menstrual symptoms which may or may not be associated with heavy blood loss involve changes in cycle pattern that may be hormonal or secondary to structural pathology. These changes include cycle irregularity, prolonged bleeding, intermenstrual bleeding (IMB) and postcoital bleeding (PCB). The term abnormal uterine bleeding (AUB),[3] favoured by the International Federation of Gynaecology and Obstetrics (FIGO), is defined as 'bleeding from the uterine corpus that is abnormal in volume, regularity and/or timing that has been present for the majority of the last 6 months'. Acute AUB, requiring immediate intervention, may occur in the context of ongoing chronic AUB or as an isolated episode.

EPIDEMIOLOGY

The reported prevalence of HMB varies between 4 per cent and 50 per cent, depending upon the population under study and the methods used.[1] In studies based on subjective self-assessment, the prevalence is around 20–25 per cent. In those using objective measurements, between 9 and 13 per cent of women have blood loss above 80 mL.[1] In an English community-based study of 1513 menstruating women[4] aged 18 to 54, the twelve-month cumulative incidence of self-reported menstrual disorders was 25 per cent for HMB, 29 per cent for changes in cycle pattern, 17 per cent for IMB, 6 per cent for PCB and 9 per cent for the occurrence of at least one prolonged period lasting 10 days or longer.

Menstrual cycle patterns change significantly with age,[1] with an overall decrease in cycle length and increase in regularity until the perimenopause, when cycle variations become more common. The incidence of HMB rises with age, as do changes in cyclical pattern, including both long and short cycles and episodes of prolonged menstruation.[4] However, the incidence of both intermenstrual and PCB declines progressively with age.[4] There is a significant association between objectively confirmed HMB and uterine fibroids, with a greater prevalence of the latter in Afro-Caribbean women (see Chapter 74). Apart from this correlation and some inherited blood disorders (see below), there are no obvious racial or genetic associations with heavy menstrual blood loss. Mental and emotional health are known to influence HMB reporting rates[1] although the relationship is not well understood.

CAUSES

A recent FIGO working party has proposed the PALM-COEIN system of classification of causes of AUB in the reproductive years (Table 75.1).[3] It is envisaged that this approach may facilitate future research into the epidemiology and treatment of menstrual disorders.

However, it is recognised that some of the conditions listed may be present in asymptomatic women, and the classification may be oversimplistic in relation to clinical management of the presenting complaint(s). Studies involving objective measurements of blood loss have shown that in a high proportion of women reporting heavy periods, the quantity of blood loss is not abnormal.[2] A study of women referred to gynaecological clinics because of excessive menstrual loss showed that more than half did not perceive this issue as severe or as their main problem.[5] There was considerable overlap between problems related to bleeding and other menstrual problems such as pain and cyclical symptoms. Psychosocial factors may also influence presentation.

Structural causes

Fibroids (leiomyomata), particularly those situated submucosally, are the most common structural cause of HMB, prevalent in around 30 per cent of women with this complaint (see Chapter 74). Heavy bleeding associated with fibroids is often painless; painful heavy periods may be secondary to

Table 75.1 FIGO classification system for causes of abnormal uterine bleeding in non-pregnant women[3]

Structural causes	Non-structural causes
Polyp	Coagulopathy
Adenomyosis	Ovulatory dysfunction
Leiomyomata – submucosal	Endometrial
Leiomyomata – other	Iatrogenic
Malignancy or hyperplasia	Not yet classified

adenomyosis (see Chapter 78). Endometrial **polyps** may cause heavy bleeding but are more often asymptomatic or associated with IMB. A retrospective review of 2500 outpatient hysteroscopies[6] reported a 17 per cent incidence of endometrial polyps in women presenting with IMB or PCB, compared with 10 per cent of those with HMB. Submucous fibroids were reported in 30 per cent of women with HMB and 20 per cent with IMB or PCB. The incidence of both polyps and fibroids rises with increasing age[1,6,10] although age alone is poorly predictive of the presence of these lesions. **Histological abnormalities** of the endometrium are usually confined to the perimenopause. They range from simple or complex hyperplasia to severe atypia and malignancy. The incidence of **malignancy** rises with age and is rare in premenopausal women. It has been estimated that the rate of endometrial cancer in women presenting with HMB in primary care is less than 1 per 10,000 below the age of 40, 3 per 10,000 between 40 and 44, and 8 per 10,000 in women of 45 to 49,[1] although these data do not relate to bleeding patterns or to those referred to secondary care. The incidence of endometrial cancer among premenstrual women undergoing endometrial investigation in secondary care is between 0.2 and 1 per cent.[1] Similarly, the probability of a woman in the community with PCB having cervical cancer is 1 in 44,000 at age 20 to 24, rising to 1 in 2800 between 35 and 44 years and 1 in 2400 at 45 to 54 years.[7]

Non-structural causes

Coagulation disorders, in particular von Willebrand's disease (vWD), have been reported in between 5 and 20 per cent of women with HMB.[1] These conditions are most prevalent among young women in whom there is likely to be a history of other bleeding problems (particularly at previous surgical or dental procedures).

Ovulatory dysfunction is common following menarche and in the lead-up to menopause. The condition is painless and in teenagers usually limited to a few cycles. During the perimenopause it may lead to any of the histological abnormalities mentioned above. Abnormal bleeding secondary to ovulatory dysfunction is also a well-recognised consequence of polycystic ovary syndrome. Irregular bleeding may be associated with other endocrine disorders, particularly thyroid disease, although the underlying mechanism is unclear. Bleeding which occurs at mid-cycle in association with the oestradiol surge is regarded as physiological.

Endometrial causes involve disorders in the local control of menstruation (see Chapter 73). A review of 20 observational and diagnostic studies[1] showed that the majority of women investigated for menstrual bleeding disorders have no histological or structural abnormality and no evidence of any abnormality of ovulation. In such cases the most likely cause of both heavy and/or irregular menstrual bleeding is endometrial dysfunction.

Iatrogenic causes include the use of hormonal contraceptive preparations, intrauterine devices and anticoagulants. Breakthrough bleeding associated with hormonal contraception is discussed in Chapter XXX). **Not yet classified** might include conditions currently poorly defined, such as bleeding from arterio-venous malformations or chronic endometritis.[3]

MANAGEMENT

Decisions regarding investigations and treatments of AUB are influenced by a number of factors, which include the age and reproductive wishes of the individual woman, the pattern and severity of her symptoms and the degree of social disruption that she experiences. Many women may simply seek reassurance. A detailed and accurate history is essential in eliciting any relevant medical problems and assessing the impact of the problem in each individual case. While simple menstrual calendars may be helpful in clarifying the pattern of bleeding, objective blood loss measurements and/or pictorial charts[8] are regarded as research tools and not recommended in routine clinical practice [E].

Investigation

History, examination and basic investigation

This is covered in the national evidence-based guideline[1] and falls within the scope of primary care. History taking should define the presenting problem, determine the impact on the wellbeing of the patient and detect abnormal bleeding patterns and/or symptoms that may require further investigation [E]. Abdominal and bimanual pelvic examinations should be performed [E]. In the absense of abnormal features no additional investigations are required prior to the initiation of medical therapy [E]. If the uterus is enlarged, an ultrasound scan is the first-line investigation for delineating fibroids or excluding other causes of a pelvic mass [A]. A full blood count should be carried out in all women with HMB [C]. Additional blood tests such as ferritin, female hormone levels and/or thyroid function are not required in the absence of specific indications [C]. Testing for coagulation disorders, in particular vWD, should be considered in young women with a personal or family history suggestive of such conditions [C].[1]

Further investigation

Endometrial biopsy should be taken to exclude endometrial cancer or atypical hyperplasia in cases of prolonged, irregular or persistent IIMB in the presence of specific risk factors (age over 45, obesity, tamoxifen therapy) [E]. It is also recommended in women over 45 if previous treatments have failed [E].[1] Various endometrial sampling devices are available for use in outpatients. The most common is the Pipelle sampler, which has been shown to have high sensitivity in the detection of both endometrial cancer and atypical hyperplasia.[1]

Endometrial biopsy does not detect polyps or fibroids[9,10] and if these are suspected on the basis of history or clinical examination then current guidance is that transvaginal ultrasound scanning (TVS) should be performed [A].[1,11] Abdominal ultrasound is required if the uterus is palpable abdominally. Hysteroscopy provides accurate visualisation of the uterine cavity and greater accuracy than TVS in distinguishing between polyps and submucosal fibroids[9,10,11] although it is more invasive and potentially more costly.[9] In centres where provision for outpatient hysteroscopy is limited, the ultrasound based technique of saline infusion sonography[11] is useful in delineating the uterine cavity, but this method is not regarded as a first line investigation [A]. Dilatation and curettage has been relaced by the clinic-based techniques described above for routine investigation and should not be used alone as a diagnostic tool [B].[1] Current guidelines[1,12] recommend that TVS should be used, together with endometrial biopsy if indicated, for the initial investigation of AUB, with hysteroscopy as a back up technique [A]. However a recent economic evaluation10 has suggested that initial investigation by hysteroscopy may be more cost effective in secondary care if contemporary 'one-stop' testing and treatment modalities are available during a single visit. .

Intermenstrual and postcoital bleeding

Careful examination of the cervix is essential, and suspicious findings are indications for colposcopy. In sexually active women, chlamydial infection should be excluded [B]. If IMB occurs only mid-cycle, then further investigation is not required. Although the incidence of structural and histological abnormalities rises with increasing age,[6,9] fibroids and polyps can cause symptoms in younger women. As discussed above, TVS is currently regarded as the primary investigation for the detection of endometrial polyps or submucosal fibroids [A], backed up by biopsy and/or hysteroscopy if additional investigations are required. In the majority of cases, no abnormality is found and spontaneous resolution of both IMB and PCB commonly occurs.[13]

MEDICAL MANAGEMENT

Non-hormonal therapy

For women with HMB who prefer to avoid hormonal treatment or who wish to conceive, antifibrinolytics (tranexamic acid)[14] or non-steroidal anti-inflammatory drugs (NSAIDs) e.g. mefenamic acid[15] are first-line drugs [A]. Both are used only during menstruation and are generally well tolerated, apart from gastrointestinal side effects which are more common with NSAIDs. Blood loss may be reduced by up to 58 per cent with tranexamic acid [A][14] but associated menstrual pain is more effectively treated with NSAIDs (see Chapter 76). Blood loss is reduced by around 29 per cent with mefenamic acid, 26 per cent with naproxen but only 16 per cent with ibuprofen.[15] There is no evidence that the long-term use of antifibrinolytics increases the incidence of thrombosis.[14] Since antifibrinolytics and NSAIDs have different mechanisms of action, they may be used in combination [E]. Ethamsylate (a drug that reduces capillary fragility) was used in the past but recent trials have shown it to be less effective than NSAIDs or tranexamic acid [A].[1] If effective, the use of tranexamic acid and/or NSAIDs can be continued in the long term, but they should be stopped if they do not improve symptoms within three menstrual cycles [E].

Combined oral contraceptive pill (COCP)

For women requiring contraception or for whom hormonal agents are acceptable, COCP preparations are effective in reducing menstrual bleeding, controlling cycle irregularities and relieving menstrual pain, although reports of efficacy have largely been based on indirect evidence from contraceptive studies and one small randomised controlled trial (RCT)[16] which reported a 43 per cent reduction in menstrual blood loss. There is some reluctance on the part of both professionals and consumers to use the COCP for the management of menstrual disorders in older women. For non-smokers with no risk factors for vascular disease, there is no upper age limit for the use of the COCP, and current guidelines recommend it as a first-line therapy for HMB [B].[1]

Progestogens

Cyclical progestogens were commonly used in the past, but the current evidence does not support the use of these treatments for HMB when given only during the luteal phase of the cycle [A].[17] They are effective when given at high doses between days 5 and 26 (e.g. norethisterone 5 mg tid) [A].[17] Cyclical progestogens are traditionally chosen for the control of bleeding secondary to ovulatory dysfunction, through their action in opposing the proliferative effects of oestrogen. Both norethisterone and medroxyprogesterone acetate, given cyclically, are generally well tolerated [C].[1] Overall reduction in blood loss is greater with the levonorgestrel-releasing intrauterine system (LNG-IUS) than with high-dose cyclical progestogen, although there is a higher incidence of breakthrough bleeding with the IUS.[17]

Progestogens at doses high enough to suppress ovulation can be given continuously by the oral route or as long-acting depot injections (e.g. Depo-Provera) to induce amenorrhoea [A].[1] However, their usefulness is limited by side effects, including bloating, fluid retention, breast tenderness and breakthrough bleeding. There is a small risk of bone mineral loss during prolonged treatment with depot preparations but this effect is reversed after treatment is stopped.

Levonorgestrel-releasing intrauterine system

The LNG-IUS is a well-established treatment for HMB. The continuous exposure of the endometrium to progestogen induces progressive atrophy, with reduction of menstrual bleeding by around 80 per cent after 3–6 months and more than 90 per cent at 12 months.[18,19] Spontaneous expulsion occurs in 3–10 per cent of women and the incidence of breakthrough bleeding is around 22–35 per cent in the initial 6–12 months.[18] There is a small (less than 1 per cent) risk of uterine perforation during insertion of the device. Progestogenic side effects of bloating, breast tenderness, headache and acne may occur although they tend to be transient. The predominant side effect which adversely affects compliance is prolonged breakthrough bleeding in up to 10 per cent of women beyond 12 months of use. Discontinuation rates of 17–20 per cent at 12 months, rising to around 28 per cent at 2 years, have been reported.[18,20] Careful counselling is therefore essential prior to insertion [E].

The LNG-IUS has been compared in three systematic reviews and a meta-analysis[18-20] with both medical and surgical treatments. The reduction of menstrual blood loss was significantly greater with the IUS than with tranexamic acid or NSAIDs.[18,19] The side effects of breakthrough bleeding and breast tenderness were more common in women with the LNG-IUS compared with high-dose cyclical norethisterone,[17,19] but overall satisfaction was greater with the LNG-IUS.

The LNG-IUS has been compared with first- and second-generation methods of endometrial ablation.[18-20] Although reduction of blood loss was greater following ablation and side effects were more common with the LNG-IUS, all studies reported that overall satisfaction rates were similar at around 83 per cent at 12 months.[20] In a study of women awaiting hysterectomy,[19,20] 64 per cent of those randomised to insertion of the LNG-IUS cancelled their operation after 6 months, compared with 14 per cent in a control group. In a direct comparison with hysterectomy,[19,20] quality-of-life assessment at 12 months was not significantly different in the two groups, although pain scores were lower after hysterectomy and 20 per cent of the group assigned to the LNG-IUS had opted for hysterectomy in the first year. Costs were three times higher in the hysterectomy group. These results indicate that the LNG-IUS is a highly effective treatment for HMB [A] that has advantages over existing medical treatments and is a potential alternative to surgery.

Other medical therapies

Second-line drugs are available for the control of severe bleeding when simpler measures have failed and, because they more reliably induce amenorrhoea, are useful in the management of severe anaemia. Androgens such as danazol and gestrinone induce amenorrhoea by a combination of negative feedback and direct effects on the endometrium, while gonadotrophin-releasing hormone (GnRH) agonists induce a hypogonadal state via their central action (see Chapter 77). While effective, these approaches are usually limited to short-term use because of their side effects [A].[1] Both danazol and GnRH analogues are of value as endometrial-thinning agents prior to first-generation methods of hysteroscopic surgery, by reducing operating times and improving ease of surgery [A].[21] GnRH analogues used prior to hysteroscopic surgery are also associated with a higher rate of postoperative amenorrhoea and improved dysmenorrhoea at 12 months,[21] although the benefits reduce with time. In cases of severe bleeding due to benign causes in which standard measures have failed, long-term therapy with a GnRH agonist plus hormonal add-back [B] (see Chapters 74 and 77) can be considered if there are contraindications to surgery.

SURGICAL MANAGEMENT

While medical treatment should normally be used as first-line therapy for HMB [E], limitations in efficacy and side effects[1] will result in many women seeking a surgical solution for their problem. The use of the diagnostic techniques described above identifies some women with benign lesions (small submucosal fibroids or endometrial polyps) that are suitable for removal by hysteroscopic surgery[1,6,12] [D] although the role of such surgery in the management of menstrual disorders has not been subjected to critical evaluation. Various methods of endometrial ablation are now well established as day-case or outpatient procedures and recent developments include second-generation techniques that are simpler and safer than older methods.

Endometrial ablation

The objective of endometrial ablation is the complete destruction of the endometrium down to the basal regenerative layer, resulting in fibrosis of the uterine cavity and amenorrhoea. In practice this is very difficult to achieve and rates of amenorrhoea are around 30 to 40 per cent.[22] However, patient satisfaction is over 80 per cent in the short term [A]. A desire for future fertility is an absolute contraindication to endometrial ablation and women must be counselled regarding the appropriate use of contraception [E].

Initially ablation techniques were carried out under direct hysteroscopic vision and involved the use of fluid for distension and irrigation. They comprised laser ablation, endometrial loop resection using electrodiathermy and rollerball electrodiathermy ablation. Of these, laser ablation was limited by its costs to a very few centres. All are operator dependent, time consuming and carry risks of systemic fluid absorption, haemorrhage and uterine perforation with heat damage to adjacent structures. The MISTLETOE Study,[23] a prospective national survey of more than 10,000 procedures in the UK, reported an immediate complication rate of 4.4 per cent which was related to the experience of the operator [C]. Increasingly these so-called first-generation methods have been replaced by the techniques described below. However, they may be carried out, if appropriate, in conjunction with hysteroscopic resection of fibroids [D] (see Chapter 74).

Second-generation endometrial ablation

Newer techniques have been developed with the goal of reducing operator dependency and minimising risk. Several are currently available, including fluid-filled thermal balloon ablation (TBA), microwave endometrial ablation (MEA) and impedance-controlled bipolar radiofrequency ablation.[1,22,24] Second-generation methods have been compared with each other,[22,24] with first-generation methods,[20,22] with abdominal and vaginal hysterectomy[25] and with the LNG-IUS,[19,20,22] in randomised trials and systematic reviews. Satisfaction rates are similar when compared with first-generation methods[20,22] but they have shorter operating times (on average 15 minutes) and fewer serious complications (Table 75.2), making them safer and more cost effective [A]. They are also more suitable for use with local rather than general anaesthesia (61 per cent compared to 21 per cent). However, they are associated with a higher incidence of technical equipment failure. Direct comparisons of different second-generation methods have shown no significant disparities in menstrual blood loss

Table 75.2 Complications of endometrial ablation. Data from systematic review of trials (n = 11) comparing 1st and 2nd generation techniques.[22]

Complication	2nd generation (%)	1st generation (%)	RR (95% CI)
Equipment failure	9.1	1.6	4.3 (1.5–12.4)
Nausea and vomiting	19.4	7.6	2.0 (1.3–3.0)
Uterine cramps	38.4	33.2	1.2 (1.0–1.4)
Fluid overload	0	3.0	0.2 (0.04–0.8)
Uterine perforation	0.3	1.3	0.3 (0.1–1.0)
Cervical lacerations	0.2	2.2	0.2 (0.08–0.6)
Haematometra	0.7	2.4	0.3 (0.1–0.9)
Haemorrhage	1.2	3.0	NS
Fever	0.1	0.1	NS
Endometritis	2.0	1.4	NS

scores, rates of amenorrhoea or patient satisfaction [B].[22,24] Second-generation methods are not suitable for women with submucosal fibroids greater than 3 cm and most are restricted to cavity lengths between 4 and 12 cm. Repeat ablation is contraindicated for most second-generation techniques. In contrast to first-generation methods, endometrial-thinning agents are not usually required [A].[21] Prophylactic antibiotics are commonly used prior to endometrial ablation procedures, although the evidence to support their use is lacking.

Despite the reduced risk of serious complications with second-generation devices, there have been reports of uterine perforation with thermal damage to nearby structures [D].[26] It is recommended that the procedures are carried out in conjunction with hysteroscopy or TVS to ensure correct placement [E]. In addition, myometrial thickness should be pre-assessed by ultrasound, particularly in women with previous uterine surgery, including caesarian section (CS), or with a small thin-walled uterus [E].[26] The presence of a fixed retroverted uterus or history of conditions which may result in adherence of the bowel to the posterior wall of the uterus, such as severe endometriosis or pelvic infection, are relative contraindications to endometrial ablation.[26]

Longer term outcome of endometrial ablation

An early life-table analysis of follow-up after endometrial resection[27] reported a cumulative hysterectomy rate of 27.4 per cent after 4 years. Data from a recent large English cohort study[28] of 114,910 women who had undergone various methods of endometrial ablation indicated that 16.7 per cent had a further procedure within 3 years and 13.5 per cent had a hysterectomy. Risk factors for further intervention in this study were younger age, lower socio-economic class and the presence of uterine fibroids [C].[28]

There is some evidence that the long-term risk of further surgery, including hysterectomy, is lower with second-generation methods.[22,28] Compared with first-generation methods, women who had radiofrequency ablation were significantly less likely to have had further surgery,[28] although outcomes after other second-generation methods were not significantly different from first-generation methods.

All methods of endometrial ablation are less effective than hysterectomy in reducing blood loss and pain.[25] However, adverse events including sepsis, pyrexia and blood transfusion are less common with endometrial ablation, and recovery time is much faster. Patient satisfaction is high with both procedures. The overall evidence is that endometrial ablation is an appropriate first-line surgical approach where medical methods have failed or are deemed inappropriate [A].

Hysterectomy

Hysterectomy provides a definitive cure for women who have completed child-bearing, but the initial costs and morbidity rates are higher than with other treatments.[1] A large cohort study of 37,298 hysterectomies performed in the UK for benign indications reported an operative complication rate of 3.5 per cent, a postoperative complication rate of 9 per cent and an overall mortality rate of 0.38 per 1000.[29] Mortality was 0.25 per 1000 in women undergoing hysterectomy for menstrual problems. The majority of hysterectomies in the latter study were performed abdominally (67 per cent) or vaginally (30 per cent), but the increasing use of laparoscopic methods

Table 75.3 Morbidity of hysterectomy

75.3A Serious morbidity related to the surgical procedure. Data from a systematic review of 34 RCTs (4495 procedures)[30]

Complication	Abdominal (%)	Vaginal (%)	Laparoscopic (%)*
Bowel injury	0.63	0	0.22
Urinary tract injury	0.94	1.21	3.24
Vascular injury	0.77	0.94	1.54
All injuries	2.34	2.15	5.00
Unintended laparotomy	–	3.02	4.30
Pelvic haematoma	5.23	4.40	3.75
Blood transfusion	4.35	3.22	3.54

75.3B Infective complications. Adapted from Table 12.2, Heavy Menstrual Bleeding Guideline: data from 27 RCTs (3643 procedures)[1]

Site	Abdominal (%)	Vaginal (%)	Laparoscopic (%)*
Abdominal wound	7.38	0	1.92
Urinary tract	4.87	1.27	4.77
Chest	4.55	6.67	0.56
Other febrile morbidity	13.15	7.73	10.01

* Any method of laparoscopic hysterectomy

has resulted in investigation of the optimal method of carrying out hysterectomy. A recent systematic review[30] of 34 RCTs which included 4495 women has concluded that laparoscopic hysterectomy is associated with a shorter hospital stay and recovery time compared with abdominal hysterectomy [A]. Blood loss and febrile morbidity were lower but the duration of operations and incidences of vascular and urinary tract injuries were significantly greater. Where significant differences were seen, all outcomes were more favourable with vaginal hysterectomy compared with both abdominal and laparoscopic hysterectomy [A] (Table 75.3). All the studies included in the systematic review used prophylactic antibiotics during surgery.

The role of subtotal hysterectomy (whether performed abdominally or laparoscopically) remains unclear. Evidence from nine RCTs[31] has failed to identify any differences in sexual, bladder or bowel functions following surgery, although the duration of operations, blood loss, febrile morbidity and urinary retention are reduced with the subtotal approach [A]. Women undergoing subtotal hysterectomy should be warned about a 7 per cent risk of occurrence of ongoing menstrual bleeding [A].[1]

Despite this evidence supporting the use of vaginal and laparoscopic routes over the abdominal route, individual assessment is essential when deciding the method of hysterectomy.[1] Factors to be considered include the size and mobility of the uterus, vaginal access, history of previous surgery and presence of other gynaecological disease(s) such as endometriosis as well as the skill and experience of the individual surgeon [E]. Patients with more complex clinical presentations may be excluded from randomised trials and/or treated by more experienced surgeons, accounting for the apparently higher morbidity seen in cohort studies compared with randomised trials.[1,29] Special training in laparoscopic surgical techniques is recommended.[32] All decisions regarding hysterectomy must be accompanied by a detailed discussion with the individual woman of the benefits, risks and future implications of the procedure [E].

Hysterectomy may have long-term implications for bladder function; a systematic review[33] estimated a 60 per cent long-term increase in the odds of developing urinary incontinence following hysterectomy. Cohort studies comparing hysterectomy with endometrial resection[1] or ablation[34] have reported a higher risk of developing urinary symptoms following hysterectomy. A recent Scottish study found an increased risk of pelvic floor or urinary incontinence surgery following hysterectomy for HMB compared with endometrial ablation.[34] This increased risk was observed to be greater in cases of vaginal compared to abdominal surgery. The results of the Scottish study are at variance with those of the large systematic review,[30] which applied a shorter period of follow-up and in which many of the studies excluded participants with prolapse and/or urinary dysfunction. The risks of subsequent adnexal surgery and genital fistula repair were also higher following hysterectomy than following endometrial ablation in the Scottish study.

Removal of healthy ovaries at the time of hysterectomy for HMB should not be undertaken without detailed discussion of the potential impact on the woman's subsequent health and wellbeing, and consideration of relevant issues including her personal and family history of breast and ovarian cancer and her attitude to the use of hormone replacement therapy [E].[1]

Economic considerations

National guidelines[1] recommend that medical treatment, in particular the LNG-IUS, should be initially offered for management of HMB, followed by endometrial ablation if medical therapy fails or is unacceptable. Hysterectomy should be considered only if these other options fail or are contraindicated. A model-based economic evaluation comparing the costs of different clinical pathways of treatment for a 42-year-old woman presenting with HMB[35] concluded that initial treatment with hysterectomy might be more cost effective than pathways starting with the LNG-IUS or with first- or second-generation endometrial ablation. This model did not take into consideration the use of the IUS in primary care. A recent literature review[36] concluded that the LNG-IUS was cost effective in various countries and settings. Factors that influence the success of endometrial ablation also need to be taken into consideration. A large English cohort study[28] found that the risk of further surgery was significantly related to patient age, with 27 per cent of women aged 35 or younger at the time of the initial ablation having further surgery, compared with only 10 per cent of those aged over 45. It is also important to consider patient choice. A survey of patient preferences[1] found that 85 per cent of women are willing to accept a 50:50 chance of treatment failure to avoid hysterectomy. Further information from long-term studies may help clinicians to target management in the most cost-effective way.

> ### EBM
>
> These recommendations for the management of heavy and irregular menstruation are based on a national evidence-based guideline, a systematic review of diagnostic procedures, seven systematic reviews of medical therapy and eight systematic reviews or meta-analyses relating to surgical management.

> ### KEY POINTS
>
> - HMB may occur alone or in combination with other symptoms and should be recognised as having a major impact on a woman's quality of life [E].
> - The initial management of AUB should take place within a primary care setting following abdominal and pelvic examination and measurement of full blood count [E].
> - Sexually active women presenting with intermenstrual or PCB should be tested for chlamydia [B].

REPRODUCTIVE GYNAECOLOGY

- If the history or clinical findings are suggestive of a structural abnormality, ultrasound should be the primary investigation [A], backed up by hysteroscopy or saline infusion sonography if the nature of an intracavity lesion is uncertain [A].
- Endometrial biopsy is indicated in cases of prolonged or irregular bleeding or treatment failure in women over 45 and those with additional risk factors for endometrial cancer, in particular obesity [E].
- NSAIDs and antifibrinolytics are effective in the management of HMB [A], but ethamsylate is ineffective [A].
- The COCP is effective for control of heavy and irregular menstrual bleeding provided there are no contraindications [B].
- Cyclical progestogens are effective for HMB when given for 21 days out of 28 and for control of bleeding associated with ovulatory dysfunction [B].
- Continuous high-dose progestogens (e.g. depot preparations) may be useful if they induce amenorrhoea [B].
- The LNG-IUS device is highly effective in reducing HMB, but adequate counselling is needed prior to insertion [A].
- Drugs that induce amenorrhoea such as GnRH analogues or danazol are useful for the short-term management of heavy bleeding associated with anaemia or for endometrial thinning prior to first-generation methods of endometrial ablation [A].
- Symptomatic endometrial polyps and small submucous fibroids should be removed hysteroscopically [D].
- Endometrial ablation is effective for the relief of HMB [A] and second-generation methods are safer and more cost effective than first-generation methods, as well as simpler and quicker to perform [A].
- Endometrial ablation is cheaper than hysterectomy in the short term but differences narrow with time [A]. Its use in women over 45 is associated with a reduced risk of further surgical intervention [C].
- Long-term satisfaction is high with hysterectomy but it is associated with significant morbidity and mortality [A] and should be offered only if simpler alternatives have failed [E].
- Healthy ovaries should not be removed at hysterectomy without detailed consideration of the risks and benefits [E].
- Vaginal hysterectomy is more cost effective than the abdominal route and should be considered as preferable to abdominal hysterectomy where possible [A].
- Laparoscopic hysterectomy is an alternative to abdominal hysterectomy but carries a greater risk of serious complications and additional specialist training is required [A].
- Subtotal hysterectomy offers no long-term advantages over abdominal hysterectomy and may be associated with continued menstrual bleeding although short-term morbidity is reduced [A].
- The route selected for hysterectomy should be determined by appropriate assessment of the individual patient as well as by the skill and experience of the gynaecologist carrying out the operation [E].

Key References

1. National Collaborating Centre for Women's and Children's Health. *Heavy menstrual bleeding*. London: RCOG Press, 2007.
2. Hallberg L, Hogdahl AM, Nilsson L, Rybo G. Menstrual blood loss – a population study. Variation at different ages and attempts to define normality. *Acta Obstet Gynaecol Scand* 1966;45:320–351.
3. Munro MG, Critchley HOD, Broder MS, Fraser IS for the FIGO Working Group on Menstrual Disorders. The FIGO classification system (PALM-COEIN) for causes of abnormal uterine bleeding in non-gravid women of reproductive age. *Int J Obstet Gynecol* 2011;113:3–13.
4. Shapley M, Jordan K, Croft PR. An epidemiological survey of symptoms of menstrual loss in the community. *Br J of Gen Pract* 2004;54:359–363.
5. Warner P, Critchley HOD, Lumsden MA, Campbell-Brown M, Douglas A, Murray G. Referral for menstrual problems: cross-sectional survey of symptoms, reasons for referral and management. *BMJ* 2001;323:24–28.
6. Nagele F, O'Connor H, Davies A, Badawy A, Mohamed H, Magos A. 2500 outpatient diagnostic hysteroscopies. *Obstet Gynecol* 1996;88:87–92.
7. Shapley M, Jordan K, Croft PR. A systematic review of postcoital bleeding and risk of cervical cancer. *Br J of Gen Pract* 2006;56:453–460.
8. Higham JM, O'Brien PM, Shaw RW. Assessment of menstrual blood loss using a pictorial chart. *Br J Obstet Gynaecol* 1990;97:734–739.
9. Critchley HO, Warner P, Lee AJ, Brechin S, Guise J, Graham B. Evaluation of abnormal uterine bleeding: comparison of three outpatient procedures within cohorts defined by age and menopausal status. *Health Tech Assess* 2004;8:iii-iv,1–139.
10. Cooper NAM, Barton PM, Breijer M et al. Cost effectiveness of diagnostic strategies for the management of abnormal uterine bleeding (heavy menstrual bleeding) and post-menopausal bleeding: a decision analysis. *Health Technology Assessment* 2014;18:24. DOI 10.3310/hta 18240..
11. Farquhar C, Ekeroma A, Furness S, Arroll B. A systematic review of transvaginal ultrasonography, sonohysterography and hysteroscopy for the investigation of abnormal uterine bleeding in premenopausal women. *Acta Obstet Gynecol Scand* 2003;82:493–504.
12. Farquhar C, Arroll B, Ekeroma A *et al.* An evidence-based guideline for the management of uterine fibroids. *Aust NZ J Obstet Gynaecol* 2001;41:125–40.
13. Shapley M, Blagojevic-Bucknall KP, Jordan PR, Croft PR. The epidemiology of self-reported intermenstrual and postcoital bleeding in the perimenopausal years. *BJOG* 2013;120:1348–1355.
14. Lethaby A, Farquhar C, Cooke I. Antifibrinolytics for heavy menstrual bleeding. *Cochrane Database of Systematic*

Reviews 2000,4:CD000249.DOI:10.1002/14651858. CD000249.

15. Lethaby A, Augood C, Duckitt K. Nonsteroidal anti-inflammatory drugs for heavy menstrual bleeding. *Cochrane Database of Systematic Reviews* 2013, Issue 1.Art.No.:CD000400. DOI:10.1002/14651858. CD000400.pub3.

16. Farquhar C, Brown J. Oral contraceptive pill for heavy menstrual bleeding. *Cochrane Database of Systematic Reviews* 2009, Issue 4. Art. No: CD000154. DOI:10.1002/14651858. CD000154.pub2.

17. Lethaby A, Irvine GA, Cameron IT. Cyclical progestogens for heavy menstrual bleeding. *Cochrane Database of Systematic Reviews* 2008, Issue 1. Art.No.:CD001016. DOI:10.1002/14651858. CD001016.pub2.

18. Lethaby A, Cooke I, Rees MC. Progesterone or progestogen-releasing intrauterine systems for heavy menstrual bleeding. *Cochrane Database of Systematic Reviews* 2005, Issue 4. Art.No.:CD002126. DOI: 10.1002/14651851858. CD002126.pub2.

19. Stewart A, Cummins C, Gold L, Jordan R, Phillips W. The effectiveness of the levonorgestrel-releasing intrauterine system in menorrhagia: a systematic review. *Br J Obstet Gynaecol* 2001;108:74–86.

20. Middleton LJ, Champaneria R, Daniels JP *et al.* Hysterectomy, endometrial destruction and levonorgestrel releasing intrauterine system (Mirena) for heavy menstrual bleeding: systematic review and meta-analysis of data from individual patients. *BMJ* 2010;341:c3929.

21. Tan YH, Lethaby A. Preoperative endometrial thinning agents before endometrial destruction for heavy menstrual bleeding. *Cochrane Database of Systematic Reviews* 2013, Issue 11.Art.No.:CD010241. DOI: 10.1002/14651858. CD010241.pub2.

22. Lethaby A, Penninx J, Hickey M, Garry R, Marjoribanks J. Endometrial resection and ablation techniques for heavy menstrual bleeding. *Cochrane Database of Systematic Reviews* 2013, Issue 8. Art.No.:CD001501. DOI:10.1002/14651858.CD001501.pub4.

23. Overton C, Hargreaves J, Maresh M. A national survey of the complications of endometrial destruction for menstrual disorders: the MISTLETOE study. *Br J Obstet Gynaecol* 1997;104:1351–1359.

24. Daniels JP, Middleton LJ, Champaniera R *et al.* International Heavy Menstrual Bleeding IPD Meta-analysis Collaborative Group. Second-generation endometrial ablation techniques for heavy menstrual bleeding: network meta-analysis. *BMJ* 2012;344:e2564.

25. Fergusson RJ, Lethaby A, Shepperd S, Farquhar C. Endometrial resection and ablation versus hysterectomy for heavy menstrual bleeding. *Cochrane Database of Systematic Reviews* 2013, Issue 11. Art.No.:CD000329. DOI:10.1002/14651858. CD000329.pub2.

26. Medicines and Healthcare Products Agency. *Medical Device Alert. Devices used for endometrial ablation. All makes and models.* MDE/2010/006.

27. Pooley AS, Ewen P, Sutton CJ. Does transcervical resection of the endometrium for menorrhagia really avoid hysterectomy? Life table analysis of a large series. *J Am Assoc Gynecol Laparosc* 1998; 5:229–235.

28. Bansi-Matharu L, Gurol-Urganci I, Mahmood T, Templeton A, van der Meulen JH, Cromwell DA. Rates of subsequent surgery following endometrial ablation among English women with menorrhagia: population-based cohort study. *BJOG* 2013;120:1500–1507.

29. Maresh MHJ, Metcalfe MA, McPherson K *et al.* The VALUE national hysterectomy study: description of the patients and their surgery. *BJOG* 2002;109:302–312.

30. Nieboer TE, Johnson N, Lethaby A *et al.* Surgical approach to hysterectomy for benign gynaecological disease. *Cochrane Database of Systematic Reviews* 2009, Issue 3. Art.No.: CD003677. DOI:10.1002/14651858. CD003677.pub4 .

31. Lethaby A, Mukhopadhyay A, Naik R. Total versus subtotal hysterectomy for benign gynaecological conditions. *Cochrane Database of Systematic Reviews* 2012, Issue 4. Art. No.:CD004993. DOI:10.1002/14651858. CD004993.pub3.

32. NICE. *Laparoscopic techniques for hysterectomy.* Interventional procedure guidance 239. November 2007.

33. Brown JS, Sawaya G, Thom DH, Grady D. Hysterectomy and urinary incontinence: a systematic review. *Lancet* 2000;356:535–539.

34. Cooper K, Lee AJ, Raja EA, Timmaraju V, Bhattacharya S. Outcomes following hysterectomy or endometrial ablation for heavy menstrual bleeding: retrospective analysis of hospital episode statistics in Scotland. *BJOG* 2011;118:1171–1179.

35. Roberts TE, Tsourapas A, Middleton LJ *et al.* Hysterectomy, endometrial ablation and levonorgestrel releasing intrauterine system (Mirena) for treatment of heavy menstrual bleeding: cost effectiveness analysis. *BMJ* 2011;342;d2202. doi:10.1136/bmj.d2202.

36. Blumenthal PD, Dawson L, Hurskainen R. Cost-effectiveness and quality of life associated with heavy menstrual bleeding among women using the levonorgestrel-releasing intrauterine system. *Int J Gynecol Obstet* 2011;112:171–178.

REPRODUCTIVE GYNAECOLOGY

Chapter 76 Dysmenorrhoea and pelvic pain

Christine P West

INTRODUCTION

Pain during menstruation is an almost universal experience among women and, when severe, it has a significant economic impact through loss of time from work or education. Recognition of the consequences of this problem has led to several large-scale reviews of treatments for dysmenorrhoea, including alternative therapies. There is thus a well-founded evidence base for its management. Pain related to or exacerbated during menstruation or sexual intercourse may be a consequence of underlying pelvic pathology, although not all women with pelvic pain have a gynaecological disorder. This chapter is mainly concerned with gynaecological causes of cyclical pelvic pain but some reference is made to the multifactorial nature of the problem and to management of symptoms of chronic pelvic pain.

DEFINITIONS

Dysmenorrhoea is a descriptive term for pain that occurs during menstruation. Primary dysmenorrhoea, also known as primary spasmodic dysmenorrhoea, is a condition of colicky, cramping, suprapubic pain that may radiate to the lower back and thighs, often associated with gastrointestinal and systemic symptoms. It typically lasts for between 8 and 72 hours, although milder manifestations are almost universally experienced by young women. Although it can cause significant morbidity, it is not associated with any pelvic abnormality.

Secondary dysmenorrhoea is menstrual pain which is secondary to identifiable pelvic pathology (e.g. endometriosis). It is often associated with deep dyspareunia. Pain which is exacerbated by menstruation and continues throughout the cycle is known as chronic cyclical pelvic pain, a subset of the condition of chronic pelvic pain in which pain of at least 6 months' duration is present continuously or intermittently, not associated exclusively with menstruation or sexual intercourse[1].

PREVALENCE

The reported prevalence of dysmenorrhoea varies widely depending on the population studied and the method of reporting. A systematic review of older studies[1] reported a prevalence of between 45 and 97 per cent. In a review of more recent community-based studies and systematic reviews,[2] the prevalence ranged between 16 and 91 per cent, with 2–29 per cent reporting severe pain. Studies of teenage or younger women generally reported a higher prevalence and a higher proportion with severe symptoms, compared with those including a wider reproductive age group. The studies did not generally distinguish between primary and secondary dysmenorrhoea. Prevalence was similar in studies from developed and developing countries.

The annual prevalence of chronic pelvic pain has been estimated at 38.3 per 1000 using consultation episodes from a large UK general practice database of women aged 12 to 70 years.[3] The 3-month prevalence among women aged 18 to 50 was 23.6 per 1000. This result is considerably lower than the 3-month prevalence of 15 per cent in a community-based US sample of women aged 15 to 50,[4] but the latter study was based on self-reported pelvic pain and only 25 per cent of the women sought medical advice for help with their symptoms.

EPIDEMIOLOGY

The general consensus in the literature[2] is that age and parity are inversely related to the incidence of dysmenorrhoea. There is generally an association with family history although it is not clear whether this is due to genetic factors or conditioning. Users of the oral contraceptive pill have a reduced prevalence, while stress is associated with increased risk. Other factors less consistently reported are low body mass index (BMI), smoking, early menarche and heavy menstrual bleeding.[5] Exercise and a high intake of fruit and vegetables have been reported as protective in some studies.

A systemic review of studies of risk factors for chronic pelvic pain[5] concluded that drug or alcohol abuse, psychological co-morbidity and a history of physical or sexual abuse are all associated with an increased risk. It also reported an association between non-cyclical pelvic pain and many gynaecological and obstetric factors including miscarriage, caesarian section (CS), heavy menstrual flow and pelvic inflammatory disease (PID). Factors such as personality traits, coping strategies, health beliefs and influences of family members may predispose an individual to the development of chronic pain.[5,6]

CAUSES

Primary dysmenorrhoea

Uterine myometrial hyperactivity has been demonstrated in women with primary dysmenorrhoea.[7] This condition is most commonly attributed to excess prostaglandin production during menstruation, resulting in increased myometrial contractions and enhancement of the normal reduction of uterine blood flow which occurs during menstruation, leading to increased ischaemia. Primary dysmenorrhoea is regarded as a physiological variant of the normal response to ovarian hormonal withdrawal and onset of menstrual bleeding and is not regarded as a pathological condition. However, in common with all painful conditions, there may be psychological, social or emotional factors that influence its impact on the individual affected.

Pain occurring at mid-cycle, known as mittelschmerz, is secondary to follicle rupture and also regarded as physiological. It may be associated with vaginal bleeding.

Secondary dysmenorrhoea

The most common cause of secondary dysmenorrhoea and chronic cyclical pelvic pain (Table 76.1) is endometriosis (see Chapter 77), which occurs in around one third of laparoscopies carried out for pelvic pain.[8] Adenomyosis is a cause of secondary dysmenorrhoea that is most commonly diagnosed in older multiparous women (Chapter 78). Unlike adenomyosis, uterine fibroids are not typically associated with pelvic pain, although dysmenorrhoea can occur with passage of clots and acute pain may be secondary to fibroid degeneration or expulsion of a submucosal fibroid through the cervix. Cervical stenosis or intrauterine adhesions secondary to surgical procedures cause dysmenorrhoea secondary to retained menstrual fluid (haematometra). Pain from trapped or residual ovaries is usually cyclical, while adhesions can cause non-cyclical

Table 76.1 Causes of dysmenorrhoea and cyclical and non-cyclical chronic pelvic pain

Physiological	Primary dysmenorrhoea
	Mittelschmerz
Gynaecological	Endometriosis
	Adenomyosis
	Uterine fibroids
	Cervical stenosis and other obstructive causes
	Pelvic venous congestion
	Residual/trapped ovary syndrome
	Pelvic adhesions
	Pelvic inflammatory disease
Gastro-intestinal	Irritable bowel syndrome
	Chronic constipation
Urinary tract	Bladder pain syndrome (interstitial cystitis)
Musculoskeletal	Pelvic floor myalgia
	Myofascial pain
Neurological	Nerve entrapment

pain due to organ distension. Secondary dysmenorrhoea is unusual in young women although both endometriosis and adenomyosis may occur. Another rare cause of the condition is pain secondary to congenital Müllerian abnormalities that are associated with obstructions to menstrual flow[7] (e.g. cryptomenorrhoea in an accessory uterine horn).

Non-gynaecological causes of pelvic pain

Around one third of laparoscopies carried out for the investigation of pelvic pain are negative.[8] Non-gynaecological conditions can be exacerbated or enhanced during menstruation and/or intercourse. In particular, irritable bowel syndrome (IBS) is commonly diagnosed following negative investigations for pelvic pain.[6,7,9] Symptoms suggestive of IBS are abdominal pain or discomfort relieved by defaecation, possibly associated with altered bowel frequency or stool form.[10] The condition is also commonly associated with abdominal bloating and other features such as lethargy, nausea, backache, dyspareunia and bladder symptoms. In a sample of 5051 UK women on a GP database with a recorded diagnosis of chronic pelvic pain,[9] 21 per cent had gastrointestinal symptoms and 29 per cent were eventually diagnosed with IBS, this diagnosis being more common in the older age group. Milder forms of inflammatory bowel disease may be confused with IBS, but in the former inflammatory markers will be raised. Bowel cancer is uncommon in the reproductive age group but symptoms such as rectal bleeding and unexplained weight loss should prompt urgent referral to a gastroenterologist.[10]

Bladder pain syndrome (BPS; formerly known as interstitial cystitis) is also commonly diagnosed in women with chronic pelvic pain.[6,7,11] Key symptoms are pain, pressure or

REPRODUCTIVE GYNAECOLOGY

discomfort, situated suprapubically, increasing as the bladder fills and relieved by voiding. Pain may radiate to the groin, vagina or rectum, and dyspareunia is frequently located over the bladder base. Two main subtypes of BPS are recognised,[11] distinguished mainly by different appearances at cystoscopy. The cause of BPS is unknown.

Chronic cyclical and non-cyclical pelvic pain

The causes of chronic pelvic pain may be less clearly defined than those of primary or secondary dysmenorrhoea, and the condition may result from more than one contributory factor. Changes in peripheral nerve function may occur following acute events such as surgery, trauma, inflammation, fibrosis or infection, resulting in altered visceral sensation and function leading to pain which persists long after the original acute episode.[6] An example of this would be pain persisting in areas affected by endometriosis after such lesions have apparently regressed or been removed. Similar changes may occur even in the absence of any such acute event. Changes in the CNS itself (central sensitisation) may modify or enhance the original signal leading to enhancement of visceral sensation, known as visceral hyperalgesia.[11] This effect causes an increased perception of pain and has been described in association with endometriosis, IBS and BPS. Viscero-visceral hyperalgesia, whereby pain from one organ can induce pain and dysfunction in others with visceral afferent nerves sharing the same distribution, may be a contributing factor.[12] This may explain why women with endometriosis-associated pain may also complain of symptoms of IBS or BPS.

As mentioned above, chronic pain has been shown to be related to CNS amplification of pain processing, which often occurs in the absence of acute injury or inflammation of peripheral structures. Reductions in the grey matter volume of brain regions involved in pain perception have been described in women with unexplained or endometriosis-associated chronic pain, but not in control groups or in women with endometriosis-associated dysmenorrhoea without chronic pain.[13] The reason for this difference is not clear but suggests that chronic pelvic pain represents some form of central maladaptation of the pain system[13] which is likely to be multifactorial in nature. Pain arising from disturbance of the central or peripheral nervous system is classified as neuropathic pain.

Pelvic venous congestion is a condition described in multiparous women of reproductive age.[14] Chronic dull, aching pain is characteristically exacerbated perimenstrually, by activity and by sexual intercourse, and relieved by lying down. It is attributed to the presence of dilated veins in the broad ligament and ovarian plexus. Typical appearances have been described at venography and reported with both ultrasound[15] and MRI, although studies reporting accuracy, sensitivity and specificity have not been undertaken and the existence of the condition as an entity distinct from unexplained chronic cyclical pelvic pain is disputed.

Musculoskeletal factors

Pain arising from the muscles or joints within the pelvis or from the muscles of the abdominal wall or pelvic floor may be a component of chronic pelvic pain, resulting from postural changes secondary to the pain[6,7] or a primary source of it. Nerve entrapment in a surgical scar and pudendal neuralgia[11] which may follow childbirth are direct causes of neuropathic pain. Spasm of the pelvic floor muscles is proposed as a secondary cause of chronic pelvic pain and dyspareunia.[6] Muscle pain and spasm may be derived from myofascial trigger points[16,17] which are specific areas of tenderness within a taut band of skeletal muscle. Hyperactivity in the nerve endings at such trigger points produces enhanced sensitivity, muscle contraction and referred pain described as deep, aching and poorly localised within the area affected. It is usually exacerbated by activity but may be relieved by pressure or stretching. Pain can be reproduced by sustained compression over the point of tenderness. The development of myofascial trigger point pain is usually secondary to physical causes such as injury, ischaemia or nerve compression, but muscle pain may also arise as a result of visceral disease[16] whereby myofascial trigger points in the zone of pain referral can become activated with the production of superimposed neuropathic pain. This could be one of the mechanisms underlying conditions such as vulvodynia as well as pelvic floor muscle spasm (myalgia).[11] Myofascial trigger points may also be detectable in muscles of the anterior abdominal wall in patients with chronic pelvic pain.

Psychological and social factors

Epidemiological studies (see above) have indicated that there is an association between chronic pelvic pain and physical and sexual abuse. There are also potential associations with drug and alcohol abuse, depression, anxiety and sleep disorders, although sleep disorders could be secondary to the pain.[6] Whilst unexplained symptoms must not be regarded as psychogenic in origin, there may be aspects of personality or past experience which render certain individuals more vulnerable to the development of chronic pain syndromes or impair their abilities to develop coping strategies.[7] The majority of women with chronic pelvic pain experience sexual dysfunction, most commonly dyspareunia, vaginismus and sexual avoidance, leading to relationship problems which contribute to psychological and social morbidity. Addressing these various issues is likely to be important in resolving the symptoms.

MANAGEMENT

Investigation

The diagnosis of primary dysmenorrhoea is based on the history of typical spasmodic, cramping, suprapubic pain, confined to menstruation and with no features suggestive of other gynaecological conditions. It should be backed up by clinical examination if appropriate and does not require investigation [E]. It is normally managed by the GP or primary care physician. Referral to a gynaecologist is required if there is a lack of response to standard therapies or if symptoms are atypical, giving rise to a suspicion of endometriosis or other pathology. Pelvic examination is not indicated in a teenager who is not sexually active [E]. A transabdominal ultrasound scan will exclude congenital uterine abnormalities or significant ovarian pathology and should provide reassurance if negative.

Gynaecological symptoms of dyspareunia, abnormal bleeding or a history of previous surgery or infection are suggestive of an underlying cause for the pain. Abdominal and pelvic examinations should be performed to assess tenderness, uterine size and the presence of any masses. Reduced uterine mobility together with tenderness and thickening or nodularity in the pouch of Douglas is suggestive of endometriosis (see Chapter 77). Tender uterine enlargement is suggestive of adenomyosis (see Chapter 78). Localised tender trigger points may be identified in the muscles of the abdominal wall or pelvic floor.

In cases of suspected PID, samples should be taken to screen for sexually transmitted infections (STIs). Ultrasound should be performed if the findings of an examination are abnormal, as it is sensitive in the detection of uterine fibroids and adenomyosis as well as ovarian cysts and endometrioma [A].[18] It has the advantage of being cheap and non-invasive. MRI scanning is useful as an additional tool if ultrasound findings are equivocal. Laparoscopy has an established role in the diagnosis and treatment of endometriosis (see Chapter 77) but is not without risk,[19] nor routinely required prior to a therapeutic trial of medical therapy [E].[6,7]

For women presenting with chronic pelvic pain, there is evidence that the quality of the initial consultation influences later progress.[6] Detailed history taking and pelvic examination (not necessarily at the same visit) are essential. The initial history should include questions about the pattern of pain and its association with other problems such as bladder and bowel symptoms and the effect of movement and posture on the pain. Psychosocial factors must be explored in detail and the woman given time to express her ideas, concerns and expectations [E]. Laparoscopy is commonly performed, but in the absence of abnormal clinical or ultrasound findings the likelihood of abnormal findings at laparoscopy is also very low.[18,20] A randomised trial comparing two therapeutic approaches to chronic pelvic pain concluded that laparoscopy played no important role in management [B].[21] Although in some cases negative findings may provide reassurance, a study assessing the value of photographic reinforcement after a negative laparoscopy showed no additional benefit.[22] However, another study showed that when pelvic ultrasound examination is accompanied by education, counselling and reassurance there is subsequent improvement in measures of pain, compared with ultrasound alone.[22]

Management of primary dysmenorrhoea

NSAIDs

These drugs inhibit prostaglandin synthesis via inhibition of the enzyme cyclooxygenase. A systematic review of 73 clinical trials[23] evaluated 21 different non-steroidal anti-inflammatory drugs (NSAIDs) including aspirin, naproxen, ibuprofen, mefenamic acid and diclofenac. All with the exception of aspirin were significantly more effective than placebo in producing moderate or excellent pain relief [A]. The NSAIDs were also more effective than paracetamol [A], but side effects included nausea, indigestion, headache, dizziness, drowsiness and dry mouth. There were not any significant disparities in the efficacy or side effects of different NSAIDs. The review included two small studies of the newer, more selective cyclooxygenase-2 (COX-2) NSAIDs, but there was no evidence favouring these over the older preparations. NSAIDs are an effective treatment for dysmenorrhoea [A] and choice will depend on clinician and patient preferences and costs [E]. NSAIDs may be used in combination with other analgesics such as paracetamol or codeine [E].

Combined oral contraceptive pill

These preparations have been widely used for the relief of primary dysmenorrhoea since before the introduction of large randomised controlled trials (RCTs). The theoretical basis for efficacy is inhibition of ovulation. A systematic review[24] concluded that combined oral contraceptive pills (COCPs) are significantly more effective than placebo for pain relief [A] although only one of the five trials included in the review was based on the low-dose formulations in current use. A small RCT comparing continuous with cyclical administration of a low-dose third-generation COCP (ethinyl estradiol 20 mcg plus gestodene 0.075 mg)[25] reported that initial pain relief was better with continuous administration, but by 6 months the methods were equally effective [B]. There are no data comparing second- and third-generation formulations but the latter are more expensive and carry a marginally higher risk of thrombotic complications. Transdermal or vaginal administration is also available. Despite the lack of high-quality evidence, combined oral contraceptive preparations should be regarded as a safe and effective therapy for the relief of primary dysmenorrhoea [A].

Other hormonal therapies

Other ovulation suppressive therapies for the treatment of menstrual pain secondary to endometriosis (see Chapter 77), such as continuous high-dose progestogens, androgens and gonadotrophin-releasing hormone (GnRH) analogues, are highly effective [A] but there is limited evidence for their long-term use. Low-dose progestogens can also be used. A prospective non-comparative multicentre study[26] of 406 women treated with the low-dose ovulation-suppressive progestogen-only contraceptive desogestrel (75 mcg per day) reported a marked reduction of moderate or severe dysmenorrhoea in

93 per cent of the women [C]. Irregular or non-cyclic bleeding was the most prevalent side effect, experienced by 24 per cent, with 3 per cent reporting prolonged bleeding. The levonorgestrel-releasing intrauterine system (LNG-IUS) is effective in the treatment of menstrual pain secondary to both endometriosis and adenomyosis (see Chapters 77 and 78), and should be regarded as another treatment option for women with primary dysmenorrhoea who are seeking contraception, and for those with contraindications to the combined pill [B]. For women whose symptoms are incompletely relieved with NSAIDs or the contraceptive preparations mentioned above, and those who develop unacceptable side effects, GnRH analogues plus add-back hormone replacement therapy (HRT) are often well tolerated and long-term safety data is reassuring (see Chapter 77).

Alternative therapies for primary and secondary dysmenorrhoea

These are popular with the public and are widely used. A recent review concluded that assessments of efficacy are limited by the poor quality of available information.[27] Interventions that have been assessed in RCTs and systematic reviews are summarised in Table 76.2. These trials were not based exclusively on women with primary dysmenorrhoea. Behavioural therapies aimed at improving coping strategies included three trials of relaxation with or without other treatment, one of pain management training and two of biofeedback.[28] All showed some evidence of benefit. Physical therapies such as TENS, exercise,[29] acupuncture[30] and topical heat appear to be of potential value. Of the herbal and dietary therapies subjected to review, only thiamine and magnesium were more effective than placebo,[31] with moderate-quality evidence for thiamine. A systematic review of 39 trials of Chinese herbal medicine[32] found promising evidence of

benefit for primary dysmenorrhoea when compared to acupuncture, heat compression and conventional medication, but (again) conclusions were limited by poor methodological quality.

Although women with chronic non-cyclical pelvic pain were not included in the studies cited above and other robust evidence is also lacking, physical, dietary and behavioural therapies are likely to be applicable as part of a multidisciplinary approach.

Secondary dysmenorrhoea and chronic pelvic pain

Causes of secondary dysmenorrhoea and cyclical and non-cyclical chronic pelvic pain are listed in Table 76.1. Management of endometriosis and adenomyosis are reviewed in detail in Chapters 77 and 78. Interventions for the management of chronic pelvic pain have been the subject of an RCOG Green-top guideline,[6] a guideline published by the European Society of Urology[11] and a systematic review.[22]

Multidisciplinary approach

One study[21] randomised 106 women with chronic pelvic pain to either standard treatment or an integrated approach. Standard treatment included comprehensive exclusion of organic causes, including routine laparoscopy, followed by attention to other causes. In the integrated approach group, laparoscopy was not performed and a gynaecologist, psychologist, physiotherapist and nutritionist assessed all the women. Management was then directed as appropriate. Evaluation 1 year later showed a significantly greater improvement in daily activities and perceptions of pain among the latter group, although pain scores were not significantly different. This

Table 76.2 Alternative therapies for dysmenorrhoea[27]

Intervention	Nature of evidence	Conclusion
TENS	Systematic review of 7 RCTs	High- but not low-frequency TENS more effective than placebo
Behavioural therapy	Systematic review of 5 RCTs	Possible benefit but data inconsistent[28]
Exercise	Systematic review of 1 RCT	Possible benefit[29]
Acupuncture or acupressure	Systematic review of 10 RCTs	Some evidence of benefit[30]
Spinal manipulation	Systematic review of 2 trials	Inconclusive
Topical heat patch/pad	2 RCTs	Similar efficacy to ibuprofen and more effective than paracetamol
Magnesium	Systematic review of 3 RCTs	Some evidence of benefit but dosage uncertain[31]
Vitamin E	Systematic review of 1 RCT	Inconclusive
Thiamine (vitamin B1)	Systematic review of 1 RCT	Some benefit with 100 mg daily
Fish oil	2 low-quality RCTs	Inconclusive
Japanese herbal therapies	Systematic review of 1 trial	Inconclusive
Chinese herbal medicine	Systematic review	Evidence of benefit[32]

REPRODUCTIVE GYNAECOLOGY

study and others[6,10,22] have highlighted the importance of a multidisciplinary approach to chronic pain [B]. A number of organisations can provide additional information and support (e.g. the Pelvic Pain Support Network; www.pelvicpain.org.uk). Pressure on multidisciplinary services may limit the availability of such facilities. A suggested plan of management for patients presenting to a general gynaecological clinic with symptoms of pelvic pain is outlined in Fig. 76.1.

Ovarian suppression

Ovarian suppression has an established role in the management of primary dysmenorrhoea and menstrual pain secondary to endometriosis and adenomyosis (see above and Chapters 77 and 78). Although there is some dispute about the existence of the condition, hormonal suppression has been advocated for women with chronic pelvic pain and dyspareunia attributed to the presence of pelvic varicosities. In a large randomised trial,[33] medroxyprogesterone acetate (MPA) (50 mg daily for 4 months), either alone or in conjunction with psychotherapy, was more effective than placebo or psychotherapy alone for the duration of therapy, but the benefit was not sustained after completion. In a subsequent study, 47 women with chronic pelvic pain and pelvic venous congestion diagnosed by venography[15] were randomised to receive a 6-month course of either the GnRH agonist goserelin or MPA (30 mg daily). Both groups had improved pain scores at the end of treatment but the improvement was sustained for 12 months afterwards only in the group who received goserelin. Ovarian suppression is also likely to benefit women with pain secondary to trapped or residual ovaries[7] and those with obstructions to menstrual flow if surgical interventions have failed or are not appropriate.

The results of a randomised placebo-controlled trial of 3 months of treatment with the GnRH agonist depot leuprolide for women with chronic pelvic pain secondary to clinically suspected endometriosis[34] showed a significantly greater reduction in dysmenorrhoea, chronic pelvic pain and dyspareunia in the active treatment group. Improvements in pain occurred in some women who were subsequently found at laparoscopy not to have endometriosis. On the basis of this evidence, there seems to be a role for a trial of empirical ovarian suppression in the management of chronic pelvic pain which is cyclically exacerbated [B].

Centrally acting drugs

Regular use of NSAIDs, together with paracetamol or codeine, forms the basis of analgesic management of chronic pain. Use of opiates is not recommended outside a specialised service.[6] Where pain control is inadequate, tricyclic antidepressants (TCAs) and anti-epileptic drugs such as gabapentinoids are commonly used in the management of chronic pain and particularly neuropathic pain.[35,36] If, as is postulated, chronic

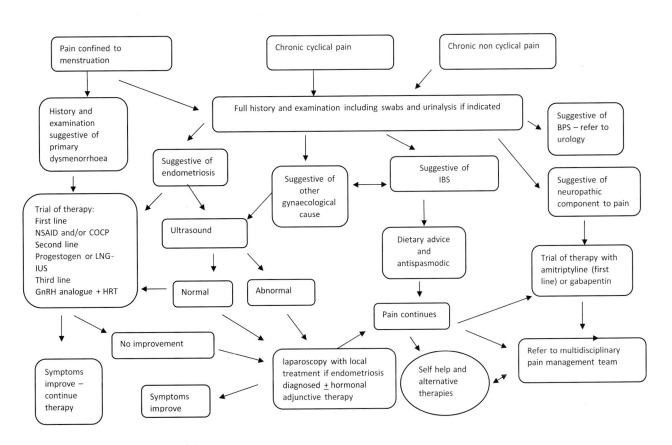

Fig. 76.1 Suggested management of dysmenorrhoea and pelvic pain in a general gynaecological setting

pelvic pain has a neuropathic component, then it is rational to try them in this setting. Amitriptyline should be started at a low dose, typically 25 mg 2 hours before bedtime (can be reduced to 10 mg if required). The drug should be slowly titrated up to effect over a period of several weeks. The target dose will be in the region of 75 mg, although many patients will not tolerate the associated side effects including dizziness, drowsiness and anti-muscarinic effects of dry mouth and blurred vision. The substitution of nortriptyline or imipramine in similar dosages may reduce the side effects, particularly sedation. The analgesic effect of amitryptyline is independent of its action as an antidepressant and other classes of antidepressants (such as selective serotonin reuptake inhibitors [SSRIs][35]) are ineffective for pain. With gabapentin, patients are typically started on 300 mg daily and slowly titrated up (over a few weeks) to a target dose of 600 mg three times a day. Side effects include dizziness, drowsiness, peripheral oedema and gait disturbance, although serious effects are rare. Pregabalin has a similar side-effect profile but may be better suited to individual patients. The starting dose is 75 mg twice a day, titrating up to a target dose of 300 mg twice a day.

There is limited evidence to support the use of these adjuvant agents to manage chronic pelvic pain. To date, only one small study (56 patients)[22,37] has compared gabapentin to amitriptyline for the treatment of chronic pelvic pain. It showed that gabapentin had greater efficacy (80 per cent compared to 70 per cent improvement in pain scores at 12 months). Unfortunately, this study had no placebo arm and the significance of the effect on quality of life was not evaluated.

Nevertheless, increasing evidence supporting a neuropathic and central sensitisation component to chronic pelvic pain has led to the prescription of these agents to good effect in general practice and in multidisciplinary settings [C]. Further studies are required to determine their true efficacy in the treatment of chronic pelvic pain.

Non-gynaecological causes of pelvic pain

Because symptoms of IBS are cyclically exacerbated and there may be associated dyspareunia, women with IBS are frequently seen in gynaecological clinics and there can be diagnostic confusion with endometriosis. The conditions may also coexist, in which case management should be directed towards both.[12] If, on the basis of history and clinical examination, IBS is considered to be the main cause of pain or a contributing factor, dietary advice [C] and a trial of treatment with an antispasmodic agent such as mebeverine hydrochloride (135 to 150 mg three times daily) is appropriate [A].[10] Dietary management should include regular meals and adequate fluid intake with restricted caffeine, alcohol and fizzy drinks.[10] Insoluble fibre such as bran should be avoided in favour of soluble fibre such as oats or ispaghula. Constipation may be managed with laxatives (avoiding lactulose) and diarrhoea with loperamide.[10] Management of IBS falls within the scope of general practice. Chronic pain associated with IBS may be resistant to these standard measures, in which case low-dose amitriptyline is a

second-line treatment [A].[10] In complex cases, multidisciplinary input should be sought.

Urinary symptoms of frequency, dysuria, urgency and nocturia are frequently present in women with chronic pelvic pain, so urinary tract infection (UTI) should be excluded. BPS is usually diagnosed by cystoscopy although appearances vary according to subtypes. Input from a urologist or urogynaecologist may be required. Symptoms of BPS associated with chronic pelvic pain may benefit from treatment with amitriptyline [B].[11]

Local treatments of myofascial trigger points and pelvic floor muscle spasms involve manual therapy by a specialist physiotherapist.[7,11,16] Local injections of botulinum toxin have also been used to relieve pelvic floor muscle spasms.[6,7]

Non-pharmacological therapies targeting the nervous system

Previous approaches to the management of dysmenorrhoea and pelvic pain involved surgical interruption of the sensory nerve pathways, either by removal of the nerve bundles of the hypogastic plexus which overlies the bodies of L 4 & 5 and the sacral promontory (presacral neurectomy – PSN) or ablation of the uterine nerves by division of the uterosacral ligaments (LUNA).[37] Both these procedures can be performed laparoscopically but PSN demands considerable surgical expertise. Although there is some evidence of benefit of PSN for uterine pain in severe endometriosis, neither technique is recommended for management of dysmenorrhoea or chronic pelvic pain, regardless of its cause[37][A].

Less invasive approaches target the nervous system by external electrical or magnetic stimulation[37] to alter neurophysiology locally at the site of pain or centrally, for example transcutaneous electrical nerve stimulation (TENS) which can be useful in the management of dysmenorrhoea. Despite some promising results, these techniques have not been fully evaluated in women with chronic pelvic pain. Direct percutaneous electrical nerve stimulation (neuromodulation) is an alternative approach which has an established role in management of overactive bladder syndrome. Both sacral nerve stimulation (SNS) and pudendal nerve stimulation (PNS) have evidence of benefit in small scale studies of women with chronic pelvic pain and one small cross-over study showed greater benefit for PNS.[37] PNS has also been used in the management of pudendal neuralgia. These data are very preliminary and long term follow up is lacking. Currently neuromodulation should only be undertaken in specialist centres which can provide multidisciplinary care [E].

Other surgical approaches for chronic pelvic pain

Adhesions may be seen in up to one quarter of laparoscopies for pelvic pain,[8] usually as a consequence of previous surgery or inflammatory conditions. The mechanism of their contribution to the pain is unclear and in many cases there may be a neuropathic component. Studies evaluating surgical division of adhesions have shown minimal or no improvement of pelvic pain[22] [A] with the exception of women undergoing laparoscopic division of severe adhesions. Hysterectomy may be beneficial for secondary dysmenorrhoea attributed to endometriosis or adenomyosis but its role in chronic pelvic pain is unclear. A trial of therapy with a GnRH agonist should be undertaken before consideration of hysterectomy in such cases [E]. A review of five studies of women undergoing hysterectomy for chronic pain presumed to be of uterine origin[39] reported that symptoms were relieved in 83 to 97 per cent of women at 12-month follow-up [D]. However, the results of these studies showed that failure of pain relief was greatest among women with no demonstrable pelvic pathology, once again emphasising the importance of a multidisciplinary approach for women with unexplained pelvic pain.

EBM

Recommendations for the management of primary and secondary dysmenorrhoea are based on eight systematic reviews, five of which address alternative therapies. The management of chronic pelvic pain has been the subject of one systematic review, an RCOG Green-top guideline and an international guideline from the European Association of Urology.

KEY POINTS

- Primary dysmenorrhoea is experienced by more than two thirds of women and a minority are severely incapacitated.
- Investigation of suspected primary dysmenorrhoea is unnecessary unless there are atypical symptoms or abnormal findings on pelvic examination [C].
- Ultrasound is a useful non-invasive method for the detection of pelvic abnormalities [A], backed up by MRI if appearances are equivocal.
- The multifactorial nature of chronic pelvic pain should be discussed and explored from the start [B].
- Pain resulting from disturbances in the central or peripheral nervous system (neuropathic pain) is an important component of chronic pelvic pain [C].
- Laparoscopy has a limited role in the investigation of chronic pelvic pain [B].
- NSAIDs are effective for the first-line management of primary dysmenorrhoea [A].
- COCPs are effective in primary dysmenorrhoea, although much of the evidence is largely based on higher-dose formulations than those in current use [A].
- Continuous progestogens at doses which suppress ovulation [C], the LNG-IUS [B] and GnRH analogues with add-back HRT [A] can be used for the relief of primary dysmenorrhoea.
- Alternative therapies, including physical and behavioural therapy, dietary supplements (magnesium, vitamin B1) and

Chinese herbal medicine may have a role in the management of dysmenorrhoea [C].
- Chronic pelvic pain which is cyclically exacerbated may be relieved by a trial of ovulation suppression [B].
- IBS, BPS and musculoskeletal abnormalities are often present in women with chronic pelvic pain and treatment should be directed towards all the components of the problem [C].
- Centrally acting drugs such as amitriptyline and gabapentin appear to have a role in the management of chronic pelvic pain [C].
- Other classes of antidepressants are not effective in the management of chronic pain [B].
- There is insufficient evidence to support the use of pelvic nerve interruption for the relief of primary or secondary dysmenorrhoea [A].
- There is no evidence that division of adhesions relieves chronic pelvic pain, with the possible exception of severe dense avascular adhesions [B].
- Where possible, chronic pelvic pain should be managed in a multidisciplinary clinic [A].

ACKNOWLEDGEMENT

With thanks to Professor Andrew W Horne for his helpful advice during the preparation of this chapter.

References

1. Zondervan KT, Yudkin PL, Vessey MP, Dawes MG, Barlow DH, Kennedy SH. The prevalence of chronic pelvic pain in women in the United Kingdom: a systematic review. *BJOG* 1998;105:93–99.
2. Hong J, Jones M, Mishra G. The prevalence and risk factors of dysmenorrhoea. *Epidemiol Rev* 2014;26:104–113.
3. Zondervan KT, Yudkin PL, Vesseyy MP, Dawes MG, Barlow DH, Kennedy SH. Prevalence and incidence of chronic pelvic pain in primary care: evidence from a national general practice database. *BJOG* 1999;106:1149–1155.
4. Mathias SD, Kuppermann M, Liberman RF, Lipschutz RC, Steege JF. Chronic pelvic pain: prevalence, health-related quality of life and economic correlates. *Obstet Gynecol* 1996;87:321–7.
5. Latthe P, Mignini L, Gray R, Hills R, Khan K. Factors predisposing women to chronic pelvic pain: systematic review. *BMJ* 2006;332:749–51.
6. RCOG. *The initial management of chronic pelvic pain.* Green-top guideline No. 41. London: RCOG, 2012.
7. Won HR, Abbott J. Optimum management of chronic cyclical pelvic pain: an evidence-based and pragmatic approach. *Int J Womens Health* 2010; 2:263–277.

8. Howard FM. The role of laparoscopy as a diagnostic tool in chronic pelvic pain. *Baillière's Clin Obstet Gynaecol* 2000;14(3):467–494.

9. Zondervan KT, Yudkin PL, Vessey MP, Dawes MG, Barlow DH, Kennedy SH. Patterns of diagnosis and referral in women consulting for chronic pelvic pain in UK primary care. *BJOG* 1999;106:1156–1161.

10. NICE. *Irritable bowel syndrome in adults. Diagnosis and management of irritable bowel syndrome in primary care* NICE Clinical Guideline 61. London: NICE, 2008. http://www.nice.org.uk/guidance/CG61/NICEGuidance.

11. Engler D, Baranowski AP, Elneil S *et al.* Guidelines on Chronic Pelvic Pain. European Association of Urology 2012. http://www.uroweb.org/gls/pdf/24_Chronic_Pelvic_Pain_LR%20March%2023th.pdf

12. Giamberardino MA, Costantini R, Affaitati G *et al.* Viscero-visceral hyperalgesia: characterization in different clinical models. *Pain* 2010;151:307–322.

13. As-Sanie S, Harris RE, Napadow V *et al.* Changes in regional gray matter volume in women with chronic pelvic pain: a voxel-based morphology study. *Pain* 2012;153:1006–1014.

14. Beard RW, Reginald PW, Wadsworth J. Clinical features of women with lower abdominal pain and pelvic congestion. *BJOG* 1988;95:153–61.

15. Soysal ME, Soysal S, Vicdan K, Ozer S, A randomized controlled trial of goserelin and medroxyprogesterone acetate in the treatment of pelvic congestion. *Hum Reprod* 2001;5:931–939.

16. Cummings M, Baldry P. Regional myofascial pain: diagnosis and management. *Best Pract Res Clin Rheumatol* 2007; 21(2):367–387.

17. Gerwin RD. Myofascial and visceral pain syndromes: visceral-somatic pain representations. *J Musculoskelet Pain* 2002;10:165–175.

18. Moore J, Copley S, Morris J, Lindsell D, Golding S, Kennedy S. A systematic review of the accuracy of ultrasound in the diagnosis of endometriosis. *Ultrasound Obstet Gynecol* 2002;20:630–4.

19. RCOG. *Diagnostic laparoscopy.* Consent Advice No. 2. London: RCOG, 2008.

20. Okaro E, Condous G, Khalid A *et al.* The use of ultrasound-based 'soft markers' for the prediction of pelvic pathology in women with chronic pelvic pain: can we reduce the need for laparoscopy? *BJOG* 2006;113:251–6.

21. Peters AA, van Dorst E, Jellis B, van Zuuren E, Hermans J, Trimbos JB. A randomized clinical trial to compare two different approaches in women with chronic pelvic pain. *Obstet Gynecol* 1991;77:740–744.

22. Cheong YC, Smotra G, Williams A C de C. Non-surgical interventions for the management of chronic pelvic pain. *Cochrane Database of Systematic Reviews* 2014;3:CD 008797. DOI: 10.1002/14651858. CD008797.pub2.

23. Marjoribanks J, Proctor M, Farquhar C, Derks RS. Nonsteroidal anti-inflammatory drugs for dysmenorrhoea. *Cochrane database of systematic reviews* 2010, Issue 1. Art.No.:CD001751. DOI:10.1002/14651858. CD001751.pub2.

24. Wong CL, Farquhar CM, Roberts H, Proctor ML. Oral contraceptive pill for primary dysmenorrhoea. *Cochrane database of systematic reviews* 2009, Issue 4. Art.No.:CD002120. DOI:10.1002/14651858. CD002120. pub3.

25. Dmitrovic R, Kunselman AR, Legro RS. Continuous compared with cyclic oral contraceptives for the treatment of primary dysmenorrhoea: a randomized controlled trial. *Obstet Gynecol* 2012;119:1143–1150.

26. Ahrendt H-J, Karck U, Pincl T, Mueller T, Ernst U. The effects of an oestrogen-free, desogestrel-containing oral contraceptive in women with cyclical symptoms: results from two studies on oestrogen-related symptoms and dysmenorrhoea. *Eur J Contracept Reprod Health Care* 2007;12:354–361.

27. Khan KS, Champaneria R, Latthe PM. How effective are non-drug, non-surgical treatments for primary dysmenorrhoea? *BMJ* 2012;344:e3011.

28. Proctor M, Murphy PA, Pattison HM, Suckling JA, Farquhar CM. Behavioural interventions for dysmenorrhoea. *Cochrane database of systematic reviews* 2007, Issue 3. Art.No.:CD002248. DOI:10.1002/14651858. CD002248.pub3.

29. Brown J, Brown S. Exercise for dysmenorrhoea. *Cochrane database of systematic reviews* 2010, Issue 2. Art. No.:CD004142. DOI:10.1002/14651858. CD004142. pub2.

30. Smith CA, Zhu X, He L, Song J. Acupuncture for dysmenorrhoea. *Cochrane database of systematic reviews* 2011, Issue 1. Art.No.:CD007854. DOI:10.1002/14651858. CD007854.pub2.

31. Proctor ML, Murphy PA. Herbal and dietary therapies for primary and secondary dysmenorrhoea. *Cochrane database of systematic reviews* 2001, Issue 2. Art. No.:CD002124. DOI:10.1002/14651858. CD002124.

32. Zhu X, Proctor M, Bensoussan A, Wu E, Smith CA. Chinese herbal medicine for primary dysmenorrhoea. *Cochrane database of systematic reviews* 2008, Issue 2. Art.No.:CD005288. DOI:10.1002/14651858. CD005288. pub3.

33. Farquhar CM, Rogers V, Franks S, Pearce S, Wadsworth J, Beard RW. A randomized controlled trial of medroxyprogesterone acetate and psychotherapy for the treatment of pelvic congestion. *BJOG* 1989;96:1153–1162.

34. Ling FW for the Pelvic Pain Study Group. Randomized controlled trial of depot leuprolide in patients with chronic pelvic pain and clinically suspected endometriosis. *Obstet Gynecol* 1999;93:51–58.

35. Onghena P, Van Houdenhove B. Antidepressant-induced analgesia in chronic non-malignant pain: a meta-analysis of 39 placebo-controlled studies. *Pain* 1992;49;205–219.

36. Moore RA, Wiffen PJ, Derry S, McQuay HJ. Gabapentin for chronic neuropathic pain and fibromyalgia in adults. *Cochrane database of systematic reviews* 2011, Issue 3.

Art.No.:CD007938. DOI:10.1002/14651858. CD007938. pub2.

37. RCOG. Therapies targeting the nervous system for chronic pelvic pain relief. Scientific Impact paper No 46. London: RCOG, 2014.

38. Swank DJ, Swank-Bordewijk SCG, Hop WCJ *et al.* Laparoscopic adhesiolysis in patients with chronic abdominal pain: a double blind randomised controlled multicentre trial. *Lancet* 2003;361: 1247-51.

39. Vercellini P, De Giorgi O, Pisacreta A, Pesole AP, Vincenti S, Crosignani PG. Surgical management of endometriosis. *Baillière's Clin Obstet Gynaecol* 2000; 14(3): 501–523.

Chapter 77 Endometriosis

Christine P West

MRCOG standards

Theoretical skills

- Understand the epidemiology, pathogenesis and clinical features of endometriosis.
- Be able to investigate suspected endometriosis and refer more complex cases where appropriate.
- Understand the nature, complications and adverse effects of medical and surgical management of endometriosis-associated pain.

Practical skills

- Understand the ultrasound diagnosis of endometrioma.
- Be familiar with the technique of diagnostic laparoscopy and staging of endometriosis.
- Understand the surgical techniques for treatment of mild to moderate endometriosis and endometrioma and be able to recognise and manage complications.

INTRODUCTION

Endometriosis is defined by the presence of ectopic endometrial tissue in extrauterine sites, usually within the pelvis. It is a common condition with many diverse manifestations and a clinical course that is highly variable and unpredictable. It may be asymptomatic, but most commonly presents with pelvic pain that is typically cyclical and in severe cases there may be associated bowel or bladder symptoms. The site of the lesions deep in the pelvis can also cause dyspareunia and there is a well-recognised but poorly understood association with subfertility. Endometriosis is usually regarded as distinct from adenomyosis (see Chapter 78), in which endometrial tissue is present within the myometrium.

Management should be individualised and will depend on the patient's symptoms, her age and reproductive plans. This chapter deals mainly with the management of pain in endometriosis, which has attracted a large literature and for which evidence-based management is relatively well developed.

PREVALENCE

Data from the UK General Practice Research Database[1] suggests that the prevalence of diagnosed endometriosis in women aged 15–55 years is 1.5 per cent. This is considerably lower than previous estimates based on series of women undergoing laparoscopy for various indications. In a prospective study of 1542 Caucasian women in a single Scottish centre[2] endometriosis was visualised in 6 per cent of women undergoing sterilisation, 21 per cent being investigated for infertility and 15 per cent being investigated for pelvic pain. Prevalence in other case series of women undergoing laparoscopy for investigation of pelvic pain has generally been higher, varying between 23 and 80 per cent.[3] Women with endometriosis are more likely to have complained of abdominopelvic pain, dysmenorrhoea, dyspareunia, subfertility and menstrual bleeding disorders compared with a control population.[1]

EPIDEMIOLOGY

Endometriosis is an oestrogen-dependent inflammatory condition and is thus a disease which affects women of reproductive age with regression after the menopause. It is most typically diagnosed in women aged 25–30 years but has been described in adolescents, in particular those with structural abnormalities of the reproductive tract. Factors which reduce menstruation, such as pregnancy and the use of oral contraceptives,[2–4] reduce its prevalence while early menarche, shorter menstrual cycles and nulliparity are associated with increased prevalence. There are also reports of reduced prevalence among current smokers and women with higher body mass index (BMI).[1] Observation of regression after pregnancy formed the basis for development of hormonal therapy for disease suppression. There are no clear racial or ethnic differences but the incidence is increased 7–10-fold among first-degree relatives.[2]

PATHOGENESIS

It is a generally accepted theory that endometrial tissue reaches the pelvis by retrograde menstruation.[3] Resulting peritoneal tissue implants release local inflammatory mediators, such as cytokines, growth factors and prostaglandins, in response to hormonal stimulation. Haematogenous or lymphatic spread in a minority of cases may account for the rare occurrence of endometriosis at distant sites. Retrograde menstruation is observed in up to 90 per cent of women but only a minority of women develop endometriosis. It is most likely that tissue implantation is a result of failure of clearance mechanisms which may be secondary to defects in the local peritoneal immune defence system in susceptible individuals. Whatever the underlying mechanisms, it is evident that the symptoms and the progression of the disease differ considerably amongst individuals, with a poor correlation between laparoscopic appearances and clinical symptoms. Results from second-look laparoscopy in treatment trials[3] have found short-term spontaneous regression of lesions in around one third of women receiving no active treatment, no change in another third and progression in the remaining third. Genetic factors appear to be relevant and these may influence local response mechanisms and the subsequent course of the disease.

Endometriomas, also known as chocolate cysts, are retention cysts which form when inflammatory adhesions develop between endometriotic deposits on the ovary and the pelvic side wall or around a superficial ovarian lesion, producing progressive inversion of the surrounding cortex. Endometriomas may be multiple and very large, when they inevitably interfere with fertility by adhesion and distortion of the Fallopian tubes.

In some women with endometriotic lesions predominantly affecting the uterosacral ligaments, marked fibrosis and scarring may develop, with infiltration of active endometriotic tissue into the rectovaginal septum or laterally to involve the ureters. Dense adhesions involving the rectum may lead to partial or complete obliteration of the pouch of Douglas. Deep infiltration may also occur on the uterovesical fold, leading to bladder involvement. It is not known why some women develop these more invasive forms of endometriosis.

The mechanism of pain in endometriosis is presumed to involve the release of inflammatory mediators. Pain related to deep lesions may be in part caused by infiltration or constriction of nerves or may be secondary to adhesions. Development of chronic pain is thought to be attributable to a mechanism whereby endometriotic lesions may develop their own nerve supply,[5] thereby creating a direct and two-way interaction between lesions and the CNS. Theories regarding the causation of chronic pelvic pain are discussed in Chapter 76.

MANAGEMENT

Investigation

The commonest presenting symptoms of endometriosis are dysmenorrhoea, chronic cyclical or non-cyclical pelvic pain, deep dyspareunia and infertility. Their non-specific nature makes diagnosis difficult and there is typically delay in referral from primary care[1] and confusion with other conditions, in particular pelvic inflammatory disease (PID) and irritable bowel syndrome (IBS). Dyschezia (pain with defaecation) and severe deep dyspareunia may be indicative of the presence of deep endometriosis.

Bimanual pelvic examination is important in facilitating diagnosis (Table 77.1) [C].[6] The posterior vaginal fornix should be inspected for the presence of visible lesions. Rectal examination is useful in cases where symptoms are suggestive of rectosigmoid involvement. In many cases the examination is unhelpful and the decision to carry out further investigation is based on the history and the wishes of the patient. Levels of serum CA-125 are likely to be raised in severe disease but there is no evidence that this is useful as a screening test [A][6] and it can lead to confusion with malignancy.

Transvaginal ultrasound is of value in detecting ovarian endometriomas (Table 77.1) [A].[7] It was also found to be accurate for pre-surgical detection of deep endometriosis of the rectosigmoid [A].[8] However, evaluation of deep lesions by ultrasound is operator dependent and considerable experience is required [E]. Other imaging techniques used in the assessment of the extent of deep endometriosis are barium studies, transrectal sonography and MRI.[6,9] Currently all appear to be

Table 77.1 Diagnosis of endometriosis

Pelvic examination findings suggestive of deep endometriosis	Ultrasound features diagnostic of endometrioma[6]	Laparoscopic appearances of endometriosis
- Palpable induration and/or nodules on vaginal walls, uterosacral ligaments or pouch of Douglas	- Ground glass echogenicity	- Red, clear or black superficial deposits or vesicles
- Visible cysts or nodules in the posterior fornix	- 1-4 compartments	- Deeper lesions of peritoneum or ovaries (endometrioma)
- Adnexal masses	- No papillary structures with detectable blood flow	- Associated adhesions
		- Reduced ovarian mobility
		- Partial or complete cul-de-sac obliteration

of value in individual cases [D]. MRI has no advantage over ultrasound in the routine assessment of endometriomas [A][6] but may assist in the evaluation of deep lesions [C].

Laparoscopy for diagnosis of endometriosis

Laparoscopy, backed up by biopsy, is regarded as the 'gold standard' investigation for diagnosis of endometriosis [E]. However there is little good-quality literature assessing the value of visual diagnosis of endometriosis at laparoscopy.[10] A systematic review of observational studies[10] comparing visual findings with biopsy results concluded that laparoscopy is highly accurate for excluding endometriosis but a positive laparoscopy is of less value in the absence of histology. Its predictive value is higher in cases of moderate/severe disease, compared with minimal/ mild disease.

Laparoscopy must involve a two-port approach with careful inspection of the uterus and adnexae, uterovesical fold, pouch of Douglas, uterosacral ligaments, pelvic side wall and ovarian fossae[E].[6] Where necessary, careful mobilisation of the ovaries should be attempted in order to inspect their anterior surface, as the presence of adhesions is strongly suggestive of endometriosis. The quality of laparoscopy is dependent on the experience of the surgeon carrying out the procedure and the operator must appreciate the varied appearances of endometriosis (Table 77.2). Visible evidence of endometriosis should be confirmed by biopsy [E],[6,10] although this procedure is not without risk in inexperienced hands. Photographs or video recordings are helpful in the documentation of disease extent and use can be made of diagrams, in particular those based on the American Society for Reproductive Medicine (ASRM) classification, previously known as the American Fertility Society (AFS) classification (Table 77.2).[11] Although useful in research and in planning surgery, ASRM scores correlate poorly with pain symptoms [C].[3] It is important to carry out

an adequate bimanual pelvic examination to detect features suggestive of deep endometriosis which may not be easily visualised laparoscopically.[6]

Laparoscopy is an invasive procedure and not without risk (Table 77.3)[12]. For some patients with pain symptoms suggestive of the disease it will be preferable to undertake a therapeutic trial of hormonal suppression as initial management.[6] All cases require an informed discussion of the various options and, for those undergoing laparoscopy, its nature and risks must be fully discussed [E]. Counselling must include discussion about the possible courses of action should endometriosis be diagnosed at the primary procedure. Best practice is to carry out surgical ablative therapy, if appropriate, at the initial laparoscopy,[6] depending on the facilities and expertise

Table 77.3 Major complications of laparoscopy (diagnostic and minor surgical interventions). Data from a case series of 29,996 procedures[12] expressed as number (rate per 1000)

Complication	Diagnostic (n = 5983)	Minor[a] (n = 5922)
Bowel damage (all)	3 (0.5)	2 (0.3)
Haemorrhage (all):	7 (1.2)	3 (0.5)
- Major vascular	1	0
- Abdominal wall/ omentum	6	3
Urological damage (all):	1 (0.2)	0
- Bladder	1	
- Ureter		
Total	11 (1.8)	5 (0.8)
Laparotomy[b]	8 (1.3)	2 (0.3)

[a] ablation of minimal/mild endometriosis, minor adhesiolysis, sterilisation, ovarian biopsy;

[b] complications requiring treatment by laparotomy.

Table 77.2 ASRM (AFS) revised classification of endometriosis[11] scoring system

Stage	Score*	Example findings
I minimal	1-5	Superficial lesions ± filmy adhesions
II mild	6-15	More extensive superficial lesions ± adhesions ± small endometrioma (less than 1 cm)
III moderate	16-40	Likely to include deep lesions e.g. endometrioma >1 cm ± partial or complete ovarian enclosure but no more than partial obliteration of the cul-de-sac (pouch of Douglas)
IV severe	>40	Extensive disease; likely to have deep lesions (± endometrioma) and dense adhesions with complete obliteration of the cul-de-sac (pouch of Douglas)

* Score based on total extent (cm) of lesions; whether superficial or deep; presence of filmy or dense adhesions; degree of ovarian enclosure; size of endometrioma; presence of partial or complete obliteration of the cul-de-sac (pouch of Douglas)
e.g. Endometrioma 1-3 cm score 16; >3 cm score 20
- Ovarian enclosure 1-2/3 score 8; >2/3 score 16
- Complete cul-de-sac obliteration score 40

available, provided that adequate informed consent has been obtained [E].

Medical management of pelvic pain associated with endometriosis

There is a large evidence base supporting the use of medical therapy in the management of endometriosis-associated pain [A]. The majority of these therapies act by ovarian suppression and induction of amenorrhoea, resulting in inactivation of local deposits. As all the hormonal therapies have similar efficacy, their tolerability in terms of immediate and long-term side effects is important when selecting the most appropriate treatment for an individual woman [A].[3,6] As discussed above, medical therapy may be initiated for the relief of pain symptoms in the absence of a definitive diagnosis of endometriosis. In women wishing to conceive, hormonal therapy is not appropriate, as it delays rather than enhances fertility [A].[6] However, medical suppression may be of value in pain control, for example in women awaiting IVF [E].

Non-steroidal anti-inflammatory drugs (NSAIDs)

These offer a non-hormonal approach that is particularly useful in women trying to conceive and they are widely used in clinical practice. However, few studies have addressed their role in management of endometriosis-associated pain[6] and evidence for their efficacy is largely based on their use in the treatment of primary dysmenorrhoea (see Chapter 76) [A].

Combined oral contraceptives

The combine oral contraceptive pill (COCP) is an effective treatment for dysmenorrhoea (see Chapter 76) and suppression or reduction of menstruation with continuous or tricyclic use of a COCP is commonly used for management of pain associated with endometriosis, although few randomised trials have addressed its use.[6,13] Cyclical administration of a low-dose COCP was as effective as a gonadotrophin-releasing hormone (GnRH) agonist[13] in the management of dysmenorrhoea and non-menstrual pain in one study, although less effective for dyspareunia [B]. Indirect evidence from a systematic review of contraceptive studies[14] showed that continuous- or extended-dose regimens are marginally more effective than cyclical therapy in improving dysmenorrhoea [A]. Reduction of endometriosis-associated pain with both cyclical and continuous use of the COCP has been reported in a systematic review comparing their efficacy with that of progestogens.[15] One randomised trial comparing 24 months of continuous or cyclical COCP use with no therapy[16] following surgical excision of endometrioma has shown significantly lower rates of recurrence of dysmenorrhoea with continuous compared with cyclical use [B]. Overall this evidence supports the use

of combined oral contraceptives for suppression of pain in endometriosis [B]. Continuous rather than cyclical use may be preferable for pain management [B]. Administration by transdermal patch or vaginal ring can also be considered [C].[6] Because of their relative safety, combined hormonal contraceptives are suitable for long-term use.

Progestogens

Progestogens given continuously inhibit ovulation, depending on dosage, and have direct antiproliferative effects on endometriotic implants, causing decidualisation and eventual atrophy. They have been widely used for the treatment of pain in endometriosis and are the subject of a systematic review.[15] No significant difference in pain scores was found in two trials comparing DMPA (Depo-Provera 150 mg 3-monthly) with GnRH analogues. Oral progestogens including medroxyprogesterone acetate 30 mg daily, dienogest 2mg daily and desogestrel 75 mcg daily were also found to have similar efficacy when compared with GnRH analogues or oral contraceptives although numbers in the individual studies were small. Cyclical administration of progestogens was ineffective. A small non-randomised study has recently shown that low-dose norethisterone acetate 2.5 mg daily may effectively relieve chronic cyclical pain and dyspareunia in women with deep endometriosis [C].[17]

The most commonly reported side effect of progestogens is breakthrough bleeding, with an overall incidence of around 33 per cent[15] which is not dose related. Other side effects which are likely to be dose related include weight gain, breast tenderness, bloating, headache, acne and nausea. On the basis of the evidence from the systematic review,[15] continuous oral or depot progestogens can be used for suppression of endometriosis-associated pain [A] although their usefulness may be limited by side effects. Further evaluation of the role of oral desogestrel 75 mcg in endometriosis would be helpful, given its popularity as a progestogen-only contraceptive.

LNG-IUS

The levonorgestrel-releasing intrauterine system (LNG-IUS) does not suppress ovulation but acts locally on the endometrium. Its effect on extrauterine endometrial tissue is therefore locally mediated. A multicentre randomised trial comparing the LNG-IUS with a GnRH agonist[18] reported no difference in pain scores after 6 months [B]. A systematic review of its use following laparoscopic treatment of endometriosis[19] reported a significantly reduced incidence of recurrence of painful periods with the LNG-IUS compared with no treatment after 12 months and no significant difference when compared with a GnRH agonist. Although bleeding scores were higher with the LNG-IUS compared with the GnRH agonist, there was no difference in pain or quality-of-life assessments between the two groups. On the basis of these results, the LNG-IUS seems to have a role in the management of pain associated with endometriosis whether as a primary treatment [B] or for prevention of recurrence of pain following surgical treatment [A].

Androgens

Gestrinone is a 19-nortestosterone derivative that also has progestogenic and antiprogestogenic actions. It has been compared with danazol and with a GnRH analogue in randomised trials.[15,20] Reduction of pain scores was not significantly different [A], but both androgenic and hypo-oestrogenic side effects were less frequent with gestrinone. Side effects of gestrinone were reduced by lowering the dose from 2.5 mg twice weekly to 1.25 mg twice weekly without a reduction in efficacy [A].[15] The reported incidence of breakthrough bleeding is much lower with gestrinone than with progestogens, making it a potentially useful alternative to other therapies [A]. However, there is a lack of information relating to its long-term safety.

Danazol is an androgenic steroid, which acts both centrally and locally to suppress steroidogenesis and induce endometrial atrophy.[6] It induces amenorrhoea and significantly improves pain at doses of 400–600 mg daily [A] but androgenic side effects such as weight gain, limb tingling, acne, greasy skin, hirsutism and deepening of the voice are common, and atherogenic effects on lipid profiles have been reported. For this reason it is not currently recommended for endometriosis if other alternatives are available.[6] Neither danazol nor gestrinone is associated with bone loss and therefore both are potential alternatives to GnRH analogues for women susceptible to bone loss and in whom oestrogenic add-back preparations are contraindicated (see below).

GnRH analogues

GnRH agonists down-regulate pituitary GnRH receptors leading to inhibition of follicle stimulating hormone and luteinising hormone production. This leads to gonadal suppression when administered by nasal spray or monthly or 3-monthly depot injection (Table 77.4). The intranasal route tends to be less costly, while depot administration improves compliance.

A summary of results of a systematic review of randomised controlled trials (RCTs) of GnRH agonist therapy have demonstrated its effectiveness in the treatment of pain associated with endometriosis [A][20] when compared with placebo or no treatment. Comparison with danazol and the LNG-IUS demonstrated no significant differences in clinical response but expected differences in side-effect profiles. The side effects of GnRH agonists include hot flushes, insomnia, vaginal dryness, reduced libido and headaches – all secondary to oestrogen suppression.

Longer-term use of GnRH analogues

It is usual to prescribe a GnRH analogue for an initial period of 3 months and, if effective, to continue for a total of at least 6 months prior to further review [E]. In common with other medical treatments, GnRH agonists do not produce permanent disease regression. A life-table analysis of follow-up of women treated with various GnRH agonists for 6–9 months[21] reported a cumulative symptomatic recurrence rate of 53.4 per cent after 7 years [C]. For severe disease, the recurrence rate was 74.4 per cent, while for minimal disease it was 36.9 per cent. Therefore many women require subsequent courses of treatment and, in some cases, treatment may be long term. In this situation loss of bone mineral density is a major concern and for this reason GnRH analogues should not be given as single agents for longer than 6 months [A]. In women needing longer-term treatment, hormonal add-back therapy can be used with the object of reducing or preventing bone loss and minimising other side effects related to oestrogen deficiency. Several continuous combined HRT regimens using oral or transdermal oestrogens in combination with various progestogens have been compared with placebo in patients treated with GnRH agonists for endometriosis.[22] All were effective in control of endometriosis-related pain while reducing vasomotor side effects and maintaining bone density during treatment and up to 12 months after discontinuation of treatment. However 2 years after discontinuation of treatment, bone density had recovered in the group treated with GnRH agonists alone.

Progestogens alone and calcium supplements are not effective in preventing bone loss.[22] For women who cannot tolerate hormonal add-back or for whom it is contraindicated, antiresorptive agents, such as bisphosphonates, have been used for bone protection but evidence of their efficacy to date is currently insufficient.[22]

Table 77.4 Gonadotrophin-releasing hormone agonists. Data from British National Formulary indicating whether each preparation is licensed for treatment of endometriosis.

Name	Monthly depot	Licensed indication	3-monthly depot	Licensed indication	Intranasal	Licensed indication
Buserelin					300 mcg tid	Yes
Goserelin	3.6 mg SC	Yes	10.8 mg	No		
Leuprorelin acetate	3.75 mg SC/IM	Yes	11.25 mg IM	Yes		
Nafarelin					200 mcg bd	Yes
Triptorelin	3.0 mg IM	Yes	11.25 mg IM	yes		

These results support the role of add-back therapy with GnRH agonists to suppress endometriosis-associated pain when given as continuous low-dose oestrogen–progestogen combinations [A]. Tibolone is licenced in the UK for bone protection when used in conjunction with GnRH analogues although there is a lack of published data to compare its effectiveness with that of other add-back therapies and it is more costly than other alternatives.

Aromatase inhibitors

Aromatase is responsible for the conversion of androgens to oestrogens and there is evidence for its expression in endometriotic tissue.[23] It has been suggested that a feedback loop involving local induction of aromatase by prostaglandin E2 may promote oestrogen production and thereby growth of lesions. There have been some reports based on individual cases or small series[23] of a positive effect of the use of aromatase inhibitors, usually in combination with another hormonal therapy, for severe or refractory pain associated with rectovaginal endometriosis. One RCT comparing a GnRH agonist alone with a GnRH agonist plus anastrazole reported a significant improvement in pain scores over 24 months with the combined therapy. However these agents are associated with hypo-oestrogenic side effects and bone loss and thus their role in management of endometriosis has yet to be established.

Choice and duration of medical therapy

As discussed above, hormonal therapies are effective for relief of endometriosis-associated pain [A]. As all appear to have similar efficacy, their use in individual patients will depend on factors such as the degree of symptom relief, side effects and cost [E]. Because hormonal suppression merely inactivates and does not remove local disease, symptoms recur after cessation in a proportion of patients and, for some, treatment may potentially be long term. COCP, progestogens and the IUS are considerably less costly than GnRH analogues but the latter have the advantage of more reliably inducing amenorrhoea with a lower incidence of hormonally related side effects such as bloating, breast tenderness, headaches and mood changes, even with the addition of low-dose HRT. The costs of hormonal therapies used to suppress ovulation are compared in Table 79.2, Chapter 79.

Treatment with an NSAID and/or a COCP could be the first-line approach in the absence of specific indications for laparoscopy,[24] with use of the IUS or a continuous progestogen if oestrogenic preparations are contraindicated or give rise to side effects [E]. There is no evidence regarding the optimum duration of these therapies for endometriosis but if effective and well tolerated, evidence from contraceptive studies [A] is that all are suitable for long-term use. Women presenting to secondary care are likely to be those whose symptoms have not responded adequately to initial therapies. In such cases, treatment with a GnRH agonist would be preferable to use of an androgenic preparation [E].[6] A 2–3 month trial of treatment with a GnRH agonist in cases of presumed endometriosis, continued for 6 months if pain symptoms are improved, is recommended as more cost effective than initial laparoscopy with local ablation in cases of clinically suspected endometriosis,[24] given that the incidence of longer-term symptom recurrence is similar. However others[25] would challenge this approach. The role of medical therapy in women who have undergone surgical treatment is discussed below.

Adjuvant therapies

Chronic pelvic pain in endometriosis may be resistant to hormonal suppression. Increasing evidence supporting a neuropathic and central sensitisation component to endometriosis-associated chronic pain has led to the use of tricyclic antidepressants such as amitryptyline and anti-epileptic drugs such as gabapentin for the management of endometriosis-associated chronic pain [C]. These therapies are discussed in Chapter 76.

Complementary therapies

Many patients with endometriosis-associated pain seek non-conventional approaches to manage their symptoms. The evidence for the use of such therapies for primary and secondary dysmenorrhoea is reviewed in Chapter 76. Few high-quality studies have specifically addressed their role in endometriosis. A systematic review of 24 studies of the use of acupuncture concluded that only one was of sufficient quality for inclusion.[26] This compared auricular acupuncture with Chinese herbal medicine and demonstrated similar efficacy for mild and moderate endometriosis-associated pain but a significantly better reduction of severe pain with acupuncture [B]. Further studies are required comparing various types of acupuncture with conventional therapy.

The role of surgery for endometriosis-associated pain

Unlike medical therapies, there have been few controlled studies of surgical approaches for the management of

Table 77.5 Major complications of laparoscopic surgical procedures. Data from a case series of 29,996 laparoscopies.[12]

Procedure	Complications	Rate (%)
Major adhesiolysis[a]	22/2665	0.83
Benign cystectomy[a]	17/3908	0.44
Ablation moderate/ severe endometriosis	3/1894	0.16
Deep endometriosis[b]	7/174	4.02

[a] Procedures not specific to endometriosis;

[b] Study published in 1998 and may not reflect current practice

endometriosis-associated pain, although the latter have gained a large literature and surgical interventions, mainly involving laparoscopy, are widely used. Because operative laparoscopy is associated with a significant risk of major complications (see Tables 77.3 and 77.5) [C][3,12] such interventions require critical review.

To date there have been only five RCTs of laparoscopic surgical treatment of endometriosis,[27] including a total of 246 women. These have compared local excision or ablation using various techniques with diagnostic laparoscopy alone (four trials) or with diagnostic laparoscopy followed by medical therapy (one trial). Presence of severe disease was generally an exclusion criterion. A systematic review of these five trials[27] reported a significant benefit from laparoscopic surgery [A]. Overall 75 per cent of the women who had active intervention reported an improvement in pain at 6 months, compared with 32 per cent of those following laparoscopy only. At 12 months, 73 per cent continued to report a benefit, compared with 21 per cent of the control group although the 12-month data were based on only one of the trials.

These small-scale studies, carried out in nationally recognised laparoscopic surgery centres, support the use of conservative laparoscopic surgery for the relief of pain in endometriosis [A] but more data are needed from larger studies to establish the duration of benefit and how this is influenced by the severity of the disease. No serious surgical complications were reported, but these results may not be reproducible in a more general context, in terms of both efficacy and safety [E].

Additional laparoscopic procedures that may be used for treatment of pain associated with endometriosis involve surgical interruption of pelvic nerve pathways. Laparoscopic uterine nerve ablation (LUNA) is a relatively simple procedure but was not found to confer any significant benefit when used as an adjunct to laparoscopic surgical treatment of endometriosis in three randomised trials [A].[28] In contrast, three trials of presacral neurectomy (PSN) as an adjunct to surgical ablation showed some benefit for dysmenorrhoea[28] but no significant difference in backache or lateral pain. Direct comparison of the two techniques in a single study also favoured PSN but side effects, in particular constipation and urinary urgency, were significantly higher with PSN. The latter procedure is technically demanding[6,28] and therefore limited to highly specialised centres.

Surgical excision or ablation at the time of the initial laparoscopy is cost effective for pain management [B][25] and also improves pregnancy rates in women with ASRM stage I or II (minimal or mild) endometriosis [A].[6] Therefore, regardless of the indication for laparoscopy for assessment of suspected endometriosis, the procedure should be carried out by a gynaecologist able to carry out ablative treatment, preceded by appropriate preoperative patient assessment, counselling and consent.

Surgical management of endometriomas

Although endometriomas may be asymptomatic, their presence in association with pain is usually regarded as an indication for laparoscopic surgical intervention. Endometriomas do not usually resolve during medical suppression, although, if small, they may reduce in size and become asymptomatic. Simple drainage of an endometrioma is followed by rapid recurrence, even if it is fenestrated and irrigated [A].[29] A systematic review of two randomised trials of laparoscopic management of endometriomas larger than 3 cm[29] has indicated a higher rate of recurrence following coagulation of the inner lining of the cyst compared with excision. Laparoscopic excision is therefore the surgical treatment of choice [A]. In women with subfertility, surgical excision of endometriomas is associated with an improved chance of spontaneous pregnancy compared with drainage and coagulation [A].[6] However cystectomy is followed by a significant and sustained fall in serum anti-Müllerian hormone,[30] indicating a reduction of ovarian reserve [A]. This reduction appears to be greater following removal of larger or bilateral lesions and has implications for the counselling of women undergoing surgical management of endometrioma.

Medical adjuncts to surgery

Surgical ablation is not curative and recurrence of pain is reported to be around 15 per cent at 1 year, 36 per cent after 5 years and 50 per cent by 7 years.[3] There have been a number of studies addressing the role of medical adjuncts to surgery for endometriosis. There is no evidence to support their use prior to surgery [A].[31] Drugs which suppress ovarian activity are frequently used following conservative surgery of endometriosis. Published evidence on their role is however conflicting. A systematic review of 12 RCTs which compared 3 or 6 months of ovarian suppression treatment with placebo or no treatment following surgery[31] reported a significant reduction of pelvic pain at 12 months but no difference in its subsequent recurrence. It was concluded that there was insufficient evidence to recommend their short-term use [A]. However a systematic review of three RCTs[18] concluded that insertion of a LNG-IUS at the time of surgery resulted in an 8.8 per cent incidence of painful symptoms after 12 months, compared with 38.3 per cent with no treatment [A]. Other studies have reported a significant reduction in frequency and severity of recurrent dysmenorrhoea and in recurrence of endometrioma but not dyspareunia with cyclical or continuous COCP given for 2 years following surgery [B].[32] Continuous use of the COCP may be more effective than cyclical use for control of dysmenorrhoea and chronic pelvic pain.[16,32] This evidence supports the longer-term use of hormonal contraceptives following surgery to prevent recurrence of endometrioma or dysmenorrhoea [B] where appropriate for individual women, in particular those needing contraception or planning to delay child-bearing.[6]

Management of pain in deep endometriosis

Surgical treatment of advanced disease where there are dense adhesions and deeply infiltrating lesions involving the rectovaginal septum can be effective in relieving pain [B] but requires advanced laparoscopic surgical skill and training and a multidisciplinary approach due to the potential need for bowel resection or excision of bladder or ureteric lesions.[3,6] Appropriate presurgical assessment by imaging[9] is essential and these procedures should only be carried out in specialist regional centres [E]. Where issues of safety arise, laparotomy still has a role in the conservative management of advanced disease [B][3,6] both for pain management and for preservation of fertility.

There is limited evidence for long-term efficacy of surgery for advanced disease in terms of recurrence of pain or subsequent pregnancy outcome. Long-term medical therapy may also be an appropriate option.[6] A review of small case series and one randomised trial[33] concluded that various forms of hormonal suppression, including the LNG-IUS, relieved pain in 60–90 per cent of women with rectovaginal endometriosis [C], thereby offering a non-invasive option for women wishing to avoid surgery or for those experiencing persistent or recurrent pain following previous surgery. Use of adjuvant therapy where chronic pain is not relieved with conventional treatment is mentioned above and discussed in Chapter 76.

Definitive surgery

For women with symptomatic endometriosis who have completed child-bearing, hysterectomy with or without bilateral salpingo-oophorectomy is frequently carried out with the objective of achieving a definitive cure. However in cases of advanced disease with dense adhesions and deep lesions in the rectovaginal septum, complete removal of the disease requires a very radical approach[6] with careful consideration of the risks. A long-term follow-up study of women undergoing surgery for pelvic pain in a regional centre where hysterectomy was accompanied by excision of all visible disease[34] reported that 23 per cent of those who had ovarian conservation required further surgery within 7 years of follow-up, compared with 8.3 per cent following ovarian removal. These results support the removal of ovaries in women undergoing hysterectomy for severe endometriosis [C]. Women should be counselled that hysterectomy may not be curative [E].[6]

Hormone replacement therapy and endometriosis

Following hysterectomy plus oophorectomy, or oophorectomy alone for severe endometriosis, there is a risk that use of hormone replacement therapy (HRT) may activate small foci of residual disease.[6] This is likely to be greater with unopposed oestrogen compared with combined oestrogen and progestogen therapy or with cyclical use of HRT. Unfortunately there is a shortage of evidence to address this issue. A systematic review[35] identified only two RCTs, neither of which included an oestrogen-only or a continuous combined preparation. In both, cyclical sequential administration of oestrogen and progestogen was compared with, in one trial, tibolone and in the other, placebo. There was a small incidence of endometriosis-related symptom recurrence with active treatment but not with the placebo. Symptom scores with tibolone were lower than with the combined preparation but none of the results reached statistical significance. The risk of symptom recurrence with HRT has to be balanced against the well-established sequelae of oestrogen deficiency in young women. Similarly the theoretical benefit of using an oestrogen–progestogen combination or tibolone rather than oestrogen alone needs to be balanced against the slightly greater risk of breast cancer with combined HRT. The consensus view is that continuous combined oestrogen–progestogen preparations or tibolone should be prescribed following oophorectomy [E][6] but individual risk factors should also be considered [E].

Psychological aspects

Addressing psychological and social issues which commonly occur in association with chronic pelvic pain may be important in resolving painful symptoms associated with endometriosis [B] (see Chapter 76). Depression, relationship breakdown and sleep disorders are common in women with chronic pain. This may be a consequence rather than a cause of their pain but specific treatment may improve the woman's ability to function. It is important that the multifactorial nature of pain is discussed and explored from the start.[36] The aim is develop a partnership between clinician and patient to plan a management programme.

Patient groups like Endometriosis UK[37] provide an excellent source of support. These groups provide self-management courses designed to teach patients how to adapt to living with a chronic condition and how to manage pain. Providing these skills may make a tangible impact on their disease and quality of life in general. These courses tackle a variety of skills including relaxation strategies, coping mechanisms for depression, cognitive symptom management skills and the role of exercise in improving symptoms. Although there is minimal evidence to support the success of a holistic approach, nutritional and exercise-based interventions are unlikely to cause detriment to patients and are associated with benefits to general health.

EBM

These recommendations are supported by one evidence-based guideline, three systematic reviews of diagnostic techniques, eight systematic reviews of medical management of endometriosis-associated pain and three systematic reviews of surgical management of endometriosis-associated pain. There have been no randomised studies comparing medical with surgical management in the relief of endometriosis-associated pain and the relative cost effectiveness of the various approaches is unclear.

KEY POINTS

- Symptoms of endometriosis include dysmenorrhoea, chronic pelvic pain, dyspareunia and infertility but are non-specific. Painful defaecation and severe dyspareunia may be indicative of deep endometriosis [C].
- Pelvic examination may be unhelpful in the presence of peritoneal disease but the presence of fixed uterine retroversion, induration, nodularity or palpable masses may be indicative of deep rectovaginal endometriosis or ovarian endometrioma [C].
- Laparoscopy is regarded as the gold standard for diagnosis of endometriosis but adequate counselling is essential prior to the procedure [E].
- Negative laparoscopy is accurate for exclusion of endometriosis but positive visual changes lack specificity unless backed up by histology [C].
- ASRM scores can be used for documentation and assessment of the extent of endometriosis but correlate poorly with pain symptoms [C].
- Where appropriate, surgical ablative therapy should be carried out at the time of the initial laparoscopy [B].
- Measurement of CA-125 is not helpful as an aid to diagnosis [A].
- Transvaginal ultrasound is useful in identifying endometriomas and can assist with detection of deep endometriosis of the recto-sigmoid [A].
- MRI should not be used routinely for assessment of endometriosis but may be useful in the assessment of deep lesions [C].
- Hormonal suppression of ovulation is effective in the management of pain associated with endometriosis [A].
- Where appropriate, a trial of empirical medical therapy can be used for symptomatic management of pain in cases of suspected endometriosis without preliminary laparoscopy [E].
- COCPs, continuous progestogens, danazol, gestrinone and GnRH agonists are all effective therapies and selection should be determined by the relative side-effect profiles [A].
- Continuous rather than cyclical use of the COCP may be more effective in control of endometriosis-associated pain. [B].
- Levonorgestrel-releasing intrauterine systems are effective for management of endometriosis-related pain [B] and for maintenance of pain control following surgical treatment [A].
- If GnRH agonists are used for longer than 6 months, add-back therapy with low-dose continuous combined HRT or tibolone should be given [A].
- Drugs used for treatment of neuropathic pain such as amitriptyline and gabapentin may have a role in the management of endometriosis-related chronic pelvic pain resistant to conventional therapies [C].
- Complementary therapies, in particular acupuncture [C], may have a role in the management of pain associated with endometriosis but evidence for their use is lacking.
- Laparoscopic surgery is effective in the treatment of pain secondary to endometriosis in experienced hands [A] but longer-term recurrence of pain occurs in around 50 per cent of women.
- LUNA is ineffective as an adjunct to surgery for the relief of endometriosis-related pain [A]. PSN may be beneficial for dysmenorrhoea but has significant side effects and should be carried out in centres with the appropriate expertise [A].
- Surgical treatment of endometriomas should be by laparoscopic cystectomy [A].
- Operative laparoscopy for advanced disease carries a significant risk [C], and cases of advanced disease should be referred to specialist centres for laparoscopic surgery [E].
- Short-term pre- or postoperative medical therapy as an adjunct to surgery is ineffective [A] but longer-term use of contraceptive preparations is effective in prevention of recurrence of endometrioma and dysmenorrhoea following surgery in women not planning to conceive [B].
- Because of a high rate of recurrence of endometriosis following both medical and surgical treatment, medical treatment may need to be intermittent or long term [C].
- If fertility is no longer an issue, hysterectomy with bilateral oophorectomy may provide a cure, but disease excision may be incomplete [C].
- Because of a risk of disease recurrence [C], low-dose combined HRT or tibolone is preferable to oestrogen-only HRT following hysterectomy with oophorectomy for endometriosis [E].
- Self-help and support groups can play an important role in pain management by teaching coping skills designed to help women adapt to living with a chronic condition [E].

ACKNOWLEDGEMENT

With thanks to Professor Andrew W Horne for his help and advice during the preparation of this chapter.

References

1. Ballard KD, Seaman HE, de Vries CS, Wright JT. Can symptomatology help in the diagnosis of endometriosis? Findings from a national case-control study: Part 1. *BJOG* 2008;115:1382–1391.
2. Mahmood TA, Templeton A. Prevalence and genesis of endometriosis. *Hum Reprod* 1991;6:544–549.

3. Falcone T, Lebovic DI. Clinical management of endometriosis. *Obstet Gynecol* 2011;118:691–705.

4. Missmer SA, Hankinson SE, Spiegelman D *et al.* Reproductive history and endometriosis among premenopausal women. *Obstet Gynecol* 2004;104:965–974.

5. Stratton P, Berkley KJ. Chronic pelvic pain and endometriosis: translational evidence of the relationship and implications. *Hum Reprod Update* 2011;17:327–346.

6. ESHRE Endometriosis Guideline Development Group. *Management of women with endometriosis*. Guideline of the European Society of Human Reproduction and Embryology, 2013.

7. Moore J, Copley S, Morris J, Lindsell D, Golding S, Kennedy S. A systematic review of the accuracy of ultrasound in the diagnosis of endometriosis. *Ultrasound Obstet Gynecol* 2002;20:630–634.

8. Hudelist G, English J, Thomas AE, Tinelli A, Singer CF, Keckstein J. Diagnostic accuracy of transvaginal ultrasound for non-invasive diagnosis of bowel endometriosis: systematic review and meta-analysis. *Ultrasound Obstet Gynecol* 2011;37:257–263.

9. Bazot M, Lafont C, Rouzier R, Roseau G, Thomassin-Naggara I, Darai E. Diagnostic accuracy of physical examination, transvaginal sonography, rectal endoscopic sonography and magnetic resonance imaging to diagnose deep infiltrating endometriosis. *Fertil Steril* 2009;92:1835–1832.

10. Wykes CB, Clark TJ, Khan KS. Accuracy of laparoscopy in the diagnosis of endometriosis; a systematic review. *BJOG* 2004;111:1204–1212.

11. American Society for Reproductive Medicine. Revised ASRM classification of endometriosis:1996. *Fertil Steril* 1997;67:817–821.

12. Chapron C, Querleu D, Bruhat M-A *et al.* Surgical complications of diagnostic and operative gynaecological laparoscopy: a case series of 29,966 cases. *Hum Reprod* 1998;13:867–872.

13. Davis L-J. Kennedy SS, Moore J, Prentice A. Oral contraceptives for pain associated with endometriosis. *Cochrane Database of Systematic Reviews* 2007, Issue 3. Art. No.: CD001019. DOI: 10.1002/1465188858. CD001019.pub2.

14. Edelman A, Gallo MF, Jensen JT, Nichols MD, Grimes DA. Continuous or extended cycle vs cyclical use of combined hormonal contraceptives for contraception. *Cochrane Database of Systematic Reviews* 2005, Issue 3. Art. No.: CD004695. DOI: 1002/14651858. CD004695.pub2.

15. Brown J, Kives S, Akhtar M. Progestagens and anti-progestagens for pain associated with endometriosis. *Cochrane Database of Systematic Reviews* 2012, Issue 3. Art. No.: CD002122. DOI: 10.1002/14651858. CD002122.pub2.

16. Seracchioli R, Mabrouk M, Frasca C, Manuzzi L, Savelli L, Venturoli S. Long-term contraceptive pills and postoperative pain management after laparoscopic excision of ovarian endometrioma: a randomized controlled trial. *Fertil Steril* 2010;94:464–471.

17. Ferrero S, Camerini G, Seracchioli R *et al.* Norethisterone acetate in the treatment of colorectal endometriosis: a pilot study. *Hum Reprod* 2010;25:94–100.

18. Petta CA, Ferriani RA, Abaro MS *et al.* Randomized clinical trial of a levonorgestrel-releasing intrauterine system and a depot GnRH analogue for the treatment of chronic pelvic pain in women with endometriosis. *Human Reproduction* 2005;20:1993–1998.

19. Abou-Setta A, Houston B, Al-Inmay HG, Farquhar C. Levonorgestrel-releasing intrauterine device (LNG-IUD) for symptomatic endometriosis following surgery. *Cochrane Database of Systematic Reviews* 2013, Issue 1. Art. No.: CD005072. DOI: 10.1002/14651858. CD005072.pub3.

20. Brown J, Pan A, Hart RJ. Gonadotropin-releasing hormone analogues for pain associated with endometriosis. *Obstet Gynecol* 2011;117:727–728.

21. Waller KG, Shaw RW. Gonadotrophin-hormone releasing hormone analogues for the treatment of endometriosis; long-term follow-up. *Fertil Steril* 1993; 59:511–515.

22. Farmer JE, Prentice A, Breeze A *et al.* Gonadotropin-releasing hormone analogues for endometriosis: bone mineral density. *Cochrane Database of Systematic Reviews* 2003, Issue 4. Art. No.: CD001297. DOI: 1002/14651858. CD001297.

23. Patwardhan S, Nawathe A, Yates D, Harrison GR, Khan KS. Systematic review of the effects of aromatase inhibitors on pain associated with endometriosis. *BJOG* 2008;115:818–822.

24. Winkel CA. A cost-effective approach to the management of endometriosis. *Curr Opin Obstet Gynaecol* 2000;12:317–320.

25. Lalchandani S, Baxter A, Phillips K. Is helium thermal coagulator therapy for the treatment of women with minimal to moderate endometriosis cost effective? A prospective randomised controlled trial. *Gynecol Surg* 2005;2:255–258.

26. Zhu X, Hamilton KD, McNicol ED. Acupuncture for pain in endometriosis. *Cochrane Database of Systematic Reviews* 2011, Issue 9. Art. No.: CD007864. DOI: 10.1002/14651858. CD007864.pub2.

27. Jacobson TZ, Duffy JMN, Barlow D, Koninckx PR, Garry R. Laparoscopic surgery for pelvic pain associated with endometriosis. *Cochrane Database of Systematic Reviews* 2009, Issue 4. Art. No.: CD001300. DOI: 10.1002/14651858. CD001300.pub2.

28. Procter M, Latthe P, Farquhar C, Khan K, Johnson N. Surgical interruption of pelvic nerve pathways for primary and secondary dysmenorrhoea. *Cochrane Database of Systematic Reviews* 2005, Issue 4. Art. No.: CD001896. DOI: 10.1002/14651858. CD001896.pub2.

29. Hart RJ, Hickey M, Maouris P, Buckett W. Excisional surgery versus ablative surgery for ovarian endometriomata. *Cochrane Database of Systematic Reviews* 2008, Issue 2. Art. No.: CD004992. DOI: 10.1002/14651858. CD004992.pub3.

30. Raffi F, Metwally M, Amer S. The impact of excision of ovarian endometrioma on ovarian reserve: a systematic review and meta-analysis. *J Clin Endocrinol Metab* 2012;97:3146–3154.

31. Furness S, Yap C, Farquhar C, Cheong YC. Pre- and postoperative medical therapy for endometriosis surgery. *Cochrane Database of Systematic Reviews* 2004, Issue 3. Art. No.: CD003678. DOI: 10.1002/14651858.CD003678.pub2.

32. Seracchioli R, Mabrouk M, Manuzzi L *et al.* Postoperative use of oral contraceptive pills for prevention of anatomical relapse or symptom recurrence after conservative surgery for endometriosis. *Hum Reprod* 2009;24:2729–2735.

33. Vercellini P, Crosignani PG, Somigliana E, Berlanda N, Barbara G, Fedele L. Medical treatment for rectovaginal endometriosis: what is the evidence? *Hum Reprod* 2009;24:2504–2514.

34. Shakiba K, Bena JF, McGill KM, Minger J, Falcone T. Surgical treatment of endometriosis. A 7-year follow-up on the requirement for further surgery. *Obstet Gynecol* 2008;111:1285–1292.

35. Al Kadri H, Hassan S, Al-Fozan HM, Hajeer A. Hormone therapy for endometriosis and surgical menopause. *Cochrane Database of Systematic Reviews* 2009, Issue 1. Art. No.: CD005997. DOI: 10.1002/14651858.CD005997.pub2.

36. RCOG. *The initial management of chronic pelvic pain.* Green-top guideline No. 41. London: RCOG, 2012.

37. Endometriosis UK. www.endometriosis-uk.org

Chapter 78 Adenomyosis

Christine P West

MRCOG standards

There are no established standards for this topic but the following are suggested

Theoretical skills

- Be aware of current understanding of the epidemiology of adenomyosis and its contribution to menstrual disorders.
- Understand the clinical features that may suggest a diagnosis of adenomyosis and the medical and surgical approaches to management.

Practical skills

- Understand the role of imaging in the diagnosis of adenomyosis.

INTRODUCTION

Adenomyosis is implicated as a cause of both heavy and painful menstruation, but because the diagnosis is most often made retrospectively and based on histological appearance, most published data relate to women who have undergone hysterectomy. Information from these studies indicates that adenomyosis is frequently asymptomatic and commonly coexists with other gynaecological conditions. Histologically, adenomyosis is characterised by the presence of endometrial glands and stroma in the uterine myometrium, with surrounding myometrial hypertrophy and hyperplasia,[1] the latter often resulting in significant uterine enlargement. The lesions are seen haphazardly and at varied depths within the myometrium. There is no current consensus regarding the exact diagnostic criteria.[2] Although histologically similar, adenomyosis is traditionally regarded as distinct from endometriosis in terms of its epidemiology (see below) although this distinction has been challenged. Recent advances in imaging have facilitated the diagnosis and study of the condition and led to greater opportunities for clinical trials of medical and conservative management. To date, such studies have been very limited and consequently the literature on adenomyosis remains small, as is the evidence base for its management.

PREVALENCE

Adenomyosis is present in 20–30 per cent of hysterectomy specimens,[2] regardless of indication. There have been some reports of a correlation between the severity of menstrual symptoms and the extent and depth of invasion of the adenomyosis but others have failed to confirm such a relationship and it seems likely that adenomyosis is commonly present as an incidental finding. A prevalence of 21 per cent was reported in an ultrasound-based study of 985 women attending a general gynaecology clinic.[3] However the median age of this population was 40 years and 54 per cent were nulligravid. Small-scale studies using imaging techniques have reported appearances consistent with adenomyosis in 12 per cent of a sample of 100 healthy women[4] and in 9 per cent of 208 women following term delivery[5] but there have been no large-scale community-based studies of adenomyosis and thus its prevalence is a normal population of women is unknown.

EPIDEMIOLOGY

Among women who have undergone hysterectomy the presence of adenomyosis is significantly associated with increasing parity.[2] In the study based on ultrasound,[3] age was also a significant factor, with the highest prevalence between 40 and 49 years. Many[2] but not all[3,6] studies have reported an increased incidence following caesarean section (CS) and surgical evacuation for abortion or management of miscarriage. There is no consistent association with ethnicity, smoking, contraceptive use or age at menarche [2,3,6,7] but increased risk in obese or overweight women has been reported.[6,7] Despite this apparent association with older reproductive age, it is known that adenomyosis can occur in adolescents and young women.[1]

Although women diagnosed with adenomyosis tend to be older and of higher parity than those with endometriosis and less likely to have a family history of the condition,[7] there have been reports of an association with endometriosis.[3,8] The presence of adenomyosis based on MRI of a population of women attending a fertility clinic[8] was increased in women with confirmed endometriosis compared with those without laparoscopic evidence of endometriosis but there have been no other studies of its prevalence in women attending for investigation of infertility.[9] There has been a report that adenomyosis may be associated with obstetric complications, in particular an increase risk of preterm delivery.[5,9]

CAUSE

The adenomyotic tissue is presumed to be derived from the endometrium by abnormal ingrowth and invagination of its basal layer[1,2] triggered by a weakness at the endometrial–myometrial junction. Disruption of this interface was previously presumed to be caused by pregnancy-related factors such as increased intrauterine pressure or surgical trauma such as curettage or CS. However recent epidemiological data[3,6] have thrown some doubt on this hypothesis. There is some evidence that endometrial cells in adenomyosis develop greater invasive potential and that this, together with altered myometrial contractility, results in disruption of the endometrial–myometrial junction. Altered myometrial contractility leading to retrograde menstruation may be a common link between adenomyosis and endometriosis[1] but this remains speculative. Angiogenic growth factors, genetic factors and hormonal influences are also likely to be involved.

MANAGEMENT

Investigation

Available evidence suggests that women with symptomatic adenomyosis are likely to present with heavy and painful menstruation.[10] Clinically, the uterus may be bulky and tender, but both the history and the clinical findings are non-specific. Further investigation is helpful in distinguishing between adenomyosis and uterine fibroids, particularly if non-medical management is considered (see below).

Reviews of diagnostic techniques[11,12] have concluded that transvaginal ultrasound scanning (TVS) should be used as a primary screening modality for the diagnosis of adenomyosis [B]. Various sonographic appearances have been described (Box 78.1).[9,11,12] These changes are usually present diffusely throughout the myometrium but discrete adenomyomata are also seen[11,12] and differ from fibroids in being elliptical rather than globular, with poorly defined borders and lack of calcification. It has been estimated that the probability of adenomyosis with an abnormal scan is 66 per cent and 9.1 per cent with a normal scan.[12]

There is no current consensus on whether one, some or all of these features should be present for diagnosis and different criteria have been used by different investigators.[9–12]

Box 78.1 Sonographic features of adenomyosis

- Heterogeneous myometrial areas
- Globular asymmetrical uterus
- Irregular cystic spaces
- Myometrial linear striations
- Parallel shadowing
- Thickening of the anterior or posterior myometrial wall with increased or decreased echogenicity

Some authorities stipulate that three or more of these features should be present for diagnosis of adenomyosis.[10,11]

Features of adenomyosis have also been described using MRI.[9,10] These include diffuse or focal widening of the junctional zone and areas of low signal intensity within the myometrium corresponding to smooth muscle hyperplasia. High signal intensity foci or linear striations are also seen. However there is disagreement between observers regarding the degree of junctional zone thickening required for diagnosis.[9] Studies comparing uterine histology with pre-surgical TVS or MRI or both have found little difference in sensitivity or specificity between the two techniques[9,10] but MRI is less observer dependent.[11] It is more accurate in distinguishing adenomyosis from fibroids in larger uteri.[11] In keeping with ultrasound, there remains some lack of consensus on diagnostic criteria.[9]

Both hysteroscopic and laparoscopic myometrial biopsy techniques have been described[1,13] but have limitations when compared with non-invasive imaging.

Medical management

Most women with menstrual disorders are managed symptomatically in the first instance and therapies which are effective in the management of heavy menstrual bleeding (Chapter 75), dysmenorrhoea (Chapter 76) and endometriosis (Chapter 77) should be beneficial for women with adenomyosis. These include non-steroidal anti-inflammatory drugs (NSAIDs), tranexamic acid, oral contraceptives and progestogens [E] but evidence relating to their use in adenomyosis is lacking.

LNG-IUS

There have been several small-scale studies reporting benefit from the use of the levonorgestrel-releasing intrauterine system (LNG-IUS) in women with adenomyosis.[13] A 3-year follow-up study of 94 women[14] reported a significant decrease in dysmenorrhoea and uterine volume with 53 per cent achieving amenorrhoea after the first year of treatment [D]. Overall satisfaction was 56 per cent at 1 year and 72.5 per cent at 3 years with a continuation rate of 66 per cent at 3 years. Expulsion was high, at 16 per cent. A prospective study of 95 women with adenomyosis treated with either LNG-IUS or expectant management following endometrial resection[15] reported a significantly lower rate of dysmenorrhoea and need for further treatment with the IUS. In a prospective study of 75 women randomised between LNG-IUS and hysterectomy[16] levels of haemoglobin were similar at 6 and 12 months. Quality-of-life assessments were marginally better in the IUS group and there was only one IUS discontinuation, due to an expulsion. This evidence, albeit limited, supports the role of the LNG-IUS in the management of adenomyosis [B] although further data based on longer term follow-up is needed.

GnRH agonists

Pituitary–ovarian suppression with a gonadotrophin-releasing hormone (GnRH) agonist causes amenorrhoea and regression of adenomyotic foci measured by MRI [D][17] but these benefits are rapidly reversed following cessation of treatment. In theory there should be a role for longer-term use in conjunction with add-back therapy to control vasomotor side effects, such as described for fibroids or endometriosis (see Chapters 74 and 77), but evidence for this is based on small case series and case reports [D].[9] There is a potential role for GnRH agonists as adjuncts to surgical excision of adenomyomata[17] (see below).

Uterine artery embolisation

Uterine artery embolisation (UAE) is established for the management of symptomatic fibroids (see Chapter 74), and as adenomyosis and uterine fibroids may coexist, this led to some early experience of UAE in cases of adenomyosis.[13] Small case series of women followed up for at least 2 years after UAE reported an early favourable response but this was sustained in less than 60 per cent of the women [D].[13,18,19] A more recent retrospective study of 40 women treated by UAE for menstrual symptoms associated with adenomyosis with or without uterine fibroids reported no significant difference in outcome between women with pure adenomyosis and those with a combination of both pathologies after a median follow-up period of 40 months.[20] Symptoms remained controlled in 72.5 per cent of the women overall. However no patients with fibroid dominance required surgical intervention for treatment failure, compared with 52 per cent of those with pure adenomyosis and 42 per cent with predominance of adenomyosis over fibroids. There was no reported correlation between the depth or extent of the adenomyosis and the clinical outcome. On the basis of this limited information it is not possible to make a recommendation regarding the role of UAE for symptomatic adenomyosis but its presence does not appear to be a contraindication to the use of UAE in women with fibroids [D]. Further data from randomised prospective trials is clearly needed.

Surgical management

Hysterectomy is regarded as the definitive treatment for adenomyosis in women who have completed child-bearing [E] although the decision to perform a hysterectomy is usually based on the presence of other pathologies such as fibroids or because of failure of conservative management of heavy and/or painful menstrual bleeding. There is some evidence that the presence of deep lesions of adenomyosis is associated with failure of endometrial ablation [D].[21] Use of the LNG-IUS may be preferred to endometrial ablation in this situation [E]. Evidence from one prospective study[13] suggested that the IUS may have a role as an adjunct to endometrial ablation in the presence of adenomyosis [C] but further studies are needed. General issues relating to hysterectomy for management of menstrual disorders are reviewed in Chapter 75.

Where preservation of fertility is desired, the role of surgery is unclear. Some superficial lesions of adenomyosis close to the endometrial–myometrial junction may be suitable for endometrial ablation or resection[21] but good-quality data are lacking. Surgical excision of adenomyomata and deeper lesions has also been described[21] although the diffuse nature of the disease makes this challenging and, in contrast to fibroids, adenomyomata cannot easily be enucleated. This highlights the importance of accurate radiological assessment prior to any form of conservative surgery for fibroids. In one large cohort study, localised excision of adenomyosis, performed by laparotomy or laparoscopy, was followed by 6 months of a GnRH agonist or no adjunct treatment.[17] The severity of menorrhagia and dysmenorrhoea declined in both groups over a 2-year follow-up period but symptom relapse was higher in the group treated with surgery alone. Pregnancy rates were over 70 per cent in both groups. However such approaches may only be applicable in specialist centres and need further evaluation.

Other treatment options

Other medical treatments including anti-progesterones and aromatase inhibitors, alone or in combination with other agents, may have a future role in management of adenomyosis but evidence is lacking. MRI-guided focused ultrasound is used successfully for treatment of fibroids (see Chapter 74) but the more diffuse nature of adenomyosis may make the application of this technique more challenging. Experience to date is based on isolated case reports[13] and small cases series[22] with varied results and it is therefore not possible to reach any conclusions about the potential use of this technique for adenomyosis.

> **EBM**
>
> There is little supporting evidence for the management of adenomyosis, and the above text relies largely on small non-randomised trials and cohort studies.

KEY POINTS

- Adenomyosis is present in 20-30 per cent of hysterectomy specimens and is a cause of uterine enlargement.
- Its prevalence in the general population is unclear and its role as a contributing factor to menstrual disorders is not well understood.
- There is a lack of consensus regarding the criteria for diagnosis of adenomyosis by histology or imaging.
- TVS backed up by MRI is of value as a diagnostic tool [B].
- Medical therapies such as oral contraceptives, progestogens and GnRH analogues that have proven value in management of painful and/or heavy menstruation and endometriosis are likely to be of value [D] but have not been adequately assessed in adenomyosis.
- The LNG-IUS appears to be effective for the medical treatment of adenomyosis [B]
- Endometrial ablation for treatment of heavy menstrual bleeding may have a greater failure rate in the presence of adenomyosis [D].
- Hysterectomy is effective for relief of menstrual symptoms associated with adenomyosis [D] in women who have completed child-bearing.
- UAE can be used in women with adenomyosis alone or in combination with fibroids but may be less effective in cases where the predominant lesions are those of adenomyosis [D].

References

1. Benagiano G, Habiba M, Brosens I. The pathophysiology of uterine adenomyosis: an update. *Fertil Steril* 2012;98:572–579.
2. Vercillini P, Vigano P, Somigliana E, Daguati R, Abbiati A, Fedele L. Adenomyosis: epidemiological factors. *Best Pract & Res Clin Obstet Gynaecol* 2006;20:465–477.
3. Naftalin J, Hoo W, Pateman K, Mavrelos D, Holland T, Jurkovic D. How common is adenomyosis? A prospective study of prevalence using transvaginal ultrasound in a gynaecology clinic. *Hum Reprod* 2012:12;3432–3439.
4. Hauth EA, Jaeger HJ, Libera H, Lange S, Forsting M. MR imaging of the uterus and cervix in healthy women: determination of normal values. *Eur Radiol* 2007;17:734–742.
5. Juang CM, Chou P, Yen M, Twu N, Horng H, Hsu W. Adenomyosis and risk of preterm delivery. *BJOG* 2007;114:165–169.
6. Trabert, B, Weiss NS, Rudra CB, Scholes D, Holt VL. A case-control investigation of adenomyosis: impact of control group selection on risk factor strength. *Women's Health Issues* 2011:21;160–164.
7. Templeman C, Marshall SF, Ursin G et al. Adenomyosis and endometriosis in the California Teachers study. *Fertil Steril* 2008:90;415–424.
8. Kunz G, Beil D, Huppert P, Noe M, Kissler S, Leyendecker G. Adenomyosis in endometriosis – prevalence and impact on fertility. Evidence from magnetic resonance imaging. *Hum Reprod* 2005; 20:2309–2316.
9. Maheshwari VA, Gurunath S, Fatima F, Bhattacharya S. Adenomyosis and subfertility: a systematic review of prevalence, diagnosis, treatment and fertility outcomes. *Hum Reprod Update* 2012;18:374–392.
10. Mehasseb MK, Habiba MA. Adenomyosis uteri: an update. *The Obstetrician and Gynaecologist* 2009;11:41–47.
11. Dueholm M. Transvaginal ultrasound for diagnosis of adenomyosis: a review. *Best Pract & Res Clin Obstet Gynaecol* 2006;20:569–582.
12. Meredith SM, Sanchez-Ramos L, Kaunitz AM. Diagnostic accuracy of transvaginal sonography for the diagnosis of adenomyosis: systematic review and metaanalysis. *Am J Obstet Gynecol* 2009;201:107. e1–6.
13. Rabinovici J, Stewart EA. New interventional techniques for adenomyosis. *Best Pract & Res Clin Obstet Gynaecol* 2006;20:617–636.
14. Sheng J, Zhang WY, Zhang JP, Lu D. The LNG-IUS study on adenomyosis: a 3-year follow-up study on the efficacy and side effects of the levonorgestrel system for the treatment of dysmenorrhoea associated with adenomyosis. *Contraception* 2009:79;189–193.
15. Maia H Jr, Maltez, Coelho G, Athayde C, Coutinho EM. Insertion of mirena after endometrial resection in patients with adenomyosis. *J Am Assoc Gynecol Laparosc* 2003;10:512–516.
16. Ozdegirmenci O, Kayikcioglu F, Akgul AM et al. Comparison of levonorgestrel intrauterine system versus hysterectomy on efficacy and quality of life in patients with adenomyosis. *Fertil Steril* 2011;95:497–502.
17. Wang P-H, Liu W-M, Fuh J-L, Cheng M-H, Chao H-T. Comparison of surgery alone and combined surgical–medical treatment in the management of symptomatic uterine adenomyomata. *Fertil Steril* 2009;92:876–885.
18. Kim MD, Kim S, Kim NK et al. Long-term results of uterine artery embolization for symptomatic adenomyosis. *Am J Roentgenol* 2007;188:176–181.
19. Bratby MJ, Walker WJ. Uterine artery embolisation for symptomatic adenomyosis – mid-term results. *Eur J Radiol* 2009;70:128–132.
20. Froeling V, Scheurig-Muenkler C, Hamm B, Kroencke TJ. Uterine artery embolization to treat uterine adenomyosis with or without uterine leiomyomata: results of symptom control and health-related quality of life 40 months after treatment. *Cardiovasc Intervent Radiol* 2012;35:523–529.
21. Farquhar C, Brosens I. Medical and surgical management of adenomyosis. *Best Pract & Res Clin Obstet Gynaecol* 2006;20:603–616.
22. Dong X, Yang Z. High-intensity focused ultrasound ablation of localized adenomyosis. *Curr Opin Gynecol Obstet* 2010;22:326–330.

Chapter 79 Premenstrual syndrome

Christine P West

Christine P West

MRCOG standards

There are no established standards for this topic but the following are suggested:

Theoretical skills

- Understand the definition of premenstrual syndrome and its variants.
- Understand the epidemiology of premenstrual disorders.
- Know how to assess a patient presenting with premenstrual symptoms.
- Be aware of non-hormonal approaches to management, including alternative therapies.
- Understand the nature and complications of hormonal approaches to management and their limitations.

INTRODUCTION

Adverse emotional and physical symptoms are experienced by the majority of women in the lead-up to menstruation, although they are usually mild and regarded as a normal physiological response to cyclical hormone changes. However, a substantial number of women are sufficiently distressed by their symptoms to seek medical help and a minority are severely incapacitated by them. Hormonal treatments were commonly used in the past, but premenstrual syndrome (PMS) is no longer regarded as a purely endocrine disorder and first-line management includes non-hormonal approaches. However, the symptoms are triggered by the endocrine changes of the menstrual cycle and women with severe premenstrual symptoms continue to be referred to gynaecologists for consideration of hormonal suppression when other therapies have failed. Assessment of the efficacy of treatment is complicated by the subjective nature of the diagnosis and the strong placebo effect. Prospective methods of symptom assessment are now well established and there is an expanding literature of randomised controlled trials (RCTs) covering various approaches to management, including several systematic reviews.

DEFINITIONS

Although the term premenstrual syndrome is generally used throughout published literature, it has been suggested that the criteria for diagnosis are too wide and the clinical syndrome should be renamed core premenstrual disorder.[1] Mild symptoms should be considered physiological and the diagnosis of core premenstrual disorder or PMS based on substantial impairment of personal or professional life. Various emotional and physical symptoms are associated with the condition (Table 79.1) but their pattern of occurrence is more important than their nature and combination. Severe symptoms which are predominantly psychological in nature are classified as premenstrual dysphoric disorder (PMDD)[1] by the American Psychiatric Association in its *Diagnostic and Statistical Manual of Mental Disorders*, Fourth Edition (DSM-IV) although this is a research criterion not in general use outside the USA.

Because of a lack of objective tests, the diagnosis is made on the basis of detailed history taking, backed up by prospective daily symptom recording over at least two cycles. Various rating scales are available for this purpose.[1] Cyclical symptoms which are present only premenstrually should be distinguished from premenstrual magnification/exacerbation of underlying psychological, psychiatric or medical disorders. Symptoms similar to those of PMS may be induced in some women by the use of progestogens[1] for contraception, hormone replacement or management of menstrual disorders.

PREVALENCE AND EPIDEMIOLOGY

In a population-based questionnaire survey of 1083 women aged 18–46 in Goteborg, Sweden[2] 92 per cent reported at least one adverse symptom in the lead-up to menstruation. Seventy per cent reported changes in mood in combination with bodily swelling, and 30–40 per cent rated their symptoms as mild to moderate in intensity. Eleven per cent felt that their symptoms were severe enough to seek medical help. Such population-based studies rely on retrospective assessment and do not distinguish between symptoms present only prior to menstruation and those that are ongoing throughout the cycle. In a recent sample of 947 UK women aged 20–34 years

Table 79.1 Criteria for diagnosis of moderate–severe PMS (core premenstrual disorder)

Symptoms	Pattern	Impact
Any combination of symptoms which may include:	Precipitated by ovulation	Substantial impairment of daily personal and professional activities
Irritability	Recur in each luteal phase	No underlying physical or psychiatric disorder
Tension	Relieved by the end of menstruation	
Depression	Followed by a symptom-free week	
Anxiety		
Fatigue		
Food cravings		
Bloating		
Breast discomfort		

assessed prospectively by symptom diaries,[3] 24 per cent were considered to have PMS, based on the presence of five or more symptoms scored as mild to moderate or two or more symptoms scored as severe, followed by a symptom-free period of at least 7 days. In the latter study prevalence was lower in women using any form of hormonal contraception and in those with higher educational attainment and lower perceived levels of stress. No association was found with alcohol, diet or exercise. Apparent association with age, smoking and body mass index (BMI) was abolished after adjustment for contraceptive use.

There are no well-defined demographic risk factors and although level of reporting may vary in different communities, a recent web-based survey showed prevalence to be similar across 19 countries.[4] Premenstrual symptoms are associated with ovulatory menstrual cycles and are reported in all reproductive age groups, including adolescence[4] although the majority of women who seek help are between 25 and 40.

CAUSES

The frequency with which these symptoms are reported by women indicate that in their milder form they are a normal manifestation of the menstrual cycle, although it is possible that those at the more extreme end of the normal range have a pathological cause. Despite their relationship with the endocrine changes of the menstrual cycle, there is no evidence for any abnormality of the hypothalamo–pituitary–ovarian axis. There have been many theories of aetiology, but current evidence suggests that PMS may be a neuroendocrine disorder caused by deficiency or abnormal function of the neurotransmitters serotonin and gamma-aminobutyric acid which may cause increased sensitivity to progesterone. This is supported by evidence that drugs which enhance serotonergic function are beneficial in its management.[5] A reported reduction of PMS symptoms with the anti-mineralocorticoid spironolactone may be suggestive of a disorder in the renin–angiotensin–aldosterone system[6] and forms the basis for the use of an oral contraceptive containing a progestogen

derived from spironolactone. Currently the nature of any underlying metabolic disorder remains unclear.

A study of prospective daily symptom self-assessment by women referred for specialist help because of cyclical symptoms found that PMS was confirmed in only one-third,[7] the remainder showing premenstrual magnification of ongoing psychological symptoms or symptoms exacerbated by menstruation itself. There was a significant relationship between menstrual and premenstrual magnification and previous psychiatric disorders, marital breakdown and increased parity. Other studies have shown a relationship between self-reported PMS and personality disorders and psychosocial stress.[8]

MANAGEMENT

A detailed history should be obtained,[1] including a description of the individual symptoms and their relationship to the menstrual cycle, together with a menstrual and reproductive history, including need for contraception. Medical, social and psychiatric history should also be explored together with details of any current or previous exposure to exogenous hormones. A diagnosis of PMS based on retrospective history taking is unreliable,[7] and prospective charting of symptoms for at least two menstrual cycles is essential in order to clarify the symptom pattern [C]. Many methods of symptom assessment are available,[1,9] but as they are time consuming to analyse, most are only suitable for use in a specialist clinic or research setting. Simple pictorial charts are available for use in primary care.

Management of PMS has been the subject of an RCOG Green-top Guideline.[9] Basic management lies within the scope of primary care.[1] Women with mild degrees of PMS may respond to reassurance and general advice about exercise, diet and stress reduction [E]. Referral for specialist help will depend on the severity of the problem, the experience of individual general practitioners and the expectations of the women involved. Many women referred for specialist help will be experiencing disruption of family or professional life and have a history of previous treatment failures. Ideally, women with severe PMS should be seen in a multidisciplinary specialist clinic or at least by a gynaecologist or a psychiatrist with a particular interest in the problem, preferably in a community-based setting [E].[9]

All RCTs of treatment for PMS have shown a very marked placebo response [A]. This emphasises the importance of critical appraisal of the evidence base before recommending specific therapies. The strength of the placebo effect may reflect the positive role of detailed history taking and a sympathetic approach.

Complementary and alternative therapies

Gynaecologists should have an awareness of the evidence underlying alternative therapies in order to advise patients appropriately. There have been three systematic reviews of trials of such therapies[10-12] and the conclusions are summarised in the RCOG Green-top Guideline.[9]

Dietary supplements

These approaches are available over the counter and may be recommended by alternative practitioners or on the internet. Beneficial effects have been reported with calcium, calcium combined with vitamin D, magnesium and isoflavones.[9-12] However, the reviewers felt that weaknesses in methodology limited recommendations of their value [E]. Similarly, studies of nutritional supplements containing high doses of vitamins and other micronutrients have yielded inconclusive results.[9-11]

Dietary supplements are popular because they are perceived to have fewer side effects than conventional medicines and are likely to be regarded as effective because of the strong placebo effect. However, interactions with conventional medicines should be considered, such as those associated with the use of St John's Wort.[9] High-dose vitamin B6, used for many years for the treatment of PMS, was reported to have neurotoxic effects.[12] Evidence from a meta-analysis suggested that low doses of vitamin B6 up to 100 mg daily may be of benefit in treating premenstrual depression [C][12] but the studies are of poor quality and other authors have challenged this conclusion.[9,10] Evening primrose oil is licensed for treatment of premenstrual mastalgia when given at high dosage but a meta-analysis failed to find sufficient evidence to support its use for PMS.[13]

Herbal medicine

The fruit of the chaste tree (*Vitex agnus-castus*) contains a mixture of iridoids and flavonoids and some compounds similar in structure to sex steroids. Evidence from a multicentre RCT[14] has shown the active treatment to be significantly more effective than placebo for the majority of the symptoms assessed (with the exception of bloating), with an overall response rate of 53 per cent for active treatment and 24 per cent for placebo. On the basis of this evidence, *Vitex*

agnus castus fruit extract seems to be a potentially useful therapy for PMS [B] although there is no standard quality-controlled preparation available. Further investigation is in progress. Similarly, reports of benefit from the use of Chinese herbal medicine[15] are limited by the lack of standard formulations. Ginkgo biloba and pollen extract have both been shown to be beneficial in small-scale studies although further data would be needed to support their use.[9]

Other alternative approaches

Massage, relaxation and aromatherapy are popular therapies for which benefit is likely to outweigh any possible harm [E], although controlled studies of their use for PMS have yielded inconclusive results.[11] Similarly, although advice about graded exercise is useful for general health and is often recommended for relief of PMS, the evidence is based on observational studies and small non-randomised trials [D].[16]

Support and self-help groups are commonly used for PMS. This approach was supported by a study in which women were managed with a package of strategies including self-monitoring, personal choice, self-regulation and environmental modification, administered within a peer support group with professional guidance.[17] The actively managed group experienced greater relief of symptoms in comparison with a control group waiting for the intervention [C]. The response was also maintained during an 18-month follow-up period.

Cognitive behavioural therapy

It has been suggested that cognitive behavioural therapy (CBT) should be routinely considered for the treatment of severe PMS.[9] A meta-analysis of five trials of CBT[18] found a significant reduction in both anxiety and depression and a possible beneficial effect on behavioural changes and interference with daily living. However, the evidence was considered to be of low quality. A subsequent meta-analysis[19] which also assessed pharmacological interventions concluded that the effect size for both interventions was small to medium and future research should focus more on a combination of both approaches. On the basis of this evidence, CBT can be considered to be effective for severe PMS [A] but such therapy is intensive, involving weekly sessions of individual cognitive therapy, and may not be available for many sufferers.

Selective serotonin reuptake inhibitors

SSRIs are now regarded as a first-line therapy for treatment of severe PMS, particularly in women who fulfil the criteria for PMDD.[9] The use of SSRIs for PMS has been the subject of a systematic review[5] of 31 trials comparing SSRIs with placebo. These included fluoxetine (n = 10), sertraline (n = 9), paroxetine (n = 9), escitalopram (n = 2) and citalopram (n = 1) given continuously (n = 20) or intermittently (n = 14) for 2–6 months. Three trials compared continuous with luteal-phase administration. The results favoured active treatment over placebo for both behavioural and physical symptoms. The onset of effectiveness was rapid and luteal-phase-only therapy was as effective as continuous treatment. Moderate doses were more effective than low doses but side effects were also dose dependent. Nausea, fatigue, insomnia, decreased libido and sweating were the most common side effects, reported by up to 20 per cent of women.

On the basis of this evidence, SSRIs can be regarded as a first-line treatment for severe PMS [A]. Low doses given during the luteal phase of the cycle (14 days premenstrually) may optimise efficacy while reducing incidence of side effects [B].[5] They can be given together with oral contraceptives[1] although there is no evidence for any synergistic effects. They may also be suitable for long-term use although their long-term effectiveness for PMS has not been established. Despite this evidence for their efficacy, side effects are a common reason for poor compliance and 30–40 per cent of women with severe PMS fail to respond to SSRIs. Use of these medications falls outwith the expertise of the average gynaecologist and should be prescribed in the context of a specialist clinic [E].

HORMONAL MANIPULATION FOR THE MANAGEMENT OF PMS

Although the majority of women with PMS have no identifiable underlying endocrine disorder, ovulation appears to act as a trigger factor and thus various strategies that suppress ovulation or abolish the cycle altogether have a potential role in management. Currently there are no preparations (hormonal or non-hormonal) licensed for the treatment of PMS. The costs of the various treatments discussed in this chapter vary widely (Table 79.2) and this, together with their side-effect profiles, should be considered alongside the evidence underlying their use.

Progesterone and progestogens

Luteal-phase supplements of progesterone were widely used in the past, based on the unproven theory that PMS was secondary to a progesterone deficiency. In the UK, progesterone is available only for vaginal or rectal administration, hence the use of synthetic progestogens for this indication. However, evidence from hormone replacement therapy (HRT) studies indicates that progestogens might actually exacerbate PMS-type symptoms in susceptible individuals.[20]

A systematic review assessed 14 RCTs of progesterone and 4 of progestogens in PMS.[21] Overall results of meta-analysis for progesterone showed no difference compared with placebo. Results with progestogens were difficult to interpret due to the small number of studies and differences in the treatment protocols. Overall odds ratios were marginally but significantly in favour of progestogens for both physical and behavioural symptoms but drop-outs due to side effects were high. The response to progestogens may have been influenced by the fact that two of the four studies used progestogens in an ovulation-suppressing regimen. However, this evidence does not support the use of either progesterone or progestogens in the management of PMS when given during the luteal phase of the cycle [A]. While the continuous use of progestogens in ovulation suppressive doses (e.g. Depo-Provera or oral desogestrel)

Table 79.2 Costs of pharmacological treatment options for PMS (data from British National Formulary – 2014 prices)[31] and evidence level for use. None of the treatments listed are licensed for this indication.

Treatment	3 monthly cost (range in £)	Evidence level
Non-hormonal:		
Pyridoxine hydrochloride 50–100 mg/day (vitamin B$_6$)	9.24–18.48	Inconclusive
Selective serotonin reuptake inhibitors	1.44–25.50	A
Hormonal:		
Ethinylestradiol 20/30 mcg plus levonorgestrel 150 mcg or norethisterone acetate 1 mg	1.89–3.76	B
Ethinylestradiol 20/30 mcg plus desogestrel 150 mcg	6.57–10.23	B
Ethinlyestradiol 30 mcg plus drospirenone 3 mg	14.20–18.93	B
Estraderm 100 mcg/24 hours + Mirena IUS	23.59	B
Estraderm 100 mcg/24 hours + oral progestogen	24.00–29.77	B
Depot medroxyprogesterone acetate	6.01	D
Desogestrel 75 mcg	4.30–8.68	None available
Danazol 200 mg bd or tid	97.32–152.10	B
Intranasal GnRH agonist + add-back HRT	157.29–174.31	A
GnRH agonist depot + add-back HRT	210.20–252.02	A

* Range covers cyclical or continuous administration (where relevant) and alternative available formulations

may be beneficial, there is lack of evidence to support this approach.

Combined oral contraceptives

The occurrence of PMS symptoms in the post-ovulatory phase of the menstrual cycle strongly suggests that any therapy that suppresses ovulation should relieve PMS. Combined oral contraceptive pills (COCPs) have the advantage of being cheap (Table 79.2) and suitable for long-term use. Earlier studies yielded varied results. Some showed a reduction in the prevalence and severity of PMS with oral contraceptive use[22,23] while others failed to show any difference in cyclical symptoms between COCP users and non-users.[24]

An oral contraceptive containing the progestogen drospirenone, which is derived from spironolactone and has anti-androgenic and anti-mineralocorticoid activities, may have advantages over older preparations. An initial placebo-controlled trial of drospirenone 3 mg in combination with ethinylestradiol (EE) 30 mcg (21 days out of 28 for 3 months) reported a non-significant improvement in symptoms of PMDD.[25]

Subsequently the authors of a systematic review[25] concluded that a combination of drospirenone 3 mg with 20 mcg EE (two studies in which the combination was given for 24 days out of 28) was significantly more effective than placebo over a 3-month period of treatment in women with a diagnosis of PMDD. However the placebo response was 36 per cent, compared with 48 per cent for the active treatment group. This drospirenone/EE combination, given cyclically for 24 days out of 28, is licensed in the USA for treatment of PMD but is not currently available in the UK.

The question remains whether other low-dose combined contraceptives, used conventionally or in extended regimens, may be effective for moderate or severe PMS. In a large multicentre study comparing desogestel 150 mcg with drospirenone 3 mg, both combined with 30 mcg EE for 21 days out of 28, there was no significant difference in premenstrual symptoms after 2 years of treatment.[25] A pre-treatment diagnosis of PMS or PMDD was not an inclusion criterion for this study. A single-centre study[26] compared desogestel 150 mcg with drospirenone 3 mg both in combination with 20 mcg EE given in extended dosage for 24 days out of 28 for 6 months. Results showed a significant improvement in premenstrual symptoms in both groups after 6 months although the response was greater in the group treated with drospirenone.

Prolongation of the contraceptive pill cycle from 21 to 24 days causes increased ovarian suppression[27] which may contribute to improvement of cyclical symptoms. Similarly, continuous administration is commonly used for relief of dysmenorrhoea and endometriosis (see Chapters 76 and 77) and may be beneficial for PMS. An overview of four studies of continuous use of levonorgestrel 90 mcg in combination with EE 20 mcg, including three placebo-controlled trials, reported a 30–59 per cent improvement in premenstrual

symptoms[28] although a large placebo effect was also observed.

Taken overall, this evidence suggests that a trial of therapy with a low-dose COCP should be considered for women with premenstrual syndrome who have no contraindications to its use [B]. Continuous use of COCP preparations may have an advantage over cyclical use [B] and both second-and third-generation formulations may be effective [B]. Strongest evidence exists for the third-generation combination of drospirenone 3 mg with 20 mcg EE administered for 24 days out of 28 for women with severe PMS [A], although evidence is limited to short-term use and this preparation is currently not available in the UK.

Transdermal oestradiol

Subcutaneous implants and transdermal estradiol patches have been used in ovulation-suppressive doses in combination with cyclical luteal-phase progestogen for the management of severe PMS. However, concerns over supraphysiological levels of estradiol due to tachyphylaxis after repeated subcutaneous implants[29] have favoured the use of transdermal patches. Both 200 mg and 100 mg estradiol patches, used twice weekly, suppressed ovulation and were more effective in symptom relief than placebo in cross-over studies but there were fewer oestrogenic side effects with the lower dosage.[30] Overall satisfaction at 8 months was around 50 per cent. Oral progestogen was given cyclically from days 17–26 for endometrial protection but information on side effects or symptom recurrence with the progestogen was lacking. These limited data support the role of ovulation-suppressive doses of transdermal estradiol for the relief of PMS [B] although information on its long-term safety in relation to breast and endometrial cancer and cardiovascular risk is required. As such preparations have not been assessed for their contraceptive efficacy, additional contraception is required [E]. Use of transdermal estradiol patches in combination with the levonorgestrel-releasing intrauterine system (LNG-IUS) for both contraception and endometrial protection is an approach that merits future investigation [E].

Oral contraceptive formulations based on estradiol (estradiol valerate or estradiol hemihydrate) in combination with newer progestogens (nomegestrol acetate or dienogest) and given in extended-dose regimens have recently become available.[31] They were developed with the objective of reducing the metabolic and thrombogenic effects of EE although their clinical relevance has yet to be established. In theory they may be useful for management of PMS although currently there are no relevant published studies. They are considerably more expensive than older oral contraceptive formulations although costs are similar to that of transdermal estradiol.

Danazol

Several studies have supported the use of danazol for PMS. At a dose of 200 mg bd in a cross-over study,[32] 44 per cent of subjects on active therapy experienced a clinically significant improvement, compared with only 8 per cent of those treated with placebo. Although effective [B], the side effects and metabolic sequelae of danazol (see Chapter 77) limit its usefulness for the long-term management of PMS.

GnRH agonists

Ovarian suppression with GnRH agonists (see Chapter 77) should eliminate PMS if the symptoms are triggered by ovulation. A meta-analysis[33] of five studies comparing a GnRH agonist with placebo reported a reduction in both physical and behavioural symptoms with the active therapy [A]. However the use of hormonal add-back is necessary for bone protection if treatment is to be long term. The meta-analysis[33] included three studies in which add-back HRT combined with a GnRH agonist was compared with the GnRH agonist alone. In two of these, add-back was with continuous oestrogen and cyclical progestogen HRT; the third used tibolone. Results showed no significant difference in efficacy with add-back HRT, although one trial reported a reduced response and a greater drop-out rate in the cyclical add-back group. On this basis, GnRH agonists should be combined with continuous combined HRT or tibolone when used for treatment of severe PMS [A].

GnRH agonists are effective in the management of severe PMS but the cost (Table 79.2) and potentially long-term nature of treatment when used with hormonal add-back should limit its use to women with severe symptoms that are socially disruptive and resistant to other forms of therapy [E].[9] Patient selection is also important. All the women included in the trials cited above had prospectively confirmed PMS. Women with premenstrual exacerbation of ongoing symptoms do not experience symptom relief.[34] GnRH agonists therefore offer a useful means of further assessment of the pattern and nature of cyclical symptoms in situations in which the diagnosis is unclear or, in particular, when oophorectomy is being considered [E].

Oophorectomy

Although there have been reports of its efficacy in the literature,[35,36] oophorectomy is not recommended for the management of PMS unless the problem is very severe and has been confirmed by prospective assessment and there has been genuine failure of conservative therapies [E].[9] It should not be considered unless supported by a trial of ovarian suppression, preferably with a GnRH agonist [E].[33] The latter also gives an opportunity to assess the response of the patient to add-back HRT. Unless there are additional indications for hysterectomy, laparoscopic oophorectomy offers a less invasive surgical approach [E]. In women undergoing hysterectomy for other indications, a history of PMS is not a sufficient indication for concurrent oophorectomy without careful assessment [E][37] as cyclical symptoms may improve following hysterectomy [B].[38,39] Indeed, improvement of premenstrual symptoms has been reported following endometrial ablation[38] and insertion of the LNG-IUS,[39] and

these options offer a less invasive approach than hysterectomy with oophorectomy in women with heavy menstrual bleeding (HMB) who also complain of mild to moderate premenstrual symptoms.

MANAGEMENT OF WOMEN WITH PREMENSTRUAL MAGNIFICATION

There is a growing evidence base for the management of premenstrual disorders. However, eligibility for treatment trials requires prospective confirmation of the diagnosis by daily self-rating, so that the majority exclude the group of women whose management tends to be most problematic: those with premenstrual magnification of underlying psychological or psychiatric problems. The presence of high baseline postmenstrual symptom scores has been identified as one factor that leads to treatment failure with SSRIs [B][40] and GnRH agonists [B][34] and to poor response with the COCP [B].[22] Women with premenstrual magnification are therefore likely to be over-represented among those who present because of treatment failure. It is important that this group is identified and the nature of the problem and the limitations of management appreciated by both the clinician and the patient so that these women are not subjected to inappropriate and over-aggressive interventions such as hormonal manipulation or even surgery. Alternative management by the multidisciplinary team or psychiatric referral may be appropriate [E].

CONCLUSION

There is a wide range of therapies that have proven efficacy for severe PMS. However, response rates to any individual therapy are rarely in excess of 50 per cent with a high response to placebo. It is important that those involved in management are aware of these limitations and of different approaches to the problem. Ideally, women with severe symptoms and those with a history of treatment failure should be managed in specialist multidisciplinary clinics. The importance of making a correct diagnosis based on adequate prospective daily symptom assessment cannot be over-emphasised.

EBM

- There are many published RCTs covering various approaches to the management of PMS, but some of those relating to alternative therapies are open to methodological criticism.
- These recommendations are based on an RCOG Green-top Guideline and nine systematic reviews or meta-analyses of PMS therapy, five of which relate to alternative or dietary approaches.

KEY POINTS

- Diagnosis of PMS should be based on detailed history taking and confirmed by at least two cycles of prospective daily symptom rating [E].
- Management of severe PMS should take place in a multidisciplinary clinic or by a specialist with a special interest in the condition [E].
- All treatment trials to date have demonstrated a strong placebo effect and the response rate to active therapy is rarely in excess of 50 per cent [A].
- Expert opinion is divided about the benefit of complementary therapies such as nutritional and herbal approaches [E]. Vitamin B_6 in doses up to 100 mg daily may be of benefit for premenstrual depression [C].
- Limited evidence supports the role of group support [C], lifestyle modification and physical interventions such as acupuncture, relaxation and exercise [D].
- Support and self-help groups are likely to have a positive role in the management of PMS [C].
- CBT is beneficial for the treatment of severe PMS [A] but availability is limited.
- SSRIs are effective for relieving both the physical and psychological symptoms of PMS [A].
- SSRIs are equally effective when given in low doses during the luteal phase of the cycle [A], and this is associated with fewer side effects [B].
- Progesterone or progestogens given during the luteal phase of the menstrual cycle are not effective for PMS [A] although ovulation suppressive regimens may be beneficial [C].
- Suppression of ovulation with a third-generation COCP containing drospirenone given for 24 days out of 28 is beneficial in the management of severe PMS [A].
- Other low-dose COCPs with both second- and third-generation progestogens may also reduce premenstrual symptoms [B], particularly if given continuously or in extended dose regimens and are cheaper than newer alternatives.
- Suppression of ovulation with transdermal estradiol combined with progestogen for endometrial protection has been shown to be beneficial in older studies [B] but information on its safety for long-term use is lacking.
- Danazol is effective for PMS [B] but is not suitable for long-term use.
- GnRH analogues are effective for severe PMS [A] and may be used in combination with low-dose continuous hormonal add-back therapy [A] but are costly and should not be used as first-line therapy [E].
- Oophorectomy may be considered in severe PMS but only when medical measures have failed, and should be preceded by a trial of GnRH agonist therapy [E].
- Women with mild to moderate premenstrual symptoms in association with HMB may benefit from use of an LUG-IUS or endometrial ablation [B].
- Lack of symptom relief following menstruation and persistence of symptoms throughout the cycle (premenstrual magnification) is an important contributor to treatment failure [B].

References

1. O'Brien S, Rapkin A, Dennerstain L, Nevatte T. Diagnosis and management of premenstrual disorders. *BMJ* 2011;342:d2994.
2. Andersch C, Wendestram L, Hahn L, Ohman R. Premenstrual complaints. 1. Prevalence of premenstrual symptoms in a Swedish urban population. *J Psychosom Obstet Gynecol* 1986;5:39–49.
3. Sadler C, Smith H, Hammond J *et al.* and Southampton Women's Survey Study Group. Lifestyle factors, hormonal contraception and premenstrual symptoms: the United Kingdom Southamptom Women's Survey. *J Womens Health (Larchmt)* 2010;19:391–396.
4. Heinemann LA, Minh TD, Heinemann K, Lindemann M, Filonenko A. Inter-country assessment of the impact of severe premenstrual disorders on work and daily activities. *Health Care Woman Int* 2012;33:109–124.
5. Marjoribanks J, Brown J, O'Brien PMS, Wyatt KM. Selective serotonin reuptake inhibitors for premenstrual syndrome. *Cochrane Database of Systematic Reviews* 2013, Issue 6. Art. No.: CD001396. DOI.1002/14651858. CD001396.pub3.
6. Wang M, Hammarback S, Lindhe BA, Backstrom T. Treatment of premenstrual syndrome by spironolactone; a double-blind, placebo-controlled study. *Acta Obstet Gynaecol Scand* 1995;74:803–808.
7. West CP. The characteristics of 100 women presenting to a gynaecological clinic with premenstrual complaints. *Acta Obstet Gynaecol Scand* 1990;68:743–747.
8. Warner P, Bancroft J. Factors related to self reporting of the premenstrual syndrome. *Br J Psychiatry* 1990;157:249–260.
9. RCOG. *The management of premenstrual syndrome.* Green-Top Guideline No. 48. London: RCOG, 2007.
10. Stevinson C, Ernst E. Complementary/alternative therapies for premenstrual syndrome: a systematic review of randomized controlled trials. *Am J Obstet Gynecol* 2001;185:227–235.
11. Carter J, Verhoef MJ. Efficacy of self-help and alternative treatments of premenstrual syndrome. *Women's Health Issues* 1994;4:130–137.
12. Wyatt KM, Dimmock PW, Jones PW, Shaughan O'Brien PM. Efficacy of vitamin B6 in the treatment of premenstrual syndrome: systematic review. *BMJ* 1999;318:1375–1381.
13. Budeiri D, Li Wan Po A, Dornan JC. Is evening primrose oil of value in the treatment of premenstrual syndrome? *Control Clin Trials* 1996; 17:60–68.
14. Schellenberg R. Treatment for the premenstrual syndrome with agnus castus fruit extract: prospective, randomised, placebo controlled study. *BMJ* 2001; 322:134–137.
15. Jing Z, Yang X, Ismail KMK Chen XY, Wu T. Chinese herbal medicine for premenstrual syndrome. *Cochrane Database of Systematic Reviews* 2009, Issue 1. Art. No.: CD006414. DOI: 10.1002/14651858. CD006414.pub2.

16. Daley A. The role of exercise in the treatment of menstrual disorders: the evidence. *Br J Gen Pract* 2009;59:241–242.

17. Taylor D. Effectiveness of professional-peer group treatment: symptom management for women with PMS. *Res Nurs Health* 1999;22:496–511.

18. Busse JW, Montori VM, Krasnik C, Patelis-Siotis I, Guyatt GH. Psychological intervention for premenstrual syndrome: a meta-analysis of randomised controlled trials. *Psychother Psychosom* 2009;78:6–15.

19. Kleinstauber M, Witthoft M, Hiller W. Cognitive-behavioral and pharmacological interventions for premenstrual syndrome or premenstrual dysphoic disorder: a meta-analysis. *J Clin Psychol Med Settings* 2012;19:308–319.

20. Bjorn I, Bixo M, Nojd KS, Nyberg S, Backstrom T. Negative mood changes during hormone replacement therapy: a comparison between two progestogens. *Am J Obstet Gynecol* 2000;183:1419–1426.

21. Wyatt K, Dimmock P, Jones P, Obhrai M, O'Brien S. Efficacy of progesterone and progestogens in management of premenstrual syndrome: systematic review. *BMJ* 2001;323:776–780.

22. Backstrom T, Hansson-Malmstrom Y, Lindhe BA, Cavalli-Bjorkman B, Nordenstrom S. Oral contraceptives in premenstrual syndrome: a randomized comparison of triphasic and monophasic preparations. *Contraception* 1992;46:253–268.

23. Serfaty D, Vree ML. A comparison of the cycle control and tolerability of two ultra low-dose oral contraceptives containing 20 micrograms ethinyloestradiol and either 150 micrograms desogestrel or 75 micrograms gestodene. *Eur J Contracep Reprod Health Care* 1998;3:179–189.

24. Bancroft J, Rennie D. The impact of oral contraceptives on the experience of perimenstrual mood, clumsiness, food craving and other symptoms. *J Psychosom Res* 1993;37:195–202.

25. Lopez LM, Kaptein AA, Helmerhorst FM. Oral contraceptives containing drospirenone for premenstrual syndrome. *Cochrane Database of Systematic Reviews* 2012, Issue 2. Art. No: CD006586. DOI:10.1002/14651858. CD006586.pub4.

26. Wichianpitaya J, Taneepanichskui S. A comparative efficacy of low-dose combined oral contraceptives containing desogestrel and drospirenone in premenstrual symptoms. *Obstet Gynecol Int* 2013; 2013:487143.

27. Sullivan H, Furniss H, Spona J, Elstein M. Effect of 21-day and 24-day oral contraceptive regimens containing gestodene (60 microg) and ethinyloestradiol (15 microg) on ovarian activity. *Fertil Steril* 1999;72:115–120.

28. Freeman EW, Halbreich U, Grubb GS *et al.* An overview of four studies of a continuous oral contraceptive (levonorgestrel 90 mcg/ethinyloestradiol 20 mcg) on premenstrual dysphoric disorder and premenstrual syndrome. *Contraception* 2012;85:437–445.

29. Garnett T, Studd JW, Henderson A, Watson N, Savvas M, Leather A. Hormone implants and tachphylaxis. *Br J Obstet Gynaecol* 1990;97:917–921.

30. Smith RN, Studd JW, Zamblera D, Holland EF. A randomised comparison over 8 months of 100 micrograms and 200 micrograms twice weekly doses of transdermal oestradiol in the treatment of severe premenstrual syndrome. *Br J Obstet Gynaecol* 1995;102:475–484.

31. British National Formulary 66, September 2013–March 2014). www.bnf.org.

32. Hahn PM, Van Vugt DA, Reid RL. A randomized, placebo-controlled, crossover trial of danazol for the treatment of premenstrual syndrome. *Psychoneuroendocrinology* 1995;20:193–209.

33. Wyatt KM, Dimmock PW, Ismail KMK, Jones PW, O'Brien PMS. The effectiveness of GnRHa with and without 'add-back' therapy in treating premenstrual syndrome: a meta analysis. *BJOG* 2004;111:585–593.

34. Freeman EW, Sondheimer SJ, Rickels K. Gonadotropin-releasing hormone agonist in the treatment of premenstrual symptoms with and without ongoing dysphoria; a controlled study. *Psychopharmacol Bull* 1997;33: 303–309.

35. Casson P, Hahn PM, Van Vugt DA, Reid RL. Lasting response to ovariectomy in severe intractable premenstrual syndrome. *Am J Obstet Gynecol* 1990;162:99–105.

36. Casper RF, Hearn MT. The effect of hysterectomy and bilateral oophorectomy in women with severe premenstrual syndrome. *Am J Obstet Gynecol* 1990;162:105–109.

37. Argent V, Woodward Z. Consent and the ovary. *Obstet Gynecol* 2001;3(4):206–210.

38. Pinion SB, Parkin DE, Abramovich DR *et al.* Randomised trial of hysterectomy, endometrial laser ablation and transcervical endometrial resection for dysfunctional uterine bleeding. *BMJ* 1994;309:979–983.

39. Leminen H, Heliovaara-Peippo S, Halmesmaki K *et al.* The effect of hysterectomy or levonorgestrel-releasing intrauterine system on premenstrual symptoms in women treated for menorrhagia: secondary analysis of a randomised contolled trial. *Acta Obstet Gynaecol Scand* 2012;91:318–325.

40. Freeman EW, Sondheimer SJ, Polansky M, Garcia-Espagna B. Predictors of response to sertraline treatment of severe premenstrual syndromes. *J Clin Psychiatry* 2000;61:579–584.

REPRODUCTIVE GYNAECOLOGY

Chapter 80 Normal conception

Yakoub Khalaf

INTRODUCTION

The fusion of the male and female gametes is the core event in reproduction. The genetic material in the two haploid gametes combines to produce a diploid zygote. In mammals, the fusion of the gametes occurs within the female reproductive tract, and is followed by implantation and the development of the embryo into a fetus in the uterus. Gametes are produced in the gonads, which also have endocrine functions that are essential for successful reproduction. It is important to explore the embryology, anatomy and some physiological aspects of the ovary and testis in order to understand conception and infertility.

THE OVARY AND FEMALE GAMETE

The functions of the ovary are to engineer the periodic release of oocytes and to produce steroid and glycoprotein hormones.

Both functions are integrated in the continuous processes of growth and maturation of the primordial to Graafian follicle, containing the oocyte, followed by ovulation and formation of the corpus luteum. The corpus luteum regresses if pregnancy does not occur, but is maintained into the first trimester if a pregnancy occurs. The human ovary consists of three major components:

1. the outer cortex, the outer part of which is the tunica albuginea, and the internal part consisting of primordial follicles embedded in stromal tissue;
2. the inner medulla;
3. the rete ovarii (hilum), which is attached to the mesovarium and contains nerves, blood vessels and hilar cells, which have the potential to become active in steroidogenesis. The hilar cells are similar to the testosterone-producing Leydig cells of the testes.

The embryonic development of the ovary passes through four stages.

1. *The indifferent gonadal stage.* This stage lasts about 7–10 days and starts at approximately 5 weeks' gestation. It starts with the development of the gonadal ridges, which consist of consolidated coelomic projections overlying the mesonephros. At this stage, the ridges are indistinguishable as testes or ovaries. By the sixth week, the indifferent stage is completed, leaving the indifferent gonads consisting of germ cells and supporting cells derived from the coelomic epithelium and the mesenchyme of the gonadal ridge.
2. *The stage of differentiation.* This occurs at 6–9 weeks if the gonad is destined to be a testis.
3. *The stage of oogonial multiplication and maturation.* This starts at 6–8 weeks and represents the first sign of ovarian differentiation. A rapid mitotic division of the germ cells takes place, giving rise to the oogonia, and by 10–12 weeks the number of oogonia reaches 6–7 million. This is the maximal oogonial content of the gonads. From this point onwards, the germ cell content will irretrievably decrease and will be exhausted approximately 50 years later. The germ cells undergo mitosis to produce the oogonia that enter the first meiotic division and arrest in the prophase to become oocytes. This process begins at 11–12 weeks, perhaps in response to a factor or factors produced by the rete ovarii. Progression of meiotic prophase to the diplotene stage takes place throughout the rest of the

intrauterine life. The completion of the first meiotic division occurs just before ovulation, and the second meiotic division takes place at sperm penetration. As a result of the two meiotic divisions, a single haploid ovum is produced and the excess genetic material is extruded as a polar body at the completion of each meiotic division.

4   *The stage of follicular formation.* This starts at 14–20 weeks, when the entire follicle undergoes various stages of maturation leading to the production of the primary follicle before atresia takes place. However, ovulation does not occur in the fetal ovary.

At the onset of puberty, the germ cell mass, incorporated into primordial follicles, is usually reduced to approximately 300,000 follicles. These regularly undergo various stages of maturation, development and atresia. In all, less than 0.1 per cent of follicles will grow beyond the pre-antral stage and develop into a dominant follicle, which ovulates. This enormous attrition of primordial follicles forms part of the process of natural selection, by which only a tiny number of germ cells pass through the reproductive cycle and form a new individual.

As the dominant follicle grows, it produces oestrogens, predominantly oestradiol, and inhibins, predominantly inhibin B. These hormones synchronise the development of the endometrial lining of the uterus with that of the follicle, and prepare the pituitary for eventual triggering of the luteinising hormone (LH0 surge. Once oestradiol production from the dominant follicle passes a threshold, a positive feedback is triggered at the pituitary and the LH surge occurs, leading to ovulation. Ovulation results in the physical release of the oocyte, allowing it to enter the Fallopian tube, with potential for fertilisation. The follicle then develops into the corpus luteum, the source of progesterone and inhibin A in the second half (luteal phase) of the cycle. Production of the sex steroids by the corpus luteum results in preparation of the uterus and the entire woman's body for the occurrence of conception. For this regular periodic process to occur, accurate communication between the ovary and the pituitary gland is essential.

THE TESTIS AND MALE GAMETE

The physiological responsibilities of the testis are, in principle, similar to those of the ovary i.e. the production of gametes (spermatozoa) and sex steroids (testosterone). However, sex steroid production in the male is a continuous, non-episodic process, which is independent of the development of gametes. The early embryonic stages of testicular development also follow those of the ovary, starting from the indifferent gonad stage. However, at 6–7 weeks of embryonic life of the male fetus, the production of testis-determining factor (TDF) results in differentiation of the gonads to testes. TDF is the product of a gene located on the Y chromosome. However, the male phenotype is dependent on the production of anti-Müllerian hormone and testosterone. The absence of these two factors leads

to the development of the female phenotype. Differentiation of the testis leads to the production of the spermatic cords, which include the Sertoli cells and primordial germ cells that later become the spermatogonia. The mature Sertoli cells produce androgen-binding protein and inhibin B. The former is responsible for maintaining the high local androgen environment necessary for spermatogenesis. The Leydig cells develop from the mesenchymal cells surrounding the spermatic cords. They produce testosterone, the secretion of which increases with the increase in the number of Leydig cells. The Leydig cell number reaches a peak at 15–18 weeks, after which they regress, leaving a restricted pool of cells present at birth. These cells become responsive to gonadotrophins at puberty, leading to the production of testosterone and the initiation of spermatogenesis. The spermatogonia divide mitotically to produce primary spermatocytes, which then divide meiotically to produce the haploid secondary spermatocytes. Secondary spermatocytes undergo a maturation process to produce the spermatids, then the mature spermatozoa.

The Sertoli cells influence the process of spermatogenesis and are directed by genes on the Y chromosome. Approximately 74 days are required to produce a mature spermatozoon, of which about 50 days are spent in the seminiferous tubules. After leaving the testicle, the sperm takes 12–21 days to travel to the epididymis and appear in the ejaculate

FOLLICULAR DEVELOPMENT, MATURATION AND OVULATION

Follicular development

This involves several stages, starting with the mobilisation of the dormant primordial follicles to form a cohort of growing follicles, which progress through the pre-antral, antral, and pre-ovulatory stages to produce (usually) one dominant follicle that reaches ovulation. The mechanism determining which primordial follicles and how many will be released into the pool of growing follicles in each menstrual cycle is not known. However, this may be regulated by an intra-ovarian mechanism. The number of primordial follicles released from quiescence to enter the pool of grow- ing follicles each cycle seems to be proportional to the size of the residual pool. Therefore, the reduction of the primordial follicle pool by total or partial unilateral oophorectomy, or towards the end of reproductive life, may result in a smaller cohort of growing follicles. The onset and the time span of folliculogenesis have been controversial. Mais *et al.*[2] suggested that the follicle destined to ovulate is recruited in the first few days of the cycle, whereas Gougeon[3] suggested that such a process occurs over a time span of several cycles, estimated to be 85 days to achieve a pre-ovulatory status. The initiation of follicular growth in the early stages is independent of pituitary control; however, without a rise in follicle stimulating hormone (FSH), these follicles are destined for atresia.

Soon after the initial resumption of maturation, the follicle develops FSH receptors and becomes capable of responding to circulating FSH. This is known as the pre-antral stage, which starts to occur towards the end of the luteal phase of the preceding cycle. FSH, aided by other autocrine/paracrine factors, initiates steroidogenesis and granulosa cell proliferation, and is also responsible for up-regulation and down-regulation of its own receptors. Therefore, the fate of each pre-antral follicle in the developing pool depends on its ability to convert an androgen microenvironment to an oestrogen microenvironment. This requires the development of aromatase within the granulosa cells that line the follicle. Once one follicle acquires sufficient aromatase to produce and secrete significant quantities of oestradiol, the remainder of the cohort stop growing and gradually become atretic.

The granulosa cell layer is separated from the stromal cells by a basement membrane called the basal lamina (lamina basalis). The surrounding stromal cells differentiate into concentric layers designated as the theca interna (closest to the basal lamina) and the theca externa (the outer portion). As the follicle develops, the theca cells develop LH receptors, leading to LH-stimulated production of androgens, which form the substrate for the production of oestrogen in the granulosa cell layer.

Under the influence of FSH and as the follicles grow, intrafollicular fluid secretion increases, to form a cavitated antral follicle. The intrafollicular fluid contains oestrogens and a variety of peptide growth factors, which provide the oocytes and the surrounding granulosa cells with an endocrine-rich environment essential for maturation and eventually ovulation.

The selection of a dominant follicle

In primates and humans, usually one follicle proceeds to ovulation and the rest of the cohort is destined for atresia. Oestradiol and inhibin B are produced in increasing amounts by the rapidly growing lead follicle in the cohort. These hormones exert a negative feedback on the pituitary, leading to a decrease in the circulating level of FSH. This in turn withdraws gonadotrophic support from the less developed follicles, but is sufficient for the continued growth of the most advanced follicle, which contains the highest number of FSH receptors. In the antral stage, the dominant follicle maintains the production of oestradiol and inhibin B, which further reduces the FSH level and seals the fate of the other less developed follicles in the cohort. The accumulation of a greater mass of granulosa cells is accompanied by advanced development of the thecal vasculature, which facilitates preferential delivery of gonadotrophins to the follicles, allowing the dominant follicle to maintain FSH responsiveness and continue to develop and function despite the decreasing levels of FSH.

In the pre-ovulatory stage, the granulosa cells enlarge, the theca cells become vacuolated and richly vascular, the oocyte resumes meiosis, and the oestradiol level continues to rise, reaching a peak approximately 24–36 hours prior to ovulation.[4]

Ovulation

The continuous production of oestradiol by the growing follicle leads to the surge in LH through a positive-feedback mechanism. The LH surge usually lasts 48–50 hours. Ovulation (follicular rupture and oocyte release) occurs 24–36 hours after the LH surge. The LH surge leads to several events essential for oocyte maturation and preparation of the endometrium for implantation. The oocyte resumes its first meiotic division, leading to the production and extrusion of the first polar body, and enters the second meiotic division, which will be completed on fusion of the sperm with the oocyte later on. This stage is essential for the oocyte to be fertilised by the sperm. Stimulation of the granulosa cells by LH leads to the production of progesterone necessary for converting the endometrium from the proliferative to the secretory phase. Furthermore, progesterone enhances the activity of proteolytic enzymes and prostaglandins to digest the follicular wall, leading to the rupture of the follicle and the release of the oocyte.

Fertilisation

The oocyte released at the time of ovulation is surrounded by granulosa cells known as the cumulus oophorus, which is separated from the actual oocyte by a layer of glycoprotein known as the zona pellucida. Within 2–3 minutes of ovulation, the oocyte (surrounded by the cumulus) is within the ampullary part of the Fallopian tube. The fertilisable life span of the human ovum is estimated to be 24–36 hours. Although several million sperm are deposited in the vagina, only about 200 will come in contact with the oocyte. For the sperm to bind with the zona pellucida, a receptor is required, which is species specific. The sperm has to undergo a process known as 'capacitation' in order to be able to bind with the receptor and penetrate the egg. The zona pellucida not only contains the receptors for the sperm, but also has a mechanism by which it prevents more than one sperm from entering the oocyte (polyspermy). This mechanism is known as the zona reaction.

IMPLANTATION

This is defined as the process by which the embryo attaches itself to the endometrial side of the uterine wall and gradually penetrates the epithelium to reach the circulatory system of the mother. This process requires preparation of both the endometrium and the embryo for a successful implantation to take place.

Embryo preparation

After ovulation, oestradiol and progesterone from the corpus luteum alter the molecular structure of the endometrium from proliferative to secretory. The individual components of the endometrium continue to grow, leading to tortuosity of the glands and coiling of the spiral arterioles. Intracytoplasmic glycogen vacuoles appear and transudation of plasma occurs, contributing to endometrial secretion. The peak secretory phase is reached by 7 days post-ovulation. At this point, the endometrial cells are rich in glycogen and lipids. The receptivity of the endometrium is limited to days 16–19 (of a 28-day cycle) and it is essential that the hatched blastocyst impacts and adheres to the surface of the endometrium during this 'implantation window' if pregnancy is to occur.

KEY POINTS

- At the onset of puberty, the size of the primordial follicles pool is approximately 300,000 follicles.
- Once oestradiol production from the dominant follicle passes a threshold, a positive feedback is triggered at the pituitary and the LH surge occurs, leading to ovulation.
- The oestradiol level continues to rise, reaching a peak leading to the LH surge, which is followed 24-36 hours later by ovulation.
- The fertilisation life span of the released ovum is 24-36 hours.
- The zona pellucida precludes more than one sperm entering the oocyte through a mechanism known as the zona reaction.
- The embryo usually reaches the blastocyst stage by day 5 post-fertilisation with a prominent inner cell mass and trophectoderm.

ACKNOWLEDGEMENT

This chapter has been revised and updated. The author and editors acknowledge the contribution of Hany AMA Lashen to the chapter on this topic in the previous edition of the book.

Key References

1. Gondos B, Westergaard L, Byskov A. Inhibition of oogenesis in the human fetal ovary: ultrasound structural and squash preparation study. *Am J Obstet Gynecol* 1986;155:189–95.
2. Mais V, Kazer RR, Cetel NS *et al.* The dependence of folliculogenesis and corpus luteum function on pulsatile gonadotrophin secretion in cycling women using a gonadotrophin-releasing hormone antagonist as a probe. *J Clin Endocrinol Metab* 1986;62:1250–55.
3. Gougeon A. Dynamics of follicular growth in the human: a model from preliminary results. *Hum Reprod* 1986;1:81–7.
4. Pauerstein CJ, Eddy CA, Croxatto HD *et al.* Temporal relationships of oestrogen, progesterone, and luteinizing hormone levels to ovulation in women and infrahuman primates. *Am J Obstet Gynecol* 1978;130:876–86.

Chapter 81 Female infertility

Yakoub Khalaf

INTRODUCTION

Infertility is defined as the inability to conceive despite regular unprotected sexual intercourse over a specific period of time, usually 1–2 years. The cumulative spontaneous pregnancy rate for a couple is approximately 57 per cent after three months, 72 per cent after six months, 85 per cent after one year and 93 per cent after two years [D].[1] Accordingly, only 50 per cent of couples failing to conceive during the first year will conceive in the second year, which justifies starting investigations for infertility after one year. However, if the physician or the patient has a reason to suspect impaired fertility, the process should be started sooner. Furthermore, if the female partner is 35 years of age or older, the investigations should not be delayed, given the rapid decline of female fecundity after this age. Over the past three decades the introduction of IVF and the wide public interest in this aspect of infertility treatment, together with the increasing ease of obtaining information, have increased patients' expectations of infertility treatment.

EPIDEMIOLOGY

It has been estimated that infertility affects 9 per cent of couples, of whom 70 per cent suffer from primary infertility i.e. no previous conception, and 30 per cent secondary infertility i.e. have achieved a previous pregnancy (regardless of the outcome of that pregnancy). Worldwide, more than 70 million couples suffer from infertility, the majority being residents of the developing countries. The recent advances in infertility treatment and the access of patients to such information have led to early presentation of these patients and their request for treatment. This may give a false impression of an increasing infertility problem.

CAUSES OF INFERTILITY

For pregnancy to occur, there must be fertile sperm and egg, a means of bringing them together and a receptive endometrium to allow the resulting embryo to implant. A defect at any of these stages can lead to subfertility. It has been estimated that in 35 per cent of cases a male factor is the reason for infertility [C]. In the remaining 65 per cent of cases, a female factor is identified in 50 per cent of couples and no cause will be identified in the remainder [C]. The most common causes of infertility in the female are ovulatory and tubal factors. Endometriosis in its moderate to severe forms has also been linked to infertility, despite a lack of clear understanding of the connection between the two phenomena [C]. Although failure of implantation will cause infertility, it is difficult to determine whether the embryo or the endometrium is at fault in such cases. The effect of age on female fertility is not a new concept, with a gradual decline in female fertility and an increase in the miscarriage rate being observed many years before the menopause [D]. As discussed earlier, women enter the reproductive age at puberty with a pool of primordial follicles of a pre-determined number. The size of this pool and the rate of follicular depletion are the deciding factors in the timing of the menopause. Female fertility declines after the age of 35 and declines more rapidly after the age of 40 [C]. The rate of follicular loss is inversely proportional to the size of the primordial pool i.e. the smaller the pool, the faster the rate. Delaying starting a family to the later years of reproductive life also increases the risk of developing endometriosis and the risk of miscarriage.

Anovulatory infertility

Anovulation is a frequent cause of infertility. Negative-feedback and positive-feedback mechanisms allow the ovaries to interact successfully with the hypothalamo–pituitary axis. The causes of anovulation can be classified according to the clinical findings when the level of disruption between the hypothalamic–pituitary axis and the ovary is assessed. This divides the causes of anovulatory infertility into three main categories – ovulatory dysfunction, hypogonadotrophic hypogonadism and hypergonadotrophic hypogonadism, with other less common causes considered separately.

Ovarian dysfunction

The most common presentation of anovulation is associated with normal gonadotrophin concentrations. Such normogonadotrophic anovulation is usually seen in polycystic ovary syndrome. PCOS is the most common endocrine disorder in women of reproductive age. In its classic form – a combination of oligomenorrhoea/anovulation and hyperandrogenism – it is estimated to affect >5 per cent of the female population. PCOS is also associated with a metabolic disturbance, central to which is peripheral insulin resistance and compensatory hyperinsulinaemia. Significant abnormalities in the very earliest stages of folliculogenesis may be the root cause of anovulation in PCOS.

Hypogonadotrophic hypogonadism

Failure of the pituitary gland to produce gonadotrophins will lead to lack of ovarian stimulation. There are a number of disorders of the anterior pituitary gland that lead to failure of production of FSH. These include destruction of the anterior pituitary by a tumour (e.g. a benign non-functioning adenoma or craniopharyngioma), by a pituitary inflammatory reaction as in tuberculosis, or following ischaemia as in Sheehan's syndrome. Rare congenital causes include Laurence–Moon–Biedl, Kallmann's and Prader–Willi syndromes. The pituitary can also be damaged by cranial irradiation or surgically at the time of hypophysectomy for a pituitary tumour.

Hypogonadotrophic hypogonadism will also occur if pulsatile secretion of GnRH is slowed or stopped. This is seen in hypothalamic dysfunction, commonly secondary to excessive exercise, psychological stress or anorexia nervosa.

Hypergonadotrophic hypogonadism

This occurs as a result of failure of the ovary to respond to gonadotrophic stimulation by the pituitary gland. The absence of negative feedback (by oestradiol and inhibin B) from a developing follicle results in excessive secretion of the gonadotrophic hormones FSH and LH. Concentrations of these hormones reach menopausal levels. Hypergonadotrophic hypogonadism classically results from premature ovarian failure with exhaustion of the ovarian follicle pool. A variant of the condition, resistant ovary syndrome, describes the occurrence of elevated levels of serum gonadotrophins in the presence of a good reserve of follicles. Abnormalities in the FSH receptor may produce this picture. Neither premature ovarian failure nor resistant ovary syndrome is treatable by FSH injection.

Other discrete causes

Endocrine disorders, most commonly hyperprolactinaemia and hypothyroidism, are possible causes of anovulation and should be excluded by appropriate biochemical testing.

Tubal infertility

Tubal damage underlies infertility in approximately 14 per cent of couples and 40 per cent of infertile women [C]. Any damage to the Fallopian tube can prevent the sperm from reaching the oocyte or the embryo from reaching the uterine cavity, leading to infertility and tubal ectopic pregnancy, respectively. The Fallopian tube is more than just a 'tube': a number of key events occur within the tube, including capacitation of the sperm, fertilisation and the early development of the zygote and embryo. Therefore, the Fallopian tube may maintain its patency but lose the ability to promote these other functions. Currently accepted investigations can only test tubal patency, and not its function.

The main causes of tubal damage are either pelvic inflammatory disease (PID) or iatrogenic causes. PID remains the major cause of tubal damage in the western world, with *Chlamydia trachomatis* infection the prime pathogen in most cases. Pelvic infection or abscess caused by appendicitis, other bowel disorders or septic abortion is responsible for a lesser proportion of cases. Fallopian tubes can be damaged iatrogenically either directly, as in tubal ligation for sterilisation, or indirectly as a consequence of pelvic surgery. Other rare causes of tubal damage include tuberculosis, schistosomiasis, viral infection and abdominal inflammatory disorders, such as Crohn's disease.

Endometriosis

It is apparent that severe endometriosis can lead to mechanical tubal damage due to adhesion formation caused by the pelvic endometrial deposits. However, it is less certain whether the lesser degrees of endometriosis can lead to infertility.

Both mild endometriosis and infertility are common, and may occur together as epiphenomena [C]. Endometriosis is discussed further in Chapter 77.

Uterine factors

Submucous leiomyomata, congenital uterine abnormalities, endometrial polyps and intrauterine adhesions are all potential causes of infertility. The presence of a fibroid that occludes or distorts the Fallopian tubes will lead to tubal infertility [D]. Fertility outcomes are decreased in women with submucosal fibroids, and removal seems to confer benefit. Subserosal fibroids do not affect fertility outcomes, and removal does not confer benefit. Intramural fibroids appear to decrease fertility, but the results of therapy are unclear. Distortion of the uterine cavity, by a fibroid, a septum or in the T-shaped uterus following exposure of the female fetus to diethystilbestrol *in utero*, can lead to implantation failure and recurrent early miscarriage [D]. Such cases should be assessed individually and the likelihood of their contribution to infertility should be examined. Excessive uterine curettage after a miscarriage or abortion, especially in the presence of uterine infection, can lead to the destruction of the strata basalis endometrium. Intrauterine scarring and synechiae develop as a result, which is known as Asherman's syndrome. This condition can also result after CS, uteroplasty or myomectomy.

It has been difficult to demonstrate a relationship between endometritis and subfertility, except when the cause of endometritis is tuberculosis. In the UK, tuberculous endometritis is a rare, but increasing, cause of infertility. The effect of chlamydial endometritis on implantation remains controversial, although there is evidence that patients with tubal disease undergoing IVF have significantly lower pregnancy and implantation rates.

Unexplained infertility

Completion of standard investigation of infertility fails to reveal a cause in 15–30 per cent of cases [C]. This does not indicate absence of a cause, but rather the inability to identify it. The results of IVF have shown that there may be undiagnosed problems of oocyte or embryo quality or of implantation failure, neither of which can easily be tested unless IVF is undertaken. Unexplained infertility causes great distress to couples, who often find it harder to bear when a cause cannot be found.

INVESTIGATION OF THE FEMALE PARTNER

Investigation of infertility will usually be initiated in general practice, frequently followed by referral to a secondary or tertiary centre, where most treatments will take place. RCOG and NICE have recently published guidelines for the management of infertility. These define the role of the medical practitioner at each level, and outline the evidence base for investigation and treatment.

History taking and examination

It is important to recognise that infertility is a problem that faces couples, and that both partners should be seen and investigated together whenever possible [E]. Consultations involving infertility require tact and sensitivity on behalf of the clinician, a quiet, private environment and sufficient clinical time to allow exploration of the couple's anxieties and explanation of available treatments, as well as classical history taking. A rapport must be established before more personal and sensitive details can be sought.

Personal and social history

The couple's ages, in particular that of the female partner, are important, as discussed earlier. The occupations of the couple, especially the male, can have an impact on their fertility. Exposure to high temperature, chemicals and ionising radiation can seriously affect sperm production [D]. If either of the partners works away from home, this may affect the frequency of sexual intercourse around the time of ovulation. Smoking, alcohol and recreational drug use can also influence fertility. Appropriate advice should be given.

Menstrual history

The age of menarche and regularity of periods are important factors. Information about the frequency and length of the menstrual cycle and any associated problems such as dysmenorrhoea or heavy menstrual loss should be sought. Irregular menstrual cycles, oligomenorrhoea and amenorrhoea are all suggestive of anovulation. If amenorrhoea is reported, enquiries should be made about any menopausal symptoms, weight loss or gain, and symptoms of hyperprolactinaemia and hypothyroidism. These patients should be investigated in specialised centres [E].

Obstetric history

The clinician should enquire about any previous pregnancies, both in the current and any previous relationships, as well as the outcome of these pregnancies. It may be wise to ask about breastfeeding and any sustained galactorrhoea at this stage. It is also important to establish if there were any difficulties encountered or treatment required prior to achieving a previous pregnancy.

Contraception

The use of the oral contraceptive pill and the long-acting progestogens can be followed by a period of amenorrhoea. In particular, use of long-acting progestogen-based contraceptives may be followed by delay in the resumption of ovulation [D]. The use of intrauterine contraceptive devices may increase the risk of pelvic infection, especially in young nulliparous women, leading to tubal disease [D].

Past medical history

It is important to establish any previous medical disorders that may affect either fertility or pregnancy. Pre-conceptional counselling may be necessary if a serious medical condition is identified. The possible impact of prescription medications on ovulation should be investigated: for example, some anti-depressants can increase prolactin secretion and NSAIDs can interfere with ovulation.

Sexual history

The clinician should enquire about the couple's frequency of sexual intercourse and associated problems, such as dyspareunia or ejaculatory dysfunction. Regular intercourse (two to three times a week) is sufficient for most couples to achieve a pregnancy. It is frequently the case that infertile couples restrict their sexual activity to the period around mid-cycle and some use commercially available ovulation detection kits to time inter-course. There is no evidence that such practices can increase fecundability, and the increase in psychological stress that results from such practices is unhelpful [C]. Sensitive enquiry concerning sexually transmitted infections should be made.

Other important points

The discussion should include advice concerning the use of folic acid and enquiry about rubella vaccination [A]. A cervical smear history should be taken and a smear offered if indicated [E]. A family history, including enquiry concerning diabetes, endometriosis and PCOS, should be taken, as this information can be useful in the diagnosis and treatment of infertility [D]. A history of familial disorder should lead to an offer of genetic counselling before starting investigation and treatment [E].

Examination of the female partner

Unless there is an indication from the patient's history that examination would be of any value in establishing the cause of infertility, there would seem to be little to be gained from rou-tine examination. Indications from the history, for example of cyclical pelvic pain or dyspareunia, should prompt pelvic examination. Other features of the physical examination, for example detection of an asymptomatic pelvic mass, have been supplanted by transvaginal ultrasound examination.

Assessment of BMI is important, as both obesity and underweight can cause anovulation [C]. If the patient is found to be obese, central obesity can be assessed by measuring the waist:hip ratio [C].

Table 81.1 Interpretation of female infertility investigations

Test	Result	Interpretation
Progesterone (mid-luteal)	<30 nmol/L	Anovulation
		Check cycle length and timing in mid-luteal phase
		Complete other endocrine tests
		Scan for PCO
		Advise re. weight gain/loss
		May need ovulation induction
		Clomiphene should not be started without test of tubal patency
FSH (early follicular)	>10 IU/L	Reduced ovarian reserve
		May respond poorly to ovulation induction
		May need egg donation
LH (early follicular)	>10 IU/L	May be PCO
		Ultrasound to confirm
Testosterone	>2.5 nmol/L	May be PCO
		Ultrasound to confirm
Prolactin	>1000 IU/L	May be pituitary adenoma
		Repeat prolactin to confirm raised level
		Exclude hypothyroidism
		Arrange MRI/CT scan
		If confirmed hyperprolactinaemia, start dopamine agonist

Test	Result	Interpretation
HSG/HyCoSy	Abnormal	May be tubal factor
		Arrange laparoscopy and dye to evaluate further
		May be intrauterine abnormality
		Evaluate further by hysteroscopy
Laparoscopy and dye	Blocked tubes	Tubal factor
		? Suitable for transcervical cannulation, surgery or IVF (also depends on semen quality)
	Endometriosis	Endometriosis
		Assess severity, may benefit from diathermy laser
		Medical suppression not helpful for fertility
		May need IVF
Rubella	Non-immune	Offer immunisation and 1 month contraception

Laboratory investigations, endoscopy and imaging

The aim of these investigations is to assess ovulation, tubal patency and uterine factors (Table 81.1).

Ovulation

A history of regular periods usually indicates ovulation. However, a reliable marker is useful to confirm that ovulation has occurred. After the release of the oocyte and the formation of the corpus luteum, progesterone levels rise sharply, reaching a peak level approximately 8 days after the LH surge. The detection of high levels of progesterone in serum or evidence of progesterone effect can be used as a secondary marker of ovulation. Historically, the effects of progesterone on basal body temperature, endometrial histology or cervical mucus were commonly used. Measuring serum progesterone at its peak in the mid-luteal phase is a reliable, safe and inexpensive test. Levels in excess of 30 nmol/L are diagnostic of ovulation [C]; however, lower (suboptimal) levels may be due to incorrect timing of blood sampling or may be caused by a luteinised unruptured follicle. It is important to remember that the mid-luteal phase is approximately 7 days before the next expected period i.e. day 21 and day 28 in 28-day and 35-day cycles, respectively.

Commercially available urinary LH detection kits can detect the LH surge and can be used to time intercourse with ovulation induction or donor insemination treatments.

Ovarian reserve tests

Another test added to the investigation of couples with infertility includes assessment of ovarian reserve. Women with advanced age or history of prior ovarian surgery are at risk for diminished ovarian function or reserve. Given the relatively non-invasive nature of the testing, several practitioners are including the evaluation of ovarian reserve as first-line work up for infertility. The testing includes a cycle day 3 serum FSH and estradiol level, AMH or an ultrasonographic ovarian antral follicle count. However, NICE guidelines recommend that women who have high levels of gonadotrophins should be informed that they are likely to have reduced fertility. The results of these tests are not absolute indicators of infertility but abnormal levels correlate with decreased response to ovulation induction medications and lowered livebirth rates after IVF.

Tubal patency tests

Although the Fallopian tube has functions other than as a conduit for the sperm, oocyte and embryo, it is not yet feasible to assess these functions in routine practice. Tubal patency can be assessed by three different methods: ultrasound scanning with hydrotubation; hysterosalpingography; and laparoscopy and dye hydrotubation [D].

Ultrasound scan and hydrotubation

HyCoSy (**hy**sterosalpingo **co**ntrast **so**nography) has recently been introduced as a method for studying tubal patency using ultrasonography. Ultrasonographic contrast medium is slowly injected into the uterine cavity under direct visualisation, with imaging of the cavity and of flow along the Fallopian tubes. This method does not require X-ray and allows the ultrasound assessment of the pelvic organs i.e. the uterus including the uterine cavity, tubes and ovaries. This screening method should be reserved for cases where history is not suggestive of tubal pathology. Finding a normal cavity and bilateral fill and spill of contrast is reassuring, but where there is doubt, hysterosalpingography or a laparoscopy and dye hydrotubation test should be performed.

Hysterosalpingography

Hysterosalpingography (HSG) is a simple, safe and inexpensive X-ray-based contrast study of the uterine cavity and the Fallopian tubes with a 65 per cent sensitivity and 83 per cent specificity for detecting tubal blockage. The principle of this test is to inject a radio-opaque contrast medium through the cervix into the uterus and take abdominal X-rays at intervals during and after the injection. The images should reveal the uterine outline and passage of contrast along the tubes, with free spill into the peritoneal cavity. HSG is usually carried out in the first 10 days of the menstrual cycle, to avoid disruption of an early pregnancy in the secretory phase of the cycle. It will cause period-like pain in most patients and may occasionally lead to a vasovagal attack. The main complication of HSG is flare-up of PID. The overall risk of infection from this test in the normal population is approximately 1 per cent, rising to 3 per cent in high-risk patients. Therefore, it is wise to carry out laparoscopy and dye test in high-risk patients and to use prophylactic antibiotics to cover the test. RCOG recommends routine screening for chlamydia in any patient before carrying out any intrauterine instrumentation [E]. HSG is recommended by RCOG as the primary screening procedure in low-risk patients [E].

Laparoscopy and dye test

A laparoscopy and dye hydrotubation ('lap and dye') test is the most reliable, albeit expensive, tool used to diagnose tubal subfertility. The principle of this procedure is to visualise the passage of methylene blue dye through the Fallopian tubes. The procedure enables inspection of the fimbrial ends of the tubes and the pelvic structures for the presence of endometriosis or adhesions. Combining this procedure with electrocoagulation of any endometriotic spots or adhesiolysis adds therapeutic value. Hence, it is advisable that such procedures are carried out in centres where the necessary expertise is available [E].

Laparoscopy and dye test requires general anaesthetic and carries the risk of bowel or visceral injury. It is therefore not recommended as a first-line screening test [E]. However, it should be considered in patients with a history suggestive of endometriosis, previous PID or previous pelvic surgery. Furthermore, if the HSG reports abnormal results, verification should be carried out with diagnostic laparoscopy [E].

When comparing HSG with laparoscopy, keep in mind that both procedures provide extra information in addition to the assessment of the Fallopian tubes. HSG provides information about the status of the uterine cavity, whereas laparoscopy allows inspection of the intra-abdominal cavity, excludes peritoneal disease and allows laparoscopic treatment of pelvic pathology.

Visualisation and assessment of the uterine cavity are not possible unless hysteroscopy is performed concurrently. However, the value of routine hysteroscopy is questionable [E], as the frequency of asymptomatic intrauterine lesions that are not seen on transvaginal ultrasound is low. Hysteroscopy should probably therefore be reserved for cases where there is an indication from the history or previous investigations.

Assessment of the uterus

Uterine anatomy can be visualised by saline hysterosonography, HSG or hysteroscopy. Conventional TVS may not always provide a good-quality image of the cavity, but 3D ultrasound, when available, can provide an accurate assessment of the uterine cavity. This may outline intrauterine polyps or synechiae. Routine hysteroscopy for infertile patients has been discouraged by RCOG [E].

Postcoital test

The postcoital test provides information concerning the ability of the sperm to penetrate and survive in cervical mucus. However, reproducibility of the test is low and the false-positive rate is high. A diagnosis of an adverse cervical factor does not alter therapeutic decisions, as both 'cervical factor' and unexplained infertility are treated with intrauterine insemination or IVF. According to NICE guidelines on the management of infertility, the routine use of postcoital testing in the investigation of fertility problems is not recommended because it has no predictive value on pregnancy rate.

Management of female infertility

Any discussion about the management of infertility should begin with an explanation of the physiology of the cycle, with information about the 'fertile period'. Among healthy women trying to conceive, nearly all pregnancies can be attributed to intercourse during a 6-day period ending on the day of ovulation.

Lifestyle issues, including advice on smoking, alcohol consumption and 'fitness for pregnancy', should be raised. Further planning of treatment protocols will depend on the presumed cause of the problem.

Management of tubal infertility

Tubal infertility can be treated with tubal surgery, IVF and embryo transfer (IVF-ET) or selective salpingography. Although tubal surgery is no longer recommended for severe tubal disease since the introduction of IVF-ET, it still has a place in less severe forms of the disorder.

Tubal surgery

Successful tubal surgery requires surgical skill and experience. The decline in the number of suitable cases has reduced training opportunities, and some advocate restriction of this practice to tertiary centres to allow concentration of expertise [E]. This permits audit of outcome and estimation of realistic, single-centre pregnancy rates. Comparison between tubal surgery and IVF is difficult. The cost, success rate, complications and benefits must be assessed in every case individually. Decision making may be altered in favour of IVF by the presence of other causes of infertility, particularly male factor and anovulation. The success rate after tubal surgery depends on the underlying disease, site of damage (proximal or distal) and patient's age. NICE guidelines have suggested that for women with mild tubal disease, tubal surgery may be more effective than no treatment. In centres where appropriate expertise is available, it may be considered as a treatment option.

The cost of a single cycle of IVF has been calculated to be comparable to that of tubal surgery and, apart from patients with mild tubal disease, the cost-effectiveness argument is in favour of IVF-ET. However, tubal surgery, if successful, offers less risk of multiple pregnancy and ovarian hyperstimulation syndrome (OHSS), and avoids the ethical issues that fertilisation *in vitro* can engender. Patients should be informed that the risk of ectopic pregnancy after tubal surgery is significantly higher than after IVF-ET [C].

Once tubal surgery is being contemplated, careful assessment of the tubes and pelvis with HSG and laparoscopy should be carried out [E]. The route of access should then be decided i.e. laparotomy or laparoscopy. Laparoscopic surgery is less costly and offers less morbidity, more technical advantages and a marginally better pregnancy rate. If pregnancy does not occur within 6–12 months of tubal surgery, reassessment of the tubes with HSG should be carried out. If the tubes remain blocked, IVF-ET is indicated. If the tubes remain patent, ovulation should be assessed and perhaps a short period of ovulation induction could be tried. This decision will depend on the patient's age and whether IVF-ET is affordable to the couple. The key issues here are to present the couple with all the available facts and to involve them in the decision-making process.

IVF-ET

Absent or irreparably damaged Fallopian tubes were the main reason for the development of IVF-ET. A lower pregnancy rate after IVF-ET in tubal-infertility couples compared to other causes of infertility has been reported. The reason is not entirely clear, but it is possible that fluid from a hydrosalpinx could be hostile to embryo development and implantation. Salpingectomy of an ultrasonographically visible hydrosalpinx should therefore be considered to improve the success rate of IVF treatment [C], although careful counselling is needed before performing salpingectomy for an infertile patient, even if the tubal damage is severe [E].

Selective salpngography and tubal cannulation

These procedures can be carried out under image intensification or at hysteroscopy. These methods were originally developed for diagnostic purposes, but were subsequently proven to be useful in treating proximal tubal damage, for which surgery yielded disappointing success rates. The outcome of these procedures in terms of regaining tubal patency is immediately known. According to NICE guidelines, for women with proximal tubal obstruction, selective salpingography plus tubal catheterisation, or hysteroscopic tubal cannulation, may be treatment options because these treatments improve the chance of pregnancy.

Management of anovulatory infertility

A number of therapeutic interventions for the induction of ovulation are available. Selecting the most appropriate method depends on the cause of anovulation. Patients with ovarian failure and resistant ovary syndrome will not respond to ovulation induction and should be offered oocyte donation [C]. Normalisation of bodyweight in underweight and obese patients can help to regain ovulation without the need for medical intervention [B]. Medical treatment of prolactinoma can also help regain normal ovulation [A]. Ovulation induction in patients with hypogonadotrophic hypogonadism can be achieved with the pulsatile administration of GnRH or by daily injection of gonadotrophin [C]. Ovulation induction in PCOS patients (80 per cent of anovular women) can be achieved by weight normalisation in obese patients [C] (40–60 per cent of PCOS patients), medical or surgical methods. The medical methods include the use of clomiphene citrate or gonadotrophins – discussed further in Chapter 84, Assisted reproduction. NICE has recommended that women with WHO group II ovulation disorders (hypothalamic pituitary gonadal dysfunction), such as PCOS, should be offered treatment with clomifene citrate (or tamoxifen) as the first line of treatment for up to 12 months because it is likely to induce ovulation [A]. Additionally, women undergoing treatment with clomifene citrate should be offered ultrasound monitoring during at least the first cycle of treatment to ensure that they receive a dose that minimises the risk of multiple pregnancy.

The surgical methods are either ovarian drilling or wedge resection. Stein and Leventhal suggested ovarian wedge resection in 1935. Their theory was that the thick tunica albugenia prevented the release of the ovum, hence the anovulation in PCOS patients. Although pregnancies resulted, the operation (performed by laparotomy) led to complications, including tubal damage and adhesion formation, and fell into disrepute. Ovarian drilling involves focal local destruction of the ovarian stroma with laser or diathermy, applied laparoscopically. The route of access reduces morbidity and postoperative complications. Ovarian drilling achieves equivalent ovulation and pregnancy rates to medical ovulation induction. Predictors of success have included LH level >10 IU/L, normal BMI and shorter duration of infertility. However, evidence suggests that ovarian drilling has less risk of multiple pregnancies and no risk of OHSS. Economic analyses of two RCTs suggest that treating women with CC-resistant PCOS by laparoscopic ovarian drilling (LOD) resulted in reduced direct and indirect costs. On the other hand, the long-term advantages and risks of ovarian drilling require further assessment. Destroying ovarian tissue inevitably leads to destruction of primordial follicles and reduction of the ovarian reserve. These anxieties have partially been resolved by studies that demonstrate that a good therapeutic response can be achieved by minimal application of energy and after reduction of the number of diathermy burns to four per ovary.

Management of endometriosis-related infertility

This depends on the severity of the condition and the presence of any other infertility factors. The two main lines of treating endometriosis are medical and surgical. Medical treatment of minimal and mild endometriosis does not enhance fertility in infertile women and should not be offered [A].

Women with minimal or mild endometriosis who undergo laparoscopy should be offered surgical ablation or resection of endometriosis plus laparoscopic adhesiolysis because this improves the chance of pregnancy [A].

As many infertile patients will undergo diagnostic laparoscopy, diathermy to endometriosis can be delivered at the same session, alleviating the need for a further anaesthetic. Women with moderate or severe endometriosis should be offered surgical treatment because it improves the chance of pregnancy [B]. Assisted reproduction has lent itself to treating endometriosis-related infertility. Whether medical or conservative surgical treatment of endometriosis before carrying out IVF-ET can improve the ovarian response and pregnancy rates remains unclear.

Management of unexplained infertility

The lack of an identifiable reason for infertility in this category makes the treatment empirical. Conservative management, ovulation induction with or without intrauterine insemination, and IVF-ET are the main approaches to managing unexplained infertility. Approximately 60 per cent of couples with unexplained secondary infertility (diagnosed after one year) achieve a pregnancy within three years of conservative management [C]. Results are less good in primary infertility. However, the woman's age should be taken into consideration when advising this line of management. Ovulation induction (or, more properly, 'augmentation') with clomiphene citrate along with timed sexual intercourse has been used frequently in patients with unexplained infertility. However, recent meta-analysis of studies in this area has not demonstrated benefit over the conservative approach [A], and treatment with clomiphene citrate carries a risk of multiple pregnancy.

A cumulative pregnancy rate of 40 per cent has been reported after controlled ovarian stimulation (COS) with gonadotrophins and intrauterine insemination [C]. The pregnancy rates after IUI alone in couples with unexplained infertility have been disappointing and its use does not appear to confer any additional benefit over expectant management. However, the advantage of IUI over timed sexual intercourse after COS has been controversial, and firm evidence is lacking. For logistic reasons, IUI may provide a better timing compared to sexual intercourse. Many centres advise two or three cycles of COS–IUI before moving to IVF-ET in this group. COS-IUI may be less stressful, less physically demanding and less costly per attempt than IVF.

IVF-ET in unexplained infertility has diagnostic as well as therapeutic value, as it provides information about fertilisation and egg and embryo quality. Owing to its high cost, IVF-ET is usually seen as a last resort in unexplained infertility. The cost of three cycles of COS-IUI is comparable to that of one IVF-ET cycle, with the latter offering a better pregnancy rate [D].

Gamete intrafallopian transfer (GIFT) used to be the treatment of choice for patients with unexplained infertility. However, IVF-ET, with its diagnostic potential, has superseded this modality. Although GIFT offered a high pregnancy rate, the ectopic pregnancy risk was also high [C], and the treatment requires general anaesthesia and laparoscopy in order for gametes to be placed within the ampulla of the Fallopian tube. This method has largely been supplanted by IVF-ET.

Management of uterine factor infertility

Congenital defects, leiomyomas and intrauterine adhesions and polyps are the only treatable uterine factors. However, before offering surgical treatment, the impact of such findings on the couple's fertility should be carefully assessed [E]. Myomectomy can be carried out either laparoscopically or by laparotomy with similar postoperative pregnancy rates [A]. Entry into the uterine cavity should be avoided if possible, and adhesion barriers and microsurgical technique should be used to reduce the risk of postoperative adhesions. The risk of a scar rupture during pregnancy is less if the endometrial cavity remains intact at myomectomy [D], although some fibroids cannot be removed without breach of the cavity. Post-operative adhesions can have a detrimental effect on tubal patency.

Submucous fibroids can successfully be resected hysteroscopically, depending on the size of the fibroid and its degree of protrusion into the uterine cavity. The risk of tubal damage with this procedure is minimal, but there is a risk of haemorrhage, uterine perforation and endometrial scarring leading to intrauterine adhesions. Hysteroscopic division of intrauterine adhesions and excision of polyps are usually straightforward, with low morbidity. Assisted reproductive technology is not applicable to uterine factor infertility. However, treatment of a uterine factor should be considered if failure of implantation seems to be the only cause of an unsuccessful IVF-ET treatment [E].

EBM

- There is no evidence that ovulation detection kits and temperature charts increase the chance of conception.
- There is no evidence that thorough physical examination of every patient is necessary.
- The postcoital test is of limited value with regard to discriminating between couples achieving and not achieving a pregnancy.
- Drug treatment is ineffective in the treatment of endometriosis-related infertility.
- Ovarian stimulation and IUI are effective in the management of mild male factor and unexplained infertility

KEY POINTS

- Around 9 per cent of couples are affected by infertility and half of them seek help.
- The most important determinant of a couple's fertility is the woman's age.
- Delaying starting a family until later life not only reduces fertility, but also increases the risk of miscarriage.
- PCOS is the most common cause of anovulatory infertility.
- Ovulatory disorders are the most common cause of female infertility.
- PID and iatrogenic causes are the main reasons for tubal infertility.
- *Chlamydia trachomatis* is the most common pathogen leading to PID in the western world.
- Unexplained infertility represents approximately 15-30 per cent of cases.
- Careful history taking is a very important starting point to the investigation of infertility.
- The mid-luteal phase is approximately 7 days from the next menstrual cycle, which is important when measuring serum progesterone levels for ovulation detection.
- Ablation of minimal and mild endometriosis adds a therapeutic dimension to a diagnostic procedure

ACKNOWLEDGEMENT

This chapter has been revised and updated. The author and editors acknowledge the contribution of Hany AMA Lashen to the chapter on this topic in the previous edition of the book.

References

1. Gutmacher AF. Factors affecting normal expectancy of conception. *J Am Med Assoc* 1956;161:855–60.
2. Boivin J, Bunting L, Collins JA, Nygren KG. International estimates of infertility prevalence and treatment-seeking: potential need and demand for infertility medical care. *Hum Reprod* 2007;22:1506–12.
3. Ombelet W, Cooke I, Dyer S *et al.* Infertility and the provision of infertility medical services in developing countries. *Hum Reprod* 2008;14:605–21.
4. Balen AH, Rutherford AJ. Management of infertility. *BMJ* 2007;335:608–11.
5. Franks S, Stark J, Hardy K. Follicle dynamics and anovulation in polycystic ovary syndrome. *Hum Reprod* 2008;14:367–78.
6. Goswami D, Conway GS. Premature ovarian failure. *Hum Reprod* 2005;11:491–510.

Chapter 82 Male infertility

Yakoub Khalaf

MRCOG standards

Theoretical skills

- Understand epidemiology, aetiology and pathogenesis of male infertility.
- Understand clinical management and prognosis of male factor infertility.
- Understand indications, limitations and interpretation of relevant investigations.

Practical skills

- Be able to take a history and examine the male partner with regard to infertility investigations.
- Be able to interpret and understand the seminal analysis report.

INTRODUCTION

The impact of male factor on a couple's fertility is difficult to quantify other than in cases of absolute azoospermia or severe oligozoospermia/asthenozoospermia. In other words, any man with motile normal spermatozoa in his ejaculate should be credited with some degree of fertility. Women undergoing donor insemination treatment have a higher probability of pregnancy if they are partners of azoospermic men than if they are partners of oligozoospermic men. This reflects the fact that a degree of compensation can exist between the female and male partners. Accordingly, in most circumstances, it is easier to define male fertility than infertility. The ability to make a woman pregnant or father a child can be considered evidence of the male's fertility. There are many causes of male infertility, although primary testicular disorders are most commonly responsible.

AETIOLOGY

Primary testicular disease

The majority of cases of male factor infertility lie in this category. The pathogenesis of testicular dysfunction is poorly understood, with no obvious predisposing factors being identifiable in more than 50 per cent of cases. Recent studies have linked azoospermia and severe oligozoospermia to microdeletions of genes on the Y chromosome, which appear to be involved in at least some cases of 'idiopathic' male infertility [D]. Other causes of failure of spermatogenesis include testicular maldescent, particularly if left uncorrected until puberty, testicular torsion, trauma or infection, neoplasm and effects of subsequent chemotherapy, haemosiderosis and Klinefelter's syndrome [D]. Mumps orchitis and severe epididymo-orchitis are the main inflammatory causes of testicular damage [D]. Other chromosomal anomalies can also lead to male infertility; however, Klinefelter's syndrome remains the only relatively commonly seen anomaly. Azoospermic and severely oligozoospermic men should have chromosomal karyotyping before their sperm is used for intracytoplasmic sperm injection (ICSI) in order to counsel the couple adequately about the risk of transmission of a chromosomal disorder (commonly deletion or translocation) to the offspring [E].

Obstructive male infertility

Obstruction can occur at any level of the male reproductive tract from the rete testis and the epididymis to the vas deferens. Obstruction can be due to congenital, inflammatory or iatrogenic causes. Desire for fertility following vasectomy is common. Congenital absence of the vas is also fairly common, being the cause of azoospermia in approximately 10 per cent of cases [D]. Bilateral congenital absence of the vas is seen in carriers of genes for cystic fibrosis [C], and pre-treatment screening of both partners is essential to avoid the possibility of cystic fibrosis in the offspring.

Endocrinological causes of male infertility

Endocrinopathies are rarely identified in cases of male infertility. The more common conditions seen in this category include hypogonadotrophic hypogonadism, and thyroid and adrenal disease [D]. Although rare, these conditions should be diagnosed, as their treatment is straightforward and can restore fertility. Hyperprolactinaemia in men can lead to impotence, but has little effect on sperm production [C].

Auto-immune causes

Approximately 12 per cent of men have anti-sperm antibodies [C]. This can lead to decreased sperm motility and may impede the binding of the spermatozoon to the zona pellucida of the oocyte, hindering fertilisation. Low levels of anti-sperm antibodies are not thought to have a significant impact on fertility [D]. The reason why some men develop anti-sperm antibodies is not known, although damage to the testis following trauma and surgery (resulting in disruption of the blood–testes barrier) can be found in many cases.

Drugs

Drugs taken for medicinal and recreational purposes can affect sperm production and/or function. Alcohol, cigarettes, opiates and marijuana can suppress spermatogenesis and affect sperm function [D]. Anabolic steroids, antifungal drugs, sulfasalazine and corticosteroids also affect spermatogenesis. The effect of most of these drugs is reversible. In contrast, chemotherapy can cause permanent damage to spermatogenesis. Other drugs, including antidepressants, sedatives and antihypertensives, can lead to male infertility by causing erectile dysfunction.

Environmental factors

Exposure to heat, chemicals and ionising irradiation can damage sperm production, and it is important to enquire about the male partner's occupation. Evidence for the extent of the effects of environmental toxins on male fertility is lacking. Although epidemiological studies have demonstrated a decline in sperm quality in the developed world, it is difficult to extrapolate from these population-based data to individual cases. However, it seems sensible to advise the avoidance of excessive heat and exposure to chemicals such as paints, organic solvents, lead-based products and pesticides in oligospermic/asthenospermic subfertile men.

Varicocele

Varicocele is a dilatation of the veins along the spermatic cord in the scrotum. Dilatation occurs when valves within the veins along the spermatic cord obstruct normal blood flow, causing a backflow of blood. The mechanisms by which varicoceles would affect fertility have not yet been explained, and neither have the mechanisms by which surgical treatment of the varicoceles might restore fertility. It occurs in both fertile and infertile men, although the incidence seems to be higher among infertile men [C]. The impact of varicocele on male fertility remains controversial. Increased testicular temperature (which is unfavourable for spermatogenesis) has been suggested as a mechanism of action in these cases, but surgical or radiological correction of the disorder is not thought to improve the chances of conception [A].[1] Additionally, there is no increase in pregnancy rates following varicocele treatment compared to no treatment in subfertile couples in whom varicoceles in the man is the only abnormal finding.

Ejaculatory disorders

Retrograde ejaculation, in which sperm enter the bladder rather than the penile urethra at ejaculation, can follow from neurological disorders, diabetes or bladder neck or prostate surgery. Failure of ejaculation due to neurological disorders, medication or psychological difficulties is a rare cause of male infertility and the most difficult to treat. Most men with such problems require sperm freezing (usually by surgical sperm retrieval) and assisted conception treatment.

INVESTIGATION OF THE MALE

All referrals to an infertility clinic should be seen as a couple, with concurrent investigation of the male and female partners. A routine semen analysis can be performed before seeing the couple in the clinic. A normal result can provide a degree of reassurance to the male partner, and erectile and ejaculatory problems can usually be excluded by a sensitively taken medical history. If the seminal parameters are abnormal, further investigations should be instigated. It is important to elicit from the history any of the causes of male infertility mentioned above. This should be followed by examination of genital development, the testicles, the epididymis and the vas deferens. Any of the aforementioned reversible causes can usually be corrected, and advice regarding smoking, alcohol and substance abuse should be given. Testicular cooling by wearing boxer shorts or taking cold baths is probably of little value, although occupational exposure to extreme heat should be avoided.

Semen analysis

The value of a diagnostic test depends on its sensitivity (ability to identify disease), specificity (ability to identify normality) and reproducibility (obtaining similar results each time the test is carried out). The wide overlap of the results of the various components of a semen analysis between fertile and infertile men reduces the sensitivity and specificity of routine semen analysis as a test of infertility. Moreover, the large biological variation seen in the quality of sperm in repeated tests on the same individual limits the reproducibility of semen analysis as a diagnostic test. Routine semen analysis should be performed according to criteria established by the WHO in order to achieve standardisation (Table 82.1). The test assesses several measures of sperm quality, some of which are more sensitive in identifying infertile men than others. The WHO-recommended method of semen analysis includes determination of the volume of ejaculate, concentration, motility and percentage of morphologically normal forms. Semen analysis can be carried out manually or using computer-assisted sperm analysis (CASA). Several population-based studies have

REPRODUCTIVE GYNAECOLOGY

Table 82.1 Reference values from the updated WHO guidelines (2010)

volume	Lower reference limit
Semen volume (ml)	1.5 (1.4–1.7)
Total sperm number (10^6 per ejaculate)	39 (33–46)
Sperm concentration (10^6 per ml)	15 (12–16)
Progressive motility (PR, %)	32 (31–34)
Sperm morphology (normal forms, %)	4 (3.0–4.0)
Vitality (live spermatozoa, %)	58 (55–63)
pH	≥7.2

Box 82.1 Sperm function tests

Objective assessment of motility

Hypo-osmotic swelling test

Tests for sperm nuclear maturity

Measure of acrosome status

Acrosome reaction and acrosin activity

Hamster zona-free oocyte penetration

Human sperm zona binding and penetration

produced statistical correlation between the different semen parameters and fertility potential in men. It is also important to remember that these values are not the minimum requirement to achieve a pregnancy; therefore they are referred to as 'reference' and not 'normal' values.

Many other tests of semen quality have been devised. These include biochemical analysis of the seminal fluid and detection of anti-sperm antibodies. Biochemical analysis of the seminal fluid can provide information about the prostate, seminal vesicles and epididymis. Zinc, fructose, carnitine and acid phosphatase have all been studied, but are not thought to impart useful diagnostic or prognostic information. The detection of anti-sperm antibodies using the immunobead or mixed antibody reaction (MAR) test may alter treatment and continues to be performed in most centres.

Sperm function tests

The functions of the sperm *in vivo* are to negotiate the cervical mucus, reach the ampullary part of the Fallopian tube in sufficient numbers, undergo capacitation and finally fertilise the egg. However, routine semen analysis does not test these functions. Therefore several tests, known as 'sperm function tests', have been developed in tertiary centres. These tests are still of academic rather than practical value and have become less significant following the introduction of IVF treatments, which circumvent most of the steps necessary for fertilisation *in vivo* Their role in routine infertility investigations has yet to be established. Some of these tests are listed in Box 82.1 and the interested reader can refer to the WHO manual for more details.

Other tests

Unexplained severe sperm abnormality including azoospermia merits further investigation. The objective of such tests is to identify whether azoospermia is due to a primary testicular disorder or an outflow obstruction. Obstructive azoospermia is usually associated with normal concentration of FSH in serum, as the testes continue to function normally. In contrast, disorders of spermatogenesis result in interruption of the gonadal–pituitary feedback loop with elevation of serum FSH. Measurement of FSH can thus be useful in the investigation of azoospermia. Testosterone, luteinising hormone and sex hormone-binding globulin (SHBG) can complement the investigations. Serum inhibin B is performed as a marker of spermatogenesis in some tertiary centres and also in research settings. Ultrasound scan of testes (with or without Doppler) can be used to rule out structural abnormalities and malignancies. Invasive investigation using testicular biopsy can assess the extent of damage to the spermatogenesis and identify whether it is possible to obtain testicular sperm for use in ICSI, even if the patient is azoospermic. Karyotyping and cystic fibrosis gene screening are necessary if a chromosomal abnormality is suspected or to assess the carrier status for cystic fibrosis genes in patients with congenital absence of the vas. However, the modern management of male infertility and the introduction of ICSI treatment has reduced the need for extensive investigations, especially in less severe cases of oligozoospermia or athenozoospermia. Where an endocrinological reason is suspected, the diagnosis should be made, as the treatment strategy in these cases differs from the usual treatment modalities for male infertility (Fig. 82.1).

Examination of the male partner

In the presence of a normal semen analysis, there is little to gain from examination of the male. On the other hand, in severe male factor infertility and especially in azoospermic men, examination is warranted to help establish the cause of the problem. Both general and genital examinations should be undertaken. The objectives of the general examination are to assess the level of masculinisation and to detect any stigmata of chromosomal abnormality, inguinal hernia or relevant surgical scars, gynaecomastia or evidence of systemic illnesses. The genital examination should include assessment of the testes, epididymis and vas deferens and detection of any scrotal swellings or varicocele. If the history suggests penile

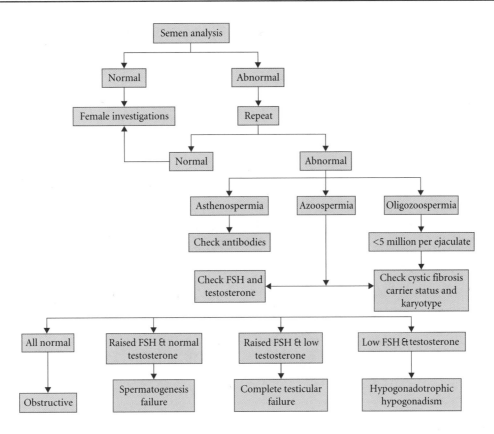

Fig. 82.1 Investigations of male infertility. FSH, follicle-stimulating hormone

or prostatic problems, it is advisable to refer for a urological opinion. The examination should be carried out in standing and supine positions in a warm private room. The testicular axis, volume and consistency should be assessed with a Prader orchiometer to measure the testicular volume. It should be noted that testicular volume is related to ethnic origin, weight and height and there is normally a small difference between the left and right testicles. For Caucasian men the normal volume is above 12 mL per testis. The consistency of the testicles can also be assessed. A soft consistency is associated with impaired spermatogenesis. Examination of the epididymis should assess its position in relation to the testicle, volume, any tenderness and any nodularity or swellings. Normally, the epididymis is small and may not be palpable. The vas should have no thickenings or nodules. Careful examination for the presence of the vasa is essential in azoospermic men, especially if the testicular volume is normal. Scrotal examination for varicocele should be carried out in the standing position. If any other scrotal swelling is palpable, the patient should be referred for a urological opinion. Testicular maldescent in infancy is associated with an increased risk of testicular cancer in later life. Such patients may present to an infertility clinic for investigation of oligospermia. They should be apprised of this risk and taught to self-examine. Similarly, tissue collected at testicular biopsy that is used to obtain sperm for ICSI in azoospermic men should also be sent for histological examination

(for example, to exclude sertoli-only syndrome). Ideally testicular sperm retrieval should be performed in an-HFEA registered clinic with facilities for cryopreservation.

MANAGEMENT OF MALE INFERTILITY

Until recently, men with primary testicular dysfunction or obstructive azoospermia were unable to reproduce. IVF and micromanipulation of sperm now offer these men the opportunity to father children and have become the mainstay in the treatment of male factor infertility. The treatment of male factor infertility, including the use of donor insemination, is discussed in Chapter 84, Assisted reproduction. However, some more traditional methods of treatment merit consideration.

Varicocelectomy

This procedure refers to the ligation of varicocele, which was carried out both prophylactically and therapeutically for many decades. Varicocele repair does not seem to be an effective treatment for male or unexplained subfertility [A]. The modern management of infertility has made the procedure redundant, removing the opportunity for further randomised trials to investigate its value.

Management of endocrine disorders

Hypogonadotrophic hypogonadism, often in association with Kallmann's syndrome, has been successfully treated with pulsatile GnRH or human menopausal gonadotrophins and hCG to restore spermatogenic drive and hence fertility. Initiation of spermatogenesis can take several months and treatment can become costly.

Men with idiopathic semen abnormalities should not be offered anti-oestrogens, gonadotrophins, androgens, bromocriptine or kinin-enhancing drugs because they have not been shown to be effective [A].

Management of anti-sperm antibodies

Many empirical therapies have been suggested for men with anti-sperm antibodies. The use of condoms and corticosteroids and intrauterine insemination of washed spermatozoa are some examples [A]. The value of all these modalities has been controversial, and IVF-ET and ICSI are currently the methods of choice in these cases. Donor insemination can be an alternative for financial reasons.

Reversal of vasectomy

Vasectomy reversal can be carried out successfully, with up to an 80 per cent chance of a subsequent pregnancy. The chance of success is inversely proportional to the length of time since the vasectomy was carried out. Although the integrity of the vas deferens can be restored in most cases, anti-sperm antibodies are common after vasectomy and reversal, and are probably the major bar to conception. In these cases and in those whose operation has failed, IVF with ICSI is the recommended treatment. A growing number of centres are offering collection and storage of sperm from the epididymis at the time of vasectomy reversal, for subsequent use in ICSI treatment if the reversal operation fails.

EBM

- The use of gonadotrophin drugs in hypogonadotrophic hypogonadal men is an effective treatment [B].
- The use of bromocriptine in men with sexual dysfunction as a result of hyperprolactinaemia is effective [B].
- Testicular biopsy should only be undertaken in tertiary centres [E].
- Vasectomy reversal is an effective treatment [A].
- Anti-oestrogens, androgens and bromocriptine are not effective in improving sperm quality [C].
- The use of steroids in the treatment of anti-sperm antibodies is ineffective and further validation is required [B].

- Surgery on the male genital tract should be undertaken only in centres where expertise is available [E].
- Men found to have abnormal chromosomal analysis (14 per cent in azoospermia and 7 per cent in severe oligozoospermia should receive genetic counselling.
- Testosterone replacement can result in oligozoospermia and/or reversible azoospermia and is therefore contraindicated in management of male infertility.

KEY POINTS

- Semen analysis is an appropriate starting point in the investigation of the male partner.
- If a severe sperm abnormality is found, clinical examination and bacteriological and endocrinological tests should be undertaken.
  - Tact and sensitivity are important when obtaining a history, examining patients and discussing abnormal results with them.
  - If reversal of vasectomy is to be undertaken, efforts should be made to obtain epididymal sperm for freezing and future use in case of operation failure.
  - There is a considerable variability in sperm quality when assessed in the same individual over time.
  - Semen analysis, unlike many modern investigative tests, is operator dependent. Adequate training of the operators is therefore essential to minimise both intra-observer and inter-observer variation.
- The andrology laboratory should be subject to external and internal quality assessments.

ACKNOWLEDGMENT

This chapter has been revised and updated. The author and editors acknowledge the contribution of Hany AMA Lashen to the chapter on this topic in the previous edition of the book.

Key Reference

1. Evers JLH, Collins JA. Assessment of efficacy of varicocele repair for male subfertility: a systematic review. *Lancet* 2003;361:1849–52.

Chapter 83 Unexplained infertility

Smriti Bhatta and Siladitya Bhattacharya

INTRODUCTION

Infertility is defined as the inability to conceive after one year of unprotected intercourse. Standard investigations performed as part of an initial work-up include semen analysis, serum mid-luteal progesterone level to confirm ovulation, and a tubal patency test. These tests are normal in about 25 per cent of couples in whom the cause of infertility is deemed to be unexplained.[1] As the decision to undergo a panel of investigations is prompted by an expectation of finding a specific cause which is amenable to targeted treatment, unexplained infertility as a concept is difficult for couples to accept.

The suitability of the term 'unexplained infertility' has been questioned as the diagnosis is dependent on the number, nature and quality of tests used. Unexplained infertility does not exclude the possibility of a number of putative causes which are undetectable by standard tests.

These include tubal transport problems, mild ovulatory dysfunction, poor gamete and embryo quality, luteal-phase deficits, implantation abnormalities and immunological causes. While absence of a precise diagnosis is intellectually and emotionally unsatisfactory, routine use of a larger panel of tests would be logistically challenging without necessarily having an impact on management, which is heavily reliant on assisted reproduction to bypass known and unknown causes.

POSSIBLE CAUSES OF UNEXPLAINED INFERTILITY

Human conception is a complex series of events that involves an interaction between the egg and sperm, fertilisation and implantation of the embryo. Any overt or hidden factors that interfere with these events can lead to infertility. A number of possible causes for unexplained infertility are listed in Box 83.1. Many of these are subtle in nature and few are actually treatable at the present time.

Box 83.1 Factors which can contribute to unexplained infertility

Ovarian
Poor ovarian reserve in older women
Poor oocyte quality
Luteinised unruptured follicle
Peritoneal
Mild endometriosis
Altered macrophage and immune activity
Endometrial
Abnormal T-cell and natural killer cell activity
Abnormal endometrial perfusion
Abnormal secretion of endometrial proteins
Male factors
Reduced acrosome reaction, oocyte binding and zona penetration
Embryo
Genetic and chromosomal abnormalities

MANAGEMENT

Absence of conception within 12 months does not equate to sterility, and in the absence of any obvious barriers to infertility, a significant proportion of couples with unexplained infertility can expect to become pregnant without active treatment.[2] In particular, where the duration of infertility is short and the female partner is young and/or has had a previous pregnancy, the prognosis is good. However, lack of a specific diagnosis has traditionally encouraged the use of a variety of empirical treatments in the management of unexplained infertility. Commonly used treatments include clomiphene citrate, intrauterine insemination with or without controlled ovarian stimulation, and IVF. Factors affecting treatment success are female age, parity and duration of infertility.

Expectant management

> **EBM**
>
> Managing the couples expectantly is the first-line approach in good-prognosis patients due to high chances of natural conception [B][2] and due to cost effectiveness [A]. However, couples prefer the treatment option [B].[4,5]

Expectant management is the first-line approach for couples with unexplained infertility of relatively short duration where the female partner is young. In an observational Dutch study, 81 per cent (356/437) of couples with unexplained infertility had an ongoing pregnancy within five years of diagnosis, with 74 per cent (263/356) of pregnancies being conceived naturally.[2]

Table 83.1 provides data from two other studies on spontaneous livebirth rates in couples undergoing expectant management in different settings.

Accurate prediction of the chances of conception can be useful in counselling patients and avoiding unnecessary treatment. A popular prediction model[3] has identified the factors associated with live birth, of which the most important are female age, duration of infertility and previous pregnancy. Female age less than 35 years and duration of infertility of less than two years are associated with higher odds of natural conception.

During expectant management, couples are advised to follow healthy lifestyle habits, maintain optimal weight and continue regular sexual intercourse in order to maximise chances of conception. However, this approach is not always appealing to many couples who equate active medical treatment with higher success rates. A Scottish RCT[4] comparing clomiphene or IUI with expectant management found that women randomised to clomiphene citrate (159/170, 94%) and IUI (155/162, 96%) found the process of treatment more acceptable than those randomised to expectant management (123/153, 80%) (p = 0.001 and p <0.001, respectively).

Expectant management is cost effective compared to active treatment. Data from a Dutch study[5] on long-term follow-up of couples with an intermediate prognosis, randomised to a six-month period of either expectant management or superovulation and IUI, found an estimated saving of 2616 euros in those managed expectantly, with no difference in pregnancy rates between the two groups. The period of expectant management needs to take into account the age of the female partner, but many would consider waiting for two years before moving on to active treatment.[1]

> **EBM**
>
> Clomiphene use is costly and does not shorten the time to pregnancy or increase the livebirth rate as compared to expectant management [A].[4,5,6]

Clomiphene citrate

Oral clomiphene citrate therapy has been commonly used for management of unexplained infertility. It is thought to correct subtle ovulatory dysfunction. Clomiphene is a selective oestrogen receptor modulator (SERM) that inhibits the negative feedback effect of oestrogen on the hypothalamus, resulting in increased gonadotrophin secretion and induction of ovulation. It can lead to multiple ovulation and is associated with a risk of multiple pregnancy. Treatment is usually initiated with a dose of 50 mg once daily from days 2–6 of a menstrual cycle, although higher doses have been used. Common side effects of clomiphene include hot flushes, abdominal discomfort or blurring of vision. Concerns regarding potential risk of ovarian cancer have not been confirmed. Clomiphene has been popular because it is inexpensive, non-invasive and needs less clinical monitoring.

In a large RCT[4] comparing clomiphene with expectant management in unexplained infertility, livebirth rates were comparable in both groups (OR 0.79, 95% CI 0.45–1.38), suggesting no benefit with clomiphene use. The number needed to treat for harm with clomiphene citrate was 33 (i.e. treating 33 more women with clomiphene would yield one less livebirth compared to expectant management). Also, there was no significant difference in time to pregnancy leading to livebirth with clomiphene (P = 0.41) compared with expectant management (Fig. 83.1).

Table 83.1 Chance of spontaneous conception

Author	Livebirth rate at 12 months	Livebirth rate at 36 months	Setting
Collins et al. 1995	14.3%	33%	Tertiary care
Snick et al. 1997	27.4%	60%	Primary care

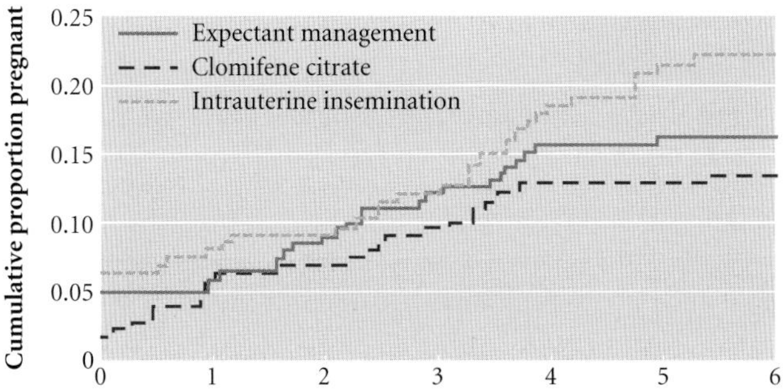

Fig. 83.1 Time to pregnancy leading to live birth in expectant management compared to treatment(clomiphene and IUI) Bhattacharya et al.[4]

A Cochrane review[5] on clomiphene use in unexplained infertility did not show any improvement in pregnancy rates with clomiphene after pooling data from two trials (OR 1.03, 95% CI 0.64–1.66).

Cost effectiveness of empirical clomiphene use has been evaluated based on data from a large trial.[6] Cost per livebirth was £72 after expectant management and £2611 after treatment with clomiphene, suggesting clomiphene to be less cost effective than expectant management.

EBM

IUI in a natural cycle does not increase the livebirth rate compared to expectant management [A].[4,7] IUI with ovarian stimulation is more effective than IUI alone but increases the risk of multiple pregnancy [A].[7]

Intrauterine insemination

Intrauterine insemination has been widely used as a fertility treatment for unexplained infertility. It involves preparation of a semen sample in the laboratory to isolate spermatozoa with high motility. The prepared sample is then loaded into a narrow catheter and introduced within the uterine cavity at around the time of ovulation. Theoretically, this allows sperm to bypass any hostile cervical factors and increases the number of motile sperm within the upper genital tract. Ovarian stimulation increases the number of available oocytes and therefore increases the risks of multiple pregnancy.

IUI in a natural cycle involves monitoring urinary or serum LH from day 10 to day 12 of the treatment cycle to detect LH surge. Insemination is performed 20–30 hours after detection of an LH surge. In stimulated cycles (IUI + ovarian stimulation [SO]), clomiphene or gonadotrophins are used to promote ovulation from more than one (ideally two) mature follicles. hCG is administered to trigger ovulation and IUI is scheduled 36–40 hours later.

A Scottish multicentre trial comparing unstimulated IUI to expectant management over a 6-month period[4] did not find a statistically significant difference in livebirth rate between the two groups (OR 1.46, 95% CI 0.88–2.43). The NNT was 17, suggesting that 17 women would need to undergo IUI over six months to achieve one extra livebirth.

Table 83.2 presents a summary of the available evidence from RCTs for the effectiveness of IUI treatment.

In an economic evaluation of a large multicentre trial,[6] the cost effectiveness of IUI was compared to expectant management. The cost per livebirth was £1487 compared to £72 for expectant management. The study concluded that IUI was unlikely to be cost effective in an NHS setting.

Stimulated IUI cycles can be associated with a high multiple pregnancy rate. A recent multicentre Dutch study10 randomised 605 couples with unexplained and mild male factor infertility to 3 cycles of IVF elective single embryo transfer (IVF e-SET), 6 cycles of modified natural cycle IVF (MNC IVF) and 6 cycles of IUI with COH to evaluate if the alternative treatment strategies have reduced multiple pregnancy rates compared to stimulated IUI. This found that the multiple pregnancy rates were low and comparable across the three groups.

IVF

IVF is increasingly used as a definitive treatment for unexplained infertility. The rationale behind using IVF is that it can bypass known and unknown causes associated with unexplained infertility, but it is expensive and is associated with the risks of multiple pregnancy and ovarian hyperstimulation syndrome.

Table 83.2 IUI in unexplained infertility compared to expectant management and IVF

Treatment	Comparison group	Study	Effectiveness (odds of livebirth)
Stimulated IUI	Natural cycle IUI	Cochrane review[7]	OR 2.07, 95% CI 1.22-3.50
Stimulated IUI	Timed intercourse in stimulated cycle	Cochrane review[7]	OR 1.59, 95% CI 0.88-2.88
Unstimulated IUI	Expectant management	Cochrane review[7]	OR 1.60, 95% CI 0.92-2.78
Stimulated IUI	Expectant management	Dutch multicentre RCT[8]	OR 0.82, 95% CI 0.45-1.49
Stimulated IUI	IVF	Cochrane review[9]	OR 1.09, 95% CI 0.74-1.59

IVF is offered to women with unresolved unexplained infertility who have been trying for more than two years. However, the contribution of IVF to pregnancy rates in couples with unexplained subfertility is around 13 per cent compared to a higher proportion of pregnancies from IVF in couples with tubal factor, endometriosis and male factor infertility (45, 45 and 37 per cent, respectively).[11] Use of ICSI technique for fertilisation has shown improved fertilisation rates when compared to conventional IVF in couples with unexplained infertility.[12]

IVF appears to be more effective compared to other treatment strategies. Table 83.3 shows data from a Cochrane review[9] to support this.

One study used a mathematical model to compare the cost effectiveness of offering primary IVF therapy with IUI cycles and IVF.[13] The study found that for a cohort of 100 couples, six cycles of IUI would cost an extra £172,200, providing an opportunity for an additional 54 IVF cycles and 14 live births. The conclusion was that a primary strategy of IVF was more cost effective than IUI followed by IVF.

PREGNANCY AFTER UNEXPLAINED INFERTILITY

Subfertile women are at a higher risk of obstetric complications even after adjusting for the influencing factors like age and parity. A study specifically investigating obstetric outcome in women with unexplained infertility found higher rates of obstetric complications in this group, including preeclampsia, preterm labour, placental abruption, and induction of labour and emergency caesarean section.[14] The explanation for this remains unclear.

Table 83.3 Efficacy of IVF compared to IUI and expectant management

Treatment	Comparison group	Study	Effectiveness (odds of live birth)
IVF	Expectant management	Cochrane review[9]	OR 22, 95%CI 2.56–189.37
IVF	IUI	Cochrane review[9]	OR 1.96, 95%CI 0.88–4.36
IVF	Stimulated IUI	Cochrane review[9]	OR 1.09, 95% CI 0.74–1.59

KEY POINTS

- Unexplained infertility is a diagnosis of exclusion after confirmation of ovulation, tubal patency and normal semen analysis.
- Introducing additional tests to identify the potential causes is not cost effective and is unlikely to change management.
- Unexplained infertility is associated with higher chances of natural conception compared with other causes of infertility.
- Expectant management is recommended in younger couples with shorter duration of infertility.
- Clomiphene and unstimulated IUI are not effective.
- IUI with ovarian stimulation is more effective than IUI alone.
- IVF may be offered after two years of expectant management and appears to be more effective in comparison with other treatment strategies.

References

1. NICE. *Fertility: assessment and treatment for people with fertility problems (update).* (Clinical guideline 156.) 2013. www.nice.org.uk/CG156.
2. Brandes M, Hamilton CJ, van der Steen JO *et al.* Unexplained infertility: overall ongoing pregnancy rate and mode of conception. *Hum Reprod* 2011;26(2): 360–8.
3. Hunault CC, Habbema JD, Eijkemans MJ *et al.* Two new prediction rules for spontaneous pregnancy leading to live birth among subfertile couples, based on the synthesis of three previous models. *Hum Reprod* 2004;19(9):2019–26.
4. Bhattacharya S, Harrild K, Mollison J *et al.* Clomifene citrate or unstimulated intrauterine insemination compared with expectant management for unexplained infertility: pragmatic randomised controlled trial. *BMJ* 2008;337:a716.
5. Hughes E, Brown J, Collins JJ *et al.* Clomiphene citrate for unexplained subfertility in women. *Cochrane Database Syst Rev* 2010;CD000057.
6. Wordsworth S, Buchanan J, Mollison J *et al.* Clomiphene citrate and intrauterine insemination as first-line treatments for unexplained infertility: are they cost-effective? *Hum Reprod* 2011;26:369–75.
7. Veltman-Verhulst SM, Cohlen BJ, Hughes E *et al.* Intrauterine insemination for unexplained subfertility. *Cochrane Database Syst Rev* 2012;9:CD001838.
8. Steures P, van der Steeg JW, Hompes PG *et al.* Intrauterine insemination with controlled ovarian hyperstimulation

versus expectant management for couples with unexplained subfertility and an intermediate prognosis: a randomised clinical trial. *Lancet* 2006;368:216–21.

9. Pandian Z, Gibreel A, Bhattacharya S. In vitro fertilisation for unexplained subfertility. *Cochrane Database Syst Rev* 2012;4:CD003357.

10. Bensdorp AJ, Tjon-Kon-Fat RI, Bossuyt PM *et al.* Prevention of multiple pregnancies in couples with unexplained or mild male subfertility: randomised controlled trial of in vitro fertilisation with single embryo transfer or in vitro fertilisation in modified natural cycle compared with intrauterine insemination with controlled ovarian hyperstimulation. *BMJ* 2015;9:350:g7771.

11. Brandes M, Hamilton CJ, de Bruin JP *et al.* The relative contribution of IVF to the total ongoing pregnancy rate in a subfertile cohort. *Hum Reprod* 2010;25(1):118–26.

12. Johnson LN, Sasson IE, Sammel MD *et al.* Does intracytoplasmic sperm injection improve the fertilization rate and decrease the total fertilization failure rate in couples with well-defined unexplained infertility? A systematic review and meta-analysis. *Fertil Steril* 2013;100(3):704–11.

13. Pashayan N, Lyratzopoulos G, Mathur R. Cost-effectiveness of primary offer of IVF vs primary offer of IUI followed by IVF (for IUI failures) in couples with unexplained or mild male factor subfertility. *BMC Health Serv Res* 2006;Jun 23;6:80.

14. Pandian Z, Bhattacharya S, Templeton A. Review of unexplained infertility and obstetric outcome: a 10 year review. *Hum Reprod* 2001;Dec; 16(12):2593–97.

Chapter 84 Assisted reproduction

Abey Eapen and Arri Coomarasamy

MRCOG standards

Theoretical skills

- Have good knowledge of the indications and treatment options for assisted reproductive techniques.
- Be aware of the risks associated with ART.
- Have a brief knowledge of the laboratory procedures.
- Appreciate the emotional, physical and financial stress involved and be aware of the social, ethical and legal implications associated with ART.
- Have a brief knowledge of the HFEA and practice code.

Practical skills

- Be able to organise appropriate investigations and offer counselling.
- Be able to identify and counsel individuals/couples regarding treatment options, risks and success rates.
- Be able to diagnose and manage ovarian hyperstimulation syndrome.
- Be able to liaise with a multidisciplinary fertility team.

INTRODUCTION

ART represents a wide range of treatment options used for management of women or couples diagnosed with infertility. The most widely used option is IVF. Human IVF treatments started as early as the 1940s, but without success. In 1976, the first IVF pregnancy was documented, albeit an ectopic.[1]

The first livebirth following 'test tube conception' occurred in 1978. Louise Brown was born in the UK following a natural cycle of IVF treatment supervised by Robert Edwards (physiologist) and Patrick Steptoe (gynaecologist). Successful IVF treatment followed in Australia, USA, Sweden and France and then worldwide.

The two major breakthroughs since inception of IVF treatment are considered to be controlled ovarian stimulation (COS) and intracytoplasmic sperm injection (ICSI). Advances in diagnosis, therapy, intervention (e.g. TVS) and laboratory techniques have resulted in a gradual increase in ART success rates over the years.

EPIDEMIOLOGY

An estimated 1 in 7 couples (approximately 3.5 million in the UK) have difficulty conceiving, and many of these couples have IVF treatment. Every year about 12,000 babies are born using assisted conception treatment in the UK,[2] representing approximately 2 per cent of all babies born every year.

Latest HFEA data show 49,636 women had a total of 64,600 cycles of IVF and 2379 women had a total of 4611 cycles of donor insemination (DI) in 2013 in the UK. Worldwide, about 1 million babies have been born as a result of ART.

INDICATIONS FOR ART

There are multiple indications for ART, including long-standing unexplained infertility (Table 84.1).

HUMAN FERTILISATION AND EMBRYOLOGY AUTHORITY

In the UK, the HFEA provides licensing and monitoring for clinical and research activities using human gametes and embryos. Clinics performing any form of assisted conception techniques will need to be registered with the HFEA and are identified by a unique HFEA reference number. The HFEA provides impartial and reliable information to the public and publishes a league table with individual clinics' success rates and statistics associated with each aspect of ART.

Table 84.1 Indications for ART

Female	Male	Couple
Tubal factor	Ejaculatory dysfunction	Long-standing primary or secondary unexplained subfertility
Moderate to severe endometriotis	Sub-optimal sperm variables	HLA matching for offspring with rare disorders
Low ovarian reserve	Azoospermia	Screening for genetic disorders (in those with a strong family history)
Age-related subfertility	Gay couples	Medical indications (surrogacy in cases of contraindications to pregnancy, anatomical abnormalities or following egg/embryo freezing in women with cancers)
Premature ovarian failure	Medical indications (malignancies or chronic debilitating illnesses)	
Single woman		
Lesbian couple		

KEY POINTS

- The HFEA replaced the Warnock committee (1982) and the HFEA 1990 Act came into force in 1991.
- Disclosure of donor information regulation (2004) allowed removal of donor anonymity allowing details about oocyte and sperm donors (registered after 1 April 2005) to be passed on to the offspring.
- As per HFEA data from 2013, a total of 78 licensed clinics conducted IVF treatment and a total of 75 conducted donor inseminations in the UK.

COUNSELLING

Counselling includes information provision by care providers and impartial advice by independent counsellors, as well as genetic and psychosexual counselling.

Counselling by clinicians: This involves explaining the options available to the couple, helping them to decide the right treatment by discussing the risks, benefits and success rates associated with the treatment options.

Counselling by a trained professional: Offering impartial advice to the individual before, during or after the assisted conception process is a requirement for ART clinics registered with HFEA. Implication counselling to help with emotional issues, to discuss needs/legal rights of donor conceived children and to help decision making is always encouraged (even though not mandatory) for individuals and couples using donor gametes or embryos. In special circumstances, counselling services are used by clinicians to assess the emotional and social circumstances of the individual or couple requesting treatment. This is an integral part of the process to ascertain the welfare of the (unborn) child.

Genetic counselling: Risk of transmission of genetic disorders through ART has implications for the welfare of the unborn child. It is important to counsel the woman or couple regarding the risk of transmission to the offspring. Some couples may benefit from pre-implantation genetic diagnosis.

KEY POINTS

- Assisted conception treatments can entail significant emotional and physical stress. Many patients make use of support services and alternative therapies such as hypnosis, holistic therapies and acupuncture (most commonly used).
- In spite of the advances in ART over the decades, the majority of treatment cycles result in a negative outcome.
- Individuals who wish to start a family after multiple failed ART attempts have the option to consider adoption or fostering.

ASSISTED REPRODUCTIVE TECHNIQUES

Although numerous options are available, the commonest assisted conception treatment is IVF. The various techniques and their indication(s) are summarised in Table 84.2.

A TYPICAL IVF TREATMENT CYCLE

A typical IVF cycle involves pituitary suppression, superovulation, monitoring ovarian stimulation and oocyte maturation, oocyte retrieval, sperm insemination and fertilisation, embryo transfer, luteal-phase support and confirming outcome of

Table 84.2 Assisted conception techniques

Technique	Explanation/indication(s)
IUI	Intrauterine insemination of sperm in the 'right place' (womb) at the 'right time' (around the time of ovulation)
	Commonly used treatment option in unexplained subfertility or in cases where the male partner is diagnosed with ejaculatory dysfunction
IUI-DS	IUI treatment using donated sperm
	Commonly used treatment option for treating single women, lesbian couples or heterosexual couples where the male partner is diagnosed with aspermia
GIFT	Gamete intra-fallopian tube transfer where retrieved oocytes and sperm are laparoscopically placed in the fallopian tubes
	Not widely used due to invasive nature, risks and low success rates
ZIFT	Zygote intra-fallopian transfer where the fertilised embryo is laparoscopically placed in the fallopian tube
	Not widely used due to invasive nature, risks and low success rates
IVF: standard insemination	Insemination of retrieved oocytes in a Petri dish using the standard insemination with sperm
	Indications: tubal factor infertility, unexplained infertility and other indications
IVF with ICSI	Intracytoplasmic sperm injection using microinjection technique where a single sperm is injected into the retrieved oocyte
	Indication: male factor infertility
IVF with ICSI using IMSI	ICSI insemination technique using morphologically selected sperm with high-magnification microscope
	Indication: severe male factor infertility
IVM	In-vitro maturation where immature oocytes are retrieved and matured in the laboratory and then inseminated with sperm using ICSI technique
	Indication: polycystic ovaries, to reduce the risk of OHSS
FET	Frozen embryo transfer where transfer of frozen embryos is performed in a natural cycle or a hormonally manipulated cycle
	Indication: in cases where the embryos were electively frozen to reduce the risk of OHSS, due to endometrial abnormalities, or for other reasons (e.g. surplus embryos after a fresh treatment cycle)
IVF with oocyte donation	IVF using donated oocytes and sperm from husband/partner
	Indications: low ovarian reserve or premature ovarian failure
IVF using sperm donation	IVF treatment using donated sperm
	Indication: male partner with aspermia
IVF using embryo donation	IVF treatment using donated embryos
	Indication: cases where there is combined female and male factor or in cases of repeated IVF failures
IVF using surrogacy	Transfer of embryos to a surrogate mother
	Indications: anatomical abnormalities or medical indications

treatment. Careful coordination of physiological events both *in vivo* and *in vitro* is crucial. A multidisciplinary team involving clinicians, nurses, embryologists and administrators is needed to provide effective care. UK regulations require an assessment of the welfare of the (unborn) child. Furthermore, it is mandatory that both partners are screened for HIV, hepatitis B surface antigen, hepatitis core antibody and hepatitis C before they undergo IVF treatment.

The most important factor determining the outcome of an IVF cycle is age of the female partner. The livebirth rate per treatment started in the UK ranges from 33 per cent (for under 35 years) to 5 per cent (43–44 years). Success rates range widely between different ART clinics.

Pituitary suppression

Pituitary suppression or 'down-regulation' is often used to prevent premature release of eggs in an IVF cycle. Pituitary suppression can be achieved with either GnRH agonists or antagonists.

GnRH agonists are synthetic peptides that interact with the GnRH receptors resulting in an initial surge in FSH and LH ('flare effect') which is followed by down-regulation once all the receptors are engaged. With continuous use ovarian down-regulation occurs in about 10–14 days resulting in endogenous gonadotrophin suppression. Side effects include hypo-oestrogenic side effects, hot flushes and headaches.

GnRH antagonists are peptide molecules which result in immediate blockage of GnRH without the flare-up effect. This helps to reduce the duration of treatment protocols. An antagonist protocol has the added advantage of enabling the use of GnRH agonists for final oocyte maturation; there is emerging evidence to suggest a reduction in the risk of OHSS with such an approach. Side effects include mild anaphylactic reactions due to release of histamine although this is rarely encountered with newer preparations.

Superovulation

The aim of superovulation is to achieve multifollicular development to allow harvesting of multiple eggs which are needed for IVF treatment. Superovulation can be achieved using various treatment protocols by prescribing combinations of hormonal preparations.

Oral medications such as clomiphene have a limited role in superovulation for IVF treatment. Natural or recombinant FSH injections are commonly used for superovulation. Human menopausal gonadotropins (hMG) contain urinary FSH and LH. Another preparation is purified urinary FSH. Technical difficulties, urinary protein contamination and initial concerns of unreliable dosing led to development of recombinant FSH (rFSH) which is 99 per cent pure FSH. Recombinant human FSH is produced from a Chinese hamster ovary cell line. The superiority of recombinant FSH versus urinary FSH is a much debated topic[3] but meta-analysis of RCTs suggests similar clinical pregnancy and livebirth rates.[4]

Recent studies suggested no increased risk of ovarian, uterine, cervical or breast cancer associated with ovarian stimulation medications. Previously some studies suggested borderline ovarian changes with long-standing high-dose clomiphene citrate; however, recently a cohort study confirmed there is no risk of borderline ovarian changes with any ovulation induction agents including clomiphene.[5,6]

Monitoring ovarian stimulation

Advances in transvaginal scanning along with Doppler assessment and 3D scanning techniques have changed ART practice significantly. Monitoring is routinely done to assess follicular response; this involves evaluating each ovary to document the number and size of growing follicles. The endometrium is also assessed to ensure appropriate endometrial development.

During this phase, there is a risk of OHSS, one of the most serious complications of IVF treatment.

Oocyte maturation

As endogenous LH release would have been suppressed in an IVF cycle (with GnRH agonist or antagonist), exogenous LH or an equivalent drug is required to achieve final oocyte maturation. The most commonly used agent is hCG, which has a similar chemical structure to LH. Recombinant LH preparations have equal efficacy to hCG but are rarely used.[7] The 'final trigger' injection of HCG or LH is administered 34–36 hours before oocyte retrieval.

Oocyte retrieval

Oocyte retrieval is generally performed via the transvaginal route under ultrasound guidance. A single or double lumen needle is passed through the lateral vaginal fornix to puncture the ovarian follicles and drain the follicular fluid. Care is taken to keep the aspirated fluid at body temperature and it is passed to the embryology lab for microscopic analysis to identify oocytes. Most frequently the risk is vaginal bleeding (venous or small arterial) which settles down with pressure. Very rarely this procedure can be associated with intraperitoneal bleeding, infection, bowel perforation and also failure to retrieve any oocytes. Oocyte retrieval can be performed using general anaesthesia or conscious sedation with or without local anaesthesia.

Sperm insemination and fertilisation

Oocytes are inseminated on the same day as oocyte retrieval using standard or ICSI techniques by using a fresh or frozen sperm sample produced by the male partner. Surgical collection of sperm is needed in cases of unexpected azoospermia in the ejaculated sample or if the male partner is unable to produce a fresh sample on the day of oocyte retrieval.

The day after insemination, oocytes are checked for presence of two pronuclei (one from the oocyte and one from the sperm) confirming normal fertilisation. Oocytes with no evidence of fertilisation or abnormal fertilisation are discarded. The remaining embryos are further incubated to allow development.

Embryo transfer

Embryos are transferred as cleavage embryos (Day 2 or Day 3) or at blastocyst stage (Day 5 or Day 6) (Fig. 84.1). Embryo transfer (ET) is done via a trans-cervical route using a polypropylene catheter and is usually straightforward, with no discomfort to the woman. Ultrasound-guided (trans-abdominal, performed by an assistant) ET provides reassurance for both the woman and the clinician. Utmost care is taken to avoid the catheter tip disturbing the uterine fundus which may trigger subendometrial–myometrial contractions. Trans-myometrial embryo transfer (TM-ET) is reserved for difficult cases. In the UK, women under the age of 40 can have a maximum of two embryos transferred and women over the age of 40 can have a maximum of three embryos transferred (using own oocytes). However the HFEA, along with NICE, recommends an elective single embryo transfer policy to reduce the risk of multiple pregnancy.

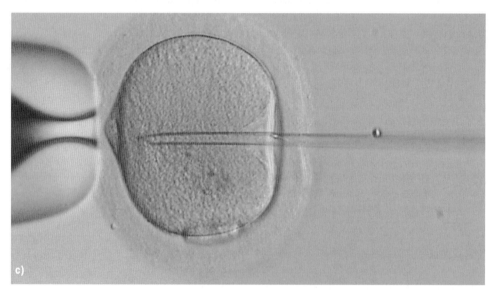
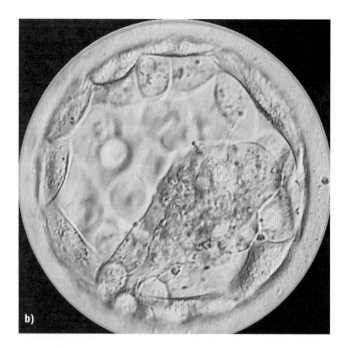

Fig. 84.1 a) Day 3 embryo with 8 cells. b) Early blastocyst. c) ICSI technique (a single sperm seen inside the pipette). (By courtesy of CARE Fertility Group, UK.)

Luteal phase support

The most commonly used medication is progesterone in the form of tablets, pessaries or injectable preparations. Even though not routinely used, some clinicians prefer to use additional hCG injections or oestrogen preparations. In cases of hormonally manipulated FET treatment, luteal-phase supplementation using progesterone and oestrogen is mandatory as the ovarian activity is suppressed by pituitary suppression. Once a pregnancy is established, luteal-phase support can be withdrawn at about 8–12 weeks when the early placenta takes over the function of pregnancy maintenance.

Confirming outcome of treatment

For those women who achieve an ET, a urinary or serum pregnancy test is performed 16 days post oocyte retrieval. If the test is positive, this corresponds to 4 weeks of gestation. In most cases luteal phase is extended until confirmation of viability which is by ultrasound assessment. In ART settings, this is routinely performed between 6 and 7 weeks of gestation (4–5 weeks after embryo transfer).

RISKS WITH ART

Other than specific procedure-related risks mentioned earlier, there may be risks for the offspring. There may be an association between ART and risks of developmental delay, low birthweight, birth defects, imprinting disorders, lower genital tract abnormalities (male offspring) and genetic transmission of Y-chromosome abnormalities. However, other factors such as maternal age, twin pregnancy and other epigenetic factors may also play a role.

A key risk of multiple ET is multiple pregnancy, which is associated with numerous obstetric and neonatal complications. ESET should be recommended whenever appropriate.

EMBRYO CRYOPRESERVATION

Women having surplus embryos can opt for embryo freezing after appropriate HFEA consents from both partners. Embryos can be frozen at the fertilisation stage, cleavage stage (Day 2/3) or at the blastocyst stage (Day 5/6). Embryo thaw survival rates are better when they are frozen at earlier stages of development. With advancement in vitrification or 'flash freezing'

KEY POINTS

- A typical IVF cycle involves pituitary suppression, superovulation, monitoring ovarian stimulation, oocyte maturation, oocyte retrieval, sperm insemination and fertilisation, embryo transfer, luteal-phase support and confirming outcome of treatment.
- Pituitary down-regulation can be achieved using GnRH agonists or antagonists.
- Superovulation can be achieved by urinary or recombinant FSH preparations.
- Trigger injection is administered 34–36 hours prior to oocyte retrieval.
- Oocyte retrieval can be performed by a transvaginal or laparoscopic approach.
- Sperm insemination is performed on the same day as oocyte retrieval.
- Embryos are transferred at cleavage or at blastocyst stage.
- In the UK, a maximum of two embryos may be transferred under the age of 40 and a maximum of three embryos over the age of 40.
- The most commonly used agent for luteal-phase support is progesterone.
- The greatest risks with ART are OHSS and multiple pregnancy.

---

process, better survival rates are observed. Women who suffer complications following oocyte retrieval, those with suboptimal endometrial quality or those at higher risk for OHSS should have their embryos frozen and should proceed with FET at a later date. They should be counselled about a small chance of a failed thawing process. Embryo cryopreservation is also undertaken to preserve fertility when one partner (in a stable relationship) is diagnosed with a significant medical condition or malignancy which may impact on their future fertility potential (Chapter 92).

References

1. Steptoe, PC, Edwards, RG. Reimplantation of a human embryo with subsequent tubal pregnancy. *Lancet* 1976;i,880–2.
2. Human Fertilisation & Embryology Authority. www.hefa.gov.uk
3. Raga F, Bonilla-Musoles F, Casan EM, Bonilla F. Recombinant follicle-stimulating hormone stimulation in poor responders with normal basal concentrations of follicle-stimulating hormone and oestradiol: improved reproductive outcome. *Human Reproduction* 1999;14:1431–4.
4. Al Inany H, Aboulghar M, Mansour R, Serour G. Meta-analysis of recombinant versus urinary-derived FSH: an update. *Hum. Reprod* 2003;18:305–13.
5. Jensen A, Sharif H, Frederiksen K, Kjaer SK. Use of fertility drugs and risk of ovarian cancer: Danish population based cohort study. *BMJ* 2009;338: b249.
6. Bjørnholt SM, Kjaer SK, Nielsen TS, Jensen A. Risk for borderline ovarian tumours after exposure to fertility drugs: results of a population-based cohort study. *Hum Reprod* 2015;30:222–31.
7. Youssef MA, Al-Inany HG, Aboulghar M, Mansour R, Abou-Setta AM. Recombinant versus urinary human chorionic gonadotrophin for final oocyte maturation triggering in IVF and ICSI cycles. *Cochrane Database Syst Rev* 2011;4:CD003719.

Chapter 85 Polycystic ovary syndrome

Adam H Balen

INTRODUCTION

Polycystic ovary syndrome is the most common endocrine disorder to affect women during their reproductive years.[1] The symptoms of PCOS include menstrual cycle disturbance and features of hyperandrogenism (hirsutism, acne, alopecia), with associated fertility problems, obesity and psychological issues. There is significant heterogeneity of presentation, such that signs and symptoms manifest across a spectrum and their severity may vary. Ovarian hyperandrogenism is thought to have genetic origins with amplification in some by hyperinsulinaemia secondary to insulin resistance, which in turn may be promoted by obesity. The primary presenting complaint itself is subject to change depending on the age and needs of the patient; for example acne may be a primary concern during adolescence whereas reduced fertility may be the main concern for an older woman. PCOS may also be associated with an increased the risk of an individual developing type 2 diabetes, the metabolic syndrome and endometrial cancer.[1,2] The symptoms of PCOS may have a profound impact on psychological well-being.[3] Options for treatment include lifestyle advice and a range of therapies depending upon the constellation of an individual's problems.[4]

PCOS appears to be underdiagnosed and, as a result, patients may not be managed appropriately.[5] Furthermore, management of PCOS may require the collaboration of a variety of healthcare professionals ranging from primary care physicians, gynaecologists, reproductive specialists, endocrinologists, diabetologists, dermatologists, dieticians and psychologists. In some clinics important components of the syndrome may not be considered; for example gynaecological problems in a dermatology clinic or metabolic problems in a gynaecology clinic. We have recently assessed a cohort of women presenting with features of PCOS in our hospital to infertility, gynaecology, dermatology and endocrine clinics.[5] Participants were assessed for symptoms and signs of PCOS and underwent a full endocrine and metabolic profile and a pelvic ultrasound scan. A significant difference between the four clinic groups existed with regards to frequency distribution of presenting symptoms as might have been expected with, for example, those in the dermatology clinic having more hirsutism and those in the gynaecology clinic a greater frequency of menstrual disturbance. It was striking that 81 per cent were overweight, 34 per cent had previously undiagnosed impaired glucose tolerance (IGT) and 9 per cent were found to be diabetic. This study emphasises the importance of understanding the full spectrum of PCOS as it presents to different specialty clinics. Not only is the syndrome underdiagnosed but so too are the significant associated morbidities such as IGT and type 2 diabetes.

DEFINING PCOS

In 2003 the European Society of Human Reproduction and Embryology (ESHRE) and the American Society of Reproductive Medicine (ASRM) held a consensus meeting in Rotterdam. They proposed that the diagnosis of PCOS should be made, once appropriate investigations have been performed to exclude other causes of menstrual disturbance and androgen excess, if two out of three criteria are met – the so-called 'Rotterdam Criteria':[1]

1 the presence of clinical or biochemical features of hyperandrogenism;
2 oligo-ovulation or anovulation (in other words a menstrual cycle disturbance);
3 polycystic ovaries on ultrasound.

This definition of PCOS requires the exclusion of specific underlying diseases of the adrenal or pituitary glands (e.g. hyperprolactinaemia, acromegaly, congenital adrenal hyperplasia, Cushing's syndrome, androgen-secreting tumors of the ovary or adrenal gland) which could predispose to similar ultrasound and biochemical features and also the exclusion of other causes of menstrual cycle irregularity secondary to hypothalamic, pituitary or ovarian dysfunction.

Box 85.1 outlines the clinical features, potential long-term sequelae and endocrine disturbances seen in women with PCOS. Tables 85.1 and 85.2 outline the investigations that are commonly performed and results expected and Table 85.3 outlines the gonadotrophin and oestradiol profiles that can be expected in different clinical scenarios.

There is considerable heterogeneity of symptoms and signs amongst women with PCOS and for an individual these may change over time. Polycystic ovaries can exist without clinical signs of the syndrome, expression of which may

Box 85.1 The spectrum of clinical manifestations of PCOS

Symptoms
- Hyperandrogenism (hirsutism, acne, alopecia)
- Menstrual disturbance
- Infertility
- Obesity
- Asymptomatic, with polycystic ovaries on ultrasound scan

Possible late sequelae
- Type 2 diabetes mellitus
- Dyslipidaemia
- Hypertension
- Cardiovascular disease
- Endometrial carcinoma

Serum endocrinology
- ↑ Androgens (testosterone and androstenedione)
- ↑ LH, normal FSH
- ↑ Fasting insulin (not routinely measured; insulin resistance assessed by GTT)
- ↓ Sex hormone binding globulin, results in elevated 'free androgen index' (FAI)
- ↑ Oestradiol, oestrone
- ↑ Anti-Müllerian hormone

Table 85.1 Investigations for PCOS

Test	Normal range (may vary with local laboratory assays)	Additional points
Testosterone (T)	0.5–1.8 nmol/L	It is unnecessary to measure other androgens unless total T >5 nmol/L
SHBG	16–119 nmol/L	Insulin suppresses SHBG, resulting in a high FAI in the presence of a normal total T
Free androgen index: T x 100/SHBG	<5	
Oestradiol	Usually normal, measurement is unhelpful to diagnosis	Oestrogenisation may be confirmed by endometrial assessment
LH	2–10 IU/L	Elevated in 40% of women with PCOS, especially those who are slim
FSH	2–8 IU/L	FSH and LH best measured during days 1–3 of a menstrual bleed. If oligo-/ amenorrhoeic then random samples are taken
Prolactin	<500 mU/L	Measure if oligo-/ amenorrhoeic
Thyroid function, TSH	0.5–5 IU/L	Measure if oligo-/ amenorrhoeic
Fasting insulin	<30 mU/L	Not routinely measured; insulin resistance assessed by GTT, see Table 85.2
Pelvic ultrasound	More than 12 follicles (cysts) 28 mm in diameter per ovary	To assess ovarian morphology and endometrial thickness; trans-abdominal scan satisfactory in women who are not sexually active
AMH	35 pmol/L	Not universally accepted and still debated; has been suggested as a biochemical marker for the polycystic ovary

Table 85.2 Definitions of glucose tolerance after a 75 g glucose tolerance test

	Diabetes mellitus	Impaired glucose tolerance	Impaired fasting glycaemia
Fasting glucose (mmol/L)	≥7.0	<7.0	≥6.1 and <7.0
2 hour glucose (mmol/L)	≥11.1	≥7.8 and ≤11.1	<7.8

Table 85.3 Gonadotrophin and oestradiol profiles in different clinical scenarios

Ovarian failure	↑ FSH	↑ LH	↓ Oestradiol
Hypothalamic or pituitary failure	↓ FSH	↓↓ LH	↓ Oestradiol
PCOS	n/↓ FSH	n/↑ LH	n/↑ Oestradiol
Mid-cycle, pre-ovulatory	↑ FSH	↑↑ LH	↑ Oestradiol

be precipitated by various factors, most predominantly an increase in bodyweight.

Debate continues regarding the reliability and reproducibility of the various tests that we have at our disposal, whether ultrasound or biochemical. Raised serum levels of LH, testosterone and androstenedione, in association with low or normal levels of FSH and abnormalities of oestrogen secretion, are variable findings and sometimes the endocrine profile may be normal. It is thought that the hyperandrogenism is driven by LH in slim women and in overweight women by insulin, which acts as a 'co-gonadotrophin' and amplifies the effect of LH.

ULTRASOUND

Polycystic ovaries are commonly detected by pelvic ultrasound, with estimates of the prevalence in the general population being in the order of 20–33 per cent.[6] The morphology of the polycystic ovary was also defined in the ESHRE/ASRM consensus as an ovary with 12 or more follicles measuring 2–9 mm in diameter and/or increased ovarian volume (>10 cm³).[7] With improvements in the resolution of ultrasound technology it has more recently been suggested that the threshold number of follicles to define a polycystic ovary should be increased and that the biochemical marker of anti-Müllerian hormone may be even more precise than ultrasound, although a figure has not been universally accepted.

EPIDEMIOLOGY AND PREVALENCE

Estimates of the prevalence of PCOS are greatly affected by the nature of the population which is being assessed. Populations of women who are selected on the basis of the presence of a symptom associated with the syndrome (e.g. hirsutism, acne and menstrual cycle disturbances) would be expected to demonstrate a prevalence greater than that which exists in the general population. The prevalence of PCOS in the general population has not been definitively determined and appears to vary considerably between populations that have been studied and the diagnostic criteria being employed and has ranged from 4 per cent to 26 per cent.[6]

PCOS tends to run in families, although there is not a single gene or pathway that causes the syndrome; however there may be genetic factors that affect expression and presentation – whether because of racial differences in the colour and distribution of hair or variations in hormone production and receptor activity. For example women from the Far East (e.g. Japan) with PCOS do not present with excess bodily or facial hair despite having dark hair and elevated testosterone levels, whereas those from Mediterranean countries or South Asia with similar hormone profiles may have profound hirsutism. There may be profound ethnic variations in the presentation of PCOS, for example South Asian women in the UK with PCOS have greater insulin resistance and more severe symptoms of the syndrome than white Caucasians with PCOS. These variations in the overt features of PCOS (symptoms of hyperandrogenism, menstrual irregularity and obesity) in women of South Asian descent are linked to the higher prevalence and degree of insulin resistance in South Asians. Type 2 diabetes and insulin resistance have a high prevalence among indigenous populations in South Asia, with a rising prevalence among women. Type 2 diabetes also has a familial basis, inherited as a complex genetic trait that interacts with environmental factors, chiefly nutrition, commencing from fetal life.[8]

PCOS AND METABOLIC ABNORMALITIES

Women with PCOS are characterised by the presence of insulin resistance, central obesity and dyslipidaemia, which appears to place them at a higher risk of developing diabetes as well as cardiovascular disease. There are a number of environmental factors that may influence the expression of the syndrome, in particular a tendency to insulin-resistant states induced by overeating and under-exercising. A plausible hypothesis for the survival of PCOS in the population is that of the 'thrifty phenotype/genotype' whereby in times of famine, individuals who have a tendency to obesity preserve the population by maintaining fertility, while those of normal bodyweight fall below the threshold bodyweight for fertility. This might explain the greater prevalence of PCOS among South Asians in the UK, where there is relatively greater nutrition and thus the right environment to express PCOS. In addition the 'thrifty phenotype' hypothesis suggests that insulin resistance *in utero* results as an adaptation to impaired nutrition and then persists through to adult life and is then amplified by overnutrition (obesity).

Women who are obese, and also many slim women with PCOS, will have insulin resistance and elevated serum concentrations of insulin (usually <30 mU/L fasting). We suggest that a 75 g oral GTT be performed in women with PCOS and a BMI >30 kg/m^2, with an assessment of the fasting and 2-hour glucose concentrations (Table 85.2). It has been suggested that South Asian women should have an assessment of glucose tolerance if their BMI is greater than 25 kg/m^2 because of the greater risk of insulin resistance at a lower BMI than seen in the Caucasian population.

Although the insulin resistance may occur irrespective of BMI, the common association of PCOS and obesity has a synergistic deleterious impact on glucose homeostasis and can worsen both hyperandrogenism and anovulation. It has been suggested that rather than BMI itself it is the distribution of fat that is important, with android obesity being more of a risk factor than gynaecoid obesity. Hence the value of measuring waist:hip ratio, or waist circumference, which detects abdominal visceral fat rather than subcutaneous fat. It is the visceral fat which is metabolically active and when increased results in increased rates of insulin resistance, type 2 diabetes, dyslipidaemia and hypertension. Waist circumference should ideally be less than 79 cm, whilst a measurement that is greater than 87 cm carries a significant risk. Exercise has a significant effect on reducing visceral fat and reducing cardiovascular risk – indeed a 10 per cent reduction in bodyweight may equate with a 30 per cent reduction in visceral fat.

HEALTH CONSEQUENCES OF PCOS

Cardiovascular disease and diabetes

Young women with PCOS who are obese have a 10–20 per cent risk of IGT and, if left untreated, have an approximately 50 per cent chance of developing type 2 diabetes in the next five years. Obesity and metabolic abnormalities are recognised risk factors for the development of ischaemic heart disease (IHD) in the general population, and these are also recognised features of PCOS. There have been a few studies that have tried to assess the long-term risk for women with PCOS and, interestingly, whilst diabetes has been associated with increase in mortality, death rates from cardiovascular disease have not been found to be higher than the normal population.[9]

Endometrial cancer

Endometrial adenocarcinoma is the second most common female genital malignancy but only 4 per cent of cases occur in women less than 40 years of age. The risk of developing endometrial cancer has been shown to be adversely influenced by a number of factors including obesity, long-term use of unopposed oestrogens, nulliparity and infertility. Women with PCOS who are amenorrhoeic have unopposed oestrogen secretion as, in the absence of ovulation, progesterone is not released by the ovary and so the endometrium is not shed as a menstrual bleed. The endometrium may then become hyperplastic and endometrial hyperplasia may progress to cystic glandular hyperplasia with atypical cellular changes and in time lead to endometrial adenocarcinoma. The true risk of carcinoma in women with PCOS, however, is difficult to ascertain but is thought to be increased approximately threefold compared with the normal population.[9] It is therefore important that women with PCOS shed their endometrium either monthly or at the very least every 3 months, which can be achieved either by cyclical administration of a progestogen or a COCP. Another option is to consider a progestogen-secreting intrauterine system such as the Mirena®.

PCOS does not appear to increase the risk for carcinoma of the breast or ovary.

MANAGEMENT OF PCOS

Psychological support and quality of life

The symptoms typically associated with the condition have also been shown to lead to a significant reduction in health-related quality of life (HRQoL). HRQoL is a multidimensional, dynamic concept that encompasses physical, psychological and social aspects that are associated with a particular disease or its treatment. Therefore any management of the woman with PCOS needs to consider and understand the negative impact this condition may have upon these psychosocial parameters. For example, although the management of hirsutism may be considered as a purely cosmetic issue, excessive facial hair has been shown to be one of the major causes of marked psychological stress in women with PCOS, often caused by embarrassment about the excessive hair growth. Infertility and weight issues have also been found to affect other social and psychological parameters. Infertility can cause tensions within the family, altered self-perception, and problems at work. Whilst obesity worsens the symptoms, the metabolic scenario conspires against weight loss and many women experience frustration in attempts to lose weight and suffer from low self-esteem and poor body image.[9]

Obesity

The management of women with PCOS should be focused on the patient's particular problems. Obesity worsens both symptomatology and the endocrine profile and so obese women (BMI >30 kg/m^2) should be encouraged to lose weight, by a combination of calorie restriction and exercise. Weight loss improves the endocrine profile and the likelihood of ovulation and a healthy pregnancy. There is no evidence that women with PCOS benefit from a specific diet compared with obese women without PCOS. The right diet for an individual is one that is practical, sustainable and compatible with her lifestyle. There does not appear to be a particular diet that is most appropriate for women with PCOS. It is sensible to reduce glycaemic load by lowering sugar content in favour of more complex carbohydrates and to avoid fatty foods. Meal replacement therapy or low-calorie diets may be appropriate; it is often helpful to refer to a dietitian, if available. An increase in physical activity is essential, preferably as part of the daily routine. Thirty minutes per day of brisk exercise is encouraged to maintain health, but to lose weight, or sustain weight loss, 60 to 90 minutes per day is advised. Concurrent behavioural therapy improves the chances of success of any method of weight loss. Furthermore there are no medications that have been shown to assist with long-term weight reduction. Bariatric surgery is used increasingly because of the global epidemic of obesity and certainly has a role in the management of obese women with PCOS. It is recommended by some that anyone with a BMI of more than 40 kg/m^2 should be referred for consideration for bariatric surgery. If there are co-morbidities, such as diabetes, then the BMI cut-off for surgery is lower at $30–35 \text{ kg/m}^2$.

Menstrual irregularity

The simplest way to control the menstrual cycle is the use of a low-dose COCP. This will result in an artificial cycle and regular shedding of the endometrium. It is also important once again to encourage weight loss. As women with PCOS are thought to be at increased risk of cardiovascular disease a 'lipid-friendly' combined contraceptive pill should be used. The third-generation oral contraceptives are lipid friendly but present the potential disadvantage of venous thromboembolism, particularly in overweight women. Dianette® and Yasmin® are both COCPs that respectively contain the anti-androgens cyproterone acetate and drospirenone, which is a derivative of spironolactone, although any COCP will help suppress ovarian hyperandrogenism and concurrently achieve an elevation in SHBG production and thereby help suppress the free androgen levels. Alternatives to the COCP include a progestogen, for example medroxyprogesterone acetate (Provera®), for 12 days every 1–3 months to induce a withdrawal bleed, or simply the insertion of a Mirena® intra-uterine system.

In women with anovulatory cycles the action of estradiol on the endometrium is unopposed because of the lack of cyclical progesterone secretion. This may result in episodes of irregular uterine bleeding, and in the long term endometrial hyperplasia and even endometrial cancer (see above). An ultrasound assessment of endometrial thickness provides a bioassay for oestradiol production by the ovaries and conversion of androgens in the peripheral fat. If the endometrium is thicker than 10 mm a withdrawal bleed should be induced and if the endometrium fails to shed then endometrial sampling is required to exclude endometrial hyperplasia or malignancy.

Hyperandrogenism and hirsutism

The bioavailability of testosterone is affected by the serum concentration of SHBG. High levels of insulin lower the production of SHBG and so increase the free fraction of androgen. Elevated serum androgen concentrations stimulate peripheral androgen receptors, resulting in an increase in 5-alpha reductase activity directly increasing the conversion of testosterone to the more potent metabolite, dihydrotestosterone. Symptoms of hyperandrogenism include hirsutism and acne, which are both distressing conditions. Hirsutism is characterised by terminal hair growth in a male pattern of distribution, including chin, upper lip, chest, upper and lower back, upper and lower abdomen, upper arm, thigh and buttocks. A standardised scoring system, such as the modified Ferriman and Gallwey score, should be used to evaluate the degree of hirsutism before and during treatments.

Treatment options include cosmetic and medical therapies. As drug therapies may take 6–9 months or longer before any improvement of hirsutism is perceived physical treatments including electrolysis, waxing and bleaching may be helpful whilst waiting for medical treatments to work. For many years the most 'permanent' physical treatment for unwanted hair has been electrolysis. It is time consuming, painful and expensive and should be performed by an expert practitioner. Regrowth is not uncommon and there is no really permanent cosmetic treatment but the last few years have seen much development in the use of laser and photothermolysis techniques. Repeated treatments are required for a near-permanent effect because only hair follicles in the growing phase are obliterated at each treatment.

Eflornithine (Vaniqua®) has been recently developed as a topical treatment for hirsutism. It works by inhibiting the enzyme ornithine decarboxylase in hair follicles and may be a useful therapy for those who wish to avoid hormonal treatments but may also be used in conjunction with hormonal therapy.

Any COCP is likely to help improve symptoms of hyperandrogenism. An effective therapy is Dianette® which contains ethinyloestradiol ($35 \mu g$) in combination with 2 mg synthetic progestogen cyproterone acetate which is antigonadotrophic and anti-androgenic. The anti-androgen effect reduces sebum excretion in 2–3 months and results in clinical improvement in acne in 4–6 months. Medical regimens should stop further progression of hirsutism and decrease the rate of hair growth. Therapy for acne should aim to lower sebum excretion, alter follicular cell desquamation, reduce propionibacteria and reduce inflammation.

Spironolactone is a weak diuretic with anti-androgenic properties and may be used in women with hirsutism and/or acne in whom the COCP is contraindicated, at a daily dose of 25–100 mg. If using anti-androgen therapy, adequate contraception is important in women of reproductive age as transplacental passage of anti-androgens may disturb the genital development of a male fetus. Other anti-androgens such as ketoconazole, finasteride and flutamide have been tried, but are not widely used in the UK for the treatment of hirsutism in women due to their adverse and potentially serious side effects.

MANAGEMENT OF INFERTILITY IN PCOS

PCOS accounts for approximately 80–90 per cent of women with anovulatory infertility, which in turn comprises about a third of those attending the infertility clinic. Various factors influence ovarian function and fertility, the most important being obesity. A patient's weight correlates with both an increased rate of cycle disturbance and infertility secondary to disturbances in insulin metabolism. Monitoring treatment is also harder in obese women because their ovaries are more difficult to see on ultrasound scans, thus raising the risk of missing multiple ovulation and multiple pregnancy. National guidelines in the UK for managing overweight women with PCOS advise weight loss, preferably to a BMI of less than 30 kg/m², before commencing drugs for ovarian stimulation. Hypersecretion of LH is found in 40 per cent of women with PCOS and is associated with a reduced chance of conception and an increased risk of miscarriage, possibly through an adverse effect of LH on oocyte maturation. Elevated LH concentrations are more often found in slim women with PCOS, whilst those who are overweight are more likely to be hyperinsulinaemic.

Strategies to induce ovulation include weight loss, oral anti-oestrogens (principally clomiphene citrate), parenteral gonadotrophin therapy and laparoscopic ovarian surgery. There have been no adequately powered RCTs to determine which of these therapies provides the best overall chance of an ongoing pregnancy when used as first-line therapy. Women with PCOS are at risk of OHSS and so ovulation induction has to be carefully monitored with serial ultrasound scans. The realisation of an association between hyperinsulinaemia and PCOS has resulted in the use of insulin-sensitising agents such as metformin, although results have been disappointing.[4,10]

Carefully conducted and monitored ovulation induction can achieve good cumulative conception rates and, furthermore, multiple pregnancy rates can be minimised with strict adherence to criteria that limit the number of follicles that are permitted to ovulate.

Clomiphene citrate therapy

Prior to commencing ovulation induction therapy it is important to comprehensively investigate the couple, with a full endocrine profile, assessment of rubella immunity and tubal patency together with a semen analysis (see Chapter 82). The anti-oestrogen clomiphene citrate (CC) has traditionally been used as first-line therapy for anovulatory PCOS. CC therapy is usually commenced on day 2 of the cycle and given for 5 days. If the patient has oligo/amenorrhoea it is necessary to exclude pregnancy and then induce a withdrawal bleed with a short course of a progestogen, such as medroxyprogesterone acetate 20 mg/day for 5 to 10 days. The starting dose of CC is 50 mg/day, for 5 days beginning on days 3–5 of the menstrual cycle (the first day of bleeding is considered day 1 of the cycle). If the patient has not menstruated by day 35 and she is not pregnant, a progestogen-induced withdrawal bleed should be initiated. The dose of CC may be increased to 100 mg if there is no response. Doses of 150 mg/day or more appear not to be of benefit. If there is an exuberant response to 50 mg/day, as in some women with PCOS, the dose can be decreased to 25 mg/day. Discontinuation of CC therapy should be considered if the patient is anovulatory after the dose has been increased up to 100 mg/day. If the patient is ovulating conception is expected to occur at a rate determined by factors such as the patient's age. CC induces ovulation in approximately 70–85 per cent of patients and approximately 60–70 per cent should be pregnant by six cycles of therapy.

CC may cause an exaggeration in the hypersecretion of LH and have anti-oestrogenic effects on the endometrium and cervical mucus. All women who are prescribed CC should be carefully monitored with a combination of endocrine and ultrasonographic assessment of follicular growth and ovulation because of the risk of multiple pregnancies, which is approximately 10 per cent. Clomiphene therapy should therefore be prescribed and managed by specialists in reproductive medicine.

If pregnancy has not occurred after 6–9 normal ovulatory cycles it is then reasonable to offer the couple assisted conception (i.e. IVF). Patients with anovulatory infertility who are resistant to anti-oestrogens may be prescribed parenteral gonadotrophin therapy or treated with laparoscopic ovarian surgery. The term 'clomiphene resistance, strictly speaking refers to a failure to ovulate rather than failure to conceive despite ovulation, which should be termed 'clomiphene failure'.

Gonadotrophin therapy

Gonadotrophin therapy is indicated for women with anovulatory PCOS who have been treated with anti-oestrogens if they have failed to ovulate or if they have a response to clomifene that is likely to reduce their chance of conception (e.g. persistent hypersecretion of LH, or anti-oestrogenic effect on cervical mucus).

In order to prevent the risks of overstimulation and multiple pregnancy, a low-dose step-up regimen should be used with a daily starting dose of 25–50 IU of FSH or hMG. This is only increased after 14 days if there is no response and then by only half an ampoule every 7 days. Treatment cycles using this approach can be quite long – up to 28–35 days – but the risk of multiple follicular growth is low and the multiple pregnancy rate should be less than 5 per cent. It can be extremely difficult to predict the response to stimulation of a woman with polycystic ovaries; indeed this is the greatest therapeutic challenge in all ovulation induction therapies. The polycystic ovary is characteristically quiescent, at least when viewed by ultrasound, before often exhibiting an exuberant and explosive response to stimulation. It can be very challenging to stimulate the development of a single dominant follicle.

Ovulation is triggered with a single subcutaneous injection of hCG 5000 units, when there has been the development of at least one follicle of at least 17 mm in its largest diameter. In order to reduce the risks of multiple pregnancy and OHSS, the exclusion criteria for hCG administration are the development of a total of two or more follicles larger than 14 mm in diameter. In overstimulated cycles hCG is withheld, and the patient counselled about the risks and advised to refrain from sexual intercourse. The cumulative conception and livebirth rates after 6 months should be 65–70 per cent and 55–60 per cent, respectively. If conception has failed to occur after six ovulatory cycles in a woman younger than 25 years or after 12 ovulatory cycles in women older than 25, then it can be assumed that anovulation is unlikely to be the cause of the couple's infertility and assisted conception (usually IVF) is now indicated.

Complications of ovulation induction

Women with PCOS are at an increased risk of developing OHSS. This occurs if many follicles are stimulated, leading to ascites, pleural and, sometimes, pericardial effusions with the symptoms of abdominal distension, discomfort, nausea, vomiting and difficult breathing. Hospitalisation is sometimes necessary in order for intravenous fluids (colloids preferable to crystalloids) and heparin to be given to prevent dehydration and thromboembolism. Although this condition is rare it is a potentially fatal complication and should be avoidable with appropriate monitoring of treatment.

Multiple pregnancy is the other undesirable side effect of fertility therapy, first because of the increased rates of perinatal morbidity and mortality and second because of the devastating effects on the family of caring for a large number of babies. High-order multiple pregnancies (quadruplets or more) result almost exclusively from ovulation induction therapies. Gonadotrophins should be given in low doses to women with anovulatory infertility and strict criteria employed before the administration of the ovulatory trigger.

Insulin-sensitising agents

It is logical to assume that therapy that achieves a fall in serum insulin concentrations should improve the symptoms of PCOS. The biguanide metformin both inhibits the production of hepatic glucose, thereby decreasing insulin secretion, and also enhances insulin sensitivity at the cellular level. In the last decade many studies have been carried out to evaluate the reproductive effects of metformin in patients with PCOS. Initial studies appeared to be promising, suggesting that metformin could improve fertility in women with PCOS; however, more recent large RCTs have observed no benefit from metformin as either first-line therapy or in combination with other drugs.[11]

Surgical ovulation induction

An alternative to gonadotrophin therapy for clomiphene-resistant PCOS is laparoscopic ovarian diathermy, which involves burning four 'holes' into each ovary with a diathermy probe. This has replaced the more invasive and damaging technique of ovarian wedge resection. Laparoscopic ovarian diathermy is free of the risks of multiple pregnancy and ovarian hyperstimulation and does not require intensive ultrasound monitoring. Furthermore, ovarian diathermy appears to be as effective as routine gonadotrophin therapy in the treatment of clomiphene-insensitive PCOS, although it does take longer to conceive and often additional therapy with CC or gonadotrophins is required after surgery if ovulation is not occuring.[12] In addition, laparoscopic ovarian surgery is a useful therapy for anovulatory women with PCOS who fail to respond to clomiphene and who persistently hypersecrete LH, or who live too far away from the hospital to be able to attend for the intensive monitoring required in gonadotrophin therapy. Surgery does, of course, carry its own risks and must be performed only by fully trained laparoscopic surgeons.

IVF in women with polycystic ovaries

IVF is not the first-line treatment for PCOS, but many patients with the syndrome may be referred for IVF, either because there is another reason for their infertility or because they fail to conceive despite ovulating (whether spontaneously or with assistance) – i.e. their infertility remains unexplained. Furthermore, approximately 30 per cent of women have polycystic ovaries as detected by ultrasound scan. Many will have little in the way of symptoms and may present for assisted conception treatment because of other reasons (for example tubal factor or male factor). When stimulated, these women with asymptomatic polycystic ovaries have a tendency to respond sensitively and are at increased risk of developing OHSS. Care must therefore be taken and there is evidence of reduced risk if protocols using a GnRH antagonist are employed .

PREGNANCY OUTCOMES

Women with PCOS may conceive naturally or, if they have anovulatory infertility, by ovulation induction (OI). In addition to anovulation there may be other factors that contribute to subfertility in women with PCOS including the effects of obesity, metabolic, inflammatory and endocrine abnormalities on oocyte quality and fetal development. Women who are obese are also more likely to experience miscarriage and pregnancy complications. A number of studies have compared pregnancy outcomes between women with PCOS and controls and have found that women with PCOS demonstrated a significantly higher risk of developing gestational diabetes, pregnancy-induced hypertension, pre-eclampsia, adverse neonatal outcomes and preterm birth.[13] Their babies had a significantly higher risk of admission to a NICU and a higher perinatal mortality, unrelated to multiple births. The potential mechanisms for these problems include obesity, altered glucose metabolism and disturbances in uterine blood flow and so careful monitoring of pregnancy is required.

CONCLUSIONS

PCOS is one of the most common endocrine disorders. It may present, at one end of the spectrum, with the single finding of polycystic ovarian morphology as detected by pelvic ultrasound. At the other end of the spectrum, symptoms such as obesity, hyperandrogenism, menstrual cycle disturbance and infertility may occur, either singly or in combination. Ovarian dysfunction leads to the main signs and symptoms and the ovary is influenced by external factors, in particular the gonadotrophins, insulin and other growth factors, which are dependent upon both genetic and environmental influences. There are long-term risks of developing diabetes and possibly cardiovascular disease in addition to the risk of endometrial hyperplasia and adenocarcinoma secondary to unopposed oestrogen. Therapy should be tailored to an individual's symptoms and needs, which may change over her lifespan.

KEY POINTS

- PCOS is the commonest endocrine disorder in women (prevalence 15-20%).
- PCOS is a heterogeneous condition. Diagnosis is made by two out of three of the following: menstrual disturbance; hyperandrogenism (clinical or biochemical); the ultrasound detection of polycystic ovaries. Appropriate investigations are required to exclude other causes of menstrual irregularity or hyperandrogenism.
- Management is symptom orientated.
- If obese, weight loss should be encouraged to improve symptoms, reproductive function and long-term health. A GTT should be performed if the BMI is >30 kg/m^2 (or >25 kg/m^2 if from South Asia).
- Menstrual cycle control is achieved by cyclical oral contraceptives or progestogens or a Mirena intrauterine system can be used to protect the endometrium.
- Ovulation induction may be difficult and require progression through various treatments which should be monitored carefully to prevent multiple pregnancy.
- Hyperandrogenism is usually managed with the COCPs Dianette or Yasmin. Alternatives include spironolactone. Flutamide and finasteride are not routinely prescribed because of potential adverse effects. Reliable contraception is required with anti-androgen therapy.
- Insulin-sensitising agents (e.g. metformin) appear to be of limited, if any, benefit may be prescribed when there is impaired glucose tolerance.

Key References

1. Rotterdam ESHRE/ASRM-Sponsored PCOS Consensus Workshop Group. Revised 2003 consensus on diagnostic criteria and long-term health risks related to polycystic ovary syndrome. *Hum Reprod* 2004;19:41–7.

2. Cussons AJ, Watts GF, Burke V, Shaw JE, Zimmet PZ, Stuckey BG. Cardiometabolic risk in polycystic ovary syndrome: a comparison of different approaches to defining the metabolic syndrome. *Hum Reprod* 2008;23:2352–8.

3. Jones GL, Hall JM, Balen AH, Ledger W. Health-related quality-of-life measurement in women with polycystic ovary syndrome: a systematic review. *Human Reproduction Update* 2008;14:15–25.

4. Balen AH, Franks S, Homburg R (eds). *Current Management of Polycystic Ovary Syndrome.* Proceedings of 59th RCOG Study Group. London: RCOG Press, 2010.

5. Sivayoganathan D, Maruthini D, Glanville JM, Balen AH. Full investigation of patients with polycystic ovary syndrome (PCOS) presenting to four different clinical specialties reveals significant differences and undiagnosed morbidity: *Human Fertility* 2011;14: 261–5.

6. Michelmore KF, Balen AH, Dunger DB, Vessey MP. Polycystic ovaries and associated clinical and biochemical features in young women. *Clin Endocrinol Oxf* 1999;51:779–86.

7. Balen AH, Laven JSE, Tan SL, Dewailly D. Ultrasound assessment of the polycystic ovary: international consensus definitions. *Human Reproduction Update* 2003;9:505–14.

8. Wijeyeratne CN, Kumarapeli V, Seneviratne Rde A *et al.* Ethnic variations in the expression of polycystic ovary syndrome. *In:* Balen AH, Franks S, Homburg R (eds). *Current Management of Polycystic Ovary Syndrome.* Proceedings of 59th RCOG Study Group. London: RCOG Press, 2010;25–46.

9. Fauser BCJM, Tarlatzis BC, Rerbar RW *et al.* Consensus on women's health aspects of polycystic ovary syndrome (PCOS): the Amsterdam ESHRE/ASRM-Sponsored 3rd PCOS Consensus Workshop Group. Simultaneous Publication *Human Reproduction* 2012;27:14–24 and *Fertility & Sterility* 2012;97:28–38.

10. ESHRE/ASRM-Sponsored PCOS Consensus Workshop Group, Thessaloniki, Greece. Tarlatzis BC (Gr), Fauser B C (Nl), Chang J (USA), Franks S (UK), Legro R (USA), Rebar RW (USA), Azziz R (USA), Balen A (UK), Bouchard P (Fr), Carr BR (USA), Casper RF (Can), Collins J (Can), Crosigniani PG (It), DeCherney A (USA), Devroey P (B), Diedrich K (G), Eijkemans R (Nl), Farquhar C (NZ), Fleming R (UK), Goulis DG (Gr), Griesinger G (Ger), Ho PC (HK), Hoeger K (USA), Homburg R (Is), Hugues JN (Fr), Kolibianakis EM (Gr), Lobo R (USA), Messinis IE(Gr), Norman RJ (Aus), Pasquali R (It), van Steirteghem A (B). Human Reproduction 2008; 23: 462–77. *Fertility and Sterility* 2008;89:505–22.

11. Tang T, Lord JM, Norman RJ, Yasmin E, Balen AH. Insulin-sensitising drugs (metformin, rosiglitazone, pioglitazone, D-chiro-inositol) for women with polycystic ovary syndrome, oligo amenorrhoea and subfertility. *Cochrane Database of Systematic Reviews* 2012,5: CD003053. DOI: 10.1002/14651858.CD003053.pub5.

12. Bayram N, van Wely M, Kaaijk EM, Bossuyt PMM, van der Veen F. Using an electrocautery strategy or recombinant FSH to induce ovulation in polycystic ovary syndrome: a randomised controlled trial. *BMJ* 2004;328:192–5.

13. Boomsma CM, Eijkemans MJ, Hughes EG, Visser GH, Fauser BC, Macklon NS. A meta-analysis of pregnancy outcomes in women with polycystic ovary syndrome. *Hum Reprod Update* 2006;12:673–83.

Chapter 86 Hirsutism and virilism

Mostafa Metwally and William Ledger

HIRSUTISM

Definition

Hirsutism is defined as male pattern hair growth in a female as a result of increased androgen production or increased skin sensitivity to circulating androgens. Hirsutism must be differentiated from hypertrichosis, which is a generalised non-sexual (vellus) hair growth that may be hereditary, or due to various medications or malignancies. It is important to recognise that hirsutism in itself is not a diagnosis but rather a manifestation of a large spectrum of abnormalities; so a careful search for the underlying cause is essential.

The physiology of hair growth

Adults have two types of hair, vellus and terminal. Vellus hair is the fine lightly pigmented hair that covers most areas of the body during the prepubertal years, while terminal hair is the thick pigmented hair normally present on the face, limbs, axilla and pubic area. It is this hair that is androgen dependent and is influenced by genetic and racial factors.

Hair growth is a dynamic process and can be divided into three distinct phases. The relative duration of these different stages influences the length and appearance of hair in different parts of the body:

1 *Anagen:* This is the growing phase during which active mitotic division occurs in the basal matrix. This stage is relatively long in areas such as the scalp where hair appears to be continuously growing. Similarly, facial hair also has a long growth phase, which is why the effects of therapy require six to nine months before becoming apparent.[1] Consequently, the focus of hirsutism treatment is to shorten this phase.[2]
2 *Catagen:* During this phase, hair growth ceases and the hair follicle prepares to enter the resting (telogen) phase.
3 *Telogen:* During this resting phase, the hair is short and loosely attached to be ultimately expelled as the follicle again enters the anagen phase and a new hair starts growing.

Incidence

It is difficult to state exactly the prevalence of hirsutism since it is highly variable depending on the studied ethnic group, being higher in those of African or Mediterranean origin. The condition, however, is believed to affect 5–10 per cent of women of reproductive age.[3]

Female androgens and hair growth

Pivotal to the understanding of hirsutism is an understanding of the metabolism of androgens in the female and how they can affect hair growth. Female androgens are produced by two sources, namely the ovaries and adrenal glands. The ovaries produce testosterone and androstenedione, whilst the adrenals produce androstenedione and dehydroepiandrosterone (DHEA). Testosterone in the ovary is produced by the theca cells under the control of LH and insulin acting through IGF-1. Testosterone is then converted by the granulosa cells to oestradiol. This transition of the ovarian environment from androgen dominant to oestrogen dominant is vital to normal ovulation and ovarian function. In conditions such as PCOS where this process is disturbed, there is a relative increase in ovarian androgen production. Adrenal androgens are also peripherally converted to testosterone, which then circulates in two forms, an inactive form bound to SHBG and a metabolically active free form. To stimulate hair growth, free testosterone needs to be further metabolised at the level of the hair follicle into a more active form, DHT, by the enzyme 5α reductase. Consequently, hirsutism can be caused by any of the following disturbances:

- Increased production of adrenal or ovarian androgens: Adrenal androgens can increase in Cushing's syndrome, delayed-onset congenital adrenal hyperplasia and androgen-producing adrenal tumours. However, the most common cause in clinical practice is an increased production of ovarian and, to a lesser extent, adrenal androgens as a result of PCOS.
- An increase in the free fraction of testosterone due to a decreased concentration of SHBG despite normal testosterone production. Decreased SHBG can occur due to increased insulin concentrations in women with insulin resistance, which again is a common finding in women with PCOS.[4]
- An increased local activity of 5α reductase. Two forms of this enzyme exist, type 1 and type 2. Type 1 is mainly present in the sebaceous gland, while type 2 is found mainly in the hair follicle. Relative activity of these isoenzymes can lead to a discrepancy between the severity of hirsutism and acne in women with hyperandrogenism.[5] In women with PCOS – especially those who are obese or are insulin resistant – insulin and IGF act to stimulate this enzyme.
- Iatrogenic hirsutism can be caused by the administration of certain medications, such as danazol, androgen therapy, sodium valporate and anabolic steroids.

Clinical assessment of hirsutism

History

A detailed history should include the following:

- The severity and duration of hirsutism, as well as the presence of any other symptoms of virilisation. Rapidly progressive virilisation or severe hirsutism point to the possibility of a more ominous cause, such as an ovarian or adrenal tumour.
- Associated menstrual disturbances or history of infertility may point to chronic anovulation as a result of PCOS.
- History suggestive of other related medical conditions, such as Cushing's syndrome or hypothyroidism.
- Medications such as steroids, androgen therapy or danazol.

Examination

- Evaluation of the severity of hirsutism is commonly performed using the Ferriman–Gallwey scoring system.

The score includes an evaluation of nine androgen-sensitive body areas. Each area is assigned a score from 0 to 4 and the scores are then added. A minimal score of 8 is required for the diagnosis of hirsutism. The disadvantages of this method are that it does not account for focal hirsutism. In addition, it ignores some androgen-sensitive areas, such as the buttocks and sideburns.[1]
- General examination may show other manifestations of androgen excess, such as acne or signs of virilisation (e.g. clitoromegaly, male pattern balding).
- The presence of velvety, pigmented skin patches (acanthosis nigricans) in the groin, neck or axillae may point to associated insulin resistance. The combination of hirsutism together with acanthosis nigricans and insulin resistance is a hereditary condition known as HAIR-AN syndrome. It is possibly due to an insulin receptor defect and can be associated with severe hirsutism.[6]
- Pelvic examination in severe cases may reveal the presence of a pelvic mass (androgen-producing ovarian tumour).

Investigations

- Testosterone concentrations: The need to measure testosterone concentrations in patients with mild isolated hirsutism is debatable, since over half of these women will have normal concentrations and results are unlikely to influence treatment.[1] Testosterone concentrations also correlate poorly with the severity of hirsutism due to individual variations in hair follicle response. Testosterone measurements are however indicated in women with other symptoms, such as menstrual irregularities, infertility, severe hirsutism or in the presence of virilism. Measurement of the free androgen index is particularly useful since it reflects changes in SHBG as well as testosterone. Obese and PCOS patients may have an elevated FAI when the testosterone concentrations are normal due to a decrease in SHBG. High testosterone concentrations (>5 mmol/L) may suggest an androgen-producing tumour. DHEA concentrations may also be measured and if markedly elevated may suggest an adrenal cause.
- Baseline 17-OH progesterone measurements should be performed to screen for suspected cases of late-onset CAH. Equivocal results will need a short Synacthen test to confirm the diagnosis. After measurement of baseline 17-OH progesterone concentrations, the patient is given an intramuscular injection of 250 mg of Synacthen and measurements are taken again after 1 hour. A significant rise in 17-OH progesterone concentrations is diagnostic of CAH.
- Tests for insulin resistance (75 g GTT and insulin concentrations) are particularly important in PCOS and obese patients.
- Dexamethasone suppression test and 24-hour urinary free cortisol for suspected cases of Cushing's syndrome.
- Pelvic imaging may show the presence of polycystic ovaries or an androgen-producing ovarian tumour. More detailed imaging (CT and MRI) may be required in cases

of suspected androgen-producing ovarian or adrenal tumours. In cases where imaging is negative, selective venous sampling from the ovarian and adrenal veins may be performed.

VIRILISM

Hirsutism may occur together with other symptoms of defeminisation in a condition known as 'virilism'. Other signs and symptoms include secondary amenorrhoea, male pattern baldness, clitoromegaly and deepening of voice. The condition usually indicates significant pathology, including the following:

- Androgen-producing ovarian and adrenal tumours: This should be suspected in the presence of progressive severe virilisation.
- Adult onset CAH: This is most commonly due to 21-hydroxylase deficiency, leading to a blockage of the production of 11-deoxycortisol from 17-OH progesterone with a consequent diversion of steroidogenesis to the androgen pathway.
- XY females with functioning testicles will usually present around the time of puberty with primary amenorrhoea and signs of virilisation. The diagnosis can be confirmed with karyotyping.
- Iatrogenic, due to androgen therapy or the use of danazol to treat endometriosis.
- Cushing's syndrome and acromegaly.

Treatment

In addition to treatment of the excessive hair growth, treatment should be directed to the likely cause. For example, weight loss in obese PCOS patients may improve hirsutism through a decrease in ovarian androgen production, an improvement in insulin resistance and an increase in SHBG (see Chapter 85, Polycystic ovary syndrome). Treatment of hirsutism can prevent or slow further hair growth but will not treat the already existent hair growth, which will need to be physically removed using a variety of methods, including electrolysis, plucking, waxing, shaving and laser removal. Targeting the hair follicles in the anagen stage can lead to permanent hair removal.[5]

Pharmacological agents

Oral contraceptive pill

The oral contraceptive pill (OCP) is usually the first line of therapy, particularly for those requiring contraception or for those with menstrual irregularities.[1] The OCP acts by increasing SHBG thus decreasing the free testosterone fraction. Other actions include antagonising LH-stimulated androgen production by the theca cells, a mild decrease in adrenal androgen production and a mild blockage of the androgen receptors.[1] Pills with an oestrogen-dominant effect, such as those containing desogesterel, gestodene or norgestimate, should be used. Levenorgestrel can oppose the

oestrogen-driven increase in SHBG, while norethisterone is an androgen derivative. Pills containing these two progestogens should therefore be avoided. Dianette® is an OCP that contains the progestogen cyproterone acetate (2 mg), which also has an anti-androgenic effect through gonadotrophin inhibition and increased hepatic clearance of androgens. Cyproterone acetate in higher doses (50–100 mg/day) can also be used, but needs to be combined with an effective contraceptive due to the risk of feminisation of a male fetus should pregnancy occur. Cyproterone acetate has a long half-life and therefore can be combined with ethinyl oestradiol in a reverse sequential regimen which involves the administration of ethinyl oestradiol 25–50 µg/day from day 5 to day 25 and cyproterone acetate in the first ten days (days 5–15). After improvement, the dose of cyproterone acetate can be decreased (5 mg/day).[1] The efficacy of cyproterone acetate combined with ethinyl oestradiol compared to placebo has been demonstrated in a Cochrane review.[7]

Similar to Dianette is Yasmin®, containing the progestogen drosperinone which has an anti-androgen effect through inhibition of ovarian androgen production, as well as blockage of androgen receptors similar to the effect of spironolactone from which it is derived.[5] A recent RCT compared two OCPs containing either drosperinone or cyproterone acetate and showed them to be similarly effective.[8]

Androgen antagonists

These medications are usually used as second-line monotherapy or in combination with the OCP in severe cases. They should be used in combination with an effective contraceptive to avoid feminisation of a male fetus. They include the following:

- Spironolactone: This is the most commonly used anti-androgen due to its relative safety and demonstrated effectiveness.[9] Spironolactone acts by blockage of the androgen receptors and by inhibition of 5α reductase. The effect of spironolactone is dose dependent[1] and side effects include diuresis and postural hypotension in early stages, as well as menstrual irregularities and, rarely, hyperkalaemia.[1]
- Flutamide: This is a potent androgen receptor antagonist that can result in hepatotoxity. Hence, it should only be used with caution and under tertiary care supervision. The dose varies from 250 to 500 mg/day.[1] Flutamide alone has been shown to have similar efficacy to a combination of spironolactone and Dianette.[10,11]
- Finasteride: This is an inhibitor of 5α reductase that is used at a dose of 5 mg/day. It can result in mild gastrointestinal disturbances, as well as dry skin and decreased libido.[5] The most important concern, however, is its teratogenicity and hence the importance of effective contraception.

Eflornithine

Eflornithine (Vaniqa®) is a topical antiprotozoal drug that acts locally to inhibit hair follicle ornithine decarboxylase enzyme that is essential for hair growth, and can result in visible improvement within a few weeks. However, on discontinuation of treatment, hair growth returns. It can also result in obstruction of the sebaceous glands and hence worsening of acne. Vaniqa has been shown to enhance the effect of laser treatment for hair removal.[12,13]

Insulin sensitising agents

Metformin has been shown to improve ovulation rates in women with PCOS (Chapter 85), and may also improve hirsutism through an improvement in insulin resistance. A recent meta-analysis has shown that metformin has similar efficacy to an OCP containing 2 mg cyproterone acetate and 35 μg of ethinyl oestradiol.[14] On the other hand, other studies have shown little or no benefit from the use of metformin.[15]

GnRH agonists

GnRH agonists can be used to suppress pituitary gonadotrophins and ovarian activity in severe resistant cases. However, treatment is associated with significant menopause-like symptoms and prolonged treatment can lead to loss of bone mineral density.

Surgical treatments

Surgical approaches include the treatment of identifiable causes, such as hypophysectomy for Cushing's syndrome, adrenal suppression for CAH and surgical removal of ovarian and adrenal tumours.

A therapeutic approach to hirsutism is summarised in Fig. 86.1.

KEY POINTS

- Polycystic ovary syndrome is the most common cause of hirsutism.
- Weight loss in obese patients may improve hirsutism.
- Virilism usually indicates significant pathology.
- The oral contraceptive pill is the most commonly used single therapy for hirsutism.

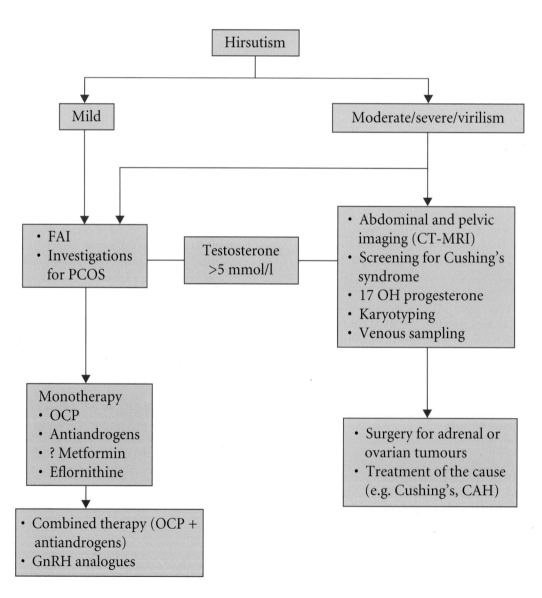

Fig. 86.1 A simplified algorithm for the management of hirsutism

Key References

1. Martin KA, Chang RJ, Ehrmann DA *et al*. Evaluation and treatment of hirsutism in premenopausal women: an Endocrine Society clinical practice guideline. *J Clin Endocrinol Metab* 2008;93:1105–20.

2. Randall VA. Androgens and hair growth. *Dermatol Ther* 2008;21:314–328.

3. Olsen EA. Evaluation and treatment of hirsutism. Introduction. *Dermatol Ther* 2008;21:313.

4. Hunter MH, Carek PJ. Evaluation and treatment of women with hirsutism. *Am Fam Physician* 2003;67:2565–72.

5. Archer JS, Chang RJ. Hirsutism and acne in polycystic ovary syndrome. *Best Pract Res Clin Obstet Gynaecol* 2004;18:737–54.

6. Somani N, Harrison S, Bergfeld WF. The clinical evaluation of hirsutism. *Dermatol Ther* 2008;21:376–391.

7. Van der Spuy ZM, le Roux PA. Cyproterone acetate for hirsutism. *Cochrane Database Syst Rev* 2003;4:CD001125.

8. van Vloten WA, van Haselen CW, van Zuuren EJ *et al*. The effect of 2 combined oral contraceptives containing either drospirenone or cyproterone acetate on acne and seborrhea. *Cutis* 2002;69:2–15.

9. Brown J, Farquhar C, Lee O *et al*. Spironolactone versus placebo or in combination with steroids for hirsutism and/or acne. *Cochrane Database Syst Rev* 2009;2:CD000194.

10. Inal MM, Yildirim Y, Taner CE. Comparison of the clinical efficacy of flutamide and spironolactone plus Diane 35 in the treatment of idiopathic hirsutism: a randomized controlled study. *Fertil Steril* 2005;84:1693–7.

11. Karakurt F, Sahin I, Guler S *et al*. Comparison of the clinical efficacy of flutamide and spironolactone plus ethinyl oestradiol/cyproterone acetate in the treatment of hirsutism: a randomised controlled study. *Adv Ther* 2008;25:321–8.

12. Hamzavi I, Tan E, Shapiro J, Lui H. A randomized bilateral vehicle-controlled study of eflornithine cream combined with laser treatment versus laser treatment alone for facial hirsutism in women. *J Am Acad Dermatol* 2007;57:54–9.

13. Smith SR, Piacquadio DJ, Beger B, Littler C. Eflornithine cream combined with laser therapy in the management of unwanted facial hair growth in women: a randomized trial. *Dermatol Surg* 2006;32:1237–43.

14. Jing Z, Liang-Zhi X, Tai-Xiang W *et al*. The effects of Diane-35 and metformin in treatment of polycystic ovary syndrome: an updated systematic review. *Gynecol Endocrinol* 2008;24: 590–600.

15. Cosma M, Swiglo BA, Flynn DN *et al*. Clinical review: Insulin sensitizers for the treatment of hirsutism: a systematic review and meta-analyses of randomized controlled trials. *J Clin Endocrinol Metab* 2008;93:1135–42.

Chapter 87 Amenorrhoea and oligomenorrhoea

Mostafa Metwally and William Ledger

DEFINITIONS

Amenorrhoea

Amenorrhoea is the absence of menses. Based on the previous occurrence of menstruation, amenorrhoea is divided into primary and secondary.

- **Primary amenorrhoea:** Menstruation has not occurred by the age of 14 in the absence of secondary sexual characters or by the age of 16, even if secondary sexual characters are present.
- **Secondary amenorrhoea:** Periods have not occurred for six months.

Oligomenorrhoea

This is defined as infrequent menstruation, where the duration between periods is more than 35 days.

CAUSES OF AMENORRHOEA

It is important to remember that amenorrhoea and oligomenorrhoea are symptoms and not a final diagnosis. The occurrence of regular menses requires a coordinated interaction between the hypothalamus, pituitary, ovaries and the outflow tract (uterus and vagina). A disturbance at any of these levels can lead to amenorrhoea (Fig. 87.1).

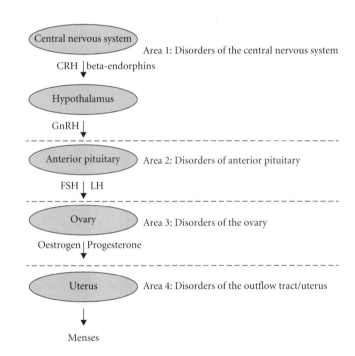

Fig. 87.1 Different compartments that may be involved in occurrence of amenorrhoea

Hypothalamus (normal or low gonadotrophins)

- **Congenital:** Kallman syndrome is a condition associated with congenital absence of GnRH secretion from the arcuate nucleus. Since GnRH-producing cells develop in the olfactory area, Kallman syndrome can be associated with defective olfactory development manifesting with anosmia.

- **Trauma:** This may be physical trauma, such as in the case of head injuries, or psychological trauma, such as in cases of severe emotional stress.
- **Inflammation:** For example, encephalitis and meningitis.
- **Neoplastic:** Hypothalamic and other brain tumours.
- **Iatrogenic:** chemotherapy or radiotherapy for malignant or auto-immune disorders
- **Weight related:** Leptin is one of the adipokines (a range of proteins secreted by white adipose tissue) that can influence the hypothalamus and is involved in various aspects of female reproductive function. Leptin has a stimulatory effect on the hypothalamus and may be responsible for signalling information to the brain on the critical amount of fat stores that are necessary for GnRH secretion and activation of the hypothalamic–pituitary–gonadal axis.[1] Rising levels of leptin have also been associated with the initiation of puberty in animals and humans, possibly acting in concert with gonadotrophins and the growth hormone axis.[2] This is further supported by the occurrence of amenorrhoea associated with a drop in body fat, seen in eating disorders such as anorexia nervosa which can affect about 0.7 per cent of teenage girls,[3] and in strenuously exercising athletes.[4]

Exogenous recombinant leptin replacement has been shown to improve reproductive and neuroendocrine function in women with hypothalamic amenorrhoea.[5]

In contrast, obesity is often associated with elevated serum or follicular fluid leptin levels, raising the possibility of relative leptin deficiency or resistance which may explain the poor reproductive performance in such conditions.[2]

Pituitary: (normal or low gonadotrophins)

- **Congenital:** Mutation of the β-subunit of FSH.[6]
- **Trauma:** After surgical removal of pituitary tumours.
- **Neoplastic:** Micro-adenomas producing prolactin, macro-adenomas or an extra-pituitary tumour compressing the pituitary stalk and hence leading to hyperprolactinaemia due to interference with dopamine (prolactin inhibitory factor).
- **Sheehan syndrome** is a condition of hypopituitarism due to ischaemic necrosis of the pituitary after massive post-partum haemorrhage. The first hormones to be affected are the gonadotrophins and growth hormone followed by ACTH and finally TSH.

Ovarian: (normal or raised gonadotrophins)

- **Congenital:** Complete androgen insensitivity in an XY female.
  - Turner syndrome (XO) presents with primary amenorrhoea, while women with mosaic Turner (XX/XO) may present with secondary amenorrhoea.

- Other forms of abnormal gonadal development may also present with primary or secondary amenorrhoea, such as cases of gonadal dysgenesis (pure or mixed).
- Resistant ovary syndrome is a condition that can present with premature menopause. The condition is characterised by a normal cohort of primordial follicles and absence of auto-immune disease. The condition can be due to a defect in the gonadotrophin receptors.[7]
- **Trauma:** Radiotherapy, chemotherapy and surgical removal.
- **Inflammation:** Rarely severe genital tuberculosis causes ovarian damage.
- **Neoplastic:** A variety of benign or malignant ovarian tumours.
- **Polycystic ovarian syndrome**: This is discussed in more detail in Chapter 85.
- **Early ovarian insufficiency (EOI, previously termed premature ovarian failure):** (see Chapter 91) This is characterised by cessation of ovarian function due to depletion of the follicular cohort before the age of 40 years. Gonadotrophins are raised in the menopausal range. The cause is usually idiopathic, in 74–90 per cent of cases,[8] but may be associated with a variety of auto-immune conditions, chromosomal abnormalities (such as mosaic Turner), galactosaemia and carriers of fragile X pre-mutation. The occurrence of premature menopause should prompt the search for chromosomal abnormalities associated with the presence of a Y chromosome due to the high risk of malignant tumours in these gonads.

Outflow tract (normal gonadotrophins)

- **Congenital:** Congenital absence of the uterus is due to faulty development of the Müllerian ducts (Meyer–Rokitansky–Kuster–Hauser syndrome). Since the Müllerian and Wolffian ducts are closely related, this condition is often associated with developmental abnormalities in the urinary tract. Other developmental abnormalities that present with primary amenorrhoea include imperforate hymen and transverse vaginal septum. These two conditions lead to cryptomenorrhoea, where cyclic bleeding and pain occur every month, but the bleeding is not revealed. Eventually haematocolpos and haematometra occur and commonly present with acute urinary retention due to stretching of the urethra.
- **Trauma:** Surgical removal (hysterectomy) or over-curettage of the endometrium.
- **Inflammation:** Postpartum or post-abortive infection.

Both surgical trauma and inflammatory destruction of the basal endometrial layer will lead to the formation of intra-uterine adhesions (Asherman syndrome).

REPRODUCTIVE GYNAECOLOGY

INVESTIGATIONS

Clinical examination, particularly in cases of primary amenorrhoea, may reveal physical characteristics of Turner syndrome, outflow obstruction and allow for examination of secondary sexual character development. According to the findings, investigations may be required at this stage including karyotyping or gonadotrophin measurement.

Other preliminary tests include exclusion of pregnancy, which is a must in all cases of secondary amenorrhoea. Thyroid function tests will exclude thyroid disorders, although it is a rare cause of amenorrhoea. Prolactin measurement is needed to exclude hyperprolactinaemia as the cause.

Progesterone challenge test

An oral progestogen given for 5–10 days will usually induce a withdrawal bleed if the endometrium has been primed by endogenous oestrogen. A positive withdrawal bleed therefore establishes the cause as anovulation (e.g. PCOS), while a negative withdrawal bleed is an indication for addition of oestrogen to the progestogen. A positive bleed with estrogen and progestogen means that the ovary is not producing adequate oestrogen (hypogonadism). This may be due to ovarian (hypergonadotrophic hypogonadism) or central deficiency of FSH/LH (hypogonadotrophic hypogonadism). The two conditions can be differentiated by measurement of gonadotrophin concentrations. On the other hand, a negative withdrawal bleed is an indication for investigation of the outflow tract (e.g. hysteroscopy to diagnose and treat Asherman syndrome, ultrasonography or MRI to investigate obstructive outflow lesions or Müllerian abnormalities).

Pituitary imaging

Imaging of the sella turcica using CT or MRI is indicated in women with significantly elevated prolactin concentrations.

Investigations for women with premature ovarian failure

The diagnosis is usually established by finding a raised FSH concentration in the menopausal range. The test should be repeated since fluctuations in FSH concentrations can occur and are associated with intermittent episodes of ovarian activity. However, other tests of ovarian reserve may be more accurate and include measuring AMH and inhibin B concentrations. Both these hormones are produced by the existing cohort of follicles and decrease with diminished ovarian reserve. However, AMH has the advantage of not fluctuating with the different phases of the cycle and therefore can be measured at any time. Other tests that may be indicated after the diagnosis is established include karyotyping, screening for autoantibodies, galactosaemia and fragile X syndrome permutations.

TREATMENT

This should be directed to the cause and depends on the patient's current desire for fertility.

Specific pathologies that will require intervention include:

- Hysteroscopic resection of intrauterine adhesions in cases with Asherman syndrome. In one series, the conception rate after treatment ranged from 33 to 58 per cent, depending on the severity of adhesions.[9]
- Removal of space-occupying pituitary or brain tumours.

The majority of pituitary micro-adenomas, however, can be managed conservatively with a dopamine agonist. For women with hyperprolactinaemia not due to a pituitary adenoma, dopamine agonists can lead to resumption of ovulation and menstruation.

- Treatment of feeding disorders and normalisation of bodyweight.
- Surgical correction of outflow tract obstruction, e.g. incision of an imperforate hymen.
- Correction of thyroid disorders.

Treatment depends on whether fertility is required. Where fertility is not required, regular withdrawal bleeds may be induced using cyclic oestrogen/progestogen therapy (e.g. oral contraceptive pill [OCP]). Women who suffer from chronic anovulation should be treated with a cyclic oestrogen/progestagen or a progestogen alone to protect the endometrium against the effects of prolonged unopposed oestrogen stimulation. The OCP or another form of combined HRT should also be used for women with POF to protect the bone density and avoid the unpleasant side effects of oestrogen deficiency.

Where fertility is required in anovulatory women, the primary method of ovulation induction depends on the level of the defect:

- PCOS (see Chapter 85).
- Oocyte donation offers the best chance for conception in women with premature ovarian failure. Natural conception, although rare (<10 per cent lifetime odds),[10] can still occur due to unpredictable late resumption of ovarian activity. There are also reports of successful ovulation induction after suppression of FSH using ethinyl oestradiol.[11–13]
- Women with pituitary or hypothalamic causes of amenorrhoea (hypogonadotrophic hypogonadism) are treated with gonadotrophins (FSH and LH) or less commonly with pulsatile GnRH administration using a subcutaneous pump.

KEY POINTS

- Amenorrhoea and oligomenorrhoea can arise from a disturbance at the level of any of the key structures controlling the menstrual cycle.
- Pregnancy should always be excluded in a patient presenting with secondary amenorrhoea.
- Premature ovarian failure should prompt the search for underlying pathologies, although most cases remain unexplained.
- In women with premature ovarian failure not requiring fertility, treatment should be directed to the prevention of the long-term health consequences of oestrogen deficiency.
- Contraception should still be advised for women with premature ovarian failure not desiring pregnancy, since spontaneous pregnancy can still occur, albeit rarely.
- Measurement of anti-Müllerian hormone (AMH) is a better test of ovarian reserve than follicle-stimulating hormone.

Key References

1. Mantzoros CS. Role of leptin in reproduction. *Ann NY Acad Sci* 2000;900:174–83.
2. Moschos S, Chan JL, Mantzoros CS. Leptin and reproduction: a review. *Fertil Steril* 2002;77:433–44.
3. Lock J, Fitzpatrick KK. Anorexia nervosa. *Clin Evid (Online)*;2009.
4. Thong FS, Graham TE. Leptin and reproduction: is it a critical link between adipose tissue, nutrition, and reproduction? *Can J Appl Physiol* 1999;24:317–36.
5. Welt CK, Chan JL, Bullen J *et al.* Recombinant human leptin in women with hypothalamic amenorrhea. *N Engl J Med* 2004;351:987–97.
6. Layman LC, McDonough PG. Mutations of follicle-stimulating hormone-beta and its receptor in human and mouse: genotype/phenotype. *Mol Cell Endocrinol* 2000;161:9–17.
7. Huhtaniemi I, Alevizaki M. Gonadotrophin resistance. *Best Pract Res Clin Endocrinol Metab* 2006;20:561–76.
8. Vujovic S. Aetiology of premature ovarian failure. *Menopause Int* 2009;15:72–5.
9. Roy KK, Baruah J, Sharma JB *et al.* Reproductive outcome following hysteroscopic adhesiolysis in patients with infertility due to Asherman's syndrome. *Arch Gynecol Obstet* 2009 [Epub ahead of print].
10. Rebar RW. Premature ovarian failure. *Obstet Gynecol* 2009;113: 1355–63.
11. Check JH. Pharmacological options in resistent ovary syndrome and premature ovarian failure. *Clin Exp Obstet Gynecol* 2006;33:71–7.
12. Blumenfeld Z. Pregnancies in patients with POF gonadotropin stimulation and pretreatment with ethinyl estradiol (author's reply). *Fertil Steril* 2007;88:763.
13. Tartagni M, Cicinelli E, De Pergola G *et al.* Effects of pretreatment with estrogens on ovarian stimulation with gonadotropins in women with premature ovarian failure: a randomized, placebo-controlled trial. *Fertil Steril* 2007;87:858–61.

Chapter 88 Menopause

Tina Sara Verghese, Jenny Williamson and Lynne Robinson

MRCOG standards

Theoretical skills

There is no established standard for this topic, but we would suggest the following points for guidance:

- Have good knowledge of the hypophyseal–pituitary–ovarian axis.
- Have knowledge of the epidemiological factors determining the age at menopause.
- Have knowledge of symptoms and health risks associated with the menopause.
- Have awareness of the risks and benefits of HRT.
- Have some knowledge of alternatives to HRT.

Practical skills

- Be able to take an appropriate history.
- Be able to diagnose menopause and arrange investigations as necessary.
- Be able to initiate referral to secondary or tertiary care for management if appropriate.

INTRODUCTION

Menopause is defined as the permanent cessation of menstruation. In the UK the mean age for menopause is 52 years. With the increase in life expectancy, a woman will live more than a third of her life beyond the menopause. Menopause is a natural phenomenon where the ovaries cease to produce significant amounts of oestrogen due to the depletion of ovarian follicles. Perimenopause is a period of change leading up to the last menstrual cycle. Menopause is retrospectively diagnosed with certainty after twelve months of amenorrhoea. The British Menopause Society and Women's Health Concern recommend that women should be able to seek advice during the climacteric and menopause periods and be able to discuss the benefits and limitations of various therapies including HRT.

EPIDEMIOLOGY

The age of menopause appears to be genetically determined. Factors that may contribute to early menopause include smoking, chemotherapy and pelvic radiation. Women who have had surgery on their ovaries or have had hysterectomy despite preservation of their ovaries may experience early menopause. Premature ovarian insufficiency is described as menopause before the age of 45 years, affecting approximately 5 per cent of the population and 1 in 100 women under the age of 40 years.

PHYSIOLOGY

Menopause is due to the depletion of ovarian follicles secondary to apoptosis or programmed cell death. Along with changes in the hypothalamic and pituitary hormones, the ovary fails to respond to the pituitary hormones (for more physiological details please refer to Chapter 91 on the subject of premature ovarian insufficiency). For more detailed description of the physiology of the reproductive tract please see Chapter X.

VASOMOTOR SYMPTOMS

The underlying cause for hot flushes during menopause is still uncertain. The hypothesis is that falling oestrogen and progesterone levels cause a change in the thermoregulatory centre of the hypothalamus.[1] This is thought to result in a transient peripheral vasodilatation mainly affecting skin blood vessels, presenting as hot flushes lasting a few seconds. If prolonged, these can progress to a sweat. Hot flushes and sweats affect approximately 75 per cent of women during perimenopause and early menopause.[2] The severity is variable. A Cochrane review incorporating 24 double-blind, randomised placebo control studies found that oral oestrogen or combined oestrogen and progestogen HRT greatly reduced the frequency and severity of these symptoms.[3] Data obtained from nine trials demonstrated a reduction in hot flush frequency for HRT compared with the placebo; the difference was statistically significant in eight of the trials.[4–7]

Women initiating HRT may experience some symptoms such as transient breast tenderness, mild headaches and fluid retention, sometimes described as bloating. The overall withdrawal rate is low.

SEXUAL FUNCTION

There is a significant decline in sexual function including libido, arousal, orgasm and satisfaction around the time of the menopause. Treatment options such as androgens may be considered in conjunction with HRT.

Tibolone has a weak androgenic effect which can have a beneficial effect on mood and libido. Tibolone exhibits a combination of oestrogenic, progestogenic and androgenic activities. In patients with a surgical menopause, RCTs have demonstrated that transdermal therapy is beneficial in improving sexual function and activity. There may also be cardiovascular benefits for women.[8] Testosterone gels are available albeit only as a male product. These are unlicensed for use in women but can be used if titrated to an appropriate dose (for more physiological details please refer to Chapter 91). Androgenic side effects and risks are minimal and reversible if testosterone levels are maintained within the female physiological range.

UROGENITAL SYMPTOMS

Oestrogen treatment can be used to reduce thinning of the vaginal and pelvic tissues. This may help to reduce or prevent symptoms of cystitis and may aid postoperative recovery after uro-gynaecological procedures. The different preparations of topical HRTs (creams, pessaries, tablets and the oestradiol vaginal ring) all appear equally effective for treating vaginal atrophy.

Estradiol vaginal tablets when used for 12 months at 10 μg daily for 2 weeks followed by twice weekly for 52 weeks resulted in a total annual oestradiol exposure of only 1.14 mg and did not stimulate the endometrium in postmenopausal women to any significant level.[9] There were no cases of endometrial hyperplasia or carcinoma in these women.[10] There is therefore no indication for the addition of progestogen treatment for endometrial protection when a twice-weekly vaginal oestrogen preparation is used.

CARDIOVASCULAR DISEASE

In the UK, one in ten women die from coronary heart disease.[11] The mortality rate from this disease is higher than from any gynaecological or breast cancers. Postmenopausal women are 2–3 times more prone to having a heart attack when compared to premenopausal women. Oestrogen reduces atheroma formation and has a favourable influence on cholesterol and lipoprotein metabolism along with maintaining the smooth muscle and collagen elasticity.

Prior to 2002, observational studies suggested that HRT was beneficial, showing a reduction in risk of cardiovascular disease, osteoporosis and colon cancer.[12] Critics suggested that the 'healthy well' were more likely to use HRT and therefore randomised trials were needed to find out if HRT was in fact cardioprotective.[12]

In 2002, the primary outcomes from the Women's Health Initiative (WHI) trial reported no cardiovascular benefit from the combined arm of HRT.[13] Subsequent analysis of this study published in 2007 now identifies that the timing of administration may be of significance.[14,15] Starting HRT many years after menopause can result in harm which is not seen when commenced in the immediate postmenopausal years. The Danish Osteoporosis Prevention study found that if HRT was started soon after menopause and continued for a prolonged period, there was no increase in adverse events such as stroke, heart failure, myocardial infarction or mortality. In addition the results also showed no increase in breast cancer or other cancers.[16] In this study, 17-beta oestradiol and norethisterone were the hormones used rather than conjugated equine oestrogen (CEE) which was used in the WHI study. 17-beta estradiol, both alone and in combination with norethisterone, appears to be less thrombogenic.[17] In contrast to CEEs which maintain the postmenopausal oestrone:oestradiol ratio, 17-beta estradiol maintains the premenopausal ratio. This may help to explain to some degree the differing results of the WHI trial compared with subsequent trials.

HRT has been found to have a positive effect on lipid metabolism. Combination therapy can lower the cholesterol levels and improve endothelial function. There is some evidence of benefit to metabolic parameters including lipids, insulin, glucose and body fat distribution with oestradiol and dydrogesterone combinations.[18] However, given the uncertainties in the evidence, HRT cannot be recommended for primary or secondary prevention of ischaemic heart disease.

STROKE

The incidence of stroke in women immediately post menopause is low but increases with age. The indication for HRT is symptom relief and studies which have identified an increased risk of stroke tend to be on women in whom HRT has been commenced later in life. The WHI study found an increase of 30–40 per cent in stroke risk in women on oestrogen alone or a combination of oestrogen with progestogens.[19] However, re-analysis of the data showed a smaller increase of stroke in women who commenced HRT aged 50–59 years. The Nurses Study, which aimed to evaluate the risk of stroke in women of various age groups on HRT, found that the age-adjusted RR of overall stroke for current users on oestrogen alone when compared with women who never used HRT was 1.33 (95% CI 1.13–1.55). In women on combined therapy, the

RR was 1.17 (95% CI 0.96–1.42).[20] The HERS study (Heart and oestrogen progestogen study) reported no increase in incidence of stroke in women on HRT and a recent open-label randomised trial found no increase in stroke after 16 years' follow-up of HRT users who commenced treatment around the time of their natural menopause.[16]

HRT, if required, should be cautiously started in low doses in women above the age of 60 with high risk for stroke or thromboembolism. This group of women may benefit from transdermal hormonal patches. Low-dose hormone therapy may be preferable for women with significant risk factors.

OSTEOPOROSIS

Osteoporosis accounts for about 35 per cent of bone fractures. Osteoporosis mainly affects the spine, hip, distal forearm and proximal humerus. In 2010, the calculated direct costs due to fractures were estimated to be €29 billion in the five largest EU countries – France, Germany, Italy, Spain and the UK.[21-23] Dual energy X-ray absorptiometry (DXA) is the most inexpensive method of measuring bone density, involving low radiation exposure. Bone mineral density (BMD) is most often described as a T- or Z-score, both of which are units of standard deviation. The T-score describes the number of SDs by which the BMD in an individual differs from the mean value expected in young healthy individuals. Osteoporosis is based on the T-score for BMD assessed at the femoral neck and is defined as a value for BMD 2.5 SD or more below the young female adult mean (T-score less than or equal to −2.5 SD).[24,25] The Z-score is mostly used in children and adolescents. A computer-based algorithm known as FRAX (www.shef.ac.uk/FRAX/) calculates the 10-year probability of a major fracture (hip, spine, humerus or wrist fracture). The variables used to calculate fracture risk are age, BMI and risk factors such as prior fragility fracture, family history, smoking, ever use of long-term oral glucocorticoids, rheumatoid arthritis, secondary causes of osteoporosis and alcohol consumption.

HRT has been shown to be very effective at maintaining and preventing bone loss in both spine and hips and should be considered in women who are at risk of osteoporosis and require symptomatic relief from climacteric symptoms.

Other drugs can be used to prevent bone density loss. Raloxifene (selective oestrogen modulator) prevents bone loss. The risk of vertebral fractures is reduced by 30–50 per cent in postmenopausal women on raloxifene (Multiple Outcomes of Raloxifene Evaluation – MORE trial).[26] However raloxifene can cause vasomotor symptoms. Bisphosphonates are also used to prevent bone loss and are inhibitors of bone resorption, acting by reducing the recruitment and activity of osteoclasts and increasing their apoptosis.

In contrast to HRT, there are no long-term outcome data with these treatments and there may be an increase in atypical fractures and osteonecrosis of the jaw with bisphosphonate use.

BREAST CANCER AND HORMONE THERAPY

Studies such as the WHI trial and the Million Women study have reported an increase in the risk of breast cancer, especially for women on combined hormone therapy.[27,28] The Million Women study stated a varied relative risk of breast cancer depending on the type of HRT used and this was significantly greater in users of combined therapy (p <0.001).[28] The study estimated that 10 years' use of HRT resulted in 5 (95% CI 3–7) additional cases of breast cancer per 1000 users of oestrogen-only preparation and 19 (95% CI 15–23) additional cases of breast cancer per 1000 users of combined HRT.[28] The study had several design flaws resulting in unreliable findings. A critique of the Million Women study identified that the participants were recruited from a national breast screening programme and this could have led to a detection bias.[29] Furthermore, cancers detected at the outset were not excluded, women on HRT were more likely to attend, and the rapid onset of breast cancer suggested by the researchers did not fit with the biological course of the disease. The findings did however indicate that the risks were greater with combined HRT than with oestrogen-only preparations or tibolone.

Women who have had a personal history of breast cancer are often the women with the most troublesome menopausal symptoms because of anti-oestrogen treatments and therefore present a real clinical dilemma. Following breast cancer treatment, many women experience hot flushes, night sweats, sexual dysfunction and poor sleep. Two thirds of breast cancers are oestrogen receptor-positive where treatment to block the effects of oestrogen results in profound vasomotor symptoms along with urogenital atrophy. Aromatase inhibitors in the postmenopausal woman inhibit the peripheral conversion of androgen to oestrogen, while tamoxifen, usually given to the pre- and perimenopausal woman, acts as an oestrogen receptor blocker.

Clonidine, a centrally acting alpha-adrenergic agonist, is the only licensed non-hormonal treatment for vasomotor symptoms. Selective serotonin reuptake inhibitors (SSRIs) and serotonin noradrenaline reuptake inhibitors (SNRIs) in low doses are unlicensed but have been evaluated and found to reduce symptoms of hot flushes to some extent. Short-term studies of women with breast cancer have found SSRIs (paroxetine, fluoxetine, citalopram) and SNRIs (venlafaxine, desvenlafaxine) more effective than placebo.[30] Some SNRIs and SSRIs induce CYP2D6 and may interfere with the breakdown of tamoxifen. Citalopram and venlafaxine may be better alternatives in breast cancer patients on tamoxifen.[30]

Gabapentin (up to 900 mg/day in divided doses) is also unlicensed for this use but can help reduce hot flushes in breast cancer patients.[31] It has a rapid onset of action. In an RCT by Reddy et al. gabapentin has exhibited equivalent efficacy to oestrogen in reducing hot flushes.[32]

For some breast cancer survivors the use of HRT will be a quality-of-life decision. The main concern of the clinician is that there may be a dormant occult breast cancer cell which would become activated by the use of oestrogenic stimulation although evidence for this is conflicting.[33-37] The stage at diagnosis, the oestrogen receptor status of the original tumour and the length of time since diagnosis are all relevant to the discussion. Patients with tiny screen-detected tumours may have an excellent prognosis and reduced incidence of disseminated metastases.[38] Initiating HRT immediately after cancer treatment would not be recommended. Patients who have suffered vasomotor symptoms relentlessly, and for whom many years have elapsed since their initial breast cancer treatment, may wish to evaluate HRT on a quality-of-life basis.[39] Discussion on the use of HRT in these women is best carried out with multidisciplinary team input. Studies on breast cancer patients using HRT have been conflicting and the use of tibolone identified recurrence in the ER+ cases but not in the ER− cases.[40]

ENDOMETRIAL CANCER

Furness *et al.*[41] reported that unopposed oestrogen therapy increases the risk of endometrial hyperplasia at any dose and duration between 1 and 3 years. The WHI study reported no increase in incidence of endometrial cancer for women on HRT (RR 0.83, 95% CI 0.29–2.32).[42] The risk is decreased by adding progestogens either sequentially or in a lower dose continuously. Sequential combined oestrogen and progestogen therapy for more than five years is associated with a very small risk of endometrial cancer and continuous combined regimens actually confer a lower risk of endometrial cancer than for non-HRT users. Combined continuous regimens are suitable for women who have had at least 12 months of sequential therapy, one year or more after their last menstrual period or two years or more if they are under 50 years. Sequential regimens are more suited to perimenopausal or prematurely menopausal women. In patients who have undergone a subtotal hysterectomy it is important to establish that there is no remaining endometrium before prescribing oestrogen-only HRT; using sequential HRT initially post surgery can help to establish this if there is doubt. In the event where there is no bleeding with a sequential regimen, unopposed oestrogen HRT is safe.

OVARIAN CANCER

The WHI study found that the there was no increased risk of incidence of ovarian cancer for women on HRT.[27] Contrary to this study, the Danish National Cancer registry reported that women on unopposed oestrogen or combined HRT for more than eight years had a small but significant increase in the incidence of ovarian cancer. Data on HRT use after ovarian cancer are limited. A systematic review including randomised and observational studies found that there was no increased risk of recurrence.[43]

CONTRAINDICATIONS TO HRT

There are few absolute contraindications to HRT. These include current breast cancer, current thromboembolism, active liver disease and SLE with renal involvement.

Conditions such as previous venous thromboembolism, hypertension, obesity and migraine can all be managed alongside prescribing HRT treatment. HRT is not known to increase blood pressure although conjugated oestrogens can be linked with an idiosyncratic rise in blood pressure. When hypertension is controlled with appropriate medication, HRT can be used concurrently.

Patients with previous thromboembolism should be adequately assessed in conjunction with a haematologist, but may be suitable for transdermal treatment started in a gradual fashion to minimise a procoagulant effect. A similar approach may be employed for migraine or seizure sufferers.

DURATION OF TREATMENT

The theory surrounding the 'window of opportunity' would suggest that HRT is most beneficial in the first 10 years after the age of natural menopause. However, many women continue to experience marked vasomotor symptoms well into their sixties and even seventies and therefore duration of treatment will vary from patient to patient. Each patient should be individually assessed and consideration should be given to their symptoms. Prolonged HRT treatment can be employed in many women safely but medication should be regularly reviewed and lower doses used if tolerated (see Table 88.1).

Table 88.1 Indications for various types of hormone replacement therapy

Type of HRT	Indications
Oestrogen only	Women without a uterus + subtotal hysterectomy (if adequate resection margin)
Sequential HRT	Premature ovarian insufficiency
	Last menstrual period (LMP) <12 months ago
Continuous combined HRT	>12 months sequential HRT
	1 year post LMP if >50 years old
	2 years post LMP if <50 years old
Oestrogen + Mirena IUS	Women with uterus preferring IUS to systemic progestogens
	Women requiring HRT + contraception
	Women with pre-existing IUS requiring HRT

A full discussion about the risks and uncertainties in the evidence is essential, particularly for women who wish to continue HRT beyond five years since treatment initiation.

NON-HORMONAL TREATMENT

There are limited clinical data on non-pharmacological treatments such as behavioural interventions, exercise and acupuncture. Acupuncture has been found to be less effective than oestrogen in management of hot flushes but more beneficial than placebo. A recent systematic review of non-hormonal therapies for hot flushes did not support the efficacy of red clover products (predominantly promensil).[44] There are mixed results on the use of soy isoflavones. Placebo-controlled RCTs of vitamin E succinate (800 IU/day) in breast cancer did not show promising results. Despite the long-term safety concerns of HRT, there are few data on non-hormonal therapies. SNRIs/SSRIs, clonidine and gabapentin are often used to control vasomotor symptoms but clonidine is the only one of these products licensed for this use.

KEY POINTS

- Menopause symptoms are often debilitating.
- It is essential that we adequately inform women of the risks and benefits of HRT.
- In recent years, lower doses of oestrogen have become available and we now know that lower doses of oestrogen adequately protect bone density.
- HRT does not appear to increase the risk of cardiovascular disease in women started on HRT within 10 years of menopause.
- Although there are uncertainties in the evidence, the available data suggest an increase in the risks of breast cancer, stroke and venous thromboembolism with HRT use.
- HRT remains one of the most effective strategies available to provide relief of vasomotor symptoms and protect bone density.

References

1. Freedman RR, Norton D, Woodward S, Cornelissen G. Core body temperature and circadian rhythm of hot flashes in menopausal women. *The Journal of Clinical Endocrinology and Metabolism* 1995;80(8):2354–8.
2. Sturdee D, Brincat M. The hot flush. *In*: Studd JWW, Whitehead MI (eds). *The Menopause.* London: Blackwell Scientific, 1988.
3. Maclennan AH, Broadbent JL, Lester S, Moore V. Oral oestrogen and combined oestrogen/progestogen therapy versus placebo for hot flushes. *The Cochrane Database of Systematic Reviews* 2004;4:CD002978.
4. Baerug U WT, Nordland G, Faber-Swensson E *et al.* Do combinations of 1 mg estradiol and low doses of NETA effectively control menopausal symptoms? *Climacteric: the Journal of the International Menopause Society.* 1998;1:219–28.
5. Conard J, Basdevant A, Thomas JL *et al.* Cardiovascular risk factors and combined estrogen-progestin replacement therapy: a placebo-controlled study with nomegestrol acetate and estradiol. *Fertility and Sterility* 1995;64(5):957–62.
6. Symons J, Kempfert N, Speroff L. Vaginal bleeding in postmenopausal women taking low-dose norethindrone acetate and ethinyl estradiol combinations. The FemHRT Study Investigators. *Obstet Gynecol* 2000;96(3):366–72.
7. Coope J. Is oestrogen therapy effective in the treatment of menopausal depression? *Journal of the Royal College of General Practitioners.* 1981;31(224):134–40.
8. Spoletini I, Caprio M, Vitale C, Rosano GM. Androgens and cardiovascular disease: gender-related differences. *Menopause International* 2013;19(2):82–6.
9. Ulrich LS, Naessen T, Elia D, Goldstein JA, Eugster-Hausmann M, investigators VAGt. Endometrial safety of ultra-low-dose Vagifem 10 microg in postmenopausal women with vaginal atrophy. *Climacteric: the Journal of the International Menopause Society.* 2010;13(3):228–37.
10. Minkin MJ, Maamari R, Reiter S. Improved compliance and patient satisfaction with estradiol vaginal tablets in postmenopausal women previously treated with another local estrogen therapy. *International Journal of Women's Health.* 2013;5:133–9.
11. British Heart Foundation. *Coronary heart disease statistics.* British Heart Foundation, 2010.
12. Grodstein F, Stampfer M. The epidemiology of coronary heart disease and estrogen replacement in postmenopausal women. *Progress in cardiovascular diseases.* 1995;38(3):199–210.
13. Hsia J, Langer RD, Manson JE, Kuller L *et al.* Conjugated equine estrogens and coronary heart disease: the Women's Health Initiative. *Archives of Internal Medicine* 2006;166(3):357–65.
14. Dubey RK, Imthurn B, Barton M, Jackson EK. Vascular consequences of menopause and hormone therapy: importance of timing of treatment and type of estrogen. *Cardiovascular research* 2005;66(2):295–306.
15. Hodis HN, Mack WJ. A 'window of opportunity': the reduction of coronary heart disease and total mortality with menopausal therapies is age- and time-dependent. *Brain Research* 2011;1379:244–52.
16. Schierbeck LL, Rejnmark L, Tofteng CL *et al.* Effect of hormone replacement therapy on cardiovascular events in recently postmenopausal women: randomised trial. *BMJ* 2012;345:e6409.

17. Norris LAJM, O'Keeffe N, Sheppard BL *et al.* Hemostatic risk factors in postmenopausal women taking hormone replacement therapy. *Maturitas* 2002;43:125–33.

18. Stevenson JC, Panay N, Pexman-Fieth C. Oral estradiol and dydrogesterone combination therapy in postmenopausal women: review of efficacy and safety. *Maturitas* 2013;76(1):10–21.

19. Wassertheil-Smoller S, Hendrix SL, Limacher M *et al.* Effect of estrogen plus progestin on stroke in postmenopausal women: the Women's Health Initiative: a randomized trial. *JAMA* 2003;289(20):2673–84.

20. Grodstein F, Manson JE, Stampfer MJ, Rexrode K. Postmenopausal hormone therapy and stroke: role of time since menopause and age at initiation of hormone therapy. *Archives of Internal Medicine* 2008;168(8):861–6.

21. Johnell O, Kanis JA. An estimate of the worldwide prevalence and disability associated with osteoporotic fractures. *Osteoporosis International* 2006;17(12):1726–33.

22. Kanis JA, Borgstrom F, De Laet C *et al.* Assessment of fracture risk. *Osteoporosis International.* 2005;16(6):581–9.

23. Strom O, Borgstrom F, Kanis JA *et al.* Osteoporosis: burden, healthcare provision and opportunities in the EU: a report prepared in collaboration with the International Osteoporosis Foundation (IOF) and the European Federation of Pharmaceutical Industry Associations (EFPIA). *Archives of Osteoporosis* 2011;6(1-2):59–155.

24. Kanis JA, Melton LJ 3rd, Christiansen C, Johnston CC, Khaltaev N. The diagnosis of osteoporosis. *Journal of Bone and Mineral Research* 1994;9(8):1137–1141.

25. Kanis JA, McCloskey EV, Johansson H, Oden A, Melton LJ 3rd, Khaltaev N. A reference standard for the description of osteoporosis. *Bone* 2008;42(3):467–75.

26. Hansdottir H. Raloxifene for older women: a review of the literature. *Clinical Interventions in Aging* 2008;3(1):45–50.

27. Rossouw JE, Anderson GL, Prentice RL *et al.* Risks and benefits of estrogen plus progestin in healthy postmenopausal women: principal results from the Women's Health Initiative randomized controlled trial. *JAMA* 2002;288(3):321–33.

28. Beral V. Million Women Study. Breast cancer and hormone-replacement therapy in the Million Women Study. *Lancet* 2003;362(9382):419–27.

29. Panay N. Commentary regarding recent Million Women Study critique and subsequent publicity. *Menopause International* 2012;18:33–5.

30. Stearns V. Clinical update: new treatments for hot flushes. *Lancet* 2007;369(9579):2062–64.

31. Pandya KJ, Morrow GR, Roscoe JA *et al.* Gabapentin for hot flashes in 420 women with breast cancer: a randomised double-blind placebo-controlled trial. *Lancet.* 2005;366(9488):818–24.

32. Reddy SY, Warner H, Guttuso T Jr *et al.* Gabapentin, estrogen, and placebo for treating hot flushes: a randomized controlled trial. *Obstet Gynecol* 2006;108(1):41–8.

33. Holmberg L, Anderson H, Steering H. HABITS (hormonal replacement therapy after breast cancer: is it safe?), a randomised comparison: trial stopped. *Lancet* 2004;363(9407):453–5.

34. Von Schoultz E, Rutqvist LE. Stockholm Breast Cancer Study. Menopausal hormone therapy after breast cancer: the Stockholm randomized trial. *Journal of the National Cancer Institute* 2005;97(7):533–5.

35. Fahlen M, Fornander T, Johansson H *et al.* Hormone replacement therapy after breast cancer: 10 year follow up of the Stockholm randomised trial. *European Journal of Cancer* 2013;49(1):52–9.

36. O'Meara ES, Rossing MA, Daling JR, Elmore JG, Barlow WE, Weiss NS. Hormone replacement therapy after a diagnosis of breast cancer in relation to recurrence and mortality. *Journal of the National Cancer Institute* 2001;93(10):754–62.

37. DiSaia PJ, Brewster WR, Ziogas A, Anton-Culver H. Breast cancer survival and hormone replacement therapy: a cohort analysis. *American Journal of Clinical Oncology* 2000;23(6):541–5.

38. Fowble B, Hanlon A, Freedman G *et al.* Postmenopausal hormone replacement therapy: effect on diagnosis and outcome in early-stage invasive breast cancer treated with conservative surgery and radiation. *Journal of Clinical Oncology* 1999;17(6):1680–8.

39. Sekar H ST, Holloway D, Rymer J. The use of hormone therapy and its alternatives in women with a history of hormone-dependent cancer. *Menopause International* 2013;19:37–42.

40. Sismondi P, Kimmig R, Kubista E *et al.* Effects of tibolone on climacteric symptoms and quality of life in breast cancer patients: data from LIBERATE trial. *Maturitas* 2011;70(4):365–72.

41. Furness S, Roberts H, Marjoribanks J, Lethaby A, Hickey M, Farquhar C. Hormone therapy in postmenopausal women and risk of endometrial hyperplasia. *Cochrane Database of Systematic Reviews* 2009;2:CD000402.

42. Anderson GL, Judd HL, Kaunitz AM *et al.* Effects of estrogen plus progestin on gynecologic cancers and associated diagnostic procedures: the Women's Health Initiative randomized trial. *JAMA* 2003;290(13):1739–48.

43. Hopkins ML, Fung MF, Le T, Shorr R. Ovarian cancer patients and hormone replacement therapy: a systematic review. *Gynecologic Oncology* 2004;92(3):827–32.

44. Nelson HD, Vesco KK, Haney E *et al.* Nonhormonal therapies for menopausal hot flashes: systematic review and meta-analysis. *JAMA* 2006;295(17):2057–71.

Chapter 89 Miscarriage

James Hounslow and Ying Cheong

MRCOG

- To have a good understanding of early pregnancy physiology and pregnancy loss.
- To be able to diagnose and treat miscarriage, both medically and surgically.
- To understand the use of ultrasound in the assessment of early pregnancy and diagnosis of miscarriage, including its limitations.
- To be able to communicate effectively and sensitively with patients.

INTRODUCTION

Miscarriage is the most common complication of early pregnancy. Its effects are both physical and psychological, and may be immediate or long term in their nature. The incidence of clinical miscarriage is around 10–15 per cent. This risk of miscarriage is highest in the first trimester of pregnancy and decreases to 2–7.5 per cent once a viable fetus is identified on ultrasound.[1-3] Recurrent miscarriage, defined as the spontaneous loss of three or more consecutive clinical pregnancies, is a separate clinical entity requiring specialist investigations and management covered elsewhere in the book and therefore will not be dealt with in this chapter.

Historically miscarriage was associated with significant maternal morbidity and mortality. Fortunately maternal death from miscarriage is rare in the developed world, with 0.3 deaths per 100,000 estimated pregnancies in the CMACE report of 2006–08.

DEFINITION AND EPIDEMIOLOGY

Seventy per cent of spontaneous human pregnancies are lost prior to live birth. From the time of conception to implantation 30 per cent of conceptions are lost, a further 30 per cent are lost between the time of implantation and the date of the first missed period, and another 10 per cent are lost as a recognised miscarriage;[4] in other words, overall only 30 per cent of conceptions will result in a live birth.

Hence, human reproduction is far from efficient. Losses from spontaneous pregnancies can be pre-clinical or clinical. Pre-clinical or occult pregnancy losses will include pregnancies where implantations were initiated with (biochemical) or without detectable circulating hCG (implantation failure).

The term 'miscarriage' refers to a spontaneous loss of pregnancy before the fetus reaches viability. The definition of viability can vary depending on the context of discussion but in the UK, miscarriage is defined as the loss of a pregnancy before 24 weeks of gestation. After 24 completed weeks, pregnancy loss is legally defined as stillbirth. The term clinical miscarriage is applied when there is either ultrasound or histological evidence that a failed intrauterine pregnancy is or has been present. Clinical miscarriage may be either early (<12 weeks' gestation) or late (>12 weeks' gestation). A pregnancy that is demonstrated by a raised urinary hCG or serum β-hCG, but that fails before ultrasound or histological evidence of the pregnancy, is defined as a biochemical loss (Table 89.1).

Table 89.1 Differential diagnosis of early pregnancy loss

Diagnosis	Presentation	Cervical findings	Ultrasound	Action
Biochemical pregnancy	Initially +ve then −ve urinary pregnancy test or serum hCG	Os closed	Not performed	No further action required
Pregnancy of unknown location (PUL)	+/− Pain; +/− bleeding	Os closed	No intra- or extrauterine pregnancy or retained products of conception (RPOC) identified	β-hCG follow up and re-scan as appropriate

Diagnosis	Presentation	Cervical findings	Ultrasound	Action
Threatened miscarriage	Bleeding; +/− pain	Os closed	Gestation sac + yolk sac +/− fetal pole/cardiac activity	Reassure, offer re-scan if fetal pole/cardiac activity not seen
Delayed miscarriage (missed miscarriage)	May be asymptomatic/ incidental finding; +/− pain or bleeding	Os closed	Gestation sac >/= 25 mm with no fetal pole OR fetal pole >/= 7 mm with no cardiac activity	Explain diagnosis of miscarriage and explain options (expectant/ medical/surgical)
Inevitable miscarriage	Bleeding; +/− pain	Os open	Gestation sac + yolk sac +/− fetal pole/cardiac activity	Explain diagnosis of miscarriage and explain options (expectant/ medical/surgical)
Incomplete miscarriage	Bleeding; +/− pain	Os open; +/− products within cervix/vagina	RPOC	Explain diagnosis of miscarriage and explain options (expectant/ medical/surgical)
Complete miscarriage	Bleeding (settling); +/− pain	Os closed	Intact midline endometrial echo or RPOC of <15 mm diameter AND previous ultrasound evidence of intrauterine pregnancy	Reassure and discharge to GP follow-up

MECHANISMS, CAUSATION AND RISK FACTORS IN EARLY CLINICAL MISCARRIAGE

The embryo or the endometrium?

It is generally accepted that sporadic early pregnancy loss represents a physiological phenomenon, selecting out conceptions which have significant and serious structural and or chromosomal problems.[4] This assumption is borne out by studies which demonstrate that a large proportion of early clinical miscarriage is affected by either an abnormal karyotype or abnormal fetal morphology, or both. One study has demonstrated that 85 per cent of fetuses observed by embryoscopy prior to uterine evacuation had fetal malformations and in the same group an abnormal karyotype was demonstrated in 75 per cent.[5]

The endometrium also contributes to embryo selection and a failure of this process can lead to implantation failure or recurrent pregnancy loss. Compared to controls, the endometrium of women with recurrent miscarriages can be overly receptive to low-quality embryos; such 'super fecundity' facilitates the implantation of embryos that normally fail to implant only to result in a clinical miscarriage further on.[6]

Risk factors for miscarriage

Various risk factors are known to modulate one's risk of miscarriage. These include high maternal[7] and/or paternal[8]

age, history of previous miscarriage,[9] history of infertility,[10] extremes of BMI, uterine malformations, alcohol consumption and a recent change of partner.[11] There is also an association of an increased risk of miscarriage with many chronic medical conditions including diabetes, epilepsy (with or without treatment), cystic fibrosis and heart disease.

Maternal age is associated with a wide variation in the incidence of clinical early miscarriage, from 10 per cent in women aged 20–24 to 51 per cent in women aged 40–44.[7] The increase in the incidence of early pregnancy loss with age is largely related to the increased rate of aneuploidy.

Alcohol consumption both pre-conception and in the first three months of pregnancy is associated with an increased risk of miscarriage.[12] Alcohol has a dose-dependent effect on the risk of miscarriage, with those drinking more than 4 drinks per week being 2.8 times more likely to miscarry.[13]

Caffeine intake has previously been implicated as a cause of miscarriage, but recent data suggest there is only an increased risk of miscarriage where the mother had been drinking >7 cups of coffee per day, which suggests moderate caffeine intake does not increase the risk of miscarriage as previously thought.[14] Unless the mother's caffeine intake is very high it is therefore unlikely that reducing or omitting intake will reduce her risk of miscarriage.

There is conflicting evidence as to whether smoking is a risk factor for miscarriage, with a large prospective study being unable to demonstrate an association,[15] although a recent study demonstrated harm.[16]

There is a three-fold increase (5–15 per cent) in the prevalence of congenital uterine malformations when comparing women with recurrent miscarriage to an unselected control group.[17] A meta-analysis has shown that a septate uterus increases the rate of first-trimester miscarriage, again nearly three-fold with an RR of 2.89.[18] It is however unclear as to whether resection of the uterine septum is beneficial.

There is an association between hypothyroidism and increased risk of miscarriage. Meta-analysis of results from 19 cohort studies showed more than a tripling in the odds of miscarriage in the presence of thyroid antibodies (OR 3.9, 95% CI 2.48–6.12).[19] It is unclear if correction of TSH by means of T_4 (levothyroxine) improves outcomes and at the time of writing the TABLET RCT is investigating whether low-dose levothyroxine improves pregnancy outcome in patients who are euthyroid but with elevated TSH.[20]

Whilst studies have suggested a biologically plausible immunological basis for miscarriage, interventions relating to immunomodulation, such as steroid immunosuppression, allogeneic lymphocyte immunisation, intravenous immunoglobulin administration, TNFα antagonists and granulocyte colony-stimulating factor, are largely non-evidence based and not recommended for standard use.

While thrombophilias are associated with an increased risk of recurrent miscarriage, it is unclear whether a causative association with sporadic miscarriage exists.

TYPES OF CLINICAL EARLY MISCARRIAGE

Until the 1990s the term 'spontaneous abortion' was in general use by gynaecologists and other medical professionals. This term can cause significant distress due to its similarity to induced abortion (termination of pregnancy) and should therefore not be used in clinical practice. The current classification of miscarriage can also cause distress to patients and relatives if care is not exercised in its explanation as part of the delivery of bad news. Terms used should be explained in language appropriate to the patient, for example avoiding the use of missed miscarriage and instead explaining a diagnosis of delayed miscarriage. The clinical presentation, examination findings and ultrasound findings are shown in Table 89.1.

A patient presenting with a suspected history of miscarriage should first be clinically assessed by way of a medical history and examination. A suggested clinical pathway for management of these patients is depicted in Fig. 89.1. It would be appropriate to arrange a transvaginal scan in order to assess the state of the pregnancy. A TVS offers a good sensitivity and specificity for the diagnosis of miscarriage although in the event that a TVS is not immediately available to the clinician, and/or the patient is cardiovascularly unstable or bleeding heavily, it is appropriate to perform, with consent, a speculum and pelvic examination to assess the severity of bleeding and to remove any products of conception from the cervical os. In rare instances, where cervical shock occurs as a result of distension of the cervix by products of conception, rapid removal of this tissue with the aid of a speculum and a pair of sponge forceps can be life saving.

A definitive diagnosis may not be made at the first ultrasound, and in such cases appropriate follow-up should be planned. If an intrauterine pregnancy is confirmed by the presence of a gestation sac and yolk sac then follow-up should be with a further ultrasound, appropriately timed to assess progression (7–14 days).

If the location of the pregnancy is uncertain then biochemical testing for serum β-hCG is appropriate. If the level of hCG rises sub-optimally, one should suspect the differential diagnosis of ectopic pregnancy (not dealt with in this chapter). A consistently declining β-hCG suggests a failing pregnancy. Serum biochemistry, either progesterone or β-hCG, should not be used to distinguish between viable and non-viable pregnancy as it is not possible to reliably discriminate between the latter two on biochemistry alone without an ultrasound diagnosis.

Provided the patient is haemodynamically stable at the time of assessment then it is appropriate to continue any further investigations required on an outpatient basis. A minority of patients will need admission to the gynaecology ward directly from their initial assessment, either for a period of observation or if immediate surgery is planned. If there is evidence of haemodynamic instability then fluid resuscitation is appropriate and consideration should be made as to the availability of blood products should they be required (Fig. 89.1).

MANAGEMENT OF DIAGNOSED MISCARRIAGE

The management of miscarriage should be individualised, taking into account the wishes of the woman as well as the clinical situation. In most instances expectant, medical or surgical management will be appropriate, although availability of these management options will depend on local provision. If the patient is haemodynamically unstable, or the pain cannot be adequately controlled, or there are concerns about infection/sepsis, then surgical management is usually indicated.

Rhesus D prophylaxis

The use of anti-D immunoglobulin for the prevention of RhD sensitisation is now well established in the UK. In order to prevent avoidable sensitisation, it is important to ascertain the patient's blood group and treat with anti-D Ig when indicated. Those opting for surgical management at any gestation, or medical or expectant management beyond 12^{+0} weeks should receive anti-D if they are rhesus negative and have not been previously sensitised. Those receiving medical management before 12^{+0} weeks' gestation should be considered for anti-D prophylaxis. Women with a diagnosis of threatened miscarriage but continued bleeding beyond 12^{+0} weeks' gestation should also be treated.[21]

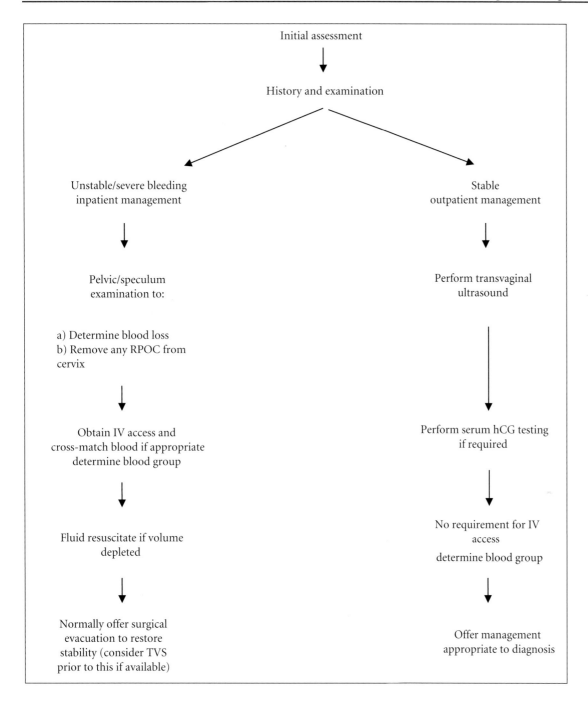

Fig. 89.1 The initial assessment of a woman with a possible diagnosis of miscarriage

Expectant management

NICE recommends that expectant management should be used for 7–14 days from a confirmed diagnosis of miscarriage unless this is unacceptable to the woman or expectant management is not clinically appropriate, for reasons such as high risk of haemorrhage or suspected infection.[22] Expectant management is an appropriate management to offer for women diagnosed with a pregnancy of uncertain viability (where the diagnosis is unclear) and threatened miscarriage.

An observational study of 1096 women diagnosed with first-trimester miscarriage evaluated the uptake and outcome of expectant management. This study demonstrated a high take-up of expectant management (70 per cent) and patient satisfaction rates of around 90 per cent with this management option.[23] The same study found that expectant management is more successful for incomplete miscarriage (84%, 185/221) compared with delayed (missed and anembryonic) miscarriage (56%, 129/230) at 14 days from diagnosis.

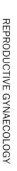

Expectant management may continue provided that the woman remains clinically well, has no signs of infection and is not compromised by the bleeding. The duration of this management can be greater than eight weeks, provided of course that the patient remains happy with this choice of management.

Follow-up is usually with ultrasound to assess whether the miscarriage has completed, as well as clinical assessment of the patient.

Medical management

Medical management involves the use of the prostaglandin analogue misoprostol to induce uterine contractions, resulting in the delivery of the pregnancy vaginally. There are several protocols being used currently regarding the dose of misoprostol used, the route of administration and whether to use mifepristone (an oral antiprogesterone). Meta-analysis of these differing protocols has allowed NICE to make the following recommendations:[22] mifepristone should not be routinely used as there is no significant increase in the success rate of treatment; misoprostol should be administered vaginally, at a dose of 800 μg for missed miscarriage or 600 μg for incomplete miscarriage; and where vaginal administration is not acceptable or wished by the patient, oral administration of the same dosage should be offered.

Success rates are similar to expectant management, with an overall success rate of around 80 per cent achieved within a shorter timescale.[24] Medical management is more likely to be successful for incomplete miscarriage than delayed miscarriage, as is the case for expectant management. It is currently uncertain as to whether expectant or surgical management is the most effective and/or cost-effective way to continue the management of patients with RPOC post medical management with misoprostol. The MisoREST trial is investigating this at the time of writing.[25]

Surgical management

Surgical management remains the treatment of choice for patients who are haemodynamically unstable, who show signs of sepsis, or who are not suitable for medical or expectant management either through patient preference or other medical co-morbidities.

Vacuum (suction) aspiration is preferable to sharp curettage as it is associated with significantly less blood loss, less postoperative pain and a shorter duration of procedure. It has a failure rate of 1–5 per cent.[26-28]

There is a risk of uterine and cervical trauma with surgical management. Uterine perforation occurs in up to 1:250 cases.[27] In such cases of suspected uterine perforation it is common to perform a laparoscopy to assess the injury and facilitate any repair that is necessary.

Intrauterine adhesions form in up to 40 per cent of patients undergoing surgical management for miscarriage[29] but it is uncommon for this to manifest in long-term fertility problems or menstrual disorders.

Which management option to recommend?

Expectant and medical management have the benefits of avoiding planned surgery and anaesthesia; however they are associated with a higher failure rate and a higher chance of needing emergency surgery due to either unacceptable bleeding or pain.[30,31]

The incidence of local pelvic infection following surgical evacuation of the uterus is around 3 per cent, and comparable with both medical and expectant management.[32]

Reassuringly the long-term follow-up of women undergoing any of the three management options for miscarriage shows no significant difference in the livebirth rate five years post miscarriage, at 79 per cent (298/454) for both medical and expectant management and 82 per cent for surgical management (192/235).[33]

There is no 'one size fits all' miscarriage management strategy, and as a result care should be individualised. Clinicians who are providing advice to patients must therefore take into account their wishes, their medical history, local provision of services and the patient's ability to access those services along with the current clinical situation.

PREVENTION OF MISCARRIAGE

1   Progesterone: Although commonly used in many countries, there is still insufficient evidence to suggest the routine use of progesterone to prevent/reduce the risk of miscarriage.[34]
2   Other pharmacological/alternative interventions: There is no evidence of reduction in the risk of miscarriage with the use of:
    – multivitamins;
    – oestrogen supplementation;
    – uterine muscle relaxants;
    – hCG;
    – complementary medicine.
3   Non-pharmacological interventions: As previously discussed, the evidence for smoking as a direct risk factor for miscarriage is inconsistent. As there are significant health benefits to stopping smoking, a recommendation that smokers stop smoking is appropriate.

Addressing concerns about maternal alcohol consumption is appropriate. Increased or even moderate alcohol intake is associated with an increased risk of miscarriage, and in an ongoing pregnancy with fetal alcohol syndrome. For those planning pregnancy the current recommendation is to avoid alcohol.[12]

Bed rest has historically been recommended as a treatment for threatened miscarriage; however there are no data to support its use.[35]

4 Embryo selection: There is currently no evidence to suggest that screening embryos prior to implantation helps with reducing the risk of miscarriage.

KEY POINTS

- Significant morbidity or indeed mortality from miscarriage is fortunately now rare in the UK.
- Diagnosis is by TVS combined (when appropriate) with hCG follow-up.
- Expectant, medical or surgical management of miscarriage will be safe management options for the majority of women with a diagnosis of miscarriage. Management will therefore depend on patient preference and local availability.
- Surgical management (evacuation of products of conception - ERPC) remains the mainstay of treatment in women who are haemodynamically unstable.

References

1. Mackenzie W, Holmes D, Newton J. Spontaneous_Abortion_Rate_in_Ultrasonographically.17.pdf. *Obstet Gynaecol* 1988; 71:1.

2. Ugwumadu A, Manyonda I, Reid F, Hay P. Effect of early oral clindamycin on late miscarriage and preterm delivery in asymptomatic women with abnormal vaginal flora and bacterial vaginosis: A randomised controlled trial. *Lancet* 2003; 361:983–8.

3. Makrydimas G, Sebire NJ, Lolis D, Vlassis N, Nicolaides KH. Fetal loss following ultrasound diagnosis of a live fetus at 6–10 weeks of gestation. *Ultrasound Obstet Gynecol* 2003; 22(4):368–732.

4. Larsen EC, Christiansen OB, Kolte AM, Macklon N. New insights into mechanisms behind miscarriage. *BMC Med* 2013;11(1):154.

5. Philipp T, Philipp K, Reiner A, Beer F, Kalousek DK. Embryoscopic and cytogenetic analysis of 233 missed abortions: factors involved in the pathogenesis of developmental defects of early failed pregnancies. *Hum Reprod* 2003;18:1724–32.

6. Weimar CHE, Kavelaars A, Brosens JJ *et al.* Endometrial stromal cells of women with recurrent miscarriage fail to discriminate between high- and low-quality human embryos. *PLoS One* 2012;7(7):e41424.

7. Andersen AN, Wohlfahrt J, Christens JP, Olsen J, Melbye M, Nybo A. General practice linkage study.

8. de la Rochebrochard E, Thonneau P. Paternal age and maternal age are risk factors for miscarriage; results of a multicentre European study. *Hum Reprod* 2002;17(6):1649–56.

9. Regan L, Braude PR, Trembath PL. Influence of past reproductive performance on risk of spontaneous abortion. *BMJ* 1989;299(6698):541–5.

10. Axmon A, Hagmar L. Time to pregnancy and pregnancy outcome. *Fertility and Sterility* 2005;84(4): 966–74.

11. Maconochie N, Doyle P, Prior S, Simmons R. Risk factors for first trimester miscarriage: results from a UK-population-based case-control study. *BJOG* 2007;114(2):170–86.

12. NICE. CG62 Antenatal care. March 2008.

13. Andersen A-M, Andersen PK, Olsen J, Grønbæk M, Strandberg-Larsen K. Moderate alcohol intake during pregnancy and risk of fetal death. *Int J Epidemiol* 2012;41:405–13.

14. Bech BH, Nohr EA, Vaeth M, Henriksen TB, Olsen J. Coffee and fetal death: a cohort study with prospective data. *Am J Epidemiol* 2005;162:983–90.

15. Wisborg K, Kesmodel U, Henriksen TB, Hedegaard M, Secher NJ. A prospective study of maternal smoking and spontaneous abortion. *Acta Obstet Gynecol Scand* 2003;82:936–41.

16. Saravelos SH, Regan L. The importance of pre-conception counseling and early pregnancy monitoring. *Semin Reprod Med* 2011;29(6):557–68.

17. Chan YY, Jayaprakasan K, Zamora J, Thornton JG, Raine-Fenning N, Coomarasamy A. The prevalence of congenital uterine anomalies in unselected and high-risk populations: a systematic review. *Hum Reprod Update* 2011;17:761–71.

18. Chan YY, Jayaprakasan K, Tan A, Thornton JG, Coomarasamy A, Raine-Fenning NJ. Reproductive outcomes in women with congenital uterine anomalies: a systematic review. *Ultrasound Obstet Gynecol* 2011;38:371–82.

19. Tan A, Knox E, Kilby MD, Franklyn J, Coomarasamy A. Association between thyroid autoantibodies and miscarriage and preterm birth: meta-analysis of evidence. *BMJ* 2011;342:d2616.

20. Coomarasamy A. Randomised Controlled Trial of the efficacy and mechanism of Levothyroxine treatment on pregnancy and neonatal outcomes in women with thyroid antibodies. Birmingham Clinical Trials Unit, University of Birmingham; ISTCTN number 15948785.

21. RCOG. *The Use of Anti-D Immunoglobulin for Rhesus D Prophylaxis.* Guideline no. 22. RCOG, 2011.

22. NICE. *ECG154 Ectopic pregnancy and miscarriage.* December 2012.

23. Luise C, Jermy K, May C. Outcome of expectant management of spontaneous first trimester miscarriage: observational study. *BMJ* 2002; 324:873–5.

24. Blohm F, Fridén BE, Milsom I, Platz-Christensen JJ, Nielsen S. A randomised double-blind trial comparing misoprostol or placebo in the management of early miscarriage. *BJOG* 2005;112(8):1090–5.

25. Verschoor MAC, Lemmers M, Bossuyt PM *et al.* Surgical versus expectant management in women with an incomplete evacuation of the uterus after treatment with

misoprostol for miscarriage: the MisoREST trial. *BMC Pregnancy Childbirth* 2013;13:102.

26. Tunçalp Ö, Am G, Jp S. Surgical procedures for evacuating incomplete miscarriage. *Cochrane Database of Systematic Reviews* 2010;9. Doi 10.1002/14651858.CD001993.pub2.

27. RCOG. *Surgical evacuation of the uterus for early pregnancy loss.* Guideline No. 10. RCOG, 2010.

28. Hassan R, Bhal K, Joseph B. The need for repeat evacuation of retained products of conception: how common is it? *J Obstet Gynaecol* 2013;33(1):75–6.

29. Westendorp IC, Ankum WM, Mol BW, Vonk J. Prevalence of Asherman's syndrome after secondary removal of placental remnants or a repeat curettage for incomplete abortion. *Hum Reprod* 1998;13(12):3347–50.

30. Nanda K, Lm L, Da G, Peloggia A, Nanda G. Expectant care versus surgical treatment for miscarriage. *Cochrane Database of Systematic Reviews*, 2012;9. Doi: 10.1002/14651858.CD003518.pub3.

31. Jp N, Gml G, Hickey M, Jc V, Dou L. Medical treatments for incomplete miscarriage. *Cochrane Database of Systematic Reviews*, 2013;3. Doi 10.1002/14651858. CD007223.pub3.

32. Trinder J, Brocklehurst P, Porter R, Read M, Vyas S, Smith L. Management of miscarriage: expectant, medical, or surgical? Results of randomised controlled trial (miscarriage treatment MIST trial). *BMJ* 2006;332(7552):1235–40.

33. Coker W, Ba S. Incidence of pregnancy after expectant, medical, or surgical management of spontaneous first trimester miscarriage: long-term follow-up of miscarriage treatment (MIST) randomised controlled trial. *BMJ* 2009;339:b3827.

34. Wahabi HA, Abed Althagafi NF, Elawad M, Al Zeidan RA. Progestogen for treating threatened miscarriage. *Cochrane Database Syst Rev* 2011;3:CD005943.

35. Aleman A, Althabe F, Jm B, Bergel E. Bed rest during pregnancy for preventing miscarriage. *Cochrane Database of Systematic Reviews* 2005;2:CD003576.

Chapter 90 Ectopic pregnancy

Ghada Salman, Davor Jurkovic

MRCOG standards

Knowledge criteria

- Understanding of epidemiology, aetiology, pathogenesis and clinical features of ectopic pregnancy.
- Prognosis after ectopic pregnancy and pregnancy of unknown location.
- Identification and assessment of evidence.

Theoretical skills

- Clinical presentation and assessment.
- Indications and limitations of investigations.
- Biochemical: serum βhCG and progesterone.
- Radiological: ultrasound.

Practical skills

Understanding of management options:
- Conservative management;
- Medical management;
- Surgical management.

INTRODUCTION

Ectopic pregnancy is a major health problem and an important cause of morbidity and mortality in women of reproductive age. Ruptured ectopic pregnancy can cause severe intra-abdominal bleeding which may require emergency life-saving surgery. The UK CEMACH reported a maternal mortality rate (MMR) of 0.2 per 1000 ectopic pregnancies or 0.3 per 100,000 maternities.[1]

Serious adverse outcomes, however, tend to occur only in a small minority of women and they are often caused by delays in reaching the correct diagnosis. Over half (54 per cent) of deaths caused by ectopic pregnancies have been attributed to substandard clinical care. It is therefore important that all health professionals are familiar with the risk factors, clinical signs and symptoms of ectopic pregnancy to ensure timely referrals to secondary care. The burden of the disease is also considerable due to the high costs of diagnostic investigations and treatment.[1,2]

Improvements in diagnosis and management are therefore needed to prevent avoidable deaths from ectopic pregnancies. Better clinical care should also help to reduce physical and psychological morbidity associated with ectopic pregnancy, improve future fertility outcomes and reduce the costs associated with repeated hospital follow-up visits and admissions.[1,3,4]

DEFINITION OF ECTOPIC PREGNANCY

Ectopic pregnancy is defined as any pregnancy that implants outside the uterine cavity. Most of the ectopic pregnancies implant within the Fallopian tubes (93–97 per cent) of which the majority are found within the ampullary part.[5] Implantation of pregnancy in the interstitial part of the Fallopian tube occurs in 2.5 per cent of cases. Despite their relative rarity, these interstitial pregnancies are responsible for about a fifth of all deaths caused by ectopic pregnancies in the UK.[1]

In about 5–7 per cent of ectopic pregnancies, the implantation occurs outside the Fallopian tubes. Most of these pregnancies are located within the uterine wall but outside the endometrial cavity and they include intramural, cervical and caesarean scar pregnancies. Other reported sites for ectopic pregnancy include ovarian and abdominal pregnancies.[6] Cornual pregnancies are those located in rudimentary, non-communicated cornua of anomalous uteri. Although these pregnancies are located within the uterine cavity, they follow the clinical course of ectopic pregnancy and they typically result in late rupture. For that reason cornual pregnancies tend to be classified as a form of ectopic pregnancy. Spontaneous heterotopic pregnancy, i.e. concomitant intra- and extrauterine pregnancy, occurs in 0.3–0.8 per cent of women of reproductive age and 1–3 per cent of pregnancies following assisted reproduction.[7]

EPIDEMIOLOGY

True prevalence of ectopic pregnancy is difficult to ascertain as the figures in the literature vary. Three commonly used denominators to express prevalence of ectopics are number of births, number of pregnancies and number of women of reproductive age (15–44 years) in the population. The reported prevalence is also influenced by the variations in diagnostic facilities between different countries. The worldwide prevalence of ectopic pregnancies is believed to be around 1–2 per cent per number of pregnancies.[8]

In the UK nearly 12,000 ectopic pregnancies are diagnosed each year, which gives an incidence of 1.1 per cent. The reported incidences in some of the other countries are shown in Table 90.1.[9-15] There are very wide variations in the reported figures which are more likely to reflect methodological differences between the studies rather than a true incidence of ectopics. The UK statistics have also suggested that the rate of hospital admission for ectopic pregnancies is around 1.5 per 100 deliveries (1.5 per cent).[1]

The UK MMR due to ectopic pregnancies is approximately 0.02 per cent, which is significantly lower compared to developing countries where the reported MMRs are between 1 per cent and 3 per cent.[1,15] Table 90.2 shows the incidence and mortality rates of ectopic pregnancies in the UK since 1991.

Table 90.1 The reported incidence of ectopic pregnancies in several countries around the world

Country	Ectopic pregnancies/1000 deliveries
UK[9]	3–16
USA[10]	4–16
Australia[11]	16–17
Norway[12]	14–22
Finland[13]	6–26
Ghana (Africa)[14,15]	11–46

AETIOLOGY AND PATHOPHYSIOLOGY

Most ectopic pregnancies develop abnormally slowly which could be due to inadequate blood supply to these gestations outside the endometrial cavity. This results in inappropriate signalling to the corpus luteum, leading to low progesterone production. Tubal ectopic pregnancies often stop growing and may eventually undergo regression and spontaneous resolution. Alternatively they may continue to develop, causing distention of the Fallopian tube accompanied by invasion of the trophoblastic tissue into the tubal mucosa. This may eventually result in tubal rupture and intra-abdominal bleeding. In some women tubal ectopic pregnancy is expelled spontaneously into the peritoneal cavity through the fimbrial end of the Fallopian tube, which is referred to as tubal miscarriage.[7]

In normal pregnancy fertilisation of the mature ovum occurs in the ampullary part of the Fallopian tubes, thus any abnormalities of the tubal morphology or function can lead to impaired migration of the fertilised egg. It has been hypothesised that damage to the tubal mucosa is the main cause of tubal ectopic pregnancy. This could result in internal scarring of the Fallopian tube that interferes with the transfer of the embryo, or to a mucosal defect that encourages implantation of the fertilised ovum in the tube. Other theories suggested that malfunction of the tubal smooth muscle because of an altered oestrogen:progesterone ratio could be a causative factor behind ectopic pregnancy.[16-18]

The pathophysiology behind ectopic pregnancies in the absence of tubal pathology remains unclear. One possible explanation is the poor quality of the morula, while others have claimed that that ectopic pregnancy might represent a chromosomally abnormal pregnancy. However a study by Goddijn *et al.*[17] has demonstrated that the rate of chromosomally abnormal ectopic pregnancy was not higher than those obtained from intrauterine pregnancies. The effect of the male factor has also been suggested in the aetiology of ectopic pregnancy but there is not enough available evidence to support this.[17,19,20]

RISK FACTORS

A number of risk factors for ectopic pregnancy have been reported in observational studies (Box 90.1). Evidence of

Table 90.2 The incidence and mortality rates of ectopic pregnancies in the UK from 1991–2008 (adapted from reference 1)

Years	Estimated pregnancies (n)	Estimated ectopic pregnancies (n)	Ectopic pregnancies/1000 pregnancies	Number of deaths	Mortality rate/10000 maternities
1991–93	3141667	30160	9.6	9	3.9
1994–96	2917391	33550	11.5	12	5.5
1997–99	2878012	31946	11.1	13	6.1
2000–02	2736364	30100	11.0	11	5.5
2003–05	2891892	32100	11.1	10	4.7
2006–08	3139315	35495	11.3	6	2.6

Box 90.1 Risk factors for ectopic pregnancies

High risks

Tubal pathology

Previous ectopic pregnancy

Previous tubal surgery

In utero diethylstilbestrol

Smoking

Moderate risks

History of pelvic infection

Infertility/sub fertility

Multiple sexual partners

Advanced age

tubal pathology, history of previous ectopic pregnancy, previous tubal surgery, and in-utero diethylstilboestrol were found to be strongly associated with ectopic pregnancy in a recent meta-analysis of studies, while previous history of genital infection (PID, chlamydia, gonorrhoea), infertility, subfertility and multiple sexual partners were moderately associated with risk of ectopic pregnancy [A].[21] Another large study of all ectopic pregnancies diagnosed in one region of France showed history of infection and smoking to be the most important risk factors; however, around 24 per cent of women who were diagnosed with ectopic pregnancy had no known risk factors [C].[22] It has been postulated that the main adverse effect of smoking is on the motility of ciliated tubal epithelium, resulting in delayed transport of the fertilised ovum, leading to implantation in the Fallopian tubes. Smoking could also affect other aspects of fertility causing delayed ovulation, fertilisation and implantation. A dose–effect relationship between smoking and ectopic pregnancy has been suggested with a higher rate of ectopic pregnancy when more than 20 cigarettes were smoked per day.[22]

It has been suggested that about a third of ectopic pregnancies are a result of tubal infection or previous surgery. Although several types of micro-organisms can cause PID, chlamydia infection appears to be the main causative agent.[21,23] The incidence of tubal damage after one episode of PID was determined to be about 8 per cent but this increases to 19.5 per cent after two episodes and 40 per cent after three episodes. The risk of tubal damage was also related to the severity of salpingitis even with one episode, increasing from 0.6 per cent for mild to 6 per cent for moderate and 21.4 per cent for severe salpingitis [C].[24]

In women with previous ectopic pregnancy, the risk of recurrent ectopic pregnancy is higher than in the general population and it increases further with every successive occurrence. In one study the ORs for having an ectopic pregnancy were 3 (95% CI 1.8–5.7) after one previous ectopic and 16 (95% CI 4.4–47.7) after two previous ectopic pregnancies.[25] An association between advanced maternal age and ectopic pregnancy has also been demonstrated in different studies. The OR for having an ectopic pregnancy can be doubled for women over 35 years of age (OR 1.4) and it is four times higher in women

over 40 (OR 2.9) when compared to younger women less than 20 years of age (OR 0.6).[22] This could be explained by potentially higher exposure to risk factors, increased incidence of chromosomal abnormalities of the conceptus and age-related changes of tubal function [C].[26,27]

Generally, the use of contraception prevents all types of pregnancy including ectopic pregnancy but failure of certain contraceptive methods is associated with increased risk of ectopic pregnancy. In women who become pregnant following tubal ligation, the risk of ectopic pregnancy is particularly high. In a multicentre prospective cohort study the 10-year cumulative probability of ectopic pregnancy after tubal sterilisation was 7.3 per 1000 procedures.[28] The risk is also significantly increased with an intrauterine contraceptive device *in situ* (IUCD). A meta-analysis of studies has shown that in women with current IUCD use, when compared to pregnant controls, there is an increased risk of ectopic pregnancy (OR 10.6, 95% CI 7.66–14.74) while past IUCD use only mildly increases the risk of ectopic pregnancy (OR 1.4, 95% CI 1.23–1.59) [A].[29] Although the risk of ectopic pregnancy is 6–10 per cent in women with failure of progesterone-only pills, the risk of ectopic pregnancy for women who have failure of oral contraceptive pills, emergency hormonal pills and the barrier method is similar to the risk of women not using any type of contraception.[30,31]

Women with a history of infertility and especially those treated with superovulatory drugs or undergoing IVF are at a higher risk of ectopic pregnancy (4–5 per cent) and heterotopic pregnancies (1–3 per cent) when compared to women conceiving naturally. The most probable explanation is the shift of the embryo from the uterine cavity back into the Fallopian tubes.[32-34]

CLINICAL PRESENTATION

Clinical presentation of ectopic pregnancy is variable and is largely determined by the location of the pregnancy. In general, ectopic pregnancies implanted closer to the uterus tend to develop further and present with more severe clinical symptoms. The more common types of tubal ectopics that develop in the ampullary part of the tube are unlikely to grow beyond the very early stages, therefore causing less serious symptoms.

The most common presentations in women with ectopic pregnancies are vaginal bleeding, pelvic pain and amenorrhoea. However in one study around one third of women did not present with this triad.[35] Vaginal bleeding is usually an early presentation that happens soon after a missed period and can vary from mild brownish vaginal spotting to period-like fresh bleeding. Occasionally vaginal bleeding may be heavy and associated with passage of a cast of endometrial tissue. This can lead to incorrect diagnosis of menstrual period or miscarriage. Abdominal pain typically occurs after the onset of vaginal bleeding. Location, type and intensity of pain can also be variable. It can be localised to one side or present as generalised abdominal pain, dull or sharp, crampy or continuous, at the ipsilateral or contralateral site to the ectopic pregnancy. Occasionally the woman might complain of upper abdominal pain or rectal pressure and/or pain on defecation. The

REPRODUCTIVE GYNAECOLOGY

pain that women with ectopic pregnancy experience usually occurs due to tubal distension, as a result of blood entering the peritoneal cavity from the fimbrial end or tubal rupture. The severity of the pain does not always correspond to the amount of blood loss into the peritoneal cavity. On the other hand, pain referred to the shoulder usually reflects irritation of the diaphragm and is a sign of a major bleed.[35-39] However, up to 9 per cent of women diagnosed with ectopic pregnancy do not complain of any abdominal pain.[40]

Nausea, vomiting and diarrhoea occasionally occur with severe intra-abdominal haemorrhage and can lead to erroneous diagnosis of gastrointestinal, urinary tract or other acute gynaecological conditions and delay the diagnosis of potentially life-threatening intra-abdominal bleeding.[1,6] Four of the six women who died from ectopic pregnancies in this last triennium complained of diarrhoea, dizziness or vomiting as the presenting symptoms.[1] A key recommendation from the 2006–2008 CEMACH report, as with the previous report, was that the diagnosis of ectopic pregnancy should be considered in all women of reproductive age with sudden onset of severe gastrointestinal symptoms.[1]

DIAGNOSIS

Physical examination

There is little evidence to support the diagnostic benefit of internal examination in women presenting in early pregnancy with abdominal pain or vaginal bleeding. In routine clinical practice, however, vaginal examination using speculum and bimanual palpation is still often used as a part of the diagnostic work-up for ectopic pregnancies. The findings of tenderness on moving the cervix or adnexal mass and/or tenderness and vaginal bleeding are all non-specific signs and can present in different early pregnancy complications, gynaecological and non-gynaecological conditions. In addition most ectopic pregnancies are too small to be felt clearly on bimanual examination and uterine size assessment is rarely helpful in making the diagnosis.[39,41,42]

Vaginal examination is generally uncomfortable for pregnant women, even for those with a normal intrauterine pregnancy. Applying pressure on a swollen Fallopian tube could result in rupture of the ectopic pregnancy; however, there is little evidence to support this assertion. In addition about 36 per cent of women will lack adnexal tenderness on pelvic examination. Referral of women with suspected ectopic pregnancies for ultrasound examination when available is suggested prior to vaginal examination. Signs of haemorrhagic shock might be also present such as high pulse rate, low blood pressure, pallor and low urine output.[35,39,41,42]

Recent NICE guidelines on the management of pain and bleeding in early pregnancy recommend that clinicians should be offering a pregnancy test to all women of reproductive age as part of their clinical assessments, even when symptoms are non-specific.[4]

Developments in ultrasound technology and improvements in the sensitivity of laboratory investigations have greatly added to the accuracy of non-invasive diagnosis of ectopic pregnancy. Ultrasound scans (especially transvaginal examination), and biochemistry investigations (quantitative serum βhCG testing and progesterone) are now considered as necessary investigations when evaluating women with pain or vaginal bleeding during early pregnancy.

Ultrasound

The first report describing ultrasound criteria for the diagnosis of ectopic pregnancy was published in 1969.[43] The introduction of the transvaginal ultrasound in the assessment of women in early pregnancy has greatly improved the diagnosis of ectopic pregnancy and it is now considered the diagnostic method of choice. In addition studies have demonstrated that it is an acceptable diagnostic tool for women presenting with early pregnancy complications such as pain or bleeding.[44,45]

A meta-analysis of the accuracy of ultrasound demonstrated a sensitivity of 99 per cent (95% CI 96.6% to 100%) with specificity of 71 per cent (95% CI 60% to 80%) when it was used as the diagnostic tool in North American emergency departments [A].[46] The presence of other factors such as increased BMI, uterine fibroids or adnexal lesions such as ovarian cysts can make visualisation of the adnexa difficult and cause delay in the diagnosis of ectopic pregnancy. NICE in its guideline has advised offering women attending an early pregnancy assessment service or emergency gynaecology service a TVS to identify the location of the pregnancy and check its viability.[4]

Despite the fact that transabdominal ultrasound is still used in some places, the benefit of using this approach is doubtful. The visualisation of intrauterine pregnancy can be challenging when the pregnancy is smaller than 6 or 7 weeks' gestation. It is also difficult for operators to clearly visualise or exclude ectopic pregnancies with certainty. It is therefore not surprising that high false-negative and false-positive rates were reported when transabdominal ultrasound examination was used in women with suspected early pregnancy complications.[41,47]

Transvaginal sonography has been shown in many studies to have a better sensitivity (87–99 per cent) and specificity (94–99 per cent) for the diagnosis of ectopic pregnancy [C].[48-50]. The additional advantage of TVS examination is that it allows guided palpation of the pelvic organs, which helps to assess their mobility and to determine the site of tenderness. The transabdominal route, however, may be helpful in women with large fibroid uteri or other pelvic pathology, such as adenomyosis or ovarian cysts.[47,51,52]

The accuracy of ultrasound examination in detecting ectopic pregnancy depends largely on the experience of the operator and the quality of the ultrasound machine. In the hands of an experienced operator, the location of pregnancy can be determined from a single ultrasound examination and about 75–80 per cent of clinically significant ectopic pregnancies are detected at the initial examination with a further 20–25 per cent detected at subsequent ultrasound scan assessments.[50,53,54] However, the detection of ectopic pregnancy on ultrasound is also dependent on its size at the time of presentation. A study comparing the diagnosis of ectopic pregnancy at first visit with serum hCG levels has shown that women with a clear diagnosis of ectopic pregnancy on TVS had a higher level of βhCG and more advanced gestational age when compared to women in whom the pregnancy could not be visualised (pregnancy of unknown location or PUL).[53]

The following morphological criteria can help to identify ectopic pregnancy when seen on ultrasound outside the uterine cavity:[55,56]

1   gestational sac surrounded by a hyperechoic ring with or without a yolk sac;
2   gestational sac with an embryo with or without cardiac activity (Fig. 90.1);
3   solid tubal swelling or inhomogeneous adnexal mass separate from the ovary.

The second morphological type is very specific to ectopic pregnancy, whilst the risk of misdiagnosis is higher when the sac is empty or in cases where there is an inhomogeneous mass. Using these criteria, the efficiency of TVS in diagnosing ectopic pregnancy was 96 per cent using diagnostic laparoscopy as the reference standard.[57] In a study by Cacciatore et al.,[58] where the visualisation of an adnexal mass was used for the diagnosis of ectopic pregnancy, a specificity of 99 per cent was demonstrated. The presence of an adnexal mass that is separate from the ovary on TVS has also been demonstrated by observational studies to be a good indicator of ectopic pregnancy.[49] This was further confirmed by a meta-analysis of studies comparing different morphological criteria for the diagnosis of ectopic pregnancy, which concluded that the presence of an inhomogeneous mass separate from the ovary had a high specificity of 98.9 per cent, a sensitivity of 84.4 per cent with a 96.3 per cent positive predictive value and negative predictive value of 94.8 per cent [A].[59]

A number of other ultrasound findings have been suggested to facilitate detection of ectopic pregnancy, but they are not specific enough to be used in clinical practice. The presence of blood or blood clots in the pelvis is highly suspicious of ruptured ectopic pregnancy and should be differentiated from free fluid in the pouch of Douglas, which is a common finding in women with a normal intrauterine pregnancy. But consideration needs to be given to other possibilities of echogenic fluid in the pelvis such as rupture of a haemorrhagic ovarian cyst. An important distinction needs also to be made between the intrauterine gestational sac in normal pregnancy and the presence of a pseudosac as a result of small bleeding within the uterine cavity in women with ectopic pregnancy. The diagnostic criteria are as listed in Table 90.3. Problems can also arise in women with congenital uterine abnormalities and large uterine fibroids. In those cases a careful and systematic approach to the ultrasound examination helps to visualise the site of the pregnancy. The use of transabdominal and 3D ultrasound may help in these cases to determine the shape of the uterine cavity. In addition, in symptomatic women, especially those who have conceived after IVF treatment or with the use of superovulation drugs, it is important to exclude the presence of heterotopic pregnancy. Heterotopic pregnancies need also to be excluded in spontaneous pregnancy when more than one corpus luteum is present.[50,60-62]

Surgical and histopathological diagnosis

Traditionally, the diagnosis of ectopic pregnancy used to be made by surgery and then confirmed by histological examination of the excised specimen, usually a Fallopian tube containing the suspected ectopic pregnancy. However, in modern practice the diagnostic role of surgery is declining as an increasing proportion of ectopic pregnancies are managed more conservatively. In recent years laparoscopy has replaced open surgery to diagnose and treat ectopic pregnancies.[63] Although laparoscopy is still perceived by many as the gold standard for the diagnosis of ectopic pregnancy, its diagnostic accuracy has never been properly tested. In an observational study 4.5 per cent (2/44) of women reported to have no evidence of ectopic

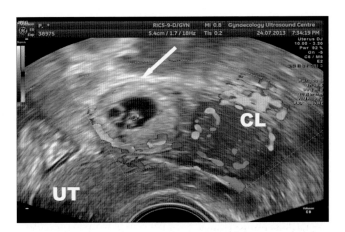

Fig. 90.1 A pelvic ultrasound image showing a gestational sac (arrow) containing an embryo with cardiac activity documented on colour Doppler examination. The sac is located behind the uterus (UT) and medial to the left ovary which contains a corpus luteum (CL)

Table 90.3 Diagnostic criteria for the distinction between intrauterine gestational sac in normal pregnancy and the presence of pseudo sac as a result of small bleeding within the uterine cavity in women with ectopic pregnancy

	Early gestational sac	Pseudo sac
Location	Eccentric, appears on one side of the cavity line within the endometrium	Central, along the endometrial cavity line
Shape	Regular, usually round	Elliptical shaped, can change contour during scan
Borders	Double decidual sign or double echogenic ring	Single layer
Colour flow pattern	Vascular peripheral flow can be demonstrated	Relatively avascular

pregnancy at the time of initial laparoscopy were subsequently diagnosed with an ectopic pregnancy [D].[64] At laparoscopy, unruptured tubal ectopic pregnancy appears as a well-defined swelling of the Fallopian tube. However, the diagnosis is not always straightforward especially in cases of small ectopic pregnancy or ectopics located in the interstitial part of the tube. The diagnosis of ectopic pregnancy can also be difficult in women with extensive pelvic adhesions that prevent clear visualisation of the tubes.[63-65] Histopathology can confirm the diagnosis of ectopic pregnancy after surgical treatment of ectopic pregnancy where chorionic villi are detected within the Fallopian tubes or other excised specimen. However, difficulty can arise when there is a complete tubal miscarriage or tubal rupture as it might not be possible to identify chorionic villi in the salpingectomy specimen and in these women, follow-up with serum βhCG measurements is advisable to ensure complete resolution of the ectopic pregnancy. A recent prospective study showed that histological examination failed to identify the presence of chorionic villi in 5 per cent of women with ultrasound, biochemical and surgical evidence of tubal ectopics.[66]

Another proposed surgical procedure to diagnose ectopic pregnancy is to perform dilatation and curettage. The theory behind it is that finding chorionic villi on histology will help to exclude ectopic pregnancy. This approach is of limited value, as although the presence of heterotopic pregnancy is uncommon, it cannot be excluded. In addition it was shown that the majority of women who had no chorionic villi on histological examination of the uterine cavity content had no ectopic pregnancies on diagnostic laparoscopy.[67]

Biochemical diagnosis

Serum human chorionic gonadotrophin

Serum βhCG is the most commonly used hormone in the assessment of women in whom ultrasound findings are non-diagnostic. Single and serial measurements of serum βhCG have been used to try to facilitate non-invasive diagnosis of ectopic pregnancy but it is rarely possible to determine the location of pregnancy on the basis of changes in maternal βhCG concentrations alone.[68,69] A single serum βhCG measurement will usually give an indication of when a singleton normal intrauterine pregnancy should be visualised on transvaginal or transabdominal ultrasound scan in a woman with a healthy uterus. Several studies have reported different discriminatory βhCG levels above which a normal intrauterine pregnancy should be detectable on ultrasound scan. The most commonly used cut-off values to detect a normal intrauterine pregnancy on TVS are 1000–1500 IU/L and 6500 IU/L when transabdominal scan is used.[47,70]

However, discriminatory or cut-off values for βhCG should be interpreted with caution. It has been shown in one study that more than 50 per cent of ectopic pregnancies detected on ultrasound had βhCG levels less than 1000 IU/L. In addition in many women who suffered complete miscarriages, serum βhCG levels remained high due to its long half-life of 24–36 hours.[71,72]

Serial βhCG measurements are considered more useful. An abnormal or slow increase in βhCG levels has been traditionally used to predict ectopic pregnancies. Although it is true that the sub-optimal βhCG rise indicates that the pregnancy is likely to be abnormal, it cannot discriminate reliably between intrauterine miscarriage and ectopic pregnancy. It has also been demonstrated in some studies that in 10–20 per cent of ectopic pregnancies, serum βhCG increases normally.[73,74]

The usefulness of measured βhCG in detecting pregnancy location was questioned in a recent meta-analysis. A single serum βhCG level was shown to be a poor test to diagnose ectopic pregnancy, and the results were only slightly better when serial measurements were performed [A].[75]

Progesterone

Progesterone production from the corpus luteum depends largely on the rate of βhCG increase in early pregnancy. The half-life of progesterone clearance is about 2 hours, which is shorter than the 24- to 36-hour half-life of βhCG. This means that it can respond rapidly to any change in the βhCG level. As a result its level can be used as an indicator of βhCG dynamics and behaviour in early pregnancy.[76]

While serum progesterone levels can be used to predict whether the pregnancy is in progression or regression, it has been shown by different studies that it should not be used to speculate about its location.[77,78] A meta-analysis by Mol et al.[79] has demonstrated that a single measurement of progesterone level can help to identify women at risk of ectopic pregnancy but it was not sufficient on its own to diagnose ectopic pregnancy [A]. It has been shown by several authors that serum progesterone <20 nmol/L reflects fast decreasing βhCG levels in maternal blood and thus can be used to predict failing pregnancy with a sensitivity of 94 per cent and specificity of 91 per cent. Progesterone levels >60 nmol/L indicate a normal increase in βhCG levels and are often associated with normal viable intrauterine pregnancy. The dilemma is when the progesterone level is between 20 and 60 as this is usually a reflection of an abnormal pregnancy that could be either ectopic or miscarriage, and further follow-up is warranted to reach the final diagnosis. The benefit of routine measurement of serum progesterone is that it can reliably diagnose pregnancies in regression and thus can reduce by 50–60 per cent the need for follow-up scans and serial βhCG measurements in pregnant women with non-diagnostic scan findings.[71,80-84]

PREGNANCY OF UNKNOWN LOCATION

Pregnancy of unknown location is a term used to describe the ultrasound scan when pregnancy is not visualised inside or outside the uterine cavity in women with a positive pregnancy test. Studies suggest that in 8–31 per cent of women presenting with mild clinical symptoms of early pregnancy complications ultrasound will not identify the location of the pregnancy. The percentage of PUL cases will depend on the skills of the ultrasound operator, the quality of the ultrasound equipment and the route of ultrasound examination (transvaginal or transabdominal).[54,85] Recent meta-analysis has concluded that the diagnostic accuracy of serum βhCG strategies in women with PUL did not provide enough data to detect the outcome of these pregnancies and whether they will end up with viable intrauterine pregnancies, failing pregnancies or ectopic pregnancies [A].[75] It has also highlighted the need for further properly conducted prospective studies.

The majority of women with PUL either have a normal pregnancy that is too small to be seen on the scan or have already suffered a miscarriage. A minority of women with PUL are eventually diagnosed with ectopic pregnancies. In about 50–70 per cent of PULs serum βhCG will decline eventually to non-pregnant level and further routine follow-up is not required.[75] Several studies have demonstrated that a declining serum βhCG level on serial measurements, or a single low initial reading of serum progesterone, can help to identify a woman in whom pregnancy is undergoing spontaneous resolution regardless of its location. When serum βhCG levels decline rapidly by >13 per cent over 48 hours or when the initial serum progesterone is ≤20 nmol/L the risk of women requiring any form of medical intervention is very low.[86-95]

In published observational studies [C–D] the outcome of 44–69 per cent of PULs was a resolution with expectant management; the remainder were early intrauterine pregnancies that miscarried. Ectopic pregnancy was eventually diagnosed in 14–28 per cent of cases.[71,96-98] Women with minimal or no symptoms of ectopic pregnancy should be managed expectantly with follow-up in two to three days. Active intervention should be considered if clinical symptoms of ectopic pregnancy occur or serum βhCG levels continue to rise. Further follow-up with ultrasound and/or repeat measurement of biochemical markers needs to continue until the correct diagnosis is reached.[75,99] If women with PULs are managed expectantly, serial serum βhCG measurements should be performed until the levels are less than 20 IU/L. In addition, women need to be given clear information regarding the follow-up plans and the importance of compliance; they also need to be within easy access of the hospital treating them. However, a very small minority of women will have the diagnosis of persistent PUL despite follow-up scans and serial βhCG measurements. The ideal management for these cases is not known but expectant management or the use of systemic methotrexate in women with mild symptoms is reported to be successful.[89,99] NICE in its recent guideline has advised that in women with PUL on scan, attention needs to focus on their symptoms more than βhCG results. Follow-up also needs to continue until the location of the pregnancy becomes known but consider a repeat scan for women with a serum βhCG level greater than or equal to 1500 IU/L.[4]

MANAGEMENT

The improvements in the quality of diagnostic ultrasound and urine pregnancy tests in recent years have facilitated early and better diagnosis of ectopic pregnancy and the development of conservative management strategies. Tubal pregnancy can be managed surgically (laparotomy or laparoscopy), medically using methotrexate (local or systemic) and more recently through the expectant approach. However, management must be tailored to the clinical condition and future fertility requirements of individual women.

Surgical management

Surgery is still considered the main treatment for tubal ectopic pregnancies in many parts of the world, especially in cases with significant internal haemorrhage. With recent advances in minimally invasive surgery, the laparoscopic approach has become the treatment modality of choice in haemodynamically stable women, over the open approach.[100,101] A meta-analysis showed that laparoscopic procedures are associated with lower blood loss during the operation, shorter operative time and hospital stay as well as less postoperative pain [A].[102] Laparotomy, however, may be safer than the laparoscopic approach if there is a major intraperitoneal bleed in which achieving immediate haemostasis is essential. An experienced laparoscopic surgeon may be able to perform the procedure and achieve haemostasis relatively quickly but this might not be applicable in all cases and laparotomy should be considered to stop the internal bleeding in a short period of time. The laparoscopic approach might also not be possible if the operator lacks surgical skills or if the approach is hampered by severe pelvic adhesions or large uterine fibroids.[103,104]

NICE and RCOG in their guidelines have advised that surgical treatment of ectopic pregnancy should be carried out laparoscopically whenever possible, taking into account the condition of the woman and the complexity of the surgical procedure. However, the surgeons providing care to women with ectopic pregnancy should be competent in performing laparoscopic surgery.[4,89]

Salpingotomy or salpingectomy

Salpingectomy (partial or complete removal of the Fallopian tube) and salpingostomy/salpingotomy (linear opening of the Fallopian tube with removal of ectopic pregnancy tissue and preservation of the tube) whether through laparoscopic approach or laparotomy can both be used to surgically treat ectopic pregnancy. Until recently there was no clear evidence whether laparoscopic salpingotomy with tubal conservation offers any advantages over salpingectomy. A recent open multicentre RCT (ESEP study)[105] analysed 446 women with tubal ectopic pregnancies who were randomly allocated over seven years to either salpingotomy or salpingectomy. The cumulative ongoing pregnancy rate by natural conception was 60.7 per cent after salpingotomy and 56.2 per cent after salpingectomy (fecundity rate ratio 1.06, 95% CI 0.81–1.38) [B]. While persistent trophoblast occurred significantly more frequently in the salpingotomy group than in the salpingectomy group, the numbers of repeat ectopic pregnancies did not differ significantly. The authors concluded that salpingotomy did not improve the cumulative rates of ongoing pregnancy by natural conception in women with tubal pregnancy and a healthy contralateral tube, but it was associated with an increased risk of persistent trophoblast. The results from another recent RCT (DEMETER trial)[106] had shown a similar result with regard to the cumulative ongoing pregnancy rates (HR 1.13, 95% CI 0.73–1.74) [B].

The choice of surgical technique is largely determined by the condition of the contralateral tube and the desire for future fertility. Currently, the consensus is that tubal conservation should be attempted if the woman desires further pregnancies and there is evidence of contralateral tubal damage at laparoscopy. In the presence of a healthy contralateral tube, salpingectomy can be performed with the woman's consent.[4,6,89] However if salpingotomy is performed, women should be informed that having a salpingotomy there is a 20 per cent chance of further treatment such as methotrexate and/or a salpingectomy and that a post-operative follow-up with serial serum βhCG measurements is required to ensure that all active tissue has been removed.[4,63]

NICE[4] also recommend offering surgery as a first-line treatment to women with ectopic pregnancies who are unable to return for follow-up after methotrexate treatment or who have any of the following:

1   significant pain;
2   adnexal mass of 35 mm or more;
3   an ectopic pregnancy with a fetal heartbeat visible on an ultrasound scan;
4   serum βhCG level of 5000 IU/L or more.

Surgery should not be delayed in women showing signs of hypovolaemic shock. TVS examination when appropriate can confirm the presence of ruptured ectopic and intra-abdominal bleeding in cases with uncertain diagnosis; however it is important to intervene rapidly in these cases to achieve haemostasis which is crucial to resuscitate and treat those women.[89,107]

Medical management with methotrexate

Methotrexate is a folic acid antagonist which interferes with DNA synthesis and inhibits cell proliferation in fast-growing tissues such as trophoblasts. Its side effects are dose related and they include conjunctivitis, inflammation of the gastrointestinal mucosa, impaired liver function and bone marrow suppression.[108]

Medical treatment with methotrexate is one of the options in treating stable asymptomatic women with small, unruptured ectopic pregnancy. In clinical practice, ectopic pregnancies suitable for methotrexate treatment usually account for about 25–30 per cent of all ectopic pregnancy cases.[109,110] However caution must be used when giving methotrexate as its use in a misdiagnosed intrauterine pregnancy can have serious adverse effects resulting in a miscarriage. Should the pregnancy continue there is a high risk that the fetus could be malformed. The other problem is the risk of tubal rupture

and the need for blood transfusion, which occur significantly more often in women treated with methotrexate than in those who had surgical treatment. This and the need to delay future pregnancy for a minimum of three months might make methotrexate a less attractive option for women.[109]

Methotrexate treatment is usually given as an injection of 50 mg/m^2 or 1 mg/kg IM. Follow-up requires women to attend for several visits and have measurements of serum hCG until they clear (<20 IU/L). Repeat ultrasound scans might also be required in women who start to experience abdominal pain to exclude ruptured ectopic and intra-abdominal haemorrhage.[89,102] This has been further enforced in the recent NICE guideline,[4] which suggests that systemic methotrexate could be offered to women who fulfil the following criteria:

1   no significant pain;
2   serum hCG level less than 1500 IU/L;
3   with unruptured ectopic pregnancy, measuring less than 35 mm and with no visible heartbeat activity;
4   no intrauterine pregnancy on ultrasound scans;
5   able to continue with follow-up visits;
6   methotrexate is an acceptable option.

Women with unruptured small ectopic pregnancies (<35 mm in size and no visible heartbeat) and with serum hCG between 1500 IU/L and 5000 IU/L can still be offered the choice of methotrexate if they have no significant pain and are able to return for follow-up visits. In addition all women who choose methotrexate treatment need to be informed that there is a chance of requiring further intervention and they may need to be urgently admitted if their symptoms worsen. Furthermore follow-up with serum βhCG measurements needs to continue after treatment until a negative result is obtained.[111]

A randomised trial of systemic methotrexate versus laparoscopic salpingostomy has shown that in haemodynamically stable women with unruptured ectopic pregnancies there is no significant difference in overall treatment success between the medical and surgical group (RR 0.98, 95% CI 0.87–1.1) [B].[109] However a meta-analysis of four randomised trials showed that a single dose of systemic methotrexate was significantly less successful than laparoscopic salpingotomy (OR 0.38, 95% CI 0.20–0.71) [A].[111] Methotrexate treatment was also cost effective only in women requiring a single injection and with initial serum βhCG concentrations <1500 IU/L but becomes more expensive in women presenting with βhCG above that level who often require multiple injections.[111,112]

In a double-blind study, more than one dose of methotrexate was required in 25–31 per cent of women [B].[113] This is in agreement with other studies which also showed that more than one dose of methotrexate was required in about 14–26 per cent of women [B–C].[110,114-116]

Expectant management

Several observational studies have suggested a high success rate for expectant management in selected cases of ectopic pregnancies that present with low βhCG levels [C].[66,117] Most clinicians however do not feel comfortable with the concept of expectant management of ectopic pregnancy and would still consider some form of treatment, whether surgical or medical. In addition there are few existing data to compare expectant management of ectopic pregnancy with other forms of treatment. The first randomised trial that compared expectant management with systemic methotrexate showed similar success rates in both arms of the study. The trial was of limited value, however, as methotrexate was administered orally at a dose much lower than that used in standard clinical practice.[118]

A more recent trial compared expectant and medical management in women diagnosed with ectopic pregnancies with serum βhCG levels <1500 IU/L and those with PULs and serum hCG 2000 IU/L. Again there was no difference in the success rate between the two arms of the study. The authors concluded that methotrexate, which is potentially a harmful drug, could be withheld in these women [B].[119]

Expectant management has important advantages over medical treatment. In addition to avoiding the side effects of methotrexate, it also follows the natural course of ectopic pregnancies which is a self-limiting process that will eventually result in tubal miscarriage or resolution. However, expectant management requires prolonged follow-up, which could lead to anxiety in the woman and her carer.[120,121]

To minimise the risk of failure, many authors have used strict criteria, such as low serum βhCG levels, to select women for expectant management, which could explain the high success rate in some of these reports, reaching 70–80 per cent [C–D].[66,122,123] Published studies have suggested that by using less strict selection criteria for expectant management, 40–49 per cent of tubal ectopics can resolve spontaneously [C].[66,117,124] This observation could reflect the increased sensitivity of modern ultrasound equipment, which enables the detection of very small ectopics that might have been missed in the past. In general, expectant management can be offered to clinically stable women with clear ultrasound diagnosis of small (<3 cm) non-ruptured ectopic pregnancy without fetal cardiac activity and with serum βhCG levels less than 1500 IU/L at the initial presentation. According to the current literature the success of expectant management in these cases can reach 67–88 per cent [C].[66,89] Clinically stable women who fit the criteria should be given the choice of surgical, medical or expectant management but their personal and medical history, in addition to their compliance with a follow-up visit, must be taken into consideration. Detailed information of the management options and their long-term outcomes will help women to choose the path of their treatment.

CONCLUSION

The diagnostic challenges and serious risks of ectopic pregnancy make this condition an important cause of maternal morbidity and mortality worldwide.

Recent advances in ultrasound diagnosis and the availability of highly sensitive urinary pregnancy tests have contributed to more accurate and timely diagnosis of ectopic pregnancies. Many of these pregnancies are small and are destined to resolve spontaneously without interventions. This has advanced the care of women with ectopic pregnancy to include non-surgical treatment options. Selection criteria when managing women conservatively, such as small ectopic pregnancy, low serum βhCG concentrations and no intraperitoneal haemorrhage, will help to avoid risk of complications. However, women with conservative management will remain at risk for tubal rupture and therefore careful follow-up including serial blood tests is important to ensure women's safety.

TVS has revolutionised the diagnosis of ectopic pregnancy and should be considered as the diagnostic test of choice for women presenting with problems such as bleeding and/or pain in early pregnancy, while serum biochemistry and laparoscopy should be considered as secondary tests in women with inconclusive findings on ultrasound scans.

RECOMMENDATIONS FOR CLINICAL PRACTICE

- When considering conservative treatment for tubal ectopic pregnancy, patients should be given detailed information about the success rate, side effects and complications.
- When considering conservative treatment, women need to comply with follow-up and adjust their lifestyle to minimise the risk of complications.
- In both medical and expectant management, follow-up with serum βhCG concentrations should continue until the level becomes undetectable.
- Anti-D prophylaxis should be given to all rhesus-negative women who require surgical treatment of ectopic pregnancy.
- Future pregnancy should be delayed for at least three months after completion of medical treatment because of the risk of teratogenicity of methotrexate.

References

1. CEMACH. *Saving mothers' lives: reviewing maternal deaths to make motherhood safer 2006–2008*. The 8th report of the Confidential Enquiries into Maternal Deaths in the United Kingdom. *BJOG* 2011;118:1–203.
2. Wedderburn CJ, Warner P, Graham B, Duncan WC, Critchley HO, Horne AW. Economic evaluation of diagnosing and excluding ectopic pregnancy. *Hum Reprod* 2010;25:328–33.
3. Lawani OL, Anozie OB, Ezeonu PO. Ectopic pregnancy: a life-threatening gynecological emergency. *Int J Womens Health* 2013;5:515–21.

4. NICE. *Ectopic pregnancy and miscarriage: diagnosis and initial management in early pregnancy of ectopic pregnancy and miscarriage.* Clinical Guideline 154. NICE, 2012.

5. Bouyer J, Cost J, Fernandez H, Pouly JL, Job Spira N. Sites of ectopic pregnancy: a 10-year population-based study of 1800 cases. *Hum Reprod* 2002;17:3224–30.

6. Jurkovic D, Wilkinson H. Diagnosis and management of ectopic pregnancy. *BMJ* 2011;342:d3397.

7. Crochet JR, Bastian LA, Chireau MV. Does this woman have an ectopic pregnancy? The rational clinical examination systematic review. *JAMA* 2013;309:1722–9.

8. Salman G, Irvine LM. Ectopic pregnancy, the need for standardisation of rate. *Journal of Obstetrics and Gynaecology* 2008;28:32–5.

9. Rajkhowa M, Rutherford AJ, Balen AH, Sharma V, Cuckle HS. Trends in the incidence of ectopic pregnancy in England and Wales from 1966 to 1996. *BJOG* 2000;107:369–74.

10. Weckstein LN. Current perspective on ectopic pregnancy. *Obstet Gynecol Surv* 1985;40:259-72.

11. Boufous S, Quartararo M, Mohsin M, Parker J. Trends in the incidence of ectopic pregnancy in New South Wales between 1990–1998. *Australian & New Zealand Journal of Obstetrics & Gynaecology* 2001;41:436–8.

12. Storeide O, Veholmen M, Eide M, Bergsjo P, Sandvei R. The incidence of ectopic pregnancy in Hordaland County, Norway 1976–1993. *Acta Obstet Gynecol Scand* 1997;76:345.

13. Makinen JI. The regional versus national incidence of ectopic pregnancy in Finland from 1966 to 1986. *Int J Gynecol Obstet* 1989;28:351–4.

14. Obed SA. Diagnosis of unruptured ectopic pregnancy is still uncommon in Ghana. *Ghana Medical Journal* 2006;40:3–7.

15. Goyaux N, Leke R, Keita N, Thonneau P. Ectopic pregnancy in African developing countries. *Acta Obstet Gynecol Scand* 2003;82:305–12.

16. Sabeer BE, Barnhart KT. Suspected ectopic pregnancy. *Obstet Gynecol* 2006;107:399–413.

17. Goddijn M, van der Veen F, Schuring-Blom GH, Ankum WM, Leschot NJ. Cytogenetic characteristics of ectopic pregnancy. *Hum Reprod* 1996;11:2769–71.

18. Horne AW, Critchley HO. Mechanisms of disease: the endocrinology of ectopic pregnancy. *Expert Reviews in Molecular Medicine* 2012;14:e7.

19. Coste J, Fernandez H, Joye N *et al*. Role of chromosome abnormalities in ectopic pregnancy. *Fertil Steril* 2000;74:1259–60.

20. Bottomley C. Epidemiology and etiology of miscarriage and ectopic pregnancy. *In*: Jurkovic D, Farquharson R (eds). *Acute Gynaecology and Early Pregnancy*. London: RCOG Press, 2011:12–23.

21. Ankum WM, Mol BW, Van der Veen F, Bossuyt PM. Risk factors for ectopic pregnancy: a meta-analysis. *Fertil Steril* 1996; 65:1093–9.

22. Bouyer J, Coste J, Shojaei T *et al*. Risk factors for ectopic pregnancy: a comprehensive analysis based on a large case-control, population-based study in France. *Am J Epidemiol* 2003;157:185–94.

23. Bjartling C, Osser S, Persson K. The frequency of salpingitis and ectopic pregnancy as epidemiologic markers of *Chlamydia trachomatis*. *Acta Obstet Gynecol Scand* 2000;79:123–8.

24. Lepine LA, Hillis SD, Marchbanks PA, Joesoef MR, Peterson HB, Westrom L. Severity of pelvic inflammatory disease as a predictor of the probability of live birth. *Am J Obstet Gynecol* 1998;178:977–81.

25. Barnhart KT, Sammel MD, Gracia CR, Chittams J, Hummel AC, Shaunik A. Risk factors for ectopic pregnancy in women with symptomatic first-trimester pregnancies. *Fertil Steril* 2006;86:36–43.

26. Goldner T, Lawson H, Xia Z, Atrash H. Surveillance for ectopic pregnancy: United States, 1970–1989. *MMWR CDC Surveill Summ* 1993;42:73–85.

27. Westrom L, Bengtsson LPH, Mardh PA. Incidence, trends and risks of ectopic pregnancy in a population of women. *Br Med J* 1981;282:15–18.

28. Peterson HB, Xia Z, Hughes JM *et al*. The risk of ectopic pregnancy after tubal sterilization. *N Engl J Med* 1997;336:762–7.

29. Xiong X, Buekens P, Wollast E. IUD use and the risk of ectopic pregnancy: a meta-analysis of case-control studies. *Contraception* 1995;52:23–34.

30. Furlong LA. Ectopic pregnancy risk when contraception fails: a review. *J Reprod Med* 2002;47:881–5.

31. McCann MF, Potter LS. Progestin-only oral contraception: a comprehensive review. *Contraception* 1994;50 (6 Suppl 1):S1–195.

32. Nazari A, Askari HA, Check JH, O'Shaughnessy AO. Embryo transfer techniques as a cause of ectopic pregnancy in in-vitro fertilization. *Fertil Steril* 1993;60:919–21.

33. Herman A, Raphael R, Golan A. The role of tubal pathology and other parameters in ectopic pregnancies occurring in in-vitro fertilization embryo transfer. *Fertil Steril* 1990;54:864–8.

34. Rojansky N, Schenker JG. Heterotopic pregnancy and assisted reproduction – an update. *J Assist Reprod Genet* 1996;13:594–601.

35. Weckstein LN, Boucher AR, Tucker H, Gibson D, Rettenmaier MA. Accurate diagnosis of early ectopic pregnancy. *Obstetrics and Gynecology* 1985;65:393–397.

36. Tay JL, Moore J, Walker JJ. Ectopic pregnancy. *BMJ* 2000;320:916–19.

37. Farquhar CM. Ectopic pregnancy. *Lancet* 2005;9485:583–91.

38. Kaplan BC, Dart RG, Moskos M *et al*. Ectopic pregnancy: prospective study with improved diagnostic accuracy. *Ann Emerg Med* 1996;28:10–17.

39. Dart RG, Kaplan B, Varaklis K. Predictive value of history and physical examination in patients with suspected ectopic pregnancy. *Ann Emerg Med* 1999;33:283–90.

40. Buckley RG, King KJ, Disney JD, Gorman JD, Klausen JH. History and physical examination to estimate the risk of

ectopic pregnancy: validation of a clinical prediction model. *Ann Emerg Med* 1999;34:589–94.

41. Jurkovic D. Ectopic pregnancy. *In*: Edmonds DK, ed. *Dewhurst's Textbook of Obstetrics and Gynaecology*. 8th edn. Wiley-Blackwell, 2012:245–54.

42. Mol BW, Hajenuis P, Engelsbel S *et al*. Should patients who are suspected of having an ectopic pregnancy undergo a physical examination? *Fertil Steril* 1999;71:155–7.

43. Kobayashi M, Hellman LM, Fillisti LP. Ultrasound: an aid in the diagnosis of ectopic pregnancy. *Am J Obstet Gynecol* 1969;103:1131–40.

44. Dutta RL, Economides DL. Patient acceptance of transvaginal sonography in the early pregnancy unit setting. *Ultrasound Obstet Gynecol* 2003;22: 503–7.

45. Basama FM, Crosfill F, Price A. Women's perception of transvaginal sonography in the first trimester; in an early pregnancy assessment unit. *Arch Gynecol Obstet* 2004;269:117–20.

46. Stein JC, Wang R, Adler N *et al*. Emergency physician ultrasonography for evaluating patients at risk for ectopic pregnancy: a meta-analysis. *Ann Emerg Med* 2010;56:674–83.

47. Cacciatore B, Stenman UH, Ylostalo P. Comparison of abdominal and vaginal sonography in suspected ectopic pregnancy. *Obstet Gynecol* 1989; 73:770–4.

48. Atri M, Valenti DA, Bret PM, Gillett P. Effect of transvaginal sonography on the use of invasive procedures for evaluating patients with a clinical diagnosis of ectopic pregnancy. *J Clin Ultrasound* 2003;31:1–8.

49. Kirk E, Papageorghiou AT, Condous G, Tan L, Bora S, Bourne T. The diagnostic effectiveness of an initial transvaginal scan in detecting ectopic pregnancy. *Hum Reprod* 2007;22:2824–8.

50. Condous G, Okaro E, Khalid A, Lu C, Van Huffel S, Bourne T. The accuracy of transvaginal ultrasonography for the diagnosis of ectopic pregnancy prior to surgery. *Hum Reprod* 2005;20:1404–9.

51. Kobayashi M, Hellman LM, Fillisti LP. Ultrasound: an aid in the diagnosis of ectopic pregnancy. *Am J Obstet Gynecol* 1969;103:1131–40.

52. Timor-Tritsch IE, Rottem S. Transvaginal ultrasonographic study of the fallopian tube. *Obstet Gynecol* 1987;70:424–8.

53. Kirk E, Daemen A, Papageorghiou AT *et al*. Why are some ectopic pregnancies characterized as pregnancies of unknown location at the initial transvaginal ultrasound examination? *Acta Obstet Gynecol Scand* 2008;87:1150–4.

54. Condous G, Timmerman D, Goldstein S, Valentin L, Jurkovic D, Bourne T. Pregnancies of unknown location: consensus statement. *Ultrasound Obstet Gynecol* 2006;28:121–2.

55. Fleischer AC, Pennell RG, McKee MS *et al*. Ectopic pregnancy: features at transvaginal sonography. *Radiology* 1990;174: 375–8.

56. de Crespigny LC. Demonstration of ectopic pregnancy by transvaginal ultrasound. *Br J Obstet Gynaecol* 1988;95:1253–6.

57. Ofili-Yebovi D, Cassik P, Lee C, Elson J, Hillaby K, Jurkovic D. The efficacy of ultrasound-based protocol for the diagnosis of tubal ectopic pregnancy. *Ultrasound Obstet Gynecol* 2003;22(S1):1–69.

58. Cacciatore B, Stenman UH, Ylostalo P. Diagnosis of ectopic pregnancy by vaginal ultrasonography in combination with a discriminatory serum hCG level of 1000 IU/L. *BJOG* 1990;97:904–8.

59. Brown DL, Doubilet PM. Transvaginal sonography for diagnosing ectopic pregnancy. *J Ultrasound Med* 1994;13:259–66.

60. Jurkovic D. Tubal ectopic pregnancy. *In*: Jurkovic D, Valentin L, Vyas S, eds. *Gynaecological Ultrasound in Clinical Practice*. RCOG Press, 2009:179–92.

61. Jansen RP, Elliot PM. Angular intrauterine pregnancy. *Obstet Gynecol* 1981; 58:167–75.

62. Salim R, Regan L, Woelfer B, Backos M, Jurkovic D. A comparative study of the morphology of congenital uterine anomalies in women with and without a history of recurrent first trimester miscarriage. *Hum Reprod* 2003;18:162–6.

63. Ehrenberg-Buchner S, Sandadi S, Moawad NS, Pinkerton JS, Hurd WW. Ectopic pregnancy: role of laparoscopic treatment. *Clin Obstet Gynecol* 2009;52:372–9.

64. Li TC, Tristram A, Hill AS, Cooke ID. A review of 254 ectopic pregnancies in a teaching hospital in the Trent Region, 1977–1990. *Hum Reprod* 1991;6:1002–7.

65. Beck P, Broslovsky L, Gal D & Tancer ML. The role of laparoscopy in the diagnosis of ectopic pregnancy. *Int J Gynaecal Obstet* 1984;22, 307–9.

66. Mavrelos H, Nicks H, Jamil A, Hoo W, Jauniaux E and Jurkovic D. Efficacy and safety of a clinical protocol for expectant management of selected women diagnosed with a tubal ectopic pregnancy. *Ultrasound Obstet Gynecol* 2013;42:102–7.

67. Lindahl B, Ahlgren M. Identification of chorion villi in abortion specimens. *Obstet Gynecol* 1986;67:79–81.

68. Murray H, Baakdah H, Bardell T, Tulandi T. Diagnosis and treatment of ectopic pregnancy. *CMAJ* 2005;173:905–12.

69. Wang R, Reynolds TA, West HH *et al*. Use of a hCG discriminatory zone with bedside pelvic ultrasonography. *Ann Emerg Med* 2011;58:12–20.

70. Kadar N, DeVore G, Romero R. Discriminatory hCG zone: its use in the sonographic evaluation for ectopic pregnancy. *Obstet Gynecol* 1981;58:156–61.

71. Banerjee S, Aslam N, Woelfer B, Lawrence A, Elson J, Jurkovic D. Expectant management of early pregnancies of unknown location: a prospective evaluation of methods to predict spontaneous resolution of pregnancy. *BJOG* 2001;108:158–63.

72. Lugt B, Drogendijk AC. The disappearance of human chorionic gonadotropin from plasma and urine following induced abortion. *Acta Obstet Gynecol Scand* 1985;64:547–52.

73. Fridstrom M, Garoff L, Sjoblom P, Hillents T. Human chorionic goandotropin patterns in early pregnancy after assisted conception. *Acta Obstet Gynecol Scand* 1995;74:534–8.

74. Silva C, Sammel MD, Zhou L, Gracia C, Hummel AC, Barnhart K. Human chorionic gonadotrophin profile for women with ectopic pregnancy. *Obstet Gynecol* 2006;107:605–10.

75. Mello V, Mol F, Opmeer BC, Ankum WM *et al.* Diagnostic value of serum hCG on the outcome of pregnancy of unknown location: a systematic review and meta-analysis. *Human Reproduction* 2012;18:603–17.

76. Hahlin M, Thorburn J, Bryman I. The expectant management of early pregnancies of uncertain site. *Hum Reprod* 1995;10:1223–7.

77. Day A, Sawyer E, Mavrelos D, Tailor A, Helmy S, Jurkovic D. Use of serum progesterone measurement to reduce need for follow-up in women with pregnancies of unknown location. *Ultrasound Obstet Gynecol* 2009;33:704–10.

78. El Bishry G, Ganta S. The role of single serum progesterone measurement in conjunction with beta hCG in the management of suspected ectopic pregnancy. *J Obstet Gynaecol* 2008;28:413–17.

79. Mol BW, Lijmer JG, Ankum W, Van der Veen F, Bossuyt PM. The accuracy of single serum progesterone measurement in the diagnosis of ectopic pregnancy: a meta-analysis. *Hum Reprod* 1998;13:3220–7.

80. Matthews CP, Coulson PB, Wild RA. Serum progesterone levels as an aid in the diagnosis of ectopic pregnancy. *Obstet Gynecol* 1986;68:390–4.

81. McCord ML, Muram D, Buster JE, Arheart KL, Stovall TG, Carson SA. Single serum progesterone as a screen for ectopic pregnancy: exchanging specificity and sensitivity to obtain optimal test performance. *Fertil Steril* 1997;67:980–1.

82. Milwidsky A, Segal S, Menashe M, Adoni A, Palti A. Corpus luteum function in ectopic pregnancy. *Int J Fertil* 1984;2:244–6.

83. Radwanska E, Frankenberg J, Allen E. Plasma progesterone levels in normal and abnormal early human pregnancy. *Fertil Steril* 1978;30:398–402.

84. Yeko TR, Gorrill MJ, Hughes LH, Rodi IA, Buster JE, Sauer MV. Timely diagnosis of early ectopic pregnancy using a single blood progesterone measurement. *Fertil Steril* 1987;48:1048–50.

85. Condous G, Kirk E, Lu C *et al.* Diagnostic accuracy of varying discriminatory zones for the prediction of ectopic pregnancy in women with a pregnancy of unknown location. *Ultrasound Obstet Gynecol* 2005;26:770–5.

86. Bignardi T, Condous G, Alhamdan D *et al.* The hCG ratio can predict the ultimate viability of the intrauterine pregnancies of uncertain viability in the pregnancy of unknown location population. *Hum Reprod* 2008;23:1964–7.

87. Cordina M, Schramm-Gajraj K, Ross JA, Lautman K, Jurkovic D. Introduction of a single visit protocol in the management of selected patients with pregnancy of unknown location: a prospective study. *BJOG* 2011;118:693–7.

88. Barnhart K, van Mello NM, Bourne T *et al.* Pregnancy of unknown location: a consensus statement of nomenclature, definitions, and outcome. *Fertil Steril* 2011;95:857–66.

89. RCOG. *The management of tubal pregnancy.* Guideline 21. London: RCOG Press, 2010.

90. Banerjee S, Aslam N, Zosmer N, Woelfer B, Jurkovic D. The expectant management of women with early pregnancy of unknown location. *Ultrasound Obstet Gynecol* 1999;14:231–6.

91. Timmerman D. Predictive models for the early diagnosis of ectopic pregnancy. *Verh K Acad Geneeskd Belg* 2004;66:155–71.

92. Condous G, Okaro E, Khalid A *et al.* The use of a new logistic regression model for predicting the outcome of pregnancies of unknown location. *Hum Reprod* 2004;19:1900–10.

93. Condous G, Okaro E, Khalid A *et al.* A prospective evaluation of a single-visit strategy to manage pregnancies of unknown location. *Hum Reprod* 2005; 20:1398–1403.

94. Gracia CR, Barnhart KT. Diagnosing ectopic pregnancy: decision analysis comparing six strategies. *Obstet Gynecol* 2001;97:464–70.

95. Jamil A, Jurkovic D. Ectopic pregnancy. *In*: Arulkumaran S, Regan L, Papageorghiou AT, Monga, Farquharson D, eds. *Oxford Desk Reference Obstetrics and Gynaecology.* Oxford University Press, 2011:490–2.

96. Hahlin M, Thorburn J, Bryman I. The expectant management of early pregnancies of uncertain site. *Hum Reprod* 1995;10:1223–7.

97. Ankum W, Van der Veen F, Hamerlynck J, Lammes F. Suspected ectopic pregnancy. What to do when human chorionic gonadotropin levels are below the discriminatory zone. *J Reprod Med* 1995;40:525–8.

98. Hajenius P, Mol B, Ankum W, Van der Veen F, Bossuyt P, Lammes F. Suspected ectopic pregnancy: expectant management in patients with negative sonographic findings and low serum βhCG concentrations. *Early Pregnancy* 1995;1:258–62.

99. Condous G, Okaro E, Bourne T. The conservative management of early pregnancy complications: a review of the literature. *Ultrasound Obstet Gynecol* 2003;22:420–30.

100. Lundorff P, Thorburn J, Hahlin M, Kallfelt B, Lindblom B. Laparoscopic surgery in ectopic pregnancy. A randomized trial versus laparotomy. *Acta Obstet Gynecol Scand* 1991;70:343–8.

101. Vermesh M, Silva PD, Rosen GF, Stein AL, Fossum GT, Sauer MV. Management of unruptured ectopic gestation by linear salpingostomy: a prospective, randomized

clinical trial of laparoscopy versus laparotomy. *Obstet Gynecol* 1989;73:400–4.

102. Mol F, Mol BWJ, Ankum WM, Van der Veen F, Hajenius PJ. Current evidence on surgery, systemic methotrexate and expectant management in the treatment of tubal ectopic pregnancy: a systematic review and meta-analysis. *Hum Reprod* 2008;14:309–19.

103. Li Z, Leng J, Lang J, Liu Z, Sun D, Zhu L. Laparoscopic surgery in patients with hypovolemic shock due to ectopic pregnancy. *Zhonghua Fu Chan Ke Za Zhi* 2002;37:653–5.

104. Ding DC, Chu TY, Kao SP, Chen PC, Wei YC. Laparoscopic management of tubal ectopic pregnancy. *JSLS* 2008;12:273–6.

105. Mol F *et al.* Salpingotomy versus salpingectomy in women with tubal pregnancy (ESEP study): an open-label, multicentre, randomised controlled trial. *Lancet* 2014;383:1483–9.

106. Fernandez H, Capmas P, Lucot JP, Resch B, Panel P, Bouyer J, for the GROG. Fertility after ectopic pregnancy: the DEMETER randomized trial. *Hum Reprod* 2013; 28:1247–53.

107. Popat R, Adams C. Diagnosis of ruptured ectopic pregnancy by bedside ultrasonography. *J Emerg Med* 2002;22:409–10.

108. Barnhart K, Coutifaris C, Esposito M. The pharmacology of methotrexate. *Expert Opin Pharmacother* 2001;2:409–17.

109. Hajenius PJ, Engelsbel S, Mol BW *et al.* Randomised trial of systemic methotrexate versus laparoscopic salpingostomy in tubal pregnancy. *Lancet* 1997;350:774–9.

110. Sowter MC, Farquhar CM, Petrie KJ, Gudex G. A randomised trial comparing single-dose systemic methotrexate and laparoscopic surgery for the treatment of unruptured tubal pregnancy. *BJOG* 2001;108:192–203.

111. Hajenius PJ, Mol F, Mol BWJ, Bossuyt PMM, Ankum WM, Van der Veen F. Interventions for tubal ectopic pregnancy. *Cochrane Database Syst Rev* 2007;1:CD000324.

112. Sowter MC, Farquhar CM, Gudex G. An economic evaluation of single-dose systemic methotrexate and laparoscopic surgery for the treatment of unruptured ectopic pregnancy. *Br J Obstet Gynaecol* 2001;108:204–12.

113. Yalcinkaya TM, Brown SE, Mertz HL, Thomas DW. A comparison of 25 mg/m² vs 50 mg/m² dose of methotrexate (MTX) for the treatment of ectopic pregnancy (EP). *J Soc Gynecol Invest* 2000;7:179.

114. Lipscomb G, Bran D, McCord M, Portera J, Ling F. Analysis of 315 ectopic pregnancies treated with single-dose methotrexate. *Am J Obstet Gynecol* 1998;178:1354–8.

115. Lipscomb G, McCord M, Stovall T, Huff G, Portera S, Ling F. Predictors of success of methotrexate treatment in women with tubal ectopic pregnancies. *N Engl J Med* 1999;341:1974–8.

116. Saraj A, Wilcox J, Najmabadi S, Stein S, Johnson M, Paulson R. Resolution of hormonal markers of ectopic gestation: a randomized trial comparing single-dose intramuscular methotrexate with salpingostomy. *Obstet Gynecol* 1998;92:989–94.

117. Elson J, Tailor A, Banerjee S, Salim R, Hillaby K, Jurkovic D. Expectant management of tubal ectopic pregnancy: prediction of successful outcome using decision tree analysis. *Ultrasound Obstet Gynecol* 2004;23:552–6.

118. Korhonen J, Stenman U, Ylostalo P. Low-dose oral methotrexate with expectant management of ectopic pregnancy. *Obstet Gynecol* 1996;88:775–8.

119. Mello NM, Mol F, Verhoeve HR *et al.* Methotrexate or expectant management in women with an ectopic pregnancy or pregnancy of unknown location and low serum hCG concentrations? A randomized comparison. *Hum Reprod* 2013;28:60–67.

120. Mashiach S, Carp HJA, Serr DM. Non-operative management of ectopic pregnancy: a preliminary report. *J Reprod Med* 1982;27:127.

121. Hajenius P, Mello N. Conservative management of tubal ectopic pregnancy. *In*: Jurkovic D, Farquharson R, eds. *Acute Gynaecology and Early Pregnancy*. RCOG Press 2011, 121–9.

122. Ylostalo P, Cacciatore B, Sjoberg J, Kaaraiannen M, Tenhunen A, Stenman UH. Expectant management of ectopic pregnancy. *Obstet Gynecol* 1992;80:345–8.

123. Makinen jI, Kivijarvi AK, Irjala KMA. Success of nonsurgical management of ectopic pregnancy. *Lancet* 1990;335:1099.

124. Rodrigues SP, Burlet KJ, Hiemstra E *et al.* Ectopic pregnancy: when is expectant management safe? *Gynecol Surg* 2012;9:421–6.

Chapter 91 Premature ovarian insufficiency

Nowmi Zaman, Jenny Williamson and Lynne Robinson

MRCOG standards

Theoretical skills

There is no established standard for this topic, but we would suggest the following points for guidance:

- Have a good knowledge of the hypophyseal–pituitary–ovarian axis.
- Understand the aetiologies which may lead to premature ovarian insufficiency (POI).
- Know about first-line investigations for POI.
- Know how to manage POI, including psychological and fertility aspects.
- Be aware of new screening techniques for POI.

Practical skills

- Be able to take an appropriate history.
- Be able to initiate appropriate investigations to enable a diagnosis and/or tertiary referral.

INTRODUCTION

Premature ovarian insufficiency is now the preferred term for a premature menopause or ovarian failure. It occurs in 1 per cent of women under 40 years.[1] The condition is characterised by primary or secondary amenorrhoea, raised gonadotrophins and hypo-oestrogenism. The British Menopause Society recommends that POI definition uses an age cut-off of less than 45 years.[1] The term 'ovarian failure' suggests that it is an irreversible condition. In fact, ovarian follicular function fluctuates in 50 per cent of women with POI and 5–10 per cent of women may eventually conceive. The term 'failure' may convey a sense of hopelessness – a better term may therefore be dysfunction or insufficiency.

The main effects of POI include subfertility, climacteric symptoms and early onset of osteoporosis and cardiovascular disease.

Over recent years there has been concern about the safety of hormone replacement therapy (HRT) and therefore many women have not received the oestrogen replacement they require. However, most of the evidence regarding HRT applies to women who achieve menopause at the usually expected age, and not those with POI. Women who suffer from POI would have normally been expected to produce endogenous oestrogen at that age and therefore it is logical to replace this until at least the age of the natural menopause.

HYPOPHYSEAL–PITUITARY–OVARIAN AXIS

The hypothalamus is part of the diencephalon at the base of the brain and forms part of the floor of the third ventricle. It synthesises hormone-releasing hormones, which are released from the median eminence into the hypophyseal portal system which carries them to the anterior pituitary gland. The releasing hormones are: thyrotropin-releasing hormone (TRH), corticotrophin-releasing hormone (CRH), dopamine, growth hormone-releasing hormone (GHRH), gonadotrophin-releasing hormone (GnRH) and somatostatin. Oxytocin and vasopressin are also released (Fig. 91.1).

GnRH is a decapeptide and is released from the medial basal hypothalamus by the process of neurosecretion (Fig. 91.1). It is released in a pulsatile manner with a pulse frequency of 90 minutes in the follicular phase and modified by the feedback of follicle-stimulating hormone (FSH) and oestrogen.

The anterior pituitary glands secrete FSH, luteinising hormone (LH), prolactin, thyroid-stimulating hormone (TSH), growth hormone (GH), corticotrophin (ACTH) and melanocyte-stimulating hormone (MSH).

FSH and LH are glycoproteins and both consist of two subunits, alpha and beta. The alpha subunit is common to FSH, LH, TSH and human chorionic gonadotrophin (HCG). The beta subunits are hormone specific although the beta subunits of LH and HCG are very similar. FSH and LH are synthesised and secreted in response to GnRH.

LH and FSH are secreted in a pulsatile manner every 1–3 hours, with the frequency and amplitude of pulses varying throughout the menstrual cycle, greatest in early follicular phase and least in luteal phase. The amplitude is maximal during the pre-ovulatory surge when the pulsatile secretion of LH is more marked than that of FSH.

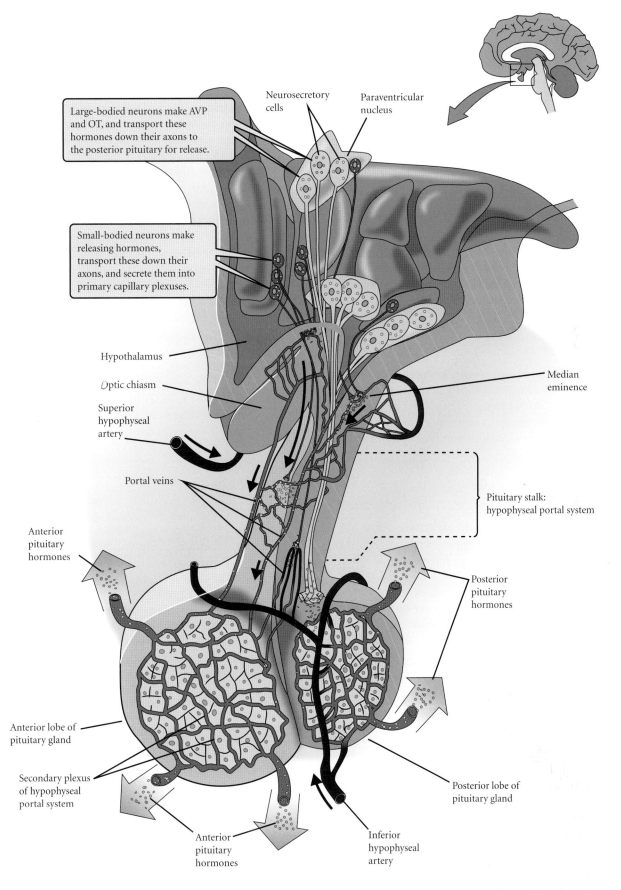

Fig. 91.1 The hormonal pathway in the hypothalamus and pituitary (reproduced from Boulpaep, Ernie, Boron, Walter. *Medical Physiology*, Elsevier, 2003, with permission)

MECHANISMS FOR CONTROL OF GONADOTROPHIN SECRETION

Gonadotrophin secretion is controlled by the positive and negative feedback of oestrogen and progesterone. During the follicular phase, oestradiol exerts a positive feedback effect and initiates the mid-cycle surge. In the luteal phase, oestradiol exerts negative feedback and suppresses gonadotrophin secretion.

Oestrogen

There are three naturally occurring oestrogens. Oestradiol is produced by the ovary, oestriol by the placenta and oestrone by peripheral conversion of androgens in the subcutaneous fat. Oestrogen has actions on the ovary, endometrium, breast, cervix and central nervous system (CNS).

Progesterone

Progesterone is produced and released by the adrenal cortex (2–3 mg/day), ovary (20–30 mg/day) and placenta. It has a very short half-life; 90 per cent is metabolised by the liver within 25 minutes. Progesterone exerts its effect throughout the reproductive tract but also increases the respiratory rate and suppresses T-cell function.

Androgens

Androgens are produced by the adrenal glands, ovary and through peripheral conversion. Dehydroepiandrostenedione, androstenedione and testosterone are produced by the ovary. The daily production of testosterone is 0.2–0.3 mg/day. Fifty per cent of this is from peripheral conversion of androstenedione, 25 per cent from the ovary and 25 per cent from the adrenals. Ovarian androgens enhance the atresia of small follicles.

FOLLICULAR DEVELOPMENT

Primordial follicles are comprised of a primary oocyte and pre-granulosa cells. Females have approximately 300,000 primordial follicles at puberty. There are three phases of follicular growth: pre-antral, peri-antral and antral.

Pre-antral and peri-antral phases occur during the three cycles before ovulation. It takes 85 days for a pre-antral follicle to develop to a mature follicle ready for ovulation. Between 10 and 30 dormant primordial follicles become active each day and they appear to be programmed to begin the maturation process on a particular day. The majority will die at some stage during development and only a small number reach the correct stage of development at the critical time to continue their development.

PREVALENCE

It is estimated that POI affects 5 per cent of women under 45 years of age,[2,5] 1 per cent of women under 40, 0.1 per cent of women under 30 and 0.01 per cent of women under 20.[1,3-5] Hispanic and African-American women reach menopause a little earlier, and Chinese and Japanese women a little later than the average Caucasian woman.[6] Steadily improving cure rates of childhood and adolescent cancers are likely to increase the numbers of young women with POI. In addition, the awareness of genetic susceptibility to cancers, such as from *BRCA1* and *BRCA2* genes, will lead to young women having prophylactic oophorectomies and therefore experiencing early menopause.

AETIOLOGY

In many women, a cause is not established. Identifiable causes of POI include genetic, infectious, autoimmune and metabolic factors. Women are born with around seven million oocytes but during their reproductive lifespan will only release up to 500 oocytes. Therefore POI may be due to a lower number of follicles present in the ovary or an increased rate of follicle loss. Another possibility is that abnormal pairing during meiosis may result in oocyte apoptosis.[7]

Genetic causes

Genetic causes of POI include X-linked, deletions and translocations, fragile X and autosomal dominant gene mutations.

The most common X-linked disorder is Turner syndrome (XO). This is rare (1:2500 female births) but is a well-recognised cause of POI. Females tend to have 'streak' ovaries due to follicular atresia.[8]

Deletions are more common than translocations and it is the proximal deletions which tend to induce ovarian failure. A deletion in Xq13 results in primary amenorrhoea while a deletion in Xp11 can lead to either primary or secondary amenorrhoea. The critical region for normal ovarian function has been proposed to be Xq13–26.[9]

Fragile X has a well-known association with POI. The *FMR1* pre-mutation is found in 5 per cent of all women with POI.[10] There is an expansion of 50–200 copies of the CGG repeats in the 5' untranslated region of the *FMR1* gene. Fragile X syndrome is due to the CGG expansion and results in POI in the female carriers and developmental deficiencies in the males.

Finally, mutations in the *FOXL2* gene can lead to POI.

Infectious causes

Viral or bacterial infection may lead to POI. Long-term ovarian function can be adversely affected by infections such as mumps, cytomegalovirus (CMV) or human immunodeficiency virus (HIV) as well as severe pelvic inflammatory disease (PID) and pelvic tuberculosis.[11]

Autoimmune causes

The prevalence of autoimmune conditions in women with POI has been reported to be 10–20 per cent,[12] suggesting an association between autoimmune conditions and POI. Anti-ovarian antibodies are occasionally detected in both type 1 (hypoparathyroidism, Addison's disease, mucocutaneous candidiasis) and type 2 (Addison's disease, hypothyroidism, type 1 diabetes) polyglandular autoimmune syndromes.[11] Autoimmune ovarian failure associated with thyroid dysfunction may occur in the absence of positive antibodies, but this may be due to lack of detection by current assays.[11]

Metabolic causes

There is a high prevalence of POI in patients with galactosaemia. Affected individuals have mutations of the galactose 1-phosphate uridyltransferase gene.[13] Ovarian insufficiency in these individuals is considered to be a result of the accumulation of galactose which disturbs the migration of the germ cells from the urogenital ridge to the gonad in fetal life.[11]

Iatrogenic causes

POI of iatrogenic origin can be as a result of ovarian damage secondary to surgery, chemotherapy or radiotherapy.[11] As more women are now surviving childhood malignancies, iatrogenic causes of POI will form a greater proportion of the causes contributing to POI in the future.

Idiopathic causes

POI is idiopathic in 74–90 per cent of cases.[3] It is unknown whether these cases are truly 'idiopathic' or due to as yet undiscovered genetic, immunological or environmental factors.[11]

HISTORY AND EXAMINATION

As with the diagnosis of any condition it is important to take a history and where appropriate carry out a physical examination of the patient.

History

- Last spontaneous menstrual cycle;
- Prior infection, surgery, radiotherapy, or chemotherapy;
- Family history of POI;
- History of autoimmune disorders;
- Symptoms of hypothyroidism;
- Symptoms of adrenal insufficiency such as hypotension and hyperpigmentation.

Physical examination

- Signs of hypo-oestrogenism such as dry skin and vaginal atrophy;
- Signs of autoimmune diseases e.g. Addison's disease and hypothyroidism.[14]

DIAGNOSIS AND INVESTIGATIONS

Diagnosis of POI can be difficult as FSH levels can fluctuate markedly. Generally, estimation of FSH levels is recommended in women with secondary amenorrhoea with or without menopausal symptoms.[5,15] Serial levels are useful and in general two or three measurements at 6-week intervals, in addition to oestradiol levels, help to confirm the diagnosis. It is important not to 'label' a young woman with the diagnosis of POI on the basis of one blood test as levels can fluctuate widely and it is a psychologically distressing diagnosis.

As autoimmune disease is linked with POI, an autoantibody screen and thyroid function tests are useful to aid diagnosis. If these show positive results, further investigation may be warranted, including tests for adrenal function, such as a synacthen test, renal function and a CT scan.

Karyotyping of the patient should be done to exclude any genetic cause of POI unless the reason for the condition is obvious e.g. previous chemotherapy or irradiation.

A pelvic ultrasound scan can be helpful as it may show small ovaries with little or no follicular activity.

A bone mineral density scan (DEXA) is a very useful investigation even if the patient is only recently menopausal. This is because the patient's peak bone mass may not have been achieved hence knowing a baseline bone density can help to counsel the patient regarding the risk of bone fractures and HRT. For those patients who are reluctant to commence HRT, it may be critical in helping them make a decision.

PREDICTION OF POI

It is currently not possible to predict which women will develop POI and therefore screening is not helpful. However, antral follicle count and anti-Müllerian hormone (AMH) are tests currently used to assess ovarian reserve. AMH, produced by developing antral follicles, is not currently used to predict or diagnose POI but a low AMH, indicating reduced ovarian reserve, may indicate that POI is more likely.[16] FSH is more commonly used to assess ovarian function with regard to the menopause but the levels fluctuate and therefore it is advisable to do several measurements.

REPRODUCTIVE GYNAECOLOGY

RISKS ASSOCIATED WITH POI

There is increasing awareness that POI can lead to earlier than expected serious health consequences contributing to increased morbidity and mortality. These include cardiovascular disease, osteoporosis, cognitive impairment including dementia and parkinsonism, psychological effects, impaired sexual function and subfertility. POI is associated with an overall 50 per cent increase in mortality when compared with women with menopause at age 52–55 years.[19] However, early menopause does appear to offer a protective effect on the development of breast malignancy.

Cardiovascular disease

Bilateral oophorectomy has been associated with increased cardiovascular risk and premature death and the younger the age at oophorectomy the greater the increase in risk.[20] In those with POI under the age of 40 years, increased risk of mortality from ischaemic heart disease is up to 50 per cent when compared with those with a menopause at the age of 52–55 years.[19] The underlying pathophysiology of this is likely to be hypo-oestrogenism contributing to enhanced progression of atherosclerosis.[21,22] Women with POI have been shown to have atherosclerosis as a result of impaired endothelial function.[23] Hypo-oestrogenism contributes to dyslipidaemia,[24] reduced insulin sensitivity[25] and metabolic syndrome.[26] A reduction in the increased risk for the development of cardiovascular disease can be achieved by commencing oestrogen replacement shortly after surgical or natural menopause at a young age.[27-29] This is usually given as HRT or synthetic ethinyl oestradiol in the form of the combined contraceptive pill.

Some progestogens have been associated with a negative impact on cardiovascular risk factors by affecting lipid profiles, vasomotion[32] and carbohydrate metabolism.[33] Micronised progesterone combined with transdermal oestrogen has been associated with a reduction in the incidence of new-onset diabetes and has a neutral or beneficial effect on blood pressure in postmenopausal women.[34] In one study, for women with a uterus, the use of micronised progesterone produced the most favourable cardiovascular effects.[35] A recent meta-analysis has also demonstrated reassuring effects on lipids, glucose, insulin and body fat distribution with oral oestradiol and dydrogestrone combinations.[36]

These studies have not been conducted on prematurely menopausal women and there is a lack of evidence to guide clinical practice in this group of patients. There is an ongoing clinical trial examining the effects of micronised progesterone and medroxyprogesterone acetate, both used with transdermal oestradiol, on the cardiovascular system, lipid profile and coagulation cascade in women with POI.[37]

Osteoporosis

Numerous studies have shown that bone loss accelerates following menopause. The earlier in life that menopause occurs, the lower the bone density will be later in life[38] and this is associated with a significantly higher overall fracture risk.[39] Even in women who undergo bilateral oophorectomy after natural menopause, the risk of osteoporotic fracture may be increased compared with women with intact ovaries.[40] This could be due to the fact that postmenopausal ovaries still secrete testosterone. Analysis of DEXA scans performed at diagnosis of POI show 3.6 per cent of women have bone density within the osteoporotic range and 25.9 per cent have osteopenia.[17] However, the usual bone density T-score classifications for osteoporosis have not been designed for use in young women and the recently developed FRAX tool (http://shef.ac.uk/FRAX/index.htm) for assessing fracture risk is not recommended for use in women under 40 years.[17]

Oestrogen therapy reduces the risk of osteoporosis and subsequent fractures.[41] All patients should also be encouraged to take regular weight-bearing exercise and have a calcium-rich diet, with consideration of calcium and vitamin D supplementation if deficient. HRT is the most effective intervention for preventing bone loss in women with POI.[17] The long-term effect of bisphosphonates and subsequent non-union of fractures is unknown as these agents have a long half-life and can affect bone metabolism for many years. Non-hormonal treatments including bisphosphonates, strontium or raloxifene can be used in women who have osteoporosis and cannot tolerate or refuse HRT but these preparations are not used or licensed to prevent bone loss in those with a normal bone density. Higher-than-usual doses of oestrogen for the relief of symptoms are often required by young women. However, adequate bone protection can be achieved with even low-dose HRT regimens.[42]

Cognitive function

It has been suggested that patients with early menopause may be at increased risk of dementia or reduced cognitive function; however, definitive conclusions regarding the risk of cognitive impairment in POI cannot yet be drawn due to a lack of data in women under the age of 40 years and in those with non-surgical causes of POI.[17] In the Mayo Clinic Cohort Study of Oophorectomy and Aging, women who underwent bilateral oophorectomy and consequently had POI had an increased risk of cognitive impairment or dementia compared with controls (hazard ratio [HR] 1.33, 95% CI 0.98–1.81; p = 0.07). The risk was greatest in the younger individuals and women under age 43 years had the highest risk (HR 1.74, 95% CI 0.97–3.14; p = 0.06).[43] Evidence suggests that there may be a neuroprotective effect of oestrogen and that the effect may be age-dependent.[43,44]

Parkinsonism

Women with a premature surgical menopause appear to have an increased risk of parkinsonism compared with controls (HR 1.80, 95% CI 1.00–3.26; p = 0.05), and the risk increased with younger age at oophorectomy (test for linear trend; p = 0.02).[45,46]

Psychological effects

The diagnosis of POI can have devastating, long-lasting psychological effects. Patients with POI have been shown to have increased levels of anxiety, depression, psychological distress and decreased overall wellbeing, compared with control groups.[47–48] They also have perceived lower levels of social support.[50] Studies have shown that in both HRT and non-HRT users there are high levels of psychological distress. This throws light on the importance of managing the psychological aspect of POI. Support groups include the Daisy Network (www.daisynetwork.org.uk) and Women's Health Concern (www.womens-health-concern.org) and patients should be made aware of these.[17]

Sexual function

Women with POI have been shown to have decreased levels of sexual fulfilment, reduced arousal, less frequent sexual encounters and increased pain.[49] Complex psychosexual impairment is likely to develop, particularly in the younger POI patients.[51] In addition to adequate oestrogen replacement and where necessary additional androgen replacement, psychosexual counselling may be required in the management of sexual dysfunction in selected cases.[17]

Associated endocrine and autoimmune conditions

POI is often associated with other autoimmune disorders, with 20 per cent of idiopathic POI patients presenting with another autoimmune condition.[52] These include hypothyroidism (25 per cent), Addison's disease (3 per cent), diabetes mellitus (2.5 per cent), Crohn's disease, vitiligo, pernicious anaemia, systemic lupus erythematosus (SLE), rheumatoid arthritis and myasthenia gravis. Patients should be tested for autoimmune antibodies, including anti-ovarian and anti-adrenal antibodies.[53]

Subfertility

Some women with POI may have irregular periods with occasional resumption of ovarian function. Spontaneous pregnancies occur in 5–10 per cent of those karyotypically normal women with idiopathic POI.[18] Although there may be future developments in fertility treatment such as storage of ovarian tissue and subsequent reimplantation of tissue or in-vitro maturation of oocytes for those who are at risk of POI, in-vitro fertilisation (IVF) using donor oocytes remains the mainstay of treatment for women who wish to conceive.[17]

MANAGEMENT

In the management of POI it is of paramount importance to provide patients with adequate information about the condition and explain the long-term health consequences, the use of oestrogen replacement and the effect of POI on the patient's fertility.[1] In idiopathic POI patients with normal karyotype there is a 5–10 per cent chance of spontaneous ovarian activity and the possibility of spontaneous pregnancy must be explained. Symptomatic women requiring HRT, yet still hoping for a natural conception, may choose sequential HRT as it is not contraceptive and in those women who wish to avoid pregnancy, effective contraceptive advice should be provided.[18] In women with POI, contraception is advised for 2 years after the last menstrual period.

The most important aspect of management is ensuring adequate hormone replacement. Oestrogen should be replaced until at least the age of 50 years and if the uterus is still present, progesterone needs to be added for endometrial protection, either as a sequential or continuous combined preparation. An alternative to this is the Mirena coil. The license for this as the progesterone arm of HRT is for 4 years in the UK (5 years in other countries).

HRT can be administered orally or transdermally and the combined oral contraceptive pill (COCP) can also be used as oestrogen replacement. There is limited evidence of the benefit of HRT over the COCP but transdermal oestrogen and micronised progesterone may confer some benefits including lowering of systolic blood pressure.[54] However, for some the COCP may be more acceptable as it makes the younger patients feel more 'normal' among their peers.

Vaginal oestrogens can be used along with HRT and this localised oestrogen can significantly help vaginal dryness and improve sexual function. Even for patients with relative contraindications to oestrogens, this can be considered as the absorbed dose is very low.

HRT in the form of oestrogen can help libido but if a trial of standard HRT adequately improves all other symptoms except libido then androgens can be considered to improve libido.[55,56] This can be administered as tibolone which is a selective oestrogenic activity regulator with oestrogenic, progestogenic and androgenic effects. Unfortunately in the UK there are no testosterone preparations licenced for use in women. However testosterone gel can be safely titrated for use in women by using one third of a 5 g tube of gel on alternate days. Implants of testosterone are scarce but can be used 6 monthly. Testosterone replacement appears to improve insulin resistance, muscle strength and functional cardiac capacity[57,58] and no adverse events. Prior to using testosterone it is best to take a thorough sexual history as lack of libido can be multifactorial.

Patients need psychological support and websites such as the Daisy Network can be useful. A repeat DEXA in 3–5 years after commencing treatment can be considered and annual follow-up should be arranged.

Fertility issues also need to be addressed and the options for fertility treatment include donor oocyte treatment, fostering and adoption. If POI can be predicted, as in the case of women undergoing cancer treatment, then oocyte preservation can be considered. The options for pre-pubertal girls are more limited but there is increasing interest in ovarian tissue freezing with a view to ovarian tissue reimplantation or in-vitro maturation but the latter is still a research tool. There have been some livebirths worldwide from ovarian tissue reimplantation.[59]

KEY POINTS

- POI is characterised by primary or secondary amenorrhoea, raised gonadotrophins and hypo-oestrogenism in women less than 45 years of age.[1]
- POI affects 5 per cent of women under 45,[2] 1 per cent of women under 40, 0.1 per cent of women under 30 and 0.01 per cent of women under 20 years.[1,3-5]
- Causes of POI include: genetic, infectious, autoimmune, metabolic, idiopathic and iatrogenic.
- In addition to FSH and oestradiol levels, important investigations at presentation include pelvic ultrasound, autoantibody screening, karyotyping and chromosomal analysis and assessment of bone density.[17]
- POI has been associated with a 50 per cent higher mortality from ischaemic heart disease when compared with women with menopause at age 52-55.[19]
- HRT relieves menopausal symptoms, conserves bone mass and there is evidence of cardiovascular benefit. It should be continued until at least the average menopausal age.
- Although ovarian follicular function fluctuates in 50 per cent of women with POI and 5-10 per cent of women may eventually conceive, IVF using donor oocytes remains the mainstay of treatment for women who wish to conceive.[17]

References

1. Pitkin J, Rees MC, Gray S et al. Management of premature menopause. Menopause International 2007;13(1):44–5.
2. Cartwright B, Robinson J, Rymer J. Treatment of premature ovarian failure trial: description of an ongoing clinical trial. Menopause International 2010;16(1):18–22.
3. Vujovic S. Aetiology of premature ovarian failure. Menopause International 2009;15(2):72–5.
4. Kalu E, Panay N. Spontaneous premature ovarian failure: management challenges. Gynecological Endocrinology 2008;24(5):273–9.
5. Panay N, Kalu E. Management of premature ovarian failure. Best Practice & Research Clinical Obstetrics & Gynaecology 2009;23(1):129–40.
6. Gold EB. Factors related to age at natural menopause: longitudinal analyses from SWAN. Am J Epidemiol 2013;178(1):70–83.
7. Schlessinger D, Herrera L, Crisponi L et al. Genes and translocations involved in POI. American Journal of Medical Genetics 2002;111(3):328–33.
8. Loughlin SA, Redha A, McIver J, Boyd E, Carothers A, Connor JM. Analysis of the origin of Turner syndrome using polymorphic DNA probes. Journal of Medical Genetics 1991;28(3):156–8.
9. Sarto GE, Therman E, Patau K. X inactivation in man: a woman with t(Xq-;12q+). American Journal of Human Genetics 1973;25(3):262–70.
10. Murray A. Premature ovarian failure and the FMR1 gene. Semin Reprod Med 2000;18:59–66.
11. Shaw RW, Luesley D, Monga A. Gynaecology. 4th edn. Churchill Livingstone Elsevier, 2010.
12. Goswami D, Conway G S. Premature ovarian failure. Hum Reprod Update 2005;11:391–410.
13. Kaufman FR, Kogut MD, Donnell GN, Goebelsmann U, March C, Koch R. Hypergonadotrophic hypogonadism in female patients with galactosemia. New England Journal of Medicine 1981;304:994–998.
14. Popat V, Nelson LM, Calis KA. Ovarian Insufficiency Clinical Presentation. Medscape. http://emedicine.medscape.com/article/271046-clinical.
15. Rebar RW. Premature ovarian failure. Obstet Gynecol 2009;113:1355–63.
16. Sowers MR, Eyvazzadeh AD, McConnell D et al. Anti-mullerian hormone and inhibin B in the definition of ovarian aging and the menopause transition. J Clin Endocrinol Metab 2008;93:3478–83.
17. Maclaran K, Horner E, Panay N. Premature ovarian failure: long-term sequelae. Menopause International 2010;16:38–41.
18. van Karseren YM, Schoemaker J. Premature ovarian failure: a systematic review on therapeutic interventions to restore ovarian function and achieve pregnancy. Hum Reprod Update 1999;5:483–92.
19. Jacobsen BK, Knutsen SF, Fraser GE. Age at natural menopause and total mortality and mortality from ischemic heart disease: the Adventist Health Study. J Clin Epidemiol 1999;52:303–7.
20. Lobo RA. Surgical menopause and cardiovascular risks. Menopause 2007;14:562–6.
21. Clarkson TB. Estrogen effects on arteries vary with stage of reproductive life and extent of subclinical atherosclerosis progression. Menopause 2007;14:373–84.
22. Merz CN, Johnson BD, Sharaf BL et al. Hypoestrogenemia of hypothalamic origin and coronary artery disease in premenopausal women: a report from the NHLBI-sponsored WISE Study. J Am Coll Cardiol 2003;41:413–19.

23. Kalantaridou SN, Naka KK, Papanikolaou E *et al.* Impaired endothelial function in young women with premature ovarian failure: normalization with hormone therapy. *J Clin Endocrinol Metab* 2004;89:3907–13.

24. Knauff EA, Westerveld HE, Goverde AJ *et al.* Lipid profile of women with premature ovarian failure. *Menopause* 2008;15:919–23.

25. Corrigan EC, Nelson LM, Bakalov VK *et al.* Effects of ovarian failure and X-chromosome deletion on body composition and insulin sensitivity in young women. *Menopause* 2006;13:911–16.

26. Eshtiaghi R, Esteghamati A, Nakhjavani M. Menopause is an independent predictor of metabolic syndrome in Iranian women. *Maturitas* 2010;65:262–6.

27. Dubey RK, Imthurn B, Barton M *et al.* Vascular consequences of menopause and hormone therapy: importance of timing of treatment and type of estrogen. *Cardiovasc Res* 2005;66:295–306.

28. Nappi RE, Sinforiani E, Mauri M *et al.* Memory functioning at menopause: impact of age in ovariectomized women. *Gynecol Obstet Invest* 1999;47:29–36.

29. Farrag AK, Khedr EM, Abdel-Aleem H, Rageh TA. Effect of surgical menopause on cognitive functions. *Dement Geriatr Cogn Disord* 2002;13:193–8.

30. Panay N, Hamoda H, Arya R *et al.* The 2013 British Menopause Society & Women's Health Concern recommendations on hormone replacement therapy. *Menopause Int* 2013;19(2):59–68.

31. Miller VT, La Rosa J, Barnabei V *et al.* Effects of estrogen or estrogen/progestin regimens on heart disease risk factors in postmenopausal women. The Postmenopausal Estrogen/Progestin Interventions (PEPI) Trial. The Writing Group for the PEPI Trial. *JAMA* 1995;273(3):199–208.

32. Sitruk-Ware R. Progestogens in hormonal replacement therapy: new molecules, risks, and benefits. *Menopause* 2002;9(1):6–15.

33. Sitruk-Ware R. Pharmacological profile of progestins. *Maturitas* 2004;47(4):277–83.

34. Mueck AO. Postmenopausal hormone replacement therapy and cardiovascular disease: the value of transdermal estradiol and micronised progesterone. *Climacteric* 2012;15(Suppl 1):11–17.

35. Manson JE, Hsia J, Johnson KC *et al.* Estrogen plus progestin and the risk of coronary heart disease. *N Engl J Med* 2003;349(6):523–34.

36. Stevenson JC, Panay N, Paxman-Fieth C. Oral estradiol and dydrogesterone combination therapy in postmenopausal women: Review of efficacy and safety. *Maturitas* 2013 Sep;76(1):10–21.

37. Mittal M, Savvas M, Arya R *et al.* A randomised controlled trial comparing the effects of micronized progesterone to medroxyprogesterone acetate on cardiovascular health, lipid metabolism and the coagulation cascade in women with premature ovarian insufficiency: study protocol and review of the literature. *Menopause Int* 2013 Sep;19(3):127–32.

38. Gallagher JC. Effect of early menopause on bone mineral density and fractures. *Menopause* 2007;14:567–71.

39. van Der Voort DJ, van Der Weijer PH, Barentsen R. Early menopause: increased fracture risk at older age. *Osteoporos Int* 2003;14:525–30.

40. Melton LJ 3rd, Khosla S, Malkasian GD *et al.* Fracture risk after bilateral oophorectomy in elderly women. *J Bone Miner Res* 2003;18:900–5.

41. MacLean C, Newberry S, Maglione M *et al.* Systematic review: comparative effectiveness of treatments to prevent fractures in men and women with low bone density or osteoporosis. *Ann Intern Med* 2008;148:197–213.

42. Gallagher JC. Moderation of the daily dose of HRT: prevention of osteoporosis. *Maturitas* 1999 Nov;33 Suppl1:S57–63.

43. Rocca WA, Bower JH, Maraganore DM *et al.* Increased risk of cognitive impairment or dementia in women who underwent oophorectomy before menopause. *Neurology* 2007;69:1074–83.

44. Henderson VW, Sherwin BB. Surgical versus natural menopause: cognitive issues. *Menopause* 2007;14:572–9.

45. Rocca WA, Bower JH, Maraganore DM *et al.* Increased risk of parkinsonism in women who underwent oophorectomy before menopause. *Neurology* 2008;70:200–9.

46. Rocca WA, Grossardt BR, Maraganore DM. The long-term effects of oophorectomy on cognitive and motor aging are age dependent. *Neurodegener Dis* 2008;5:257–60.

47. Schmidt PJ, Cardoso GM, Ross JL, Haq N, Rubinow DR, Bondy CA. Shyness, social anxiety, and impaired self-esteem in Turner syndrome and premature ovarian failure. *JAMA* 2006;295:1374–6.

48. Liao KL, Wood N, Conway GS. Premature menopause and psychological well-being. *J Psychosom Obstet Gynaecol* 2000;21:167–74.

49. van der Stege JG, Groen H, van Zadelhoff SJ *et al.* Decreased androgen concentrations and diminishes general and sexual wellbeing in women with premature ovarian failure. *Menopause* 2008;15:23–31.

50. Orshan SA, Ventura JL, Covington SN *et al.* Women with spontaneous 46,XX primary ovarian insufficiency (hypergonadotropic hypogonadism) have lower perceived social support than control women. *Fertil Steril* 2009;92:688–93.

51. Graziottin A, Basson R. Sexual dysfunction in women with premature menopause. *Menopause* 2004;11:766–77.

52. LaBarbera AR, Miller MM, Ober C *et al.* Autoimmune etiology in premature ovarian failure. *Am J Reprod Immunol Microbiol* 1988;16:115–22.

53. Betterle C, Volpato M, Rees Smith B *et al.* Adrenal cortex and steroid 21-hydroxylase autoantibodies in adult patients with organ-specific autoimmune

diseases: markers of low progression to clinical Addison's disease. *J Clin Endocrinol Metab* 1997;82:932–8.

54. Langrish JP, Mills NL, Bath LE *et al.* Cardiovascular effects of physiological and standard sex steroid replacement regimens in premature ovarian failure. *Hypertension* Epub 2009 May;53(5):80511.

55. Buster JE, Kingsburg SA, Aguirre O *et al.* Testosterone patch for low sexual desire in surgically menopausal women: A randomized trial. *Obstetrics and Gynecology* 2005;105,944–52.

56. Simon J, Braunstein G, Nachtigall L *et al.* Testosterone patch increases sexual activity and desire in surgically menopausal women with hypoactive sexual desire disorder. *J Clin Endocrinol Metab* 2005;90(9):5226–5233.

57. Volterrani M, Rosano G, Iellamo F. Testosterone and heart failure. *Endocrine* 2012;42(2):272–277.

58. Saccà L. Heart failure as a multiple hormonal deficiency syndrome. *Circ Heart Fail* 2009;2(2):151–6.

59. Donnez J, Silber S, Andersen CY *et al.* Children born after autotransplantation of cryopreserved ovarian tissue. A review of 13 live births. *Ann Med* 2011;43(6):437–50.

Chapter 92 Fertility preservation

Hoda Harb and Arri Coomarasamy

MRCOG standards

There are currently no MRCOG standards for this subject. The following are suggested:
- Understand who should be offered cryopreservation of sperm, oocytes, embryos and ovarian tissue.
- Be able to counsel patients on options for fertility preservation.

INTRODUCTION

It is estimated that currently 1 in 1000 young adults (25–35 years) have survived childhood cancer. The five-year survival rates with haematological malignancies, breast cancer, testicular cancer and other cancers that affect young people are in the range of 90–95 per cent. Treatment for these cancers, however, is often highly detrimental to both female and male reproductive function. Thus the concern is no longer only to save lives from cancer, but also to ensure improved quality of life, which often includes preserving fertility.[1,2]

Although this chapter will focus mainly on patients with cancer, some treatments for non-cancerous conditions (e.g. long-term methotrexate therapy) can result in damage to reproductive organs, and the options discussed for fertility preservation should therefore also be considered for these patients.

There are two key aspects to fertility preservation:

1 Minimisation of the effect of cancer treatment on fertility;
2 Provision of effective options for storage of gametes, embryos or indeed germinal (e.g. ovarian) tissues.

The commonest cancer in women of reproductive age is breast cancer; other cancers of note in this age group are leukaemia, lymphoma, melanoma, cervical and ovarian cancers. In men, the commonest cancers during reproductive years are leukaemia, Hodgkin's lymphomas and testicular germ cell tumours.[3] Semen analysis may be abnormal in men with germ cell tumours. Furthermore, there is evidence that the integrity of sperm DNA is affected even before initiation of cancer therapy in men with Hodgkin's lymphomas and testicular cancers.[4]

The type of cancer, its stage, its biological features and patient factors have an influence on prognosis and treatment. The treatment may be a combination of surgery, chemotherapy and radiotherapy.

CHEMOTHERAPY

Chemotherapy and the ovary

Chemotherapy, particularly with alkylating agents like cyclophosphamide, is highly toxic to the primordial follicles in the ovary (Table 92.1). Histological studies of human ovaries following chemotherapy treatment have shown ovarian atrophy and global loss of primordial follicles.[5,6] The ovarian cortical stromal cells are mostly replaced with collagen and the ovary shrinks in size. The extent of the effect of chemotherapy on ovarian reserve will depend on the drug(s) used, dose, age and the baseline ovarian reserve of the patient. Factors associated with the development of acute ovarian failure are increased age at the time of treatment, diagnosis of Hodgkin's

Table 92.1 Drugs associated with significant gonadotoxic effects

Group	Drug
Alkylating agents	Cyclophosphamide
	Chlorambucil
	Mustine
	Melphalan
Vinca alkaloids	Vincristine
	Vinblastine
Antimetabolites	Cytarabine
Others	Cisplatin

disease, increased radiation doses (particularly >10 Gy), and exposure to alkylating agents (specifically procarbazine and cyclophosphamide).

Chemotherapy and the testis

Germinal epithelium of the testis is very sensitive to the detrimental effects of chemotherapy. Men can be rendered oligospermic or azoospermic. The degree to which the testicular function is affected is dose and agent dependent. Following higher cumulative doses of gonadotoxic chemotherapy, Leydig cell dysfunction may also become apparent.[7] As a result, testosterone production is affected, with the risk of developing osteoporosis, erectile dysfunction and cardiovascular disease.

RADIOTHERAPY

Radiation and the ovaries

Radiotherapy, particularly if directed to the pelvis, can adversely affect ovarian reserve. The extent of damage is related to the radiation dose, age at the time of treatment and fractionation schedule.[8,9]

Radiation and the uterus

Uterine function may be impaired following radiation to the pelvis as a consequence of disruption to uterine vasculature and musculature elasticity, impaired blood flow and endometrial damage. The clinical consequences are increased risk of miscarriage, lower birthweight, premature delivery and fewer livebirths.[10,11]

Radiation and the testis

Radiation doses as low as 0.1–1.2 Gy can impair spermatogenesis, with doses over 4 Gy causing permanent azoospermia.[12]

MANAGEMENT

Management of cancer patients requires a multidisciplinary approach consisting of a close partnership between the oncologist and fertility specialists, with the patient, partner and family at the centre of a treatment plan that prioritises not only the prolongation of life, but which considers quality of life and the psychological, physical and social wellbeing of the patient. The role of counsellors in supporting patients and family is important.

Oncologists and medical specialists should:

- be aware of options for fertility preservation;
- offer referral to a fertility specialist for counselling prior to commencement of treatment.

Once a referral is received, a fertility specialist will consider the following issues:

1 history: including age, menstrual history, pregnancies, fertility wishes, and whether or not the patient has a partner/spouse;
2 cancer: location, biology of the tumour, stage, prognosis, potential for metastasis in ovary, proposed treatment, and foreseeable long-term effects;
3 time available for fertility preservation – possibility or impossibility of delaying the start of treatment;
4 patient's general condition;
5 baseline ovarian reserve.

Conservative fertility-sparing treatment for early invasive disease, such as hormonal treatment of early endometrial cancer, may be possible in some patients. Ovarian transposition can be considered where irradiation of the pelvis becomes necessary, for example in the management of cervical cancer, to reduce the dose of radiation to the ovaries.

Controlled ovarian stimulation and cryopreservation of oocytes or embryos

This is the most established female fertility preservation method (Table 92.2). It requires approximately 2 weeks to complete the treatment to the oocyte retrieval stage. A working partnership with a fertility clinic should be established so that rapid referral can be made and the patient seen expeditiously to avoid delay (RCOG Scientific Impact Paper No. 35, 2013).

Cryopreservation of embryos

Embryo cryopreservation following IVF is a routine procedure in fertility clinics and is the method of choice with the greatest chance of success; however it is only an option if there is a male partner or if donor sperm is acceptable to the woman or couple. It is estimated that of the 3 million children born by IVF, 15–20 per cent were conceived following transfer of cryopreserved embryos. However, there are limited data on its success rates in the context of fertility preservation in women with gynaecological cancers.

Cryopreservation of oocytes

When embryo cryopreservation is not feasible or desired, women who have the time to undergo a stimulation cycle should be offered oocyte cryopreservation. Oocyte cryopreservation is technically challenging due to the size and structural complexities of oocytes. Effectiveness of oocyte preservation is limited by the number of oocytes that can be obtained, as *each* oocyte carries a 3–5 per cent chance of resulting in a successful pregnancy. A recent meta-analysis evaluating the age-specific probability of livebirth with oocyte cryopreservation found that livebirths continued to occur as late as ages 42 and 44 years with slowly frozen and vitrified oocytes, respectively.[13]

Table 92.2 Fertility preservation options available for girls and women

Group	Pre-pubertal girls	Post-pubertal girls	Women
Fertility preservation options	Cryopreservation of ovarian tissue and ovarian transplantation when fertility is required	COS and preservation of oocytes	COS and preservation of embryos
		Cryopreservation of ovarian tissue and ovarian transplantation	COS and preservation of oocytes
		GnRH agonist co-treatment during chemotherapy	Cryopreservation of ovarian tissue and ovarian transplantation
			GnRH agonist co-treatment during chemotherapy
Considerations	Transplantation carries the potential risk of reintroduction of cancer cells	COS introduces delay in cancer treatment	For creation of embryos, sperm is required
	IVM may become an option in the future	Oocyte cryopreservation may not be as effective as embryo cryopreservation	If the male withdraws consent in the future, the woman is unlikely to be able to use the embryos
	Consenting issues		

COS, controlled ovarian stimulation; IVM, in-vitro maturation.

Cryopreservation of ovarian tissue

Cryopreservation and transplantation of ovarian cortex may be the only option for fertility preservation in pre-pubertal girls or in women who need cancer treatment within the minimum of 2 weeks required for COS. With several live-births reported from various countries, this option is gradually moving from the experimental phase to clinical practice.[14] Generally, no more than 50 per cent of one of the ovaries is removed in a day-case laparoscopic procedure, and thin slivers of the cortex are prepared and cryopreserved.[14] If the woman becomes menopausal following her cancer treatment, she may have the ovarian cortical tissue transplanted when she decides to try to conceive a pregnancy.

Cryopreservation and transplantation of ovarian tissues are best carried out in specialised and centralised facilities. One of the major concerns regarding cryopreservation of ovarian tissue is the risk of ischaemic damage to the tissue pending transplant and revascularisation. Also, there is a theoretical possibility of transplantation reintroducing malignant tumour cells. IVM and xenotransplantation are both experimental, but may offer a way of dealing with this risk in the future.

GnRH agonist co-treatment during chemotherapy

Suppression of folliculogenesis with GnRH analogue during chemotherapy has been proposed to provide ovarian protection. Research evidence on the effects of GnRHa co-treatment during chemotherapy has yielded conflicting results.[15–18]

A systematic review on this subject identified 16 controlled studies, of which 5 were of randomised design.[15] Meta-analysis of all the studies found a statistically significant reduction in the risk of premature ovarian failure with GnRHa co-treatment (RR 0.26, 95% CI 0.14–0.49). However, the advantage of GnRHa was primarily found in the non-randomised studies, with the randomised studies showing conflicting results, with only 3/5 studies indicating benefit with the use of GnRHa co-treatment. A more recent meta-analysis of seven randomised trials[19] comparing GnRHa co-treatment with chemotherapy in premenopausal women found that the number of patients with resumption of spontaneous menstruation was statistically significantly greater in the GnRHa co-treatment patients (OR 2.83, 95% CI: 1.52–5.25).

There are at least three ongoing randomised studies that may allow us to draw a firm inference on the role of GnRHa co-treatment in the future. In the meantime, it would be reasonable to offer a woman GnRHa treatment during chemotherapy.

Sperm banking

Men should be offered the opportunity to bank sperm before cancer treatment (Table 92.3). Spermache occurs at a median age of 13.4 (range 11.7–15.3) years. Post-pubertal males will ordinarily be capable of ejaculation and can provide sperm for storage. In males who cannot ejaculate or who are too young, electro-ejaculation, epididymal sperm aspiration or testicular sperm extraction may be performed. Cryopreserved material is usually stored for an initial period of 10 years; however,

Table 92.3 Fertility preservation options available for boys and men

Group	Pre-pubertal boys	Post-pubertal boys	Men
Fertility preservation options	There are no established procedures	Electro-ejaculation or masturbatory ejaculation and sperm banking	Ejaculatory sperm banking
		SSR and sperm banking	SSR and sperm banking
Considerations	Experimental: stem cell extraction and later repopulation of the testis	Consenting issues	
SSR, surgical sperm retrieval.			

continued storage of cryopreserved sperm, beyond 10 years, should be offered to men who remain at risk of significant infertility. Testicular tissue cryopreservation from prepubescent males remains experimental.

Pregnancy in cancer survivors

Depending on the type of cancer and gonadotoxic treatment the patient received, oncologists may recommend that cancer survivors wait at least a year before attempting pregnancy,[20] although optimal timing of conception after treatment remains uncertain.[21]

The Childhood Cancer Survivor Study (CCSS),[22] including 3531 survivors and 1366 female sibling controls, found that 292 (64 per cent) of 455 participants with self-reported clinical infertility achieved a pregnancy, although survivors had an increased time to pregnancy compared with their siblings. The analysis, however, did not include women with ovarian failure and the proportion of infertile survivors achieving pregnancy is expected to have been lower if this group was included. The study also showed that the risk of non-surgical premature menopause in childhood cancer survivors was higher in survivors than in their siblings, with a cumulative incidence of 8 per cent by 40 years of age.[23]

Fertility after chemotherapy depends primarily on ovarian reserve for a woman. Ovarian assessment can be performed in a number of ways (Box 92.1). The most commonly used test is the FSH level, although AMH and antral follicle count (AFC) are increasingly being used.

Women should be counselled regarding reproductive options including natural conception, or assisted reproduction using stored gametes or donor gametes. If a woman is found to have a reduced ovarian reserve, or if natural conception does not occur, fertility specialists should have a low threshold to move to assisted reproduction. Women should also be counselled about other options including surrogacy and adoption.

Box 92.1 Assessment of ovarian reserve

Assessment of ovarian reserve

- Follicle-stimulating hormone, measured between day 2 and day 5 of cycle
- Serum anti-Müllerian hormone, at any stage of the menstrual cycle
- Sonography: total antral follicle count
- Sonography: ovarian volume
- Response to ovarian stimulation

KEY POINTS

Background:
- Young patients with many cancers have excellent survival prognosis, and may request fertility preservation.
- The effect of chemotherapy on ovarian function and fertility will depend on the drug(s) used, dose, duration of treatment, age of the patient and baseline ovarian reserve.
- Radiotherapy, particularly if directed to the pelvis, can affect fertility.

Management:
- Multidisciplinary team approach.
- Fertility preservation options will be determined by the pubertal stage of the patient, baseline ovarian reserve, time available for fertility preservation, and whether the patient is in a stable relationship with a partner who can offer sperm for the creation of embryos.
- Clinicians should inform patients about options for fertility preservation *prior* to starting potentially gonadotoxic treatment.
- Fertility preservation options are:
  - Pre-pubertal girls: ovarian tissue storage and transplantation;
  - Post-pubertal girls: COS and oocyte storage; ovarian tissue storage; GnRHa co-treatment during chemotherapy;

- • Women: COS and embryo storage; COS and oocyte storage; GnRHa co-treatment during chemotherapy;
  - • Pre-pubertal boys: no established options;
  - • Post-pubertal boys: sperm banking (sperm obtained from masturbation, electro-ejaculation or surgical sperm retrieval);
  - • Men: sperm banking.
- • Ovarian tissue storage and transplantation: generally no more than 50 per cent of one ovary is removed for storage; storage and transplantation should be carried out in specialised and centralised facilities.
- • COS: requires approximately 2 weeks to complete treatment to the oocyte retrieval stage.
- • There is contradictory evidence on the role of GnRHa co-treatment to reduce gonadal toxicity during chemotherapy. Results of on-going randomised trials are awaited.

References

1. Jeruss JS, Woodruff TK. Preservation of fertility in patients with cancer. *N Engl J Med* 2009;360(9):902–11.
2. Lee SJ, Schover LR, Partridge AH *et al.* American Society of Clinical Oncology recommendations on fertility preservation in cancer patients. *J Clin Oncol* 2006;24(18):2917–31.
3. Dohle GR. Male infertility in cancer patients: Review of the literature. *Int J Urol* 2010;17(4):327–31.
4. Jeruss JS, Woodruff TK. Preservation of fertility in patients with cancer. *N Engl J Med* 2009;360(9):902–11.
5. Himelstein-Braw R, Peters H, Faber M. Morphological study of the ovaries of leukaemic children. *Br J Cancer* 1978;38(1):82–7.
6. Familiari G, Caggiati A, Nottola SA, Ermini M, Di Benedetto MR, Motta PM. Ultrastructure of human ovarian primordial follicles after combination chemotherapy for Hodgkin's disease. *Hum Reprod* 1993;8(12):2080–7.
7. Gerl A, Muhlbayer D, Hansmann G, Mraz W, Hiddemann W. The impact of chemotherapy on Leydig cell function in long-term survivors of germ cell tumors. *Cancer* 2001;91(7):1297–303.
8. Meirow D, Nugent D. The effects of radiotherapy and chemotherapy on female reproduction. *Hum Reprod Update* 2001;7(6):535–43.
9. Whitehead E, Shalet SM, Blackledge G, Todd I, Crowther D, Beardwell CG. The effect of combination chemotherapy on ovarian function in women treated for Hodgkin's disease. *Cancer* 1983;52(6):988–93.
10. Critchley HO, Wallace WH, Shalet SM, Mamtora H, Higginson J, Anderson DC. Abdominal irradiation

in childhood; the potential for pregnancy. *Br J Obstet Gynaecol* 1992;99(5):392–4.
11. Signorello LB, Mulvihill JJ, Green DM *et al.* Stillbirth and neonatal death in relation to radiation exposure before conception: a retrospective cohort study. *Lancet* 2010;376(9741):624–30.
12. Shalet SM, Tsatsoulis A, Whitehead E, Read G. Vulnerability of the human Leydig cell to radiation damage is dependent upon age. *J Endocrinol* 1989;120(1):161–5.
13. Cil AP, Bang H, Oktay K. Age-specific probability of live birth with oocyte cryopreservation: an individual patient data meta-analysis. *Fertil Steril* 2013;100(2):492–9.
14. von WM, Donnez J, Hovatta O *et al.* Cryopreservation and autotransplantation of human ovarian tissue prior to cytotoxic therapy: a technique in its infancy but already successful in fertility preservation. *Eur J Cancer* 2009;45(9):1547–53.
15. Ben-Aharon I, Gafter-Gvili A, Leibovici L, Stemmer SM. Pharmacological interventions for fertility preservation during chemotherapy: a systematic review and meta-analysis. *Breast Cancer Res Treat* 2010;122(3):803–11.
16. Clowse ME, Behera MA, Anders CK *et al.* Ovarian preservation by GnRH agonists during chemotherapy: a meta-analysis. *J Womens Health* (Larchmt) 2009;18(3):311–19.
17. Blumenfeld Z, von WM. GnRH-analogues and oral contraceptives for fertility preservation in women during chemotherapy. *Hum Reprod Update* 2008;14(6):543–52.
18. Beck-Fruchter R, Weiss A, Shalev E. GnRH agonist therapy as ovarian protectants in female patients undergoing chemotherapy: a review of the clinical data. *Hum Reprod Update* 2008;14(6):553–61.
19. Wang C, Chen M, Fu F, Huang M. Gonadotropin-releasing hormone analog cotreatment for the preservation of ovarian function during gonadotoxic chemotherapy for breast cancer: a meta-analysis. *PLoS One* 2013;8(6):e66360.
20. Del ML, Catzeddu T, Venturini M. Infertility and pregnancy after breast cancer: current knowledge and future perspectives. *Cancer Treat Rev* 2006;32(6):417–22.
21. The Ethics Committee of the American Society for Reproductive Medicine. Fertility preservation and reproduction in patients facing gonadotoxic therapies: a committee opinion. *Fertil Steril* 2013;100(5):1224–31.
22. Barton SE, Najita JS, Ginsburg ES *et al.* Infertility, infertility treatment, and achievement of pregnancy in female survivors of childhood cancer: a report from the Childhood Cancer Survivor Study cohort. *Lancet Oncol* 2013;14(9):873–81.
23. Sklar CA, Mertens AC, Mitby P *et al.* Premature menopause in survivors of childhood cancer: a report from the childhood cancer survivor study. *J Natl Cancer Inst* 2006;98(13):890–6.

Chapter 93   Psychosexual medicine

Susan V Carr

INTRODUCTION

Women's sexual difficulties include problems of function, such as pain on intercourse and dyspareunia, and problems of desire, such as loss of libido. Any woman presenting to a gynaecologist complaining of a sexual problem should have a routine clinical history and examination and any indicated tests, followed by treatment. There are, however, a significant number of women who have no organic lesions, yet continue to experience sexual difficulties which have major negative effect on their lives.

Psychosexual medicine is the area of medicine which deals with sexual difficulties in patients, recognising the emotional and relationship aspects of the problem.[1]

WHAT IS SEXUALITY?

Sexuality is a biopsychosocial phenomenon. It is composed of gender identity, sexual orientation and sexual knowledge, attitudes and behaviour. Gender identity and sexual orientation are mainly organically determined, but sexual knowledge, attitudes and behaviour are shaped by many external factors, and can change over the course of a woman's lifetime.

THE HUMAN SEXUAL RESPONSE

The physiological sexual response depends not only on intact vascular, endocrine and neurological pathways, but also on sensory input. Bancroft[2] describes this as the 'Psychosomatic Circle of Sex', the fundamental concept of mind–body interaction, on which the discipline of psychosexual medicine is based. Female responsiveness is a result of sensory input through the peripheral nerves of the somatic and autonomous nervous systems, as well as through the cranial nerves and psychogenic stimulation. The frontal and temporal lobes all have a role to play in mediating the sexual response. The precise details of the processing of afferent information within the spinal cord and brain still remain unclear.[3]

Genital motor responses include vasocongestion and vaginal lubrication. During sexual penetration the vagina lengthens, the labia increase in fullness, the uterus draws back and the clitoris retracts. At orgasm there is also contraction of the uterine and pelvic muscles.

PREVALENCE OF SEXUAL PROBLEMS

According to Laumann,[4] in a US-based population study, 43 per cent of females and 37 per cent of men at some time have a problem with sex. Of these, a third of women had loss of libido, 25 per cent were inorgasmic and around 20 per cent had loss of vaginal lubrication and did not enjoy sex. In 2004 similar figures were reported, also showing that the incidence of these problems increases with age.[5] This is shown in another study where 26.7 per cent of pre-menopausal women had low sexual desire, but that figure increased to 52.4 per cent in naturally menopausal women.[6] Menopausal women comprise the group who have the highest prevalence of sexual problems worldwide. Roos in 2012 reported that 37 per cent of women in a general gynaecology/urogynaecology clinic had sexual problems but only 17 per cent volunteered this information spontaneously.[7]

There is also a high prevalence of sexual problems in women with gynaecological cancer, significantly more than in a control population.[8] These problems are multifactorial and, of necessity, require a multimodal treatment approach.[9]

VAGINISMUS

In a population-based survey, vaginismus was seen in 6 per cent of the 37.9 per cent of women who reported sexual problems[10] (see Box 93.1).

Box 93.1 Case scenario: clinical presentation of vaginismus

> *Lucy, age 32, had been married for 5 years to James. She presented at her GP surgery saying that she hadn't been able to become pregnant. The GP noticed that she had never had a smear test. She said she would make an appointment to have it done. She was in good health, had a regular menstrual cycle and was not using contraception. All blood tests were normal. He referred her to the local hospital for investigations.*
>
> *When Lucy attended the hospital she became very distressed at the mention of a vaginal examination or scans, and was unable to tolerate any form of genital examination.*
>
> *It then became clear that she had never had sex, and had primary vaginismus.*
>
> *After psychosexual counselling and physiotherapist-guided vaginal trainer therapy (dilators), she was able to have penetrative sex.*

Vaginismus is defined as recurrent involuntary spasm of the musculature of the outer third of the vagina which interferes with sexual penetration of any kind. Primary vaginismus is diagnosed when nothing has ever entered the vagina. In this condition the vagina is healthy, and a deep-seated fear of sexual penetration triggers involuntary muscle contraction, making penetration impossible. The vaginismus precedes the pain, which only occurs on attempted penetration.

Secondary vaginismus occurs often after vulvovaginal trauma such as infection, childbirth, malignancy or its treatment, or sexual trauma such as rape or abuse. It is thought that the memory or expectation of pain on penetration causes involuntary muscle spasm resulting in vaginismus.

Although vaginismus is classified as a pain disorder, its clinical presentation is very different. Women with vaginismus can often orgasm easily, and express desire for sex. They report more sexual desire and less difficulty with lubrication compared to women with dyspareunia.[11]

Diagnosis of vaginismus

Primary vaginismus will be diagnosed mainly on the history. A good general and gynaecological history should be taken. A woman who has never had penetration of any kind, despite wishing to, may have vaginismus. These women may be 'cervical smear avoiders'. They are frequently too embarrassed to disclose that they are unable to have sex.

Good questions to ask include 'Have you ever used tampons?' and 'Have you ever had sex?'

A vaginal examination should then be offered, to assess not only the degree of vaginismus but also the acceptability of any vaginal examination.

1 Offer vaginal examination, and observe the woman's reaction to this offer.
2 If refused, then accept her decision.
3 If accepted, proceed with single digital examination only, not a speculum examination.
4 Only proceed if the patient is comfortable, and assess the degree of vaginal spasm.

In most cases even digital examination at this stage is unsuccessful. This is a positive diagnostic sign for vaginismus.

Treatment of vaginismus

A recent Cochrane review on the subject of interventions for vaginismus was only able to include five controlled trials. The authors stated that, although uncontrolled case series of sex therapy and desensitisation appear promising, in controlled trials there was no difference between systematic desensitisation and any of the control interventions.[12] They also highlighted the lack of research in this area.

There are excellent psychodynamic and behavioural treatment options which are widely accepted by specialists working in the field, but due to the paucity of research, most evidence is derived from expert opinion, based on grading of available research, committee discussion, public presentations and debate.

There are various modes of treatment for this condition, which is mainly of psychogenic origin.

Psychosexual therapy

Using short-term, focused and reflective doctor–patient interactions, the psychosexual approach offers a starting point for assessment of the problem, and addresses emotional aspects of the condition. It is the mainstay of treatment, and can be used in conjunction with other treatment options. A multidisciplinary approach is frequently recommended[13] in order to simultaneously address the psychogenic as well as the physical aspects of the condition.

Behavioural therapy

Sex therapy is a commonly used form of treatment for women with a partner.[14] This approach follows modified Masters and Johnson programmes of couple therapy.[15] The technique 'reteaches' a couple how to touch and interact sexually, sets boundaries which facilitate trust and acts as a vehicle for communication about intimate issues. This approach is useful to both heterosexual and same-sex couples. A success rate of over 90 per cent is reported in those who continue therapy.[16]

Biofeedback therapy

Physiotherapist-aided vaginal training and biofeedback therapy are effective.[17] A combination of increasing knowledge and awareness of genital anatomy combined with vaginal self-insertion of graduated trainers can prove very effective but may take up to 2 years to achieve success; there is rarely a quick fix.

Cognitive behavioural therapy

CBT is also an effective mode of treatment[18] which can achieve positive effects on sexual intimacy and communication, and has been successfully conducted online.[19]

Botulinum toxin A therapy

There is some evidence of success in using intravaginal injections of botulinum toxin for vaginismus. This may hold true for treatment of refactory patients,[20] but to date there is a lack of placebo-controlled randomised clinical trials on which to base the approach.

Individual case treatment is usually dependent on what options are available locally. If the condition is accurately diagnosed and referred appropriately to a relevant trained professional, the cure rate is over 90 per cent.

DYSPAREUNIA

Dyspareunia is pain on sexual intercourse (see Box 93.2). This applies to any form of sexual vaginal penetration, not only with the penis, but other objects such as fingers or sex toys. Deep dyspareunia is more likely to have an organic cause and should be thoroughly investigated before psychosexual diagnosis is considered.

Vulvar pain syndromes, such as vulvodynia and vestibulodynia, may also present as dyspareunia.

In many women there may be a clear organic explanation, such as post-menopausal vaginal dryness, vulvar skin lesions, endometriosis, infection or the physical sequelae of childbirth. In cases where any obvious physical or hormonal

disruption has been treated but the pain on sex persists, then a psychogenic element must be considered.

Treatment of dyspareunia

1   Take a careful history including sexual and psychosocial issues.
2   Treat any underlying condition.
3   If the problem remains unresolved then consider a psychogenic origin and offer psychosexual assessment.
4   Refer the patient to a physiotherapist experienced in sexual difficulties if necessary following psychosexual assessment.

LOSS OF LIBIDO

There are no physiological markers for the loss of libido (loss of sexual interest and desire). The severity of the condition may be judged by the attitude of the patient towards her lack of sexual feelings. To some women, the loss of libido causes no difficulty; it is only those who would like to recover who are likely to seek clinical assistance (see Box 93.3, 93.4).

Loss of libido is associated with menopause, and post-menopausal women worldwide are the population group most likely to suffer from sexual problems. This is especially true in young women with acute, surgical menopause.

Treatment of loss of libido

1   Elicit and listen to the patient history, including sexual, social and relationship issues. The timing of presentation may be important.
2   Treat any underlying clinical condition, including any menopausal effects.
3   If anything in the history is suggestive of psychosocial problems underlying the loss of libido, or if hormonal treatment is unsuccessful, then offer referral for psychosexual counselling.

Box 93.2 Case scenario: clinical presentation of dyspareunia

> *Maya, age 28 and para 0+1, had been treated for chlamydia. She had been living with Carlos for 6 months when she was referred to the gynaecologist, saying that sex, particularly on penetration, had become painful. This difficulty was beginning to negatively affect their relationship. She said there were no other problems.*
>
> *Indications from clinical and bacteriological examinations were normal. The gynaecologist expected Maya to be relieved by these results, but when she was discharged from the gynaecology clinic she began to cry. After further discussion she was referred to a sexual difficulties clinic, where she was able to discuss the underlying, unresolved emotional issues about her previous pregnancy loss, sexual infection and current relationship.*
>
> *She cancelled her gynaecology review appointment, because the dyspareunia had resolved.*

Box 93.3 Case scenario: clinical presentation of loss of libido

> *Renee is a 54-year-old woman and has been with her current partner, Louisa, for the past 7 years. Previously she was married to Tom and has 3 children in their 20s. At first Renee was embarrassed to disclose her sexual orientation to her gynaecologist, but after careful prompting she became comfortable in discussing her loss of libido.*
>
> *Renee had experienced a very active sex life with Louisa, but since menopause 2 years ago her vagina had been dry, and she began to avoid sex because of vaginal discomfort. She lost any interest in sex. She wanted to improve sexual relations for both of them although Louisa insisted that the problem did not affect her commitment to a life together.*
>
> *The gynaecologist treated Renee with vaginal oestrogen. Sex became more comfortable, and the situation resolved.*

Box 93.4 Case scenario: clinical presentation of loss of libido

Marina, in good health at age 54 and para 4+0, presented at the menopause clinic with loss of libido.

She said things were difficult with Robert, her husband of 30 years, since she experienced menopause.

She requested 'Tablets and a check-up, please.'

After many repeat appointments and changes of HRT, the loss of libido did not improve. When asked if there was anything else wrong, Marina finally broke down and admitted there were other problems with her and Robert. She was offered the opportunity to see a psychosexual counsellor, with whom she admitted longstanding inter-relationship violence. Marina's loss of libido resulted from this difficulty and was further exacerbated by the menopause.

Marina persuaded her husband to engage in couple counselling, and things improved a little.

The only strong evidence for the use of testosterone to recover libido is confined to post-menopausal women also receiving HRT and with no previous underlying problems.[21] Transdermal testosterone is effective, but any additional treatment such as oral or vaginal dehydroepiandrosterone remains controversial.[22]

ORGASMIC DISORDERS

The female orgasm is defined as a sensation of intense pleasure creating an altered state of consciousness accompanied by the contraction of pelvic striated circumvaginal musculature, uterine/anal contractions and myotonia that resolves sexually induced vasocongestion and induces feelings of wellbeing and contentment.[23]

Orgasmic disorder, or anorgasmia, is the absence of orgasm following a phase of normal sexual excitement, causing frustration[24] which can lead to distress. Commonly psychological, cultural and emotional factors are at play. A patient may maintain a good libido and interest in sex, yet be unable to 'let go' and lose herself in the sexual act.

Female orgasmic disorder is reportedly the second most common female sexual disorder worldwide, with a prevalence of 24 per cent in the US.[23]

Treatment of orgasmic disorders

1 Take a comprehensive sexual and psychosocial history, and determine the time of onset and circumstance of the condition.
2 Exclude any rare organic causes, such as multiple sclerosis; if there are any indicators of an organic cause,

such as gradual onset in a previously orgasmic woman, then indicated investigations should be conducted.
3 Refer the patient for psychosexual assessment.
4 Treatments such as basic sexual education, simple masturbation techniques and Kegel exercises may be helpful.
5 CBT may alleviate the anxiety of the patient, and assist the behavioural route to cure.

To date, no pharmacological agents have been proven to cure anorgasmia.[23]

COMMUNICATION

It is impossible to diagnose and treat a sexual problem if neither the gynaecologist nor the patient will mention it. Studies indicate that as many as 80 per cent of non-oncology general gynaecology patients would like the subject to be broached, but the enquiry is made by practitioners in only around one third of cases.[25] It may be difficult for a patient to ask about sex, especially as a result of gender, age and cultural barriers.[26] It is therefore up to the gynaecologist to make a simple enquiry about sex as part of the routine consultation. Simple questions such as 'Do you have a partner?', 'Are they male or female?' and 'Do you have any problems with sex?' will give the patient 'permission' to discuss the subject if she wishes.

KEY POINTS

- Sexual problems are common and amenable to treatment (options are varied).
- Patients may be reluctant to bring up the topic but good communication with the patient is essential.
- Psychosexual medicine addresses emotional as well as physical aspects of the problem.
- Treatment for vaginismus should be based on available research evidence and expert opinion, committee consensus and public debate: there is no good evidence for surgical intervention.
- Dyspareunia is multifactorial: emotional as well as organic causes must be considered and a multidisciplinary approach is optimal.
- Post-menopausal women worldwide are the population group most likely to suffer from loss of libido, but menopause is not the only cause.
- Orgasmic disorders may result from psychological, cultural and emotional factors.
- Good communication skills and knowledge of conditions, treatment and referral options will enhance practitioner confidence in the field of sexual problems, leading to good patient outcomes.

References

1. Skrine R (ed). *Introduction to Psychosexual Medicine.* London: Chapman and Hall, 1989.
2. Bancroft J. *Human Sexuality and its Origins.* Edinburgh: Churchill Livingstone, 2008.
3. Yang H, Toy E, Baker B. Sexual dysfunction in the elderly patient. *1y care update for OG/GYN* 2000;7(6):269-74
4. Laumann EO, Paik A, Rosen RC. Sexual dysfunction in the United States: prevalence and predictors. *JAMA* 1999;281:537–44.
5. Lewis RW, Fugl-Meyer KS, Bosch R *et al.* Epidemiology/risk factors of sexual dysfunction. *Journal of Sexual Medicine* 2004;1:35–9.
6. West SL, D'Aloisio AA, Agans RP, Kalsboek WD, Borisov NN Thorp JM. Prevalence of low sexual desire and hypoactive desire disorder in a nationally representative sample of US women. *Archives of Internal Medicine* 2008;168:1441–9.
7. Roos AM, Sultan AH, Thakar R. Sexual problems in the gynaecology clinic: are we making a mountain out of a molehill? *Int Urogynaecol J* 2012;23(2):145–52.
8. Aerts L, Enzlin P, Verhaeghe J, Vergote I, Amant F. Sexual and psychological functioning in women after pelvic surgery for gynaecological cancer. *Eur J Gynaeol Oncol* 2009;30(6):652–6.
9. Krychman M, Millheiser LS. Sexual health issues in women with cancer. *J Sex Med* 2013;10 Suppl.1:5.doi:10.1111/jsm.12034.
10. Peixolo MM *et al.* Prevalence and sociodemographic predictors of sexual problems in Portugal: a population-based study with women aged 18–79 years. *J Sex Marital Therapy* 2013; Oct 28. Epub ahead of print.
11. Cherner RA *et al.* A comparative study of sexual function, behaviour and cognitions of women with lifelong vaginismus. *Arch Sex Behav* 2013;42(8):1605–14.
12. Melnik T *et al.* Interventions for vaginismus. *Cochrane Database System Review* 2012;12:12.
13. Reissing ED. Consultation and treatment history and causal attributions in an online sample of women with lifelong and acquired vaginismus. *J Sex Med* 2012;9(1):251–8.
14. Pereira VM, Arias-Carrion O, Machado S, Nardi AE, Silva AC. Sex therapy for sexual dysfunction. *Int Arch Med* 2013:6(1):37.
15. Gunzler C, Berner MM.Efficacy of psychosocial interventions in men and womenwith sexual dysfunctions–a systematic review of controlled clinical trials:part 2–the efficacy of psychosocial interventions for female sexual dysfunction. *J Sex Med* 2012;9(12):3108-25.
16. Jeng CJ, Wang LR, Chou CS Shen J, Tzeng CR. Management and outcome of primary vaginismus. *J Sex Marital Ther* 2006;32(5):379–387.
17. Reissing E, Armstrong HL, Allen C. Pelvic floor physical therapy for lifelong vaginismus: a retrospective chart review and interview study. *J Sex Marital Ther* 2013;39(4):306–320.
18. Kabakci E, Batur S.Who benefits from cognitive behavioural therapy for vaginismus? *J Sexual Marital Ther* 2003;29(4):277–288.
19. Hucker A, McCabe MP. An online, mindfulness based, cognitive behavioural therapy for female sexual difficulties: impact on relationship functioning. *J Sex Marital Ther* 2013;Oct 10 (epub).
20. Ferreira JR, Souza RP. Botulinum toxin for vaginismus treatment. *Pharmacology* 2012;89(5-6):256–9.
21. Blumel JE, Del Pino M, Aprikaian D, Vallejo S, Sarra S, Castelo-branco C. Effect of androgens combined with hormone therapy on quality of life in post-menopausal women with sexual dysfunction. *Gynecol Endocrinol* 2008;24(12):691-5.
22. Pluchino N, Carmigiani A, Cubeddu A, Santoro A, Cela V, Errasti T. Androgen therapy for women: for whom and when? *Arch Gynecol Obstet* 2013;288(4):731–7.
23. Meston CM, Hull E, Levin RJ, Sipski M. Disorders of orgasm in women. *J Sex Med* 2004;1(1):66–8.
24. Kingsberg SA, Tkachenko N, Lucas J, Burbrink A, Kreppner W, Dickstein JB. Characterisation of orgasmic difficulties by women: focus group evaluation. *J Sex Med* 2013;10(9):2242–50.
25. Breidite I. *et al.* Insufficient assessment of sexual dysfunction: a problem in gynaecological practice. *Medicina (Kaunas)*2013;49(7):315–20.
26. Burd ID, Nevadunsky N, Bachmann G. 2006 Impact of physician gender in sexual history taking in a multispecialty practice. *J Sex Med* 2006;3(2):194–200.

SECTION NINE

Urogynaecology and Sexual Health and Wellbeing

Chapter 94 Assessment of lower urinary tract function

Angie Rantell

INTRODUCTION

Lower urinary tract symptoms (LUTS) are common and can be due to a wide variety of underlying mechanisms. It is therefore important to approach the investigation of such symptoms in a logical and objective manner. An accurate and detailed history and examination provide a framework for diagnosis. However, it is important to recognise that different underlying conditions can cause the same urinary symptoms and that the medical history alone is a poor predictor of pathophysiology.

HISTORY

According to the International Continence Society (ICS)/ International Urogynaecology Association (IUGA) (2010), symptoms are any morbid phenomenon or departure from the normal in structure, function or sensation, experienced by the woman and indicative of disease[1] or a health problem that may lead her to seek help from healthcare professionals.[1] Symptoms may be volunteered by the patient or described during the patient interview. In general, LUTS cannot be used to make a definitive diagnosis.

Although urinary symptoms alone do not lead directly to a diagnosis, this should in no way detract from the central importance of the medical history in assessing a woman who presents with urinary problems. Listening to any patient is important, and an appropriate history should be obtained in a targeted and methodical manner. Not only will this enable the woman's own words to be turned into a graduated list of symptoms, but it will also provide information about how the woman's quality of life is affected by the condition. There are a number of ways in which a woman can ameliorate her urinary symptoms through behavioural changes. When taking a history, it is important to elucidate these restrictions and adaptations in order to gain a proper impression of the morbidity of the disorder. For example, by severely restricting fluid intake and never venturing far from a toilet, it is possible that a woman could greatly reduce the number of episodes of leaking. However, these adaptations do not lessen the severity of the disorder, or the need for appropriate treatment that will reduce this social restriction.

Urinary symptoms are valuable in directing further management by guiding the investigator in his or her choice of additional tests. Investigations may produce a diagnosis that is inconsistent with the problems complained of by the woman. It is very important to establish which problems bother her most, so that management can be targeted at these problems. This can only be done by taking the time to listen to the patient's description of her urinary symptoms in her own words. To ensure that a complete picture of lower urinary tract symptoms is gained, it is often useful to question the patient about individual symptoms. This can take the form of a questionnaire or a series of structured questions, and ensures that important features of the history are not omitted because the woman is unable to describe a symptom or is too embarrassed to mention it.

LUTS can be grouped into three main areas. These reflect disorders of different aspects of bladder and urethral function. That function is to store urine in a low-pressure reservoir until such time as it is socially convenient to void, when the bladder should be efficiently emptied to completion. The first group of symptoms reflects abnormal storage, the second group includes symptoms associated with abnormal voiding or post-micturition symptoms and the final group relates to abnormal bladder sensations (Table 94.1).

Table 94.1 Classification of urinary symptoms into groups

Group	Symptoms
Urinary incontinence symptoms	Stress urinary incontinence
	Urgency urinary incontinence
	Postural urinary incontinence
	Nocturnal enuresis
	Mixed urinary incontinence
	Continuous urinary incontinence
	Insensible urinary incontinence
	Coital incontinence
Bladder storage symptoms	Increased daytime urinary frequency
	Nocturia
	Urgency
	Overactive bladder syndrome
Sensory symptoms	Increased bladder sensation
	Reduced bladder sensation
	Absent bladder sensation
Voiding and post-micturition symptoms	Hesitancy
	Slow stream
	Intermittency
	Straining to void
	Spraying (spitting) of urinary stream
	Feeling of incomplete bladder emptying
	Need to immediately re-void
	Post-micturition leakage
	Position-dependent micturition
	Dysuria
	Urinary retention

URINARY SYMPTOMS

All the following definitions are as defined by ICS/ IUGA (2010).[1]

Urinary incontinence symptoms

Urinary incontinence
Urinary incontinence is the complaint of any involuntary leakage of urine. It is important to consider factors such as type, frequency, severity, precipitating factors, social impact, effect on hygiene and quality of life, the measures used to contain the leakage and whether or not the individual seeks or desires help because of urinary incontinence. Urinary leakage may need to be distinguished from sweating or vaginal discharge.

Stress urinary incontinence
Stress urinary incontinence is the complaint of involuntary loss of urine on effort or physical exertion (e.g. sporting activities), or on sneezing or coughing. The leakage of urine is usually in small, discrete amounts, coinciding with the physical activity. It is important to distinguish the subjective symptom of stress incontinence from the objectively demonstrated diagnosis of urodynamic stress incontinence, which can only be made following urodynamic assessment.

Urgency urinary incontinence
Urgency urinary incontinence is the complaint of involuntary loss of urine associated with urgency. It is frequently described as an inability to reach the toilet in time, and women suffering from this symptom often restrict their social activities to ensure that they are constantly near a toilet. Typical triggers for urgency incontinence include hearing running water, opening the front door (latch-key incontinence) and sudden changes in temperature. Urgency incontinence can present in different symptomatic forms e.g. as frequent small losses between micturitions or as a catastrophic leak with complete bladder emptying.

Postural urinary incontinence
The complaint of involuntary loss of urine associated with a change of body position, for example, on standing from a seated or lying position. This is a common symptom, the mechanism of which is not fully understood. It is uncertain whether it should be linked to stress urinary incontinence or urgency urinary incontinence.

Nocturnal enuresis
Enuresis means any involuntary loss of urine. Nocturnal enuresis is the complaint of loss of urine occurring during sleep. It can be primary or secondary. Primary nocturnal enuresis starts in infancy and can persist in adulthood. Secondary nocturnal enuresis occurs when the nocturnal incontinence restarts following a period of night-time continence. It is

important to distinguish enuresis from night-time urgency incontinence, in which the woman is awoken by urgency and leaks before reaching the toilet.

Mixed urinary incontinence

Mixed urinary incontinence is the complaint of involuntary leakage associated with urgency and also with effort or physical exertion or on sneezing or coughing. It is important to differentiate urodynamic mixed incontinence (the presence of urodynamic stress incontinence and detrusor overactivity based on urodynamic observations) from the symptoms of overactive bladder with stress or urgency incontinence.

Continuous urinary incontinence

The complaint of continuous involuntary loss of urine. This is a common symptom, the mechanism of which has not been adequately researched and it is uncertain whether it is linked to stress or urgency incontinence.

Insensible urinary incontinence

The complaint of urinary incontinence where the woman has been unaware of how it occurred. This can often be confused with a watery vaginal discharge or increased sweating in the vulval area.

Coital incontinence

The complaint of involuntary loss of urine with coitus. This can be further divided into incontinence occurring with penetration, with intromission and at orgasm.

Bladder storage symptoms

Increased daytime frequency

Increased daytime frequency is the complaint by the patient that micturition occurs more frequently during waking hours than previously deemed normal by the woman. A normal frequency is around four to seven times per day but this symptom is subjective to the patient and a frequency of six voids a day may be normal for one woman, but bothersome for another.

Nocturia

Nocturia is the complaint of interruption of sleep one or more times because of the need to micturate. Each void is preceded by and followed by sleep. It is important to establish whether the woman wakes due to the desire to pass urine or for other reasons (e.g. insomnia, breathing problems) and is going to the toilet as she is awake.

Urgency

Urgency is the complaint of a sudden compelling desire to pass urine which is difficult to defer. If this desire is not relieved it may result in urgency incontinence.

Overactive bladder syndrome

Overactive bladder syndrome (OAB) can be defined as urinary urgency, usually accompanied by frequency and nocturia, with or without urgency incontinence, in the absence of urinary tract infection or other obvious pathology.

Sensory symptoms

Increased bladder sensation

The complaint that the desire to void during bladder filling occurs earlier or is more persistent than that previously experienced. Suprapubic bladder pain on filling is a significant symptom and, if it persists, it is an indication for a cystoscopy and bladder biopsy. Inflammation of the bladder, such as bladder pain syndrome, stones, bladder tumours, endometriosis and pelvic infections are associated with this symptom.

Decreased bladder sensation

The complaint that the definite desire to void occurs later than that previously experienced despite awareness that the bladder is filling. This can lead to bladder over-distension, if women are not advised to void at regular intervals.

Absent bladder sensation

The complaint of both the absence of the sensation of bladder filling and a definite desire to void. It is usually due to denervation caused by spinal injury or pelvic trauma. It leads to infrequent micturition and a large-capacity bladder and is often associated with overflow incontinence.

Voiding and post-micturition symptoms

Hesitancy

Hesitancy is the term used when an individual describes difficulty or delay in initiating micturition. It is not uncommon for most women to experience this occasionally. Even in those women who complain of persistent hesitancy, only a small minority are found to have outflow obstruction. The other causes of persistent hesitancy include poor detrusor contractility and a lack of coordination in the normal neurological control of micturition (detrusor sphincter dyssynergia).

Slow stream

Slow stream is the complaint that the urinary stream is perceived as slower compared to previous performance or in comparison with others. Urinary flow rate is dependent on the total volume voided, the pressure generated by the detrusor muscle, and outflow resistance. In order to differentiate between these causes, urodynamic investigations need to be undertaken. Bladder outflow obstruction is rare in women who have not undergone previous surgery. Other causes of poor urinary stream include an underlying neurological condition and a pelvic mass.

Intermittency

This is the term used when the individual describes urine flow which stops and starts, on one or more occasions, during micturition.

Straining to void

Straining to void describes the intensive effort needed (by abdominal straining, Valsalva or suprapubic pressure) to either initiate, maintain or improve the urinary stream. Straining to empty the bladder is suggestive of voiding difficulty. Like the other symptoms in this category, it can be the result of a number of different disorders affecting bladder contractility, as well as outflow resistance. Raising intra-abdominal pressure by a Valsalva manoeuvre exerts increased intravesical pressure to aid bladder emptying. Suprapubic pressure may be used to initiate or maintain urine flow. The Credé manoeuvre is used by some spinal cord injury patients. The urinary flow produced is characteristically intermittent and prolonged.

Spraying (splitting) of the urinary stream

The complaint that the urine passage is a spray or split rather than a single discrete stream. For women who describe this symptom it is important to perform a vaginal examination to rule out pelvic organ prolapse and labial hypertrophy.

Feeling of incomplete bladder emptying

Feeling of incomplete emptying is the complaint that the bladder does not feel empty after micturition. It does not always correlate with the presence of a significant urinary residual. Similarly, women with large residuals are often unaware of it. This sensation can also arise as a result of an open bladder neck, abnormal bladder sensation, and a cystocele acting as a urinary sump.

Need to immediately re-void

The complaint that further micturition is necessary soon after passing urine. This is slightly different from double voiding which occurs at the same visit to the toilet to ensure compete bladder emptying.

Post-micturition leakage

The term used when an individual describes the involuntary loss of urine immediately after she has finished passing urine, usually after rising from the toilet in women. This symptom is associated with a collection of fluid left in the bladder after voiding, such as is found with a cystocele. It is also seen where there is a separate reservoir of urine, such as a urethral diverticulum, which fills up during voiding and subsequently drains.

Position-dependent micturition

The complaint of having to take specific positions to be able to micturate spontaneously or to improve bladder emptying e.g. leaning forwards or backwards on the toilet or voiding in the semi-standing position. This can be particularly common in women with a large cystocele or after incontinence surgery.

Dysuria

Dysuria is described as burning or other discomfort during micturition. It is most frequently associated with a UTI or urethritis, but can also be caused by inflammatory bladder conditions such as bladder pain syndrome. The discomfort can also be external such as vulvar dysuria.

Urinary retention

The inability to pass urine despite persistent effort. This can be a chronic or acute condition and can be due to many reasons such as constipation/faecal impaction, pelvic mass (e.g. large fibroid uterus) or an acontractile or underactive detrusor muscle. It should be managed with either intermittent catheterisation or in the short term an indwelling catheter, and an underlying cause should be sought and treated.

Other urinary symptoms

Haematuria

The presence of blood in the urine is always significant and should not be ignored. The commonest cause is a UTI but if it persists after appropriate antibiotic treatment it warrants investigation of the upper urinary tract with ultrasound or an intravenous urogram (IVU) and of the lower tract with cystoscopy and urine cytology.

PHYSICAL EXAMINATION

Abdominal and pelvic examinations form an essential part of the assessment of any woman who presents with urinary tract symptoms. Depending upon the medical history, there may be certain additional aspects of the physical examination that require particular attention. If there are any symptoms that point to a possible neurological cause, it is important to perform a screening neurological examination. The patient's mobility and mental state affect her ability to react to her symptoms and it may be appropriate to test these formally as part of the examination, as they will influence management. Similarly, an assessment of motivation and manual dexterity is important in determining the treatment most likely to prove effective.

As part of the gynaecological examination, the condition of the vulval skin should be noted. There may be signs of erythema, oedema and inflammation from chronic exposure to urine (incontinence-associated dermatitis). This can cause pain and discomfort and increase the risk of developing pressure sores. Vulval and vaginal atrophy may also be noted. Because of the close proximity of the lower urinary and genital tracts in the female, the presence of pelvic organ prolapse can have an important bearing on urinary symptoms and their management. This is best assessed in the left lateral position, using a Sims' speculum and asking the patient to cough and bear down. It is important to note that in order to demonstrate stress incontinence during examination, the bladder needs to be reasonably full, which is often not the case. Speculum examination should be complemented by performing a digital examination with the woman standing, legs abducted and performing a Valsalva manoeuvre. This gives a more accurate impression of the size and origin of any prolapse that is present. The grade of prolapse can be classified subjectively as mild, moderate or severe or graded according to the ICS pelvic organ prolapse quantification (POP-Q) score. While performing a vaginal examination in a woman who complains of leaking urine, it is important to assess the degree of anterior vaginal wall mobility and note any scarring that may be present, as this will influence the most appropriate choice of continence surgery. In addition, the anterior vaginal wall should be examined for any mass that may be a urethral diverticulum or cyst. Pelvic masses, such as ovarian cysts or uterine enlargement, can cause urinary symptoms and need to be excluded by bimanual examination. If this cannot be done with confidence, for example in the obese patient, a transvaginal ultrasound scan should be considered. For some women, a rectal examination may be indicated to further assess pelvic organ prolapse and to rule out faecal impaction.

It is important to ensure that informed consent has been gained and that all examinations are performed in line with RCOG guidelines.[2]

INVESTIGATIONS

The bladder has been described as an 'unreliable witness'. Although urinary symptoms provide a framework for diagnosis, they do not on their own allow an accurate impression to be formed of the underlying pathology. This may lead to inappropriate treatment being given and is especially important if surgical management is being considered, as the effects of surgery are irreversible. Investigations can be divided into

Table 94.2 Investigations of lower urinary tract disorders

Basic investigations	Midstream urine specimen
	Frequency–volume chart
	Pad test
Specialist investigations	Uroflowmetry
	Subtracted cystometry
	Videourodynamics
	Ambulatory urodynamics
	Urethral pressure profilometry
	Leak-point pressures
	Neurophysiological studies
	Radiological imaging
	Ultrasonography
	Endoscopy

basic tests, which all gynaecologists should be capable of performing and interpreting, and more complex investigations that require specialist expertise to perform (Table 94.2).

Midstream urine specimen

A midstream urine specimen must be taken for microscopy, culture and sensitivity from all women presenting with urinary symptoms. Bacteriuria is considered to be significant if >105 organisms/mL of urine are reported. It is important to rule out a UTI before going on to perform more invasive investigations. The presenting LUTS can be exacerbated or entirely caused by a bacterial infection, and effective treatment with appropriate antibiotics may be all that is required. If it proves necessary to proceed to urodynamic studies, it is important to ensure that there is not an infection already present, which would lead to unrepresentative findings and the risk of an ascending urinary infection of the upper tracts. In some situations, such as investigating a patient with recurrent UTIs, it is necessary to request cultures for 'fastidious organisms' such as *Mycoplasma hominis*, *Ureaplasma urelyticum* and *Chlamydia trachomatis*.

Frequency–volume chart

This is also known as a bladder diary or micturition time chart (Fig. 94.1). The patient is asked to record on a standard time sheet the volume of all fluid consumed and of all urine passed, as well as indicating any episodes of urgency and incontinence. The value of this simple, non-invasive tool is often overlooked, which is unfortunate as, if filled in conscientiously, it provides a good indication of fluid input and a natural volumetric record of bladder function.

An accurately filled-out chart provides invaluable information about the patient's voiding function in her natural environment and adds objectivity to the medical history (Box 94.1).

Frequency–volume charts can be completed prior to the initial hospital consultation to triage care and determine the urgency and complexity of the condition. They provide a useful form of feedback to the practitioner and the patient so that they can objectively evaluate the effectiveness of any therapy, for example in women undergoing bladder training for

Box 94.1 Information that can be derived from a frequency–volume chart

An idea of the normal functional bladder capacity, which should be fairly consistently around 300–500 mL. Frequent voids of variable amounts throughout the day imply bladder overactivity or behavioural adaptation to symptoms

A volumetric summary of diurnal urinary frequency and nocturia

Quantification of total fluid intake and its distribution throughout the day

A semi-objective evaluation of the severity of urinary incontinence and associated or provocative events

(a)

Bladder Diary
IMPORTANT – PLEASE READ INSTRUCTIONS CAREFULLY

It is very important that you fill in the chart overleaf as accurately as possible over a 3 day period prior to attending your test.

It is designed to help us take a closer look at your fluid intake and output, and leakage if any. It also helps us to plan the right treatment for you.

For each day, record *how much* (mL if possible) and *what time* you drink and write it down in the *IN* column.

When you go the toilet, measure the urine you pass using a jug (mL if possible) and write it down in the *OUT* column.

If you leak urine, put an X, yes or ✓ in the *WET* column. If you experience urgency i.e a sudden desire to pass urine that is difficult to defer please score 0, 1, 2, 3 or 4 according to the urge score that is described on the next page. Then according to how severe your urgency was please enter the appropriate number in the URGE SCORE column.

FOR EXAMPLE:

Time	DAY 1			
	IN	OUT	WET	URGE SCORE
07:10 am		140 mL		
08:30 am	250 mL			
10:40 am		90	Yes	
12:00 noon		150		2
12:45 pm	200 mL			
02:00 pm		60		0

This means that you passed 140 mL at 07:10 am and had 250 mL of a drink (maybe a cup of tea with breakfast). At 10:40 you leaked urine and passed 90 mL. At 12:00 noon you had 'moderate urgency' with a score of 2 which according to the urgency score means 'you could postpone voiding for a short while without fear of wetting yourself'.

Please write the time you got up and time you went to bed at the top and bottom of the chart for each day. This allows us to see the difference between what is happening during the day and during the night.

(b) Urogynaecology Department, King's College Hospital Bladder Diary

Time got up: Time got up: Time got up:

TIME	DAY 1				DAY 2				DAY 3			
	IN	OUT	WET	URGE SCORE	IN	OUT	WET	URGE SCORE	IN	OUT	WET	URGE SCORE

Time went to bed: Time went to bed: Time went to bed:

Urge score

0	No urgency: I felt no need to empty my bladder but did so for other reasons
1	Mild Urgency: I could postpone voiding for as long as necessary without fear of wetting myself
2	Moderate Urgency: I could postpone voiding for a short while without fear of wetting myself
3	Severe Urgency: I could not postpone voiding but had to rush to the toilet in order not to wet myself
4	Urge Incontinence: I leaked before arriving at the toilet

Fig. 94.1 Bladder diary. (a) Instructions for patient (b) Three-day frequency–volume chart for patient to fill in

detrusor overactivity. In addition, they can also aid diagnosis for conditions such as nocturnal polyuria. A frequency–volume chart should always be completed prior to urodynamic testing so that the patient's functional bladder capacity is known. This prevents over-distension during filling cystometry. There is no standardised format for frequency–volume charts; the duration varies between 48 hours and 7 days in different centres. In addition to the standard volumetric information, the patient may be asked to quantitate incontinent episodes, note associated or provocative activities, and state the number of pads used per day. Measures of urinary urgency e.g. the patient perception of intensity of urgency scale (PPIUS) can provide additional information on a bladder diary.

Quality-of-life assessment

Symptom and quality-of-life (QoL) scoring is used to give some quantification of the impact of urinary symptoms and provides a measure that can be used to assess outcomes of treatment at a later stage.[1] This employs carefully designed and validated patient-assessed health questionnaires.

Traditionally, doctors have categorised the severity of a condition using objective clinical measures. However, the impact of a disease and the success of any treatment should no longer be measured purely in terms of 'doctor-centred' clinical parameters alone. It is increasingly recognised that a patient's quality of life and psychosocial adjustment to an illness are equally as important as the status of their physical disease. Two major types of QoL questionnaire are available: generic questionnaires, which can be used across a range of medical conditions, and disease-specific questionnaires, which focus on the likely impacts of a particular disorder. It is very important that any questionnaires used for this form of assessment have been subjected to rigorous reliability testing and validation in order to derive meaningful data from them. QoL assessment is particularly useful in determining the response of patients to treatment. It gives useful information about therapeutic effects as seen from the patient's perspective across a range of different domains. This form of patient assessment has many applications. It is now widely used as an outcome measure in the evaluation of clinical practice and in research trials. There are many disease-specific questionnaires to assess women with urinary incontinence. These include the King's

Health Questionnaire (KHQ), International Consultation on Incontinence Questionnaire (ICIQ), Bristol Female Urinary Tract Symptoms (BFLUTS), Overactive Bladder Questionnaire (OAB), Urogenital Distress Inventory (UDI) and Incontinence Impact Questionnaire (IIQ). These are available through the International Consultation on Incontinence website[3] and further information is available in the RCOG document on measuring outcomes in gynaecology.[4]

Pad test

The objective demonstration of leaking is essential in reaching a diagnosis of urinary incontinence. A pad test provides a simple, non-invasive, objective method for detecting and quantifying urinary leakage. Various protocols exist for performing a pad test. To obtain a representative result, especially for those who have variable or intermittent urinary incontinence, the test should be as long as possible in circumstances that approximate those of everyday life. It should be conducted in a standardised fashion so that results are comparable and reproducible. This allows the effect of treatment to be objectively assessed in a non-invasive manner.

The ICS has produced guidelines for a standardised 1-hour pad test.[5] The patient wears a pre-weighed pad or sanitary towel, drinks 500 mL of water and rests for 15 minutes. She then performs 30 minutes of moderate exercise, such as stair climbing and walking. The remaining 15 minutes are spent performing more provocative exercises, including coughing vigorously, bending over, hand washing and running. At the end of 1 hour, the pad is removed and re-weighed. An increase of >2 g is considered a significant loss. A weight gain of >10 g is categorised as severe incontinence.

The standard 1-hour ICS pad test has been shown to have good reproducibility, and reliably differentiates normal from abnormal continence mechanisms. However, the short period of study and lack of a standardised bladder volume before starting the test mean that there is a significant false-negative rate.

Long-term protocols also exist in which the patient is given several pre-weighed pads to be worn at home for periods of 12, 24 or 48 hours. The used pads are collected in sealed plastic bags and reweighed at the end of the specified period to determine total urine loss. The extended pad test is particularly useful to confirm or refute leakage in those patients complaining of incontinence that has not been demonstrated on urodynamic studies.

Recent studies have shown that pad tests bear little relationship to the underlying urodynamic diagnosis but there is a positive relationship with symptom severity.[5] According to NICE guidelines the pad test should not be used for routine assessment of urinary incontinence.[6]

Methylene blue test

For women who are unable to differentiate urinary leakage from vaginal discharge, or in cases of possible vesico-vaginal or urethra-vaginal fistula, a methylene blue test can be performed. During this test, a solution of 0.9% saline and methylene blue is instilled into the patient's bladder to half the cystometric capacity. Gauze swabs are then placed into the upper, mid- and lower vagina and a pre-weighed pad into the patient's underwear. They are then asked to mobilise for 1 hour and perform provocative exercises. At the end of the test, patients are asked to void and then each vaginal swab is removed. Staining on the pad represents urinary leakage. Blue on the lower vaginal swab may represent urethro-vaginal reflux or contamination from the test. Blue on the mid-vaginal swab may be indicative of a urethro-vaginal fistula and on the upper vaginal swab could suggest a vesico-vaginal fistula. A heavy vaginal discharge can also be assessed from this test. During the instillation of methylene blue into the bladder, it is important to ensure that there is no contamination of dye on to the labia or vagina as this will give false-positive results from the test. Fig. 94.2 demonstrates the placement of swabs during the test.

Uroflowmetry

Uroflowmetry is the simplest and one of the most useful investigations in the assessment of voiding dysfunction. It consists simply of measuring urinary flow over time and allows a rapid and non-invasive analysis of the normality or otherwise of flow rate. When combined with the measurement of residual urine volume by ultrasound or catheterisation, it provides information on the efficiency of micturition in emptying the bladder. One or more symptoms of voiding disorder are commonly described in women complaining of urinary tract disorders, and it is important to diagnose or eliminate voiding difficulty. This is particularly so when treatment is being considered for incontinence. Both surgical treatment of urodynamic stress incontinence and drug treatment for detrusor overactivity have the potential to cause voiding difficulty. Therefore pre-treatment uroflowmetry and the measurement of residual urine are essential.

Indications

Uroflowmetry should be regarded as a screening test for voiding difficulty in all women with symptoms of lower urinary tract dysfunction. It is important to appreciate that urinary

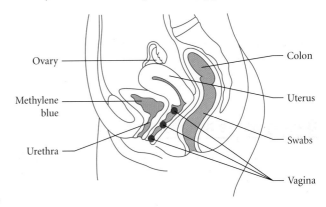

Fig. 94.2 Diagrammatic representation of methylene blue test

Ovary

Methylene blue

Urethra

Colon

Uterus

Swabs

Vagina

flow is dependent upon a number of factors, including detrusor contractility, neurological coordination of sphincter relaxation, and outflow patency. Uroflowmetry on its own cannot successfully distinguish between the causes of voiding dysfunction.

Methods

There are several different physical principles that can be utilised to provide an accurate assessment of flow. The following three methods are in common use.

1   *Gravimetric method.* The rate of change of the weight of the voided urine in the collecting jug is converted into a flow rate (Fig. 94.3).
2   *Rotating disc method.* A known amount of power is required to keep a rotating disc spinning at a constant rate. Voided fluid is directed onto the disc, increasing its inertia. The flow rate is proportional to the amount of extra power that is required to keep the disc spinning at a constant rate.
3   *Capacitance dipstick.* A metal capacitor strip is attached to the side of the flowmeter. As urine accumulates in the container, the electrical capacitance of the dipstick changes and from this the rate of flow can be calculated. It should be noted that the environment in which the woman performs the flow rate recording will have a considerable influence on the results. It is important that every effort is made to make the patient feel as comfortable and relaxed as possible, and that privacy and dignity are maintained at all times.

Interpretation

The definitions for urine flow rate measurements have been standardized by the ICS and should be expressed in millilitres per second (Fig. 94.4).

The two most useful parameters are the maximum flow rate and the voided volume. The maximum flow rate is partially dependent on the voided volume, as this determines how distended the bladder muscle fibres are. For this reason, small voided volumes of less than 150 mL are insufficient to obtain an accurate impression of flow, and the test needs to be repeated.

The third major factor to consider when interpreting flow rate is the pattern of flow, in particular whether flow is continuous or intermittent. A normal flow curve is bell shaped and characterised by a rapid rise to maximal flow. A prolonged, intermittent flow curve is suggestive of voiding dysfunction, with the patient using abdominal straining to achieve bladder emptying. The results must always be interpreted within the context of the clinical situation, and the limitations of the study should be recognised. These include the reliability of the apparatus, and the ability of the staff interpreting the trace in recognising artefact. More information concerning the cause of voiding difficulty is provided by the addition of simultaneous pressure measurements as part of cystometry (pressure flow studies).

Factors influencing urine flow rate

The peak flow rate (PFR) is highly dependent on voided volume, as has already been discussed. Most commonly, a minimum accepted PFR of 15 mL/s is used. Urine flow rates are higher in women than in men for a comparable voided volume. Age and parity have not been shown to have a significant effect on urine flow rates in asymptomatic women. As might be expected, there is a progressive decline in flow rate with increasing grades of pelvic floor prolapse, especially uterine prolapse and cystourethrocele.

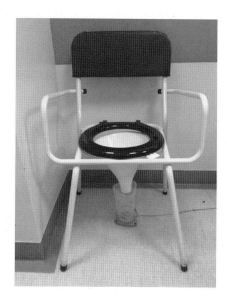

Fig. 94.3 (a) Gravimetric flow meter

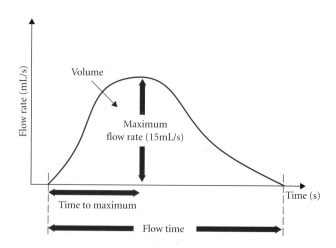

Fig. 94.4 Diagrammatic representation of urinary flow rate with standardised ICS terminology. Voided volume: total volume expelled via the urethra; the area beneath the flow–time curve. Maximum flow rate: maximum measured value of the flow rate. Flow time: the time over which measurable flow actually occurs. If flow is intermittent, the time intervals between flow episodes are not included. Average flow rate: volume voided divided by the flow time. Time to maximum flow: elapsed time from onset of flow to maximum flow

Altered detrusor function influences flow rate by determining the contractile force with which urine is expelled. In addition, bladder neck and urethral anatomy influence urine flow by affecting outflow resistance. To distinguish between these two major causes of voiding dysfunction, more complex urodynamic tests are required in which simultaneous pressure/flow measurements are taken.

Subtracted cystometry

Cystometry is the method by which the pressure–volume relationship of the bladder is assessed during filling and voiding. It involves the simultaneous measurement of intravesical and intra-abdominal pressures. Electronic subtraction of the intra-abdominal pressure from the intravesical pressure enables the detrusor pressure to be calculated and compared with changes in bladder volume and flow rate. Cystometry aims to characterise detrusor and urethral function during the filling and voiding phases (Table 94.3). It can be useful, when learning to interpret cystometrograms, to break down the functions of the detrusor and urethra by phases of the micturition cycle.

Indications

When access to investigations is limited, it is reasonable to manage patients with clear-cut symptoms empirically with conservative treatment, provided that cystometry is subsequently performed in those in whom empirical treatment fails. Certainly surgical treatments should never be considered without urodynamic assessment, as the inappropriate selection of surgery can have disastrous and largely irreversible consequences for the patient. If a policy of urodynamic screening on all women with lower urinary tract symptoms is not practised, selective testing should certainly be considered in the investigation of:

- symptoms that have failed to respond to empirical conservative measures;
- a patient being considered for any form of incontinence surgery if there is a clinical suspicion of detrusor overactivity;

- voiding difficulties;
- mixed symptoms e.g. frequency, urgency and stress incontinence;
- previous unsuccessful incontinence surgery;
- suspected neuropathic bladder disorders.

The last two complex groups are better investigated by videourodynamics, as this yields valuable information about the anatomical structure of the urinary tract, as well as the dynamic function.

A good urodynamic practice comprises three main elements:[7]

1 A clear indication for and appropriate selection of relevant measurements and procedures;
2 Precise measurement with data quality control and complete documentation;
3 Accurate analysis and critical reporting of results.

There is a document available detailing minimum standards for urodynamic practice in the UK.[8]

Methods

It is important that cystometric diagnoses are related to the patient's symptoms and physical findings at the time of the investigation. The aim is to reproduce the presenting symptoms that cause the woman concern, so that a diagnosis can be made and appropriate treatment planned. Terminology and standards are defined by ICS/IUGA.[1] This allows cystometric data to be compared among different centres and used in research trials.

Modern multichannel cystometry requires two pressure transducers (to measure the abdominal and intravesical pressures), an electronic subtraction unit (to derive the detrusor pressure), an amplifying unit and a display or printout (Fig. 94.5). Three types of pressure transducers are available: a fluid-filled or air-charged pressure line inserted into the bladder or rectum and connected to an external transducer, and a solid microtip pressure transducer placed directly inside the body. The difference between the two is largely cost and convenience of use. Fluid-filled lines are generally disposable, whereas microtip pressure transducers are reusable and need sterilisation between patients. Local infection control policies

Table 94.3 Cystometry

Phases of cycle	Urethra	Detrusor
Filling	Should remain closed and competent but can: be incompetent due to physical stress, but without an associated rise in detrusor pressure (stress incontinence); be incompetent as a direct result of an involuntary rise in detrusor pressure (detrusor overactivity)	Should remain relaxed/stable throughout filling but can: show abnormal involuntary contractions (detrusor overactivity); show a gradual rise in pressure with filling (low compliance)
Voiding	Should be appropriately relaxed but can: be constricted, leading to outflow obstruction (obstructed cause)	Should contract efficiently under voluntary instruction but can: be under-active or acontractile (possible neuropathic cause); show high-pressure contractions (if overactive or needing to overcome an outflow obstruction)

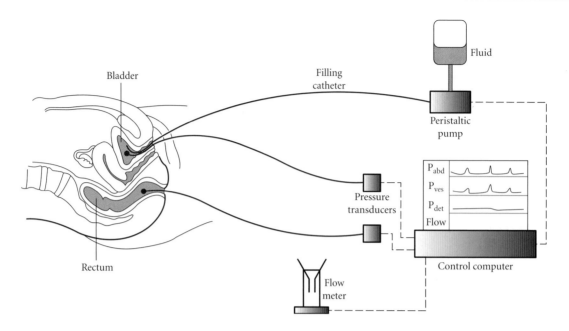

Fig. 94.5 Schematic diagram showing the position of the pressure catheters and the measurements recorded during subtracted cystometry. The following measurements are made:

- Free-flow rate and residual urine are measured at the start of the test by means of a flow meter and subsequent urethral catheterisation.
- Intra-abdominal pressure (Pabd) is measured with the rectal pressure catheter. Alternatively, this could be measured with a pressure catheter in the vagina or colostomy stoma.
- Intravesical pressure (Pves) is measured with a pressure catheter in the bladder via the urethra or suprapubic route.
- Detrusor pressure (Pdet) is derived from continuous electronic subtraction of intra-abdominal from intravesical pressure (Pdet = Pves − Pabd) and displayed concomitantly.
- Filling volume is recorded by a peristaltic pump connected to the system or calculated manually.
- Flow rate is measured by a flow meter allowing simultaneous pressure–flow analysis.
- During filling, the patient is asked to indicate her first FDV and when she experiences an SDV. This is taken as bladder capacity.
- In addition, it is important to explain to the patient the relevance of expressing her sensations (such as urgency) during the test so that the cystometry trace can be annotated. This helps to interpret the findings

should be adhered to. All pressure measurements are made in centimetres of water (cmH$_2$O).

Prior to inserting the pressure catheters, the patient is asked to void on the flow meter to allow the measurement of a free flow rate. The presence of any residual urine on subsequent urethral catheterisation is noted. The pressure catheters are then inserted and calibrated. Quality control is an essential part of performing cystometry if valid conclusions are to be drawn from the investigation. The system is checked for adequate subtraction by asking the patient to cough at regular intervals. An equal pressure rise should be observed in both the abdominal and intravesical pressure traces, which should cancel out to leave the detrusor pressure unchanged. Once the integrity of the pressure readings has been checked and the system zeroed to atmospheric pressure, filling can commence.

0.9% saline at room temperature is instilled into the bladder at a predetermined rate under the control of a peristaltic pump. This is usually in the range of 25–100 mL/min, depending on the indication for cystometry. This rate should be reduced to a slower filling rate closer to the normal physiological range when assessing patients with neuropathic bladders. During filling, the patient is asked to indicate her first

desire to void (FDV) and when she experiences an uncontrollable strong desire to void (SDV). Any rise in detrusor pressure is noted and whether this is associated with the sensation of urgency or leaking. Filling is discontinued once there is a sustained SDV. This volume is taken as cystometric bladder capacity and is usually in the range 400–600 mL. Filling can occur when the patient is in the supine, sitting or standing position.

At the end of filling, the patient is asked to stand, to assess whether there is a postural rise in detrusor pressure, and to cough several times. More strenuous stimuli, such as star jumps, can be performed if leakage is not demonstrated by coughing in women who complain of this symptom in their history. The presence of any leakage is noted and whether a stable trace or an associated rise in detrusor pressure accompanies this. Provocative tests for detrusor overactivity are performed at this stage and the patient may be asked to listen to running water, wash her hands or heel bounce to try to induce leakage. Finally, the patient transfers back on to the flow meter, with the pressure catheters still *in situ*. She is instructed to void and the detrusor pressure and urine flow rate are measured simultaneously to provide a simultaneous pressure/flow analysis.

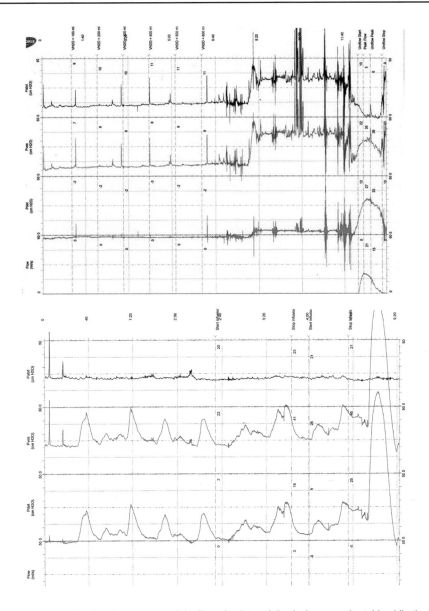

Fig. 94.6 Part of a cystometrogram trace showing detrusor overactivity. Note that intra-abdominal pressure is stable while the intravesical pressure line shows an involuntary detrusor contraction

Interpretation

As has been previously discussed, it is vital that the cystometric findings are evaluated in the light of the woman's symptomatology. The following are normal cystometric parameters:

- Filling cystometry:
  - residual urine <50 mL;
  - capacity (taken as SDV) >400 mL;
  - absence of uninhibited detrusor contractions during filling;
  - negligible rise in detrusor pressure on filling: this should be <15 cm H_2O for a filling volume of 500 mL.
- Voiding cystometry:
  - no leakage on coughing or performing exercise;
  - no provoked detrusor contractions as a result of precipitating factors, such as postural changes, hand washing or coughing;

  - a maximum voiding detrusor pressure of <50 cm H_2O, with a maximum flow rate >15 mL/s for a volume voided of >150 mL.

By considering urethral and detrusor function during the filling and voiding phases of cystometry, abnormalities can be systematically classified (Fig. 94.6). The presence of involuntary detrusor contractions, during filling or on provocation, that the patient cannot suppress is diagnostic of detrusor overactivity. If there is a gradual rise in detrusor pressure during filling to >15 cm H_2O, but without phasic contractions, this is termed 'low compliance'. This can be artefactual owing to superphysiological or fast bladder filling. If there is a neurological condition present, such as multiple sclerosis, this is often accompanied by marked low compliance. If leakage occurs on coughing, with an associated rise in intra-abdominal pressure but in the absence of abnormal detrusor activity, urodynamic stress incontinence is diagnosed.

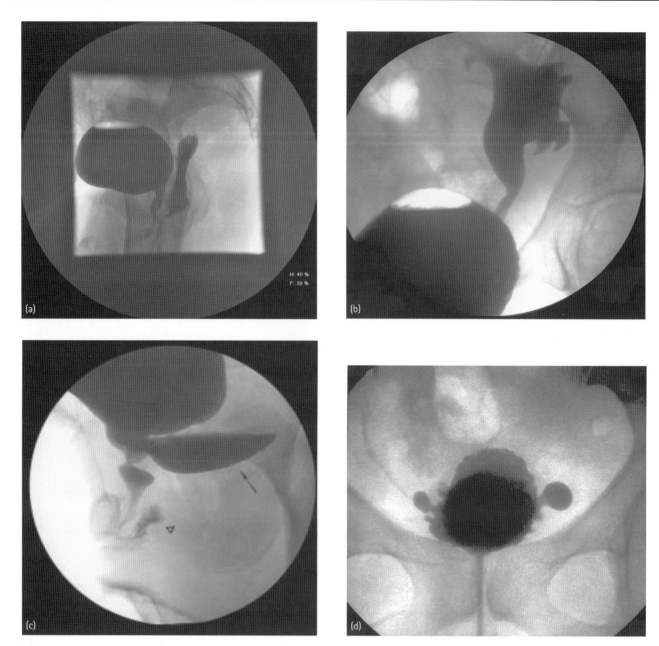

Fig. 94.7 Examples of structural and functional abnormalities seen by fluroscopy. a) urethro-vaginal reflux, b) vesico-uretic reflux into a transplanted kidney, c) urethral diverticulum, d) multiple bladder diverticulae, trabeculation and right sided vesico-ureteric reflux, suggestive of a neurogenic bladder

Videourodynamics

Videourodynamics offers the facility to simultaneously study the anatomical structure and the pressure/flow characteristics of the lower urinary tract. This is achieved by using contrast medium rather than saline to fill the bladder during cystometry, and radiologically screening the bladder and urethra intermittently throughout the procedure. The combination of these approaches results in the videocystourethrogram (VCU), which is regarded as the 'gold standard' for assessing lower urinary tract disorders. Most patients can be adequately investigated using simpler techniques, but VCU does offer several advantages over cystometry alone for the investigation of complex cases in tertiary centres. The addition of radiological screening provides valuable additional information relating to bladder morphology, the degree of bladder base support and function of the bladder neck during coughing, the presence of vesico-ureteric reflux (which may be present in up to 7 per cent of incontinent patients) and the site of outflow obstruction (Fig. 94.7).

Clinical situations in which VCU offers significant advantages over simple cystometry include the following:

- Women in whom previous incontinence surgery has failed, as the position and mobility of the bladder neck can be assessed at rest and on straining. When combined with urethral pressure profilometry (UPP), an experienced investigator can infer information about the relative contributions of bladder neck hypermobility and sphincter deficiency as the causes of continued stress incontinence.

- Neurological lower urinary tract dysfunction. VCU is required to adequately assess the complex dysfunction seen in neuropathic bladders and to provide a framework for treatment. It is important to look for the presence of vesico-ureteric reflux in this group of women.
- Assessment of voiding difficulties or symptoms suggestive of an anatomical lesion, such as a urethral diverticulum.

Technique

The technique is identical to that used for routine subtracted cystometry, except that the investigation is performed in a room set up for radiological X-ray screening. Uroflowmetry, measurement of urinary residual and the insertion of pressure catheters are the same as for subtracted cystometry. Radio-opaque contrast is used to fill the bladder. X-ray screening takes place if the woman complains of leaking during filling and then during provocative coughing. This allows assessment of the degree of bladder neck opening, the severity of leakage and the extent of bladder-base descent. The presence of vesico-ureteric reflux, bladder trabeculation and diverticulae is noted. The woman then commences voiding and, once normal flow has been established, she is asked to interrupt it. This should result in cessation of flow and urine being 'milked back' from the proximal urethra into the bladder. Finally, the presence of a post-void residual can be determined.

Ambulatory urodynamic monitoring

Ambulatory urodynamic monitoring (AUM) is of particular use in the investigation of detrusor overactivity, where standard laboratory urodynamics have failed to replicate the symptoms that are experienced by the patient in her normal environment. Although laboratory urodynamics forms the standard method of objectively investigating bladder and urethral function, it is by design unphysiological. This is because relatively fast retrograde filling of the bladder is employed rather than slower filling from the kidneys via the ureters. In addition, the environment in which the test is performed and the focus of attention directed towards the subject are far removed from her everyday activities. In an attempt to study bladder function in circumstances that more closely approximate those in which the subject normally finds herself, ambulatory urodynamics has been developed.

AUM uses natural anterograde bladder filling and allows the patient to reproduce her normal daily activities, including those that commonly provoke symptoms e.g. exercise.

Technique

Ambulatory systems have three main components:

1 Pressure transducers are placed in the bladder and rectum as in laboratory urodynamics.
2 A portable recording system allows several channels of data to be recorded simultaneously. This should include an event marker, to enable the patient to mark particular activities on the trace, and a method quantifying urine leakage, such as an electronic pad.
3 An analysing system is needed to retrieve and process the data. All traces are interpreted with the patient present so that more information can be obtained about particular events.

The ICS has standardised the terminology and methodology of AUM,[9] allowing the comparison of results from different centres.

The investigation is usually carried out over a 4-hour time period. Once the transducers have been inserted into the bladder and rectum and the system has been calibrated, the patient is encouraged to drink normally and perform normal activities. During the investigation, the patient is asked to keep a careful record of symptoms and events, and the position of the catheters is checked periodically. At the conclusion of the test, provocative manoeuvres are carried out with a full bladder prior to removing the transducers and analysing the results. Significantly more detrusor overactivity is diagnosed using AUM than with conventional laboratory urodynamics. However, it is uncertain whether this is due to a higher sensitivity or whether AUM simply has a high false-positive rate for diagnosing detrusor overactivity. Ambulatory urodynamics is subject to significant artefact, but this can be greatly reduced by rigorous methodology.

Urethral pressure profilometry

The relationship between intravesical pressure and urethral pressure is the key to maintaining continence. Normally, urethral pressure exceeds intravesical pressure at all times, except during voluntary relaxation of the bladder neck leading to micturition. UPP can assess this ability of the urethra to exert a positive closure pressure in order to prevent leakage. This is done by simultaneously measuring the intravesical and urethral pressures using a catheter with two pressure transducers set 6 cm apart.

Technique

The pressure catheter is inserted into the bladder with the distal pressure transducer inside the bladder and the proximal transducer near the bladder neck. It is then withdrawn at a standard speed by a mechanical retractor, allowing pressure measurements to be made along the functional length of the urethra to give a graph of pressure over distance travelled along the urethra. The ICS has also standardised the terminology and methodology of urethral pressure measurement.[10] Two types of UPP may be measured:

1 resting UPP, with the patient at rest in a supine position;
2 stress UPP, with the patient coughing throughout the test to see if the intravesical pressure exceeds the urethral pressure during increases in intra-abdominal pressure – this would result in a negative closure pressure and leakage of urine per urethram.

Although the closure pressures in women with urodynamic stress incontinence are generally less than in their dry counterparts, this test is not sufficiently discriminatory to be used in the diagnosis of urodynamic stress incontinence. However, it is often useful in understanding the pathophysiology of urodynamic stress incontinence and in planning the most appropriate intervention, especially in women who have had previous failed surgery for incontinence. A low maximum urethral closure pressure correlates with a poor outcome for incontinence surgery. The other group of patients in whom UPP can be useful is women with voiding difficulties. An increased maximum urethral closure pressure indicates outflow obstruction, sometimes as the result of previous surgery or a stricture. In these women, urethral dilatation or urethrotomy may be appropriate.

NEUROPHYSIOLOGICAL INVESTIGATION

The normal coordinated functions of the bladder and urethra are controlled by a complex set of central and peripheral neurological reflexes. In an effort to understand these mechanisms better and to evaluate patients with lower urinary tract dysfunction, a whole range of neurophysiological tests have evolved. These techniques stimulate and record activity at different levels of the neurological pathways that control bladder and urethral function. The most commonly employed techniques in clinical neurophysiological testing are electromyography (EMG), in which recordings of bioelectrical potentials in muscles are studied, and nerve conduction studies. The latter examine the capacity of a nerve to transmit a test electrical stimulus along its length.

Electromyography

Electromyography is the study of bioelectrical potentials generated by the depolarisation of muscle fibres. It is predominantly used to study striated muscle, in particular the urethral sphincter and the pelvic floor muscles. The functional unit studied is called a motor unit and consists of the muscle fibres innervated by branches from the motor neuron of a single anterior horn cell. The potential it generates during contraction is called the motor nerve unit potential (MUP). This can be measured by means of surface electrodes or various types of needle electrode. By measuring the amplitude, duration and number of phases of the action potential, the extent of neurological denervation and subsequent re-innervation in the target muscle can be inferred. This is a highly specialist investigation and a skilled investigator is required to interpret the results. While EMG studies have greatly improved our understanding of pelvic floor, lower urinary tract and bowel function in health and disease, the results to date have had little effect on clinical management. The main clinical indication for EMG studies is as an adjunct to videourodynamics to distinguish between striated and smooth muscle in neuropathic urethral obstruction.

Nerve conduction studies

A number of different techniques have been employed to study the conduction of central and peripheral nerve pathways to the bladder and urethra. These examine the capacity of a nerve to transmit a test electrical signal along its length. If the pathway being tested is damaged, there will be a delay in conduction time and thus a prolonged latency between the stimulus and the muscular response. In addition, the amplitude of the muscle response will be reduced. A wide range of neurological pathways have been investigated using variations of this technique, including the sacral reflex arc, pudendal terminal motor latencies, transcutaneous spinal stimulation and cortical evoked responses. As with EMG studies, these investigations have improved our understanding of the neurophysiological control of the normal and dysfunctional bladder, but are of limited use in the clinical investigation of most patients.

RADIOLOGICAL IMAGING

Radiological imaging of the urinary tract is not justified as a routine investigation in all women presenting with urinary symptoms, but instead should be targeted at specific indications. The diagnostic procedures available include plain abdominal films, intravenous urography and various contrast studies of the lower urinary tracts.

Plain X-ray

A plain abdominal film may be a useful screening investigation for a variety of conditions that affect lower urinary tract function. Foreign bodies and bladder calculi causing outflow obstruction can be diagnosed. Bladder wall calcification is rare in the UK but is seen more frequently worldwide as a result of tuberculosis and schistosomiasis. Probably the most useful indication for plain radiographic films is to investigate spinal abnormalities, such as spina bifida or sacral agenesis, as a cause of neuropathic bladder disorder.

Intravenous urography

This is not a routine investigation of lower urinary tract dysfunction. It provides anatomical and some functional information on the kidneys, ureters and bladder. IVU is indicated in women with neuropathic bladders, suspected congenital or acquired abnormalities (such as uterovaginal fistulae), haematuria and suspected ureteric compromise secondary to the effects of a pelvic mass (e.g. large fibroids or a procidentia) or trauma. A CT urogram or MR urinary tract can often give the same information and discussion with the local radiologist regarding the preferred examination method is advised.

Micturating cystourethrography

This investigation requires instillation of radio-opaque contrast medium into the bladder and then screening with fluoroscopy as the patient voids. It is similar to the X-ray screening performed as part of a videocystometrogram, but without any pressure–flow information. Its main value is to demonstrate bladder and urethral fistulae, vesico-ureteric reflux and anatomical abnormalities of the lower tracts, such as urethral diverticulae.

ULTRASONOGRAPHY

Ultrasound provides a relatively non-invasive method of imaging the urinary tract in real time, without exposing the patient to ionising radiation. There is an ever-increasing range of applications for ultrasound imaging in the investigation of urinary tract dysfunction. As well as the lack of radiation exposure, ultrasound has the advantage of having significantly lower operating costs than comparable radiological investigation. The main disadvantage is that ultrasound waves do not penetrate as far and so the probe has to be held close to the target. The field of view is more limited than X-rays, so that only one part of the urinary tract can be viewed at a time. Ultrasound imaging depends on the different echogenicity of tissues to form a picture. It is especially well suited for visualizing fluid-filled and air-filled cystic structures.

Post-micturition residual volume

Ultrasonography is widely used to estimate residual urine volumes. This obviates the need for urethral catheterisation, with its concomitant risk of infection. This is particularly useful in the assessment of women with voiding difficulties. It can also be used following post-operative catheter removal or in women in labour as an alternative to repeated catheterisation to ensure that the bladder is not allowed to overdistend. There are many methods of estimating bladder volume from real-time scanning; however, most portable bladder scanners presently available automatically calculate the volume of urine in the bladder.

Assessing lower urinary tract structure

Ultrasound offers an inexpensive, non-invasive method of assessing the structure of the lower urinary tract and is advocated as an alternative to cystourethroscopy for many indications. The arguments in favour of each technique are similar to those proposed for the use of transvaginal ultrasonography and hysteroscopy for the assessment of the reproductive organs. The sensitivity of ultrasonography and endoscopy in different disorders varies, largely according to the experience of the operator and the quality of the equipment used. The majority of bladder tumours are exophytic and papillary in

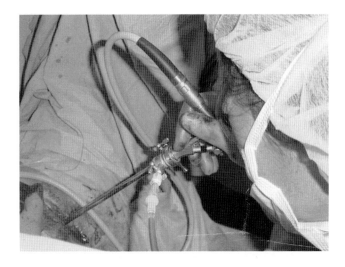

Fig. 94.8 Rigid cystometry with multiple bladder biopsies being performed under general anaesthesia in a patient with a history of recurrent UTIs

shape and are well visualised by ultrasound. Similarly, bladder diverticulae and calculi are easily detected.

Transabdominal ultrasound does not provide satisfactory imaging of the bladder neck and urethra, owing to their position behind the symphysis pubis. These are visualised better with the use of a transvaginal, transrectal or perineal probe. Ultrasonography is a very sensitive method of detecting urethral diverticulae and their relation to the urethral sphincter. Differentiation from para-urethral cysts may be difficult if a connection cannot be visualised. Three dimensional ultrasound has been used as a research tool to determine urethral sphincter volumes as part of the assessment of women presenting with incontinence.

Another technique is the measurement of bladder wall thickness. This is performed using the transvaginal approach when the bladder is empty and offers a reproducible, sensitive method of screening for detrusor overactivity.[8]

IMAGING

CT and MRI can provide confirmation of alternative pelvic pathology, by means of cross-sectional imaging e.g. urethral diverticulae. It can be used to characterise the extent and anatomical contents of a pelvic organ prolapse, especially in the standing position with MRI.[11]

CYSTOURETHROSCOPY

Cystourethroscopy enables the inside of the bladder and urethra to be visualised (Fig. 94.8). It is an invasive but relatively low-risk procedure that can be undertaken for women of any age as a day case. The choice between a rigid or flexible cystoscope and the anaesthetic used will depend on the individual case and the preferences of the operator. Modern cystoscopes consist of at least three elements.

1 An optical system for transmitting the image to a video monitor with maximum clarity and resolution. In a rigid endoscope this is performed by a rod–lens system, and in a flexible endoscope by a bundle of optical fibres.
2 Another system of optical fibres is needed to transmit light into the bladder.
3 An irrigating channel is needed to flush away blood and debris, and dilate the bladder under direct vision.

Most operating cystoscopes also have an outflow channel to carry debris away. Cystourethroscopy is an invaluable tool in investigating the lower urinary tract, as it provides detailed anatomical information. It is not usually performed as part of the routine investigation of women with incontinence, but there are many indications for which direct visual inspection and targeted biopsies of the bladder and urethra are important in establishing a diagnosis.

Indications

Cystourethroscopy is indicated:

- to investigate haematuria not related to UTI;
- when a reduced bladder capacity or painful filling is found at cystometry;
- to exclude bladder tumours and stones as a cause of recurrent or persistent UTI;
- if a lower urinary tract fistula is suspected;
- if interstitial cystitis is suspected;
- following failed incontinence surgery when the patient complains of voiding difficulty, overactive symptoms or persistent incontinence;
- to provide certain treatments e.g. intradetrusor injections of botulinum toxin A.

Technique

The majority of cystourethroscopies undertaken by gynaecologists are performed under a general anaesthetic with a rigid scope. The advantage of a rigid cystoscope is that biopsies and other manipulative procedures are relatively easily carried out through the large instrument channel. Flexible cystoscopes offer the advantage of use in the outpatient setting, with topical anaesthetic only, and the view is often better that that of a

> ### KEY POINTS
>
> - Investigations of lower urinary tract dysfunction vary from simple tests that can easily be performed in an office setting to complex investigations available in tertiary centres.
> - As the correlation between lower urinary tract symptoms and underlying diagnosis is poor, early investigation is desirable so that a firm diagnosis can be established and rational treatment instigated.

> - Thorough assessment, including urodynamics, is mandatory prior to considering surgical treatment.
> - The choice of investigations performed should be individualised according to the patient's presenting symptoms and past medical history.

rigid scope. However, the instrumentation that can be used is slightly more limited. This and the fact that only a topical anaesthetic is used can make it difficult to take histologically valid biopsy specimens.

Rigid cystoscopes are available with several viewing angles, including 0° (straight), 12°, 30° and 70°. Angled telescopes have a field marker, which appears as a notch at the edge of the field of view and helps to maintain orientation. The choice of telescope depends on the procedure being performed and the operator's preference. The cystoscope is placed into the urethral meatus and advanced towards the bladder under direct vision with the irrigation fluid running. Sterile saline is usually used as the irrigating fluid unless diathermy is planned, in which case a non-ionic solution, such as glycine, is required. Once the bladder is sufficiently distended to allow inspection of the folds of mucosa (200–400 mL), the irrigation can be switched off. The careful inspection of the urethra is a vital part of the investigation and should not be neglected. This is most commonly done while withdrawing the instrument at the end of the procedure. The trigone and the position of the ureteric orifices should be noted. Next, the mucosa is examined for colour, vascularity, trabeculation and abnormal lesions. Orientation is easily established by identifying the air bubble at the dome of the bladder. This serves as a landmark during inspection of the bladder mucosa, which is conventionally performed by going around clockwise in a series of 12 sweeps, coming back to the bubble after each one. Visualisation of the bladder base can be difficult if a large cystocele is present. This is made easier by inserting a finger in the vagina to correct the prolapse.

NATIONAL POLICIES AND GUIDANCE

In 2013 NICE published guidelines on the management of urinary incontinence in women.[6] It provided recommendations and practice algorithms on assessment and investigations of LUTS. The Fifth International Consultation on Incontinence (Paris 2013) has recently published recommendations and guidance on the assessment of urinary incontinence.[12]

ACKNOWLEDGEMENT

This chapter has been revised and updated. The author and editors acknowledge the contribution of James Balmforth to the chapter on this topic in the previous editions of the book.

References

1. Haylen B, Riddler D, Freeman R *et al*. An IUGA/ICS joint report on the terminology for female pelvic floor dysfunction. *Int Urogynaecol J* 2010;21:5–26.

2. RCOG. *Gynaecological Examinations: Guidelines for Specialist Practice*. London: RCOG, 2002.

3. International Consultation on Incontinence Modular Questionnaire (ICIQ) homepage (http://iciq.net/index.html)

4. RCOG. *Patient-reported Outcome Measures in Gynaecology*. Scientific Impact paper 31. London: RCOG, 2012.

5. Matharu GS, Assandra RP, Williams KS *et al*. Objective assessment of urinary incontinence in women: comparison of the 1-hour and 24-hour pad test. *Eur Urol* 2004;45:208–12.

6. NICE. *Urinary Incontinence: The Management of Urinary Incontinence in Women*. Clinical Guideline 171. Implementation advice. London: NICE, 2013.

7. Schafer W, Abrams P, Lioa L. Good urodynamic practices: uroflowmetry, filling cystometry and pressure flow studies. *Neurolurol Urodyn* 2002;21: 261–74.

8. UK Continence Society. Joint statement on minimum standards for urodynamic practice in the UK, 2009. http://www.ukcs.uk.net/docs/joint_statement.pdf.

9. van Waalwijk, van Doorn E, Anders K *et al*. Standardisation of ambulatory urodynamic monitoring: report of the Standardisation Sub-committee of the International Continence Society for ambulatory urodynamic studies. *Neurourol Urodyn* 2000;19:113–25.

10. Lose G, Griffiths D, Hosker G *et al*. Standardisation of urethral measurement: report from the Standardisation Sub-Committee of the International Continence Society. *Neurourol Urodyn* 2002;21:258–60.

11. Robinson D, Anders K, Cadozo L *et al*. Can ultrasound replace ambulatory urodynamics when investigating women with irritative urinary symptoms? *BJOG* 2002;109:145–8.

12. Abrams P, Cardozo L, Khoury S, Wein A (eds). *Incontinence*. 5th edn. Paris: Health Publication, 2013.

Chapter 95 Urinary Incontinence

Dudley Robinson and Linda Cardozo

INTRODUCTION

Urinary incontinence is defined by the International Continence Society as 'the complaint of any involuntary leakage of urine'.[1] Whilst not life threatening it is known to be a cause of considerable morbidity and has a considerable impact on quality of life.[2]

PREVALENCE

Urinary incontinence is known to be a prevalent and often under-reported condition. A large epidemiological study of urinary incontinence has been reported in 27,936 women from Norway.[3] Overall 25 per cent of women reported urinary incontinence of whom 7 per cent felt it to be significant and the prevalence of incontinence was found to increase with age. When considering the type of incontinence 50 per cent of women complained of stress, 11 per cent urge and 36 per cent mixed incontinence. Further analysis has also investigated the effect of age and parity. The prevalence of urinary incontinence among nulliparous women ranged from 8 per cent to 32 per cent and increased with age. In general parity was associated with incontinence and the first delivery was the most significant. When considering stress incontinence in the age group 20–34 years the relative risk was 2.7 (95% CI 2.0–3.5) for primiparous women and 4.0 (95% CI 2.5–6.4) for multiparous women. There was a similar association for mixed incontinence although not for urge incontinence.[4]

Evidence would suggest that incontinence is often under-reported. In a large study of patients assessed after tertiary referral 60 per cent of women were found to have delayed seeking treatment for more than one year from the time their symptoms became severe. Of these women 50 per cent claimed that this was because they were too embarrassed to discuss the problem with their doctor, and 17 per cent said that they thought the problem was normal for their age.[5]

EPIDEMIOLOGY

Age

The incidence of urinary incontinence increases with increasing age. Elderly women have been found to have a reduced flow rate, increased urinary residuals, higher filling pressures, reduced bladder capacity and lower maximum voiding pressures. In a large study of 842 women aged 17–64 years the prevalence rates of urinary incontinence increased progressively over seven birth cohorts (1900–1940) from 12 per cent to 25 per cent. These findings agree with those of a large telephone survey in the USA which reported a prevalence of urge incontinence of 5 per cent in the 18–44 age group rising to 19 per cent in women over 65 years of age.[6] Conversely, as mobility and physical exercise decrease with advancing age so does the prevalence of stress urinary incontinence.

Race

Several studies have been performed examining the impact of racial differences on the prevalence of urinary incontinence in women. In general there is evidence that there is a lower incidence of both urinary incontinence and urogenital prolapse in black women and North American studies have found a larger proportion of white than African-American women reported symptoms of stress incontinence (31 per cent vs 7 per cent) and a larger proportion were found to have demonstrable stress incontinence on objective assessment (61 per cent vs 27 per cent). Overall white women had a prevalence of urodynamic stress incontinence 2.3 times higher than African-American women.[7] Whilst most studies confirm these findings there is little evidence regarding the prevalence of urge incontinence or mixed incontinence.

Pregnancy

Pregnancy is responsible for marked changes in the urinary tract and consequently lower urinary tract symptoms are more common and many are simply a reflection of normal physiological change. Urine production increases in pregnancy due to increasing cardiac output and a 25 per cent increase in renal perfusion and glomerular filtration rate.

Frequency of micturition is one of the earliest symptoms of pregnancy affecting approximately 60 per cent in the first trimester and middle trimester and 81 per cent in the final trimester. Nocturia is also a common symptom although it was only thought to be a nuisance in 4 per cent of cases. Overall frequency occurs in over 90 per cent of women in pregnancy.

Urgency and urge incontinence have also been shown to increase in pregnancy. Urge incontinence has been shown to have a peak incidence of 19 per cent in multiparous women whilst other authors have reported a rate of urge incontinence of 10 per cent and urgency of 60 per cent. The incidence of detrusor overactivity and low compliance in pregnancy has been reported as 24 per cent and 31 per cent respectively. The cause of the former may be high progesterone levels whilst the latter is probably a consequence of pressure from the gravid uterus.

Stress incontinence has also been reported to be more common in pregnancy, with 28 per cent of women complaining of symptoms although only 12 per cent remained symptomatic following delivery. The long-term prognosis for this group of women remains guarded. Continent women delivered vaginally have been compared to those who had a caesarean section. Whilst there was initially a difference in favour of CS this effect was insignificant by three months following delivery.[8]

Childbirth

Childbirth may result in damage to the pelvic floor musculature as well as injury to the pudendal and pelvic nerves. The association between increasing parity and urinary incontinence has been reported in several studies. Some authorities have found this relationship to be linear whilst others have demonstrated a threshold at the first delivery and some have shown that increasing age at first delivery is significant. A large Australian study has demonstrated a strong relationship between urinary incontinence and parity in young women (18–23 years) although in middle age (45–50 years) there was only a modest association and this was lost in older women (70–75 years).[9]

Obstetric factors themselves may also have a direct effect on continence following delivery. The risk of incontinence increases 5.7-fold in women who have had a previous vaginal delivery although a previous CS did not increase the risk.[10] In addition an increased risk of urinary incontinence has been associated with increased exposure to oxytocic drugs, vacuum extraction, forceps delivery and fetal macrosomia.

Mode of delivery has also been investigated in a large population-based cohort study of 5236 primiparous women in Sweden followed up over 20 years after a single delivery. Overall the prevalence of stress incontinence, urgency incontinence and mixed incontinence was 15.3 per cent, 6.1 per cent and 14.4 per cent respectively and was higher in all types of incontinence following vaginal delivery when compared to CS. Moderate to severe incontinence was more prevalent after vaginal delivery than after CS (21.3 per cent vs 13.5 per cent; OR 1.68, 95% CI 1.40–2.03). In addition the prevalence of bothersome urinary incontinence was also greater after vaginal delivery (11.2 per cent vs 16.3 per cent; OR 1.85, 95% CI 1.42–2.39).[11]

Menopause

The urogenital tract and lower urinary tract are sensitive to the effects of oestrogen and progesterone throughout adult life. Epidemiological studies have implicated oestrogen deficiency in the aetiology of lower urinary tract symptoms occurring following the menopause with 70 per cent of women relating the onset of urinary incontinence to their final menstrual period.[12] LUTS have been shown to be common in post-menopausal women attending a menopause clinic with 20 per cent complaining of severe urgency and almost 50 per cent complaining of stress incontinence.[13] Urge incontinence in particular is more prevalent following the menopause and the prevalence would appear to rise with increasing years of oestrogen deficiency. Some studies have shown a peak incidence in perimenopausal women whilst other evidence suggests that many women develop incontinence at least 10 years prior to the cessation of menstruation with significantly more pre-menopausal women than post-menopausal women being affected.

THE CAUSES OF URINARY INCONTINENCE

1   Urodynamic stress incontinence (USI);
2   Detrusor overactivity;

Table 95.1 Symptoms and definitions

Definition	Symptoms
Daytime frequency	Complaint by the patient who considers that she voids too often by day
Urgency	Sudden and compelling desire to pass urine, which is difficult to defer
Noctural enuresis	Complaint of loss of urine occurring during sleep
Continuous urinary incontinence	Complaint of continuous leakage
Stress urinary incontinence	Complaint of involuntary leakage on effort or exertion, or on sneezing or coughing
Urgency Incontinence	Complaint of involuntary leakage accompanied by or immediately preceded by urgency
Mixed Incontinence	Complaint of involuntary leakage associated with urgency and also with exertion, effort, sneezing or coughing

3   Overflow incontinence;
4   Fistulae (vesicovaginal, ureterovaginal, urethrovaginal);
5   Congenital (e.g. ectopic ureter);
6   Urethral diverticulum;
7   Other (e.g. UTI, faecal impaction, medication);
8   Functional (e.g. immobility).

Urinary symptoms can be broadly divided. Detrusor over-activity is classically associated with frequency, urgency, urge incontinence, nocturia and nocturnal enuresis. Urodynamic stress incontinence is classically associated with involuntary leakage on effort or on exertion or on coughing or sneezing (Table 95.1).

Continuous incontinence and/or post-micturition dribbling are more likely to be associated with neurological disorders, overflow, urethral diverticulae or a fistula. However, there are problems with making a presumptive diagnosis on the basis of symptoms alone. Many women complain of a mixture of symptoms. For instance those women who are found to have USI often complain of frequency, as they are going to the toilet more often in order to avoid leaking. One study found that even an experienced clinician made the correct diagnosis only 65 per cent of the time when relying on symptoms only.[14]

URODYNAMIC STRESS INCONTINENCE

Definition

Urodynamic Stress Incontinence (USI) is noted during filling cystometry and is defined as 'the involuntary leakage of urine during increased abdominal pressure, in the absence of a detrusor contraction'.

Incidence

Urodynamic stress incontinence is the commonest cause of incontinence in women. It is difficult to assess the true incidence, as many women suffer in silence and consider it an inevitable consequence of childbirth and ageing. However, conservative estimates are that 1 in 10 women will suffer from USI at some point in their lives.

Aetiology

There are various factors that are thought to predispose to the development of USI.

1   Increased intra-abdominal pressure:
    – pregnancy
    – chronic cough
    – abdominal, pelvic mass
    – constipation
    – ascites.
2   Damage to the pelvic floor:
    – childbirth
    – radical pelvic surgery.
3   Fixed, scarred urethra:
    – previous surgery
    – radiotherapy.

Pathophysiology

The exact pathophysiology is unclear, but several hypotheses have been put forward.

1   Failure of the supporting structures such as the pubo-urethral and pubovesical ligaments.
2   Failure of the intrinsic sphincter mechanism as a result of damage to the rhabdosphincter, poor collagen or reduced urethral vascularity (intrinsic sphincter deficiency – ISD).
3   Failure of the extrinsic sphincter mechanism as a result of weakness or damage to the pelvic floor musculature. This allows displacement of the bladder neck from within the intra-abdominal pressure zone.

More recently the 'integral theory' has been described by Petros and Ulmsten.[15] This hypothesises that the distal and mid urethra have an important role in the continence mechanism[16] and that maximal urethral closure pressure is controlled at the mid-urethral point.[17] The theory also proposes that damage to the pubo-urethral ligaments, which support the urethra, impaired support of the anterior vaginal wall to the mid urethra, and weakened function of part of the pubococcygeal muscles, which insert adjacent to the urethra, are responsible for causing stress incontinence.

MANAGEMENT OF USI

Conservative management

USI interferes with a woman's quality of life but it is not a life-threatening condition and therefore conservative measures should be tried in every woman prior to resorting to surgical treatment.

Conservative treatment is effective, has few complications and does not compromise further surgical procedures.[18] It is particularly useful in those women who are medically unfit for surgery and those who have not completed their family, are breastfeeding or are less than six months postpartum.

Conservative measures include:

1. pelvic floor exercises;
2. biofeedback;
3. electrical stimulation;
4. vaginal cones;
5. urethral devices.

In order to maximise the benefits that can be obtained using these techniques, it is vital to ensure that the treatment is tailored to the individual and that it is properly taught.

Pelvic floor muscle training

Pelvic floor muscle training (PFMT) and pelvic floor physiotherapy have been the first-line conservative measure since their introduction in 1948.[19] PFMT appears to work in a number of different ways:

- women learn to consciously pre-contract the pelvic floor muscles before and during increases in abdominal pressure to prevent leakage ('the knack');
- strength training builds up long-lasting muscle volume and thus provides structural support;
- abdominal muscle training indirectly strengthens the pelvic floor muscles.[20]

In addition during a contraction the urethra may also be pressed against the posterior aspect of the symphysis pubis producing a mechanical rise in urethral pressure.[21] Since up to 30 per cent of women with stress incontinence are unable to contract their pelvic floor correctly at presentation,[22] some patients may simply need to be re-taught the 'knack' of squeezing the appropriate muscles at the correct time.[23]

PFMT remains integral to the management of women with stress urinary incontinence with level 1, grade A evidence from five prospective RCTs with short-term cure rates between 35 per cent and 80 per cent.[24] Supervised training is generally felt to be more effective than unsupervised training[25] although benefits of biofeedback and electrical stimulation are less clear.[26] Consequently the International Consultation on Incontinence (ICI)[27] recommends that PFMT should be considered as first-line treatment in all women with stress urinary incontinence. In addition there is no evidence to suggest that age is a factor when determining outcome of PFMT.

There is also good evidence to support the use of PFMT for the prevention of urinary incontinence in antenatal and postnatal women in a systematic review of 15 studies including 6181 women.[28] Pregnant women without prior urinary incontinence who were randomised to antenatal PFMT were less likely than those who had no PFMT to report urinary incontinence in late pregnancy (RR 0.44, 95% CI 0.30–0.65) and immediately postpartum (RR 0.71, 95% CI 0.52–0.97). In addition postnatal women who had received PFMT with persistent urinary incontinence three months after delivery were less likely to report urinary incontinence at 12 months (RR 0.79, 95% CI 0.70–0.90). Consequently the evidence would suggest that PFMT in women during pregnancy may be useful in the prevention of incontinence.

Biofeedback

Biofeedback is used to augment the effect of pelvic floor exercises. It can range in complexity from the very simple, such as a vaginal examination measuring the strength of the squeeze, which the woman can perform herself at home, to the much more sophisticated electromyography, which is usually used in a clinic. Biofeedback has not been shown to be superior to pelvic floor exercises alone.

Electrical Stimulation

Electrical stimulation uses an electrical pulse to augment the ability to produce a voluntary contraction. A probe is put into the vagina near the muscles of the pelvic floor and a pulse of electricity is passed. The pulse frequency is debated, but it is usually in the 35–40 Hz range. This method cannot be used in pregnancy or in those with an IUCD *in situ*. It is not suitable for most women as it is excessively time consuming.

Vaginal cones and urethral devices

Vaginal cones or weights are now used infrequently, as the results are no better than those of pelvic floor exercises alone.

Many women find a tampon or an intravaginal device very helpful. These devices elevate the bladder neck and in some cases partially obstruct the flow of urine. They are particularly suitable for women who find they are incontinent only at specific times, for instance during aerobics or playing tennis. Several urethral support devices are available such as Conveen or Contrelle, although these are now very rarely used.

Pharmacological management

Whilst various agents such as α_1-adrenoceptor agonists, oestrogens and tricyclic antidepressants have all been used anecdotally in the past for the treatment of stress incontinence, duloxetine is the first drug to be specifically developed and licensed for this indication.

Duloxetine is a potent and balanced serotonin (5-hydroxytryptamine) and noradrenaline re-uptake inhibitor (SNRI) which enhances urethral striated sphincter activity via a centrally mediated pathway.[29] The efficacy and safety of duloxetine has been evaluated in a double-blind randomised parallel group placebo-controlled phase II dose-finding study in the US involving 553 women with stress incontinence.[30] Duloxetine was associated with significant and dose-dependent decrease in incontinence episode frequency whilst the most frequently reported adverse event was nausea.

A further global phase III study of 458 women has also recently been reported.[31] There was a significant decrease in incontinence episode frequency and improvement in quality of life with duloxetine compared to placebo. Once again nausea was the most frequently reported adverse event, occurring in 25.1 per cent of women receiving duloxetine compared to a rate of 3.9 per cent in those taking placebo.

Duloxetine may also be useful in those women awaiting continence surgery. In a further double-blind, placebo-controlled study of 109 women awaiting surgery for stress incontinence[32] there was a significant improvement in incontinence episode frequency and quality of life when compared to placebo. Furthermore, 20 per cent of women who were awaiting continence surgery changed their mind whilst taking duloxetine.

In addition the role of synergistic therapy with PFMT and duloxetine has been examined in a prospective study of 201 women with stress incontinence. Women were randomised to one of four treatments: duloxetine, PFMT, combination therapy or placebo. Overall duloxetine, with or without PFMT, was found to be superior to placebo or PFMT alone whilst pad test results and QoL analysis favoured combination therapy to single treatment.[33]

Surgical procedures

More than 200 operative procedures for the treatment of USI have been described. Many of these are modifications of similar procedures, but there is not one definitive operation. The first operative procedure offers the best chance of cure and therefore it is very important to select the appropriate procedure for each patient.

Historically colposuspension, originally described by Burch in 1961,[34] has been regarded as the operation of choice in cases of primary stress incontinence. However, with the description of the 'mid-urethral theory' or 'integral theory' by Petros and Ulmsten the rationale behind surgery for stress incontinence has changed and has led directly to the development of both the retropubic and trans-obturator mid-urethral tape procedures and these new, minimally invasive procedures have now largely replaced retropubic suspensions and sling procedures.

For those women who may not be suitable for a mid-urethral tape procedure, urethral bulking agents may also be considered and many of these may now be performed under local anaesthesia in the ambulatory setting.

Colposuspension

The patient is placed in the modified lithotomy position using Lloyd–Davies stirrups. A Foley catheter is inserted into the bladder and allowed to drain freely. A low transverse incision is made just above the symphysis pubis (i.e. lower than a pfannenstiel). The retropubic space is dissected until the white paravaginal tissue lateral to the bladder neck is exposed. Two to four polydioxanone (PDS), Ethibond or polyglycolic acid sutures are inserted into the paravaginal fascia. Each suture is tied and the needle is then re-inserted into the ipsilateral iliopectineal ligament. The first suture is placed at the level of the bladder neck and the subsequent sutures are placed 1 cm laterally and 1 cm cranially (Fig. 95.1). When all the sutures have been inserted, an assistant elevates the lateral fornix on each side to allow the sutures to be tied without tension (Fig. 95.2).

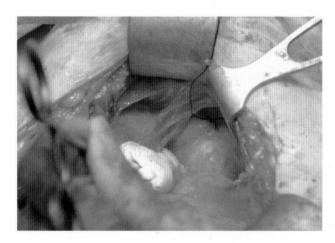

Fig. 95.1 Colposuspension: the bladder neck is mobilised medially and the first suture placed in the white paravaginal tissue

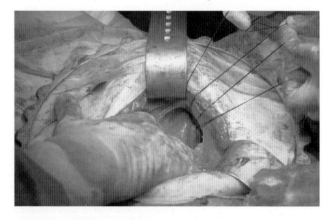

Fig. 95.2 Colposuspension: four sutures are placed on each side to elevate the paravaginal tissue to the ipsilateral pectineal ligament

A suction drain is left in the retropubic space, a suprapubic catheter is inserted and the urethral catheter is removed.

The suprapubic catheter is left on free drainage for at least two days and then a clamping regimen is initiated. This usually entails clamping the catheter at a set time and allowing the patient to void normally. Initially, the residual is checked after each void or, if the patient experiences discomfort, the clamp is released and the residual measured. If the patient is passing good volumes of urine with small residuals, the time between unclamping can be extended to 12 hours and then 24 hours. When the residuals are persistently under 100 mL, the suprapubic catheter can be removed.

Post-operative complications

Voiding difficulties are the main complication following a colposuspension. Overall the incidence of voiding difficulties lasting over one month is reported as 5 per cent (CI 3–5)[35] although other series have reported rates as high as 21 per cent.[36]

These women are initially managed by allowing them to go home with their suprapubic catheter *in situ*, leaving it on free drainage. Two weeks later they are re-admitted and a further trial of clamping is attempted. The majority of women will be able to void spontaneously at this stage. About 2 per cent will continue to complain of voiding difficulties, and these women are usually taught clean intermittent self-catheterisation.

Detrusor overactivity arises *de novo* in between 12 per cent and 18.5 per cent of women who have undergone a colposuspension.[37] It seems to occur more commonly after previous continence surgery. It may be that a number of cases reflect pre-existing detrusor overactivity that went undetected at pre-operative cystometry. Alternatively, the autonomic nerve supply may be damaged when the bladder is medially displaced at the time of surgery.[38]

A longer-term complication is the development of prolapse. Enterocele and rectocele formation is thought to occur as a result of elevation of the anterior vaginal wall creating a posterior defect and causing intra-abdominal pressure to be transmitted directly to the posterior vaginal wall. The incidence is estimated to be between 7 per cent and 17 per cent.[39] It is unclear whether these represent new defects or merely a pre-existing defect becoming symptomatic once the support of the anterior vaginal wall has been rectified.

Outcome

Historically there have been many prospective case series and cohort studies assessing the efficacy of colposuspension with some studies providing long-term follow-up data for up to 20 years and cure rates of 80[40]–94[41] per cent.

In addition there have also been three reported meta-analyses. The first of these was reported by Jarvis in 1994[42] who reviewed 1726 women with follow-up of at least one year and a mean objective success rate of 84.3 per cent. Very similar results were reported from a meta-analysis of 2196 women reported by the American Urological Association

in 1997. Overall mean objective cure rates were 84 per cent at 48 months (CI 79–88%) with follow-up to at least four years. More recently the Cochrane group has published a meta-analysis of 39 RCTs involving 2403 women with a mean follow-up of one year. Objective cure rates were found to be 85–90 per cent and there was a slow decline in cure rates to 70 per cent over five years.[43]

Laparoscopic colposuspension

Minimally invasive surgery is attractive and this trend has extended to surgery for stress incontinence. Although many authors have reported excellent short-term subjective results from laparoscopic colposuspension, early studies have shown inferior results to the open procedure.

Two large prospective RCTs have been reported from Australia and the UK comparing laparoscopic and open colposuspension. In the Australian study 200 women with USI were randomised to either laparoscopic or open colposuspension.[44] Overall there were no significant differences in objective and subjective measures of cure or in patient satisfaction at 6 months, 24 months or 3–5 years. Whilst the laparoscopic approach took longer it was associated with less blood loss and a quicker return to normal activities.

These findings are supported by the UK multicentre RCT of 291 women with USI comparing laparoscopic to open colposuspension.[45] At 24 months intention to treat analysis showed no significant difference in cure rates between the procedures. Objective cure rates for open and laparoscopic colposuspension were 70.1 per cent and 79.7 per cent respectively whilst subjective cure rates were 54.6 per cent and 54.9 per cent respectively.

These studies have confirmed that the clinical effectiveness of the two operations is comparable although the cost effectiveness of laparoscopic colposuspension remains unproven. A cost analysis comparing laparoscopic to open colposuspension was also performed alongside the UK study.[46] Healthcare resource use over the first six-month follow-up period translated into costs of £1805 for the laparoscopic group versus £1433 for the open group.

Post-operative complications

The incidence of urinary tract injury has been found to be higher during laparoscopic colposuspension than during the open operation. A 1–10 per cent rate of bladder injury has been reported, and although the rate of ureteric injury or kinking is less than 0.1 per cent, this is significantly higher than at the open procedure. Operative morbidity has also been extensively studied, with intra-operative blood loss, febrile morbidity and length of hospital stay all higher in the open colposuspension group.[47]

Pubovaginal sling

Sling procedures are often performed as secondary operations where there is scarring and narrowing of the vagina.

The sling material can either be organic (rectus fascia, porcine dermis) or inorganic (Prolene, Mersilene, Marlex or Silastic). The sling may be inserted either abdominally, vaginally or by a combination of both. Normally the sling is used to elevate and support the bladder neck and proximal urethra, but not intentionally to obstruct it.

Sling procedures may be associated with a high incidence of side effects and complications. It is often difficult to decide how tight to make the sling. If it is too loose, incontinence will persist and if it is too tight, voiding difficulties may be permanent. Women who are going to undergo insertion of a sling must be prepared to perform clean intermittent self-catheterisation post-operatively. In addition, there is a risk of infection, especially if inorganic material is used. The sling may erode into the urethra, bladder or vagina, in which case it must be removed and this can be exceedingly difficult.

Mid-urethral tape procedures

Retropubic approach: tension-free vaginal tape

The tension-free vaginal tape (TVT, Gynaecare), first described by Ulmsten in 1996,[48] is now the most commonly performed procedure for stress urinary incontinence in the UK and more than two million procedures have been performed worldwide.

A knitted 11 mm × 40 cm polypropylene mesh tape is inserted transvaginally at the level of the mid urethra, using two 5 mm trochars (Fig. 95.3). The procedure may be performed under local, spinal or general anaesthesia.

Technique

The procedure may be performed under local or general anaesthesia. The patient is placed in the dorsal lithotomy position and having prepared the vagina and suprapubic area an indwelling 18 Fr Foley catheter is inserted into the bladder. Once the bladder has been emptied a rigid catheter guide is then inserted down the catheter in order to deflect the bladder away from the passage of the needle introducers. The use of local anaesthesia (20 mL bupivacaine 0.5% with 1 in 200,000 adrenaline – diluted in 100 mL normal saline) allows effective hydrodissection and vasoconstriction whilst at the same time providing effective intra-operative and post-operative analgesia. 20 mL of dilute local anaesthetic is injected on each side retropubically immediately behind the pubic tubercle. In addition a further 20 mL is injected para-urethrally on each side up to the level of the urogenital diaphragm and 5 mL sub-urethrally.

A 2 cm midline sub-urethral vaginal incision is made and para-urethral dissection performed using sharp dissection with McIndoe scissors between the vaginal mucosa and pubo-cervical fascia to the level of the inferior pubic ramus and the urogenital diaphragm. Two small 0.5 cm suprapubic incisions at the upper border of the pubic tubercle 2 cm lateral to the midline may be made to facilitate needle passage through the skin.

The TVT needle is then placed in the starting position within the dissected para-urethral tunnel with the tip of the needle between the index finger (in the vagina) and the lower border of the pubic ramus. Prior to the passage of the needle the bladder is pushed away from the track of the needle using the rigid catheter guide. In a controlled movement the needle is then pushed through the urogenital diaphragm, the retropubic space and the rectus fascia keeping in close contact to the dorsal aspect of the pubic bone. The procedure is then repeated on the contralateral side.

With the needles still in position a cystoscopy using a 70° cystoscope is performed to check that there is no bladder injury (Fig. 95.4). Should a bladder perforation be noted the needle is withdrawn, replaced, passed once again and the cystoscopy repeated. Once the integrity of the bladder is confirmed the bladder is again emptied completely and the tape pulled through.

In those centres which continue to use the cough stress test the bladder is then refilled with 300 mL normal saline and the patient asked to cough vigorously. The tape may then be adjusted to a point where there is only a drop of leakage from the urethral meatus. After this final adjustment the

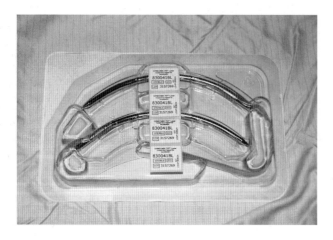

Fig. 95.3 TVT: tension-free vaginal tape

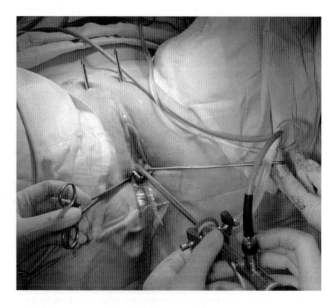

Fig. 95.4 TVT trochars inserted and check cystoscopy to exclude bladder perforation

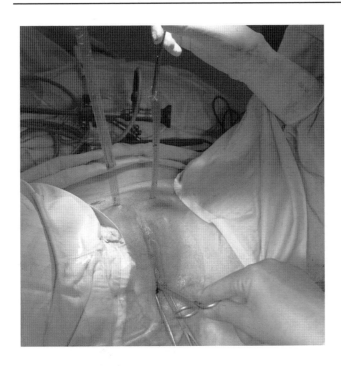

Fig. 95.5 TVT: adjusting the tension of the tape

tape is held in position beneath the urethra using a pair of McIndoe scissors whilst the plastic sheaths are removed on each side (Fig. 95.5).

In those centres where a cough stress test is no longer used the tape is positioned loosely below the mid-urethra without tension. Finally the vaginal incision is closed using an absorbable suture and the suprapubic incisions are closed with steri-strips. Whilst an indwelling catheter is not required in all cases a urethral catheter should be left on free drainage for 48 hours following a bladder injury.

Outcome

The initial multicentre study carried out in six centres in Sweden reported a 90 per cent cure rate at one year in women undergoing their first operation for USI, without any major complications.[49] Long-term results would confirm durability of the technique with success rates of 86 per cent at 3 years,[50] 84.7 per cent at 5 years,[51] 81.3 per cent at 7 years,[52] 90 per cent at 11 years[53] and 90 per cent at 17 years.[54]

The TVT has also been compared to open colposuspension in a multicentre prospective randomised trial of 344 women with USI.[55] Overall there was no significant difference in terms of objective cure; 66 per cent in the TVT group and 57 per cent in the colposuspension group. However, operation time, postoperative stay and return to normal activity were all longer in the colposuspension arm. Analysis of the long-term results at 24 months using a pad test, QoL assessment and symptom questionnaires showed an objective cure rate of 63 per cent in the TVT arm and 51 per cent in the colposuspension arm.[56] At five years there were no differences in subjective cure (63 per cent in the TVT group and 70 per cent in the colposuspension group), patient satisfaction and QoL assessment. However, whilst there was a significant reduction in cystocele in both groups there was a higher incidence of enterocele,

rectocele and apical prolapse in the colposuspension group.[57] Furthermore, cost utility analysis has also shown that at six months follow-up TVT resulted in a mean cost saving of £243 when compared to colposuspension.[58]

A smaller randomised study has also compared TVT to laparoscopic colposuspension in 72 women with USI. At a mean follow-up of 20 months objective cure rates were higher in the TVT group when compared to the laparoscopic colposuspension group: 96.8 per cent vs 71.2 per cent respectively.[59]

Post-operative complications

Following the procedure most women can go home the same day, although some do require catheterisation for short-term voiding difficulties (2.5–19.7 per cent). Other complications include bladder perforation (2.7–5.8 per cent), de-novo urgency (0.2–15 per cent) and bleeding (0.9–2.3 per cent).[60]

SPARC: mid-urethral sling suspension system

The SPARC sling system (American Medical Systems) is a minimally invasive sling procedure using a knitted 10 mm-wide polypropylene mesh which is placed at the level of the mid urethra by passing the needle via a suprapubic to vaginal approach.[61] The procedure may be performed under local, regional or general anaesthetic. A prospective multicentre study of 104 women with USI has been reported from France.[62] At a mean follow-up of 11.9 months the objective cure rate was 90.4 per cent and subjective cure 72 per cent. There was a 10.5 per cent incidence of bladder perforation and 11.5 per cent of women complained of de-novo urgency following the procedure. More recently SPARC has been compared to TVT in a prospective randomised trial of 301 women.[63] At short-term follow-up there were no significant differences in cure rates, bladder perforation rates and de-novo urgency. There was, however, a higher incidence of voiding difficulties and vaginal erosions in the SPARC group.

Trans-obturator sling procedures

The trans-obturator route for the placement of synthetic mid-urethral slings was first described in 2001.[64] As with the retropubic sling procedures trans-obturator tapes may be performed under local, regional or general anaesthetic and have the theoretical advantage of eliminating some of the complications associated with the retropubic route such as bladder and urethral perforation.

The trans-obturator approach may be used as an 'inside-out' (TVT-O, Gynaecare) or alternatively an 'outside-in' (Monarc, American Medical Systems) technique. To date there have been several studies documenting the short-term efficacy of trans-obturator procedures.

Trans-obturator 'inside-out'

The TVT-O device consists of an 11 mm × 40 cm tape of polypropylene mesh, both ends of which are attached to a plastic sheath which threads over the helical needle introducer. A winged needle guide is also provided to facilitate passage of the needle through the obturator membrane (Fig. 95.6).

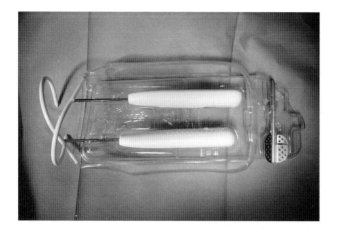

Fig. 95.6 TVT-O: tension-free vaginal tape – obturator

The procedure may be performed under local or general anaesthesia. The patient is placed in the dorsal lithotomy position in 120° hyperflexion. The vagina and thighs are then prepared and an indwelling 12 Fr Foley catheter is inserted into the bladder. Next two 0.5 cm incisions are made 2 cm superior to a horizontal line level with the urethra and 2 cm lateral to the thigh folds. This marks the exit point for the helical needle introducer.

The use of local anaesthesia (20 mL bupivacaine 0.5% with 1 in 200,000 adrenaline – diluted in 100 mL normal saline) allows effective hydrodissection and vasoconstriction whilst at the same time providing effective intra-operative and post-operative analgesia. 20 mL of dilute local anaesthetic is injected para-urethrally on each side in the direction of the inferior pubic ramus.

A midline sub-urethral incision is then made at the level of the mid urethra prior to para-urethral sharp dissection between the vaginal epithelium and peri-urethral fascia using McIndoe scissors. Dissection is continued laterally to the inferior border of the pubic ramus at the level of the mid-urethra and the medial aspect of the obturator membrane is perforated.

The winged needle guide is then passed at 45° relative to the saggital plane of the urethra until reaching the posterior aspect of the inferior pubic ramus and perforating the obturator membrane. Having mounted the tape onto the helical introducer the tip is then placed along the guide channel in the winged guide to pass through the obturator membrane and is then rotated so as to exit through the inner thigh incision. The tip of the tubing is then clamped and the helical introducer withdrawn. The procedure is then repeated on the contralateral side (Fig. 95.7). Once both needles have been passed and the tape inserted a cystoscopy may be performed to exclude bladder or urethral injury.

The tape is then held loosely in position beneath the urethra using a pair of McIndoe scissors whilst the protective plastic sheaths are removed ensuring that there is no tension on the urethra and the tape is lying flat (Fig. 95.8). The vaginal incision is then closed using an absorbable suture and steristrips are used to close the two small incisions on the thighs. Whilst an indwelling catheter is not required in all cases a urethral

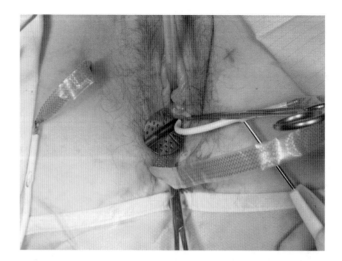

Fig. 95.7 TVT-O: insertion of TVT-O using the winged guide

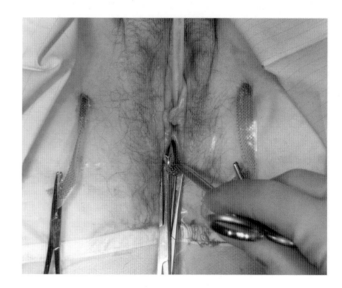

Fig. 95.8 TVT-O: adjusting the tension of the tape

catheter should be left on free drainage for 48 hours following a bladder injury.

Trans-obturator 'outside-in'

The procedure may be performed under local or general anaesthesia. The patient is placed in the dorsal lithotomy position in 120° hyperflexion. The vagina and thighs are then prepared and an indwelling 12 Fr Foley catheter is inserted into the bladder. The use of local anaesthesia (20 mL bupivacaine 0.5% with 1 in 200,000 adrenaline – diluted in 100 mL normal saline) allows effective hydrodissection and vasoconstriction whilst at the same time providing effective intra-operative and post-operative analgesia. 20 mL of dilute local anaesthetic is injected para-urethrally on each side in the direction of the inferior pubic ramus.

A midline sub-urethral incision is then made at the level of the mid urethra prior to para-urethral sharp dissection between the vaginal epithelium and peri-urethral fascia using McIndoe scissors. Dissection is continued laterally to the inferior border of the pubic ramus at the level of the mid urethra and the medial aspect of the obturator membrane is perforated. Next a small incision is made 1.5 cm lateral to the ischiopubic ramus on each side at the level of the clitoris. The helical needle introducer is then passed 'outside-in' through the incision to perforate the medial aspect of the obturator membrane. With the index finger in the vaginal incision palpating the ischiopubic ramus and obturator internus muscle the tip of the helical needle may then be guided through to the vaginal incision. Care should be taken to avoid perforating the lateral vaginal fornix and the urethra is guarded by the operator's finger. Once the tip of the needle has been passed through the vaginal incision the tape may then be attached to the needle and pulled through to exit through the thigh incision. The procedure is then repeated on the contralateral side.

The tape is then held loosely in position beneath the urethra using a pair of McIndoe scissors whilst the protective plastic sheaths are removed ensuring that there is no tension on the urethra and the tape is lying flat. The vaginal incision is then closed using an absorbable suture and steristrips are used to close the two small incisions on the thighs. Whilst an indwelling catheter is not required in all cases a urethral catheter should be left on free drainage for 48 hours following a bladder injury.

Outcome

Initial studies have reported cure and improved rates of 80.5 per cent and 7.5 per cent respectively at 7 months[65] and 90.6 per cent and 9.4 per cent respectively at 17 months.[66]

More recently the trans-obturator approach (TVT-O) has been compared to the retropubic approach (TVT) in an Italian prospective multicentre randomised study of 231 women with urodynamic stress incontinence.[35] At a mean of nine months subjectively 92 per cent of women in the TVT group were cured compared to 87 per cent in the TVT-O group. Objectively, on pad test, cure rates were 92 per cent and 89 per cent respectively. There were no differences in voiding difficulties and length of stay although there were more bladder perforations in the TVT group; 4 per cent vs none in the TVT-O group. A further multicentre prospective randomised trial comparing TVT and TVT-O has also recently been reported from Finland in 267 women complaining of stress urinary incontinence.[68] Objective cure rates at nine weeks were 98.5 per cent in the TVT group and 95.4 per cent in the TVT-O group. Whilst complication rates were low and similar in both arms of the study there was a higher incidence of groin pain in the TVT-O group.

These data are supported by a recent meta-analysis of the five randomised trials comparing TVT-O with TVT and six randomised trials comparing TOT with TVT.[69] Overall subjective cure rates were identical with the retropubic and trans-obturator routes. However, adverse events such as bladder injuries (OR 0.12, 95% CI 0.05–0.33) and voiding difficulties (OR 0.55, 95% CI 0.31–0.98) were less common, whereas groin pain (OR 8.28, 95% CI 2.7–25.4) and vaginal erosions (OR 1.96, 95% CI 0.87–4.39) were more common after the trans-obturator approach.

Long-term data would also seem to support the durability and efficacy of the trans-obturator approach. A three-year follow-up study of a prospective observational study evaluating the use of TVT-O has been reported (Waltregny et al. 2008).[70] Of the 102 patients recruited 91 (89.2 per cent) were available for follow-up at a minimum of three years. The objective cure rate was 88.4 per cent with an improvement in 9.3 per cent of cases and there was no statistical difference in outcome as compared to the results reported at one year.

Post-operative complications

Whilst the trans-obturator route may be associated with a lower risk of bladder injury there is a risk of damage to the obturator nerve and vessels. In an anatomical dissection model the tape passes 3.4–4.8 cm from the anterior and posterior branches of the obturator nerve respectively and 1.1 cm from the most medial branch of the obturator vessels.[71] Consequently nerve and vessel injury in addition to buttock pain, bladder injury and vaginal erosion remain potential complications of the procedure.

Urethral bulking agents

Urethral bulking agents are a minimally invasive surgical procedure for the treatment of USI and may be useful in the elderly and those women who have undergone previous operations and have a fixed, scarred, fibrosed urethra.

Although the actual substance which is injected may differ the principle is the same. It is injected either peri-urethrally or transurethrally on either side of the bladder neck under cystoscopic control and is intended to 'bulk' the bladder neck, in order to stop premature bladder neck opening, without causing outflow obstruction. The procedure may be performed under local, regional or general anaesthesia. There are now several different products available (Table 95.2). The use of minimally invasive implantation systems has also allowed some of these procedures to be performed in the office setting without the need for cystoscopy (Fig. 95.9).

Outcome

In the first reported series 81 per cent of 68 women were dry following two injections of collagen.[72] There have been longer-term follow-up studies, most of which give a less than 50 per cent objective cure rate at two years but a subjective improvement rate of about 70 per cent.[73,74,75] Macroplastique has been compared to Contigen in a recent North American study of 248 women with USI. Outcome was assessed objectively using pad tests and subjectively at 12 months. Overall objective cure and improvement rates favoured Macroplastique over Contigen (74 per cent vs 65 per cent; p = 0.13). Whilst this difference was not significant subjective cure rates were higher in the Macroplastique group (41 per cent vs 29 per cent; p = 0.07).[76]

The role of Bulkamid in the management of women with USI has been investigated in an open-label multicentre European study of 135 women.[77] At 12 months the subjective

Table 95.2 Urethral bulking agents

Urethral bulking agent	Application technique
Gluteraldehyde crosslinked bovine collagen (Contigen)	Cystoscopic
Polydimethylsiloxane (Macroplastique)	Cystoscopic (MIS implantation system)
Pyrolytic carbon-coated zirconium oxide beads in β-glucan gel (Durasphrere)	Cystoscopic
Calcium hydroxylapatite in carboxymethylcellulose gel (Coaptite)	Cystoscopic
Polyacrylamide hydrogel (Bulkamid)	Cystoscopic

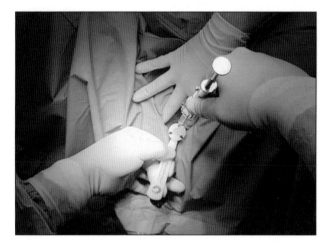

Fig. 95.9 Macroplastique: use of the Macroplastique implantation system under local anaesthesia

response rate was 66 per cent and there was a significant reduction in incontinence episodes (from 3.0 to 0.7 episodes per day) and pad test loss (from 29 g to 4 g). In addition the procedures were well tolerated and there was a corresponding improvement in QoL. The re-injection rate was 35 per cent. More recently a two-year follow-up has been reported documenting a subjective responder rate of 64 per cent and no deterioration in terms of objective outcomes. Reassuringly there were no reported safety concerns.[78]

Whilst success rates with urethral bulking agents are generally lower than those with conventional continence surgery they are minimally invasive and have lower complication rates meaning that they remain a useful alternative in selected older women or those with significant co-morbidities.

Single-incision mid-urethral tape procedures

Whilst the development of mid-urethral retropubic and trans-obturator tapes has transformed the surgical approach to stress urinary incontinence by offering a minimally invasive day-case procedure, there has recently been interest in

developing a new type of 'mini sling' which may offer a truly office-based approach. A number of single-incision tapes have been developed including the TVT Secur (Gynaecare) Fig. 95.10, MiniArc (American Medical Systems) and Ophira (Promedon) although the former has now been withdrawn.

Whilst there is an increasing evidence base to support their use at present there is a paucity of long-term efficacy data. A systematic review and meta-analysis has compared single-incision tapes with mid-urethral tapes in nine RCTs in 758 women.[79] Overall the single-incision tapes were associated with significantly lower patient-reported and objective cure rates (RR 0.83, 95% CI 0.70–0.99 and RR 0.85, 95% CI 0.74–0.97 respectively) although there was no difference in QoL improvement.

Consequently, whilst the single-incision mini tapes may offer a minimally invasive alternative to standard mid-urethral tapes, current evidence would suggest that efficacy may be inferior and further long-term studies are required.

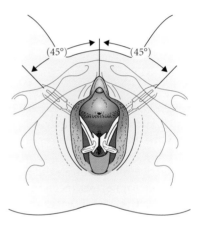

Fig. 95.10 Single incision tape (TVT Secur)

KEY POINTS

- Conservative measures should be offered prior to surgical intervention.
- Duloxetine may be used in conjunction with conservative measures.
- Mid-urethral tape procedures have largely replaced colposuspension as the operation of choice in primary continence surgery.
- Laparoscopic colposuspension has a comparable outcome to open colposuspension and TVT.
- Retropubic mid-urethral tape procedures and transobturator mid-urethral tape procedures have similar success rates.
- Urethral bulking agents offer an alternative minimally invasive approach to continence surgery.
- The role of single-incision mini tapes remains under investigation.

Nice guidelines

The management of stress urinary incontinence has recently been reviewed by NICE.[80]

- A trial of supervised PFMT of at least three months' duration should be offered as first-line treatment to all women with stress or mixed urinary incontinence.
- Retropubic mid-urethral tape procedures using a 'bottom-up' approach with macroporous (type 1) polypropylene meshes are recommended as treatment options for stress urinary incontinence where conservative management has failed.
- Open colposuspension and autologous rectus fascial sling procedures are recommended alternatives where clinically appropriate.
- Laparoscopic colposuspension should only be performed by experienced laparoscopic surgeons.
- Single-incision mini slings (SIMS) should only be used within the setting of a clinical trial.
- Intramural bulking agents (silicone, carbon-coated zirconium beads, hyaluronic acid/dextran copolymer) should be considered for the management of stress urinary incontinence if conservative management has failed although women should be made aware that repeat injections may be required, the efficacy diminishes with time and it is inferior to that of a retropubic suspension or mid-urethral tape.
- Anterior colporrhaphy, needle suspension procedures, paravaginal defect repair and the Marshall–Marchetti–Krantz procedure are not recommended.

OVERACTIVE BLADDER

Overactive bladder is the term used to describe the symptom complex of urgency with or without urge incontinence, usually with frequency and nocturia, in the absence of UTI or any other obvious cause.[1]

The symptoms of OAB are due to involuntary contractions of the detrusor muscle during the filling phase of the micturition cycle. These involuntary contractions are termed detrusor overactivity[1] and are mediated by acetylcholine-induced stimulation of bladder muscarinic receptors.[81] It has been estimated that 64 per cent of patients with OAB have urodynamically proven detrusor overactivity and that 83 per cent of patients with detrusor overactivity have symptoms suggestive of OAB.[82]

Detrusor overactivity

Detrusor overactivity is defined as 'a urodynamic observation characterised by involuntary detrusor contractions during the filling phase which may be spontaneous or provoked' (Fig. 95.11). The detrusor is shown objectively to contract (either spontaneously or with provocation) during bladder filling whilst the subject is attempting to inhibit micturition.[1] Detrusor overactivity is a urodynamic diagnosis and usually presents with symptoms of frequency, urgency, urge incontinence, nocturia, nocturnal enuresis and sometimes incontinence at orgasm.

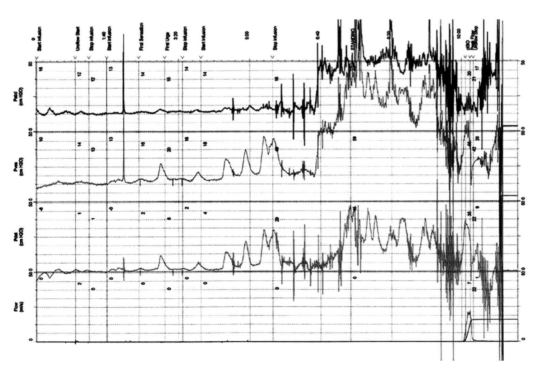

Fig. 95.11 Urodynamic trace showing detrusor overactivity

Prevalence

Epidemiological studies have reported the overall prevalence of OAB in women to be 16.9 per cent, suggesting that there could be 17.5 million women in the US who suffer from the condition. The prevalence increases with age, from 4.8 per cent in women under 25 years to 30.9 per cent in those over the age of 65 years.[83] This is supported by recent prevalence data from Europe in which 16,776 interviews were conducted in a population-based survey.[84] The overall prevalence of overactive bladder in individuals 40 years and above was 16.6 per cent and increased with age. Frequency was the most commonly reported symptom (85 per cent) whilst 54 per cent complained of urgency and 36 per cent urge incontinence. When considering management 60 per cent had consulted a doctor although only 27 per cent were currently receiving treatment.

More recently a further population-based survey of lower urinary tract symptoms in Canada, Germany, Italy, Sweden and the UK has reported on 19,165 men and women over the age of 18 years.[85] Overall 11.8 per cent were found to complain of symptoms suggestive of OAB and 64.3 per cent reported at least one urinary symptom. Nocturia was the most prevalent lower urinary tract symptom being reported by 48.6 per cent of men and 54.5 per cent of women.

Muscarinic receptors

Molecular cloning studies have revealed five distinct genes for muscarinic acetylcholine receptors in rats and humans and it has been shown that there are five receptor sub-types (M_1–M_5). In the human bladder there are M_2 and M_3 receptors and the latter is thought to cause a direct smooth muscle contraction. Whilst the role of the M_2 receptor has not yet been clarified it may oppose sympathetically mediated smooth muscle relaxation. In general it is thought that the M_3 receptor is responsible for the normal micturition contraction although in certain disease states, such as neurogenic bladder dysfunction, the M_2 receptors may become more important in mediating detrusor contractions.

Pathophysiology

A detrusor contraction is initiated in the rostral pons. Efferent pathways emerge from the sacral spinal cord as the pelvic parasympathetic nerves (S2, S3, S4) and run forwards to the bladder. Whilst preganglionic neurotransmission is predominantly mediated by acetylcholine acting on nicotinic receptors transmission may also be modulated by adrenergic, muscarinic, purinergic and peptidergic presynaptic receptors.

Acetylcholine is released by the post-ganglionic nerves at the neuromuscular junction and results in a coordinated detrusor contraction mediated through muscarinic receptors. However ATP also has a role,[86] mediated through non-adrenergic, non-cholinergic (NANC) receptors.

Conversely sympathetic innervation is from the hypogastric and pelvic nerves acting on β-adrenoreceptors causing relaxation of the detrusor muscle. Thus a balance between sympathetic and parasympathetic stimulation is required for normal detrusor function.

Detrusor overactivity a: outflow obstruction hypothesis

The association of detrusor overactivity with outflow obstruction has been recognised for some time[87] although it is more important in men than in women.

Outflow obstruction may lead to partial denervation and morphological studies have demonstrated a reduction in acetylcholine esterase staining nerves in obstructed human bladder.[88] In addition pharmacological studies have shown that muscle strips from patients with detrusor overactivity exhibit supersensitivity to acetylcholine.[89]

In addition outflow obstruction may alter the contraction properties of the detrusor muscle[90] leading to changes in cell-to-cell propagation of electrical activity and this in turn may lead to a higher incidence of instability of membrane potential.[91] These findings suggest that individual cells are more irritable when synchronous activation is damaged.

Outflow obstruction has also been shown to lead to the facilitation of the spinal reflex[92] mediated by C-fibres with increased expression of nerve growth factor (NGF) and tachykinins.[93] The latter have been shown to have an effect on spinal and supraspinal control of the bladder via neurokinin receptors.[94]

Detrusor overactivity b: neurogenic hypothesis

The pathophysiology of detrusor overactivity remains unclear. In-vitro studies have shown that the detrusor muscle in cases of idiopathic detrusor overactivity contracts more than normal detrusor muscle. These detrusor contractions are not nerve mediated and can be inhibited by the neuropeptide vasoactive intestinal polypeptide.[95] Other studies have shown that increased α-adrenergic activity causes increased detrusor contractility.[96]

There is evidence to suggest that the pathophysiology of idiopathic and obstructive overactive bladder is different. From animal and human studies on obstructive overactivity, it would seem that the detrusor develops postjunctional supersensitivity, possibly due to partial denervation,[97] with reduced sensitivity to electrical stimulation of its nerve supply but a greater sensitivity to stimulation with acetylcholine.[98] If outflow obstruction is relieved the detrusor can return to normal behaviour and re-innervation may occur.[99]

Detrusor overactivity c: urethral reflex

Relaxation of the urethra is known to precede contraction of the detrusor in a proportion of women with detrusor overactivity.[100] This may represent primary pathology in the urethra which triggers a detrusor contraction or may merely be part of a complex sequence of events which originate elsewhere. It has been postulated that incompetence of the bladder neck, allowing passage of urine into the proximal urethra, may result in an uninhibited contraction of the detrusor. However, Sutherst and Brown[101] were unable to provoke a detrusor contraction in 50 women by rapidly infusing saline into the posterior urethra using modified urodynamic equipment.

Detrusor overactivity d: myogenic hypothesis

Brading and Turner[102] have suggested that the common feature in all cases of detrusor overactivity is partial denervation of the detrusor which may be responsible for altering the properties of the smooth muscle, leading to increased excitability and increased ability of activity to spread between cells, resulting in coordinated myogenic contractions of the whole detrusor.[103] They dispute the concept of neurogenic detrusor overactivity, that is, increased motor activity to the detrusor, as the underlying mechanism in detrusor overactivity, proposing that there is a fundamental abnormality at the level of the bladder wall with evidence of altered spontaneous contractile activity consistent with increased electrical coupling of cells, a patchy denervation of the detrusor and a supersensitivity to potassium.[104] Charlton et al.[105] suggest that the primary defect in the idiopathic and neuropathic bladders is a loss of nerves accompanied by hypertrophy of the cells and an increased production of elastin and collagen within the muscle fascicles.

Detrusor overactivity e: urothelial afferent hypothesis

More recently the role of afferent activation in the urothelium and sub-urothelial myofibroblasts has been investigated as a factor in the pathophysiology of detrusor overactivity. C-fibre afferents are known to have nerve endings in the sub-urothelial layer of the bladder wall as well as in the urothelium. Studies have revealed that ATP is released from the urothelium by bladder distension[106] and this may lead to activation of purinergic receptors on afferent nerve terminals which in turn evokes a neuronal discharge leading to bladder contraction.

In addition prostanoids[107] and nitric oxide[108] are synthesised locally in the urothelium and are also released by bladder distension. It is probable that a cascade of stimulatory (ATP, prostanoids, tachykinins) and inhibitory (nitric oxide) mediators are involved in the activation of sensory pathways during bladder filling.[109] The role of C-fibres in the pathophysiology of detrusor contractions is also supported by the use of intravesical vanilloids (capsaicin and resiniferatoxin) in patients with idiopathic detrusor overactivity and hypersensitivity disorders.[110]

Management of detrusor overactivity

The treatment options for detrusor overactivity can be divided into conservative, pharmacological, neuromodulation and surgical options.

Conservative management

Conservative measures include advice regarding fluid intake. It may be that simply cutting down on the volume of fluid consumed throughout the day or altering the times at which drinks are taken will be enough to reduce the symptoms and improve QoL. Women should be advised to consume between 1 L and 1.5 L in any 24-hour period. It is not advisable to restrict fluid intake severely, as a low urine output together with frequent voiding can lead to a reduction in the bladder's functional capacity. Caffeine and alcohol are known to irritate the bladder, and women should be advised to try to avoid caffeine-based drinks or substitute them with decaffeinated drinks.

Bladder retraining

The principles of bladder retraining are based on the ability to suppress urinary urge and to extend the intervals between voiding. The regimen is generally initiated at set voiding intervals and the patient is not allowed to void between these predetermined times, even if she is incontinent. When she remains dry, the time interval is lengthened. This continues until a suitable time span is achieved, usually around 3–4 hours. Cure rates using bladder retraining alone and no pharmacological agents have been reported between 44 and 90 per cent.[111] Many professionals advise the combined use of pelvic floor exercises with bladder retraining, as this can help suppress the symptom of urinary urgency.

Pharmacology

Drug therapy has an important role in the management of women with urinary symptoms caused by OAB although there are none which specifically act on the bladder and urethra which do not have systemic effects. The large number of drugs available is indicative of the fact that none is ideal and it is often their systemic adverse effects which limit their use in terms of efficacy and compliance. The pharmacology of drugs and recommendations for usage has recently been reviewed by the 5th ICI[112] (Table 95.3).

Antimuscarinic drugs

The detrusor is innervated by the parasympathetic nervous system (pelvic nerve), the sympathetic nervous system (hypogastric nerve) and by NANC neurones. The motor supply arises from S2, 3 and 4 and is conveyed by the pelvic nerve. The neurotransmitter at the neuromuscular junction is acetylcholine, which acts upon muscarinic receptors. Antimuscarinic drugs should therefore be of use in the treatment of detrusor overactivity. Atropine is the classic

Table 95.3 Drugs used in the treatment of overactive bladder

	Level of evidence	Grade of recommendation
Antimuscarinic drugs		
Tolterodine	1	A
Trospium	1	A
Solifenacin	1	A
Darifenacin	1	A
Fesoterodine	1	A
Propantheline	2	B
Atropine, hyoscamine	3	C
Drugs acting on membrane channels		
Calcium channel antagonists	2	D
Potassium channel openers	2	D
Drugs with mixed actions		
Oxybutynin	1	A
Propiverine	1	A
Flavoxate	2	D
Alpha-antagonists		
Alfuzosin	3	C
Doxazosin	3	C
Prazosin	3	C
Terazosin	3	C
Tamsulosin	3	C
Beta-agonists		
Mirabegron	1	B
Terbutaline	3	C
Salbutamol	3	C
Antidepressants		
Imipramine	3	C
Duloxetine	2	C
Prostaglandin synthesis inhibitors		
Indomethacin	2	C
Flurbiprofen	2	C
Vasopressin analogues		
Desmopressin	1	A
Other drugs		
Baclofen	3	C (intrathecal)
Capsaicin	2	C (intravesical)
Resiniferatoxin	2	C (intravesical)
Botulinum toxin (idiopathic)	3	B (intravesical)
Botulinum toxin (neurogenic)	2	A (intravesical)

Reference: Andersson KE, Chapple CR, Cardozo L *et al.* Pharmacological treatment of urinary incontinence. *In*: Abrams P, Cardozo L, Khoury S, Wein A (eds). *Incontinence*. 5th edn. Paris: Health Publication Ltd, 2013, 623-728.

non-selective anticholinergic drug with antimuscarinic activity; however, its non-specific mode of action makes it unacceptable for clinical use because of the high incidence of side effects. All antimuscarinic agents produce competitive blockade of acetylcholine receptors at postganglionic parasympathetic receptor sites. They all, to a greater or lesser extent, have the typical side effects of dry mouth, blurred vision, tachycardia, drowsiness and constipation. Unfortunately, virtually all the drugs which are truly beneficial in the management of OAB produce these unwanted systemic side effects.

Tolterodine

Tolterodine is a competitive muscarinic receptor antagonist with relative functional selectivity for bladder muscarinic receptors. Whilst it shows no specificity for receptor subtypes it does target the bladder muscarinic receptors rather than those in the salivary glands. Several randomised, double-blind, placebo-controlled trials have demonstrated a significant reduction in incontinent episodes and micturition frequency[113] whilst the incidence of adverse effects has been shown to be no different to placebo. When compared to oxybutynin in a randomised double-blind placebo-controlled parallel group study, it was found to be equally efficacious and to have a lower incidence of side effects, notably dry mouth.[114]

Tolterodine has also been developed as an extended-release once-daily preparation. A double-blind multicentre trial of 1235 women has compared extended-release tolterodine to immediate-release tolterodine and placebo. Whilst both formulations were found to reduce the mean number of urge incontinence episodes per week the extended-release preparation was found to be significantly more effective.[115]

Extended release (ER) oxybutynin and ER tolterodine have also been compared. In the OPERA (Overactive bladder: Performance of Extended Release Agents) study, which involved 71 centres in the US, improvements in episodes of urge incontinence were similar for the two drugs although oxybutynin ER was significantly more effective than tolterodine ER in reducing frequency of micturition.[116]

In summary, the available evidence would suggest that tolterodine is as effective as oxybutynin although since it has fewer adverse effects patient tolerability and compliance are improved.

Trospium chloride

Trospium chloride is a quaternary ammonium compound which is non-selective for muscarinic receptor subtypes and shows low biological availability. It crosses the blood–brain barrier to a limited extent and hence would appear to have few cognitive effects.[117] A placebo-controlled, randomised, double-blind multicentre trial has shown trospium to increase cystometric capacity and bladder volume at first unstable contraction, leading to significant clinical improvement without an increase in adverse effects over placebo.[118] When compared to oxybutynin it was found to have comparable efficacy although was associated with a lower incidence of dry mouth and patient withdrawal.[119] At present trospium chloride

would appear to be as effective as oxybutynin although it may be associated with fewer adverse effects.

Solifenacin

Solifenacin is a potent M_3 receptor antagonist that has selectivity for the M_3 receptors over M_2 receptors and has much higher potency against M_3 receptors in smooth muscle than it does against M_3 receptors in salivary glands.

The clinical efficacy of solifenacin has been assessed in a multicentre, randomised, double-blind, parallel-group placebo-controlled study of solifenacin 5 mg and 10 mg once daily in patients with OAB.[120] The primary efficacy analysis showed a statistically significant reduction of the micturition frequency following treatment with both 5 mg and 10 mg doses when compared with placebo, although the largest effect was with the higher dose. The most frequently reported adverse events leading to discontinuation were dry mouth and constipation. These were also found to be dose related.

In order to assess the long-term safety and efficacy of solifenacin a multicentre open-label long-term follow-up study has been reported. This was essentially an extension of two previous double-blind placebo-controlled studies in 1637 patients.[121] Overall the efficacy of solifenacin was maintained in the extension study with a sustained improvement in symptoms of urgency, urge incontinence, frequency and nocturia over the 12-month study period. The most commonly reported adverse events were dry mouth (20.5 per cent), constipation (9.2 per cent) and blurred vision (6.6 per cent) and these were the primary reasons for discontinuation in 4.7 per cent of patients.

Solifenacin has also been compared with tolterodine ER in the Solifenacin (flexible dosing) od and Tolterodine ER as an Active comparator in a Randomised trial (STAR).[122] This was a prospective double-blind, double-dummy, two-arm, parallel-group, 12-week study of 1200 patients with the primary aim of demonstrating non-inferiority of solifenacin to tolterodine ER. Solifenacin was non-inferior to tolterodine ER with respect to change from baseline in the mean number of micturitions per 24 hours. In addition solifenacin resulted in a statistically significant improvement in urgency, urge incontinence and overall incontinence when compared with tolterodine ER. The most commonly reported adverse events were dry mouth, constipation and blurred vision and they were mostly mild to moderate in severity. The number of patients discontinuing medication was similar in both treatment arms (3.5 per cent in the solifenacin arm vs 3.0 per cent in the tolterodine arm).

Darifenacin

Darifenacin is a tertiary amine with moderate lipophilicity and is a highly selective M_3 receptor antagonist which has been found to have a 5-fold higher affinity for the human M_3 receptor relative to the M_1 receptor.

A review of the pooled darifenacin data from the three phase III, multicentre, double-blind clinical trials in patients with OAB has been reported in 1059 patients.[123] Darifenacin resulted in a dose-related significant reduction in median number of incontinence episodes per week. Significant decreases in the frequency and severity of urgency, micturition frequency and number of incontinence episodes resulting in a change of clothing or pads were also apparent, along with an increase in bladder capacity. Darifenacin was well tolerated. The most common treatment-related adverse events were dry mouth and constipation, although together these resulted in few discontinuations. The incidence of CNS and cardiovascular adverse events was comparable to placebo.

Fesoterodine

Fesoterodine is a novel derivative of 3,3-diphenylpropyl-amine which is a potent antimuscarinic agent that has more recently been developed for the management of OAB. A phase II dose-finding study was conducted in 728 patients in Europe and South Africa.[124] Fesoterodine 4 mg, 8 mg and 12 mg were all found to show significantly greater decreases in micturition frequency than placebo. The most commonly reported side effect was dry mouth with an incidence of 25 per cent in the 4 mg group, rising to 34 per cent in the 12 mg group. Discontinuation rates were 6 per cent and 12 per cent respectively. Subsequently a phase III randomised placebo-controlled trial has been reported comparing fesoterodine 4 mg and 8 mg with tolterodine ER 4 mg in patients complaining of OAB in 1135 patients at 150 sites throughout Australia, New Zealand, South Africa and Europe.[125] Both doses of fesoterodine demonstrated significant improvements over placebo in reduction of daytime frequency and number of urge incontinence episodes per day and were found to be superior to tolterodine. The current evidence from two large phase IV studies would support these findings and suggest that fesoterodine may offer some advantages over tolterodine in terms of efficacy and flexible dosing regimens.[126,127]

Drugs that have a mixed action

Oxybutynin

Oxybutynin is a tertiary amine that undergoes extensive first-pass metabolism to an active metabolite, N-desmethyl oxybutynin, which occurs in high concentrations and is thought to be responsible for a significant part of the action of the parent drug. It has a mixed action consisting of both an antimuscarinic and a direct muscle relaxant effect in addition to local anaesthetic properties. Oxybutynin has been shown to have a high affinity for muscarinic receptors in the bladder and has a higher affinity for M_1 and M_3 receptors over M_2.

The effectiveness of oxybutynin in the management of patients with detrusor overactivity is well documented. A double-blind placebo-controlled trial found oxybutynin to be significantly better than placebo in improving LUTS although 80 per cent of patients complained of significant adverse effects, principally dry mouth or dry skin.[128]

The antimuscarinic adverse effects of oxybutynin are well documented and are often dose limiting, with 10–23 per cent of women discontinuing medication.[129] Using an intravesical route of administration higher local levels of oxybutynin can be achieved whilst limiting the systemic adverse effects. Intravesical administration of oxybutynin is an effective and useful alternative for patients with neurogenic detrusor overactivity who need to self-catheterise or who suffer from 'bypassing' an indwelling catheter.

In order to improve tolerability a controlled-release oxybutynin preparation using an osmotic system (OROS) has been developed which has been shown to have comparable efficacy when compared with immediate-release oxybutynin but is associated with fewer adverse effects.[130] In order to maximise efficacy and minimise adverse effects alternative delivery systems are currently under evaluation. An oxybutynin transdermal delivery system has recently been developed and compared with extended-release tolterodine in 361 patients with mixed urinary incontinence. Both agents significantly reduced incontinence episodes, increased volume voided and led to an improvement in QoL when compared to placebo. The most common adverse event in the oxybutynin patch arm was application site pruritus in 14 per cent although the incidence of dry mouth was reduced to 4.1 per cent compared to 7.3 per cent in the tolterodine arm.[131]

More recently a large prospective multicentre, randomised, double-blind placebo-controlled study has been reported investigating the use of oxybutynin gel in the management of OAB in 704 patients.[132] Overall there was a significant reduction in urge incontinence episodes in the gel arm compared to placebo, a significant reduction in daytime frequency and an increase in volume voided. When considering adverse events dry mouth was more common in the treatment arm when compared to placebo (6.9 per cent vs 2.8 per cent) and skin site reactions were infrequent in both arms – 5.4 per cent and 1.0 per cent respectively. Consequently oxybutynin gel may represent an important development over the oxybutynin patch in terms of patient acceptability.

In summary, the efficacy of oxybutynin is well documented although very often its clinical usefulness is limited by adverse effects. Alternative routes and methods of administration may produce better patient acceptability and compliance.

Propiverine

Propiverine has both antimuscarinic and calcium channel-blocking actions. Open studies have demonstrated a beneficial effect in patients with overactive bladder[133] and neurogenic detrusor overactivity.[134] Dry mouth was experienced by 37 per cent in the treatment group as opposed to 8 per cent in those taking placebo, with dropout rates being 7 per cent and 4.5 per cent respectively. Overall propiverine was found to have comparable efficacy to oxybutynin but was better tolerated in terms of adverse effects.

More recently propiverine extended release has been introduced and been shown to be as effective as the immediate-release preparation in the management of overactive bladder.[135]

β₃ Adrenoceptor agonists

β₃ Adrenoceptor agonists have been shown to be effective in the management of OAB and mirabegron[136] has been recently been launched in the UK. β₃ adrenoceptor agonists induce bladder relaxation by the activation of adenyl cyclase with the subsequent formation of cyclic adenyl monophosphate (cAMP) and have been shown to increase bladder capacity with no change in micturition pressure and residual urine volumes.[137] β₃ adrenoceptor agonists may offer an alternative to antimuscarinic therapy whilst at the same time offering a better side-effect profile.[138] In addition the introduction of a new class of drug may offer the possibility of combination therapy which may minimise adverse events whilst maximising efficacy.

Tricyclic antidepressants

These drugs have a complex pharmacological action. Imipramine has antimuscarinic, antihistamine and local anaesthetic properties. It may increase outlet resistance by peripheral blockage of noradrenaline uptake and it also acts as a sedative. The side effects are antimuscarinic, together with tremor and fatigue. Imipramine is particularly useful for the treatment of nocturia and nocturnal enuresis. In light of relatively poor evidence and the serious adverse effects associated with tricyclic antidepressants their role in detrusor overactivity remains of uncertain benefit although they are often useful in patients complaining of nocturia or bladder pain.

Anti-diuretic agents

Desmopressin

Desmopressin (1-desamino-8-D-arginine vasopressin; DDAVP) a synthetic analogue of vasopressin has been shown to reduce nocturnal urine production by up to 50 per cent. It can be used for children or adults with nocturia or nocturnal enuresis,[139] but must be avoided in patients with hypertension, ischaemic heart disease or congestive cardiac failure. There is good evidence to show that it is safe to use in the long term and it may be given orally or as a buccal preparation. Desmopressin has also been used as a 'designer drug' for daytime incontinence[140] and also in the treatment of OAB.[141]

Desmopressin is safe for long-term use, however the drug should be used with care in the elderly due to the risk of hyponatraemia and the current recommendations are that serum sodium should be checked in the first week following the start of treatment.

Oestrogens in the management of overactive bladder

Whilst the effect of oestrogens on lower urinary tract function remains controversial there is evidence to show that oestrogen deficiency may increase the risk of developing OAB following the menopause. Animal data would suggest that oestrogen might inhibit the function of Rho-kinase in bladder smooth muscle, and hence effect smooth muscle contraction, whilst having no effect on its expression. Consequently oestrogen deprivation following the menopause may lead to the development of OAB symptoms.[142] In vitro work has has demonstrated that ovariectomised rats showed a significant decrease in voided volume and an increase in 24 hour frequency with an increase in basal and stretch-induced acetylcholine release. Conversely there was a reduction in acetylcholine release from nerve fibres. This may explain why there is a decrease in detrusor contractility following the menopause with a corresponding increase in the development of OAB symptoms. Interestingly oestrogen replacement therapy reversed these changes.[143]

Based on these findings oestrogen replacement following the menopause may lead to an improvement in physiological voiding function whilst at the same time reducing the risk of developing symptoms of OAB. Given the concerns regarding the use of systemic oestrogen replacement therapy the vaginal route of administration may offer a better treatment approach.

Oestrogens have been used in the treatment of urinary urgency and urgency incontinence for many years although there have been few controlled trials to confirm their efficacy. A double-blind placebo-controlled crossover study using oral oestriol in 34 post-menopausal women produced subjective improvement in symptoms,[144] although a double-blind multicentre study of the use of oestriol in post-menopausal women complaining of urgency has failed to confirm these findings.[145]

There is some evidence to show that vaginal 17β-oestradiol tablets (Vagifem) therapy may be useful in managing the symptoms of OAB and in particular improving the symptom of urgency.[146] A further double-blind, randomised, placebo-controlled trial has shown LUTS of frequency, urge, urgency and stress incontinence to be significantly improved although there was no objective urodynamic assessment performed.[147] However, some of the subjective improvement in these symptoms may simply represent local oestrogenic effects reversing urogenital atrophy rather than a direct effect on lower urinary tract function.

In a review of 10 randomised placebo-controlled trials oestrogen was found to be superior to placebo when considering symptoms of urgency incontinence, frequency and nocturia although vaginal oestrogen administration was found to be superior to placebo for the symptom of urgency.[148] Consequently the implications of these findings are that exogenous oestrogen therapy, particularly using the vaginal route of administration, may be useful in the management of OAB.

Intravesical therapy

Capsaicin

This is the pungent ingredient found in red chillies and is a neurotoxin of substance P-containing (C) nerve fibres. Patients with neurogenic detrusor overactivity secondary to multiple

UROGYNAECOLOGY AND SEXUAL HEALTH AND WELLBEING

sclerosis appear to have abnormal C-fibre sensory innervation of the detrusor, which leads to premature activation of the holding reflex arc during bladder filling. Intravesical application of capsaicin dissolved in 30 per cent alcohol solution can be effective for up to six months. The effects are variable (Chandiramani *et al* 1994) and the long-term safety of this treatment has not yet been evaluated.

Resiniferatoxin

This is a phorbol-related diterpene isolated from cactus and is a potent analogue of capsaicin that appears to have similar efficacy but with fewer side effects of pain and burning during intravesical instillation. It is 1000 times more potent than capsaicin at stimulating bladder activity. As with capsaicin, the currently available evidence does not support the routine clinical use of the agents although they may prove to have a role as an intravesical preparation in neurological patients with neurogenic detrusor overactivity.

Botulinum toxin

The use of intravesical botulinum toxin type A (onobotulinumtoxin) was first described in the management of patients with neurogenic detrusor overactivity[149] although there is now considerable evidence to support its usage in patients with idiopathic detrusor overactivity as well.

A randomised double-blind placebo-controlled trial of onobotulinumtoxin 200 IU has demonstrated a significantly greater improvement in urgency episodes, incontinence episodes and urinary frequency with onobotulinumtoxin when compared to placebo. The commonest side effects were UTI in 31 per cent of patients and voiding dysfunction necessitating self-catheterisation in 16 per cent of cases.[150]

These results are supported by a large phase III randomised double-blind placebo-controlled trial of onobotulinumtoxin 100 IU in 557 patients with idiopathic OAB. There was a significantly greater decrease in incontinence episodes with onobotulinumtoxin when compared to placebo (-2.65 vs -0.87, p <0.001) and incontinence resolved in 22.9 per cent vs 6.5 per cent of patients respectively. Once again UTI was the most commonly reported adverse event although the rate of urinary retention was found to be reduced to 5.4 per cent with the lower dose of onobotulinumtoxin.[151]

The efficacy of onabotulinumtoxin 100 IU has also been compared to antimuscarinic therapy (solifenacin 5 mg escalating to 10 mg and trospium chloride 60 mg) in a randomised double-blind placebo-controlled trial in 249 women. There was no difference between groups in the mean reduction of urgency incontinence episodes between the antimuscarinic arm and the onobotulinumtoxin arm (3.4 vs 3.3; p=0.81) and resolution of incontinence was reported by 13 per cent and 27 per cent of the women, respectively (p = 0.003). Whilst QoL improved in both groups, the antimuscarinic group had a higher rate of dry mouth (46 per cent

vs 31 per cent, p = 0.02) but lower rates of self-catheterisation at two months (0 per cent vs 5 per cent, p = 0.01) and UTIs (13 per cent vs 33 per cent, p <0.001).[152]

Consequently onobotulinumtoxin may be effective in managing women with refractory OAB symptoms and may be administered either under general anesthetic with a rigid cystoscope or under local anaesthetic with a flexible cystoscope. Whilst botulinum toxin type A (Botox®) is currently licensed in the UK for the treatment of neurogenic detrusor overactivity it is not currently licensed for the management of idiopathic OAB.

Neuromodulation

Sacral neuromodulation

Stimulation of the dorsal sacral nerve root using a permanent implantable device in the S3 sacral foramen has been developed for use in patients with OAB and neurogenic detrusor overactivity. The sacral nerves contain nerve fibres of the parasympathetic and sympathetic systems providing innervation to the bladder as well as somatic fibres providing innervation to the muscles of the pelvic floor. The latter are larger in diameter and hence have a lower threshold of activation, meaning that the pelvic floor may be stimulated selectively without causing bladder activity.

Prior to implantation temporary cutaneous sacral nerve stimulation is performed to check for a response and if successful, a permanent implant is inserted under general anaesthesia. Initial studies in patients with OAB refractory to medical and behavioural therapy have demonstrated that after three years, 59 per cent of 41 urinary urge incontinent patients showed greater than 50 per cent reduction in incontinence episodes, with 46 per cent of patients being completely dry.[153]

Whilst neuromodulation remains an invasive and expensive procedure, it does offer a useful alternative to medical and surgical therapies in patients with severe, intractable OAB prior to considering reconstructive surgery although technical failure may often necessitate surgical revisions.

Peripheral neuromodulation

Stimulation of the posterior tibial nerve in patients with urge incontinence was first reported in 1983[154] and has also been proposed for pelvic floor dysfunction.[155] The tibial nerve is a mixed nerve containing L4–S3 fibres and originates from the same spinal cord segments as the innervation to the bladder and pelvic floor. Consequently peripheral neural modulation may have a role in the management of urinary symptoms.

Posterior tibial nerve stimulation (PTNS) is performed by the insertion of a needle in the lower leg posterior to the tibia and two finger widths above the medial malleolus. Treatment is performed in the outpatient setting weekly for the first 12 weeks and then monthly maintenance therapy with each session lasting 30 minutes.

In a prospective multicentre study 35 patients with urge incontinence underwent 12 weekly sessions of PTNS with 70 per cent of patients reporting a greater than 50 per cent reduction in urinary symptoms and 46 per cent being completely cured.[156] In addition a randomised trial of PTNS vs sham stimulation has demonstrated improvement in 54.5 per cent of the active arm compared to 20.9 per cent in the sham arm.[157]

More recently a prospective randomised multicentre North American study has been reported comparing PTNS with tolterodine 4 mg ER in 100 patients. Overall there was an improvement in 75 per cent of patients with PTNS compared to 55.8 per cent with tolterodine ER and there was a significant improvement in QoL in both groups.[158] Furthermore a recent systematic review and meta-analysis has reported a subjective success rate of 61.4 per cent (95% CI 57.5–71.8) and objective success rate of 60.6 per cent (95% CI 49.2–74.7) and also demonstrated similar efficacy to antimuscarinic therapy.[159]

Consequently peripheral neuromodulation may offer an alternative therapeutic option for those patients with intractable OAB who have failed to respond to medical therapy.

Surgery

Approximately 10 per cent of women with OAB remain refractory to medical and behavioural therapy and may be considered for surgery. Various different surgical techniques have been developed although currently augmentation is the most commonly performed technique using a clam cystoplasty or auto-augmentation using detrusor myectomy.

Clam cystoplasty

In the clam cystoplasty[160] the bladder is bisected almost completely and a patch of gut (usually ileum) equal in length to the circumference of the bisected bladder (about 25 cm) is sewn in place. This often cures the symptoms of overactive bladder by converting a high-pressure system into a low-pressure system although inefficient voiding may result. Patients have to learn to strain to void or may have to resort to clean intermittent self-catheterisation, sometimes permanently. In addition, mucus retention in the bladder may be a problem and chronic exposure of the ileal mucosa to urine may lead to malignant change.

Detrusor myectomy

Detrusor myectomy offers an alternative to clam cystoplasty by increasing functional bladder capacity without the complications of bowel interposition. In this procedure the whole thickness of the detrusor muscle is excised from the dome of the bladder, thereby creating a large bladder diverticulum with no intrinsic contractility.[161] Whilst there is a reduction in episodes of incontinence there is little improvement in functional capacity and thus frequency remains problematic.[162]

Urinary diversion

As a last resort, for those women with severe overactive bladder or neurogenic detrusor overactivity who cannot manage clean intermittent catheterisation, it may be more appropriate to perform a urinary diversion. Usually this will utilise an ileal conduit to create an incontinent abdominal stoma for urinary diversion. An alternative is to form a continent diversion using the appendix (Mitrofanoff) or ileum (Koch pouch) which may then be drained using self-catheterisation.

KEY POINTS

- Bladder retraining should be considered as first-line therapy although it has high recurrence rates.
- There is a marked placebo effect associated with all pharmacological interventions.
- Oxybutinin is effective, although it may have significant adverse side effects.
- More specific antimuscarinic agents may have similar efficacy to oxybutynin but with fewer side effects.
- The beta 3 agonists are a new class of drug for treating OAB and have been shown to have similar efficacy with fewer adverse effects.
- Oestrogens are frequently prescribed, although there is little objective evidence to support their use.
- Botulinum toxin may offer a useful therapeutic option in patients with intractable detrusor overactivity.
- Neuromodulation may be an alternative to reconstructive surgery.
- Surgical interventions such as diversion are reserved for cases for which no other treatment has succeeded and quality of life is poor.

Nice guidelines

The medical management of OAB has recently been reviewed by NICE.[80]

- Patients should be counselled regarding caffeine and fluid intake.
- Those who are overweight (BMI >30) should be encouraged to lose weight.
- PFMT lasting for a minimum of three months should be offered to all women with mixed incontinence.
- Bladder retraining lasting for a minimum of six weeks should be offered to all women with mixed or urge incontinence.
- In those women who do not achieve satisfactory benefit from bladder retraining alone the combination of an antimuscarinic agent, in addition to bladder retraining, should be considered.

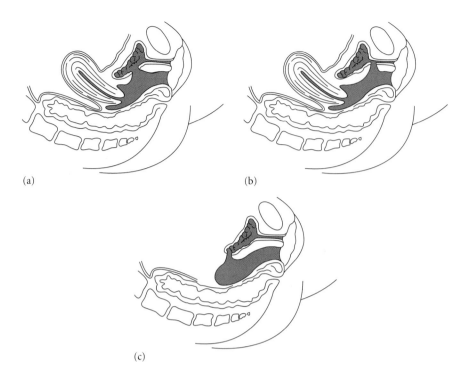

Fig. 95.12 Genitourinary fistulae. (a) Mid-vaginal fistula. (b) Urethral fistula. (c) Post-hysterectomy vesicovaginal fistula.

- Immediate-release non-propriety oxybutynin, tolterodine or darifenacin should be offered to women with OAB or mixed urinary incontinence as first-line drug treatment if bladder retraining has been ineffective.
- If first-line therapy is not well tolerated the drug with the lowest acquisition cost should be used as second-line therapy. Transdermal oxybutynin and mirabegron may also be used in patients who have had significant adverse effects with antimuscarinics. In addition women should be counselled regarding the adverse effects of antimuscarinic drugs.
- A medication review should be performed at four weeks. If there is clinical improvement then treatment should continue. If there is lack of efficacy or troublesome side effects then an alternative drug should be prescribed.
- Patients on medication should be followed up at 12 months. Those over the age of 75 years should be followed up at six months.
- Referral to secondary care should be considered if symptoms do not improve with primary or secondary therapy.
- Systemic HRT should not be recommended although intravaginal oestrogens are recommended for the treatment of OAB in postmenopausal women with urogenital atrophy.
- Patients referred to secondary care should be investigated with urodynamic investigations and their medical management discussed at a multidisciplinary team meeting.
- Patients who are happy to self-catheterise, have been taught how to do so, and have a diagnosis of detrusor overactivity, should be offered botulinum toxin.

- Sacral neuromodulation may be offered to patients who are unable to self-catheterise or who have failed on botulinum toxin.
- PTNS should be considered in women when botulinum toxin or sacral neuromodulation are not appropriate.
- If conservative measures fail those patients who are able to self-catheterise should be offered augmentation cystoplasty. Those who are unable to self-catheterise should be offered a urinary diversion.

URINARY FISTULAE

The development of a genitourinary fistula has profound effects on both the physical and psychological health of a woman. The most common simple genitourinary fistulae are (Fig. 95.12):

- vesicovaginal (42 per cent);
- ureterovaginal (34 per cent);
- urethrovaginal (11 per cent);
- vesicocervical (3 per cent).

The development of a fistula following surgery has considerable legal implications. Whilst most gynaecologists accept that the development of a fistula is deeply regrettable, it was generally thought that this was, on occasion, unavoidable. However, more recent legal cases involving ureteric injury would seem to refute that. There is a body of opinion that holds the view that ureteric damage can always be avoided and that not to do so constitutes negligence.

Vesicovaginal fistulae

Aetiology

The most common cause of vesicovaginal fistulae in the developed world is gynaecological surgery. The procedure with the highest incidence of post-operative fistula formation is a hysterectomy, either abdominal or vaginal. This accounts for about 75 per cent of cases. Particular risk factors include distorted anatomy, for example previous surgery, fibroids or endometriosis. Other procedures associated with fistula formation include anterior colporrhaphy, laparoscopic pelvic surgery and urological surgery. Fistula formation has also been associated with pelvic malignancy, pelvic trauma and radiotherapy.

In the developing world, the most common cause remains obstetric trauma. It is estimated that the incidence is 1–3/1000 deliveries in West Africa.

Presentation

The majority of women with a vesicovaginal fistula present with continuous leakage of urine, both day and night. This leads to discomfort and excoriation in the genital region as the urine irritates the skin of the vulva and thighs. However, if the fistula is relatively small, a woman may complain of increased vaginal discharge. The timing of presentation is variable, although the most common time to present is 5–10 days following surgery.

Diagnosis

A large fistula is usually obvious, and may easily be seen by examining the woman in the left lateral position using a Simms' speculum. Urine may be seen pooling in the vagina. If no fistula can be seen, useful diagnostic tests include the introduction of methylene blue into the bladder, via a urethral catheter. The blue dye may then be seen draining into the vagina. Alternatively, Bonney's 'three swab test', in which three swabs are placed in the vagina prior to instilling the dye, may help to locate the site of the fistula, which is indicated by the swab that emerges with the most dye. However, this may mask the presence of multiple fistulae. Intravenous urogram is not usually helpful in the diagnosis of a vesicovaginal fistula, but it is mandatory to rule out a ureterovaginal fistula or ureteric obstruction, which is seen concurrently in as many as 12 per cent of cases and is obviously very important when planning future treatment. If an IVU has failed to elucidate the ureteric anatomy, retrograde ureteropyelography should be undertaken at the same time as a cystoscopy and examination under general anaesthesia.

When the woman is anaesthetised, it is often possible to palpate the vaginal opening of the fistula tract. The vesical opening may be seen at cystoscopy, usually on the posterior wall or at the bladder base. If the fistula is not related to recent gynaecological surgery for a benign condition, both the vaginal and the vesical openings should be biopsied to exclude the possibility of malignancy.

Treatment

Treatment options range from simple conservative measures to more complex surgical procedures using either an abdominal or vaginal approach. In addition it is important to give general advice regarding the management of symptoms experienced as a result of the fistula. Barrier creams may help prevent the skin becoming sore and excoriated. Advice about incontinence pads, the increased risk of UTI and the need in some cases for prophylactic antibiotics may be required.

Urethrovaginal fistulae

In the developed world, these occur most commonly following an anterior repair with or without a vaginal hysterectomy. However, they may develop as a result of a urethral diverticulum or its repair or following bladder neck suspension procedures. In the developing world, the overwhelming majority are again caused by childbirth.

Symptoms vary depending on the site of the fistula. With a fistula higher up in the urethra there may be continuous incontinence; a fistula nearer the bladder neck may present with stress incontinence and recurrent UTIs; and one lower down may cause symptoms of spraying of urine at micturition or post-micturition dribble.

Women should initially be managed using a conservative approach with a urethral catheter, although almost all patients will need surgical repair. Due to the complex nature of such procedures this should be performed in a specialist centre.

KEY POINTS

- In the developed world, gynaecological surgery is the most common cause, with 75 per cent being attributable to hysterectomy.
- Obstetric trauma is the most common cause in the developing world.
- Most present between 5 and 10 days post surgery.
- Presentation varies from a mild discharge with small fistulae to continuous urine loss with larger fistulae.
- IVU is mandatory as part of the assessment because of high ureteric co-morbidity.

OVERFLOW INCONTINENCE AND VOIDING DYSFUNCTION

Symptoms

These may be a result of the voiding difficulty, such as:

- poor stream;
- prolonged voiding time;
- double void;
- incomplete emptying;

- hesitancy;
- frequency;
- nocturia;
- urgency;
- pain;
- abdominal distension;

or may reflect the underlying disease:

- abdominal distension, due to a mass such as fibroids or an ovarian cyst;
- pregnancy;
- peri-anal pain;
- peripheral paraesthesia;
- herpetic rash;

or a consequence of the voiding difficulties:

- recurrent urinary tract infections.

Aetiology

Neurological

The aetiology depends on the underlying neurological condition and the level at which the anatomy is affected. CNS conditions that commonly cause voiding difficulties include multiple sclerosis, spinal injuries, cerebrovascular accidents and brain tumours. Peripheral lesions include lesions at the sacral outflow, for instance a prolapsed intervertebral disc, cauda equina syndrome or herpes zoster.

Myogenic

This usually results from ischaemia due to acute retention, for example after an epidural block or spinal shock.

Iatrogenic

Post-operative retention is relatively common and may be associated with long operation times, epidural anaesthesia, patient-controlled analgesia, high doses of opiates and large volumes of intravenous fluids. It may also be associated with obstructive outflow procedures such as continence procedures.

Obstructive

This may be extrinsic, for example pregnancy or a large fibroid uterus, or intrinsic, such as a urethral stricture or foreign body. Alternatively, it may be as a result of kinking of the urethra, as can occur with a large prolapse.

Inflammatory

Any lesion may be sufficiently painful to inhibit the voiding reflex. This is seen, for instance, with vulval abscess or acute herpetic infections.

Diagnosis

Voiding difficulties should be suspected if a pelvic mass that is dull to percussion is palpable on clinical examination. The diagnosis can be confirmed using ultrasound. The patient is asked to empty her bladder and then an abdominal ultrasound scan can easily be performed to assess the residual urine. Alternatively, a urethral catheter can be inserted to assess the residual urine. In either case, it is very important that the residual volume is measured and accurately recorded.

Management

It is vital that all clinicians are aware of the complications associated with an episode of acute retention and that all possible steps are taken to avoid it happening. If it does occur, catheterisation should be undertaken as soon as possible and the catheter should be left in for at least two days, after which it is reasonable to undertake a trial without catheter, but only under strict supervision. If there is a further episode of retention, this should be managed with a suprapubic catheter and the bladder allowed to rest for a period of 2–6 weeks.

Medical therapy

Bethanechol 25 mg twice daily has been shown to enhance bladder emptying providing there is no evidence of outflow obstruction, although it is seldom useful clinically.

Surgery

If the voiding difficulties are a result of extrinsic compression, this is usually best treated by removing the underlying cause, for example a hysterectomy or myomectomy in the case of fibroids. However, in the case of pregnancy causing obstruction, supportive measures are usually used in the form of a urethral catheter until the uterus has grown a little more and the obstruction relieves itself.

If the obstruction is intrinsic, this may be treated by the removal of a foreign body or offending material. Alternatively, if a urethral stricture is suspected, a cystoscopy and an Otis urethrotomy may be required, in which case the patient would need to be counselled about having a urethral catheter on free drainage for two weeks on discharge from hospital and the possibility of post-operative urinary incontinence.

In the long term, intractable voiding difficulties may need to be treated with clean intermittent self-catheterisation. The patient needs to be able to perform the technique, and this usually requires a degree of manual dexterity in addition to willingness to undertake it.

CONCLUSION

Urinary incontinence is common and, whilst not life threatening, is known to have a significant effect on quality of life. Appropriate investigation and management allows an accurate diagnosis and avoids inappropriate treatment. Whilst many forms of conservative therapy may be initiated in primary care, continence surgery and the investigation of more complex and recurrent cases of incontinence should be performed in specialist secondary and tertiary referral units. Ultimately, an integrated pathway utilising a multidisciplinary team approach including specialist nurses, continence advisors, physiotherapists, urologists and colorectal surgeons will ensure the best possible outcomes in terms of 'cure' and patient satisfaction.

References

1. Haylen BT, de Ridder D, Freeman RM, Swift SE, Berghmans B, Lee J, Monga A, Petri P, Rizk DE, Sand PK, Schaer GN. An International Urogynaecological Association (IUGA)/International Continence Society (ICS) joint report on the terminology for female pelvic floor dysfunction. *Int Urogynecol J* 2010;21:5–26.

2. Kelleher CJ, Cardozo LD, Khullar V, Salvatore S. A new questionnaire to assess the quality of life of urinary incontinent women. *Br J Obstet Gynaecol* 1997;104:1374–9.

3. Hannestad YS, Rortveit G, Sandvik H, Hunskar S. A community-based epidemiological survey of female urinary incontinence: The Norwegian EPINCONT Study. *J Clin Epidem* 2000;53:1150–7.

4. Rortveit G, Hannnestad YS, Daltveit AK, Hunskaar S. Age and type dependent effects of parity on urinary incontinence: the Norwegian EPINCONT study. *Obstet Gynaecol* 2001;98:1004–10.

5. Norton PA, MacDonald LD, Sedgwick PM, Stanton SL. Distress and delay associated with urinary incontinence, frequency, and urgency in women. *Br Med J* 1988;297:1187–9.

6. Stewart WF, Corey R, Herzog AR et al. Prevalence of overactive bladder in women: results from the NOBLE program. *Int Urogynaecol. J.* 2001;12 (3):S66.

7. Bump RC. Racial comparisons and contrasts in urinary incontinence and pelvic organ prolapse. *Obstet Gynaecol* 1993;81:421.

8. Viktrup L. Lose G, Rolff M, Farfoed K. The symptom of stress incontinence caused by pregnancy or delivery in primiparas. *Obstet Gynaecol* 1992;79:945.

9. Chairelli P, Brown W, Mcelduff P. Leaking urine: prevalence and associated factors in Australian women. *Neurourol Urodyn* 1999;18:567

10. Hojerberg KE, Salvig JD, Winslow NA, Lose G, Secher NJ. Urinary incontinence; prevalence and risk factors at 16 weeks of gestation. *Br J Obstet Gynaecol* 1999;106:842

11. Gyhagen M, Bullarbo M, Nielsen T, Milsom I. A comparison of the long-term consequences of vaginal delivery versus caesarean section on the prevalence, severity and bothersomeness of urinary incontinence subtypes: a national cohort study in primiparous women. *BJOG* 2013;Jun 21.Epub.

12. Iosif C, Bekassy Z. Prevalence of genitourinary symptoms in the late menopause. *Acta Obstet Gynaecol Scan.* 1984; 63:257–60.

13. Cardozo LD, Tapp A, Versi E, Samsioe G, Bonne Erickson P (eds.). The lower urinary tract in peri- and postmenopausal women. In The urogenital Defiency Syndrome. *Bagsverd, Denmark: Novo Industri* AS;1987:10–17.

14. Jarvis GJ, Hall S, Stamp S, Miller DR, Johnson A. An assessment of urodynamic examination in incontinent women. *Br J Obstet Gynaecol* 1980;87:893–6.

15. Petros P & Ulmsten U. An integral theory of female urinary incontinence. Experimental and clinical considerations. *Acta Obstet Gynaecol Scand* 1990;153:(Suppl), 7–31.

16. Ingelman-Sundberg A. Urinary incontinence in women, excluding fistulas. *Acta Obstet Gynaecol Scand* 1953; 3:266-95.

17. Westbury M, Asmussen M & Ulmsten U. Location of maximal intraurethral pressure related to urogenital diaphragm in the female subject as studied by simultaneous urethra-cystometry and voiding urethrocystography. *Am J Obstet Gynaecol* 1982;144:408–12.

18. Berghmans LCM, Hendriks HJM, Bo K et al. Conservative treatment of stress urinary incontinence in women: a systematic review of randomised clinical trials. *Br J Urol* 1998; 82:181–91.

19. Kegel AH. Progressive resistance exercise in the functional restoration of the perineal muscles. *Am J Obstet Gynaecol* 1948;56:238–49.

20. Bo K. Pelvic floor muscle training is effective in treatment of female stress urinary incontinence, but how does it work? *Int Urogynaecol J Pelvic Floor Dysfunct* 2004;15:76–84.

21. DeLancey JOL. Anatomy and mechanics of structures around the vesical neck: how vesical position may affect its closure. *Neurourol Urodyn* 1988;7:161–2.

22. Bo K, Larsen S, Oseid S, Kvarstein B, Hagen RH. Knowledge about and ability to correct pelvic floor muscle exercises in women wit urinary stress incontinence. *Neurourol Urodyn* 1988;7:261–2

23. Miller JM, Ashton Miller JA, DeLancey JOL. A pelvic muscle precontraction can reduce cough-related urine loss in selected women with mild SUI. *J Am Geriatric Soc* 1998;46:870–4.

24. Bo K. Pelvic Floor muscle training in treatment of female stress urinary incontinence, pelvic organ prolapse and sexual dysfunction. *World J Urol* 2012;30(4):437–43.

25. Hay-Smith EJ, Herderschee R, Dumoulin C, Herbison GP. Comparisons of approaches to pelvic floor muscle training for urinary incontinence in women. *Cochrane Database Syst Rev* 2011;7:CD 009508

26. Herderschee R, Hay-Smith EJ, Herbison GP, Roovers JP, Heineman MJ. Feedback or biofeedback to augment pelvic floor muscle training for urinary incontinence in women. *Cochrane Database Syst Rev* 2011;7:CD 009252

27. Moore K, Dumoulin C, Bradley C, Burgio K, Chambers T, Hagen S, Hunter K, Imamura M, Thakar R, Williams K, Vale, L. Adult Conservative Management. Incontinence, 5th Edition. 2013. Eds Abrams P, Cardozo L, Khoury

S, Wein A. Health Publication Ltd, Editions 21, Paris, France. 1101–228.

28. Hay Smith J, Morkved S, Fairbrother KA, Herbison GP. Pelvic floor muscle training for prevention and treatment of urinary and faecal incontinence in antenatal and postnatal women. *Cochrane Database Syst Rev* 2008 Oct 8;(4):CD007471

29. Thor KB, Katofiasc MA. Effects of Duloxetine, a combined serotonin and norepineephrine reuptake inhibitor, on central neural control of lower urinary tract function in the chloralose-anesthetised female cat. *J pharmacol Exp Ther* 1995;274:1014–24.

30. Norton PA, Zinner NR, Yalcin I, Bump RC; Duloxetine Urinary Incontinence Study Group. Duloxetine versus placebo in the treatment of stress urinary incontinence. *Am J Obstet Gynaecol.* 2002;187(1):40–8.

31. Millard R, Moore K, Yalcin I, Bump R. Duloxetine vs. placebo in the treatment of stress urinary incontinence: a global phase III study. *Neurourol Urodynam* 2003;22:482–3.

32. Cardozo L, Drutz HP, Baygani SK, Bump RC. Pharmacological treatment of women waiting surgery for stress urinary incontinence. *Obstet Gynaecol* 2004;104:511–19.

33. Ghoniem GM, Van Leeuwen JS, Elser DM *et al.* Duloxetine/Pelvic Floor Muscle Training Clinical Trial Group. A randomised controlled trial of duloxetine alone, pelvic floor muscle training alone, combined treatment and no active treatment in women with stress urinary incontinence. *J Urol* 2005;173:1453–4.

34. Burch JC. Urethrovaginal fixation to Cooper's ligament for correction of stress incontinence, cystocele and prolapse. *Am J Obstet Gynaecol* 1961;81:281–90.

35. Leach GE, Dmochowski RR, Appell RA *et al.* Female Stress Urinary Incontinence Clinical Guidelines Panel summary report on surgical management of female stress urinary incontinence. The American Urological Association. *J Urol* 1997;158:875–80.

36. Ward KL, Hilton P. On behalf of the UK and Ireland TVT Trial Group. Prospective multicentre randomised trial of tension free vaginal tape and colposuspension as a primary treatment for stress incontinence. *Br Med J* 2002;325:67–70.

37. Alcalay M, Monga A, Stanton SL. Burch colposuspension: a 10–20 year follow up. *Br J Obstet Gynaecol* 1995;102:740–5.

38. Cardozo LD, Stanton SL, Williams JE. Detrusor instability following surgery for GSI. *Br J Urol* 1979;**58**:138–42.

39. Burch JC. Cooper's ligament urethrovesical suspension for urinary stress incontinence. *Am J Obstet Gynecol* 1968;100:764–72.

40. Cardozo L, Cutner A. Surgical management of incontinence. *Contemporary Reviews in Obsterics and Gynaecology* 1992;4:36–41.

41. Langer R, Lipshitz Y, Halperin R et al. Longterm (10-15 years) follow up after Burch colposuspension for urinary stress incontinence. *Int Urogynecol J Pelvic Floor Dysfunct* 2001;12: 323–6.

42. Jarvis GJ. Surgery for genuine stress incontinence. *Br J Obstet Gynaecol* 1994;101:371–4.

43. Lapitan MC, Cody DJ, Grant AM. Open retropubic colposuspension for urinary incontinence in women. *Cochrane Database of Systematic Reviews* 2005; Issue 3, Art.No.CD002912. DOI: 10.1002/1465 1858.CD002912.pub2.

44. Carey MP, Goh JT, Rosamilia A *et al.* Laparoscopic versus open Burch colposuspension: a randomised controlled trial. *BJOG* 2006;113:999–1006.

45. Kitchener HC, Dunn G, Lawton V, Reid F, Nelson L, Smith ARB on behalf of the COLPO study group. Laparoscopic versus open colposuspension – results of a prospective randomised controlled trial. *BJOG* 2006;113:1007–13.

46. Dumville JC, Manca A, Kitchener HC, Smith ARB, Nelson L, Torgerson DJ, on behalf of the COLPO study group. Cost effectiveness analysis of open colposuspension versus laparoscopic colposuspension in the treatment of urodynamic stress incontinence. *BJOG* 2006;113:1014–22.

47. Lyons TL, Winner WK. Clinical outcomes with laparoscopic and open Burch procedures for urinary stress incontinence. *J Am Assoc Gynecol Laparosc* 1995;2:193–8.

48. Ulmsten U, Henriksson L, Johnson P, Varhos G. An ambulatory surgical procedure under local anesthetic for treatment of female urinary incontinence. *Int Urogynaecol J* 1996;7:81–6.

49. Ulmsten U, Falconer C, Johnson P *et al.* A multicentre study of Tension Free Vaginal Tape (TVT) for surgical treatment of stress urinary incontinence. *Int Urogynecol J* 1998;9:210–13.

50. Ulmsten U, Johnson P, Rezapour M. A three year follow up of tension free vaginal tape for surgical treatment of female stress urinary incontinence. *BJOG* 1999;106:345–50.

51. Nilsson CG, Kuuva N, Falconer C *et al.* Long term results of the tension free vaginal tape (TVT) procedure for surgical treatment of female stress urinary incontinence. *Int Urogynaecol J* 2001;12 (suppl):5–8.

52. Nilsson CG, Falconer C, Rezapour M. Seven year follow up of the tension free vaginal tape procedure for the treatment of urinary incontinence. *Obstet Gynaecol* 2004;104:1259–62.

53. Nilsson CG, Palva K, Rezapour M, Falconer C. Eleven years prospective follow up of the tension free vaginal tape procedure for the treatment of stress urinary incontinence. *Int Urogynaecol J Pelvic Floor Dysfunct* 2008;19:1043–7.

54. Nilsson CG, Palva K, Aarnio R, Morcos E, Falconer C. Seventeen years' follow up of the tension free vaginal tape procedure for female stress urinary incontinence. *Int Urogynaecol J* 2013;24:1265–9.

55. Ward K, Hilton P, United Kingdom and Ireland Tension Free Vaginal Tape Trial Group. Prospective multicentre randomised trial of tension free vaginal tape and colposuspension as primary treatment for stress incontinence. *BMJ* 2002;325:67.

56. Ward KL, Hilton P, UK and Ireland TVT Trial Group. A prospective multicentre randomised trial of tension free vaginal tape and colposuspension for primary urodynamic stress incontinence: two-year follow up. *Am J Obstet Gyanecol* 2004;190:324–31.

57. Ward K, Hilton P; UK and Ireland TVT Trial Group. Tension-free vaginal tape versus colposuspension for primary urodynamic stress incontinence: 5 year follow up. *BJOG* 2008;115:226–33.

58. Manca A, Sculpher MJ, Ward K, Hilton P. A cost utility analysis of tension free vaginal tape versus colposuspension for primary urodynamic stress incontinence. *BJOG* 2003;110:255–62.

59. Paraiso MF, Walters MD, Karram MM, Barber MD. Laparoscopic Burch colposuspension versus tension free vaginal tape: a randomised trial. *Obstet Gyanecol* 2004;104:1249–58.

60. Nilsson CG. Tension free vaginal tape procedure for treatment of female urinary stress incontinence. *In*: Cardozo L, Staskin D (eds). *Textbook of Female Urology and Urogynaecology*. Abingdon: Informa Healthcare, 2010: 917-23.

61. Staskin DR, Tyagi R. The SPARC sling system. *Atlas Urol Clinic* 2004;12:185–95.

62. Deval B, Levardon M, Samain E *et al.* A French multicentre clinical trial of SPARC for stress urinary incontinence. *Eur Urol* 2003;44:254–8.

63. Lord HE, Taylor JD, Finn JC *et al.* A randomised controlled equivalence trial of short term complications and efficacy of tension free vaginal tape and suprapubic urethral support sling for treating stress incontinence. *BJU Int* 2006;98:367–76.

64. Delorme E. Trans-obturator urethral suspension: mini-invasive procedure in the treatment of stress urinary incontinence in women. *Prog Urol* 2001;11:1306–13.

65. Costa P, Grise P, Droupy S *et al.* Surgical treatment of female stress urinary incontinence with a trans-obturator tape (TOT). Uratape: short term results of a prospective multicentric study. *Eur Urol* 2004;46: 102–6.

66. Delorme E, Droupy S, De Tayrac R *et al.* Trans-obturator tape (Uratape) : a new minimally invasive procedure to treat female urinary incontinence. *Eur Urol* 2004;45:203–7.

67. Meschia M, Pifarotti P, Bernasconi F *et al.* Multicentre randomised trial of tension free vaginal tape (TVT) and trans-obturator tape in out technique (TVT-O) for the treatment of stress urinary incontinence. *Int Urogynaecol J Pelvic Floor Dysfunct* 2006;17:S92–3.

68. Laurikainen EH, Valpas A, Kiiholma P *et al.* A prospective randomised trial comparing TVT and TVT-O procedures for treatment of SUI: Immediate outcome and complications. *Int Urogynaecol J Pelvic Floor Dysfunct* 2006;17:S104–5.

69. Latthe PM, Foon R, Toozs-Hobson P. Trans-obturator and retropubic tape procedures in stress urinary incontinence: a systematic review and meta-analysis of effectiveness and complications. *BJOG* 2007;114:522–31.

70. Waltregny D, Gaspar Y, Reul O, Hamida W, Bonnet P, de Leval J. TVT-O for the treatment of female stress urinary incontinence: results of a prospective study after a 3 year minimum follow up. *Eur Urol* 2008;53:401–8.

71. Whiteside JL, Walters MD. Anatomy of the obturator region: relations to a trans-obturator sling. *Int Urogynaecol J Pelvic Floor Dysfunct* 2004;15:223-6.

72. Appell RA. New developments: injectables for urethral incompetence in women. *Int Urogynaecol* 1990;1,117–19.

73. Harris DR, Iacovou JW, Lemberger RJ. Peri-urethral silicone micro implants (Macroplastique) for the treatment of genuine stress incontinence. *Br J Urol* 1976;78:722–8.

74. Khullar V, Cardozo LD, Abbot D, Anders K. GAX collagen in the treatment of urinary incontinence in elderly women: a 2 year follow-up. *Br J Obstet Gynaecol* 1997;104:96–9.

75. Stanton SL, Monga AK. Incontinence in elderly women: is periurethral collagen an advance? *Br J Obstet Gynaecol* 1997;104:154–7.

76. Ghoniem G, Bernhard P, Corcos J *et al.* Multicentre randomised controlled trial to evaluate Macroplastique urethral bulking agent for the treatment of female stress urinary incontinence. *Int Urogynaecol J* 2005;16(2):S129–30.

77. Lose G, Sorensen HC, Axelsen Sm, Falconer C, Lobodasch K, Safwat T. An open multicentre study of polyacrylamide hydrogel (Bulkamid) for female stress and mixed incontinence. *Int Urogynaecol J* 2010;21:1471–7.

78. Toozs-Hobson P, Al-Singary W, Fynes M, Tegerstedt G, Lose G. Two year follow up of an open label multicentre study of polyacrylamide hydogel (Bulkamid) for female stress and stress predominant mixed incontinence. *Int Urogynaecol J* 2012;23:1373–8.

79. Abdel- Fattah M, Ford JA, Lim CP, Madhuvrata P. Single incision mini slings versus standard mid-urethral slings in surgical management of female stress urinary incontinence: a meta-analysis of effectiveness and complications. *Eur Urol* 2011;60:468–80.

80. NICE Clinical Guideline 171. Issued September 2013.

81. Andersson K-E. The overactive bladder: Pharmacologic basis of drug treatment. *Urology* 1997;50(6A Suppl.):74–84.

82. Hashim H, Abrams P. Do symptoms of overactive bladder predict urodynamic detrusor overactivity? *Neurorol Urodyn* 2004;23:484.

83. Stewart WF, Corey R, Herzog AR *et al.* Prevalence of overactive bladder in women: results from the NOBLE program. *Int Urogynaecol J* 2001;12(3):S66.

84. Milsom I, Abrams P, Cardozo L, Roberts RG, Thuroff J, Wein AJ. How widespread are the symptoms of overactive bladder and how are they managed? A population-based prevalence study. *BJU Int* 2001;87(9):760–6.

85. Irwin DE, Milsom I, Hunskaar S *et al.* Population-based survey of urinary incontinence, overactive bladder and other lower urinary tract symptoms in five countries; results of the EPIC study. *Eur Urol* 2006;50: 1306–15.

UROGYNAECOLOGY AND SEXUAL HEALTH AND WELLBEING

86. Burnstock G. Purinergic signaling in lower urinary tract. *In*: Abbracchio MP, Williams M (eds). *Purinergic and Pyrimidinergic Signalling I: Molecular, Nervous and Urogenitary System Function*. Berlin: Springer, 2001;151:423–515.

87. Abrams P. Detrusor instability and bladder outlet obstruction. *Neurourol Urodyn* 1985;4:317.

88. Gosling JA. Decrease in the autonomic innervation of human detrusor muscle in outflow obstruction. *J Urol* 1986;136:501–4.

89. Harrison SC *et al*. Bladder instability and denervation in patients with bladder outflow obstruction. *Br J Urol* 1987;60:519–22.

90. Van Koeveringe GA *et al*. Effect of partial urethral obstruction on force development of the guinea pig bladder. *Neurourol Urodyn* 1993;12:555–6.

91. Seki N, Karim OM, Mostwin JL. The effect of experimental urethral obstruction and its reversal on changes in passive electrical properties of detrusor muscle. *J Urol* 1992;148:1957–61.

92. Steers WD, De Groat WC. Effect of bladder outlet obstruction on micturition reflex pathways in the rat. *J Urol* 1988;140:864–71.

93. Steers WD *et al*. Nerve growth factor in the urinary bladder of the adult regulates neuronal form and function. *J Clin Invest* 1991;88:1709–15.

94. Ishizuka O *et al*. Role of intrathecal tachykinins for micturition in unanaesthetised rats with and without bladder outlet obstruction. *Br J Pharmacol* 1994;113:111–16.

95. Kinder RB, Mundy AR. Pathophysiology of idiopathic overactive bladder and detrusor hyperreflexia - an *in vitro* study of human detrusor muscle. *British Journal of Urology* 1987;60:509–15.

96. Eaton AC, Bates CP. An *in vitro* physiological, study of normal and unstable human detrusor muscle *British Journal of Urology* 1982;54:653–7

97. Sibley GN. Developments in our understanding of overactive bladder. *British Journal of Urology* 1997;80:54–61.

98. Sibley GNA. An experimental model of overactive bladder in the obstructed pig. *British Journal of Urology* 1985;57:292–8.

99. Speakman MJ, Brading AF, Gilpin CJ, Dixon JS, Gilpin SA, Gosling JA. Bladder outflow obstruction - cause of denervation supersensitivity. *Journal of Urology* 1987;183:1461–6.

100. Wise BG, Cardozo LD, Cutner A, Benness CJ, Burton G. The prevalence and significance of urethral instability in women with overactive bladder. *British Journal of Urology* 1993;72:26–9.

101. Sutherst JR, Brown M. The effect on the bladder pressure of sudden entry of fluid into the posterior urethra. *British Journal of Urology* 1978;50:406–9.

102. Brading AF, Turner WH. The unstable bladder: towards a common mechanism. *British Journal of Urology* 1994;73:3–8.

103. Brading AF. A myogenic basis for the overactive bladder. *Urology* 1997;50:57–67.

104. Mills IW, Greenland JE, McMurray G *et al*. Studies of the pathophysiology of idiopathic overactive bladder: the physiological properties of the detrusor smooth muscle and its pattern of innervation. *Journal of Urology* 2000;163(2):646–51.

105. Charlton RG, Morley AR, Chambers P, Gillespie JI. Focal changes in nerve, muscle and connective tissue in normal and unstable human bladder. *British Journal of Urology International* 1999;84(9):953–60.

106. Ferguson DR, Kennedy I, Burton TJ. ATP is released from rabbit urinary bladder epithelial cells by hydrostatic pressure changes – a possible sensory mechanism? *J Physiol* 1997;505:503–11.

107. Maggi CA. Prostanoids as local modulators of reflex micturition. *Pharmacol Res* 1992;25:13–20.

108. Birder LA. Adrenergic and capsaicin evoked nitric oxide release from urothelium and afferent nerves in urinary bladder. *Am J Physiol* 1998;275:F226–9.

109. Andersson KE. Bladder activation: afferent mechanisms. *Urology* 2002;59:43–50.

110. Silva C, Ribero MJ, Cruz F. The effect of intravesical Resiniferatoxin in patients with idiopathic detrusor instability suggests that involuntary detrusor contractions are triggered by C-fibre input. *J Urol* 2002;168:575–5.

111. Jarvis GJ, Millar DR. Controlled trial of bladder drill for detrusor instability. *Br Med J* 1980;281:1322–3.

112. Andersson KE, Chapple CR, Cardozo L, Cruz F, Gratzke, Lee KS, Tannenbaum C, Wein AJ. Pharmacological treatment of urinary incontinence. In Incontinence, 5th Edition. 2013. Eds Abrams P, Cardozo L, Khoury S, Wein A. Health Publication Ltd, Editions 21, Paris, France. 631–700.

113. Millard R, Tuttle J, Moore K *et al*. Clinical efficacy and safety of tolterodine compared to placebo in detrusor overactivity. *Journal of Urology* 1999:161:1551–5.

114. Abrams P, Freeman R, Anderstrom C, Mattiasson A. Tolterodine, a new antimuscarinic agent: as effective but better tolerated than oxybutynin in patients with an overactive bladder. *British Journal of Urology* 1998;81:801–10.

115. Swift S, Garely A, Dimpfl T, Payne C. Tolterodine Study Group. A new once daily formulation of tolterodine provides superior efficacy and is well tolerated in women with overactive bladder. *Int J Pelvic Floor Dysfunct* 2003;14(1):50–4.

116. Diokno AC, Appell RA, Sand PK *et al*. OPERA Study Group. Prospective, randomised, double blind study of the efficacy and tolerability of the extended-release formulations of oxybutynin and tolterodine for overactive bladder: results of the OPERA trial. *Mayo Clin Proc* 2003;78(6):687–95.

117. Fusgen I, Hauri D. Trospium chloride: an effective option for medical treatment of bladder overactivity. *Int J Clin Pharmacol Ther* 2000;38(5):223–34.

118. Cardozo LD, Chapple CR, Toozs-Hobson P *et al.* Efficacy of trospium chloride in patients with overactive bladder: a placebo-controlled, randomized, double-blind, multicentre clinical trial. *British Journal of Urology International* 2000;85:659–64.

119. Madersbacher H, Stoher M, Richter R *et al.* Trospium chloride versus oxybutynin: a randomised, double-blind multicentre trial in the treatment of detrusor hyperrflexia. *British Journal of Urology* 1995;75:452–6.

120. Cardozo L, Lisec M, Millard R *et al.* Randomised, double blind placebo controlled trial of the once daily antimuscarinic agent solifenacin succinate in patients with overactive bladder. *J Urol* 2004;172:1919–24.

121. Haab F, Cardozo L, Chapple C, Ridder AM, Solifenacin Study Group. Long-term open label solifenacin treatment associated with persistence with therapy in patients with overactive bladder syndrome. *Eur Urol* 2005;47:376–84.

122. Chapple CR, Martinez-Garcia R, Selvaggi L et al.; for the STAR study group. A comparison of the efficacy and tolerability of solifenacin succinate and extended release tolterodine at treating overactive bladder syndrome: results of the STAR trial. *Eur Urol* 2005;48:464–70.

123. Chapple CR, Steers W, Norton P *et al.* A pooled analysis of three phase III studies to investigate the efficacy, tolerability and safety of darifenacin, a muscarinic M3 selective receptor antagonist, in the treatment of overactive bladder. *BJU Int* 2005;95:993–1001.

124. Chapple C. Fesoterodine: A new effective and well tolerated antimuscarinic for the treatment of urgency-frequency syndrome: results of a phase II controlled study. *Neurourol Urodyn* 2004;23(5/6):598–9.

125. Chapple CR, Van Kerrebroeck PE, Junemann KP, Wang JT, Brodsky M. Comparison of fesoterodine and tolterodine in patients with overactive bladder. *BJU Int* 2008;102:1128–32.

126. Herschorn S, Swift S, Guan Z *et al.* Comparison of fesoterodine and tolterodine extended release for the treatment of overactive bladder: a head-to head placebo controlled trial. *BJU Int* 2010;105:58–66.

127. Kaplan SA, Schneider T, Foote JE, Guan Z, Carlsson M, Gong J. Superior efficacy of fesoterodine over tolterodine extended release with rapid onset: a prospective, head-to-head placebo controlled trial. *BJU Int* 2011;107:1432–40.

128. Cardozo LD, Cooper D, Versi E. Oxybutynin chloride in the management of idiopathic overactive bladder. *Neurourology and Urodynamics* 1987:6:256–7.

129. Kelleher CJ, Cardozo LD, Khullar V, Salvatore S, Hill S. Anticholinergic therapy: the need for continued surveillance. *Neurourology and Urodynamics* 1994;13:432–3.

130. Anderson RU, Mobley D, Blank B, Saltzstein D, Susset J, Brown JS. Once daily controlled versus immediate release oxybutynin chloride for urge urinary incontinence. OROS Oxybutynin Study Group. *J Urol* 1999;161(6):1809–12.

131. Dmochowski RR, Sand PK, Zinner NR, Gittelman MC, Davila GW, Sanders SW; Transdermal Oxybutynin Study Group. Comparative efficacy and safety of transdermal oxybutynin and oral tolterodine versus placebo in previously treated patients with urge and mixed urinary incontinence. *Urology* 2003;62(2):237–42.

132. Staskin DR, Dmochowski RR, Sand PK *et al.* Efficacy and safety of oxybutynin chloride topical gel for overactive bladder: a randomised double-blind, placebo controlled, multicentre study. *J Urol* 2009;181:1764–72.

133. Mazur D, Wehnert J, Dorschner W, Schubert G, Herfurth G, Alken RG. Clinical and urodynamic effects of propiverine in patients suffering from urgency and urge incontinence. *Scandinavian Journal of Urology and Nephrology* 1995;29:289–94.

134. Stoher M, Madersbacher H, Richter R, Wehnert J, Dreikorn K. Efficacy and safety of propiverine in SCI-patients suffering from detrusor hyperreflexia: a double-blind, placebo-controlled clinical trial. *Spinal Cord* 1999:37:196–200.

135. Junneman KP, Hessdorfer E, Unamba-Oparah I *et al.* Propiverine hydrochloride immediate and extended release: comparison of efficacy and tolerability in patients with overactive bladder. *Urol Int* 2006;77:334–49.

136. Khullar V, Amarenco G, Angulo JC *et al.* Efficacy and tolerability of mirabegron, a β_3 adrenceptor agonist, in patients with overactive bladder: results from a randomised European-Australian phase III trial. *Eur Urol* 2013;63:283–95.*Pivitol Phase III study of the new β_3 adrenceptor agonist, Mirabegron.

137. Igawa Y, Yamazaki Y, Takeda H *et al.* Relaxant effects of isoproterenol and selective beta3-adrenoceptor agonists on normal, low compliant and hyperreflexic human bladders. *J Urol* 2001;165:240.

138. Chapple CR, Kaplan SA, Mitcheson D *et al.* Randomised double-blind, active-controlled phase III study to assess 12 month safety and efficacy of mirabegron, a β_3 adrenceptor agonist, in overactive bladder. *Eur Urol* 2013;63:296–305.

139. Norgaard JP, Rillig S, Djurhuus JC. Nocturnal enuresis: an approach to treatment based on pathogenesis. *Journal of Pediatrics* 1989;114:705–9.

140. Robinson D, Cardozo L, Akeson M, Hvistendahl G, Riis A, Norgaard J. Anti-diuresis – A new concept in the management of daytime urinary incontinence. *BJU International* 2004;93:996–1000.

141. Hashim H, Malmberg L, Graugaard-Jensen C, Abrams P. Desmopressin as a 'designer-drug' in the treatment of overactive bladder syndrome. *Neurourol Urodyn* 2009;28:40–6.

UROGYNAECOLOGY AND SEXUAL HEALTH AND WELLBEING

142. Hong SK, Yang JH, Kim TB, Kim SW, Paick JS. Effects of ovariectomy and oestrogen replacement on the function and expression of Rho-kinase in rat bladder smooth muscle. *BJU Int* 2006;98:1114–17.

143. Yoshida J, Aikawa K, Yoshimura Y, Shishido K, Yanagida T, Yamaguchi O. The effects of ovariectomy and oestrogen replacement on acetylcholine release from nerve fibres and passive stretch induced acetylcholine release in female rats. *Neurourol Urodyn* 2007;26:1050–5.

144. Samsicoe G, Jansson I, Mellstrom D, Svanberg A. Urinary incontinence in 75 year old women. Effects of oestriol. *Acta Obstet Gynaecol Scand* 1985;93:57.

145. Cardozo LD, Rekers H, Tapp A *et al.* Oestriol in the treatment of postmenopausal urgency: a multicentre study. *Maturitas* 1993;18:47–53.

146. Benness C, Wise BG, Cutner A, Cardozo LD. Does low dose vaginal oestradiol improve frequency and urgency in postmenopausal women? *Int Urogynaecol J* 1992;3(2):281.

147. Eriksen PS, Rasmussen H. Low dose 17β-oestradiol vaginal tablets in the treatment of atrophic vaginitis: a double-blind placebo controlled study. *Eur J Obstet Gynaecol Reprod Biol* 1992;44:137–44.

148. Cardozo L, Lose G, McClish D, Versi E. Estrogen treatment for symptoms of an overactive bladder, results of a meta-analysis. *Int J Urogynaecol* 2001;12(3):V.

149. Schurch B, de Seze M, Denys P *et al.* Botox Detrusor Hyperreflexia Study Team. Botulinum Toxin Type A is a safe and effective treatment for neurogenic urinary incontinence: results of a single treatment, randomised, placebo contolled 6-month study. *J Urol* 2005;174:196–200.

150. Tincello DG, Kenyon S, Abrams KR *et al.* Botulinum Toxin A versus placebo for refractory detrusor overactivity in women: a randomised blinded placebo controlled trial of 240 women (the RELAX Study). *Eur Urol* 2012;62:507–14.

151. Nitti VW, Dmochowski R, Herschorn S *et al.*; EMBARK Study Group. Onabotulinumtoxin A for the treatment of patients with overactive bladder and urinary incontinence: results of a phase 3, randomized, placebo controlled trial. *J Urol* 2013 Jun;189:2186–93.*Large Phase III study investigating the use of Botulinum Toxin

152. Visco AG, Brubaker L, Richter HE *et al.* Pelvic Floor Disorders Network. Anticholinergic therapy vs. onabotulinumtoxin a for urgency urinary incontinence. *N Engl J Med* 2012 Nov 8;367:1803–13.

153. Seigel SW, Cantanzaro F, Dijkema H *et al.* Long-term results of a multicentre study on sacral nerve stimulation for treatment of urinary urge incontinence, urgency-frequency and retention. *Urology* 2000;56:87–91.

154. McGuire EJ, Shi-Chun Z, Horwinski ER *et al.* Treatment of motor and sensory detrusor instability by electrical stimulation. *J Urol* 1983;129:78.

155. Stoller ML. Afferent nerve stimulation for pelvic floor dysfunction. *Eur Urol* 1999;135:32.

156. Vandoninick V, van Balken MR, Finazzi Agro E *et al.* Posterior tibial nerve stimulation in the treatment of urge incontinence. *Neurourol Urodyn* 2003;22:17–23.

157. Peters KM, Carrico DJ, Perez- Marrero RA *et al.* Randomised trial of percutaneous tibial nerve stimulation versus sham efficacy in the treatment of overactive bladder syndrome: results from the SUmit trial. *J Urol* 2010;183:1438–43.

158. Peters KM, Macdiarmid SA, Wooldridge LS *et al.* Randomised trial of percutaneous tibial nerve stimulation versus extended-release tolterodine: results from the overactive bladder innovative therapy trial. *J Urol* 2009;182:1055–61.

159. Burton C, Sajja A, Latthe PM. Effectiveness of percutaneous posterior tibial nerve stimulation for overactive bladder: a systematic review and meta-analysis. *Neurourol Urodyn* 2012;31(8):1206–16.

160. Bramble FJ. The clam cystoplasty. *British Journal of Urology* 1990;66:337–41.

161. Cartwright PC, Snow BW. Bladder autoaugmentation: partial detrusor excision to augment the bladder without use of bowel. *Journal of Urology* 1989;142:1050–3.

162. Snow BW, Cartwright PC. Bladder autoaugmentation. *Urologic Clinics of North America* 1996;23:323–31.

Chapter 96 Other lower urinary tract disorders

Ganesh Thiagamoorthy and Sushma Srikrishna

INTRODUCTION

This chapter includes some disorders of the lower urinary tract which are seen less often. These are not necessarily well understood and there may be little evidence-based information regarding diagnosis or management. The established management is based largely on non-randomised, observational data and expert opinion.

BLADDER PAIN SYNDROME

Bladder pain syndrome (BPS), previously referred to as interstitial cystitis (IC), is defined as chronic pelvic pain, pressure or discomfort of greater than six months' duration, perceived to be related to the urinary bladder. This is usually accompanied by at least one other urinary symptom, such as persistent urge to void or urinary frequency.[1] BPS has a strong relationship with other pain syndromes, such as irritable bowel syndrome, fibromyalgia and chronic fatigue syndrome. Therefore, other diseases which may cause symptoms which are similar to those of BPS must be excluded (see Table 96.1). Based on this, a comprehensive article has been published by the European Society for the Study of Bladder Pain Syndrome/Interstitial Cystitis (ESSIC).[2]

The presence of other cognitive, behavioural, emotional and sexual symptoms should also be addressed. The diagnosis may change after findings at cystoscopy or bladder biopsies.

Historically, IC has been seen as a chronic severe inflammatory disease of the bladder that is difficult to diagnose and treat. It has been agreed by the members of the ICI that the term 'bladder pain syndrome' complies with the current knowledge and understanding of this syndrome.[3] However, BPS and IC are being used in parallel for the time being, as IC is a well-known term and omitting the name 'Interstitial cystitis' might cause reimbursement problems in different health systems.

PREVALENCE

The prevalence of chronic bladder pain in the general population due to benign conditions is at least 19 per cent.[4] The lack of a clear definition and valid diagnostic criteria have been deterrents to epidemiological studies of BPS. There is also an overlap of lower urinary tract symptoms such as frequency and urgency in conditions like overactive bladder and BPS.[5] In one study, 15 per cent of BPS patients also demonstrated detrusor overactivity at urodynamics.[6] This makes it difficult to estimate the true incidence. OAB however is not usually associated with pain, unlike BPS. The prevalence of painful bladder syndrome symptoms is 2.7–6.5 per cent in women depending on the sensitivity and specificity of the definition used.[7] Painful bladder symptoms are more common than suggested by coded physician diagnoses and show a female preponderance of 5:1 or more.[8] The presence of BPS is associated with a significant adverse impact on quality of life. There is a higher incidence of co-morbidities like anxiety, depression and overall mental health problems in BPS sufferers. Consequently, there is a six-fold increase in absenteeism from work due to sickness, over the general population.[9]

AETIOLOGY

Due to the lack of consensus relating to the definition and classification of BPS, the aetiology still remains obscure. However, there are several hypotheses with little evidence to support them. Inflammation and mast cell activation have been put forward as factors in ulcerative BPS. A defect in the glycosaminoglycan (GAG) layer has been proposed by some[10] and bladder epithelial dysfunction by others.[11] Although certain histopathological characteristics present in BPS patients are similar to autoimmune diseases, only a portion of BPS patients have auto-antibodies. Infection, autonomic nerve changes, disorders of nitric oxide metabolism, toxic agents, hypoxia and genetic susceptibility are other factors that are considered as possible aetiologies. Numerous propositions without solid evidence show that the aetiology of BPS is more complex than previously believed.

MANAGEMENT

History

Patients presenting with frequency and urgency need to be carefully questioned about other urinary symptoms. Associated urgency incontinence, dysuria or suprapubic pain may be relevant. If haematuria is reported, this must be investigated further. The presence of a UTI, bladder carcinoma, calculus or a lesion of the upper urinary tracts needs to be excluded. A thorough history should be undertaken with special emphasis on previous pelvic surgery, UTIs and urological diseases. Characteristics of pain including onset, correlation with events, description, location and relation to bladder filling and emptying must be sought. History of previous pelvic radiation treatment, chemotherapy and autoimmune diseases is also important.

Examination

Examination should be undertaken in the standing position for kyphosis, scars and hernia and in the supine position to assess abduction/adduction of the hips and hyperaesthetic areas. A neurological assessment is important to exclude an upper motor neuron lesion. The S2, S3, S4 nerve roots innervate the bladder and particular regard should be paid to these dermatomes. An abdominal examination will rule out a mass or large distended bladder. Vaginal examination should be performed with pain mapping of the vulvar region and vaginal palpation for tenderness of the bladder, urethra, levator and adductor muscles of the pelvic floor. Tenderness might be graded as mild, moderate or severe. Assessment of prolapse should also carried out via vaginal examination in the supine and standing positions.

Investigation

Initial investigation should always include a midstream urine sample for culture and sensitivity. If the woman is over 40 years of age with microscopic haematuria, or of any age with macroscopic haematuria, urine should also be sent for cytology. Appropriate cultures for 'fastidious organisms' (*Mycoplasma hominis*, *Ureaplasma urealyticum* and *Chlamydia trachomatis*), tuberculosis and schistosomiasis may be indicated.

A completed frequency–volume chart is an invaluable tool, providing useful information on fluid input and output, drinking habits, voided volumes and the episodes of urgency and incontinence. (Fig. 96.1 shows the frequency–volume chart used at King's College Hospital.) When the cause for the symptoms is not revealed by such assessment, more specialist investigations should be considered. Ultrasound scan can be used to assess residual bladder volumes accurately and to give more information on any masses detected on pelvic examination. Once a UTI has been ruled out, uroflowmetry, post-void residual urine volume and pressure–flow study may be performed.

In 1914, Hunner described the classic cystoscopic picture of a bladder ulcer with a corresponding appearance of patches of red epithelium exhibiting small vessels radiating to a central pale scar in patients with BPS.[12] Glomerulations, described as punctuate petechial haemorrhages observed after hydrodistension, have become the primary cystoscopic feature of BPS. However, these findings are not always present and do not correlate with the severity of the disease. There is also evidence that the cystoscopic appearance of the bladder wall after hydrodistension may not be constant over time and the absence of the initial findings of glomerulations or haematuria does not preclude further developments of these features on subsequent evaluation.[13]

There is also a considerable variation in the procedure of cystoscopy and hydrodistension. The ICI has recently recommended a standardised procedure using a rigid cystoscope to enable biopsies to be performed at the same time.[3] The bladder is filled using a dripping chamber at 80 cm above the symphysis pubis and filling is stopped after fluid dribbling stops. Continuous inspection is necessary to view the epithelium for radiating vessels, hyperaemia, oedema, cracks, scars or any other changes. When maximum capacity is reached, the distension should be maintained for 3 minutes. The bladder is then emptied and the degree of bleeding, if any, is noted. The total volume drained is the measured maximum bladder capacity. The bladder is then refilled to a third or two thirds of the capacity to look for changes and perform biopsies. At least two biopsies including detrusor muscle should be taken and used for mast cell counting in addition to biopsies taken from abnormal areas. Only the biopsy with the highest number of mast cells/mm^2 should be reported and 27 mast cells/mm^2 is considered indicative of mastocytosis.[14]

Confusable diseases can be mistaken for BPS or BPS may coexist together with other disorders,[15] such as chronic or remitting urinary infections or endometriosis. Endometriosis accounts for 70–90 per cent of pelvic pain in pre-menopausal women referred to a gynaecological pain unit and 93 per cent had some urinary symptoms as well.[16,17] The diagnosis of BPS is usually made on the basis of exclusion of these disorders. If the main urinary symptoms are not explained by a single diagnosis, the presence of a second diagnosis should be considered. Table 96.1 lists some of these confusable diseases related to BPS and the diagnostic procedures to exclude them.

TREATMENT

Conservative treatment

In motivated patients, behavioural therapy has been noted to be efficacious in treating urinary frequency and urgency without any side effects. Behavioural therapy includes timed voiding, controlled fluid intake, pelvic floor muscle training and bladder training. Physical therapy for the pelvic floor is effective for genitourinary and anorectal disorders. Biofeedback and soft tissue massage may help in the relaxation of the pelvic

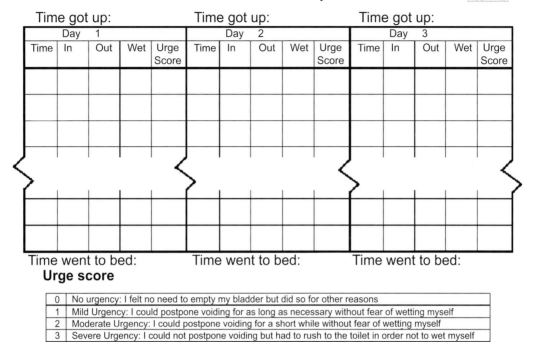

KING'S
College
LONDON
Founded 1829

Urogynaecology Department
Bladder Diary

Time got up: _____   **Time got up:** _____   **Time got up:** _____

Day 1					Day 2					Day 3				
Time	In	Out	Wet	Urge Score	Time	In	Out	Wet	Urge Score	Time	In	Out	Wet	Urge Score

Time went to bed: _____   **Time went to bed:** _____   **Time went to bed:** _____

Urge score

0	No urgency: I felt no need to empty my bladder but did so for other reasons
1	Mild Urgency: I could postpone voiding for as long as necessary without fear of wetting myself
2	Moderate Urgency: I could postpone voiding for a short while without fear of wetting myself
3	Severe Urgency: I could not postpone voiding but had to rush to the toilet in order not to wet myself
4	Urge Incontinence: I leaked before arriving at the toilet

Fig. 96.1 An example frequency–volume chart with an urgency scale

Table 96.1 'Confusable diseases' and the diagnostic procedures to exclude them

Confusable disease	Exclude or confirm by:
Carcinoma	Cystoscopy and biopsy, MRI
Common intestinal bacteria	Routine bacterial culture
Chlamydia trachomatis, Ureaplasma urealyticum	Special cultures *Mycoplasma hominis, Mycoplasma genitalium, Corynebacterium urealyticum, Candida* sp.
Mycobacterium tuberculosis	If dipstick shows sterile pyuria culture
Herpes simplex virus and human papilloma virus	Physical examination
Radiation	Medical history
Chemotherapy	Medical history
Bladder neck obstruction	Uroflowmetry and ultrasound
Bladder stone	Imaging or cystoscopy
Urethral diverticulum	History, examination, micturating cysto-urethrogram (video-urodynamics), MRI
Urogenital prolapse	History and examination
Endometriosis	History, examination, transvaginal ultrasound scan and laparoscopy
Cervical, uterine and ovarian cancer	History, examination/colposcopy/hysteroscopy, transvaginal ultrasound scan and CT/MRI
Incomplete bladder emptying	History and ultrasound
Overactive bladder	Urodynamics
Pudendal nerve entrapment	History and examination
Pelvic floor muscle-related pain	History and examination

UROGYNAECOLOGY AND SEXUAL HEALTH AND WELLBEING

floor muscles. Stress reduction and dietary manipulation are other methods of conservative management which have been shown to be effective.[18]

Oral medications

Several groups of drugs have been used in the management of BPS. These include non-opioid analgesics e.g. paracetamol and NSAIDs, gabapentin and pregabalin. Opioid analgesics are used as a last resort and better administered in a pain clinic to reduce the incidence of addiction. Amitriptyline is a tricyclic antidepressant with the property of blocking H1-histaminergic receptors. It stabilises mast cells, inhibits painful nociception from the bladder and facilitates urine storage.

The most widely used antihistamine for BPS is hydroxyzine. It also inhibits bladder mast cell activation and has anticholinergic and anxiolytic properties.[19] In addition, it has a good safety profile which makes it desirable. Sodium pentosanpolysulphate (PPS) is the most intensively studied treatment for BPS and is the only medication approved by the Food and Drug Administration for the pain of interstitial cystitis. A defective GAG layer is hypothesised to be one of the important causes of BPS and PPS may replenish it.[20]

Intravesical medications

Intravesical therapies are the next line of treatment in patients in whom oral medications have failed. DMSO (dimethyl sulphoxide) has been used as a therapy for BPS for a long time. It is believed to reduce inflammation, degranulate mast cells, relax muscles and eliminate pain.[21] The exact mechanism of action, however, is not known. The instillation is performed weekly for 6–8 weeks and treatment is suspended after an initial course until symptoms recur. A further 6-week course with monthly maintenance can be initiated if the results are good. Heparin, hyaluronic acid, chondroitin sulphate, PPS, capsaicin, resiniferatoxin, BCG, oxybutynin and lidocaine are other agents used.

Cystoscopic hydrodistension has been shown to have variable benefit but this is short lived and bladder rupture and voiding dysfunction are possible risks.[22] Fulguration of Hunner's ulcers has been shown to improve symptoms in patients with repeat treatments required within 11–23 months.[23] Intravesical botulinum toxin type A injections have been shown to improve symptoms of BPS but patients must be monitored due to significant risk of urinary retention and UTIs.[24]

Surgical treatment

Although BPS is a chronic and debilitating disease, surgical management should only be considered when other conservative and medical therapies have been unsuccessful. Bladder augmentation cystoplasty has been used for refractory BPS for 50 years.[25] Urinary diversion with or without total cystectomy and urethrectomy is the ultimate, final and most invasive option. It should be used as a last therapeutic resort in selected patients. Urinary diversion with formation of an ileal conduit is the most common surgical treatment for BPS/IC. Initially, diversion can be performed without cystectomy, and only when bladder pain is persistent, cystectomy may be considered. To avoid further bowel resection, a bowel segment used for cystoplasty can often be converted to a conduit.

KEY POINTS

- BPS is defined as chronic pelvic pain, pressure or discomfort, related to the urinary bladder accompanied by urgency and/or urinary frequency.
- 'Confusable diseases' as the cause of the symptoms must be excluded.
- The initial assessment should consist of a frequency-volume chart, focused physical examination, urinalysis and urine culture.
- Urine cytology and cystoscopy are recommended.
- Patient education, dietary manipulation and pelvic floor relaxation techniques comprise the initial treatment of BPS.
- When conservative therapy fails oral medication, intravesical treatment should be offered.
- If medical therapy fails, further evaluation should include urodynamics, pelvic imaging and cystoscopy with distension, and biopsy under anaesthesia.
- Urinary diversion with or without cystectomy may be the ultimate option for refractory patients.

URETHRAL CARUNCLES

Urethral caruncles are found only in women, typically in post-menopausal women and pre-pubertal girls. They usually represent ectropion of the urethral wall secondary to hypo-oestrogenic regression of the vaginal epithelium. Urethral prolapse may be mistakenly diagnosed as a caruncle in a child. On physical examination, a urethral caruncle is seen as a solitary red polypoid lesion protruding from one segment of the urethral meatus, usually the posterior aspect. Most caruncles measure only a few millimetres in diameter. The caruncle consists of well-vascularised transitional epithelium and is sometimes uncomfortable during voiding, but more often does not give rise to any urinary symptoms. The patient may alternatively present with post-menopausal 'spotting'. Initial treatment is with topical oestrogen therapy. If the lesion does not respond to oestrogen, it is important to biopsy it to exclude more serious pathology. Once malignancy is ruled out, it can be treated by either excision or cautery. There is a high rate of recurrence.

URETHRAL PROBLEMS

The female urethra is a complex muscular tube, approximately 4 cm in length. It is composed of several layers of muscle, the richly vascular submucosa and the urothelium. There is considerable debate regarding the relative roles of different components of the muscles, both within the wall of the urethra and surrounding it, in maintaining continence. A number of changes occur to the urethra with age. The strength and the amount of urethral connective tissue fall as a result of oestrogen deficiency. This causes the support of the urethrovesical junction to weaken. In addition, urethral vascular pulsations in the submucosal plexus gradually decrease with age.

Urethritis

Urethritis is inflammation of the urethra leading to symptoms of frequency, urgency, dysuria and localised urethral pain. It is caused either by an infectious pathogen or by chemical irritation. Evidence of the use of causative chemical agents, such as bubble baths, vaginal deodorants and perfumed cosmetics, should be sought as part of the medical history in women with such symptoms. Responsible infectious agents include many of the microorganisms associated with sexually transmitted infections, such as herpes simplex virus, *Neisseria gonorrhoeae* and *Chlamydia*. The group of organisms that typically cause acute bacterial cystitis, such as *Escherichia coli*, may also cause urethritis. Where urethritis is suspected, appropriate cultures should be taken from the urethra and vagina, as well as a midstream urine culture. Urine microscopy typically shows evidence of pyuria and bacteria.

Acute urinary retention can occur secondary to urethritis and needs to be considered. Prompt treatment with an indwelling catheter until symptoms have resolved is important in order to prevent overdistension of the bladder. The initiation of treatment with the appropriate antibiotic usually results in a rapid recovery, but scarring of the urethra can result in strictures and subsequent voiding difficulties. Referral to a genito-urinary medicine clinic for contact tracing and treatment of partners is important if sexually transmitted organisms are responsible. Cessation of the use of the offending chemical agent results in fairly rapid resolution of symptoms without the need for further treatment.

Urethral diverticulum

A urethral diverticulum is usually found on the anterior vaginal wall along the distal two thirds of the urethra, bulging into the vagina. They are occasionally found congenitally, but thought to arise more often from repeated inflammation of the para-urethral glands. Urethral diverticula are formed as a consequence of infected peri-urethral glands or cysts rupturing into the urethral lumen.[26] Common organisms include *Escherichia coli*, *Gonococcus* and *Chlamydia*. The presenting symptoms vary, but usually include frequency, dysuria, dyspareunia, voiding difficulties and recurrent UTIs. The classical symptom associated with this condition is post-micturition dribble, caused by the delay in the diverticulum draining after voiding.

On vaginal examination, it is sometimes possible to palpate a sub-urethral mass or even a calculus that has formed in the diverticulum. An infected urethral diverticulum is tender on examination and clear urine or purulent material can be expressed from the urethral meatus on compression. Alternatively, there may be no physical signs. However, Neitlich *et al.* demonstrated that high-resolution, fast-spin echo MRI has a higher sensitivity for detecting diverticula and has a higher negative predictive rate than double-balloon urethrography.[27]

Sometimes, a urethral diverticulum may be found incidentally as part of X-ray screening during videourodynamics (Fig. 96.2). Similarly, they may be seen on transvaginal ultrasound examination. Urethral pressure profilometry shows a characteristic 'saddle-shaped dip' in urethral closure pressure and gives useful information about the position of the opening of the diverticulum relative to the urethral sphincter and bladder neck. If a patient has symptoms suggestive of a diverticulum and a diagnosis is required, a voiding cystourethrogram or a positive-pressure double-balloon urethrography using a Trattner catheter will give useful information about the size and position of the defect prior to surgery. These lesions are not always easy to see on cystourethroscopy unless the opening into the diverticulum is large.

Surgical repair is usually undertaken if the patient has related symptoms, such as suffering from recurrent urinary infections. Endoscopic incision has been described, but transvaginal excision is the preferred treatment.[28] The techniques described include marsupialisation and vaginal diverticulectomy. There are no good long-term studies to guide clinicians as

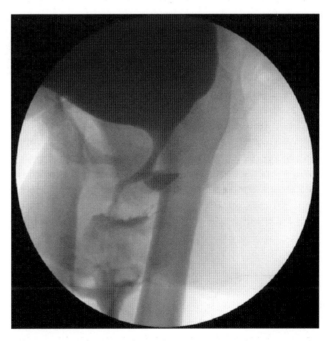

Fig. 96.2 A urethral diverticulum is clearly seen during the voiding phase of videourodynamic assessment

to the best surgical techniques for treating urethral diverticula. Recurrence is fairly common, especially if there has been failure to remove the whole sac. If the diverticulum is small and not causing any problems, it is better left alone.

Iatrogenic urinary tract injury

Damage to the urinary tract at the time of pelvic surgery is an important consideration for all gynaecological surgeons. It is estimated to occur in 0.5–2.5 per cent of routine pelvic operations and in as many as 30 per cent of radical pelvic procedures for malignancy.[29] Common types of iatrogenic ureteric injuries, in descending order of frequency, are ligation, kinking by suture, transection/avulsion, partial transection, crush and devascularisation.[30] Although relatively uncommon, when ureteric injury does occur, it presents a difficult challenge both to identify the injury and then to repair the damage. A good understanding of female pelvic anatomy and how this may be altered as the result of previous surgery or pelvic pathology is essential in order to minimise the risk of inadvertently damaging the urinary tract. Prompt recognition of the injury and the early involvement of an experienced urologist are important in ensuring a good outcome.

Aetiology

There are three common sites of ureteric injury during gynaecological surgery:

1 at the point where the ureters cross over the pelvic brim and enter the pelvis in close proximity to the ovarian vessels;

2 as the ureters course medially in the base of the broad ligament with the uterine artery crossing directly over the top of them; this is the site at which the ureters may be crushed by a clamp or divided while taking the uterine pedicle at hysterectomy;

3 at the ureterovesical junction as the ureters sweep medially to enter the bladder.

Any disease process that alters the normal anatomical course of the ureters or that makes their intraoperative identification more difficult increases the risk of injury. Malignant disease, advanced-stage endometriosis and previous abdominal surgery or radiotherapy all make it more difficult to predict the path of the ureters. Similarly, the normal anatomical relations of the bladder are often distorted in these circumstances. It is often wise to consider the use of a pre-operative intravenous urogram or the placement of ureteric stents at cystoscopy before proceeding to complex pelvic surgery. The path of the ureters should always be identified prior to any extensive pelvic dissection.

Management

A keen awareness of the proximity of the lower urinary tract during gynaecological surgery is the key to preventing these injuries. Such damage is largely preventable and forms an ever-increasing source of medical litigation. The success of managing these problems once they occur is largely dependent on whether the injury was detected at the time of operation and on close liaison with urological colleagues. Most bladder injuries are relatively straightforward to repair, provided they are identified intraoperatively.

Methylene blue dye instilled into the bladder via a urethral catheter can aid in the identification of bladder injuries. If damage is found, associated ureteric injury should also be borne in mind. The bladder can be satisfactorily repaired with two layers of absorbable suture and left to drain freely with an indwelling catheter for 10–14 days. The bladder heals well and the prognosis for such repairs is extremely good.

If ureteric injury is suspected intra-operatively, the advice of a urologist should be sought. The course of the ureter above and below the area of concern needs to be demonstrated. Indigo carmine dye can be given intravenously to aid in checking the integrity of the ureters. The most appropriate method of repairing damage to the ureter depends largely on the site of the injury and should only ever be undertaken by an experienced surgeon with appropriate urological training. It is not appropriate for a gynaecologist who has not received such training to embark on these procedures. The most commonly employed techniques for repair of injuries to the mid-ureter are summarised in Box 96.1.

In those cases in which injury to the lower urinary tract goes unnoticed at the time of operation, the patient is likely to develop symptoms and signs within a few days postoperatively. These may include fever, abdominal or flank pain, abdominal distension, sepsis, decreased urine output and rising serum creatinine and leukocytosis. These result from the extravasation of urine into the peritoneal cavity or from ureteric obstruction. However, the presentation may be delayed and the patient subsequently complains of persistent discharge from a fistula or abdominal wound. Anuria may occur if there is bilateral ureteric injury. Sometimes, ureteric obstruction is only discovered many years later as an incidental finding.

If damage to the bladder or ureters is suspected post-operatively, an intravenous urogram is the diagnostic study of choice.[31] Repair of the damaged bladder is dependent upon the extent of urinary leakage. Extraperitoneal injuries and small leaks in women who are still voiding spontaneously can be managed with a trial of catheter drainage for 10–14 days

---

Box 96.1 Possible methods of repair

- Mid-ureteric injuries
  - Boari flap
  - Primary ureteric anastomosis (uretero-ureterostomy)
  - Ureteric anastomosis to the contralateral ureter (transuretero-ureterostomy)
- Lower ureter (distal 4 cm of the ureter)
  - Primary ureteric anastomosis (uretero-ureterostomy)
  - Psoas hitch
  - Ureteric reimplantation into the bladder

in order to rest the bladder. In patients with more extensive bladder damage, intraperitoneal injuries with physical signs and in those in whom conservative management has failed, surgical exploration and repair of the defect are required. In cases where ureteric injury is recognised post-operatively, it is important to identify the site of damage in order to plan the most appropriate course of action. A retrograde urogram can give more information regarding the precise location of the injury. If the patient is septic or not well enough to undergo immediate surgical re-exploration, a nephrostomy tube can be inserted to improve renal function to the point at which surgery is a more realistic alternative. In a small minority of cases where ureteric obstruction is caused by suture entrapment, nephrostomy drainage alone may resolve the damage. More often, surgical intervention is required. The techniques available are the same as those discussed previously for performing an intra-operative repair at the time of the initial injury.

KEY POINTS

- The ureters and bladder should always be respected by gynaecologists operating in the pelvis.
- A thorough knowledge of their anatomical relationships and of how these may be modified by pathological processes is important in order to minimise the risk of inadvertently damaging the lower urinary tract.
- The possibility of such an injury should always be borne in mind, both at the time of surgery and in the post-operative period.

ACKNOWLEDGEMENT

This chapter has been revised and updated. The author and editors acknowledge the contribution of James Balmforth and Arasee Renganathan to the chapter on this topic in previous editions of this book.

Key References

1. Fall M, Baranowski AP, Elneil S *et al.* EAU guidelines on chronic pelvic pain. *Eur Urol* 2010;57:35–48.

2. Van De Merwe J, Nordling J, Bouchelouche K *et al.* Diagnostic criteria, classification, and nomenclature for painful bladder syndrome/interstitial cystitis: an essic proposal. *Eur Urol* 2008;53:60–7.

3. Hanno P, Dinis, Lin A *et al.* Bladder pain syndrome. International consultation on incontinence. *In:* Abrams P, Cardozo L, Khoury S, Wein A (eds). *Incontinence.* Paris: Health Publications, 2013:1581–650.

4. Breivik H, Collett B, Ventafridda V *et al.* Survey of chronic pain in Europe: Prevalence, impact on daily life, and treatment. *European Journal of Pain* 2006;287–333.

5. Castro-Diaz D, Cardozo L, Chapple CR *et al.* Urgency and pain in patients with overactive bladder and bladder pain syndrome. What are the differences? *Int J Clin Pract* 2013: Dec 22. [Epub ahead of print].

6. Kirkermo A, Peabody M, Diokno A *et al.* Associations among urodynamic findings and symptoms in women enrolled in the interstitial cystitis database (ICDB) study. *Urology* 1997;49(Suppl. 5A):76–80.

7. Berry SH, Elliott MN, Suttorp M *et al.* Prevalence of symptoms of bladder pain syndrome/interstitial cystitis among adult females in the United States. *J Urol* 2011;186(2):540–4.

8. Clemens JQ, Link CL, Eggers PW *et al.* Prevalence of painful bladder symptoms and effect on quality of life in black, Hispanic and white men and women. *J Urol* 2007;177:1390–4.

9. Michael YL, Kawachi I, Stampfer MJ *et al.* Quality of life among women with interstitial cystitis. *J Urol* 2000;164:423–427.

10. Parsons CL, Lilly JD, Stein P. Epithelial dysfunction in nonbacterial cystitis (interstitial cystitis). *J Urol* 1991;145:732–5.

11. Keay S, Kleinberg M, Zhang CO *et al.* Bladder epithelial cells from patients with interstitial cystitis produce an inhibitor of heparin-binding epidermal growth factor-like growth factor production. *J Urol* 2000;164:2112–18.

12. Hunner GL. A rare type of bladder ulcer in women; report of cases. *Boston Med Surg J* 1915;172:660–4.

13. Shear S, Mayer R. Development of glomerulations in younger women with interstitial cystitis. *Urology* 2006;68(2):253–6.

14. Larsen MS, Mortensen S, Nordling J *et al.* Quantifying mast cells in bladder pain syndrome by immunohistochemical analysis. *BJU Int* 2008;102:204–7.

15. Fries J, Hochberg M, Medsger T *et al.* Criteria for rheumatic disease. Different types and different functions. *Arthr Rheum* 1994;37:454–62.

16. Gambone J, Mittman B, Munro M *et al.* Chronic pelvic pain and endometriosis: proceedings of an expert panel consensus process. *Fertil Steril* 2002;78:961–72.

17. Cheng C, Rosamilia A, Healey M. Diagnosis of interstitial cystitis/bladder pain syndrome in women with chronic pelvic pain: a prospective observational study. *Int Urogynecol J* 2012;23(10):1361–6.

18. Tirlapur S, Khan S. Grading of evidence for bladder pain syndrome: a comparative review of study quality assessment methods. *Int Urogynecol J* 2013 Nov 23. [Epub ahead of print].

19. Minogiannis P, El Mansoury M, Betances JA *et al.* Hydroxyzine inhibits neurogenic bladder mast cell activation. *Int J Immunopharmacol* 1998;20:553–63.

20. Parsons CL, Schmidt JD, Pollen JJ. Successful treatment of interstitial cystitis with sodium pentosanpolysulfate. *J Urol* 1983;130:51–7.

21. Peeker R, Haghsheno MA, Holmang S, Fall M. Intravesical bacillus Calmette-Guerin and dimethyl sulfoxide for treatment of classic and non-ulcer interstitial cystitis:

a prospective, randomized double-blind study. *J Urol* 2000;164:1912–15.

22. Ottem DP, Teichman JM. What is the value of cystoscopy with hydrodistension for interstitial cystitis? *Urology* 2005;66(3):494–9.

23. Jeman R, Sahyun P, Miho S *et al.* Elimination of Hunner's ulcers by fulguration in patients with interstitial cystitis: is it effective and long lasting? *Korean J Urol* 2013;54(11):767–71.

24. Kuo H-C, Chancellor M. Comparison of intravesical botulinum toxin type A injections plus hydrodistension with hydrodistension alone for the treatment of refractory interstitial cystitis/painful bladder syndrome. *BJU Int* 2009;104(5):657–61.

25. Dounis A, Gow JG. Bladder augmentation – a long-term review. *Br J Urol* 1979;51:264–8.

26. Foley C, Greenwell T, Gardiner R. Urethral diverticula in females. *BJU Int* 2011;108 Suppl 2:20–3.

27. Neitlich J, Foster H Jr, Glickman M *et al.* Detection of urethral diverticula in women: comparison of a high-resolution fast-spin echo technique with double-balloon urethrography. *J Urol* 1998;159:408–10.

28. Ockrim JL, Allen DJ, Shah PJ *et al.* A tertiary experience of urethral diverticulectomy: diagnosis, imaging and surgical outcomes. *BJU Int* 2009;103:1550–4.

29. Mariotti G, Natale F, Trucchi A *et al.* Ureteral injuries during gynecologic procedures. *Minerva Urol Nefrol* 1997;49:95–8.

30. Brandes S, Coburn M, Armenakas N *et al.* Diagnosis and management of ureteric injury: an evidence-based analysis. *BJU Int* 2004;94(3):277–89.

31. Mann WJ. Intentional and unintentional ureteral surgical treatment in gynaecologic procedures. *Surg Gynecol Obstet* 1991;17:453–6.

Chapter 97 Lower urinary tract infections

Ilias Giarenis and Dudley Robinson

MRCOG standards

- Have comprehensive knowledge of lower urinary tract infections affecting pregnant and non-pregnant women.
- Appreciate the pathogenesis of lower UTI.
- Identify those at risk of developing UTI and those at risk of recurrence.
- Collect appropriate specimens, use the laboratory appropriately and order additional investigations when necessary.
- Make accurate diagnoses and appreciate definition of different terms.
- Successfully manage uncomplicated and complicated UTI and its recurrence.
- Make recommendations for follow-up care.

INTRODUCTION

'Urinary tract infection' is a term that is used to describe various infections involving the urinary tract. The spectrum ranges from asymptomatic bacteriuria to severe pyelonephritis.

There are different classifications for UTI and these can be divided into lower UTI, i.e infection involving the urethra and bladder, or upper UTI, mainly involving the kidneys. UTI may also be classified as uncomplicated, when the infection happens without underlying structural or functional abnormalities, or complicated, when several anatomical abnormalities predispose to UTI. The classification system is important in patient management as it provides a guide to investigation, treatment and prophylaxis.

DEFINITIONS

Bacteriuria

This is used to describe the presence of small numbers of bacteria in the urine. In a clean-catch freshly voided sample, this represents 10,000 colony-forming units (CFU)/mL.

Significant bacteriuria

This term is used to describe the presence of at least 100,000 CFU/mL of urine in a voided midstream clean-catch specimen, or at least 100 CFU/mL of urine from a catheterised specimen.[1] While 20–40 per cent of women with symptomatic UTIs may present with bacterial counts of 100,000 CFU/mL,[2] bacterial counts of 100–10,000 CFU/mL have also been associated with symptoms of cystitis. This may represent the early stages of infection.

Asymptomatic bacteriuria

This is used to describe the presence of bacteria in the urine of an asymptomatic woman. Asymptomatic bacteriuria is common; the prevalence depends on age, sex, sexual activity and the presence of urological abnormalities. In women it is only diagnosed if the same organism is present in quantities of at least 100,000 CFU/mL of urine in at least two consecutive voided specimens.

Whilst the organisms causing asymptomatic bacteriuria and symptomatic UTI are the same, it is not fully understood why patients with asymptomatic bacteriuria do not develop symptoms. This is probably related to organism virulence, where organisms with decreased virulence may only colonise the urine, without causing symptoms.

Complicated lower UTI

This term is used to describe UTIs that may be related to other pathology (Table 97.1). One of the most common forms of complicated UTI is related to the use of urinary catheters. The incidence of bacteriuria associated with an indwelling urinary catheter is 3–10 per cent per day, and the duration of catheterisation is the most important risk factor for developing UTI. They represent a huge reservoir of resistant bacteria in the hospital environment.

Recurrent lower UTI

This is defined as three or more episodes of UTI during a 12-month period,[3] or two infections in a six-month period. Recurrent UTI with the same organism following adequate therapy is termed a relapse. Reinfection is a recurrent UTI caused by bacteria previously isolated after treatment and a

Table 97.1 Conditions associated with complicated lower UTI

Type	Condition
Structural	Urolithiasis
	Malignancy
	Ureteric stricture
	Urethral stricture
	Bladder diverticula
	Renal cysts
	Fistulae
	Urinary diversions
Functional	Neurogenic bladder
	Vesico-ureteric reflux
	Voiding difficulties (incomplete bladder emptying)
Foreign bodies	Indwelling catheter
	Ureteric stent
	Nephrostomy tube
	Mid-urethral tapes for incontinence surgery
Other	Diabetes mellitus
	Pregnancy
	Renal failure
	Renal transplant
	Immunosuppression
	Multidrug resistance
	Hospital-acquired (nosocomial) infection

negative intervening urine culture or a recurrent UTI caused by a second isolate.[4] In a study involving college students with their first UTI, Foxman *et al.*[5] have shown that 27 per cent had at least one culture-confirmed recurrence within the six months following the initial infection, and 2.7 per cent had a second recurrence over the same period of time. The risk of recurrence of UTI is age related. In a study of women with age range between 17 and 82 years with *E. coli* cystitis, 44 per cent had a recurrence within one year, and recurrence is more common in older than younger women.[6]

EPIDEMIOLOGY

UTIs are common medical conditions. In the US, they account for 7–8 million clinic visits and more than 100,000 hospital admissions, mainly due to pyelonephritis.[7] They are more common in females than males with a female-to-male ratio of 14:1. The reasons are probably related to anatomical and functional differences; the female urethra is shorter with the distal third contaminated by bacteria from the vagina and rectum. In addition, during intercourse, bacteria are introduced into the urethra and bladder, and also female bladder emptying may be incomplete compared with males.

The woman's lifetime risk of at least one UTI is around 20 per cent, with a prevalence that is age related, and increases by 1 per cent per decade of life.

RISK FACTORS FOR LOWER UTI

Risk factors for UTI seem to vary according to age. Data regarding recurrent UTIs are scarce. Tables 97.2 and 97.3 summarise congenital and acquired risk factors for urinary tract infection.

Table 97.2 Congenital risk factors for urinary tract infection

Location	Risk factor
Urethra	Hypospadias
	Epispadias
Bladder	Vesico-ureteric reflux
	Ectopic ureters
	Obstructive mega-ureter
Pelvis	Pelvic-ureteric junction obstruction
Central nervous system	Meningomyelocele
	Tethered cord syndrome

Table 97.3 Acquired causes of urinary tract infection

Type	Cause
Traumatic	Surgery (urinary diversion, clam cystoplasty)
	Sexual intercourse
	Sexual abuse
	Foreign bodies (catheters, stents)
	Contraceptive diaphragm
Inflammatory	Vulvo-urethritis
	Chronic inflammation (tuberculosis, syphilis, schistosomiasis)
	Interstitial cystitis
	Radiotherapy
	Fistulae
Metabolic	Calculi
	Diabetes mellitus
Drugs	Cyclophosphamide
	Tioprofenic acid
Anatomical	Cystocele
	Urethral diverticula
Functional	Detrusor hypotonia
	Detrusor dyssynergia
	Constipation
Malignancy	Bladder tumours
	Other pelvic tumours (cervix, uterus, ovary)

Pre-menopausal women

Behavioural factors are thought to increase the risk of UTI. In a large case–control study of women with and without a history of recurrent UTI, the strongest risk factor for recurrent UTI was the frequency of sexual intercourse. Other risk factors include spermicidal use during the past year, having a new sexual partner during the past year, having a first UTI at or before 15 years of age, and having a mother with a history of UTIs.[8]

Post-menopausal women

Anatomical and functional factors are thought to increase the risk of UTI. Raz et al.[9] have shown that in healthy post-menopausal women with a history of recurrent UTI, when compared with a control group, three factors were found to be strongly associated with recurrent UTI; namely urinary incontinence, cystocele and post-void residual urine.

PATHOGENESIS

UTIs are the result of a complex interaction between several factors related to both the host and the uropathogens.

Host factors

The main route of bacterial entry into the urethra and bladder is ascending from the bowel to the vaginal vestibule, and then to the urethra and bladder. In support of that, it has been shown that the vaginal vestibule of women with recurrent UTI had higher enterobacterial colonisation than women with no recurrent UTI. Changes in the vaginal microflora are important in the aetiology. These changes may be caused by the use of spermicides, antibiotics and lack of oestrogen.

Host defence

There are several protective mechanisms against UTI; the main function is to prevent colonisation with uropathogens.[10] These mechanisms include:

- Urinary hydrodynamics: urine production and micturition provide a washout mechanism to prevent uropathogens from colonising the urinary tract; if this mechanism is impaired, a significant post-void residual urine may result in increased risk of UTI.
- Urine biochemical characteristics; namely, high osmolality and low pH prevent bacterial multiplication.
- Urinary tract epithelium has bactericidal activities.
- Inhibitors of bacterial adherence: several protective mechanisms work to prevent bacterial adherence to the urinary tract epithelium which is a prerequisite for infection. The factors that prevent bacterial adherence include

Tamm–Horsfall protein, bladder mucopolysaccharides and oligosaccharides and lactoferrin.
- Inflammatory response will take effect when bacteria adhere to epithelium. The inflammatory response includes polymorphonuclear leukocytes and cytokines.
- Both humoral and cell-mediated arms of the immune system play an important part in the resistance against bacterial infection of the urinary tract.

Virulence factor

Microorganisms have the ability to survive and multiply in the bladder and are able to adhere to the bladder epithelium.[11] E. coli is responsible for 80 per cent of UTIs and this is why most virulence studies have focused on it. The virulence factors that are thought to play a role in the pathogenesis of UTI include:

- *Adherence factors*: The two most important fimbriae thought to play a role in the E. coli UTI are type P and type 1. These fimbriae will bind to specific receptors on the urinary tract epithelium, and eventually provoke an inflammatory reaction. It seems that they are site specific, where type 1 is present in the majority of E. coli causing lower UTI, and type P is mostly found in E. coli causing pyelonephritis.
- *Invasion factors*: Uropathogens produce substances that aid in the direct invasion of the urinary tract mucosa with subsequent systemic dissemination. The most important bacterial toxins are lipopolysaccharides and haemolysins.
- *Bacterial resistance*: This represents a microorganism defence mechanism against antimicrobials.

ORGANISMS OF LOWER URINARY TRACT INFECTION

The organisms responsible for UTI are well-established and consistent. *Escherichia coli* is responsible for almost 80 per cent of acute community-acquired uncomplicated infections. *Klebsiella*, *Proteus* and enterococci are infrequent causes of uncomplicated UTI. The commonly occurring organisms in community practice differ when compared to those found within the hospital environment (Table 97.4).[12]

Table 97.4 Common uropathogens in general practice and hospital

Organism	Community (%)	Hospital (%)
Escherichia coli	77.3	56.3
Proteus mirabilis	4.3	6.3
Enterococcus faecalis	3.8	8.4
Klebsiella pneumoniae	3.5	6.9
Pseudomonas aeruginosa	1.8	3.8

UROGYNAECOLOGY AND SEXUAL HEALTH AND WELLBEING

Viral UTIs

Lower UTIs are most often caused by bacteria; however, in the immunocompromised host, viruses are being increasingly recognised as a cause, especially in haemorrhagic cystitis. Predominant viruses include the BK virus (a type of polyomavirus that infects most people, but generally causes no symptoms), adenovirus and cytomegalovirus. The diagnosis is based on molecular techniques. Cidofovir is becoming a drug of choice in viral UTIs.[13]

MANAGEMENT

The management of lower urinary tract infection is aimed at treating the current infection and preventing further recurrences. The aims of treatment may be summarised as follows:

- symptomatic relief;
- microbiological cure;
- detection of predisposing factors;
- prevention of upper urinary tract involvement;
- management of recurrence.

DIAGNOSIS

Symptoms and signs

Women with lower UTIs typically complain of symptoms of cystitis i.e. dysuria, suprapubic discomfort, frequency, urgency and nocturia. While the diagnostic accuracy of clinical assessment of UTI is uncertain, the presence of both dysuria and frequency increases the probability of UTI by 90 per cent. Of these women, approximately 30 per cent will also have an upper UTI, which may present as loin pain and tenderness. Whilst young children may present with general malaise and pyrexia, in the elderly, UTIs may present with atypical symptoms, such as confusion and falls. History is also important in the differentiation between uncomplicated and complicated UTI.

Physical examination is usually unremarkable; however, suprapubic or loin tenderness may be the only physical signs.

INVESTIGATIONS

In the majority of women with simple acute lower UTI, there is no need for further investigation. However, some cases do warrant further investigation in order to exclude an underlying cause.

Indications for investigation include:

- children;
- proven recurrent UTI;
- adults with a childhood history of UTI;
- persistent haematuria;

- atypical organism such as *Proteus, Pseudomonas, Enterobacter* and *Klebsiella*;
- persistent infection despite appropriate antibiotic therapy.

Basic investigations

- Urine appearance. Whilst urine turbidity has been shown to have a specificity of 66.4 per cent and sensitivity of 90.4 per cent for predicting symptomatic UTI, it is prone to observer error.[14]
- Urine microscopy has a sensitivity of 60–100 per cent and specificity of 49–100 per cent for predicting significant bacteriuria in women.[15]
- Urine dipstick for nitrites and leukocytes. If the test is positive for both, then the probability of UTI is higher than each alone; however if both are negative, the likelihood of UTI is less than 20 per cent.[16]
- Urine culture will isolate the causative organism and provide antibiotic sensitivities that should guide antimicrobial treatment.

Other investigations

- In women who have recurrent or complicated urinary infections, renal function should be assessed with serum creatinine, urea and electrolytes.
- For persistent or recurrent infections, urine should be sent for culture of fastidious organisms (*Mycoplasma hominis, Ureaplasma urealyticum, Chlamydia trachomatis*) to rule out less common causes of infection.
- Ultrasound of the upper urinary tract will exclude renal causes, such as hydronephrosis or calculi, and a postmicturition bladder scan will rule out a significant urinary residual.
- An alternative is radiological imaging using an intravenous urogram or CT urogram. These involve exposure to ionising radiation and influence treatment in limited cases.
- A transvaginal ultrasound can exclude the possibility of a pelvic mass.
- Cystourethroscopy will exclude an intravesical lesion, such as a bladder tumour, and anomalies, such as diverticula and calculi, and also synthetic tapes eroding through the bladder wall or the urethra. A bladder biopsy may show evidence of chronic follicular or interstitial cystitis.

TREATMENT

General measures

Patients with cystitis should be encouraged to increase their fluid intake in order to achieve a short voiding interval and a high flow rate, which will help to dilute and flush out the infecting organism. Using potassium citrate preparations may provide symptomatic relief; it is thought to act by reducing urinary pH.

Antimicrobials

When treating UTI, an antimicrobial should be selected that has the appropriate sensitivity and is also able to achieve a high concentration within the urinary tract. Drugs should be safe, efficacious and have few side effects. Ideally, the drugs should be rapidly absorbed and not induce bacterial resistance. Some antimicrobials are particularly useful when treating urinary infections. Nitrofurantoin is specific to the urinary tract and therefore has little effect on bowel and vaginal flora. It is bactericidal to most common uropathogens, but it is contraindicated in cases of renal failure. Trimethoprim, primarily bacteriostatic, is also useful in the treatment of urinary tract infection.

Antimicrobial therapy should ideally be based upon culture and sensitivity results from a midstream specimen of urine, although initially empirical treatment often needs to be on a 'best guess' basis. The choice of empirical treatment should be based on local guidelines considering the frequency and resistance of different uropathogens. In the lack of local guidance, international clinical practice guidelines could be followed (Table 97.5).[17,18]

Duration

Compliance with therapy may be improved by using shorter courses of antimicrobial therapy which also have the advantage of reducing the effect on faecal and vaginal flora and may help in reducing the emergence of resistant organisms. Several studies have documented the dosing and effectiveness of antimicrobial regimens for uncomplicated UTI. A Cochrane review concluded that three days of antibiotic therapy is similar to 5–10 days in achieving symptomatic cure during uncomplicated UTI treatment, while the longer treatment is more effective in obtaining bacteriological cure.[19]

PREVENTION OF RECURRENT URINARY TRACT INFECTION

Women with recurrent UTI, who use spermicides mainly in conjunction with contraceptive diaphragms, should be advised about their association with recurrent UTI, and hence a reduction in use or elimination would be expected to reduce recurrence. Early post-coital voiding and increased fluid intake might be helpful.

Methenamine hippurate may be effective for preventing UTI in patients without renal tract abnormalities, particularly when used for short-term prophylaxis. It does not appear to work in patients with a neuropathic bladder or in patients who have renal tract abnormalities.[20]

Cranberry juice has been used for many years for the prevention and treatment of UTIs. It is thought to act by preventing bacterial adherence to bladder epithelium. A recent Cochrane review showed that cranberry juice is less effective than previously indicated by small studies.[21] For patients interested in taking cranberry prophylaxis, cranberry tablets have been shown to be more cost effective than cranberry juice.

The use of probiotics, especially lactobacilli, can be beneficial for preventing recurrent UTI in women; they also have a good safety profile.[22] Vitamin C is often recommended as a supplement that can prevent recurrent UTI. In-vitro data suggest that it can have a bacteriostatic effect in the urine, but there is a lack of strong clinical evidence.[23]

In post-menopausal women, the prevalence rate for having one episode of UTI in a given year varies from 8 to 10 per cent. This increased risk is associated with a decrease in oestrogen levels. Vaginal oestrogens, but not oral oestrogens, have been shown to reduce the number of UTIs in post-menopausal women with recurrent UTI.[24] Local preparations, such as vaginal oestriol cream 0.1%, vaginal oestradiol tablets or oestradiol-releasing vaginal ring, should be considered in post-menopausal women with signs of urogenital atrophy.

When compared to placebo, continuous antibiotic prophylaxis for 6–12 months reduces the rate of UTI; however, there was no difference in the UTI incidence upon discontinuation of therapy.[3] In women with recurrent UTI related to intercourse, post-coital prophylaxis is as effective as continuous daily therapy in preventing UTI with fewer side effects. Another alternative option is self-start therapy which involves providing patients with instructions and materials (urine reagent strips and antibiotics) that allow them to both diagnose and treat their UTI at the onset of symptoms. This strategy should be restricted to women who are motivated, compliant and have a good relationship with a doctor. Regimens for antibiotic prophylaxis are presented in Table 97.6.[25]

Table 97.5 Recommended treatment for acute uncomplicated cystitis

1st choice	Nitrofurantointoin 50 mg every 6 hours for 7 days
2nd choice	Trimethoprim 200 mg twice daily for 5 days (if local *E. coli* resistance is <20%)
3rd choice	Ciprofloxacin 250 mg twice daily for 3 days OR Norfloxacin* 400 mg twice daily for 3 days
4th choice	Co-amoxiclav 500/125 mg every 8 hours for 3 days OR Cefaclor 500 mg every 8 hours for 3 days

*Unavailable in the UK at time of print

Table 97.6 Prophylaxis regimens for women with recurrent UTI

Continuous prophylaxis	Cefaclor 250 mg daily
	Cephalexin 125–250 mg daily
	Ciprofloxacin 125 mg daily
	Nitrofurantoin 50–100 mg daily
	Norfloxacin* 200 mg daily
	Trimethoprim 100 mg daily
Post-coital prophylaxis (single dose)	Cephalexin 125–250 mg
	Ciprofloxacin 125 mg
	Nitrofurantoin 50–100 mg
	Norfloxacin* 200 mg
	Trimethoprim 100 mg
Self-start treatment	Ciprofloxacin 250 mg twice daily for 3 days
	Norfloxacin* 200 mg twice daily for 3 days
	Trimethoprim 200 mg twice daily for 3 days

*Unavailable in the UK at time of print

URINARY TRACT INFECTION IN PREGNANCY

UTIs are the most common medical complication of pregnancy.

The incidence of asymptomatic bacteriuria in pregnancy is 2–5 per cent.[26] If not treated, up to 20 per cent will develop lower UTI. The overall incidence of UTI in pregnancy is 8 per cent and the incidence of acute pyelonephritis is 2 per cent.

Aetiology

The increased susceptibility in pregnancy is due to a number of physiological changes that make asymptomatic bacteriuria progress to symptomatic UTI. These include changes in bladder volume, decreased bladder tone and ureteric dilatation secondary to an increased level of progesterone. This will lead to urinary stasis and chronic residual urine with subsequent UTI.

A review of randomised, controlled studies has found good evidence that urine culture and dipstick testing for leukocytes and nitrites reduced the risk of pyelonephritis and was cost effective, thus offering a rationale for screening.[27]

Uropathogens responsible for UTI in pregnancy are similar to those in non-pregnant women, with *E. coli* responsible for over 80 per cent of the cases.

Maternal/fetal complication

UTIs in pregnancy have been associated with increased risks of chorioamnionitis and endometritis. With regard to the fetus, it has been shown that UTI is associated with fetal growth restriction, stillbirth, preterm labour and delivery, increased perinatal mortality, mental retardation and developmental delay.[28]

Treatment

Asymptomatic bacteriuria

Treatment of asymptomatic bacteriuria reduces the risk of pyelonephritis and, consequently, the risks of preterm delivery and low birthweight.

Symptomatic UTI

Treatment is directed by urine culture and sensitivity. Although antibiotic treatment is effective for the cure of UTIs, there are insufficient data to recommend any specific drug regimen for treatment of symptomatic UTIs during pregnancy.[29] An antibiotic course for 7 days would be appropriate, although in an attempt to increase patient compliance and reduce side effects shorter courses could be considered. It is of paramount importance to repeat urine culture after treatment to confirm bacteriological cure.

Penicillins and cephalosporins have been shown to be safe in the first and second trimesters. As it is a folate antagonist, trimethoprim should be avoided in the first trimester, although it may be used safely in late pregnancy. Conversely, nitrofurantoin and sulphonamides are safe in early pregnancy, although they should be avoided in the third trimester when the former may cause a haemolytic anaemia and the latter hyperbilirubinaemia and kernicterus. Tetracyclines should be avoided because of their chelating action, which will lead to hypoplasia and staining of the teeth. While in general erythromycin is considered safe, the estolate salt may be associated with cholestatic jaundice. Finally, fluoroquinolones may affect fetal cartilage formation, and chloramphenicol may be associated with neonatal cardiovascular collapse.

Recurrent UTI in pregnancy

The risk of recurrence in pregnancy is 4–5 per cent. While the exact aetiology of recurrence is uncertain, it is believed that the causes of the first infection are likely to cause recurrence. Postpartum urological investigation to exclude urinary anomalies should be considered. Long-term, low-dose antimicrobial cover and single-dose antimicrobial in intercourse-related UTI are suggested as prophylactic measures.[30]

KEY POINTS

- Lower UTIs are a common cause of morbidity.
- Risks of lower UTI are related to behavioural, anatomical and functional factors.
- Community-acquired infections may be caused by different organisms from those acquired in hospital.

- In the majority of women with uncomplicated cystitis, there is no indication for further investigation.
- Antimicrobial therapy should be based upon culture and sensitivity results, although often initial treatment is on a 'best guess' basis.
- Short- and low-dose antibiotics may be used as prophylaxis and reduce infection rates by 95 per cent, compared with placebo.
- UTI in pregnancy may be associated with pyelonephritis, preterm delivery and low birthweight.

Key References

1. Saint S, Chenoweth CE. Biofilms and catheter-associated urinary tract infections. *Infect Dis Clin North Am* 2003;17:411–32.
2. Hanson LA. Prognostic indicators in childhood urinary infection. *Kidney Int* 1982;21:659–67.
3. Albert X, Huertas I, Pereiro I *et al*. Antibiotics for preventing recurrent urinary tract infection in non-pregnant women. *Cochrane Database Syst Rev* 2004;3:CD001209.
4. American College of Obstetricians and Gynecologists. ACOG Practice Bulletin No. 91: Treatment of urinary tract infections in non-pregnant women. *Obstet Gynecol* 2008;111:785–94.
5. Foxman B. Recurring urinary tract infection: incidence and risk factors. *Am J Public Health* 1990;80:331–3.
6. Ikaheimo R, Sutonen A, Heiskanen T *et al*. Recurrence of urinary tract infection in a primary care setting: analysis of a 1-year follow-up of 179 women. *Clin Infect Dis* 1996;22:91–9.
7. Stamm WE, Hooton TM. Management of urinary tract infections in adults. *N Engl J Med* 1993;329:1328–34.
8. Scholes D, Hooton TM, Roberts PL *et al*. Risk factors for recurrent UTI in young women. *J Infect Dis* 2000;182:1177–82.
9. Raz R, Stamm WE. A controlled trial of intravaginal estriol in postmenopausal women with recurrent urinary tract infections. *N Engl J Med* 1993;329:753–6.
10. Sobel JD. Pathogenesis of UTI. Role of host defences. *Infect Dis North Am* 1997;11:531–49.
11. Svanborg C, Godaly G. Bacterial virulence in urinary tract infection. *Infect Dis Clin N Am* 1997;11:513–29.
12. Farrell DJ, Morrissey I, De Rubeis D *et al*. A UK multicentre study of the antimicrobial susceptibility of bacterial pathogens causing urinary tract infection. *J Infect* 2003;46:94–100.
13. Paduch DA. Viral lower urinary tract infections. *Curr Urol Rep* 2007;8:324–35.
14. Flanagan PG, Rooney PG, Davies EA, Stout RW. Evaluation of four screening tests for bacteriuria in elderly people. *Lancet* 1989;1:1117–19.
15. Jenkins RD, Fenn JP, Matsen JM. Review of urine microscopy for bacteriuria. *JAMA* 1986;255:3397–403.
16. Hurlbut TA 3rd, Littenberg B. The diagnostic accuracy of rapid dipstick tests to predict urinary tract infection. *Am J Clin Pathol* 1991;96:582–8.
17. Gupta K, Hooton TM, Naber KG *et al*. International clinical practice guidelines for the treatment of acute uncomplicated cystitis and pyelonephritis in women: A 2010 update by the Infectious Diseases Society of America and the European Society for Microbiology and Infectious Diseases. *Clin Infect Dis* 2011;52:e103–20.
18. European Association of Urology. *Guidelines on urological infections*. 2010. http://www.uroweb.org/
19. Milo G, Katchman E, Paul M *et al*. Duration of antibacterial treatment for uncomplicated urinary tract infection in women. *Cochrane Database Syst Rev* 2005;2:CD004682.
20. Lee BSB, Bhuta T, Simpson JM *et al*. Methenamine hippurate for preventing urinary tract infections. *Cochrane Database Syst Rev* 2012;10:CD003265.
21. Jepson RG, Williams G, Craig JC. Cranberries for preventing urinary tract infections. *Cochrane Database Syst Rev* 2012;10:CD001321.
22. Falagas ME, Betsi GI, Tokas T *et al*. Probiotics for prevention of recurrent urinary tract infections in women: a review of the evidence from microbiological and clinical studies. *Drugs* 2006;66:1253–61.
23. Hickling D, Nitti V. Management of recurrent urinary tract infections in healthy adult women. *Rev Urol* 2013;15:41–8.
24. Perrotta C, Aznar M, Mejia R *et al*. Oestrogens for preventing recurrent urinary tract infection in post-menopausal women. *Cochrane Database Syst Rev* 2008;2:CD005131.
25. Society of Obstetricians and Gynaecologists of Canada (SOGC). Recurrent urinary tract infection. *J Obstet Gynaecol Can* 2010;32:1082–90.
26. Foley ME, Farquharson R, Stronge JM. Is screening for bacteriuria in pregnancy worthwhile? *BMJ* 1987;295:270.
27. Villar J, Bergsjo P. Scientific basis for the content of routine antenatal care. *Acta Obstet Gynaecol Scand* 1997;76:1–14.
28. McCormick T, Ashe RG, Kearney PM. Urinary tract infection in pregnancy. *Obstet Gynaecol* 2008;10:156–62.
29. Vazquez JC, Abalos E. Treatments for symptomatic urinary tract infections during pregnancy. *Cochrane Database Syst Rev* 2011;1:CD002256.
30. Romero R, Oyarzun E, Mazor M *et al*. Meta-analysis of the relationship between asymptomatic bacteriuria and preterm delivery/low birthweight. *Obstet Gynecol* 1989;73:576–82.

Chapter 98 Urogenital prolapse

Sushma Srikrishna and Dudley Robinson

MRCOG standards

Theoretical skills

- Have comprehensive knowledge of the functional pelvic anatomy as applied to gynaecological surgery.
- Understand the aetiology of urogenital prolapse.
- Understand preventative measures.

Practical skills

- Know how to clinically assess women presenting with urogenital prolapse.
- Be able to undertake conservative management of prolapse.
- Be able to undertake surgical management of urogenital prolapse.

STRAT OG: Learning objectives

To achieve a better understanding of:

- the incidence and epidemiology of urogenital prolapse;
- the classification and grading scales to indicate the severity of the prolapse;
- means of preventing urogenital prolapse;
- management procedures;
- non-surgical;
- surgical.

INTRODUCTION

Urogenital prolapse occurs when there is a weakness in the supporting structures of the pelvic floor allowing the pelvic viscera to descend and ultimately fall through the anatomical defect.

While usually not life threatening, prolapse is often symptomatic and is associated with a deterioration in quality of life and may be the cause of bladder and bowel dysfunction.

Increased life expectancy and an expanding elderly population mean that prolapse remains an important condition, especially since the majority of women may now spend a third of their lives in the post-menopausal state. Surgery for urogenital prolapse accounts for approximately 20 per cent of elective major gynaecological surgery and this increases to 59 per cent in elderly women. The lifetime risk of having surgery for prolapse is 11 per cent; a third of these procedures are operations for recurrent prolapse.

The economic cost of urogenital prolapse is considerable, with figures from the US revealing a total expenditure of $1012 million in 1997: vaginal hysterectomy accounted for 49 per cent, pelvic floor repairs for 28 per cent and abdominal hysterectomy for 13 per cent of costs.[1]

EPIDEMIOLOGY

Age

The incidence of urogenital prolapse increases with increasing age, with approximately 60 per cent of elderly women having some degree of prolapse and up to half of all women over the age of 50 years complaining of symptomatic prolapse. In a study of women with severe vaginal vault prolapse following hysterectomy, 60 per cent were over the age of 60 years.

Parity

Urogenital prolapse is more common following childbirth, although it may be asymptomatic. Studies have estimated that 50 per cent of parous women have some degree of urogenital prolapse and, of these, 10–20 per cent are symptomatic. Only 2 per cent of nulliparous women are reported to have prolapse.

Race

Prolapse is generally thought to be more common in Caucasian women and less common in women of Afro-Caribbean origin. However, a study examining racial differences in North America has shown that this may not be the case, as there was little racial variation noted, although this may simply reflect cultural differences in reporting.

CLASSIFICATION

Urogenital prolapse is classified anatomically depending on the site of the defect and the pelvic viscera that are involved.

- *Urethrocele:* prolapse of the lower anterior vaginal wall involving the urethra only.
- *Cystocele:* prolapse of the upper anterior vaginal wall involving the bladder. Generally, there is also associated prolapse of the urethra and hence the term cystourethrocele is used.
- *Uterovaginal prolapse:* this term is used to describe prolapse of the uterus, cervix and upper vagina.
- *Enterocele:* prolapse of the upper posterior wall of the vagina, usually containing loops of small bowel. A traction enterocele is secondary to uterovaginal prolapse, a pulsion enterocele is secondary to chronically raised intra-abdominal pressure, and an iatrogenic enterocele is caused by previous pelvic surgery. An anterior enterocele may be used to describe prolapse of the upper anterior vaginal wall following hysterectomy.
- *Rectocele:* prolapse of the lower posterior wall of the vagina involving the anterior wall of the rectum.

GRADING OF UROGENITAL PROLAPSE

- *First degree:* The lowest part of the prolapse descends halfway down the vaginal axis to the introitus.
- *Second degree:* The lowest part of the prolapse extends to the level of the introitus and through the introitus on straining.
- *Third degree:* The lowest part of the prolapse extends through the introitus and lies outside the vagina. Procidentia describes a third-degree uterine prolapse.

PROLAPSE SCORING SYSTEM

Recently, the International Continence Society produced a standardisation document in order to assess urogenital prolapse more objectively.[2] The ICS Prolapse Scoring System (POPQ) allows the measurement of fixed points on the anterior and posterior vaginal walls, cervix and perineal body against a fixed reference point, the genital hiatus (Fig. 98.1). Measurements are performed in the left lateral position at rest and at maximal valsalva, thus providing an accurate and reproducible method of quantifying urogenital prolapse.

ANATOMY OF THE PELVIC FLOOR

The pelvic floor provides support to the pelvic viscera and consists of the levator ani muscles, urogenital diaphragm, endopelvic fascia and perineal body. The levator

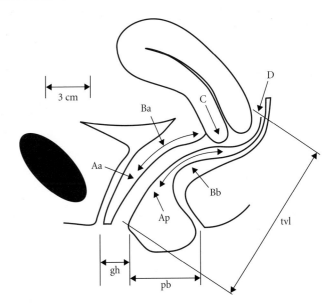

Fig. 98.1 ICS Prolapse Scoring System (POPQ)

ani, when considered with its associated fascia, is termed the 'pelvic diaphragm'.

The muscle fibres of the pelvic diaphragm are arranged to form a broad U-shaped layer of muscle with a defect anteriorly. This physiological defect is the urogenital hiatus and allows the passage of the urethra, vagina and rectum through the pelvic floor.

Pelvic floor musculature

The muscles of the pelvic floor are composed of the levator ani and coccygeus, which form a cradle within the bony pelvis supporting the pelvic organs. The levator ani originate on each side from the pelvic sidewall, arising anteriorly just above the arcus tendineus fasciae pelvis (the white line) and inserting posteriorly into the arcus tendineus levator ani. The arcus tendineus fasciae pelvis and arcus tendineus levator ani fuse near the ischial spine; the levator ani unite in the midline to form the anococcygeal raphe (Fig. 98.2).

The levator ani has three divisions: the pubococcygeus, iliococcygeus and puborectalis muscles (Fig. 98.3). The iliococcygeus and pubococcygeus arise from the arcus tendineus levator ani fascia overlying the obturator internus and insert into the midline anococcygeal raphe and the coccyx, while the latter forms the inner fibres of the pelvic floor musculature inserting into the rectum and perineal body. Posteriorly, the coccygeus arises from the ischial spine and sacrospinous ligament and inserts into the coccyx and sacrum.

The striated muscle of the pelvic floor is composed of both slow- and fast-twitch muscle fibres. The slow-twitch fibres provide muscle tone over a long period of time, thus supporting the pelvic viscera, while the fast-twitch fibres react to sudden increases in intra-abdominal pressure.

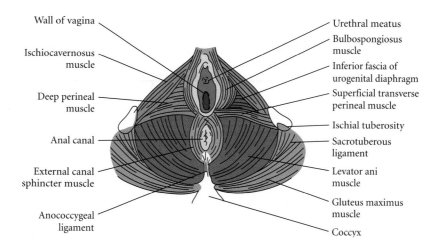

Fig. 98.2 Anatomy of the pelvic floor

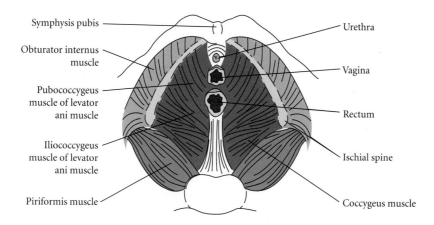

Fig. 98.3 Anatomy of the pelvic floor showing the divisions of levator ani

Urogenital diaphragm

The urogenital diaphragm (perineal membrane) is a triangular sheet of dense fibrous tissue spanning the anterior half of the pelvic outlet, which is pierced by the vagina and urethra. It arises from the inferior ischiopubic rami and attaches medially to the urethra, vagina and perineal body, thus supporting the pelvic floor.

Perineal body

The perineal body lies between the vagina and the rectum and provides a point of insertion for the muscles of the pelvic floor. It is attached to the inferior pubic rami and ischial tuberosities through the urogenital diaphragm and superficial transverse perineal muscles. Laterally, it is attached to the fibres of the pelvic diaphragm; posteriorly, it inserts into the external anal sphincter and coccyx.

Pelvic fascia

The endopelvic fascia is a meshwork of collagen and elastin that represents the fused adventitial layers of the visceral structures and pelvic wall musculature. Condensations of the pelvic fascia are termed 'ligaments' and these have an important part in the supportive role of the pelvic floor.

Uterine support

The parametrium, composed of the uterosacral and cardinal ligaments, attaches the cervix and upper vagina to the pelvic sidewall. The uterosacral ligament forms the medial margin bordering the pouch of Douglas; the cardinal ligaments attach the lateral aspects of the cervix and vagina to the pelvic sidewall over the sacrum. The former is composed mostly of smooth muscle, whereas the cardinal ligaments contain mostly connective tissue and the pelvic blood vessels. The round ligaments are not thought to have a role in supporting the uterus, although they may help to maintain anteversion and anteflexion; the broad ligaments are simply folds of peritoneum and provide no support.

Vaginal support

Support to the upper third of the vagina is provided principally by the downward extension of the cardinal ligaments; the middle third is supported by lateral attachments to the arcus tendineus fasciae pelvis, a condensation of the obturator and levator fasciae. These supports suspend the anterior vaginal wall across the pelvis, the layer of fascia anterior to the vagina being called the 'pubocervical fascia'. Posterolaterally, the vagina is attached to the endopelvic fascia over the pelvic diaphragm and sacrum by the rectovaginal septum (fascia of Denonvilliers), which extends caudally into the perineal body and cranially into the peritoneum of the pouch of Douglas. The lower third is attached anteriorly to the pubic arch by the perineal membrane, posteriorly to the perineal body and laterally to the medial aspect of levator ani.

Urethral support

The proximal urethra is supported by a sling of endopelvic fascia and the anterior vaginal wall, which is stabilised by lateral attachments to the arcus tendineus fasciae pelvis, and medial border of the levator ani. Contraction and relaxation of the levator muscles allows elevation or descent of the urethra, respectively, which is important in the control of voiding. In addition, an increase in intra-abdominal pressure causes compression of the urethra against the fixed anterior vaginal wall, thus maintaining continence. Bladder neck mobility and the stress continence mechanism are thus dependent on fascial integrity and connective tissue elasticity.

AETIOLOGY

Pregnancy and childbirth

The increased incidence of prolapse in multiparous women would suggest that pregnancy and childbirth have an important impact on the supporting function of the pelvic floor. Damage to the muscular and fascial supports of the pelvic floor and changes in innervation contribute to the development of prolapse.

The pelvic floor may be damaged during childbirth, causing the axis of the levator muscles to become more oblique and creating a funnel that allows the uterus, vagina and rectum to fall through the urogenital hiatus. In addition, the proportion of fascia to muscle within the pelvic floor tends to increase with increasing age, and thus once damaged by childbirth, muscle may never regain its full strength. This is supported by studies showing decreased cellularity and increased collagen content in 70 per cent of women with urogenital prolapse, compared to 20 per cent of normal controls.

Mechanical changes within the pelvic fascia have also been implicated in the causation of urogenital prolapse. During pregnancy, the fascia becomes more elastic and thus more likely to fail. This may explain the increased incidence of stress incontinence observed in pregnancy and the increased incidence of prolapse with multiparity.

Denervation of the pelvic musculature has been shown to occur following childbirth, although gradual denervation has also been demonstrated in nulliparous women with increasing age. However, the effects were greatest in those women who had documented stress incontinence or prolapse.[3] Furthermore, histological studies have revealed changes in muscle fibre type and distribution, suggesting denervation injury associated with ageing and also following childbirth. In conclusion, it would appear that partial denervation of the pelvic floor is part of the normal ageing process, although pregnancy and childbirth accelerate these changes.

The biochemical properties of connective tissue may also play an important role in the development of prolapse. Changes in collagen content have been identified, the hydroxyproline content in connective tissue from women with stress incontinence being 40 per cent lower than in continent controls. In addition, changes in collagen metabolism may be associated with the development of urogenital prolapse, increased levels of collagenases being associated with weakened pelvic support and stress incontinence.

Hormonal factors

The effects of ageing and those of oestrogen withdrawal at the time of the menopause are often difficult to separate. Rectus muscle fascia has been shown to become less elastic with increasing age, and less energy is required to produce irreversible damage. Furthermore, there is also a reduction in skin collagen content following the menopause. Both of these factors lead to a reduction in the strength of the pelvic connective tissue.

More recently, oestrogen receptors, alpha and beta, have been demonstrated in the vaginal walls and the utero-sacral ligaments of pre-menopausal women, although the beta receptor was absent from the vaginal walls in post-menopausal women. However, a further study was unable to identify oestrogen receptors in biopsies from the levator ani muscles in urinary incontinent women participating in pelvic floor exercises. In conclusion, it would appear that oestrogens and oestrogen withdrawal have a role in the development of urogenital prolapse, although the precise mechanism has yet to be established.

Smoking

Chronic chest disease resulting in a chronic cough leads to an increase in the intra-abdominal pressure and thus exposes the pelvic floor to greater strain. Over a period of time this will exacerbate any defects in the pelvic floor musculature and fascia, leading to prolapse.

UROGYNAECOLOGY AND SEXUAL HEALTH AND WELLBEING

Constipation

Chronically increased intra-abdominal pressure caused by repetitive straining will exacerbate any potential weaknesses in the pelvic floor and is also associated with an increased risk of prolapse.

Obesity

Although obesity has been linked to urogenital prolapse due to a potential increase in intra-abdominal pressure, there has been no good evidence to support this theory.

Exercise

Increased stress placed on the musculature of the pelvic floor will exacerbate pelvic floor defects and weakness, thus increasing the incidence of prolapse. Consequently, heavy lifting and exercise, as well as sports such as weight lifting, high-impact aerobics and long-distance running, increase the risk of urogenital prolapse.

Surgery

Pelvic surgery may also have an effect on the occurrence of urogenital prolapse. Continence procedures, while elevating the bladder neck, may lead to defects in other pelvic compartments. At Burch colposuspension, the fixing of the lateral vaginal fornices to the ipsilateral ileopectineal ligaments leaves a potential defect in the posterior vaginal wall that predisposes to rectocele and enterocele formation. In a five-year follow-up study of women, 36 per cent had cystoceles, 66 per cent rectocele, 32 per cent enterocele and 38 per cent uterine prolapse. A further study of 109 women with vaginal vault prolapse reported that 43 per cent had previously undergone Burch colposuspension. Overall, 25 per cent of the women who had had Burch colposuspension required further surgery for prolapse.

Needle suspension procedures, such as the Pereyra or Stamey endoscopically guided bladder neck suspension, are also associated with an increased incidence of recurrent cystocele, although this is not the case following sling procedures. In addition, there is an increased incidence of posterior compartment defects, such as enterocele and rectocele, after Manchester repair, caused by the anterior plication of the uterosacral and cardinal ligaments, which leaves a large posterior hiatus.

The association between prolapse and prior hysterectomy is not as clear. One large study reporting on this followed up 184 women over a median of 11.3 years. Less than 3% had stage-3 prolapse. No significant difference was found in the presence of stage-2 or higher stage prolapse between the two hysterectomy groups (39% in subtotal hysterectomy versus 37% in Total Hysterectomy; OR 1.28, 95% CI 0.59–2.80). There was also no significant difference in the quality-of-life measurement between the two groups.[4] However, other factors, such as the ageing process and oestrogen withdrawal following the menopause, may also have an important role. Prolapse of the vaginal vault may present following either vaginal or abdominal hysterectomy, although the incidence is low, with only 0.5 per cent of women who have had a hysterectomy requiring further surgical intervention for vaginal vault prolapse.

CLINICAL SYMPTOMS

Most women complain of a feeling of discomfort or heaviness within the pelvis in addition to a 'lump coming down'. Symptoms tend to become worse with prolonged standing and towards the end of the day. Women may also complain of dyspareunia, difficulty in inserting tampons and chronic lower backache. In cases of third-degree prolapse, there may be mucosal ulceration and lichenification, which results in a symptomatic vaginal discharge or bleeding.

A cystocele may be associated with LUTS of urgency and frequency of micturition in addition to a sensation of incomplete emptying, which may be relieved by digitally reducing the prolapse. Recurrent UTIs may also be associated with a chronic urinary residual. While less than 2 per cent of mild cystoceles are associated with ureteric obstruction, severe prolapse may lead to hydronephrosis and chronic renal damage. Between 33 and 92 per cent of cases of complete procidentia are associated with some degree of ureteric obstruction.

A rectocele may be associated with difficulty in opening the bowels, some women complaining of tenesmus and having to digitate to defaecate.

CLINICAL SIGNS

Women are generally examined in the left lateral position using a Simms' speculum, although digital examination when standing allows more accurate assessment of the degree of urogenital prolapse and, in particular, vaginal vault support. An abdominal examination should also be performed to exclude the presence of an abdominal or pelvic tumour that may be responsible for the vaginal findings.

Differential diagnosis includes:

- vaginal cysts;
- pendunculated fibroid polyp;
- urethral diverticulum;
- chronic uterine inversion.

INVESTIGATION

In women who also complain of concomitant LUTS, urodynamic studies or a post-micturition bladder ultrasound should be performed in order to exclude a chronic residual due to associated voiding difficulties. In such cases, a midstream specimen of urine should be sent for culture and sensitivity.

Subtracted cystometry, with or without videocystoure-throgography, will allow the identification of underlying detrusor overactivity, which is important to exclude prior to surgical repair. In cases of significant cystocele, stress testing should be carried out by asking the patient to cough while standing. Since occult urodynamic stress incontinence may be unmasked by straightening the urethra following anterior colporrhaphy, this should be simulated by the insertion of a ring pessary or tampon to reduce the cystocele. If stress incontinence is demonstrated, a continence procedure such as colposuspension or insertion of tension-free vaginal tape may be a more appropriate procedure.

In cases of severe prolapse in which there may be a degree of ureteric obstruction, it is important to evaluate the upper urinary tract with either a renal tract ultrasound or an intravenous urogram.

Although a cystocele itself may be responsible for irritative urinary symptoms, if these are unusually severe cystoscopy should be performed to exclude a chronic follicular or interstitial cystitis.

MANAGEMENT

Prevention

In general, any factor that leads to chronic increases in intra-abdominal pressure should be avoided. Consequently, care should be taken to avoid constipation, which has been implicated as a major contributing factor to urogenital prolapse in Western society. In addition, the risk of prolapse in patients with chronic chest pathology, such as obstructive airways disease and asthma, should be reduced by effective management of these conditions. Hormone replacement therapy may also decrease the incidence of prolapse, although to date there are no studies that have tested this effect.

Maintaining an ideal BMI during pregnancy, smaller family size and improvements in antenatal and intrapartum care have also been implicated in the primary prevention of urogenital prolapse. A large national cohort study investigating the prevalence and risk factors for symptomatic pelvic organ prolapse women 20 years after one vaginal delivery or one caesarean delivery found that the prevalence of symptomatic prolapse was doubled after vaginal delivery compared with caesarean section, two decades after one birth. Infant birthweight and current BMI were implicated as risk factors for prolapse after vaginal delivery.[5] The role of caesarean section may also be important, although studies examining the outcome in terms of incontinence and symptomatic prolapse have had mixed results. Equally, antenatal and postnatal pelvic floor exercises have not yet been shown conclusively to reduce the incidence of prolapse, although they may be protective.

Physiotherapy

Pelvic floor exercises may have a role in the treatment of women with symptomatic prolapse, although there are no objective evidence-based studies to support this. Education about pelvic floor exercises may be supplemented with the use of a perineometer and biofeedback, allowing quantification of pelvic floor contractions. In addition, vaginal cones and electrical stimulation may also be used, although again, while they have been shown to be effective in the treatment of urodynamic stress incontinence, there are no data to support their use in the management of urogenital prolapse.

In summary, physiotherapy probably has a role in cases of mild prolapse in younger women who find an intravaginal device unacceptable and are not yet willing to consider definitive surgical treatment, especially if they have not yet completed their family.

Intravaginal devices

The use of intravaginal devices offers a further conservative line of therapy for those women who are not candidates for surgery. Consequently, they may be used in younger women who have not yet completed their family, during pregnancy and the puerperium, and also for those women who may be unfit for surgery. Clearly, this last group of women may include the elderly, although age alone should not be seen as a contraindication to surgery. In addition, a pessary may offer symptomatic relief while awaiting surgery.

Ring pessaries made of silicone or polythene are currently most frequently used. They are available in a number of different sizes (52–120 mm) and are designed to lie horizontally in the pelvis with one side in the posterior fornix and the other just behind the pubis, hence providing support to the uterus and upper vagina. Pessaries should be changed every six months; long-term use may be complicated by vaginal ulceration and therefore a low-dose topical oestrogen may be helpful in post-menopausal women.

Ring pessaries may be useful in the management of minor degrees of urogenital prolapse, although in severe cases, and for vaginal vault prolapse, a shelf pessary may be more appropriate. These may be difficult to insert and remove and their use is becoming less common, especially as they preclude coitus.

SURGERY

Surgery offers definitive treatment of urogenital prolapse. As in other forms of pelvic surgery, patients should receive prophylactic antibiotics to cover both Gram-negative and Gram-positive organisms, as well as thromboembolic prophylaxis in the form of low-dose heparin, and thromboembolic deterrent (TED) stockings.

All patients should also have a urethral catheter inserted at the time of the procedure unless there is a particular history of voiding dysfunction, in which case a suprapubic catheter may be more appropriate. This allows the residual urine volume to be checked following a void without the need for recatheterisation.

Patients having pelvic surgery are positioned in lithotomy with the hips abducted and flexed. To minimise blood loss, local infiltration of the vaginal epithelium is performed using 0.5 per cent xylocaine and 1/200,000 adrenaline, although care should be taken in patients with coexistent cardiac disease. A vaginal pack may be inserted at the end of the procedure, and removed on the first postoperative day.

Anterior compartment defects

Anterior colporrhaphy

Indication
Anterior colporrhaphy is indicated for the correction of cystourethrocele.

Procedure
A midline incision is made in the vaginal epithelium from 1 cm below the urethral meatus to the cervix or vaginal vault. The cystocele is dissected off the overlying epithelium using sharp and blunt dissection and is secured using two poly-glycolic (Vicryl, Ethicon) or polydioxanone (PDS, Ethicon) purse-string sutures. The redundant skin edges are then trimmed and the epithelium and fascia closed using interrupted polyglycolic (Vicryl, Ethicon) sutures.

In patients who have mild concurrent stress incontinence, a 'Kelly' mattress suture[6] may be placed under the urethrovesical junction, although colposuspension is preferable in cases of severe stress incontinence and will also cure a mild to moderate cystocele.

Lower urinary tract injury is uncommon. However, should a bladder or urethral injury occur, the defect can be repaired in layers using absorbable sutures and the bladder left on free drainage for ten days.

Paravaginal repair

Indication
Paravaginal repair is indicated for correction of cystourethrocele.

Procedure
First described in 1909, this offers an abdominal approach to correct an anterior compartment defect. The retropubic space (cave of Retzius) is opened through a Pfannenstiel incision and the bladder swept medially, exposing the pelvic sidewall. The lateral sulcus of the vagina is elevated with the overlying pubocervical fascia and reattached to the pelvic sidewall using interrupted polydioxanone (PDS, Ethicon) sutures from the pubis to just anterior to the ischial spine. Long-term follow up in a series of 800 patients reported a cure rate of more than 95 per cent.[7]

Posterior compartment defects

Posterior colporrhaphy

Indication
Posterior colporrhaphy is indicated for the correction of rectocele and deficient perineum.

Procedure
Two Allis forceps are first placed on the perineum at the level of the hymenal remnants, allowing the calibre of the introitus to be estimated. Following infiltration, the perineal scarring is excised and the posterior vaginal wall opened using a longitudinal incision. The rectocele is mobilised from the vaginal epithelium by blunt and sharp dissection and secured using two or more polyglycolic (Vicryl, Ethicon) or polydioxanone (PDS, Ethicon) purse-string sutures. The redundant skin edges are then trimmed, taking care not to remove too much tissue and thus narrow the vagina. The pararectal and rectovaginal fasciae from each side are approximated using interrupted polyglycolic (Vicryl, Ethicon) sutures incorporating the vaginal epithelium, and the posterior wall is closed with a continuous polyglycolic (Vicryl, Ethicon) suture. Care should be taken not to create a constriction ring in the vagina, which will result in dyspareunia. Finally, a perineoplasty is performed by placing deeper absorbable sutures into the perineal muscles and fascia, thus building up the perineal body to provide additional support to the posterior vaginal wall and lengthening the vagina.

Injury to the rectum is unusual, but should be identified at the time of the procedure so that the defect can be closed in layers using an absorbable suture and the patient managed with prophylactic antibiotics, low-residue diet and faecal softening agents to avoid constipation.

Pelvic floor surgery may also have an adverse effect on sexual function. Following pelvic floor repairs with or without vaginal hysterectomy, 50 per cent of women reported sexual dysfunction, nearly half of the cases being due to shortening of the vagina, dyspareunia or fear of injury.[8]

These findings have been confirmed more recently in a follow-up study of women undergoing posterior repair.[9] This series reported an increase in sexual dysfunction from 11 per cent pre-operatively to 27 per cent following surgery. In addition, 22 per cent of women complained of vaginal pain, 11 per cent had incontinence of faeces and 33 per cent had constipation.

Enterocele repair

Indication
Enterocele repair is indicated for the correction of enterocele.

Procedure
An enterocele repair is normally performed using a vaginal approach similar to that of posterior colporrhaphy. The vaginal epithelium is dissected off the enterocele sac, which is then secured using two or more polyglycolic (Vicryl, Ethicon) or polydioxanone (PDS, Ethicon) purse-string sutures. It is not

essential to open the enterocele sac, although care should be taken not to damage any loops of small bowel that it may contain. The posterior vaginal wall is then closed as described for posterior colporrhaphy.

An abdominal approach may also be used, although this is much less common. The Moschowitz procedure[10] is performed by inserting concentric purse-string sutures around the peritoneum in the pouch of Douglas, thus preventing enterocele formation.

Uterovaginal prolapse

Vaginal hysterectomy

Indication

Vaginal hysterectomy is indicated for uterovaginal prolapse. This procedure may be combined with anterior and posterior colporrhaphy.

Contraindications (relative)

- Uterine size >14 weeks' gestation, although morcellation[11] or uterine bisection may be used;
- Two or more caesarean sections;
- Endometriosis;
- PID;
- Suspected malignancy (uterine or ovarian).

Procedure

A cervical incision is performed and the uterovesical fold and pouch of Douglas opened. The uterosacral and cardinal ligaments are divided and ligated first, followed by the uterine pedicles and finally the tubo-ovarian and round ligament pedicles. In cases of procidentia, care should be taken to avoid kinking of the ureters, which are often dragged into a lower position than normal. After closure of the pelvic peritoneum, the upper pedicles are tied in the midline to provide support for the vaginal vault, while the uterosacral ligaments are tied posteriorly to obliterate the potential enterocele space. In addition, a McCall suture[12] may be performed, bringing the two uterosacral ligaments together in the midline as a further precaution against enterocele formation. Inclusion of the upper posterior vaginal wall also provides additional vault support. The vaginal epithelium is then closed with interrupted sutures.

Uterine preserving surgery

Uterine prolapse can also be treated with 'uterus sparing' procedures where an attempt is made to suspend the uterus rather than remove it through a hysterectomy. The evidence base for such procedures is very limited and largely anecdotal. The indications to preserve the uterus may be as follows:

- preservation of fertility;
- role of uterus in orgasm and female sexuality;
- influence on female sexual identity;
- lack of uterine pathology.

Routes

- Abdominal: Sacrospinous hysteropexy, Shirodkar's sling, pectineal ligament suspension;
- Vaginal: Manchester repair, sacrospinous hysteropexy and uterosacral ligament plication have been described;
- Laparoscopic: Round ligament plication, sacrohysteropexy, uterosacral plication.

Manchester repair (Fothergill repair)

Procedure

This procedure is only rarely performed nowadays. Cervical amputation is followed by approximating and shortening the cardinal ligaments anterior to the cervical stump and elevating the uterus. This is combined with an anterior and posterior colporrhaphy. The operation has fallen from favour, as the long-term complications include fertility problems in addition to recurrent uterovaginal prolapse and enterocele formation.

Vaginal vault prolapse

Vaginal vault prolapse occurs equally commonly following vaginal or abdominal hysterectomy, with an incidence of approximately 5 per cent, although only 0.5 per cent of women require further surgery.

Sacrospinous ligament fixation

Indication

Sacrospinous ligament fixation is indicated for vaginal vault prolapse.

Procedure

A longitudinal posterior vaginal wall incision is performed to expose the rectovaginal space. The right ischial spine is then identified and exposed using sharp and blunt dissection. The sacrospinous ligament may then be palpated running from the ischial spine to the lower aspect of the sacrum. An absorbable braided polyglycolic suture (Dexon, Davies + Geck) is passed through the ligament using a Miya hook ligature carrier and then through the vaginal vault. Care must be taken to avoid the sacral plexus and sciatic nerve, which are superior, and the pudendal vessels and nerve, which are lateral to the ischial spine. Once the enterocele has been secured using two purse-string sutures, the upper third of the vagina is closed as previously described. The sacrospinous sutures are then tied to support the vaginal vault from the sacrospinous ligament, following which a perineorrhaphy is performed.

Success rates of 98 per cent have been reported,[13] although posterior fixation of the posterior vaginal wall increases the incidence of anterior compartment defects. For this reason, it should not be performed routinely at vaginal hysterectomy. As the vaginal axis is changed by the procedure, there is a risk of post-operative dyspareunia and development of stress incontinence.

Abdominal sacrocolpopexy

Indication

Abdominal sacrocolpopexy is indicated for vaginal vault prolapse.

Procedure

This procedure may be performed through a lower midline or Pfannenstiel incision after packing the vagina. The apex of the vagina and sacral promontory are identified and a retroperitoneal tunnel is created between the two just to the right of the midline and medial to the right ureter. A strip of Mersilene tape is then passed through the peritoneal tunnel and sutured to the vaginal vault and posterior vaginal wall using interrupted, non-absorbable ethylene sutures (Ethibond, Ethicon). Once the other end of the tape has been secured to the periosteum overlying the sacral promontory, the sutures are tied, allowing gentle elevation of the vaginal vault towards the sacrum, but without tension. The peritoneum is then closed over the vaginal vault and sacral promontory. Complications include bleeding from the presacral venous plexus and sacral artery and damage to the right ureter and sigmoid colon.

A 93 per cent success rate has been reported,[14] although associated cystocele or rectocele may still require a vaginal colporrhaphy. In addition, since the vaginal axis is changed, there is also the risk of developing dyspareunia and stress incontinence following the procedure. Mesh erosion into the vagina, and rarely into the bladder or bowel, is a possible late complication.

A recent Cochrane review into surgical management of prolapse showed that abdominal sacrocolpopexy is associated with a lower rate of recurrent vault prolapse and dyspareunia than the vaginal sacrospinous colpopexy. These benefits must be balanced against a longer operating time, longer time to return to activities of daily living and increased cost of the abdominal approach.[15]

Posterior intravaginal slingplasty

Indication

Posterior intravaginal slingplasty (IVS) is indicated for vaginal vault prolapse.

Procedure

Posterior IVS using an 8-mm polypropylene tape has been described as a minimally invasive procedure for the treatment of vaginal vault prolapse. Under tension, a 5-cm transverse full-thickness incision is made in the posterior vaginal wall 1.5 cm below the scar line at the vaginal vault. Adjacent rectocele and enterocele are than dissected out so as to avoid accidental damage while passing the IVS tunneller (Tyco Healthcare, Mansfield, MA, USA) needle. Bilateral 1-cm perineal skin incisions are then made 2 cm lateral and below the external anal sphincter at the 4 and 8 o'clock positions.

Next, the IVS tunneller is advanced 4 cm into the ischirectal fossa before being turned inwards and guided using a finger through the rectovaginal fascia so as to exit through the

transverse vaginal incision. The procedure is then repeated on the contralateral side and a rectal examination performed to exclude bowel injury. The tape is then secured to the vaginal vault using polydioxanone (PDS, Ethicon) and the vagina closed with interrupted polyglycolic (Vicryl, Ethicon) sutures. A posterior colpoperineorrhaphy is then performed as previously described. Finally, the polypropylene tape is pulled posteriorly through the bilateral buttock incisions pulling the vaginal vault in a postero-superior direction. The tape is then cut flush with the skin and incisions closed using interrupted sutures.

To date, only one retrospective series of posterior IVS has been reported[16] with symptomatic cure rates of 91 per cent. However, there were five cases of tape rejection, one rectal tape erosion and one rectal perforation. Consequently, while early data would appear to be encouraging, more studies are required to determine its role in the management of vaginal vault prolapse.

Recurrent urogenital prolapse

Approximately one third of operations for urogenital prolapse are for recurrent defects. Recurrent prolapse may occur following both abdominal and vaginal hysterectomy, previous vaginal repairs and continence surgery. In addition, women with intrinsically weak connective tissue, such as patients with Ehlers Danlos syndrome, are at increased risk.

In such cases, the vaginal epithelium may be scarred and atrophic, making surgical correction technically more difficult and increasing the risk of damage to the bladder and bowel. The risk of post-operative complications, such as dyspareunia secondary to vaginal shortening and stenosis, is also increased. In those women who have had a previous continence operation, such as colposuspension, there is an increased risk of recurrent incontinence that may require further surgical correction.

Mesh repair

The use of synthetic mesh is becoming increasingly common in patients with prolapse, and may offer further support in cases in which the endopelvic fascia and vaginal epithelium are felt to be deficient. The ideal mesh should be strong and flexible, allowing ease of use. In addition, woven meshes should have an adequate pore size to allow the ingrowth of fibroblasts so as to minimise the risks of erosion and rejection.

Vaginal mesh kits are being used to surgically treat apical vaginal prolapse; however, their safety and efficacy are currently unknown. Several companies now market these 'mesh kits' despite lack of robust evidence regarding their safety and efficacy. A recent systematic review of these kits suggests that although they are associated with high objective cure rates between 87 and 95 per cent, they have a high risk of mesh erosion (4.6–10.7 per cent) and re-operation rates of up to 6 per cent.[17]

Recent guidelines by NICE and the MHRA suggest more stringent regulation on the use of mesh for prolapse surgery. The guidelines advise that mesh should only be considered for recurrent prolapse, and that all patients being considered for such surgery need to be discussed at the multidisciplinary team meeting, and only operated on a by surgeon with a special interest in surgery for pelvic organ prolapse.[18,19]

Dyspareunia is a common complication associated with the use of synthetic mesh and may be associated with erosion into the vagina, lower urinary tract and rectum. Although the use of mesh is becoming more common, it should be reserved for those patients with recurrent defects in specialist pelvic floor reconstructive surgery units.

CONCLUSION

Although not life threatening, urogenital prolapse is responsible for a significant degree of morbidity and impairment of quality of life. With approximately half of elective gynaecological operations being performed for correction of urogenital prolapse, the economic considerations are also considerable. In common with continence procedures, the initial procedure offers the greatest probability of success, and therefore patients should be carefully assessed with regard to their symptoms and investigations prior to surgery.

KEY POINTS

- Urogenital prolapse is a common condition associated with a high degree of morbidity.
- Incidence increases with increasing age and parity.
- Lifetime risk of surgery for urogenital prolapse is 11 per cent.
- Urogenital prolapse may be associated with concomitant urinary and faecal incontinence.
- Conservative management involves pelvic floor exercises and the use of vaginal pessaries.
- Surgery should be tailored to the needs of the individual patient.
- The use of synthetic mesh should be reserved for repeat procedures only.
- There is a high risk of recurrence following surgery, with a third of women requiring a further procedure.
- Complicated or recurrent cases are best managed using a multidisciplinary approach

Although conservative measures may be useful in the management of mild symptomatic prolapse, surgery offers the definitive treatment. The number of surgical procedures described is indicative of the fact that there is no perfect solution, and this is reflected in the number of patients who complain of recurrent prolapse. Such women should be managed in tertiary units by surgeons with a specialist interest in pelvic floor reconstructive surgery.

Key References

1. Subak LL, Waetjen E, van den Eeden S *et al.* Cost of pelvic organ prolapse surgery in the United States. *Obstet Gynecol* 2001;98:646–51.

2. Abrams P, Blaivas JG, Stanton SL, Andersen JT. The International Continence Society Committee on Standardization of Terminology. The standardization of terminology of lower urinary tract function. *Scand J Urol Nephrol* 1988;114S:5–19.

3. Smith ARB, Hosker GL, Warrell DW. The role of partial denervation of the pelvic floor in the aetiology of genito-urinary prolapse and stress incontinence. A neurophysiological study. *Br J Obstet Gynaecol* 1989;96:24–8.

4. Persson P1, Brynhildsen J, Kjølhede P; Hysterectomy Multicentre Study Group in South-East Sweden. *BJOG*. 2013;120:1556-65.

5. Gyhagen M, Bullarbo M, Nielsen TF, Milsom I. Prevalence and risk factors for pelvic organ prolapse 20 years after childbirth: a national cohort study in singleton primiparae after vaginal or caesarean delivery. *BJOG* 2013;120(2):152–60. doi: 10.1111/1471-0528.12020. Epub 2012 Nov 2.

6. Kelly HA. Incontinence of urine in women. *Urol Cutan Rev* 1913;17:291–7.

7. Richardson AC. Paravaginal repair. *In*: Benson JT (ed.). *Female Pelvic Floor Disorders*. New York: Norton, 1992: 280–7.

8. Francis WJA, Jeffcoate TNA. Dyspareunia following vaginal operations. *Br J Obstet Gynaecol* 1961;68:1.

9. Kahn MA, Stanton SL. Posterior colporrhaphy: its effects on bowel and sexual function. *Br J Obstet Gynaecol* 1997;104:82–6.

10. Muschovitz AV. The pathogenesis, anatomy and cure of prolapse of the rectum. *Surg Gynecol Obstet* 1912;15:7.

11. Magos A, Bournas N, Sinha R *et al.* Vaginal hysterectomy for the large uterus. *Br J Obstet Gynaecol* 1996;103:246–51.

12. McCall ML. Posterior culdoplasty. *Obstet Gynecol* 1957;10:595.

13. Shull BL, Capen CV, Riggs MW, Kuehl TJ. Preoperative and postoperative analysis of site-specific pelvic support defects in 81 women treated with sacrospinous ligament suspension and pelvic reconstruction. *Am J Obstet Gynecol* 1992;166:1764–71.

14. Addison WA, Livergood CH, Parker RT. Post hysterectomy vaginal vault prolapse with emphasis on management by transabdominal sacral colpopexy. *Post Grad Obstet Gynaecol* 1988;81.

15. Maher C, Baessler K, Glazener CM *et al.* Surgical management of pelvic organ prolapse in women: a short version Cochrane review. *Neurourol Urodyn* 2008;27:3–12.

16. Farnsworth BN. Posterior intravaginal slingplasty (infracoccygeal sacrocolpopexy) for severe post-hysterectomy vaginal vault prolapse – a preliminary report on efficacy and safety. *Int Urogynecol J* 2002;13:4–8.

17. Feiner B, Jelovsek JE, Maher C. Efficacy and safety of transvaginal mesh kits in the treatment of prolapse of the vaginal apex: a systematic review. *BJOG* 2009;116:15–24.

18. MHRA. *Vaginal mesh for pelvic organ prolapse.* MHRA, 2013.

19. NICE. *Surgical repair of vaginal wall prolapse using mesh (IPG267).* NICE, 2008.

Chapter 99 Infection and sexual health

Melanie Mann

PELVIC INFLAMMATORY DISEASE

This section covers the diagnosis, treatment and follow-up of PID. PID is important because it can have serious long-term sequelae such as pelvic pain, ectopic pregnancy and infertility. It is the result of post-infection scarring that is normally associated with healing. The virulence of the infection and the host-immune factors both determine the extent of the damage caused. There may be complete tubal closure, extensive peritubal adhesions, intratubal adhesions and mucosal and cilial damage, all of which can cause ectopic pregnancy and infertility (including interference with ovum transport and sperm migration). In a large, multicentre WHO study of more than 8000 couples in 25 countries investigated for infertility, approximately 32 per cent of diagnoses were tubal factor infertility in the female.

Incidence

The incidence of PID is unknown, as many cases go unnoticed until investigations for infertility are performed. There is no record of cases of PID held nationally apart from diagnosed records of all attendances at genito-urinary (GUM) clinics. Approximately 1 in 60 consultations in general practice is for women less than 45 years for suspected PID.

Aetiology

Neisseria gonorrhoeae and *Chlamydia trachomatis* are the most important organisms (but only account for a quarter of cases in the UK), although *Gardnerella vaginalis*, anaerobes and other organisms, such as mycoplasmas commonly found in the vagina, may also be implicated. Other factors associated with PID include:

- young age (<25 years);
- multiple sexual partners;
- past history of STI (in the patient or her partners);
- termination of pregnancy;
- insertion of an IUD in the previous six weeks;
- hysterosalpingography;
- IVF procedure;
- postpartum endometritis;
- bacterial vaginosis;
- a new sexual partner (within the previous three months).

Diagnosis

PID can be symptomatic or asymptomatic. Even in symptomatic patients, clinical symptoms and signs lack sensitivity and specificity. The positive predictive value of a clinical diagnosis is 65–90 per cent compared to laparoscopic diagnosis in experienced hands. The symptoms suggestive of PID include:

- lower abdominal pain;
- fever >38°C;
- dyspareunia;
- unscheduled vaginal bleeding;
- abnormal vaginal discharge.

The signs associated with PID are usually also non-specific. Pyrexia may be present, but not exclusively. Lower abdominal and adnexal tenderness on bimanual examination, as well as cervical excitation (cervical motion tenderness) on bimanual examination, are indicative of acute inflammation affecting the pelvic peritoneum. However, they are not specific for PID. Other conditions that should be considered when assessing lower abdominal pain in a young woman include:

- ectopic pregnancy;
- acute appendicitis;
- urinary tract infection;
- endometriosis;
- complications of an ovarian cyst (torsion or rupture);
- constipation;
- functional pain (pain of unknown origin).

Investigation of suspected PID

Testing for gonorrhoea and chlamydia in the lower genital tract is recommended, as positive results support a diagnosis (see p. 796-797 for details on testing for gonorrhoea and chlamydia). However, the absence of infection at this site does not exclude PID. Absence of cultured organisms may be due to poor sampling technique, inadequate storage and/or transportation of swabs or the presence of organisms that cannot easily be cultured in the laboratory, such as mycoplasmas. An elevated erythrocyte sedimentation rate (ESR) or C-reactive protein (CRP) can support the diagnosis. Laparoscopy may strongly support the diagnosis of PID, but is not justified routinely on the basis of cost and invasiveness. Furthermore, even laparoscopy lacks the sensitivity to identify mild intratubal inflammation or endometritis reliably. Endometrial biopsy and ultrasound scanning may also be helpful when there is diagnostic difficulty, but there is insufficient evidence to support their routine use at present.

Management

It is likely that delay in treatment increases the risk of the development of long-term sequelae of PID, such as ectopic pregnancy, pelvic pain and infertility. Owing to this, and to the lack of definitive diagnostic criteria, it is recommended that clinicians have a low threshold for treating empirically. It is also important that women are not labelled with the wrong diagnosis just because they appear to be in a high-risk group for having PID. Effort must be made to confirm the correct diagnosis, particularly in difficult or recurrent episodes of lower abdominal pain. It is also important in the gynaecological setting not to forget to investigate and treat the sexual partner(s), in order to prevent reinfection.

General measures

- Rest is advised for severe disease (preferably as an in-patient for observation to check that there is resolution of symptoms and signs) [C].
- A pregnancy test should be performed [C].
- Appropriate analgesia is advised [C].
- Parenteral therapy as an inpatient is advised for those with severe disease [C].
- Patients should avoid sexual intercourse until they and their partners have been fully treated and contact traced [C].

A full explanation should be given to the patient regarding the short- and long-term issues associated with PID. Leaflets to clarify and back up verbal explanation should be given to the client and her partner, if present. All patients should be offered full STI screening and HIV testing at some point in the management [C]. Good links with local GUM clinics are essential.

Antibiotic treatment

Broad-spectrum antibiotics are needed that will cover gonorrhoea and chlamydia. This treatment should be commenced as soon as possible. Information on recent and current medications should be obtained and appropriate advice given regarding any interactions. Latest evidence is that antibiotics (unless liver enzyme inducing e.g. rifampicin) do not affect the efficacy of hormonal contraception. There is a lack of evidence regarding antibiotic use and the prevention of long-term complications and fewer data on oral than parenteral regimens. There are important factors to be considered when choosing a regimen:

- local antimicrobial sensitivities (especially gonorrhoea);
- local epidemiology of infections (knowing where there are high-prevalence areas for gonorrhoea);
- cost;
- patient preference and likelihood of compliance;
- severity of disease.

When considering selection for inpatient treatment, the uncertainty of the diagnosis and severity of the disease will usually be sufficient to identify those who require inpatient observation. Other cases for which inpatient supervision is advised include women who have failed to respond to orally administered outpatient therapy, those who are suspected of having a tubo-ovarian mass and those who are unable to tolerate oral therapy. Two special subgroups might also be considered for inpatient treatment: those known to have an immunodeficiency problem (where a much more severe disease situation can develop quickly) and those who are pregnant – PID can occur up to about 12 weeks of pregnancy.

Recommended regimens

The following are evidence based. Intravenous therapy should be continued until 24 hours after clinical improvement and then switched to oral treatment [B].

Outpatient regimens

- Oral ofloxacin 400 mg twice daily plus oral metronidazole 400 mg twice daily for 14 days [A].
- Intramuscular ceftriaxone 500 mg single dose followed by oral doxycycline 100 mg daily plus metronidazole 400 mg twice daily for 14 days [A].
- Ofloxacin should be avoided in women at high risk of gonococcal PID due to increased quinolone resistance in the UK.

There is no evidence of one antibiotic regime listed above being superior to the others.

Inpatient regimens

Inpatient antibiotic treatment should be based on intravenous therapy which should be continued until 24 hours after clinical improvement and followed by oral therapy. Recommended regimens are:

- ceftriaxone 2 g by intravenous infusion daily plus intravenous doxycycline 100 mg twice daily, followed by oral doxycycline 100 mg twice daily plus oral metronidazole 400 mg twice daily for a total of 14 days;

- oral doxycycline may be used, if tolerated, while on intravenous ceftriaxone;
  or
- intravenous clindamycin 900 mg three times daily plus intravenous gentamicin, followed by either – oral clindamycin 450 mg four times daily to complete 14 days or – oral doxycycline 100 mg twice daily plus oral metronidazole 400 mg twice daily to complete 14 days.
- Gentamicin should be given as a 2 mg/kg loading dose followed by 1.5 mg/kg three times daily (or a single daily dose of 7 mg/kg may be substituted).
- Intravenous ofloxacin 400 mg twice daily plus intravenous metronidazole 500 mg three times daily for 14 days.

The clinical trial data support the use of cefoxitin for the treatment of PID, but this agent is not easily available in the UK so ceftriaxone, which has a similar spectrum of activity, is recommended. An alternative third-generation cephalosporin would also be acceptable. If parenteral gentamicin is used, then serum drug levels and renal function should be monitored. The choice of an appropriate treatment regimen will be influenced by robust evidence on local antimicrobial sensitivity patterns, robust evidence on the local epidemiology of specific infections, cost, the woman's preference and compliance, and severity of disease. Evidence of the efficacy of antibiotic therapy in preventing the long-term complications of PID is currently limited. Metronidazole may be discontinued in those women with mild or moderate PID who are unable to tolerate it, since its addition provides uncertain additional efficacy in this patient group.

Other important situations

Women with PID who are also infected with HIV should be treated with the same antibiotic regimens as women who are HIV-negative. Hospital admission and parenteral treatment is only required for those with clinically severe disease. Potential interactions between antibiotics and antiretroviral drugs should be considered.

The risk of giving any of the recommended antibiotic regimens in very early pregnancy (before a positive pregnancy test) is low, since significant drug toxicity results in failed implantation.

Pregnant women should ideally receive IV therapy, as PID is associated with higher maternal and fetal morbidity. (However, PID in pregnancy is rare except for septic abortion.) None of the regimens above is of proven safety in this group. There is insufficient evidence in pregnant women to suggest one treatment over another as long as the appropriate organisms are covered for 14 days' treatment and this is parenteral, if possible.

Consideration should be given to removing an IUD in women presenting with PID, if symptoms have not resolved within 72 hours [A] of starting antibiotics. The RCT evidence for whether an IUD should be left in place or removed in women presenting with PID is limited. Removal of the IUD should be considered and may be associated with better short-term clinical outcomes, but the decision to remove it needs to be balanced against the risk of pregnancy in those who have had unprotected intercourse in the preceding seven days. Emergency hormonal contraception may be appropriate for some women in this situation.

Fitz–Hugh–Curtis syndrome comprises right upper quadrant pain associated with perihepatitis, which occurs in up to 10–20 per cent of women with PID and may be the most obvious symptom. There is insufficient evidence to recommend laparoscopic adhesiolysis in this situation.

Management of partners should be by testing and treatment, ideally in a GUM clinic. Empirical treatment should be given. Broad-spectrum antibiotic treatment should be offered to male partners e.g. azithromycin 1 g single dose [C]. Contact tracing of all partners in the previous six months is recommended. Partners should avoid sexual intercourse until they and the index patient have completed the treatment course [C].

Follow-up

All patients should be followed up at three days to check improvement and exclude the need for parenteral or surgical treatment. Further review at four weeks is recommended to check resolution of symptoms, pregnancy test where appropriate and to discuss long-term issues. It is also an ideal time to check up on partner notification and treatment.

Management of vaginal discharge in women of reproductive years

The commonest cause of vaginal discharge is bacterial vaginosis (BV), which is not an STI. Candidiasis is the next commonest but is overdiagnosed by both women and their healthcare professionals. It is not an STI either. *Trichomonas vaginalis* (TV) *is* sexually transmitted and, if diagnosed, contact tracing needs to be done. Other causes of abnormal vaginal discharge can be infective (chlamydia or gonorrhoea) or non-infective such as foreign bodies, malignancies, fistulae, cervical ectopy or physiological (a diagnosis of exclusion).

Taking a good history is vital including a sexual history to pick up those at higher risk of an STI (under 25 years, previous STI, recent change in sexual partner or more than one partner in the previous year). Questions need to be asked regarding whether there has been unscheduled bleeding, upper reproductive tract symptoms (such as pelvic pain/deep dyspareunia), pregnancy/recent termination of pregnancy/recent instrumentation and whether these are recurrent symptoms and treatment has failed. In these situations, a full STI screen and examination should be carried out and referral to GUM may be necessary. It is useful to ask about medication already/recently used such as antibiotics.

The most important questions about the discharge then need to be asked: is there associated itch (candida) or malodour (BV or TV)? Is the discharge lumpy (? candida) or thin (BV) or frothy (TV)? Does anything make the symptoms worse (e.g. sex/menses/bathing make BV worse)? Has any treatment been tried (e.g. antifungals) and does it help?

If a woman is at low risk of STI and has no other concerning symptoms/history it is reasonable to examine and also test the vaginal pH. If the pH is >4.5 and the symptoms fit with BV, then she can be treated as such. If the symptoms are of candida and the clinical picture fits, then she can be treated with oral or topical antifungals. A high vaginal swab is not necessary unless there are recurrent or worrying symptoms or failure of therapy.

SEXUALLY TRANSMITTED INFECTIONS

This section focuses generally on the management of women, but one should not forget to consider partners and to think about them when talking about this aspect of gynaecology. Talking about these very personal aspects of a woman's life is very important and all gynaecologists need to be able to talk about sex sensitively and non-judgementally in order to do the best for the patient. It is therefore important that clinicians practise taking a sexual history to achieve this (Box 99.1). Clinician communication skills are very important.

Sexually transmitted infections are an important part of the everyday work of a gynaecologist and these conditions can have long-term sequelae for the patient if not managed promptly and thoroughly. The majority of large towns and cities in the UK have a department of GUM with at least one

Box 99.1 Taking a sexual history to assess the risk of STI

Preface by warning the patient that you need to ask some personal questions to do with her relationships with partners:

> *I need to ask you some personal questions now. Are you in a sexual relationship?*

You need to find out if this is a heterosexual or homosexual relationship. This is one of the most difficult questions. You can ask the first name of the partner and then clarify whether male or female if the first name is equivocal e.g. Nicky or Chris. Or you can say:

> *Can I just check, is your partner male or female? How long have you been with your partner?*

Avoid the term 'steady' or 'long term' as these have different meanings for different people.

> *Do you or your partner have any other partners, as far as you are aware?*

In some situations, it is important to ask about different sexual practices, such as oral or anal sex. Sometimes patients may volunteer the information that sex in a particular position causes discomfort, so it is important to be able to discuss this openly. Consideration should be given to asking about intimate partner violence and alcohol and recreational drug history.

specialist employed. It is good practice to develop strong links with this local department to improve the overall management of STIs within each gynaecology unit. This will ensure that patients receive optimum evidence-based treatment and that contact tracing and partner notification are performed according to approved guidelines.

Basic tenets of GUM

- The patient's confidentiality is paramount and patient details are not given to other patients or other healthcare professionals without the patient's informed consent (see below). Sexual history taking should take place in a private environment.
- If a patient has an STI, at least one other person is also carrying it and needs to be sought, treated and contact traced.
- If a patient has one STI, she must be at risk of all other STIs. She should therefore be offered screening for all other infections. This may be carried out in a GUM clinic.
- When swabs for STI are taken, it is important to obtain informed consent about the nature of the tests and explain what the follow-up procedure will be if the test is positive for an STI.
- Patients diagnosed with an STI should be advised not to have sexual intercourse until they and their partners have completed treatment and follow-up. This is to minimise further spread or reinfection.
- Patients should be given a detailed account of their condition, with particular emphasis on the long-term implications for themselves and their partner(s). This should be reinforced with clear and accurate written information.

Law relating to STIs

All NHS employees are required to adhere to the Caldicott principles for confidentiality and there is also explicit guidance from the General Medical Council to emphasise the importance. Confidentiality is a common-law duty and is absolute except in special circumstances such as when breaking confidentiality would be in the patient's or the public's best interests e.g. child protection cases.

The Venereal Diseases Act 1917 applies to GUM clinics and makes the rules of confidentiality even stricter: patient records are locked away and are not accessible to other clinicians outside the department, including the GP, without the express consent of the patient.

Terms used in GUM clinics

Partner notification
Contact slips, with a nationally agreed code for each STI, are given to patients to pass on to their sexual contacts. Contacts can then present the slip at any GUM clinic in the UK, where the infection will be managed appropriately. This is because there is communication between GUM clinics regarding partner notification.

Contact tracing
This involves finding the sexual contacts of the index patient carrying an infection and managing them appropriately, including ongoing partner notification if possible.

Health advisors
These are specially trained professionals whose job is to educate patients in the GUM clinics about STIs. They are also responsible for most partner notification and contact tracing.

Gonorrhoea

Gonorrhoea is an STI caused by the Gram-negative diplococcus *N. gonorrhoeae*. The primary sites of infection are the mucous membranes of the urethra, endocervix, rectum, pharynx and conjunctiva. Transmission occurs as a result of direct inoculation of secretions from one mucous membrane to another. Vertical transmission from mother to fetus may also occur during labour.

Clinical features
Up to 50 per cent of women are asymptomatic. In those who do have symptoms, the most common are an increased or altered vaginal discharge (up to 50 per cent) and lower abdominal pain (up to 25 per cent). Urethral infection may cause dysuria (12 per cent), but not usually frequency. Gonorrhoea is a rare cause of intermenstrual bleeding or menorrhagia and this is due to infection of the endometrium (endometritis). Infection in the pharynx is usually asymptomatic. Coexistent pathogens may be responsible for symptoms e.g. candida or trichomonas.

In men, the infection may also be asymptomatic (10 per cent), but generally causes urethral discharge (80 per cent) or dysuria (50 per cent).

Clinical signs
Less than 50 per cent of women will present with mucopurulent endocervical discharge and easily induced endocervical bleeding, and less than 5 per cent will present with pelvic or lower abdominal tenderness. Commonly, no abnormal findings are present on clinical examination. In men, there is usually a purulent urethral discharge present. Epididymal tenderness or balanitis, although reported, is rare. Gonorrhoea is also transmitted vertically to the fetus. It can cause severe conjunctivitis (ophthalmia neonatorum) and this is a notifiable disease in the UK. Neonatal infections can be severe and should be managed systemically by a paediatrician/ophthalmologist.

Complications
Transluminal spread of *N. gonorrhoeae* may occur, causing PID (<10 per cent) and epididymo-orchitis (<1 per cent) in men. Haematogenous dissemination can also occur, causing skin lesions, arthralgia, arthritis and tenosynovitis. Disseminated gonococcal infection is rare (<1 per cent).

Diagnosis

Detection of *N.gonorroeae* can be achieved by nucleic acid amplification tests (NAATs) or culture. NAATs are generally more sensitive than culture and offer testing on a wider range of specimen types. NAATs show a higher sensitivity (>96 per cent) in both symptomatic and asymptomatic infection; they are therefore the test of choice for asymptomatic individuals. Positive NAATs from low-prevalence populations need confirmation by supplementary testing that uses a different nucleic acid target. There is equal sensitivity of the test whether a vaginal swab or an endocervical swab is used. The sensitivity of urine NAATs in women is significantly lower and it is not the optimal specimen in women [B]. In men there is equal sensitivity in testing both urine and urethral swabs.

Positive NAATs should be confirmed by culture on selective medium which has been impregnated with antibiotics to prevent overgrowth of unwanted organisms. Gonorrhoea, under different circumstances, may not be cultured easily and so refrigeration of swabs prior to transport to the laboratory is recommended and sensitivities to antibiotics checked. Culture requires an endocervical and urethral swab specimen for maximal sensitivity. The collection of rectal and pharyngeal swab specimens should be directed by sexual history and symptoms and considered in women who are sexual contacts of gonorrhoea. Rectal gonorrhoea in women can be caused by tracking of discharge posteriorly. It is important to follow local guidance and liaise with the laboratory.

Management

All patients should be treated if they have a positive test result (NAAT or culture, if NAAT positive then culture too to confirm infection especially in low-prevalence areas and to check antibiotic sensitivities) or if a recent partner has confirmed gonococcal disease and testing of the patient is not possible. Consider treating epidemiologically after sexual assault. Referral to GUM is highly recommended [B]. There have been clinical reports of treatment failures using many recommended treatments and there is increasing concern about reduced sensitivity of *N. Gonorrhoeae* to third-generation cephalosporins.

Recommended treatments

Uncomplicated anogenital infection in adults:

- Ceftriaxone 500 mg IM as a single dose plus azithromycin 1 g oral as a single dose (Grade C recommendation). This is first-line treatment due to concerns around drug resistance and drug failures. Azithromycin is always recommended as a co-treatment to epidemiologically treat chlamydia, but even if chlamydia negative there is evidence that it might delay the widespread onset of cephalosporin resistance.
- Cefixime 400 mg oral as a single dose. Only if there are contraindications to an IM injection or refused (Grade A recommendation)
  or
- Spectinomycin 2 g IM as a single dose (Grade A recommendation).

Surveillance data for 2009 show significant levels of *N. gonorrhoeae* resistance to penicillin (22 per cent), tetracyclines (68 per cent) and ciprofloxacin (35 per cent) in the UK. Most resistant infections are acquired in the UK.

Antimicrobial therapy should take account of local patterns of antimicrobial sensitivity to *N. gonorrhoeae*. The chosen regimen should eliminate infection in at least 95 per cent of those presenting in the local community. This issue of local resistance patterns is another reason why all cases should be referred to GUM in the UK.

Treatment of gonorrhoea when pregnant or breastfeeding

Pregnant women should not be treated with quinolone or tetracycline antibiotics. Azithromycin: manufacturer advises use only if adequate alternatives are not available.

Recommended regimes

- Ceftriaxone 500 mg IM as a single dose with azithromycin 1 g orally as a single dose [C]
  or
- Spectinomycin 2 mg IM as a single dose with azithromycin 1 g stat orally [A].

In the case of allergy, the above regimes can be used.

Co-infection with *C. trachomatis* is common (up to 41 per cent of women) and therefore screening and, if positive, treatment should always be performed. In many departments, epidemiological treatment for chlamydia is given at the same time as gonococcal disease is treated.

Partner notification using national recommendations and contact tracing should be performed as described previously [B].

Follow-up and test of cure

At least one follow-up visit is recommended to confirm compliance with therapy, resolution of symptoms and partner notification. A test of cure is now recommended because of the concerns around antibiotic resistance. Test of cure should be done by NAAT ideally 2 weeks after treatment is completed. Infection identified at this point may be due to reinfection. All cases of gonorrhoea should be seen by a trained person (ideally a GUM health advisor) for partner notification and contact tracing.

Chlamydia trachomatis

National Chlamydia Screening Programme

The National Chlamydia Screening Programme (NCSP) is a control-and-prevention programme in the UK, targeted at sexually active young people under 25 years of age. Chlamydia is the most common bacterial STI in the UK, affecting both men and women, with sexually active young people at highest risk, with equal frequency in men and women. Most people with chlamydia have no symptoms but left untreated, chlamydia in women can lead to tubal factor infertility, ectopic pregnancy and chronic pelvic pain. In men, it may cause urethritis and epididimitis. In both sexes, it can cause arthritis.

The Chief Medical Officer's Expert Advisory Group on *Chlamydia trachomatis* (1998) considered the evidence base associated with screening for genital chlamydial infection. This group concluded that chlamydia screening met the criteria for a screening programme and recommended that one be established. Since then, the evidence base for chlamydial screening has continued to develop. Self-collected first-void urine specimens and vulvovaginal swabs have been found suitable samples for testing with NAATs. RCTs have demonstrated reductions in PID among women screened for chlamydia. There is considerable uncertainty and scientific debate about the mathematical models of screening effectiveness. The studies have predicted more moderate reductions in prevalence following the introduction of chlamydia screening than before screening. The NCSP facilitates the provision of screening in core sexual health services (community contraceptive services, general practice, abortion services and community pharmacies). Tests are also available via internet request and samples can be sent to the test provider in the mail.

It is recommended that young people are tested annually or when they change partner. If a young person has a positive test it is recommended that they are retested at three months as there is evidence that this group are at higher risk of being reinfected with higher risk of longer-term sequelae.

Screening for chlamydia should be promoted in young people, especially those who are pregnant (antenatal and those seeking abortion) and those attending GUM clinics, where the incidence varies between 5 and 16 per cent. Infection is sustained by unrecognised and untreated, symptomless chlamydial infection. It is now thought that overall the complications of this infection cost at least £50 million annually in the UK.

Clinical features

Eighty per cent of infected women are asymptomatic. When symptoms are present, they include post-coital or intermenstrual bleeding, lower abdominal pain, purulent vaginal discharge, mucopurulent cervicitis and/or contact bleeding. Fifty per cent of men are asymptomatic, with urethral discharge and dysuria being the most common symptoms. The risk factors associated with chlamydial infection include young age (<25 years), new sexual partner or more than one sexual partner in recent years. There is also an association with contraceptive practice, with infection being less common in barrier contraception users and more common in those using combined oral contraception. Women undergoing termination of pregnancy also appear to have a higher association with chlamydial infection. Prophylactic antibiotic use and screening for infection reduce the risk of post-abortion infection [B].

Complications

One of the immediate complications is developing PID. In chlamydial PID, perihepatitis can also occur; this is known as Fitz–Hugh–Curtis syndrome. As with other types of PID, the long-term sequelae include tubal damage resulting in an increased risk of infertility and ectopic pregnancy and chronic pelvic pain. Less common outcomes include adult conjunctivitis and sexually acquired reactive arthritis or Reiter's syndrome. This is more common in men who have chronic chlamydial infection.

Chlamydia can be transmitted to the neonate at the time of delivery, causing neonatal conjunctivitis (ophthalmia neonatorum) and pneumonitis. The risk of transmission is about 20–50 per cent for eye infections and 10–20 per cent for lung infections. The mother may also be at increased risk of infection of the uterus.

Specimen collection and laboratory tests for chlamydia

With the advent of NAATs reliable specimens are both self-taken vulvovaginal swabs (first choice) and also first-catch urine samples. Endocervical tests can also be taken, if a speculum examination is being done anyway. There are also assays which test for chlamydia and gonorrhoea detection in the same assay. It is recommended that patients are tested for chlamydia (using a NAAT) when they first present but that they are made aware of the two-week 'window period' and are advised to return for a repeat NAAT two weeks after the last exposure.

The current standard is to use NAAT testing which is highly sensitive for all cases including medico-legal cases. Enzyme immunoassay is now not recommended and culture is now not available.

In general, NAATs are 90–95 per cent sensitive with the majority of studies indicating that as either the number of sites sampled increases, or the number of different NAAT used increases, the greater the detection of *C. trachomatis* in any given population. Both first-catch urine (65–100 per cent sensitivity) and self-taken vulvovaginal swabs (90–95 per cent sensitivity) are suitable for testing and for screening. However, first-catch urine samples may be less sensitive than vulvovaginal or cervical samples for detecting infection with *C. trachomatis*.

General management

Women should be advised to take the treatment (see below under Treatment) and avoid sexual intercourse (including oral sex) for the duration of the treatment, or for one week after taking the stat dose of azithromycin. Men and women with a positive chlamydia test should be offered a full STI screen and this may require a visit to the local GUM department. All contacts of positive chlamydia tests should be tested and treated epidemiologically and also offered a full STI screen. Uncomplicated chlamydia is not an indication to remove an IUD or IUS. All patients with a positive test for chlamydia should be given written information regarding the infection.

Treatment

The recommended treatment of uncomplicated chlamydial infection is with azithromycin 1 g stat as a single dose or doxycycline 100 mg twice a day for seven days. Alternative

UROGYNAECOLOGY AND SEXUAL HEALTH AND WELLBEING

regimens include erythromycin 500 mg four times a day for seven days or erythromycin 500 mg twice a day for 14 days. However, erythromycin has a significant side-effect profile and is less than 95 per cent effective. Ofloxacin 400 mg once a day for one week can also be used. The majority of studies are flawed in design, small and give no details regarding the treatment of sexual partners. Doxycycline and azithromycin have been the most rigorously tested. Women using combined hormonal contraception should be advised there is no interaction between these antibiotics and their contraception and they should use as normal. Follow-up of chlamydial infection is recommended to check partner notification, reinforce health education, assess treatment efficacy and exclude reinfection [B].

Treating *Chlamydia trachomatis* in pregnancy: Quinolones and tetracyclines should not be used in pregnancy.

Amoxicillin appears to be an acceptable alternative to erythromycin in achieving microbiological cure (amoxicillin 500 mg three times a day for seven days) and is better tolerated. Clindamycin and azithromycin may be considered. Azithromycin is recommended for treatment by WHO, but is not licensed in the UK for use in pregnancy. The British National Formulary (BNF) says it can be used if no other alternative is available. However, Scottish guidelines recommend azithromycin as first-line treatment in pregnancy [A] (1 g as a single oral dose).

Test of cure

A test of cure is not routinely recommended but should be performed in pregnancy or if non-compliance or re-exposure is suspected. It should be deferred for five weeks (six weeks if azithromycin has been given) after treatment is completed.

Trichomonal infection

The causative organism is *Trichomonas vaginalis*. This is a flagellated protozoon which is found in the vagina, urethra and para-urethral glands. Transmission is almost exclusively sexual in adults. It can be acquired perinatally and occurs in 5 per cent of babies born to infected mothers. If infection is found after the first year, sexual contact is implied, although other modes of transmission are postulated.

Clinical features

Between 10 and 50 per cent of women are asymptomatic [B]; among the remainder, the most common symptoms are vaginal discharge, vulval itching, dysuria and offensive odour. Occasionally, lower abdominal pain may be present. Seventy per cent of infected women have a vaginal discharge, which can vary in consistency from thin and scanty to profuse and thick. The classical frothy yellow discharge occurs in 10–30 per cent. Vulvitis, vaginitis and cervicitis are associated with trichomonal infection. A 'strawberry cervix' appearance is visible to the naked eye in approximately 2 per cent of cases

and in more women on colposcopy. No abnormalities are found in 10–15 per cent of women.

Complications

There is increasing evidence that trichomonal infection can have a detrimental effect on pregnancy and is associated with preterm delivery and low-birthweight infants [B].

Diagnosis

Direct observation of a wet smear from the posterior fornix will diagnose 40–80 per cent of cases, whereas culture of the organism will correctly diagnose 95 per cent of infected women. Trichomonads are no longer reported by the national cervical screening programme which is now mainly using liquid-based cytology methods. There may be NAATs in future.

Treatment

Systemic chemotherapy is recommended, as urethral and para-urethral glands are frequently infected. Most strains of TV are highly sensitive to metronidazole and related drugs (approximately 95 per cent cure rate). There is a spontaneous cure rate in 20–25 per cent.

The recommended regimens for treating trichomonal infection include metronidazole 2 g orally in a single dose (avoid in pregnancy and breastfeeding) or metronidazole 400–500 mg twice daily for 5–7 days [A]. The single dose is cheaper with better compliance, but there is evidence that there may be a higher failure rate, especially if partners are not treated concurrently. Patients should be advised not to drink alcohol for the duration of, and for 48 hours after completion of, treatment due to the disulfiram-like effect (severe sickness).

Treatment failures should be referred to GUM to assess the possible reasons, such as poor compliance, re-infection, co-infection and/or resistance. There is no evidence that metronidazole is teratogenic in the first trimester of pregnancy [A], although the BNF warns against high-dose regimens. In breastfeeding women, metronidazole may change the taste of breast milk. High doses should be avoided.

Genital herpes

Genital herpes is acquired by sexually transmitted infection with either herpes simplex type 1 virus (HSV-1) – which is the usual cause of orolabial herpes – or herpes simplex type 2 virus (HSV-2). The infection may be primary or non-primary and disease episodes may be initial or recurrent and symptomatic or asymptomatic. Severe primary attacks of herpes constitute a genito-urinary emergency and patients should be dealt with quickly and referred to a department of GUM for ongoing support and partner notification. After childhood, symptomatic primary infection with HSV-1 is equally likely to be acquired in the genital or oral areas. After primary infection, the virus becomes latent in local sensory ganglia, periodically reactivating to cause symptomatic lesions or asymptomatic but infectious viral shedding. This may be important in the acquisition of infection in long-term relationships where there has been primary infection with no history of a new partner. New diagnoses of genital herpes are equally likely to be caused by HSV-1 or HSV-2; however, HSV-2 is more likely to recur than HSV-1. Median recurrence rates per month after a first episode are 0.34 for HSV-2 (approximately 4 episodes a year) and 0.08 for HSV-1 (approximately 1 episode a year). Recurrence rates generally reduce over time.

Clinical features of genital herpes in women

The most common symptoms are those of vulval pain, which is usually associated with ulcers that are preceded by blisters (Table 99.1). In a primary infection, this can be quite severe and the whole vulva can become swollen, ulcerated and infected. This, in turn, can cause discharge and dysuria and in severe cases urinary retention. The cervix may also become ulcerated. Tender inguinal lymphadenopathy is also a feature of the primary infection, although this may be the result of secondary infection. More generalised features of a viral illness may also be present, particularly in primary infections. These include fever and myalgia. Herpetic infection can be asymptomatic; this is more likely in recurrent episodes.

Complications

Urinary retention can occur as a result of autonomic neuropathy, or because of the severe pain caused by the local reaction around the urethra and vulva. It has also been postulated that chronic vulval pain may also be a result of post-herpetic neuralgia.

Diagnosis

HSV confirmation and typing are important for diagnosis, prognosis and counselling [C]. Swabs must be taken from the base of a lesion, kept cold and transported directly to the laboratory in the viral culture medium. Serology is not commonly used to make the diagnosis. Given the implications of the diagnosis and potential for recurrent infections, it is vital that an accurate diagnosis be made at the outset. It cannot be assumed that vulval ulceration is herpetic until so proven by viral culture. HSV NAAT/PCR (polymerase chain reaction for HSV DNA) for herpes diagnosis has a higher sensitivity (71 per cent) than virus culture (11 per cent).

Table 99.1 Clinical features of acute herpes infections in women

Symptoms	Signs
Painful ulceration, dysuria, vaginal discharge	Blistering and ulceration of vulva ± cervix, preceded by vesicles
Fever, myalgia (flu-like symptoms) – more common in primary infections	Inguinal lymphadenopathy
May be asymptomatic	

Management

Primary genital herpes

General advice includes drinking large quantities of fluids to make the urine less concentrated and therefore reduce the pain on micturition, saline bathing and analgesia with a combination of NSAIDs and topical anaesthetic gels. Antiviral drugs are indicated if commenced within five days of the start of the episode and if lesions are still developing. Aciclovir (200 mg five times daily), valaciclovir (500 mg twice daily) and famciclovir (250 mg three times daily) all reduce the severity and duration of episodes [A], but they do not alter the natural history of the infection. Topical agents are less effective than oral agents, and intravenous therapy is only indicated when the patient cannot tolerate oral medication.

Management of complications

Hospitalisation may be required because of urinary retention, meningism and severe constitutional symptoms. If catheterisation is required, it is recommended that the suprapubic approach be used [C] to prevent the theoretical risk of ascending infection, reduce the painfulness of the procedure and allow normal micturition to take place without multiple attempts at recatheterisation.

Recurrent genital herpes

Recurrent attacks of genital herpes are generally less severe than primary attacks and are self-limiting. It is important to make management decisions together with the patient, and advice should be given with regard to sexual activity while potentially infective. However, not all patients will be aware of their potential infective state, particularly those who do not have symptoms or a prodrome (disordered local vulval sensations prior to the onset of a recurrent attack). Supportive and episodic antiviral therapy may be given [A], but if individuals suffer more than six attacks each year, suppressive therapy using antiviral agents and under the supervision of a genitourinary physician should be considered. Counselling may be required for those with problems adapting to the diagnosis.

Management in pregnancy

Referral of a woman with suspected herpes in pregnancy to a GUM physician is recommended. The main concern is the risk of neonatal HSV acquired during delivery from maternal viral shedding. This is most likely to occur with new maternal acquisition in the third trimester.

First-episode genital herpes

First- and second-trimester acquisition: Diagnosis in pregnancy is as described above. Serological testing of HSV-1 and -2 (IgG) has not been fully evaluated. First-trimester herpes has been associated with miscarriage, but there is no evidence of increased risk of fetal abnormality if the pregnancy continues. It is not an indication for termination of pregnancy.

Management should be as above, with oral or intravenous aciclovir in standard doses. Aciclovir is not licensed in pregnancy, but there is substantial clinical evidence supporting its safety. Unless there are other complications, vaginal delivery can be anticipated. Continuous aciclovir in the last 4 weeks of pregnancy (aciclovir 400 mg tds) reduces the risk of both clinical recurrences at term and the need for caesarean section [A]. However, this point is contentious as other RCOG guidance quotes a study which did not demonstrate that aciclovir in the last 4 weeks of pregnancy gave any further protection.

Third trimester acquisition: Caesarean section should be considered for those developing symptoms after 34 weeks, as the risk of viral shedding during labour is very high, and thus also the risk of vertical transmission to the neonate (risk of neonatal herpes 41 per cent). If it is difficult to differentiate between a primary and a recurrent attack, it may be helpful to take viral swabs as well as serum (IgG) and if the HSV is the same type then CS may be avoided. If membranes have been ruptured for more than 4 hours, then CS may not prevent vertical transmission. The paediatricians should be informed. Neonatal herpes carries a mortality of 30 per cent for disseminated herpes infection and 17 per cent have long-term neurological sequelae. Caesarean section for the prevention of neonatal herpes has not been evaluated in RCTs and may not be completely protective against neonatal herpes. If CS does not take place, prolonged rupture of membranes and invasive monitoring should be avoided, intrapartum antivirals should be given and the baby treated postnatally.

Recurrent genital herpes

Sequential cultures in late pregnancy do not predict viral shedding at term. If there are no lesions at delivery, CS should not be performed, even if there has been a brief recurrence during the third trimester. Continuous aciclovir in the last four weeks of pregnancy may be cost effective compared with no therapy or CS. It may not reduce the risk of CS, as it does not eliminate viral shedding completely. There is no proven benefit in taking swabs for viral cultures at delivery to assess asymptomatic shedding.

Genital lesions (recurrent herpes) at delivery

The current British Association for Sexual Health and HIV (BASHH) consensus is that a caesarean section should be performed, despite lack of evidence for its effectiveness. The current RCOG consensus is that mode of delivery and pros and cons should be discussed with the mother, but that CS is not necessary as recurrent lesions are associated with a much lower risk of neonatal herpes (1–3 per cent). Therefore, the risks for the fetus at vaginal delivery may be small and need to be compared to the risks to the mother of caesarean section.

Prevention of acquisition of infection

All women should be asked about genital herpes in themselves or in their partners. The asymptomatic female partners of men known to have genital herpes should be advised to avoid sexual contact during recurrences [C]. Conscientious use of condoms during pregnancy may reduce the risk of acquisition, but this is unproven. Pregnant women should be advised about the risk of orogenital contact for acquiring HSV-1. The identification of susceptible women by means of type-specific antibody testing has not been shown to be cost effective. All women, not just those with a history of genital herpes, should undergo careful inspection of the vulva at the onset of labour to look for clinical signs of herpes infection. Mothers, staff and other relatives and friends with active oral lesions should be advised about the risk of postnatal transmission.

Bacterial vaginosis

Bacterial vaginosis is not regarded as an STI and its aetiology is unknown. It is the most common cause of vaginal discharge in women of child-bearing age. The reported prevalence varies from 5 per cent in a group of asymptomatic college students to 50 per cent of women in Uganda. It has been reported in 12 per cent of pregnant women and in 30 per cent of women undergoing termination of pregnancy in the UK.

BV is characterised by an overgrowth of predominantly anaerobic organisms (*Gardnerella vaginalis*, *Prevotella* spp., *Mycoplasma hominis*, *Mobiluncus* spp.) in the vagina. This leads to replacement of lactobacilli and an increase in pH from a normal of 4.5 to 7. BV can arise and remit spontaneously in sexually active and non-sexually active women. It is more common in black than in white women, in those with an IUD and in those who smoke cigarettes.

Clinical features

In approximately 50 per cent of confirmed cases, there are no volunteered symptoms. Those with symptoms usually complain of an offensive, fishy-smelling vaginal discharge, not usually associated with vulvovaginitis. There is also a thin, white, homogeneous discharge coating the walls of the vagina and vestibule.

Complications

Although the incidence of BV is high in women with PID, there are no prospective studies investigating whether treating asymptomatic women for bacterial vaginosis reduces their risk of developing it subsequently. The condition is common in some populations of women undergoing elective termination of pregnancy and is associated with post-termination endometritis and PID [A]. In pregnancy, BV is associated with late miscarriage, preterm birth, preterm premature rupture of the membranes and postpartum endometritis [A]. It has been associated with an increased incidence of vaginal cuff cellulitis and abscess formation following transvaginal hysterectomy [B]. It is unclear how important this is in the UK, where antibiotic prophylaxis is routine practice. There are no studies investigating the role of BV in the development of PID following IUD insertion.

Diagnosis

Amsel's criteria for diagnosing bacterial vaginosis

At least three out of these four should be present for the diagnosis to be confirmed:

- thin, white, homogeneous discharge;
- clue cells on microscopy;

- pH of vaginal fluid >4.5;
- release of a fishy odour on adding alkali (10 per cent potassium hydroxide). (This test is rarely performed these days.)

Routine use of a high vaginal swab may not be useful, as culture of *G. vaginalis* can be possible in more than 50 per of normal women [B]. However, criteria can be used to judge whether a vaginal smear that has been Gram-stained shows features consistent with a diagnosis of BV. Realistically, if a woman has typical symptoms, history and signs together with a raised pH (>4.5), a presumptive diagnosis can be made and the woman treated.

Management

Initially, simple advice should be offered; this includes advice against the practice of vaginal douching, use of shower gels and antiseptic bath agents [C].

Antibiotic treatment is recommended for symptomatic women [A], women undergoing surgical procedures [A] and some pregnant women [A]. Studies support screening and treating BV with either metronidazole or clindamycin cream, to reduce the incidence of endometritis and PID post abortion. Using the oral route of administration, recommended regimens for treating BV include metronidazole 400–500 mg twice daily for 5–7 days [A] or metronidazole 2 g as a single dose [A]. An alternative approach is to use the vaginal route, with intravaginal metronidazole gel (0.75 per cent) once daily for five days [A] or intravaginal clindamycin cream (2 per cent) once daily for seven days [A]. All these treatments have been shown to achieve cure rates of 70–80 per cent after four weeks in controlled trials using placebo or comparing with oral metronidazole.

No reduction in relapse rates has been reported in studies in which the male partners were treated, and therefore there is no indication to treat the male partners of women with BV.

Follow-up is only required if symptoms recur, although a more cautious approach should be employed in pregnancy where recurrent infection may be associated with adverse outcomes.

The optimal management of those who have recurrent episodes of bacterial vaginosis remains unresolved.

EBM: Pregnancy and bacterial vaginosis

- Meta-analyses have concluded that there is no evidence for teratogenicity from the use of metronidazole in pregnancy [A].
- The results of clinical trials investigating the value of screening for and treating BV in pregnancy are conflicting, and it is therefore difficult to make firm recommendations.

In summary, symptomatic pregnant women should be treated in the normal way and there is insufficient evidence to treat asymptomatic women. Breastfeeding women might be better treated intravaginally as metronidazole affects the taste of the milk.

Anogenital warts

Aetiology

Warts are benign epithelial skin tumours that are caused by the human papillomavirus (HPV), of which there are more than 100 genotypes. The mode of transmission is most often sexual, but it may be transmitted perinatally and also from digital lesions (more commonly in children). Although the majority are benign and caused by HPV sub-types 6 and 11, others may contain oncogenic subtypes that are associated with genital tract dysplasia and cancer. Warts are just one manifestation of HPV infection of the genital tract, as there may also be subclinical and latent infection. Men and women with warts are best treated in a GUM department and also screened for other STIs.

Clinical features

Anogenital warts may cause irritation, but generally present as 'lumps' which may be found disfiguring and psychologically distressing. They can occur at any site in the genital area including perianally, which does not imply anal intercourse. Lesions can be flat or raised, single or multiple, soft or keratotic, small or 'cauliflower like', flesh-coloured or pigmented.

Occult lesions may also occur in the vagina and cervix. Extra-genital lesions may occur on the oral mucosa, larynx, conjunctiva and nasal cavity. Warts may be exophytic, single or multiple, keratinised and non-keratinised, broad based or pedunculated, and some are pigmented.

Diagnosis is mainly by naked-eye examination, although any doubt about the diagnosis should prompt biopsy under local anaesthetic. Speculum examination should be performed to look for cervical and vaginal lesions.

Management

General advice

Condom usage with regular partners has not been shown to affect the treatment outcome of anogenital warts. However, using condoms may result in both partners feeling more comfortable and may prevent the transmission of HPV to uninfected partners and therefore should be encouraged.

Treatment (see Box 99.2)

Treatment is generally uncomfortable and can be painful, and patients should be made aware that all treatments have

Box 99.2 HPV vaccination for genital wart protection

In the UK, young women at the age of 12 and 13 are offered Gardasil (from September 2012), a quadrivalent vaccine, meaning it protects against four strains of HPV. Gardasil protects against HPV-16, HPV-18 (high-risk HPV strains that are responsible for 70 per cent of cervical cancers in Europe) and HPV-6 and HPV-11, the strains responsible for 99 per cent of genital warts in young women. It is likely that genital warts will become far less frequent. In France the quadrivalent vaccine accounted for between 37 and 56 per cent cost savings in terms of genital wart protection.

significant failure and relapse rates. Warts may regress and disappear spontaneously; one third of all visible warts will disappear by six months. The choice of treatment depends on the morphology, number and distribution of the warts. First- and second-line treatments are not based upon robust evidence.

Soft, poorly keratinised warts respond well to podophyllin, podophyllotoxin (an antimitotic agent)and trichloroacetic acid, whereas keratinised lesions are better treated with physical ablative therapies, such as cryotherapy (causes cytolysis at dermal/epidermal junction), excision and electrocautery. Imiquimod, an immune modulating agent, may be suitable for both types. Podophyllotoxin is usually administered over a four week cycle and imiquimod for up to 16 weeks, and both are suitable for self-application at home after appropriate instruction and screening for other sexually transmitted infections. This is best supervised from a GUM clinic, as are most anogenital wart treatments. Adequate contraception must be ensured prior to the use of podophyllin-type chemicals because of the known teratogenic effect in animals.

Cervical warts can be removed by a variety of methods. Colposcopy is recommended if there is any doubt as to the diagnosis, but otherwise warts on the cervix are not an indication for colposcopy in themselves.

Anogenital warts in pregnancy

Podophyllin and podophyllotoxin should be avoided because of their possible teratogenic effects, and currently imiquimod does not have approval for use in pregnancy. The objectives of treatment in pregnancy are to minimise the number of lesions present at delivery and to reduce neonatal exposure to the virus. Potential problems in the neonate are the development of laryngeal papillomatosis and anogenital warts. Very rarely, a caesarean section is indicated due to blockage of the vaginal outlet.

Cervical cytology

The National Health Service Cervical Screening Programme (NHSCSP) recommends no changes to screening intervals for women with anogenital warts. Furthermore, developing anogenital warts prior to the age when screening would normally start is not an indication to commence cervical screening.

Immunosuppressed women

This category includes women with impaired cell-mediated immunity (renal transplant patients and those infected with HIV), who are likely to have poor treatment responses, increased relapse rates and dysplasia. Careful follow-up is required.

Syphilis

Aetiology

Treponema pallidum, the spirochaete responsible for sexually acquired syphilis, causes one type of treponemal disease.

The pathological strains also cause non-sexually transmitted tropical diseases, such as yaws, endemic syphilis, bejel and pinta. These organisms are serologically and morphologically similar and cannot be grown on artificial media. Occasionally, saprophytic strains, found in the mouth in dental sepsis, can cause diagnostic confusion.

Syphilis is transmitted sexually, via blood products and vertically in pregnancy; therefore, the condition can be acquired and congenital. Syphilis is a treatable but complicated infection, best managed by GUM.

Epidemiology

Syphilis first became widespread and epidemic at the end of the fifteenth century in Europe. Syphilis and gonorrhoea were recognised as STIs in the eighteenth century, but were thought to be the same disease, until they were finally shown to be separate infections in the mid-nineteenth century. Until recently, syphilis was in a steady decline in the West, but over the last 20 years the incidence has begun to increase together with HIV infection.

Classification

Acquired syphilis can be divided into early and late infections. Early syphilis is further subdivided into primary, secondary and early latent (less than two years of infection). The subdivisions of late infection include late latent (greater than two years of infection) and tertiary, which includes gummatous, cardiovascular and neurological involvement. Cardiovascular and neurological involvement is sometimes classified as quaternary syphilis.

Congenital syphilis is divided into early (first two years) and late, which includes the classical stigmata of congenital syphilis.

Clinical features

Primary syphilis is characterised by an ulcer (the chancre) and regional lymphadenopathy. The chancre is classically a single, painless and indurated ulcer with a clean base discharging clear serum and is usually found in the anogenital region. However, it may also be atypical, multiple, painful, purulent and destructive and occur at extra-genital sites. The ulcer(s) of primary syphilis should not be confused with other genital ulcerative disorders (Box 99.3).

Box 99.3 Aetiology of anogenital ulceration

- Herpes simplex
- Syphilis
- Chancroid
- Lymphogranuloma venereum
- Donovanosis
- Candidiasis (severe)
- Behçet's disease
- Scabies-excoriated

Secondary syphilis is characterised by multisystem involvement occurring within the first two years of infection. The features include a generalised polymorphic rash, often affecting the palms and soles, condylomata lata (moist warty lesions at sites of skin friction such as vulva, under breasts, axillae) mucocutaneous lesions, generalised lymphadenopathy and other rare multisystem manifestations. Early latent syphilis is characterised by positive serological tests for syphilis with no clinical evidence of treponemal infection, again within the first two years of infection. In cases testing positive serologically for treponemal infection in the absence of clinical signs, it is important to exclude other infections such as yaws, particularly in people of Caribbean origin. All women with positive treponemal serology should be investigated and treated in a GUM department.

Diagnosis

The diagnosis can be made by direct demonstration of *Treponema pallidum* from lesions or infected lymph nodes in early syphilis by dark-field microscopy, direct fluorescent antibody testing and tests based upon the PCR.

Serological tests include:

- cardiolipin (reaginic) tests: Venereal Disease Research Laboratory;
- carbon antigen test/rapid plasma reagin (RPR) test;
- specific tests: treponemal enzyme immunoassay (EIA) to detect IgG, IgG and IgM; *T. pallidum* haemagglutination assay (TPHA) and others.

Treatment

All treatment should be managed in a GUM clinic.

The mainstay of treatment is parenteral penicillin as it is given under supervision, therefore ensuring compliance, and has bioavailability guaranteed.

Early syphilis is treated with benzathine penicillin G with a single dose, which is unlicensed in the UK. Azithromycin single dose can be used as second line.

Late syphilis is treated with benzathine penicillin G at three-weekly doses, except for neurosyphilis where procaine penicillin G with concomitant oral probenicid is used as first line. All patients should be offered screening for other STIs, including HIV.

Approximately 40 per cent of those treated will have a reaction to the penicillin treatment called the Jarisch–Herxheimer reaction. In pregnancy this also occurs in the same frequency and in addition to the fever the pregnant woman may experience uterine contractions, which resolve in 24 hours. Fetal heart rate decelerations may also occur. As described below these cases should be managed with obstetric and paediatric colleagues.

Pregnancy

All pregnant women should be screened for syphilis at the initial antenatal visit. Syphilis may be transmitted transplacentally at any stage of pregnancy and may lead to polyhydramnios, miscarriage, preterm labour, stillbirth, hydrops and congenital syphilis.

Sixty to ninety per cent of the infants of pregnant women with untreated primary or secondary syphilis will be infected and one third will be stillborn. Mother-to-child transmission is lower (40 per cent) in early latent and decreases to less than 10 per cent in late latent syphilis.

Patients should be jointly managed with GUM physicians and treated as above, but in the third trimester be given a second dose of benzathine penicillin G one week after the first dose. Ceftriaxone 500 mg IM for 10 days should be added to alternatives. When pregnant women are treated for syphilis after 26 weeks, the fetus should be investigated for infection and distress during treatment in a department of fetal medicine. All neonates should be treated at birth.

Congenital syphilis

Babies of mothers with positive serology for syphilis and treated antenatally should be managed jointly by a GUM physician and a paediatrician. Laboratory blood tests should be performed on the infant's (not cord) blood. In view of the highly treatable nature of the disease and the high perinatal morbidity and mortality of congenital syphilis, it is extremely important to continue with antenatal testing.

Human immunodeficiency virus

There are two strains of HIV, types 1 and 2, of which HIV-1 is responsible for most HIV infections. HIV carries its genetic code as RNA; this is translated by an enzyme present in the virus (reverse transcriptase) into DNA, which then integrates into the host's target cells, including CD4 T-lymphocytes, and other cells of the immune system. This results in a decline in CD4 cells and progression to AIDS. HIV infection can cause a decline in CD4 counts from a normal level of about $1000/\mu L$ to $<200/\mu L$. The infected person then becomes susceptible to the opportunistic infections and malignancies characteristic of AIDS.

HIV disease is an extremely important, fatal disease worldwide. It is currently estimated that approximately 40 million people are infected. HIV infection increases the susceptibility to other infectious diseases, such as tuberculosis, with a huge impact on morbidity and mortality. HIV is most prevalent in economically deprived areas in the developing world where people are less likely to be able to afford the expensive antiretroviral drugs that can limit disease progression and spread. HIV is transmitted sexually, in blood products and to the fetus vertically and through breastfeeding. In developed countries such as the UK, infected people have access to the latest evidence-based treatments and are managed by GUM physicians.

With the currently available antiretroviral agents, eradication of HIV infection is not likely to be possible. The aims of treatment are to prolong life and improve quality of life by maintaining suppression of virus replication for as long as possible. Antiretroviral therapy is monitored by measurements of viral load together with CD4 counts. The aim of therapy is to decrease the viral load to less than 50 copies per mL within four to six months of commencing therapy. Treatment is recommended for patients with primary HIV infection, asymptomatic HIV infection and symptomatic HIV infection or AIDS. However, treatment should be commenced in patients when their CD4 count is <350 cells mL. There is overwhelming evidence from cohort studies to show that the dramatic fall in AIDS-related mortality seen in the developed world coincided with the introduction of anti retroviral therapy (ART). ART regimens should be individualised to achieve the best potency, minimise toxicity and avoid drug interactions. Prior to commencing therapy, individuals should have full tests for HIV drug resistance, and be screened for hepatitis B and C infections.

The primary aim of ART is the prevention of morbidity and mortality associated with chronic HIV infection at low cost of drug toxicity. The effectiveness and tolerability of ART has improved over the last 15 years and the majority of patients attending HIV services in the UK and receiving ART experience long-term virological suppression and good treatment outcomes, which compare with other developed countries. Recent life-expectancy data have are still about 13 years less than that of the UK population as a whole. Other aims of ART are to reduce sexual transmission of HIV and also to prevent mother-to-child transmission.

ART consists of three drugs which can be from a variety of types: protease inhibitors, non-nucleoside reverse transcriptase inhibitors, or nucleoside reverse transcriptase inhibitors. Issues to be considered during therapy are adherence, toxicity, resistance, long-term safety, clinical trial data and stage of disease. Change of therapy is advocated for virological failure diagnosed by viral load testing. Up-to-date guidance should be sought on which drugs are suitable for which group of people based on evidence.

Therapy-naive patients should start ART containing two nucleoside reverse transcriptase inhibitors (NRTIs) plus one of the following: a ritonavir-boosted protease inhibitor (PI/r), an NNRTI or an integrase inhibitor (INI) [A]. It is recommended that patients are given the opportunity to be involved in making decisions about their treatment.

HIV testing

A significant number of people are unaware of their HIV infection and they are at risk from HIV-related infections leading to an increase in morbidity and mortality. They are also at risk of transmitting the infection both sexually and vertically (to a fetus). HIV testing should be encouraged in a variety of settings and healthcare professionals should obtain consent for testing in the same way as for any other investigation. Lengthy pre-test counselling is not necessary, simply discussion of the benefits of early diagnosis and how the results will be given. Concerns about insurance applications should be discussed; insurance companies are not allowed to ask if an individual has been tested for HIV.

However, applicants should declare HIV positivity in the same way as any other medical condition.

Fourth-generation assays test for HIV antibodies and p24 antigen simultaneously and they will detect the vast majority of individuals who have been infected with HIV at four weeks after specific exposure. An additional HIV test should be offered at 12 weeks to definitively exclude HIV infection and this test alone is sufficient for people at lower risk to avoid the need for HIV testing twice.

Post-exposure prophylaxis for HIV following sexual exposure (PEPSE)

There is evidence that HIV infection can be aborted after sexual exposure if antiretrovirals are given as soon as possible after exposure. Delays in commencing PEP can adversely affect its efficacy and certainly after 72 hours PEP may be ineffective and is not recommended. Ideally it should be started as soon as possible, ideally within 1 hour. This works by inhibiting viral replication once the virus has crossed the mucosal barrier. It then takes five days before HIV can be detected in the blood. PEPSE drugs need to be given as soon as possible and only up to 72 hours after initial exposure. The risk of acquisition needs to be assessed depending on the HIV risk or status of the contact and the type of sexual contact that has taken place. For example, receptive vaginal intercourse from a known HIV-positive individual carries a median risk of 0.1 per cent and receptive oral sex of 0.02 per cent.It is recommended that PEPSE is indicated if the risk is 1 in 1000 or greater. There is evidence of greater risk of HIV acquisition if the source has a known or high risk of other STIs. Clinicians may consider PEPSE more readily in cases of sexual assault as it is believed that there is a higher risk of HIV transmission where sex is aggravated. Informed consent must be taken following full discussion including the possible side effects (mainly gastrointestinal) and the need for blood tests at the time, and at three and six months after the event. Hepatitis B screening, immunoglobulin and accelerated vaccination should also be considered. Twenty-four hour access to starter packs for treatment (in Accident and Emergency and GUM departments) should be available, following GUM advice and arrangement for at least four weeks of ongoing treatment.

Risk assessment for HIV testing/other blood-borne viruses (for women)

Several questions can be asked which enable some assessment of the risks of HIV/other blood-borne viruses, and these questions are asked routinely in GUM:

- Have you or any of your partners ever injected (recreational) drugs (injecting drug user, IDU)?
- Have you ever had any partners who come from another country? If yes, ask where and assess whether this may pose an extra risk e.g. sub-Saharan Africa.
- Have any of your partners also had sex with men?

- Do you have any tattoos which were done in unlicensed premises without adequate precautions for sterility?
- Have you ever been paid for sex?

HIV and sexual and reproductive health

There can be huge psychosocial issues for women with HIV, especially around conception and pregnancy. All women with HIV should be offered an annual sexual health check to include screening for STIs and contraceptive advice, where appropriate. The majority of STIs can be treated in the same way as in the non-HIV-positive woman. If considering conception, pre-conception counselling should be given especially carefully and if possible should include written consent in non sero-same couples, regarding the small risk of HIV transmission. This guidance should be led by an HIV expert.

Women with HIV on ART have a decreased risk of HIV sexual transmission. Those whose viral loads are very low for long periods of time may have almost negligible risks of transmission, especially in the absence of any STIs. Counselling and advice to continue to use condoms should take place. In those who wish to have unprotected sex, detailed counselling by experts should be offered.

HIV and contraception

It is important that HIV-positive women are open about their infection so that they receive the best advice. Safer sex is to be encouraged, with the concomitant use of condoms, as well as a reliable hormonal method to prevent pregnancy. For HIV-positive women not on ART, all methods of contraception can be used.

Methods of contraception adversely affected by ART are combined hormonal contraception and progestogen-only pills, if on PI/rs. Antiretroviral drugs have the potential to either decrease or increase the bioavailability of steroid hormones in hormonal contraceptives. However, DMPA, the LNG-IUS and IUDs can all be used by HIV-positive women on ART without increased failure rates.

Where emergency contraception is required for a woman on ART or other liver enzyme-inducing drugs, then an emergency IUD is preferable. If progesterone-only emergency contraception is requested, then a 3 mg (double stat dose) is recommended. Ulipristal acetate cannot be used by women using liver enzyme-inducing drugs.

HIV and cervical screening, colposcopy and cervical cancer

Cervical cancer is an AIDS-defining illness. Women with HIV need to have regular cervical cytology and all women with cervical cancer should be offered an HIV test. The current NHSCSP guidelines on screening suggest that HIV-positive women should have an annual smear. Any cytological abnormality, however minor, should be taken as an indication for colposcopy. As there is a higher incidence of inflammatory vaginocervical disorders in HIV-positive women, the accuracy of both cytology and colposcopy is less than in non-HIV-infected women.

Women with proven cervical intraepithelial neoplasia (CIN) require treatment, although the results of treatment of CIN are significantly worse than in non-HIV women. Data also suggest that HIV-positive women with normal CD4 counts have better outcomes than those who have low CD4 counts. This observation supports the concept that the host cell-mediated immune system is implicated in the eradication of CIN following local treatments.

HIV infection and pregnancy

The prevalence of HIV in pregnancy varies over the UK. For example, in 2009, a large survey of over 400,000 livebirths estimated HIV prevalence as 1 in 449, about 1 in 250 in London, about 1 in 700 elsewhere. The majority of these women are from sub-Saharan Africa. The risk of transmission is related to maternal health, obstetric factors and infant prematurity. There appears to be a linear correlation between maternal viral load and risk of transmission. Antenatal testing is carried out in all units in the UK, and there is a recommendation to repeat test women at increased risk of acquisition during the pregnancy. Near-patient testing is also recommended in untested women in labour. Checking documentation of HIV testing is important, as well as communicating results to labour ward staff. Uptake of antenatal screening for HIV was >80 per cent in over two thirds of maternity units, in 2003. There is a greater diversity of clinical situations for women with HIV and each scenario may need individual clinical guidance.

Viral load is important in terms of transmission and should be measured every three months, at 36 weeks or two weeks after changing therapy, and at delivery. Any opportunistic infections suspected should be investigated and managed as in non-pregnant women. Pregnant women with HIV should be managed jointly by obstetric and HIV specialists according to British HIV Association (BHIVA) guidelines to optimise up-to-date treatment.

Fetal ultrasound scanning should be performed as per national guidelines regardless of maternal HIV status [D]. Invasive prenatal diagnostic testing should not be performed until the HIV status of the woman is known and should be deferred until the viral load is adequately suppressed, if HIV positive.

Obstetric factors in untested women that consistently show an association with risk of transmission are mode of delivery and duration of membrane rupture. It is suggested that invasive monitoring of babies and artificial rupture of membranes is avoided in HIV-positive women. Delivery should be expedited for term pre-labour rupture of membranes. If maternal viral load is >1000 RNA copies per mL, then immediate CS is recommended. Delivery before 34 weeks has been shown to be associated with an increased risk of transmission. There is an untreated vertical transmission risk of 25 per cent. The findings of the first RCT in 1994 showed that the use of zidovudine (AZT) could reduce transmission from 25 to 8 per cent. This has since been confirmed by multiple smaller observational studies. Vaginal delivery is recommended for women on ART with a very low viral load (<50) at 36 weeks. Neonatal PEP should be given in untreated HIV-positive mothers. Exclusive formula feeding is still recommended in all HIV-positive women in the UK. Elsewhere in the world, where formula feeding poses extra risks to the infant because of unsafe water, breastfeeding is recommended. Highly active ART (HAART) started before pregnancy can be continued throughout pregnancy. There is no evidence for teratogenicity of any retroviral drugs, but there is an increased risk of preterm delivery. Zidovudine monotherapy should commence by 28 weeks and remains a valid option in women who do not wish to use HAART in pregnancy, or do not need to.

There should be clear local referral pathways for HIV-positive pregnant women, including specialist nurses and social workers where available. Information for the woman concerning follow-up for the baby needs to be given. Use of ART in pregnant women with HIV is both to prevent mother-to-child transmission and also for the welfare of the mother herself. Pregnant women with HIV should be screened for all STIs, including syphilis (and again in the third trimester or if clinically indicated) and hepatitis B. Genital tract infections should be treated according to BASHH guidelines [B]. There should be social assessment of all women with HIV in pregnancy by the multidisciplinary team.

Preconception and fertility management in men and women with HIV

There are three groups to consider:

1 HIV-positive men and negative female partners;
2 HIV-positive women and negative male partners;
3 HIV-positive couples.

All three groups may have fertility problems, but for the first two groups there is also the risk of HIV transmission.

Positive man, negative woman

The risk of transmission to the woman is approximately 1:500 per sexual encounter and until recently this was the only way couples could conceive. Limiting exposure to the most fertile period only has been shown to reduce the risk of transmission. In one study, four of 103 women seroconverted using this method. In 1992, Semprini et al.[2] invented the technique of 'sperm washing' – a process whereby spermatozoa are removed from the surrounding seminal plasma. (HIV is found in the seminal plasma, but not bound to the spermatozoa themselves.) There have not so far been any seroconversions of women after they have been inseminated with washed sperm. The technique of sperm washing is only available in a few centres in the UK and is funded by the couple in more than 50 per cent of cases.

Positive woman, negative man

Couples are advised to use condoms and then to practise self-insemination around ovulation to minimise the risk of transmission to the man.

Positive couples

These couples are recommended to practise safer sex (condoms) in order to reduce the risk of transmission of viral variants. It is advisable that the couple are in the best possible health before embarking on a pregnancy and are under specialist care. The woman should have normal up-to-date cervical cytology before becoming pregnant. They are advised to have unprotected sex around ovulation. There has been considerable debate concerning HIV-infected couples and IVF; it is now ethically acceptable as the vertical transmission rate is less than 1 per cent and there is an increased life expectancy for parents on treatment.

HEPATITIS

Hepatitis A

Hepatitis A is caused by a picorna virus (RNA) and is common in areas of the world where there is poor sanitation and mainly affects children in those areas. There were only 367 cases in England and Wales in 2010 in all age groups. (Hepatitis A is a notifiable disease.) Transmission is by the faeco-oral route or close personal contact and there have been outbreaks in men who have sex with men (MSM), and in those who have multiple partners and group sex. There are also increased risks among IDUs and haemophiliacs (cases of contamination of factor VIII) and vaccination may be important in these groups. The incubation period is 15–45 days and people are most infectious two weeks before the jaundice when they are asymptomatic or not yet diagnosed. Many people have no symptoms at all, but the typical illness is characterised by a prodromal flu-like illness with possible right upper quadrant pain, followed by an icteric illness with jaundice (mixed hepatic and cholestatic, with symptoms of pale stools and dark urine) associated with nausea, anorexia and fatigue which can go on for 1–3 weeks or even longer. Hepatitis A is rarely complicated by acute liver failure (ALF, 0.4 per cent). This is more common in those with chronic other liver disease, including hepatitis B and C. Mortality rates are very low (0.1 per cent), except those complicated by ALF.

There is no evidence that hepatitis A is teratogenic, but there is an increased risk of miscarriage and premature labour.

There have been cases of possible vertical transmission. Breastfeeding can be continued and most children will have mild or asymptomatic infection. The diagnosis can be confirmed by positive serum hepatitis A-specific IgM and can remain positive for six months or more. If the hepatitis A was acquired sexually, then tests for other STIs should be undertaken.

General advice for women should include avoiding food handling and refraining from unprotected sex. Rest and fluids are advised together with advice to seek medical help if there is a deterioration in health. A full explanation including a patient information leaflet should be given.

Vaccination is recommended to travellers to developing countries, haemophiliacs and for people at risk in an outbreak.

Hepatitis B

Hepatitis B is a hepadna virus (DNA). It is endemic worldwide with high carriage rates of up to 20 per cent in high-risk areas, such as South and East Asia, Central and South America, Africa and Eastern Europe. In the UK, 0.01–0.04 per cent of blood donors have evidence of hepatitis B infection. In 2010, there were 5805 cases notified in England and Wales. Transmission is sexual, parenteral and vertical. The incubation is 40–160 days. It is mainly asymptomatic in children and in 10–50 per cent of adults and is especially likely in coexistent HIV infection. The prodrome and icteric phases are similar to hepatitis A. Fulminant hepatitis can occur in <1 per cent. Chronic infection (greater than six months) occurs in 5–10 per cent and is more likely in HIV patients. Chronic active hepatitis can proceed to cirrhosis and liver cancer. Concurrent infection with HIV or hepatitis C worsens the disease. It is important to screen for other STIs, to check liver function and to advise to avoid sexual intercourse.

In pregnancy, there is an increased risk of miscarriage and premature labour in acute infection and there is a risk of vertical transmission in >90 per cent. Infants born to infected mothers are vaccinated at birth, usually in conjunction with hep B-specific antigen, which decreases transmission by 90 per cent. Women can continue to breastfeed as there is no additional risk of transmission. Partner notification should take place and all children not vaccinated at birth should be screened.

Specific hepatitis B Ig (HBIg) can be administered to a non-immune contact after sexual exposure from a known infective contact. This needs to be done before 48 hours, but works for up to 7 days and should be followed up by an accelerated course of hep B vaccine (0, 7 and 21 days). Hep B vaccine should be given to MSM, sex workers, IDUs, victims of sexual assault and needle-stick injury and sex partners of high-risk patients.

All those with active infection should be referred to a hepatologist (HbsAg-positive). All should also have an HIV test, as well as a full STI screen. The screening test for hepatitis B is anti-HBc. Those who have been vaccinated will have anti-HBs detectable in the blood.

All hepatitis B patients should be considered for hepatitis D testing which can coincide and make patients worse. Hepatitis D occurs in IDUs and sex workers.

Hepatitis C

Hepatitis C is an RNA virus and is prevalent (1–4.5 per cent) in Europe, Africa, the Pacific and the Eastern Mediterranean. UK prevalence is 0.53 per cent in adults but is >40 in IDUs. There were 8147 cases in England in 2010. Transmission is parenteral via shared needles, transfusion pre-1990s and in renal dialysis. There are low rates of sexual transmission (<1 per cent per year in relationships). There are also increased levels in MSM, female sex workers and tattoo recipients. Vertical transmission takes place in only 5 per cent, but is increased in HIV co-infection. Incubation is 7–140 days and serology may take three months to show.

More than 60 per cent will be asymptomatic with occasional icteric phase. There can also be chronic infections in hepatitis B. Acute fulminant hepatitis is rare. Of these, 50–85 per cent become chronic carriers and 30 per cent of these will develop severe liver disease after long periods of up to 30 years with an increased risk of liver cancer. Pregnant patients should be treated as for hepatitis A.

Screening of blood is by EIA then confirmed with PCR.

General advice would be to not donate blood, semen or organs.

KEY POINTS

- Pelvic inflammatory disease is most commonly caused by *Chlamydia trachomatis* and *Neisseria gonorrhoeae*; the long-term sequelae include infertility, ectopic pregnancy and chronic pelvic pain.
- The symptoms and signs of PID can be non-specific and treatment may have to be initiated empirically.
- PID should be considered as a sexually transmitted infection and therefore contact tracing, treating partners and liaison with GUM departments are important features of management.
- Gynaecologists should take sexual histories where indicated and apply the basic tenets of GUM practice.
- Many patients will have concurrent sexually transmitted infections; therefore genito-urinary screening is recommended.
- For better patient care, it is recommended that each clinician should have a thorough understanding of the chlamydia test used in his/her clinical setting, and encourage women under 25 years to take part in the NCSP.
- Testing for chlamydial infection should be considered when undertaking any procedure that entails instrumentation of the upper genital tract, such as hysteroscopy and IUD insertion, because of the serious possible complications.
- The only way to assess the risk of infection is to take a sexual history, as outlined above.
- The vulva should be carefully examined in all women – not just those at high risk of genital herpes – at the onset of labour.
- The aetiology of bacterial vaginosis is unknown; it is not sexually transmitted.
- Anogenital warts are the most common STI in the UK; they do not indicate the need for cervical screening outwith the NHSCSP.
- All women with positive tests for syphilis should be referred to GUM departments to confirm or exclude neurological, cardiovascular and ophthalmic involvement.
- There has been a significant improvement in survival and quality of life for HIV-infected women treated with ART.

UROGYNAECOLOGY AND SEXUAL HEALTH AND WELLBEING

Refer all HCV positive patients to liver specialist. In both the acute and chronic phases, they may respond to interferon. Interferon is also used in some hepatitis B patients. All hepatitis C patients should be vaccinated against hepatitis A and B to decrease the chances of fulminant hepatitis co-infection. There is no firm evidence that breastfeeding increases the risk of transmission, except if the woman is very ill. Sexual contacts and children should be tested. There is no vaccine or immunoglobulin preparation that will prevent transmission. All IDUs, haemophiliacs and people receiving blood pre-1990 should be tested, as well as sex workers and tattoo recipients.

EBM

Evidence in this chapter is taken from peer-reviewed national guidance as shown below under Published Guidelines and is accessible to all on the internet.

Published Guidelines

BHIVA Guidelines for the Treatment of HIV1-infected Adults with Antiretroviral Therapy. BHIVA Guidelines Writing Group. London: BHIVA, 2012, updated November 2013.

BASHH. Statement on HIV window period. March 2010.

Emergency Contraception. Faculty of Sexual and Reproductive Health Clinical Effectiveness Unit. RCOG, August 2011, updated January 2012.

UK Medical Eligibility Criteria for Contraceptive Use and Selected Practice Recommendations 2010. Faculty of Sexual and Reproductive Healthcare, RCOG.

Drug interactions with hormonal contraception, updated 2012. Clinical Effectiveness Committee, FSRH.

Guidelines for the Management of HIV Infection in Pregnant Women. BHIVA, 2012.

Guidelines for the Management of the Sexual and Reproductive Health of People Living with HIV Infection. Fakoya A on behalf of British HIV Association, BASHH and FSRH, 2008.

Intrauterine Contraception. Faculty of Sexual and Reproductive Health Clinical Effectiveness Unit. London: RCOG, November 2007.

UK National Guideline for the Management of Gonorrhoea in Adults. Clinical Effectiveness Group. London: BASHH, 2011.

UK National Guideline for Gonorrhoea Testing 2012. Clinical Effectiveness Group BASHH National Guideline for the Management of Bacterial Vaginosis. Hay P for the Clinical Effectiveness Group. London: BASHH, 2012.

National Guideline for the Management of Chlamydia trachomatis Genital Tract Infection. Horner PJ and Boag F for the Clinical Effectiveness Group. London: BASHH, 2006.

Chlamydia window period statement. Radcliffe K on behalf of Clinical Effectiveness Group, BASHH, 2008.

Chlamydia trachomatis UK Testing Guidelines. Clinical Effectiveness Group, BASHH, 2010.

Management of vaginal discharge in non-genito-urinary medicine settings 2012. FSRH, Clinical Effectiveness Unit, 2012.

National Chlamydia Screening Programme Patient Information Leaflet (August 2013).

Sexually Transmitted Infections in Primary Care 2013. (RCGP/BASHH) by Lazaro N. Available at www.rcgp.org and www.bashh.org/guidelines.

Scottish Intercollegiate Guidelines network: SIGN 109 Management of Genital Chlamydia trachomatis infection, March 2009.

National Guideline for the Management of Genital Herpes. Herpes Simplex Advisory Panel for the Clinical Effectiveness Group. London: BASHH, 2007.

National Guideline for the Management of Trichomonas vaginalis. Sherrard J for the Clinical Effectiveness Group. London: BASHH, 2007.

National Guideline for Consultations Requiring Sexual History taking. Clinical Effectiveness Group, BASHH. London: BASHH, 2013.

RCOG Green-top Guideline No. 30. Management of Genital Herpes in Pregnancy. London: RCOG, 2007.

RCOG Green-top Guideline No. 32. Management of Acute Pelvic Inflammatory Disease. London: RCOG, 2008.

UKMEC, 2009. Available from www.fsrh.org/guidelines.

RCOG guideline: The Care of Women Requesting Induced Abortion. November 2011.

UK National Guideline for the Management of PID. Ross J and McCarthy for the Clinical Effectiveness Group. London: BASHH, 2011.

UK National Guideline for the Management of Syphilis. Kingston M for the Clinical Effectiveness Group. London: BASHH, 2008.

Update on management of syphilis in pregnancy. Kingston M and McAuliffe F for the BASHH Statement Clinical Effectiveness Group, August 2011.

UK National Guideline for the Management of Viral Hepatides. Brook G et al. for the Clinical Effectiveness Group. London: BASHH, 2008.

UK National Guideline for the Use of Post-exposure Prophylaxis for HIV Following Sexual Exposure. Clinical Effectiveness Group. London: BASHH, 2011.

UK National Guideline on the Management of Anogenital Warts. Sonnex C et al. for the Clinical Effectiveness Group. London: BASHH, 2007.

UK National Guidelines for HIV testing. BHIVA and BASHH. London: BASHH, 2008.

All the BASHH guidelines and patient information leaflets are available at www.bashh.org.uk. All HIV guidance is available at www.bhiva.org.uk. All FSRH guidelines are available at www.fsrh.org.uk. All RCOG guidelines are available at www.rcog.org.uk. Information (including patient information) and references regarding Chlamydia screening and prevalence are available at ‹www.chlamydiascreening.nhs.uk›. All SIGN guidelines are available at www.sign.ac.uk.

Key References

1. Villa LL. Overview of the clinical development and results of a quadrivalent vaccine against HPV (types 6, 11, 16 and 18). *Int J Infect Dis* 2007;11(Suppl. 2):S17–25.

2. Semprini AE, Levi-Setti P, Bozzo M *et al.* Insemination of HIV-negative women with processed semen of HIV-positive partners. *Lancet* 1992; 340:1317–19.

3. Garland SM, Hernandez-Avila M, Wheeler CM *et al.* Females United to Unilaterally Reduce Endo/Ectocervical Disease (FUTURE). Quadrivalent vaccine against human papillomavirus to prevent anogenital diseases. *N Engl J Med* 2007;356(19):1928–43.

4. Bresse X, Adam M, Largeron N, Roze S, Marty R A. Comparative analysis of the epidemiological impact and disease cost savings of HPV vaccines in France. *Hum Vaccin Immunother* 2013;9(4):823–33.

Chapter 100 Dyspareunia and other psychosexual problems

Melanie Mann

DYSPAREUNIA

This is recurrent genital pain associated with sexual activity, usually penetration, although it can refer to any genital stimulation. Dyspareunia can be primary, where pain has always occurred, or secondary, where it occurs after a period of pain-free sexual activity. It is important to classify it further in terms of the site of pain: i.e. superficial or deep. Dyspareunia can itself lead to relationship difficulties due to the cycle of fear. Pain at intercourse can lead to problems of sexual arousal, causing further sexual pain and then avoidance of sexual activity.

Talking to patients about the exact site, nature and other features of the pain is important. It is also important to be comfortable talking about aspects of the sexual act, especially as some dyspareunia may be position related. Remember that patients are usually more embarrassed mentioning these aspects to us and may expect us to bring up the subject. Most of these causes (see Box 100.1) are dealt with in more detail in other sections of this book.

It is important to confirm diagnoses as far as possible with diagnostic tests, such as pelvic ultrasonography, microbiological swabs, laparoscopy or vulval biopsy where appropriate. Some diagnoses or problems are best dealt with by general practitioners or other specialists, such as gastroenterologists.

If an organic cause for dyspareunia is found, it does not necessarily exclude emotional and/or psychological sequelae for the woman. The aetiology of dyspareunia should be viewed on a continuum from primarily physical to primarily psychological, with many women exhibiting components of both.

HUMAN SEXUAL RESPONSE

According to Masters and Johnson,[1] there are classically four phases in the human sexual response:

1 Excitement: This is the first part of arousal and is caused by physical stimulation, especially clitoral stimulation, thoughts of sex and emotions. It leads to vasodilatation in the genitals causing swelling of the labia and the tissues surrounding the vagina resulting in heightened labial colouring and increased vaginal lubrication. Excitement can be enhanced or inhibited by signals from the brain, which are in turn influenced by previous experience. Oestrogen affects vaginal lubrication by enhancing the vascular bed beneath the epithelium. The clitoris becomes swollen and erect, the skin flushed and the nipples erect.

Box 100.1 Causes of dyspareunia

Main causes of superficial dyspareunia (superficial vulval and vaginal pain at intercourse)
Vulvitis and vulvovaginitis (infection, hypo-oestrogenic)
Vestibulodynia (provoked vulval pain)
Vulvodynia (unprovoked vulval pain)
Topical irritants/dermatitis
Urethral disorders and cystitis
Vaginismus
Lack of vaginal lubrication (arousal problems)
Obstetric perineal trauma, mainly episiotomy
Radiation vaginitis
Main causes of deep dyspareunia
Pelvic inflammatory disease
Endometriosis
Genital or pelvic masses e.g. ovarian cyst
Pelvic congestion syndrome
Urinary tract infection
Retroverted uterus in some women
Irritable bowel syndrome
Psychosexual issues

2 Plateau: There is intensification of the above changes with increased blood flow to the genitals accompanied by increases in heart rate, blood pressure and breathing rates. The vagina lengthens and balloons with engorgement.

3 Orgasm: This is a genital reflex controlled by spinal neural centres (spinal injuries to vertebrae T11 to L2 can lead to orgasmic problems). There is reflex contraction of pelvic muscles located around the vaginal introitus together with release of vaginal fluids. Orgasm is the highest point of pleasure. Orgasm can last longer in women and be multiple.

4 Resolution: There is a feeling of satisfaction and wellbeing together with a return to the pre-arousal state. Men experience a refractory phase during which they cannot have another orgasm, but women do not.

There is also another phase which is necessary before the classic phases described above and this is known as desire or libido. This varies from one person to another and during the life cycle. It is also subject to changes in oestrogen and testosterone. A newer model, 'the sexual response cycle', describes physical, emotional and cognitive feedback. A variety of biological, social and psychological factors can affect the cycle.[2]

Educating patients regarding the phases above is really important. The most important of these is giving sufficient time for foreplay and relaxation to be sufficiently aroused and lubricated prior to penetration, together with the importance of stimulating the clitoris to achieve orgasm. Women often feel they are failing in some way if they cannot achieve orgasm with vaginal intercourse alone and may need to be reassured.

PSYCHOSEXUAL PROBLEMS

Physiological events, such as pregnancy, childbirth, menopause and ageing, as well as gynaecological conditions, such as infertility, prolapse, urinary incontinence and gynaecological cancers, can have an impact on sexual wellbeing. Sexual activity in later life remains taboo, but a large number of women remain sexually active beyond 70 years. It must also be remembered that intercourse is only one way for couples to be sexual and there are other ways that sexual intimacy can be maintained at different times of the life cycle.

Psychosexual problems may present to the gynaecologist as part of general history taking for a variety of presenting complaints, and it is sometimes difficult to disentangle how much of the gynaecological complaint is due to the psychosexual problem, or whether the gynaecological problem has caused the psychosexual issue. It is therefore extremely important that the clinician feels comfortable asking about sexual problems, especially in relation to gynaecological problems, for which there is a good chance of concomitant psychosexual issues, such as vulval disorders and dyspareunia. However, there may also be circumstances in which it is important to establish sexual habits and issues, for example prior to gynaecological surgery when any interference with sexual function can cause problems within a sexual relationship. It is also very important to have an open and non-judgemental attitude to people's sexual practices (as long as they are not causing or suffering harm) and this includes those in same sex relationships.

Psychosexual history taking

Each clinician needs to find his/her own words that feel comfortable to use when talking about sex with the patient. There is no substitute for practice, and the more you use the words and ask the difficult questions, the more comfortable you will feel. Open-ended questions are useful in order to encourage the patient to talk; for example: 'Tell me a little bit about …'. The clinician's body language is also extremely influential to the way the patient will feel about opening up in this very intimate part of history taking. For example, sitting back in the chair, putting down your pen and not having a large expanse of desk between you and the patient will go a long way towards making her feel more comfortable.

Some drugs will also affect sexual function such as antidepressants, antipsychotics, antihypertensives, corticosteroids and hormones including contraception and HRT.

Typical questions for use in psychosexual history taking

Not all the questions need to be asked or are appropriate to ask every time.

- 'Are you in a sexual relationship?'
- 'Is sex comfortable for you?'
- 'Are there any problems with sex?'
- 'Do you get any pain with sex?'
- 'Where exactly does it hurt during sex – on the outside or the inside?'
- 'Is there anything that makes the pain worse; any position, for example?'
- 'Are you able to have an orgasm during sex?'
- 'Have you ever masturbated? Do you get an orgasm during masturbation?'
- 'Tell me a little bit about your relationship with your partner.'
- 'Tell me a little bit about what happens when you try to have sex with your partner.'

Most gynaecologists would refer a patient on to an expert in psychosexual medicine for further treatment. There will be local variation in availability and waiting time.

SEXUAL PAIN DISORDERS

Dyspareunia

Dyspareunia is recurrent or permanent genital pain associated with sexual intercourse. This is the only sexual disorder in which physical factors are thought to play a major aetiological role. However, the psychological and interpersonal factors are significant.[3] The organic causes for this condition are discussed above. In addition to gynaecological treatment approaches, women may require an adjunctive course of cognitive–behavioural sex therapy to ensure good outcomes.[4]

Vaginismus

Vaginismus is the involuntary spasm of the pubococcygeal and associated muscles causing painful and difficult penetration of the vagina, during sex, tampon insertion or clinical examination. Primary vaginismus occurs when a woman has never experienced vaginal penetration; secondary vaginismus is diagnosed when the problem occurs after previous successful vaginal penetration.

Usually at the root of vaginismus is a combination of physical or non-physical triggers that cause the body to anticipate pain. The body reacts to this by automatically tightening the vaginal muscles, which makes sex more painful and this response becomes the 'cycle of pain'.

The patient may present with a painful vulva at intercourse. The differential diagnosis is then of organic vulval disorders, such as vulval vestibulitis. However, there is likely to be some degree of vaginismus in all women with organic vulval disease. The skill is in trying to work out whether the vaginismus is the primary problem or is a result of organic disease. The 'Q-tip' test can be helpful to elucidate the exact site of pain and whether it is in the contracted muscles or in the tender epithelium of the vestibule. (The 'Q-tip' test involves the use of a moistened cotton bud to elicit the exact site and degree of discomfort or vulval pain.) The other main form of presentation is admission of non-consummation of a relationship in the fertility clinic setting.

Aetiology

Vaginismus is a conditioned (learned) response that often results from associating sexual activity with pain and fear. It can occur together with a phobia of all sexual contact or as the only problem within an otherwise normal sexual relationship. Typical phrases used by the patient include: 'There's a block'; 'He just can't seem to get it (his penis) in'; 'It's as if it (her vaginal opening) is too small'.

Vaginal examination is important in diagnosing vaginismus but is not always straightforward. What happens at the point of vaginal examination might be significant in terms of what happens with the woman's partner and sometimes reflecting feelings felt by the doctor or observations can help elucidate the psychosexual problem. Sometimes the doctor may be able to feed back to the patient that she appears to be disassociated from that area of her body, and further questioning often confirms that she does not touch that area much herself due to concerns with cleanliness, smell or religious beliefs.

Causes of vaginismus

- No cause found
- Sexual abuse
- Physical abuse
- Painful medical procedure in the perineal area
- Painful first intercourse
- Relationship problems/anger between couples ('I won't let him in' – subconsciously)
- Fear of pregnancy/labour
- Religious orthodoxy
- Poor sexual education
- Sexual inhibition.

Treatment

There needs to be discussion around the main issues in the relationship and how the woman feels about touching her own genitalia. Behavioural therapy comprising systematic desensitisation, pubococcygeal muscle training and the use of vaginal trainers works well. The response to this therapy for this group is good, with complete resolution for most couples, especially if the origin is uncomplicated in nature.[5] The phobia of penetration needs to be explored so that the woman reaches a situation in which she feels in control of her vagina and can enjoy sex when and how she wishes.

A Cochrane systematic review of the different interventions for vaginismus such as sex therapy and desensitisation could not rule out a clinically relevant effect of systematic desensitisation when compared to any control interventions. However the findings were very limited by the evidence available and so conclusions about the efficacy of interventions for the treatment of vaginismus should be drawn cautiously. Further larger studies are needed.[6]

Treatment includes:

- discussion and education about sex and the condition;
- teaching the location and control of the vaginal (pubococcygeal) muscles;
- self-examination of the vulva and vagina when alone and relaxed e.g. in the bath (beginning of systematic desensitisation);
- insertion of her own finger, then fingers or plastic vaginal trainers;
- doing the above in a sexual situation with her partner present;
- the woman inserting her partner's finger, then penis, with her in control;
- insertion of the penis with her partner in control, but with the woman on top so that it is less threatening;
- sexual intercourse as the couple would wish.

EBM

There have been no RCTs on vaginismus. Observational studies indicate that treatment is generally very successful for women with vaginismus.

SEXUAL DESIRE DISORDERS

This is now often referred to as hypoactive sexual desire disorder (HSDD). This usually presents as loss of libido (loss of interest in sex). It should also be remembered that there is huge variability between individuals and within the normal range. Interest in sex declines in both sexes with increasing age, but this change is more pronounced in women. The prevalence of 'low sexual desire' is about 30 per cent but the personal distress is about 20 per cent from this problem and is highest in middle-aged women. Sometimes it is the disparity between partners that leads a woman or couple to seek help. Risk factors for female sexual dysfunction may be non-hormonal (e.g. conflict between partners, insomnia, inadequate stimulation, life stress, depression and other medical disorders such as hypothyroidism/diabetes) or hormonal (oestrogen and androgen deficiency). Testosterone deficiency can be considered among the underlying causes of desire disorders in post-menopausal women but no level of a single androgen is predictive of low sexual function in women. However, post-menopausal oestrogen deficiency does cause atrophic changes and lead to painful sex, which can in itself lead to a decrease in desire as well as any direct effect of oestrogen within the brain. Testosterone should only be replaced together with oestrogens.

Specific pathways for sexual arousal, desire, reward and inhibition exist in the brain and are altered by hormones and experience. Hypothalamic, limbic and dopamine systems are important for desire as are certain neuropeptic systems.[6]

There is also controversy about what comes first in women, arousal or desire.

The prognosis is variable, but is better when it is the female with the initial problem. One study examined 60 couples presenting with the female partner's loss of interest as the major problem. There was only modest success, with 56 per cent experiencing a relatively good outcome at the end of treatment.[7]

These problems are usually the symptom of a generally poor relationship overall, and the sexual disorder is only part of the whole problem. Sexual wellbeing is related to a woman's subjective happiness and wellbeing.

SEXUAL AROUSAL DISORDER

It is difficult to separate sexual arousal disorder from sexual desire disorder and female orgasm disorder due to the close relationship of the three conditions in women. Causes of lack of arousal are numerous. They can be psychological (distractions, childhood loss, low self-esteem), endocrine (lack of oestrogen), neurological (e.g. multiple sclerosis) or drug induced (e.g. antihistamines). Additionally, the widespread use of vaginal lubricants/vaginal oestrogens may mask or alleviate the disorder.

There have been cases of persistent sexual arousal syndrome, where women with no conscious desire for sexual expression are overwhelmed by continual sensations in the genitals. This is differentiated from hypersexuality, a syndrome which does involve a high level of desire for sexual activity. Little is known about these disorders, but psychological/cognitive–behavioural treatment does seem to confer some benefit.[8]

FEMALE ORGASMIC DISORDER (ANORGASMIA)

This is the term used for failure to achieve orgasm due to inhibition of the orgasmic reflex or poor sexual technique/ignorance.

Aetiology

There may be holding back and fear of losing control. It may be situational, in that the woman can achieve orgasm by masturbation or with the aid of sex toys, but not during sexual intercourse. Sometimes, realistic ideas and the discussion of what most women achieve are necessary. For example, many women do not experience orgasm by penetration alone and do need other clitoral stimulation at the same time. Education regarding sexual positions to enhance clitoral stimulation and education about the clitoris itself may be required. There may be unrealistic expectations on the part of the partner, who may equate the female orgasm with his own and will not be happy unless his female partner also has one during penetration.

This pressure on the female can lead to faking of orgasm to keep the partner happy and a premature end to the sexual act and frustration on the part of the female, who has not actually achieved orgasm. Drugs, such as antipsychotics, can also cause orgasm problems.[9]

Treatment of anorgasmia

- Encourage self-exploration and what is pleasurable when she is alone.
- Sensate focus – concentration on the sensual pleasure of touching her partner, but avoiding the genitals.
- Masturbation.
- Use of sex toys such as vibrators, if helpful; use of DVDs to help arousal and provide ideas (e.g. *The Lovers' Guide* series by Dr Andrew Stanway).
- Discussion and resolution of unconscious fears of orgasm, if present.
- Heightening sexual arousal so that the woman is close to orgasm before penetration.

Hysterectomy and sexual function

There has been debate in the literature about the role of hysterectomy in sexual function. This has become more important now that women are more involved in their own treatment choices and feel more able to demand a good outcome from surgery. It has also become more pertinent since there have been more non-surgical (e.g. the levonorgestrel intrauterine system) and less complicated (e.g. endometrial destruction methods) procedures to treat one of the most common reasons for hysterectomy, namely menorrhagia. There has been a steady rise in some countries in the number of supracervical hysterectomies performed for benign conditions. The ratio of subtotal to total hysterectomies in Scandinavia is high at 0.56 compared to the UK where in 2005 it was reported as 0.04.[10] This may reflect the changing attitudes of surgeons and women towards a less invasive procedure, which was believed to have a reduced operative morbidity and reduced the risk of urinary and sexual dysfunction. Various mechanisms have been proposed to explain why cervical conservation may have a less detrimental effect on sexual function than total abdominal hysterectomy. Early pioneering work[1] described elevation of both the cervix and uterus during excitement and the plateau phase, followed by fundal uterine contractions progressively involving the lower uterine segment as orgasm developed. Cervical os dilatation occurred immediately afterwards, implicating a role for the cervix in the female sexual response. Another theory postulates that the ability to achieve orgasm depends on the nerve endings of the uterovaginal (cervical) plexus of Frankenhauser.[11] This plexus is a matrix of nerve fibres intimately surrounding the cervix. Stimulation of the cervix may contribute to a pleasurable sensation ultimately experienced as orgasm. However, the most recent evidence does not support superiority of subtotal over

total hysterectomy and instead the most rigorous studies show that the majority of women experience no negative impact on sexual satisfaction, whatever the method and whether subtotal or not [A]. In a Cochrane review of total versus subtotal hysterectomy for benign gynaecological conditions, subtotal hysterectomy did not offer an improved outcome for sexual function.[12] Most of the studies demonstrate improvement in sexual function in general after hysterectomy, because there is relief from dyspareunia and menstrual bleeding.[13]

OESTROGEN REPLACEMENT THERAPY AND SEXUAL FUNCTION

Women often complain about changes in sexual function after a natural or iatrogenic menopause (bilateral salpingo-oopherectomy). Oestrogens appear to be an important part of the sexual response and loss of libido is a recognised symptom of the menopause.[14] Systemic oestrogens (e.g. oral, transdermal, subcutaneous) can be used following full discussion of the pros and cons. Testosterone may also be used, but should always be used in conjunction with systemic oestrogens.

If the main problem with sex is due to vaginal dryness causing dyspareunia and diminishing sexual pleasure and desire, it may also be useful to use local oestrogens in the form of cream or pessaries (let the woman try both to see what suits her best). Even if a woman is using systemic oestrogens she may also require local therapy, especially if she has ongoing symptoms of hypo-oestrogenism (soreness, dryness, dyspareunia). Care with the type of vaginal oestrogens should be taken with longer-term use to prevent endometrial hyperplasia in the woman with an intact uterus (only use oestriol cream or oestradiol pessaries).

TESTOSTERONE THERAPY AND SEXUAL FUNCTION

Testosterone is produced in the ovaries and in the adrenal glands in women. Testosterone has been used in women with various sexual disorders and testosterone deficiency disorders since the 1930s. Despite this, the use of testosterone therapy is still controversial. Circulating testosterone declines in the late reproductive years so that healthy women in their forties have half the level compared to women in their twenties. A direct link between sexual dysfunction and endogenous testosterone levels has not been clearly found in pre-menopausal women. Research on testosterone levels is mainly confined to post-menopausal women so the place of testosterone therapy in pre-menopausal women with low libido is not currently known. The generalised use of testosterone by women has been advised against because of inadequate indications and long-term data.

Decreased levels of testosterone in post-menopausal women may lead to decreased levels of libido, sexual activity and physical wellbeing. Bilateral salpingo-oopherectomy (BSO) causes a decrease in sex drive by 50 per cent, by removing ovarian contribution of testosterone. Many gynaecologists have used subcutaneous implants for testosterone replacement after BSO, for many years. There is also another form of hormone replacement therapy used in post-menopausal women which is licensed for libido problems, called tibolone. It has some androgen-like properties.

Transdermal patches and gels or creams are preferred over oral products because of first-pass hepatic effects documented with oral formulations. Monitoring should include assessments of sexual response as well as (usually reversible) side effects of hirsutism and acne. It is also good practice to measure fasting lipid and glucose levels after six months of therapy. More recently, transdermal testosterone therapy has been shown to increase sexual activity and satisfaction in at least 51 per cent of women in randomised double-blind trials compared to placebo. The patches are well tolerated with the main side effect being atopic site reactions. Testosterone therapy overdose can also cause acne, hirsutism and lowered voice.[15]

Psychosexual dysfunction in women treated for gynaecological cancer

There is no convincing evidence to support the use of any interventions for psychosexual dysfunction in women treated for gynaecological cancer. This is mainly due to the lack of studies of high methodological quality. However one trial did suggest short-term benefit from vaginal oestrogens after pelvic radiotherapy.[16]

PLACES TO REFER WOMEN/COUPLES WITH PSYCHOSEXUAL PROBLEMS

- Relate – provides counselling for all relationship and psychosexual problems (there may be a fee).
- Local contraceptive/reproductive healthcare services may have a psychosexual service (contact your local consultant).
- Local hospital-based psychosexual services – may be within urology, gynaecology, genito-urinary medicine or psychiatry departments.
- Private sex therapists (contact via the British Association for Sexual and Relationship Therapists or the British Association for Counselling).
- Doctors trained by the Institute of Psychosexual Medicine (contact the institute directly).

KEY POINTS

- It is important to classify further the site of pain: superficial or deep.

- Pain at intercourse can lead to problems of sexual arousal causing further sexual pain and then avoidance of sexual activity.
- If an organic cause for dyspareunia is found, it does not necessarily exclude emotional and/or psychological sequelae for the woman.
- In assessing gynaecological problems where there is a good chance of concomitant psychosexual issues, such as vulval disorders and dyspareunia, it is extremely important that the clinician feels comfortable to ask about sexual problems.
- Dyspareunia is the only sexual disorder in which physical factors are thought to play a major aetiological role. However, the psychological and interpersonal factors are significant.
- Observational studies indicate that treatment is generally very successful for women with vaginismus.[17]

Key References

1. Masters WH, Johnson VE. *Human Sexual Response.* Boston: Little, Brown, 1966.
2. Mokate T, Wright C, Mander T. Hysterectomy and sexual function. *J Br Menopause Soc* 2006;12:153–7.
3. Rosen RC, Leiblum SR. The treatment of sexual disorders in the 1990s: an integrated approach. *J Consul Clin Psychol* 1995;65:877–90.
4. Schover LP, Youngs DD, Cannata R. Psychosexual aspects of the evaluation and management of vulvar vestibulitis. *Am J Obstet Gynecol* 1992;167:630–6.
5. Hawton K, Catalan J, Martin P, Fagg J. Long-term outcome of sex therapy. *Behav Res Ther* 1986;24:665–75.
6. Basson R. Biopsychosocial models of women's sexual response: applications to management of 'desire disorders'. *Sex Relations Ther* 2003;18:107–15.
7. Hawton K, Catalan J, Fagg J. Low sexual desire: sex therapy results and prognostic factors. *Behav Res Ther* 1991;47:832–8.
8. Hiller J, Hekster B. Couple therapy with cognitive behavioural techniques for persistent sexual arousal syndrome. *Sex Relations Ther* 2007;22:91–6.
9. Murthy S, Wylie K. Sexual problems in patients on antipsychotic medication. *Sex Relations Ther* 2007;22:97–107.
10. Garry R. The place of subtotal/supracervical hysterectomy in current practice. *BJOG* 2008;115:1597–600.
11. Hanson HM. Cervical removal at hysterectomy for benign disease, risks and benefits. *J Reprod Med* 1993;38:781–90.
12. Lethaby A, Mukhopadhyay A, Naik R. Total versus subtotal hysterectomy for benign gynaecological conditions. *Cochrane Database of Systematic Reviews* 2012;Issue 4.Art.No.:CD004993.
13. Kupperman M, Summitt RL Jr, Varner RE *et al.* Total or Supracervical Hysterectomy Research Group. Sexual functioning after total compared to supracervical

hysterectomy: a randomised trial. *Obstet Gynecol* 2005;105:1309–18.

14. Wylie KR. Sexuality and the menopause. *J Br Menopause Soc* 2006;12:149–52.

15. Kingsberg S. Testosterone treatment for HSDD in post-menopausal women. *J Sex Med* 2007;4 (Suppl. 3):227–34.

16. Flynn P, Kew F, Kiseley SR. Interventions for psychosexual dysfunction in women treated for gynaecological malignancy. *Cochrane Database of Systematic Reviews* 2009;Issue 2.Art No.CD004708.

17. Melnik T, Hawton K, McGuire H. Interventions for vaginismus. *Cochrane Database of Systematic Reviews* 2012;Issue 12.Art.No.CD001760

Help and further information for both patients and healthcare professionals: www.vaginismus.com

Evidence-based guideline: Guidelines on the management of sexual problems in women: the role of androgens. 2010 British Society of Sexual Medicine, available at www.bashh.org.

Chapter 101 Child sexual abuse

Catherine White

INTRODUCTION

Child sexual abuse (CSA) can take on many forms. WHO defines child sexual abuse as:

The involvement of a child in sexual activity that he or she does not fully comprehend, is unable to give informed consent to, or for which the child is not developmentally prepared, or else that violate the laws or social taboos of society. Children can be sexually abused by adults or other children who are – by virtue of their age or stage of development – in a position of responsibility, trust, or power over the victim.

WHO, 2006.

Working Together to Safeguard Children, 2013[1] states that sexual abuse:

…involves forcing or enticing a child or young person to take part in sexual activities, not necessarily involving a high level of violence, whether or not the child is aware of what is happening. The activities may involve physical contact, including assault by penetration (for example, rape or oral sex) or non-penetrative acts such as masturbation, kissing, rubbing and touching outside of clothing. They may also include non-contact activities, such as involving children in looking at, or in the production of, sexual images, watching sexual activities, encouraging children to behave in sexually inappropriate ways, or grooming a child in preparation for abuse (including via the internet). Sexual abuse is not solely perpetrated by adult males. Women can also commit acts of sexual abuse, as can other children.

HM Government, 2013.

DEFINITION OF A CHILD

There is no single law that defines the age of a child across the UK. The UN Convention on the Rights of the Child, ratified by the UK government in 1991, states that a child 'means every human being below the age of eighteen years unless, under the law applicable to the child, majority is attained earlier' (Article 1, **Convention on the Rights of the Child**, 1989). That a healthcare worker may be dealing with a child that has reached the age of 16, may be living independently, etc. does not change his/her status or entitlements to services or protection.

THE LAW

The **Sexual Offences Act 2003**[2] states that the age of consent for sex is 16 years in England and Wales. In order to protect younger children, the law says that children aged under 13 years can never legally give consent. The Sexual Offences Act 2003 covers a variety of offences against children. These include offences such as:

- sexual activity with a child;
- causing or inciting a child to engage in sexual activity;
- meeting a child following sexual grooming.

In addition the Female Genital Mutilation Act 2003 covers FGM.

PREVALENCE OF CHILD SEXUAL ABUSE

According to WHO[3] approximately 20 per cent of women and 5–10 per cent of men report being sexually abused as children, while 23 per cent of people report being physically abused as children.

Research done by the NSPCC[4] in 2011 involved interviewing over 6000 young adults, adolescents and parents of younger children. Participants were asked whether anyone had tried to make them do anything sexual whilst they were under the age of 18 years. Parents of children aged under 11 years responded on their child's behalf. Older teenagers and young adults were also asked if they had done sexual things with an adult when they were still under 16 years or with an adult in a position of trust whilst they were still under 18 years. This research used a definition of sexual abuse that included any unwanted sexual activity, as well as criminal sexual activity with an adult, where physical contact took place. It excluded non-contact sexual abuse (such as flashing or saying sexual things) as well as 'consensual' sexual activity between adolescents. The figures below are all based on the reports from young people aged 11–17 years.

- One in 20 children (4.8 per cent) have experienced contact sexual abuse.
- Over 90 per cent of children who experienced sexual abuse were abused by someone they knew.
- More than one in three children (34 per cent) who experienced contact sexual abuse by an adult did not tell anyone else about it.
- Four out of five children (82.7 per cent) who experienced contact sexual abuse from a peer did not tell anyone else about it.

There have been many recent changes in the recognition of how children may be victims of sexual abuse. For example, there has been much publicity about historical disclosures of institutional CSA. In addition, the arrival of new technologies has seen the development of new practices such as online grooming and abuse, sexting, etc. Child sexual exploitation is something that will have been happening throughout the centuries and yet is only now beginning to be recognised. Recent inquiries have shown that these children were often failed by professionals, who had been judgemental in their assessment of the behaviour and circumstances of the children and had failed to pick up on the signs and symptoms of sexual abuse.

RISK FACTORS FOR CHILD SEXUAL ABUSE

Whilst all children may be a victim of sexual abuse, research shows that certain children are more at risk than others.

Girls seem to be more at risk than boys. Children with disabilities are particularly vulnerable. A 2012 WHO-funded systematic review[5] indicated that children with disabilities are 3.7 times more likely than non-disabled children to be victims of any sort of violence, 3.6 times more likely to be victims of physical violence, and 2.9 times more likely to be victims of sexual violence. Children with mental or intellectual impairments appear to be among the most vulnerable, with 4.6 times the risk of sexual violence than their non-disabled peers. It may be that they have fewer people to tell, are less able to communicate what is happening to them or that when they do tell, they are less likely to receive adequate protection.

Sexual abuse is only one form of child abuse, the others being physical, emotional and neglect. Often a child will be subjected to more than one type of abuse, highlighting the need to undertake a holistic assessment of the child.

Whilst a common myth about CSA is that perpetrators are strangers, the reality is that most children will be abused by someone that they know. Therefore much of the risk for children will be determined by who their carers are and who has access to them. Educating children about such issues should help empower them. There have been a variety of campaigns with this in mind.[6]

MANAGEMENT

For the clinician, the management of CSA will vary case by case, dependent upon the age of the child, the nature of the abuse, the wishes of the child, etc. (See Table 102.1, Things to consider when someone discloses acute rape/sexual assault, in Chapter 102.)

Many children, particularly younger children, may not present with a direct disclosure. For example they may present with vaginal bleeding, genital soreness, STIs or behavioural changes. It is therefore incumbent upon the clinician to have a high level of suspicion of CSA when formulating a differential diagnosis. Where abuse is suspected it is important that there is an opportunity for the child to disclose what is happening, bearing in mind that the child may be reluctant to provide details within earshot of carers in attendance. In addition a child may have been manipulated or threatened by the abuser not to tell.

The assessment of a child where CSA is suspected should always be a holistic one, not merely a preoccupation with the genitalia. That said, knowledge of normal genital anatomy, including prepubertal genitalia, is a prerequisite for the clinician in order to be able to identify anything abnormal (Fig. 101.1).

Key messages for the generalist would be to have a high level of suspicion and to involve senior colleagues at an early stage. The Royal College of Paediatrics and Child Health (RCPCH) and the Faculty of Forensic and Legal Medicine (FFLM) have produced guidance[7] on paediatric forensic examinations for CSA. Information regarding injury documentation and the

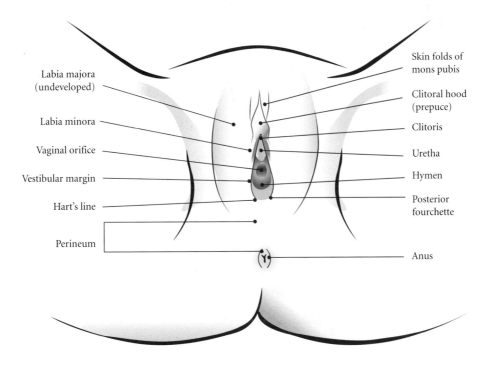

Fig. 101.1 Prepubertal female genitalia. Taken from *Sexual Assault, A Forensic Physician's Practice Guide*. Dr Catherine White. 2010. ISBN 978-0-9564737-0-7.

gathering of forensic samples is included in Chapter 102, Rape and sexual assault.

Any examination should be preceded by a careful discussion with the child and/or carer that covers issues around consent for the examination, the limitations of confidentiality, disclosure of information for safeguarding purposes, etc. as well as the nature of the examination. Given that sexual abuse is about the disregard of consent and the abuse of power, great care must be taken by healthcare workers not to repeat this process.

Careful consideration must be given by the doctor to balance what may sometimes seem to be competing pressures, such as the child requesting information regarding sexual activity not be shared, the need to protect a child from the risk of ongoing abuse and the need to protect other children from serial offenders. Readers are advised that they should be well versed on GMC guidance on these matters.[8]

ANOGENITAL INJURY RATES

The common misconception is that there would be a high injury rate for child victims of sexual abuse. Whilst this may sometimes be the case it is not the norm. Many forms of abuse will not result in any injury and even when anogenital injuries are sustained they tend to heal quickly and completely. It is important to appreciate that for many cases the absence of injury does not necessarily negate the allegation of abuse. The RCPCH in collaboration with the FFLM has produced an evidence-based review of the physical signs of CSA.[9]

VIRGINITY TESTING

Many cultures place a very high value on virginity. There may be a great deal of pressure exerted on a clinician to say if a child is a virgin or not; indeed there may even be requests for certificates of virginity.

Doctors should not get involved in such practice. Apart from the myriad of associated ethical issues there is no evidence base to determine with accuracy if a person has been sexually active or not.

MEDICAL AFTERCARE

This should include consideration of the risk of STIs (including post-exposure prophylaxis and screening), emergency contraception, pregnancy testing as well as psychological care.

Where samples are taken for STI screening, it may be appropriate to do so employing chain of custody so that the results may be submitted as evidence in any subsequent court process.

UROGYNAECOLOGY AND SEXUAL HEALTH AND WELLBEING

Advice around HIV PEP and hepatitis B PEP is available from BASHH (www.BASHH.org) and also the Children's HIV Association (CHIVA, www.chiva.org.uk).

A risk assessment for safeguarding with the appropriate referrals should be made.

Psychological follow-up will vary from child to child. Not all children will need the services of mental health teams. Some units e.g. some Sexual Assault Referral Centres (SARCs) have dedicated staff specialising in the follow-up care of these children. Knowledge of what services are available in the local area is important to ensure timely smooth referrals and ensure seamless care for this very vulnerable group.

CHILD SEXUAL EXPLOITATION

There are various definitions of child sexual exploitation (CSE); the following is used by BASHH in its guidance:

CSE involves those under 18 in exploitative situations, contexts and relationships where young people (or a third person or persons) receive something (for example food, alcohol, cigarettes, affection, gifts) as a result of them and/ or another or others engaging in sexual activities. It is an abuse of power by those exploiting by virtue of their age, gender, intellect and physical strength and/or economic or other resources.

CSE encompasses both gang-related and other sexual violence and exploitation.

A *pro forma, Spotting the Signs,*[10] has been developed to help health professionals across the UK to identify young people attending sexual health services who may be at risk of or experiencing sexual exploitation.

As well as professionals being alert to the warning signs that a child is either a victim of exploitation or at risk of such, it is also crucial that the child or young person is not alienated by an interrogative style of history taking and any suggestion that they may to blame for what has happened to them by the decisions they have made.

SAFEGUARDING

The 2013 Working Together to Safeguard Children[1] guide sets out the legislative requirements and expectations on individual services to safeguard and promote the welfare of children. It states:

This guidance aims to help professionals understand what they need to do, and what they can expect of one another, to safeguard children. It focuses on core legal requirements and it makes clear what individuals and organisations should do to keep children safe. In doing so, it seeks

to emphasise that effective safeguarding systems are those where:

*   *the child's needs are paramount, and the needs and wishes of each child, be they a baby or infant, or an older child, should be put first, so that every child receives the support they need before a problem escalates;*
*   *all professionals who come into contact with children and families are alert to their needs and any risks of harm that individual abusers, or potential abusers, may pose to children;*
*   *all professionals share appropriate information in a timely way and can discuss any concerns about an individual child with colleagues and local authority children's social care.*

Section 11 of the **Children Act 2004**[11] places duties on a range of professionals including healthcare workers. It is clear that health professionals are in a strong position to identify welfare needs or safeguarding concerns regarding individual children and, where appropriate, provide support. This includes understanding risk factors, communicating effectively with children and families, liaising with other agencies, assessing needs and capacity, responding to those needs and contributing to multi-agency assessments and reviews.

Clinicians should be familiar with the intercollegiate document, March 2014, *Safeguarding children and young people: roles and competences for health care staff.*[12]

EFFECTS OF CHILD SEXUAL ABUSE

As in all aspects of life where individuals respond to events, situations and stresses in their own way the same is true for CSA. The impact will depend upon many factors such as the nature of the abuse, who the abuser was, in terms of the abuse of power and trust, how long the abuse went on for, what other disadvantages a child was subject to, etc. Therefore victims will show a range of symptoms as a result of their abuse, with some seemingly having no long-term ill effects. Whilst much is often made of physical sequelae it is often the psychological effects that affect a victim the most.[13] Some children will have been told that the abuse was their fault and this will have an impact on their psychological recovery. Some victims may suffer with low self-esteem, underperformance at school, self-harm or suicide. Feelings of shame and guilt are frequent and can have devastating effects on a victim's ability to go on to have healthy relationships later in life.

In addition to this some longer-term studies are revealing that child victims are at increased risk of physical illness including cardiovascular disease in adulthood.[14]

KEY POINTS

- Child abuse involving boys and girls is common although many victims do not disclose their abuse.
- Clinicians should have a high level of suspicion for CSA and must facilitate disclosure by empowering the child.
- Safeguarding is everyone's responsibility. Knowledge of local safeguarding procedures is vital.
- Absence of injury does not negate the possibility of abuse.
- Virginity testing has no basis in evidence-based medicine.
- The long-term health consequences of CSA can be massive. Prevention and early detection are key.
- SARCs can provide holistic, medical, forensic and psychological care for victims.

CONCLUSIONS

All doctors will be exposed to the consequences of CSA no matter what speciality they practice in. A society is judged by its treatment of its most vulnerable. Doctors must play a central role in this, acting as advocates for those without a voice, challenging myths and stereotypes, raising awareness of issues however unpalatable and seeking to eradicate the causes and perpetuation of the circumstances that allow such abuse to flourish.

Key References

1. HM Government. *Working Together To Safeguard Children: A guide to interagency working to safeguard and promote the welfare of children.* March 2013; DFE-00030-2013. https://www.gov.uk/government/uploads/system/uploads/attachment_data/file/281368/Working_together_to_safeguard_children.pdf
2. Sexual Offences Act 2003. Legislation.gov.uk. http://www.legislation.gov.uk/ukpga/2003/42/contents.
3. World Health Organization. Child Maltreatment Factsheet 150. Last updated January 2014. http://www.who.int/mediacentre/factsheets/fs150/en/. Accessed September 2014.
4. Radford L, Corral S, Bradley C *et al. Child abuse and neglect in the UK today.* London: NSPCC, 2011.
5. Jones L, Bellis M *et al.* Prevalence and risk of violence against children with disabilities: a systematic review and meta-analysis of observational studies. *Lancet.* Published online July 12, 2012 http://dx.doi.org/10.1016/S0140-6736(12)60692-8
6. This is Abuse. http://thisisabuse.direct.gov.uk/. The NSPCC Underwear Rule campaign http://www.nspcc.org.uk/news-and-views/media-centre/press-releases/2013/underwear-rule/campaign-teach-underwear-rule_wdn97140.html
7. Guidelines on Paediatric Forensic Examinations in Relation to Possible Child Sexual Abuse October 2012. http://fflm.ac.uk/upload/documents/1352802061.pdf.
8. General Medical Council. 0–18 years: guidance for all doctors. http://www.gmc-uk.org/guidance/ethical_guidance/children_guidance_index.asp.
9. RCPCH. The Physical Signs of Child Sexual Abuse. An evidence-based review and guidance for best practice. http://www.rcpch.ac.uk/physical-signs-child-sexual-abuse.
10. British Association for Sexual Health and HIV. CSE: Spotting the Signs. www.BASHH.org. http://www.bashh.org/documents/Spotting-the-signs-CSE-20a%20national%20proforma%20April%202014%20online.pdf
11. The Children Act 2004. http://www.legislation.gov.uk/ukpga/2004/31/contents.
12. FFLM. Safeguarding children and young people: roles and competences for health care staff. Intercollegiate Document, 3rd edn. March 2014. http://fflm.ac.uk/upload/documents/1396609235.pdf.
13. NSPCC. Child Sexual Abuse research Briefing. July 2013. http://www.nspcc.org.uk/Inform/resourcesforprofessionals/sexualabuse/child-sexual-abuse-briefing_wda96887.html#effect.
14. Rich-Edwards *et al.* Physical and sexual abuse in childhood as predictors of early-onset cardiovascular events in women. *Circulation* 2012;126:920–7.

Chapter 102 Rape and sexual assault

Catherine White

MRCOG standards

Core Module 15: Sexual and Reproductive Health
Knowledge criteria

- Mental Capacity Act 2005
- Sexual Offences Act 2003
- Recognise the sexual health needs of vulnerable groups.
- Emergency contraception: mode of action and efficacy, methods, indications, contraindications and complications.
- Recognise and manage the sexual healthcare needs of vulnerable groups e.g. young people, asylum seekers, commercial sex workers, drug users and prisoners.

Forensic Gynaecology (2011)

This ATSM is designed to create departmental and regional leaders who can structure a successful multiprofessional service to manage the victims of domestic violence and sexual assault.

Section 1 covers the law and the basic competencies for the initial contact, management, examination, evidence collection and subsequent follow-up.

Completion of the Diploma of the Faculty of Sexual and Reproductive Healthcare (DFSRH) prior to the ATSM is recommended but not mandatory.

Training to child protection level 3 is required. This may be undertaken either prior to or during the ATSM.

The ATSM must be undertaken under the supervision of an identified preceptor who must be in a position to directly supervise and assess competency. In order to ensure exposure to the required case mix the unit must be of a sufficient size to ensure completion of the training.

Once trained, individuals should:

- be clinically competent and confident in all aspects of domestic violence and forensic services;
- be competent to lead the provision of domestic violence and forensic services in a unit or region;
- work well as part of a multidisciplinary team;
- be clinically competent in understanding police processes and know how the Police Criminal Evidence Act 1984 might have an impact on the process of forensic medical examination;
- be competent and confident to write a statement which is an accurate account based on contemporaneous evidence;
- be able to define and identify different types of injury by undertaking full examination;
- be able to undertake and use clinical audit;
- be able to write protocols and evidence-based guidelines.

INTRODUCTION

The worldwide prevalence of sexual violence is high. Frequently it remains a hidden problem and yet the sequalae may have profound effects on the physical and psychological health of the victim, both in the short and long term. This in turn may have an impact on subsequent generations. Victims of sexual violence can be of any age, gender and sexuality. Those who are already vulnerable e.g. the elderly and those with learning disorders or physical disabilities are often targeted.

It is important for clinicians to have an awareness of the scale of the problem, how it may present and then how to manage the situation. They should be able to respond to a direct disclosure of rape or sexual violence and also, perhaps more importantly, they should be alert to the possibility of sexual violence as the root cause of other presentations e.g. chronic pelvic pain, STIs, requests for emergency contraception, unplanned pregnancy and mental health problems including depression, self-harm and substance misuse and be able to respond appropriately.

Interpersonal violence may also cause ethical dilemmas for the clinician. There may be a need to balance the competing requirements and demands of respecting the autonomy of a victim versus public interest issues. Therefore thorough knowledge and understanding of the relevant laws, for example the Mental Capacity Act 2005, professional guidelines (for example GMC guidelines), and ethical principles are vital.

This chapter will cover the immediate management of a patient who discloses rape/sexual assault and also cover some of the possible long-term consequences.

There are many **myths and stereotypes** held by professionals and public alike regarding sexual violence. For example:

- *Most victims will be raped by a stranger.*
- *Men cannot be raped.*
- *A rape victim would put up a struggle and try to fight off the assailant.*
- *A rape victim would report the assault immediately.*
- *A female who was raped, especially if she was a virgin, would always have genital injuries as a result.*

These can act as a barrier for victims to seek and subsequently receive the help that they require. The aim is to highlight and hopefully dispel some of these.

PREVALENCE (BOX 102.1)

Box 102.1 Statistics on the prevalence of sexual violence

Statistics on sexual violence from the UK

- 28% of women aged 16–59 have experienced abuse in their lifetime.[1]
- 3.1 million women have been sexually assaulted since the age of 16.[2]
- 70% of women with mental health problems have experienced physical or sexual abuse.[3]
- 40–50% of women who have experienced domestic violence are raped within their physically abusive relationship.[4]
- Just under 50% of mental health service users have been subject to sexual abuse and around 50% to physical abuse in childhood, notwithstanding adult abuse which they may also be surviving.[5]
- 23% of women and 3% of men experience sexual assault as an adult.[6]
- Around 21% of girls and 11% of boys experience some form of childhood sexual abuse.[7]
- 2.5% of women aged 16–59 and 0.5% of men had experienced a sexual assault (including attempts) in 2010–2011.[8]

International key facts[9]

- Violence against women – particularly intimate partner violence and sexual violence against women – is a major public health problem and violation of women's human rights.
- Recent global prevalence figures indicate that 35% of women worldwide have experienced either intimate partner violence or non-partner sexual violence in their lifetime.
- On average, 30% of women who have been in a relationship report that they have experienced some form of physical or sexual violence by their partner.
- Globally, as many as 38% of murders of women are committed by an intimate partner.
- Violence can result in physical, mental, sexual, reproductive health and other health problems, and may increase vulnerability to HIV.
- Risk factors for being a perpetrator include low education, exposure to child maltreatment or witnessing violence in the family, harmful use of alcohol, attitudes accepting of violence and gender inequality.
- Risk factors for being a victim of intimate partner and sexual violence include low education, witnessing violence between parents, exposure to abuse during childhood and attitudes accepting violence and gender inequality.
- In high-income settings, school-based programmes to prevent relationship violence among young people (or dating violence) are supported by some evidence of effectiveness.
- In low-income settings, other primary prevention strategies, such as microfinance combined with gender equality training and community-based initiatives that address gender inequality and communication and relationship skills, hold promise.
- Situations of conflict, post-conflict and displacement may exacerbate existing violence and present new forms of violence against women.

UROGYNAECOLOGY AND SEXUAL HEALTH AND WELLBEING

THE LAW

The Sexual Offences Act (SOA) 2003 deals with offences that have taken place in England and Wales and applies to offences committed after 1 May 2004. Prior to that the Sexual Offences Act 1956 would apply.

Northern Ireland (The Sexual Offences (Northern Ireland) Order 2008) and Scotland are covered by similar legislation.

The SOA 2003 covers over 50 sexual offences. Box 102.2 sets out the definitions of two of the main sections.

Box 102.2 The Sexual Offences Act 2003

Sexual Offences Act 2003[10]
Section 1 (Statutory definition of rape)
1. A person (A) commits an offence if:
(a) he intentionally penetrates the vagina, anus or mouth of another person (B) with his penis.
(b) B does not consent to the penetration, and
(c) A does not reasonably believe that B consents.
2. Whether a belief is reasonable is to be determined having regard to all the circumstances, including any steps A has taken to ascertain whether B consents.
Section 5 (Statutory definition of rape of a child under 13 years)
1. A person commits an offence if:
(a) he intentionally penetrates the vagina, anus or mouth of another person with his penis, and
(b) the other person is under 13 years.

MANAGEMENT

Given the prevalence of sexual violence *all* obstetricians and gynaecologists will be seeing rape victims on a regular basis. Only the best doctors will have any inkling of how many they see.

The management of a complaint of rape or sexual violence will depend on several factors. One of the main issues is how a rape victim presents (see Fig. 102.1).

A key issue when dealing with any victim is to understand that sexual violence is fundamentally about power and control: the loss of it for the victim, and the exertion of it by the assailant. It is important not to replicate this. Wherever possible give back power and control to the patient. Know and then outline to them their options, given their particular circumstances, allow them to make choices and then respect their decisions (Table 102.1).

Up to date, comprehensive knowledge of local resources and referral pathways is necessary.

Ideally a rape victim would have the option of being seen in a Sexual Assault Referral Centre. SARCs offer medical, forensic, practical and emotional support to anyone who has been sexually assaulted or raped. They have specially trained doctors, support workers and counsellors to care for victims.

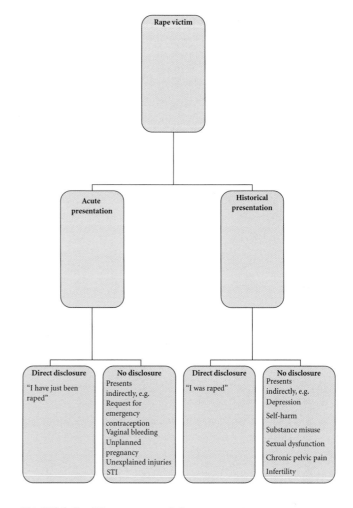

Fig. 102.1 Possible ways a rape victim may present

Many SARCs, as well as seeing victims who have made a report to the police, will offer the option of seeing victims as 'self-referrals' i.e. those who are not willing to report to the police.

In the UK contact details for SARCs can be found on the NHS Choices website http://www.nhs.uk/Pages/HomePage.aspx.

Table 102.1 Things to consider when someone discloses acute rape/sexual assault

Immediate safety	Are they safe?
	Are there any third parties to consider e.g. children, other dependants?
	Are any safeguarding referrals required?
	Are you safe?
Medical needs	Injuries, assessment and treatment
	Emergency contraception
	HIV PEPSE
	Hepatitis B PEPSE
	Screening for STIs
	Pregnancy testing

Forensic needs	Preservation of evidence
	Documentation of injuries including photography where necessary
	Documentation of allegations
	All to be done in a manner that makes evidence admissible to court
Psychological needs	Of the complainant (including risk of self-harm, suicide)
	Of other witnesses
	Of you

Safeguarding

Remember that safeguarding issues, for both children and vulnerable adults, are the responsibility of *every* healthcare worker, not the remit of only the specialists.[11] All clinicians must be alert to safeguarding issues and know how to respond when a concern arises, always considering both the patient in front of them and also any of their dependants.

In the O&G setting there are numerous situations where the doctor may be faced with safeguarding problems, for example:

- domestic violence during pregnancy;
- substance misuse in pregnancy;
- termination services;
- contraception and women with learning difficulties;
- female genital mutilation;
- 'honour'-based violence.

Consent

Consent is important in all patient–doctor interactions. For the reasons discussed already, it is especially important with victims of sexual violence. A thorough understanding of the Mental Capacity Act 2005 is needed.

Capacity and the Mental Capacity Act

The definition of, assessment of and responsibilities in relation to capacity (also known as mental capacity) in England and Wales are laid out in the Mental Capacity Act (MCA) 2005.

The MCA applies to all adults aged 16+.

The MCA defines capacity as the ability to make a decision. It relates to the *process* of making a decision and not to the *outcome* of the decision. It is not limited to medical decisions, but can apply to any decision-making process e.g. financial or social choices.

Capacity is task specific. A person may be capable of deciding one issue but not another.

Capacity is also time specific. A person's capacity may alter with time.

The MCA defines the lack of capacity thus: if, at the time the decision needs to be made, patients are unable to make the decision because of an 'impairment of, or a disturbance in the functioning of, the mind or brain', they are deemed incapable.

The term 'capacity' was previously used interchangeably with the term 'competence'. Since the MCA 2005 'capacity' is the preferred term.

The MCA lays out five statutory principles:

1. A person must be assumed to have capacity unless it is established that s/he lacks capacity.
2. A person is not to be treated as unable to make a decision unless all practicable steps to help him or her to do so have been taken without success. *(This includes communicating in an appropriate way. In forensic practice the clinician may need to arrange for interpreters or signers to be present or to use visual aids.)*
3. A person is not to be treated as unable to make a decision merely because s/he makes an unwise decision.
4. An act done, or a decision made, under this Act for or on behalf of a person who lacks capacity must be done, or made, in his or her best interests.
5. Before the act is done, or the decision is made, regard must be had as to whether the purpose for which it is needed can be as effectively achieved in a way that is less restrictive of the person's rights and freedom of action.

Healthcare professionals are warned that a person cannot be judged to lack capacity simply because of age, appearance or behaviour.

Assessment of capacity

All adults are presumed to have capacity unless there is evidence to the contrary.

In order to assess someone's capacity to make a valid treatment decision, two criteria have to be considered:

1. Do they have an impairment of mind or brain (temporary or permanent)?
2. Does the impairment mean that the person is unable to make the decision in question, at the time it needs to be made?

Where the patient is less than 16 years old they are still able to make autonomous decisions independent of those with parental responsibility provided that they have the capacity to do so. The term 'Gillick competence' is often used here following on from a particular court case where Victoria Gillick had a legal challenge against the NHS providing contraceptive advice to girls under the age of 16 years.[12] The outcome was a judicial decision that, provided the child was competent to make the decisions in question, then they were able to do so without involving their parents, although medical best practice would be to encourage parental involvement where possible.

There has been some confusion over the years with the terminology, in particular with what became known as the Fraser Guidelines. These too were related to the Gillick case but deal specifically with prescribing contraception to this age group (as opposed to a general assessment of capacity where 'Gillick competency' is used.

History taking

Ideally this will be done by a forensic physician.

The information gathered and note keeping must be:

1 Comprehensive
2 Comprehensible
3 Correct
4 Contemporaneous

When making enquiries about the details of the assault, open rather than closed questions should be used. Sometimes direct questions may need to be employed but these should be recorded verbatim as should their answers. Accusations of 'contaminating' evidence may otherwise be levied.

Injuries

There are several key points regarding injuries as the result of sexual violence:

- The majority of victims will not have any injuries.
- Should any injuries be sustained they tend to be minor.
- Many of the usual injuries sustained in sexual violence will heal quickly and rarely will they leave any scars.
- Where possible they should be documented by a trained forensic physician specialising in sexual assault.
- Documentation must be accurate and may include photo documentation.

Although some rape victims may suffer extensive, possibly even fatal, injuries, many will have none. They should be reassured that lack of injuries is common and does not negate their allegations.

Any injuries that are found, however small, should be documented accurately to help aid subsequent interpretation (e.g. age of injury and possible causation). Objective findings must be distinguished from subjective descriptions or conclusions.

Injuries can be subdivided into:

- bruises;
- abrasions;
- lacerations;
- incisions;
- burns.

Bites are not unusual in sexual assault and may contain a mixture of injuries including bruises, abrasions and lacerations.

More information regarding the interpretation of injuries (or the lack of them) can be found elsewhere.[13]

Forensic samples

Dependent upon a number of factors including the nature of the assault and the time elapsed, there may be an opportunity for a forensic physician to gather forensic samples. The FFLM has produced *Recommendations for the Collection of Forensic Specimens from Complainants and Suspects*. These are updated twice a year and available on their website[14] along with numerous other guidelines, *pro formae* and body maps to aid the documentation of injuries. These give guidance regarding samples in terms of what to take, when to take, how to take and how to store.

When dealing with an acute rape victim, urgent medical considerations should always take precedence over the preservation of forensic evidence, but where possible both should be achieved. If in doubt seek advice. Where there may be a delay to a patient being seen by a forensic physician seek advice from them on the best way to minimise destruction of any forensic evidence and how to gather and store any possible evidence source (e.g. underwear) in a way that will be most useful and also admissible in any subsequent criminal investigation.

It must be remembered that forensic evidence is not restricted to forensic samples e.g. DNA evidence. It may be possible to collect forensic evidence such as documentation of injuries and scars long after any trace evidence has been lost. The concept of a 'forensic window' is sometimes referred to but should be avoided as it is often restricted to trace evidence and an opportunity to gather other types of evidence, offer support and reassurance is then lost.

Emergency contraception

Where the sexual assault is such that pregnancy is a possibility then a risk assessment for the need for emergency contraception should be done as soon as possible.

Given the nature of what has happened, possible injuries and risk of STIs, hormonal methods are often preferable to using a copper coil, but the pros and cons of the different methods should be evaluated on a case-by-case basis. Prophylactic use of antibiotics if inserting a coil is recommended.

For emergency contraception, see Chapter 72.

Pregnancy and paternity analysis

Where it is believed that a pregnancy has been the result of a rape paternity analysis can be carried out to establish the identity of the father. This may be done when a child is born or using the products of conception following a termination. Guidance has been produced to assist this process.[15]

HIV and hepatitis B post-exposure prophylaxis

A risk assessment should be undertaken to assess the need for PEP for blood-borne viruses e.g. HIV and hepatitis B. Risks will be dependent upon assailant factors and the nature of the assault. Detailed guidance on this has been developed.[16]

When it is required HIV PEP should be started as soon as possible and certainly within 72 hours. Specialist advice from GUM should be sought if one is not familiar with its use. Usually a SARC would prescribe a 5-day starter pack with follow-up by the GUM clinic.

Hepatitis B PEP can be started within 6 weeks although in some circumstances immunoglobulins may be required soon after the assault.

Suicide/self-harm risk

Mental health problems are not unusual in complainants of sexual violence. This may be as a consequence of the assault, or the case that having such problems makes them vulnerable and therefore a target for perpetrators. Often it can be a mixture of both.

The clinician must be able to undertake a preliminary screening of the mental health assessment including suicide risk of the victim and then manage the situation accordingly (Box 102.3).

Box 102.3 Suicide risk assessment[17]

High-risk indicators are in red print
1. Do you have thoughts about harming yourself?
2. Are you thinking about suicide?
3. Do you have a specific plan to kill yourself?
4. What methods have you considered?
5. Do you have access to any of these methods?
6. Do you have a date or place in mind?
7. Have you ever self-harmed or attempted suicide in the past?
8. Has anyone in your family died by suicide?
9. Are you suffering from mental health problems?
10. Have you suffered from mental health problems in the past?
11. Have you ever had contact with mental health services or seen your GP in relation to psychological or psychiatric problems?
12. Are you taking any medication for mental health problems?
13. Do you have a problem with drugs or alcohol?
14. Have you been drinking in the past few hours?
15. Are you experiencing particular difficulties in your life or struggling to deal with difficult past events (e.g. bereavement, divorce, running away from home)?
16. Do you have friends or family you can turn to for help?
17. Do you feel that the future is hopeless and that things cannot improve?

STI screening

Given the incubation times for most STIs, usual practice would be for the patient to be screened at 2 weeks post assault and then at 3 months for blood-borne viruses.

ISVAs

Independent Sexual Violence Advisors (ISVAs) are victim-focused advocates who help people who have experienced sexual violence to access the services they need. Most SARCs and some voluntary organisations will have access to them. Many will see victims even in cases where the police are not involved. They will be able to support the victim with practical issues and offer support through the criminal justice process. Should counselling be required they will be able to facilitate this.

LONG-TERM CONSEQUENCES OF SEXUAL VIOLENCE

In a national cross-sectional study of reported health outcomes and exposure to violence, Black *et al.* (2011)[18] found a statistically significant (p <0.001) higher prevalence of adverse physical and mental health outcomes for nine out of the ten measured health outcomes in women with a history of rape, stalking, or physical violence by an intimate partner in comparison with women with no reported exposure to these forms of gender-based violence. The health outcomes measured in the study were: asthma, irritable bowel syndrome, diabetes, high blood pressure, frequent headaches, chronic pain, difficulty sleeping, activity limitations, poor physical health and poor mental health; the only measured outcome with non-significant difference was high blood pressure.

Psychological sequlae of sexual violence

Sexual violence is likely to have an impact on a victim. The level of impact will depend upon a number of factors, including the baseline mental health, nature of the assault, chronicity of the violence and subsequent support and safety for the victim. Early intervention has been found to be protective in reducing the risk of longer-term psychological problems. There is no one 'uniform' response. Judgemental response by professionals when dealing with victims can be immensely damaging.

Many victims will suffer initial symptoms, both physical and mental. They should be reassured that this is a normal response to an abnormal event. Some will go on to develop more long-term problems.[19] Rape victims are more at risk of developing PTSD than other victims of violence.

MALE RAPE

Male rape is a not uncommon problem. For the O&G specialist it may present as an issue in settings such as patients with psychosexual problems or investigations of fertility. There are many excellent resources for male victims and the clinician should have up-to-date local knowledge of such.[20]

FEMALE GENITAL MUTILATION

FGM describes any deliberate, non-medical removal or cutting of female genitalia. Different regions and communities practise various forms of mutilation.

FGM includes procedures that intentionally alter or cause injury to the female genital organs for non-medical reasons.

A review by WHO in 2000[21] and a more recent review in 2008 showed that FGM has significant health consequences for a woman's physical, mental, gynaecological and reproductive health.[22,23]

HONOUR-BASED CRIMES

Honour-based violence (HBV) is a form of domestic abuse which is perpetrated in the name of so-called 'honour'. The honour code which it refers to is set at the discretion of a family or community. Those who do not abide by the 'rules' may be punished for bringing shame on the family. Infringements may include a girl or woman having a boyfriend; rejecting a forced marriage; pregnancy outside marriage; interfaith relationships; seeking divorce; inappropriate dress or make-up and even kissing in a public place.

Forced marriage is a component of honour-based crime. Women may present in a healthcare setting as a result. The clinician should be alert to possibility that this is a problem and be able to deal with it sensitively and safely. More information and resources can be found at Honour-Based Violence Awareness Network, http://hbv-awareness.com.

Advice regarding the law can be found at http://www.cps.gov.uk/legal/h_to_k/honour_based_violence_and_forced_marriage/#a02.

DOMESTIC VIOLENCE

- Domestic sexual violence is common and frequently is not disclosed.
- Patients may present in a healthcare setting with sexual violence-related problems.
- Domestic sexual violence can have an impact on the physical and mental health of victims, both in the immediate and long term.

- Deal with victims in a sensitive, non-judgemental manner.
- Have a thorough and up-to-date knowledge of local resources.

CONCLUSIONS

Sexual violence continues to be a worldwide problem of high prevalence. All ages can be victims.

The clinician must keep an open mind as to its possibility. The response of the clinician may be crucial in reducing the impact of an assault and indeed preventing further victimisation.

Key References

1. The British Crime Survey (BCS) 2008/09. Self Completion Module on Sexual and Domestic Violence. http://www.homeoffice.gov.uk/publications/science-research-statistics/research-statistics/crime-research/hosb1210/
2. Homicides, Firearm Offences and Intimate Violence 2008/09: Supplementary Volume 2 to Crime in England and Wales 2008/09. http://data.gov.uk/dataset/crime_in_england_and_wales_-_supplementary_volume_2
3. The British Crime Survey (BCS) 2008/09. Self Completion Module on Sexual and Domestic Violence. http://www.homeoffice.gov.uk/publications/science-research-statistics/research-statistics/crime-research/hosb1210/
4. Martin EK, Taft CT, Resick PA. A review of marital rape. *Aggression and Violent Behavior* 2007;12(3):329–47.
5. Implementation Guidance; Mainstreaming Gender and Women's Health, DH 03. http://www.dh.gov.uk/en/Publicationsandstatistics/Publications/PublicationsPolicyAndGuidance/DH_4072067 and Refocusing the Care Programme Approach Policy and Practice Guidance, DH 08. http://www.dh.gov.uk/en/Publicationsandstatistics/Publications/PublicationsPolicyAndGuidance/DH_083647
6. BCS 2005/06.
7. NSPCC research.
8. BCS 2010/11. http://www.homeoffice.gov.uk/publications/science-research-statistics/research-statistics/crime-research/hosb1011/.
9. WHO Fact sheet Number 239 (updated October 2013). http://www.who.int/mediacentre/factsheets/fs239/en/index.html.
10. http://www.legislation.gov.uk/ukpga/2003/42/pdfs/ukpga_20030042_en.pdf.
11. Protecting children and young people. The responsibilities of all doctors. GMC. http://www.gmc-uk.org/static/documents/content/Child_protection_guidance.pdf.

12. *Gillick v West Norfolk and Wisbech AHA and DHSS* 1985;3 WLR (HL).

13. Dalton M. Clinical obstetrics and gynaecology, clinical aspects of sexual violence. *Best Practice and Research* 2013;27(1):ISSN 1521-6934.

14. Faculty of Forensic and Legal Medicine. http://fflm.ac.uk/

15. ACPO/FSS/FFLM Guidance in Criminal Paternity Cases, 2010. http://fflm.ac.uk/upload/documents/1280843586.pdf.

16. UK National Guidelines on the management of Adult and Adolescent Complainants of Sexual Assault. Reviewed 2012. Cybulska. http://www.bashh.org/documents/4450.pdf.

17. Adapted from British Transport Police and Oxford University.

18. Black MC, Basile KC, Breiding MJ *et al. The National Intimate Partner and Sexual Violence Survey (NISVS): 2010 Summary Report.* Atlanta, Georgia: National Center for Injury Prevention and Control, Centers for Disease Control and Prevention, 2011. Available at: http://www.cdc.gov/ViolencePrevention/pdf/NISVS Report2010-a.pdf.

19. Royal College of Psychiatrists. *Post-traumatic Stress Disorder.* http://www.rcpsych.ac.uk/healthadvice/problemsdisorders/ptsdkeyfacts.aspx.

20. For example Survivors UK. http://www.survivorsuk.org/

21. WHO. *A systematic review of the health complications of female genital mutilation including sequelae in childbirth.* Geneva: Department of Women's Health, Family and Community Health, WHO, 2000.

22. Utz-Billing I, Kentenich H. Female genital mutilation: an injury, physical and mental harm. *J Psychosom Obstet Gynaecol* 2008;29:225–9.

23. https://www.gov.uk/government/uploads/system/uploads/attachment_data/file/416323/Fact_sheet_-_FGM_-_Act.pdf

Further Reading

From Report to Court: A handbook for adult survivors of sexual violence. 2011. Rights of women is an excellent free resource that explains in plain language the legal process around sexual violence. Available from www.rightsofwomen.org.uk.

Overview of the worldwide best practices for rape prevention and for assisting women victims of rape. 2013. At: http://www.europarl.europa.eu/studies.

Best Practice and Research. Clinical Obstetrics and Gynaecology, Clinical Aspects of Sexual Violence. Guest Editor M Dalton. Volume 27 Number 1 February 2013. (ISSN 1521-6934)

GMC documents. http://www.gmc-uk.org/publications/standards_guidance_for_doctors.asp#0-18. a. Consent. 2008 b. 0–18 years: Guidance for all doctors. 2007.

Chapter 103 Female genital mutilation

Ben Chisnall and Janice Rymer

MRCOG standards

- Core Curriculum 4 (Ethics and Legal Issues): Demonstrate the ability to discuss issues surrounding female genital mutilation with patients in a sensitive manner.
- Core Curriculum 8 (Antenatal Care): Counsel about defibulation in cases of female genital mutilation.
- Core Curriculum 11 (Delivery): Management of female genital mutilation.

Additional competencies

- Knowledge of the short-term and long-term physical and psychological consequences of FGM.
- Identification of girls who may be at high risk of FGM.
- Understanding of the legal context around FGM and the statutory duty of health professionals if FGM is encountered.

EBM

A 2013 Cochrane review found no suitable studies for inclusion in a meta-analysis of interventions to improve obstetric outcomes in women who have undergone FGM.

INTRODUCTION

Female genital mutilation (FGM) comprises all procedures involving partial or total removal of the external female genitalia or other injury to the female genital organs for non-medical reasons. FGM has been documented in at least 29 countries in Africa, where it is most prevalent, as well as in countries in Asia and the Middle East.[1]

FGM is carried out for traditional and cultural reasons. There may be involvement of religious leaders in communities which practise FGM, even though FGM pre-dates Christianity, Islam and Judaism, and is not advocated in any religious scripture.[2]

DEFINITION

Normal female anatomy is illustrated in Fig. 103.1. FGM is classified by the WHO into four types:

- Type 1: Clitoridectomy (Fig. 103.2a): Partial or total removal of the clitoris and/or prepuce;
- Type 2: Excision (Fig. 103.2b,c): partial or total removal of the clitoris and labia minora, +/- excision of the labia majora;
- Type 3: Infibulation (Fig. 103.2d): narrowing of the vaginal orifice with creation of a covering seal by cutting and opposing the labia majora and /or minora with/without excision of the clitoris;
- Type 4: Other: all other harmful procedures to the female genitalia for non-medical purposes, for example pricking, piercing, cutting. This is also called 'symbolic circumcision'.

Current estimates indicate that around 90 per cent of FGM includes Types 1, 2 or 4, and about 10 per cent are Type 3.[1]

TERMINOLOGY

The term 'female genital mutilation' has been used by the WHO to describe the practice since 1991. The practice had previously been referred to as 'female circumcision', and the new terminology was chosen to differentiate FGM from male circumcision. UNICEF and the UN currently use the term 'female genital mutilation/cutting' (FGM/C) which they feel reflects the practice's violation of women's and girls' rights, but also allows respectful terminology to be used amongst practising communities. The 2011 Department of Health report on FGM includes a useful list of terms used for FGM in different languages.[2]

PREVALENCE

The WHO estimates that FGM affects around 140 million women worldwide, and that 3 million women in Africa are at risk of FGM each year.[1] Girls are most likely to be subjected to FGM between infancy and age 15, and although the average age at which FGM occurs differs between countries the most common age is thought to be between 5 and 8 years.[3]

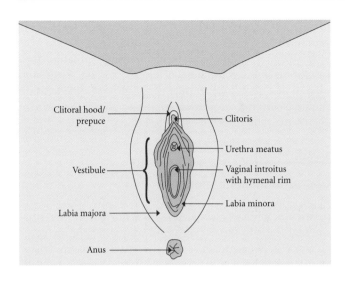

Fig. 103.1 Unaltered female genitalia. Simpson J, *et al*. Female genital mutilation: the role of health professionals in prevention, assessment, and management. *BMJ* 2012;344:e1361

Countries where the prevalence of FGM amongst women is estimated at over 90 per cent are Somalia, Guinea, Djibouti, Sierra Leone and Egypt, and over 80 per cent in Sudan, Eritrea and Mali.[2]

In England and Wales nearly 66,000 women are estimated to be living with the consequences of FGM, and over 20,000 girls under the age of 15 could be at risk of FGM each year.[2] As these figures are based on 2001 census data they may underestimate the scale of FGM in the UK, and a study began in October 2013 to establish figures based on the 2011 census. Women who come to Britain from high-prevalence countries are likely to have undergone FGM, and their daughters may be at risk of mutilation in future.

There are certain regions of the UK where FGM is more prevalent, due to large populations of communities from high-prevalence countries residing within these areas. These are London, Cardiff, Manchester, Sheffield, Northampton, Birmingham, Oxford, Crawley, Reading, Slough and Milton Keynes.[2]

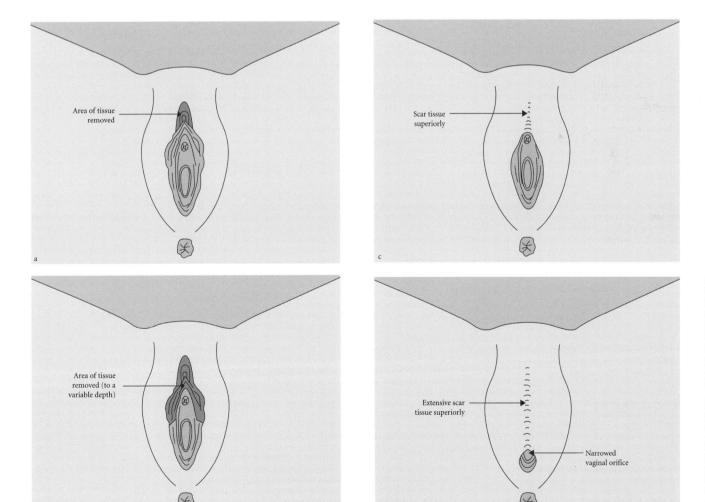

Fig. 103.2 Tissue removed in type 1 female genital mutilation (a); type 2 female genital mutilation (b,c); type 3 female genital mutilation (d). Simpson J, *et al*. Female genital mutilation: the role of health professionals in prevention, assessment, and management. *BMJ* 2012;344:e1361

UROGYNAECOLOGY AND SEXUAL HEALTH AND WELLBEING

CULTURAL AND TRADITIONAL BACKGROUND TO FGM

In some cultures it is believed that FGM will preserve a girl's virginity until marriage.[5] Another view in practising communities is that mutilation makes girls 'clean' or beautiful by removing the 'masculine' parts of the female vulva (such as the clitoris), and that infibulation creates a 'smoothness' which is aesthetically pleasing.[6]

FGM is considered necessary to raise a girl properly and to prepare her for adulthood and marriage in practising cultures. It is performed to secure a girl's status in society, and although mothers may feel uncomfortable about hurting their daughters they perceive the social advantages for the girl to outweigh the risks of the practice.[7] Girls may themselves desire to undergo FGM, due to family and community expectations, and the promise of rewards and gifts afterwards.

The position of men with regard to FGM is complex. A belief sometimes held by women is that FGM enhances men's sexual pleasure. Although some men in practising cultures express a preference for women who have undergone FGM, a study of Sudanese men found that many preferred sex with women who hadn't been mutilated, and experienced discomfort during sex with a woman with FGM [D].[8] As FGM is largely performed and encouraged by women, men in these cultures may not be fully aware of the procedure and potential complications. A recent study amongst Gambian men showed that 77 per cent did not realise that FGM had a negative impact on women's health, and 60 per cent thought it was equivalent to male circumcision [D].[9] Younger men, with more knowledge of FGM and its effects, are more receptive to banning it.[5]

Women are more likely to support the continuation of FGM if they are uneducated, married, living in a rural area, and lacking exposure to the media. A Nigerian study found that educating mothers and their daughters over a 10-year period reduced the prevalence of FGM [C].[10] Recent data suggest that FGM is becoming less prevalent over time, with 36 per cent of girls aged 15–19 in practising countries having undergone FGM compared to 53 per cent of women aged 45–49 [C].[3]

HEALTH CONSEQUENCES OF FGM

Short term

The procedure of FGM is traumatic, often being performed by 'traditional circumcisers' in non-sterile conditions with no anaesthetic, and requiring girls to be physically restrained. As a result, there are a number of immediate complications including severe pain, haemorrhage, infection (including tetanus) and sepsis, transmission of blood-borne viruses including hepatitis B and C and HIV, urinary retention, damage to adjacent tissues, and fracture or dislocation from being restrained.

If a woman is admitted acutely following mutilation, they should be assessed for signs of blood loss and sepsis, and offered analgesia and tetanus vaccination. Consideration should be given to prophylactic antibiotics in the absence of overt sepsis, and to urinary catheterisation.[4]

Long term

Obstetric complications

FGM causes scar tissue formation around the vulva and perineum, which is less elastic than normal perineal tissue and leads to obstetric complications. These include a greater risk of caesarean section, postpartum haemorrhage and extended hospital stay correlated with the severity of the mutilation [C].[13] Additionally, type 3 FGM requires anterior episiotomy (defibulation) either antenatally or at the time of delivery, which carries risks of infection, bleeding and damage to the genital and urinary tracts.

Although FGM has been linked with obstructed labour in studies conducted in African countries, this does not seem to be the case in countries with more developed obstetric care and facilities.[4] A case–control study carried out in Sweden in 2005 found that women requiring defibulation had shorter labours than Swedish controls who had not undergone FGM [C].[11] Perineal tears are more common in women with FGM, but evidence suggests that types 1 and 2 FGM are not independent risk factors for obstetric fistula formation [C].[4,12]

Perinatal mortality

The 2006 WHO Study Group on FGM and Obstetric Outcome in six African countries found increased rates of perinatal mortality of around 1–2 per 100 deliveries amongst babies born to mothers who had undergone FGM [C].[13] Death rates were 15 per cent higher for those whose mothers had type 1, 32 per cent higher for type 2 and 55 per cent higher for type 3 FGM. Babies born to mothers with FGM were also more likely to need resuscitation after delivery, but no association was found between neonatal birthweight and maternal FGM [C].

Urinary symptoms

FGM can alter the structure of the urinary tract, predisposing women to recurrent UTIs as well as urethral strictures and peri-urethral tears. This altered anatomy may impair women's ability to detect dysuria; a study from Khartoum showed that only 8 per cent of women and girls with FGM diagnosed with UTI on urine testing reported experiencing urinary symptoms [D].[14] Although FGM can cause urinary retention and poor flow, and UTIs can predispose to urinary incontinence, FGM does not seem to be implicated as a direct causal factor of incontinence.

Genital and pelvic infections

An increased frequency of bacterial vaginosis, genital herpes and candidiasis has been found amongst women subjected to FGM, correlating with the extent of their mutilation and the amount of labia majora removed [C].[1] The prevalence of chronic pelvic disease is higher in women who have undergone FGM than in non-mutilated women, and women with FGM have higher rates of primary infertility associated with the extent of their FGM [C].[15]

HIV transmission

Although there is no epidemiological evidence linking FGM to HIV transmission, some studies have suggested possible associations between the two. These include the increased likelihood of coital bleeding in women who have undergone FGM; the increased need for blood products perinatally; the repeated use of FGM equipment between numerous girls; and the increased likelihood of anal intercourse occurring in infibulated women [E].[16]

Cyst formation

Epidermal inclusion cysts may occur in around 5 per cent of women who undergo type 2 FGM, and in around 0.6 per cent with type 3 [C].[17] These are caused by excision of tissue and growth of epidermal elements in the dermal layer. Inclusion cysts grow slowly but become symptomatic when infected. Treatment requires excision and drainage of the cyst, with removal of the excess skin and re-approximation of the skin edges.

Chronic pain

Infibulated women may experience pelvic pain from haematocolpos, if the passage of menses is blocked, and dyspareunia, if the vaginal opening is not sufficient to allow intercourse. The mutilation itself can cause chronic neuropathic vulval pain from severed nerve endings, and women may also experience pain from chronic pelvic and urinary infections.

Psychological consequences

Women who have been subjected to FGM have significantly higher rates of PTSD and other psychiatric conditions than women who have not undergone mutilation [C].[18] Women who have undergone FGM may experience lower rates of orgasm and reduced orgasmic functioning, with lower sexual quality of life scores the greater the extent of their FGM [C].[19]

IDENTIFYING GIRLS AT RISK

Risk factors for FGM include a low level of family integration into British society; a family history of FGM, including within the extended family; withdrawal from school; or withdrawal from Personal, Social and Health Education lessons at school.[2]

FGM may also be imminent if a female family elder is visiting the UK, or if a girl mentions that she is about to have a 'special procedure' or 'become a woman'.

If FGM has already taken place, the girl may show obvious signs of trauma such as difficulty walking, standing or sitting; urinary or menstrual difficulties; prolonged or repeated absences from school; noticeable behaviour changes, such as depression or withdrawal; or reluctance to undergo medical examinations.[2]

THE CONSULTATION

RCOG Guidelines on FGM state that any woman from a country which practises FGM – especially where prevalence is high – should be asked about her mutilation status.[4] In antenatal care, this can be incorporated into the family origin questioning used for haemoglobinopathy screening. Alongside those from high-prevalence African countries, the possibility of FGM should be considered in women from Yemen and from Iraq, where prevalence is around 23 per cent and 8 per cent respectively [D].[3]

A female member of staff should be available, should the girl or woman prefer this. It is important to be sensitive; loaded terms such as 'mutilation' should be avoided, and instead questions like 'Have you been closed/cut?' should be used. It is equally important, however, to ascertain if she or any other female in her family has been subjected to or is at risk of FGM. Symptoms indicative of FGM such as dyspareunia, dysuria, voiding difficulties, pelvic pain, dysmenorrhoea or other menstrual symptoms, and obstetric difficulties, should be explored.

Explain that FGM is illegal, and that the law can be used to protect them and other family members from being mutilated. If the woman is worried about her immigration status, reassurance must be given that any treatment for FGM will not affect this.[20]

In cases where a girl has already been subjected to or is at risk of FGM, a referral to children's services and to the police must be made.[21] For women who have undergone FGM, an individual risk assessment should be made using an FGM safeguarding risk tool, and a referral to the police should be considered, with the woman's consent.[2] In both cases a detailed history should be taken and clearly documented, including the nature of their mutilation, where and when it was carried out and by whom, and any immediate complications. The woman should be asked about symptoms or complications resulting from FGM, as listed above. Blood and urine should be tested for infection, including a screen for blood-borne viruses.

If a child is at risk of FGM, her parents may be asked to sign a contract prohibiting FGM, and carry a 'health passport' which states the law around FGM and can be used to resist pressure to undergo FGM in their home country.[22]

Examination, where required for girls, should be performed by a consultant paediatrician or gynaecologist with experience of dealing with FGM.[2] For adult women, the use

UROGYNAECOLOGY AND SEXUAL HEALTH AND WELLBEING

of a speculum should be determined by the size of the vaginal opening. A paediatric speculum is preferable, but if the women is not be able to tolerate this then a bimanual examination may be performed with one finger. The nature of the injuries should be documented, either as diagrams or clinical photographs, to reduce the need for repeat examinations.[4] If necessary, vaginal swabs should be taken as the incidence of STIs is higher in women with FGM.[1]

Women with FGM should be involved in planning their delivery; the RCOG suggests that FGM is not an absolute indication for caesarean section, unless their anatomy is severely distorted. A referral to a local African Well Woman clinic can be made, to advise on suitability for vaginal delivery. If a vaginal birth is planned, a low threshold for episiotomy should be maintained due to the risk of prolonged labour and perineal tears [D].[4]

The British Medical Association has published guidance for health professionals on the ethical considerations involved in managing women already subjected to, or at risk of, FGM.[23]

DE-INFIBULATION

The WHO recommends that defibulation should be offered to women as soon as possible, as it may reduce some of the complications of FGM [D].[1] When a women with FGM wishes to become pregnant, defibulation should be recommended before conception, especially if difficult surgery is anticipated. If the woman is already pregnant, defibulation should be performed before 20 weeks to allow adequate healing time [D].[4] Caution should be exercised at later gestations as the gravid uterus may cause hypotension during the procedure. Guidance should be sought from an obstetrician or centre with experience of managing FGM. Urine should be screened for bacteria before surgery, and bloods should be sent for group and save because of the risk of bleeding. The procedure itself can be carried out in a suitable outpatients' room or operating theatre under local or general anaesthesia.[4]

The defibulation procedure requires the operator to identify the urethra, incise the vulval scar with cutting diathermy to reduce risk of bleeding, and to use fine absorbable sutures (e.g. Vicryl Rapide) to suture raw edges. Prophylactic antibiotics should be considered.[4]

If vaginal access is adequate then intrapartum defibulation may be performed, either in the first stage of labour by anterior midline episiotomy with epidural, or during the second stage at crowning of the baby's head. Defibulation can also be performed following a Caesarian section.

Re-infibulation, or re-closing a woman, is illegal and must not be performed after birth or at any other time. In the repair of birth trauma after FGM, the WHO recommends suturing any raw edges to prevent re-infibulation passively occurring through the healing process.[24]

Women who have undergone FGM should be offered counselling after childbirth.[2] The woman should be told the benefits of not being re-infibulated, which include better hygiene, less pelvic pain and dyspareunia, fewer obstetric complications and better fertility outcomes.[2] Where the mother has given birth to a girl, she should have the reasons for not having her daughter subjected to FGM explained to her.

THE LAW AND FGM

The Prohibition of Female Circumcision Act (1985) made FGM illegal in Britain. The Female Genital Mutilation Act (2003) made it illegal to take girls out of the UK to undergo FGM, or to assist someone with this. The maximum sentence for carrying out or assisting in FGM is 14 years in prison. Re-infibulation is also illegal in the UK and should never be performed by any health professional. To date, three doctors have been struck off the medical register by the GMC for serious professional misconduct relating to FGM, and in 2014 two individuals were charged and subsequently acquitted by the Crown Prosecution Service under the FGM Act 2003 for carrying out and aiding FGM.[19]

Under the Children Act of 1989, local authorities can apply to the courts to prevent a child being taken abroad for mutilation. Section 47 of the Act states the requirement of health professionals to inform social care or the police if they believe a child to be actually or potentially at risk. This also includes if the ill treatment of a child is seen or heard of, through the Adoption and Children Act 2002.

Other relevant legislation includes the Children Act 2004 (England and Wales), the Human Rights Act 1998, and the European Convention on Human Rights.

ELIMINATING FGM

FGM is already illegal in developed nations, and 26 countries in Africa and the Middle East have passed laws or constitutional decrees against FGM. This legislation ranges in scope, from the prohibition of health professionals carrying out FGM in Mauritania, to complete prohibition in Burkina Faso and Kenya, which includes fines for failing to report knowledge of others carrying out the procedure.

Internationally, efforts are being made to eliminate FGM. The WHO published *Eliminating Female Genital Mutilation: An Interagency Statement* in 2008 and *A Global Strategy to Stop Healthcare Providers from Performing Female Genital Mutilation* in 2010. In 2012 the UN General Assembly passed a resolution to ban FGM. The UK Department for International Development (DFID) has committed £35 million over 5 years to support African communities to eliminate FGM.

The 2013 report *Tackling FGM in the UK: Intercollegiate recommendations for identifying, recording and reporting* sets out a number of steps towards eliminating FGM in the UK. These include treating FGM as child abuse and integrating its management into current safeguarding frameworks; multi-agency collaboration, documentation and data sharing; education of frontline staff; reporting cases of FGM; and education and empowerment of girls at risk of FGM. The report identifies a lack of knowledge amongst healthcare professionals and concerns about offending cultural groups as barriers to the detection of FGM. In May 2012 the Chief Medical Officer wrote to all clinical staff to request that they know about FGM, and what action is to be taken if it is discovered or suspected. Consequently, it is vital that all NHS staff have good knowledge of FGM, and understand the importance of asking women whether they have been subjected to mutilation. Partnerships between health organisations and community groups or educational institutions are crucial to raise awareness of FGM amongst girls who may be at risk, and to ensure that they are aware of the help available.

KEY POINTS

- FGM is conducted in at least 29 countries in Africa, as well as in Asia and the Middle East.
- 140 million women have been subjected to FGM, and 3 million are at risk each year, but its global prevalence may be decreasing.
- Many cultural, social and traditional factors lie behind FGM.
- It is illegal to perform or assist FGM in the UK, or to take a UK citizen abroad for the purposes of FGM.
- Short-term complications: pain, infection, haemorrhage, and damage to adjacent structures.
- Long-term complications: infertility, chronic pain, cyst formation, obstetric complications, neonatal mortality, recurrent UTIs, PID and psychosexual trauma.
- Defibulation may be required antenatally or during labour, but is most beneficial prior to conception and should be offered routinely.
- All women from high-prevalence countries should be asked about FGM.
- FGM should be addressed sensitively and findings should be clearly documented.
- If a girl is at risk of, or has already undergone, FGM, child protection services and the police must be informed.
- Indications that a girl is at risk are poor family integration, family history of FGM, and withdrawal from school or from certain lessons at school.
- A multi-agency approach is needed including education, information sharing, and community programmes to raise awareness of FGM.

RESOURCES

Training video for MRCOG: http://www.fgmnationalgroup.org/

DoH report with terms for FGM in different languages: https://www.gov.uk/government/uploads/system/uploads/attachment_data/file/216669/dh_124588.pdf

References

1. WHO. *Eliminating female genital mutilation: An interagency statement.* WHO, 2008.
2. HM Government. *Multi-Agency Practice Guidelines: Female Genital Mutilation.* 2011.
3. UNICEF. *Female Genital Mutilation/Cutting: A statistical overview and exploration of the dynamics of change.* 2013.
4. RCOG. *Female Genital Mutilation and its Management* (Green-top Guideline 53). RCOG, 2015.
5. Rymer J, O'Flynn N. Female genital mutilation: everyone's problem. *Br J Gen Pract* 2013 Oct;63(615):515–16.
6. Gruenbaum E. Sexuality issues in the movement to abolish female genital cutting in Sudan. *Medical Anthropology Quarterly* 2006;20:121.
7. UNICEF. *Battling an ancient tradition: Female genital mutilation in Ethiopia.* UNICEF, 2006.
8. Almroth L, Almroth-Berggren V, Hassanein OM *et al.* Male complications of female genital mutilation. *Soc Sci Med* 2001;53(11):1455–60.
9. Kaplan A, Cham B, Njie LA *et al.* Female genital mutilation/cutting: the secret world of women as seen by men. *Obstet Gynecol Int* 2013;2013:643780.
10. Adeokun L, Oduwole M, Oronsave F *et al.* Trends in female circumcision between 1933 and 2003 in Osun and Ogun States in Nigeria (a cohort analysis). *Afr J Reprod Health* 2006;10(2):48–55.
11. Essen B, Sjoberg NO, Gudmundsson S, Ostergren PO, Lindqvist PG. No association between female circumcision and prolonged labour: a case-control study of immigrant women giving birth in Sweden. *Eur J Obstet Gynecol Reprod Biol* 2005;121:182–85.
12. Browning A, Allsworth JE, Wall LL. The relationship between female genital cutting and obstetric fistulae. *Obstet Gynecol* 2010;115(3):578–83.
13. Banks E, Meirik O, Fairley T *et al.* Female genital mutilation and obstetric outcome: WHO collaborative prospective study in six African countries. WHO study group on female genital mutilation and obstetric outcome. *Lancet* 2006;367(9525):1835–41.

14. Almroth L, Bedri H, El Musharaf S *et al.* Urogenital complications among girls with genital mutilation: a hospital-based study in Khartoum. *Afr J Reprod Health* 2005;9(2):118–24.

15. Almroth L, Elmusharaf S, El Hadi N *et al.* Primary infertility after genital mutilation in girlhood in Sudan: a case-control study. *Lancet* 2005;366(9483): 385–91.

16. Brady M. Female genital mutilation: complications and risk of HIV transmission. *AIDS Patient Care and STIs* 1999;(13)12:709–16.

17. Shell-Duncan B. The medicalization of female 'circumcision': harm reduction or promotion of a dangerous practice? *Soc Sci Med* 2001;52:1013–28.

18. Andersson SH, Rymer J, Joyce DW, Momoh C, Gayle CM. Sexual quality of life in women who have undergone female genital mutilation: a case–control study. *BJOG* 2012;119(13):1606–11.

19. Royal College of Midwives. *Tackling FGM in the UK: Intercollegiate recommendations for identifying, recording and reporting.* RCM, 2013.

20. WHO. *Management of Pregnancy, Childbirth and Postpartum Period in the Presence of Female Genital Mutilation.* Geneva: WHO, 2001.

21. Berendt A, Moritz S. Post-traumatic stress disorder and memory problems after female genital mutilation. *Am J Psychiatry* 2005;162:1000–2.

22. UK Government. *A Statement Opposing Female Genital Mutilation.* 2012. www.gov.uk/government/uploads/system/uploads/attachment_data/file/208440/fgm-v12-web.pdf.

23. British Medical Association. *Female Genital Mutilation: Caring for patients and safeguarding children.* BMA, 2011.

24. Simpson J, Robinson K, Creighton SM, Hodes D. Female genital mutilation: the role of health professionals in prevention, assessment, and management. *BMJ* 2012;14;344:e1361.

SECTION TEN

LOWER GENITAL TRACT

Chapter 104 Benign vulval problems

Lubna Haque and Margaret Cruickshank

INTRODUCTION

Benign vulval skin disorders are common. Vulval itch, pain or skin changes are commonly experienced. Community-based surveys indicate that about 20 per cent of women have significant vulval symptoms. Of women who are referred on to a gynaecology clinic, the most common causes seen are dermatitis, lichen simplex, vulval candidiasis, lichen sclerosus and lichen planus. This chapter relates to the initial assessment and care of women with vulval disorders expected in the RCOG core curriculum by the general gynaecologist.

ANATOMY

The vulva consists of the external genital organs of the female (Fig. 104.1).

Major structures of the vulva are:

- the mons pubis;
- the labia, consisting of the labia majora and the labia minora;
- the external portion of the clitoris, consisting of the clitoral glans and the clitoral hood;

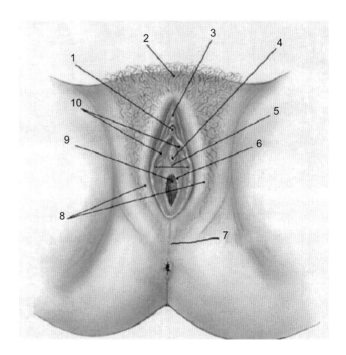

Fig. 104.1 Anatomical landmarks of the vulva: 1, clitoris; 2, mons pubis; 3, clitoral hood; 4, urethral meatus; 5, vestibule; 6, hymen (torn); 7, perineum; 8, labia majora; 9, vaginal opening; 10, labia minora

- the urinary meatus;
- the vaginal orifice;
- the hymen.

The mons pubis is the soft mound of the anterior vulva formed by fatty tissue covering the pubic bone. This separates into two folds known as the labia majora. Between the labia majora is the pudendal cleft and posteriorly between the pudendal cleft and the anus is the flat hairless area of the perineum. The labia minora are two folds of skin within the labia majora which originate with the covering of the clitoris, the clitoral hood. Between the labia minora is the vestibule which contains the urethral and vaginal openings. The opening of the vagina is known as the introitus. This may be partly covered by the hymen, a mucosal membrane or, more commonly, its remnants known as carunculae myrtiformes which can be mistaken for skin tags or polyps. Posteriolateral on the left and right of the introitus are two

Bartholin glands and the ducts from these open into the lower, posterior vagina.

ASSESSMENT

A standard gynaecological history will not identify all relevant symptoms and potential causes of vulva skin disorders. In addition to factors that relate to the presenting vulval symptoms, the patient should be asked specifically about symptoms at other skin sites, other medical problems, and recent or current drug history and family history.

History

Non-specific symptoms such as pruritus and pain are the common presenting symptoms in vulval skin disorders but they are not diagnostic. The pattern of intensity and flare-up of symptoms should be explored during the day and over the menstrual cycle, and aggravating and relieving factors such as urinary or faecal incontinence. The use of self-medication or previous inadequate or inappropriate treatments may contribute to symptoms. It is not unusual for vulval skin to come into contact with potential allergens and irritants such as sanitary products, textile dyes, perfumes and preservatives.

Examination

It is important to examine the vulva with an adequate light source and a systematic approach. Colposcopy is not necessary as the use of a gynaecology couch allows visualisation of the whole anogenital region. It is important to ask the patient to identify the symptomatic area. If vulval intraepithelial neoplasia (VIN) is suspected, it is important to examine other lower genital tract sites including the vagina, cervix and perianal skin. Consider examination of other skin sites including the mouth for signs of lichen planus or ulcers and the scalp, elbows, knees and nails for psoriasis. Eczema can involve any site but is more commonly found on the scalp, neck, and elbow and knee flexor surfaces.

Investigations

Routine investigations in the initial assessment of women with vulval symptoms should only be performed if clinically indicated. These include thyroid function tests and random blood glucose,[1] a vulval skin swab for culture or an STI screen [D]. In addition, serum ferritin and skin patch testing should be considered in women with vulval dermatitis [D].[2] Specific allergic reactions are often identified in women with pruritus vulvae. The most common relevant allergens are cosmetics, medicaments and preservatives. Others include fragrances, preservatives in topical treatments, rubber and textile dyes. Washing powder, fabric conditioners, sanitary towels or panty liners and synthetic underwear may also be irritants and secondary sensitisation to multiple products is common.

Selectiveness in the use of skin biopsy is advised as a diagnosis can usually be made on clinical examination. Many vulval dermatoses can be recognised from history and classical features on examination. Biopsy is required if the woman fails to respond to treatment, there is diagnostic uncertainty of skin changes or there is clinical suspicion of VIN or cancer [E].

General measures

General measures are a key component of the management of vulval dermatoses in addition to condition-specific management. Emollients protect the skin and restore skin barrier function. General vulval care includes avoiding potential irritants that may worsen vulval symptoms, reducing symptoms and resolving contact dermatitis and lichen simplex. Avoiding soap and detergents and using soap substitutes instead can be soothing and protective to the skin. The combined use of emollients and soap substitutes helps maintain symptom relief[3] and reduce use of topical steroids making this approach safe and inexpensive [C]. (See Box 104.1 on general measures.)

Box 104.1 General measures for vulval care

General measures which can help improve symptoms of vulval discomfort and irritation.

- Use a soap substitute to clean the vulva area. Water on its own tends to cause dry skin and lead to soreness.
- Shower rather than bathe and clean the vulval area only once a day. Overwashing can aggravate vulva symptoms.
- Wear loose-fitting natural fabric (silk/cotton) underwear.
- Sleep without underwear.
- Avoid fabric conditioners and biological washing powders.
- Avoid soaps, shower gel, scrubs, bubble baths, deodorants, baby wipes or douches in the vulval area.
- Some over-the-counter creams including baby or nappy creams, herbal creams (e.g. tea tree oil/aloe vera) and 'thrush' treatments may include possible irritants.
- Avoid wearing panty liners or sanitary towels on a regular basis.
- Avoid antiseptic (as a cream or added to bath water) in the vulval area.
- Wear white or light colours of underwear. Dark textile dyes (black, navy) may irritate sensitive skin.
- Use white or pastel toilet paper and avoid strong colours such as blue, green and peach.

DERMATOSES

The term 'dermatosis' covers any skin disorder and those most commonly seen in anogenital skin are covered below but the complete classification has been developed by the

Box 104.2 Summary of 2011 ISSVD clinical classification of vulvar dermatological disorders[5]

1. Skin-coloured lesions

A. Skin-coloured papules and nodules

    e.g. Bartholin gland cyst, warts, skin tags

B. Skin-coloured plaques

    1. Lichen simplex chronicus (LSC)

    2. Vulvar intraepithelial neoplasia

2. Red lesions: patches and plaques

A. Eczematous and lichenified diseases

    e.g. dermatitis, lichen simplex

B. Red patches and plaques

    e.g. candidiasis, psoriasis, plasma cell (Zoon's) vulvitis, extramammary Paget's disease

3. Red lesions: papules and nodules

A. Red papules

    e.g. hidradenitis suppurativa

B. Red nodules

    e.g. urethral caruncle, Bartholin's abscess

4. White lesions

A. White papules and nodules

    e.g. warts, scars

B. White patches and plaques

    e.g. lichen sclerosus, lichen planus, VIN, vitiligo

5. Dark coloured lesions

A. Dark coloured patches

    e.g. melanocytic naevus

B. Dark coloured papules and nodules

    e.g. VIN, melanoma

6. Blisters

A. Vesicles and bullae

    e.g. herpes simplex, pemphigoid

B. Pustules

    e.g. candidiasis, folliculitis

7. Erosions and ulcers

A. Erosions

    e.g. erosive lichen planus

B. Ulcers

    e.g. chancre, Beçhet's

8. Oedema

A. Skin coloured oedema

    e.g. Crohn's disease, post-radiation lymphatic obstruction

B. Pink or red oedema

    e.g. cellulitis, Bartholin's abscess

International Society for the Study of Vulvovaginal Disease (ISSVD).[5] The ISSVD terminology was designed to enable clinicians to describe skin features in a consistent and systematic way with the intention of aiding the diagnosis and care of women (Box 104.2).

Lichen sclerosus

Lichen sclerosus (LS) is a chronic inflammatory dermatosis that is commonly seen in post-menopausal women but can present at any age. Women complain bitterly of severe pruritus that often follows a fluctuating pattern of symptoms but may be worse at night. The vulval and perianal area is usually affected in a typical figure-of-eight distribution although occasionally it can be localised. Scratching causes skin trauma with symptoms of discomfort, pain and dyspareunia.

Pruritus is related to active inflammation with erythema and keratinisation of the skin. The skin is often atrophic and erythematous, classically demonstrating sub-epithelial haemorrhages (ecchymoses), and fissuring. Hyperkeratosis may be marked with thickened white skin. Continuing inflammation results in inflammatory adhesions. Lateral fusion of the labia minora starts with adherence to the outer mucosa and increasing agglutination can eventually result in complete reabsorption. The hood of the clitoris and its lateral margins may fuse, burying the clitoris. The accumulation of underlying skin debris and secretions can form a painful retention cyst often described as the sensation of 'walking on a pebble'. Midline fusion produces webbing at the fourchette and narrowing of the introitus, making intercourse painful and eventually penetration impossible. Occasionally the labia minora fuse together medially causing difficulty with micturition, dribbling incontinence and eventually acute urinary retention.

Aetiology

The aetiology of LS is unknown but it does not appear to be linked to female hormone changes, contraceptives, HRT or the menopause. Evidence suggests that it is an autoimmune condition with around 40 per cent of women with LS having or going on to develop another autoimmune condition.[6]

Prognosis

Prepubescent LS often improves at puberty but can recur in adulthood. It is a lifelong condition but good symptom control and prevention of tissue destruction can be achieved with ultrapotent topical steroids. LS is associated with a 4 per cent lifetime risk of squamous cell carcinoma (SCC) of the vulva[7] and women need to know the signs or symptoms of malignant change to look out for.

Management

The treatment of LS should control symptoms, prevent further skin damage and reduce the risk of developing cancer. Ultrapotent corticosteroids are the cornerstone of treatment for most women with LS. Clobetasol propionate is the most potent topical corticosteroid available and recommended as first-line treatment. Response rates are high with either complete or partial resolution of symptoms [A].[8] Relapse of symptoms is common although improved response rates are seen with longer regular use on an ultrapotent steroid, usually on a reducing regime before returning to 'as required' use. Lower-potency steroids and topical testosterone are not advocated. The British Association of Dermatology has detailed guidelines based on the best available evidence for the management of LS (see Box 104.3 for summary points) [A].[9] Women need clear information and directions on the use of their medicaments. Underuse of topical steroids is a more common problem than overuse. However there are no RCTS to support the frequency and duration of use of topical steroids. A widely used regime is daily clobetasol propionate for one month followed by a gradual reducing regime [E].[4]

Box 104.3 British Association of Dermatologists' guidelines for the management of lichen sclerosus 2010:[9] Recommendations and conclusions

1. An ultrapotent topical corticosteroid is the first-line treatment for LS in either sex or age group, at any site, but there are no RCTs comparing steroid potency, frequency of application and duration of treatment.

2. Asymptomatic patients with evidence of clinically active LS (ecchymosis, hyperkeratosis and progressing atrophy) should be treated.

3. Anogenital LS is associated with SCC but the development of this complication is rare in clinical practice, <5%. It is not yet known whether treatment lessens the long-term risk of malignant change.

4. Long-term follow-up in a specialised clinic is unnecessary for uncomplicated disease that is well-controlled clinically using small amounts of a topical corticosteroid i.e. <60 g in 12 months.

5. Secondary care follow-up should be reserved for patients with complicated LS that is unresponsive to treatment and those patients who have persistent disease with a history of a previous SCC.

6. A dermatology opinion should be sought in any patient with atypical or poorly controlled LS.

7. Surgical intervention is only indicated in women for the complications of scarring, premalignant change or an invasive SCC.

8. If psychosexual issues arise, these should be addressed and, if appropriate, referral made to a practitioner experienced in this field.

Second-line treatment

Approximately 5–10 per cent of women with LS will have symptoms that do not improve with topical ultrapotent steroids (steroid-resistant disease). The recommended second-line treatment is topical tacrolimus under the supervision of a specialist clinic.[9] Tacrolimus and pimicrolimus belong to the class of immunosuppressant drugs known as calcineurin inhibitors. Their mode of action differs from corticosteroids, mainly reducing inflammation by suppressing the T-lymphocyte responses. Tacrolimus and pimicrolimus have both been shown to be effective in controlling the symptoms of LS[8] although less effective in reversing changes in the skin appearance [A]. In a phase II study, maximal effects were seen after 10–24 weeks of treatment and 77 per cent of women had a full or partial response.[10] Calcineurin inhibitors are well tolerated and avoid steroid side effects. However use in LS is off licence and should be monitored in a specialist clinic. Local side effects such as burning are usually short lived. They may also cause heat sensitivity and increase the risk of herpes. Tacrolimus cannot be used in pregnancy due to teratogenic effects. The long-term safety of topical calcineurin inhibitors is not established although based on reports from extensive use, this would appear to be low. Whilst long-term data are awaited, use for longer than two years is not recommended due to concerns about potential malignant transformation [E].

It is important to consider other factors which may contribute to failure to respond to first-line treatment: poor compliance with treatment; inability to comply e.g. due to poor eyesight or mobility problems; superimposed secondary condition such as infection; contact allergy to medicaments; urinary or faecal incontinence; development of vulvodynia secondary to tissue damage.[9]

Surgery

Surgery and CO_2 laser vaporisation do not relieve the symptoms of LS but have a role in restoring function impaired by agglutination and adhesion of vulva skin or mucosal surfaces. This can result in partial or complete urinary retention or narrowing of the vaginal introitus with altered body image or impaired sexual function. Prior to surgery, the skin should be pre-treated with daily clobetasol propionate to ensure that there is no active inflammation at the time of surgery. Simple procedures such as modified Fenton's procedure can be effective in releasing webbing to allow restoration of sexual function [D].[11]

Follow-up

Women who achieve good symptom control on 'as required' regimes of topical ultrapotent steroids do not require follow-up at a gynaecology clinic. They should have information on suspicious symptoms and continue to use general measures to improve skin care. There are no clinical trials on self-examination or the frequency or duration of monitoring. However patient support groups and specialist societies do advocate self-examination to detect any suspicious areas.[12] Self-examination techniques are provided by these groups and may have a role in follow-up [E].

Lichen planus

Lichen planus (LP) is a common dermatosis which may affect the skin anywhere on the body. LP usually affects mucosal surfaces and is more commonly seen in oral mucosa. LP presents with polygonal purple plaques and papules with a fine white reticular pattern (Wickham's striae). However, in the vulva it is more likely to be erosive LP and associated with pain rather than pruritus. Erosive LP appears as a well demarcated, glazed erythema around the introitus. It can extend into the vagina as a painful desquamative vaginitis[13] which can cause dyspareunia and apareunia from stenosis and even vaginal obliteration.

Aetiology

The aetiology of LP is unknown but it may be an autoimmune condition. It can affect all ages, although it is more common after the menopause, and is not linked to hormonal status.[6]

Prognosis

Like LS, LP is thought to have a small lifetime risk of SCC of the vulva, but the small number of reported cases makes the level of risk unclear. A UK-wide audit suggests a similar rate to LS of 2.3 per cent although this may be confounded by case collection from specialist centres.[13]

Management

High-potency topical corticosteroids are first-line therapy for all forms of LP although there have been no RCTs to support this widely accepted practice which include anogenital LP [A].[15] It needs to be recognised that this is indirect evidence as this systematic review identified only RCTs of the management of LP in oral disease. In addition to clobetasol, topical tacrolimus appears to be an effective treatment for vulvovaginal LP. A number of different treatments are reported for women when LP does not respond to topical treatment, or symptoms are severe or widespread. The most common is oral steroids until disease remission is reached.[14] Evidence is limited for vulval LP refractory to topical steriods but a multicentre UK CRS trial completed recruitment in July 2015 and is still to report. The hELP study (systemic therapy for vulval erosive lichen planus) compares methotrexate, hydoxychloroquine and mycophenolate mofetil[16] along with general supportive measures and topical ultrapotent steroids and oral steroids if required. (Further information can be found at http://public.ukcrn.org.uk/search/StudyDetail.aspx?StudyID=16788)

Prognosis

LP may resolve spontaneously within one to two years, although recurrences are common. However, LP involving mucous membranes may be more persistent and resistant to treatment.

Lichen simplex

Women with sensitive skin, dermatitis or eczema can present with vulval symptoms of dermatitis which can result in lichen simplex, a common chronic inflammatory skin condition. This presents with severe intractable pruritus, especially at night. Non-specific inflammation often involves the labia majora but can extend to the mons pubis and inner thighs. There may be erythema and oedematous swelling with discrete areas of thickening and lichenification often secondary to scratching. This can be exacerbated by chemical or contact dermatitis and is sometimes linked to stress or low body iron stores.

Management

The mainstay of treatment is general care of the vulva avoiding potential irritants and use of emollients and soap substitutes. Antihistamines or other antipruritics may be helpful, especially if sleep is disturbed. However, moderate or ultrapotent topical steroids may be necessary to break the itch–scratch cycle.

Vulval candidiasis

Vulval candidiasis tends to present with irritation and soreness of the vulva and anus rather than discharge. Diabetes, obesity and antibiotic use may be contributory factors. Vulval candidiasis may become chronic. On examination, a leading edge of inflammation with satellite lesions may be seen extending out from the labia majora to the inner thighs or mons pubis. There may be oedema, fissuring and excoriation from inflammation and scratching.

Management

Prolonged topical antifungal therapy may be necessary to clear a skin infection with oral or topical preparations. A small prospective case series suggests that a combined approach with oral fluconazole and topical antifungal cream may increase clearance and reduce recurrence [D].[17] In non-responsive cases, identification of the candida type and sensitivity may help to guide treatment.

Extramammary Paget's disease

Extramammary Paget's disease of the vulva is a rare condition seen in post-menopausal women. The main symptom is pruritus. On examination, discrete lesions usually affect hair-bearing skin and not the mucosa, and have a florid eczematous appearance with lichenification, erythema and excoriation. Extramammary Paget's disease can be associated with an underlying adenocarcinoma. Imaging is recommended for the GI and urinary tracts and breasts but there is insufficient evidence to advocate best practice.

Management

Surgical excision is recommended to exclude adenocarcinoma arising locally from a skin appendage and a case series of 76 cases pooled by BSSVD[18-19] indicated that this is the treatment option of choice. Photodynamic therapy, radiotherapy and topical imiquimod have been used with some success in case reports [D]. Despite what appear to be obvious clinical features, surgical margins are difficult to achieve due to subclinical disease and recurrence is common. However the margin status and lesion size did not appear to correlate with progression-free interval in a retrospective cohort study from a single institution.[19]

Psoriasis

Psoriasis can involve the skin of the vulva but not vaginal mucosa. The appearance differs from the typical scale of non-genital sites. It often appears as smooth, non-scaly red or pink discrete lesions. Scratching may cause infection, dryness and skin thickening. Examination of other sites including nails and scalp may be helpful in making a diagnosis.

Management

Emollients, soap substitutes, topical steroids and calcipotriene are useful for symptom control but cold tar preparations should not be used in genital sites.

Plasma cell vulvitis (Zoon's vulvitis)

Zoon's vulvitis is a rare benign chronic inflammatory condition of the vulva which presents with symptoms of pruritus, burning, dyspareunia and dysuria. It usually presents in postmenopausal women and its appearance is similar to erosive LP with glazed erythema often involving the introitus and labia minora. Zoon's vulvitis is diagnosed histologically and is characterised by dermal infiltration with plasma cells, vessel dilatation and haemosiderin deposition. The aetiology of this condition is unknown; one theory is that it is an autoimmune disorder. There have been case reports favouring successful treatment with topical ultrapotent steroids and surgical excision.[20]

Blistering and ulcerative conditions

Herpes

Genital herpes usually presents with acute vulva pain and asymptomatic episodes with genital blisters or ulcers are more likely to be seen with recurrence than primary infection. Swabs should be taken for confirmation and typing when herpes infection is suspected as it is essential to have an accurate diagnosis.

Beçhet's disease

Beçhet's disease is a chronic multisystem disease characterised by recurrent oral and genital ulcers. In women, ulcers can involve the cervix, vulva or vagina. These are usually recurrent, painful and can leave scarring. Treatment to control flare-ups and reduce symptoms is based on topical or systemic immunosuppressants.

Vulval Crohn's disease

Crohn's disease is a chronic inflammatory bowel disorder. It can involve the vulva by direct extension from involved bowel or 'metastatic' granulomas. Rarely it is seen without known bowel disease or preceding the presentation of bowel disease. The vulva is often swollen and oedematous with granulomas, abscesses, draining sinuses and ulceration. Surgery can result in sinus and fistula formation and tissue breakdown and therefore should be avoided. Treatments include metronidazole and oral immunomodulators and so care needs to involve liaison with medical and surgical gastrointestinal specialists.

Pemphigoid and pemphigus

Pemphigoid is a rare blistering disorder which usually occurs in later life, the average age of onset for vulval disease being over 70 years. Pemphigoid is classified as a connective tissue autoimmune disease. Prior to blister development or with atypical disease, there may be non-specific pruritic papules, eczematous or urticarial rash with marked itch. The blisters are large tense fluid-filled bullae.

Pemphigus vulgaris is a rare autoimmune disease that causes severe blistering of the skin and of the mucous membranes lining the mouth, nose, throat and genitals. The fragile blisters break down to painful ulcers and itching is unusual. Treatment is with topical or oral steroids. Vulval rather than vaginal involvement is more common and is almost always associated with mouth and skin lesions. The bullae are usually large and tense. Treatment is important because secondary infection can lead to sepsis. Pemphigus vulgaris is usually treated with oral corticosteroids.

If pemphigoid or pemphigus is suspected, the diagnosis can usually be made on the clinical appearance of the preceding rash or large fluid-filled bullae. Biopsies of the blister and adjacent normal skin should be taken for histological examination and a fresh sample in 0.9% saline for direct immunofluorescence. Dermatological opinion on atypical blistering rashes and the treatment is essential.

Vulva lumps and bumps

Lumps and bumps are common in the vulva area and normal anatomical features such as carunculae myrtiformes or papillomatosis may be mistaken by the patient (or their doctor) for pathology. Vulval cysts are usually benign and can be treated conservatively.

Sebaceous cyst

Sebaceous cysts are generally mobile masses that can consist of fibrous tissue filled with inspissated sebaceous material. They are more common in hair-bearing areas, are smooth in appearance and to the touch, and vary greatly in size. They can be multiple and widespread involving the labia majora. Infection is uncommon but can recur. Excision of a sebaceous cyst scan be done under local anaesthetic. It is important to remove the central punctum to prevent recurrence. With multiple cysts, it is possible to treat by laser ablation to avoid scarring and extensive skin excision.[21]

Epithelial inclusion cyst

This benign cyst is usually found on the skin of the labia majora or minora. The appearance is similar to a sebaceous cyst. The cyst may be asymptomatic but can also become infected. The management is the same as for a sebaceous cyst.

Bartholin's cyst

A Bartholin's cyst is formed when the duct from the Bartholin's gland to the vaginal opening becomes blocked, causing a fluid-filled cyst to develop. Infection of the duct and/or gland results in a Bartholin's abscess. Bartholin's cysts are most likely to occur in women of child-bearing age and can grow from the size of a pea to the size of a golf ball. This is usually smooth and well localised but when infected, there may be surrounding oedema and induration. Marsupialisation is more effective than simple incision and drainage for cysts and abscesses as it allows the gland to drain and reduces the risk of recurrence. A cruciate incision is performed over the dome of the abscess, the cavity drained and the wound edges are sutured apart to ensure drainage. An alternative procedure is to insert a balloon catheter under local anaesthetic. The catheter stays in place using a saline-filled balloon, usually for up to 4 weeks. This is to allow epithelialisation of the tract, after which it is deflated and removed if it has not fallen out spontaneously. This procedure is recommended by a NICE review[22] which identified from a small number of case series that insertion is almost always successful, most women find this procedure acceptable and the recurrence rate is 3–17 per cent [C] even if the catheter falls out in a shorter time [D].

Papillomatosis

Papillomatosis describes a benign epithelial tumour, growing exophytically with often finger-like fronds. Vulvar vestibular papillomatosis is considered an anatomical variant of the vulva, characterised by pink, asymptomatic, fine projections.[9] Recognition of this condition is important to distinguish it from warts and therefore avoid unnecessary biopsy or treatment. Papillomatosis may be more pronounced with inflammation of the vulval mucosa.

Dermatofibroma

Dermatofibromas are classed as benign, often pigmented, skin lesions forming firm solitary papules. They can be elevated or pedunculated. Dermatofibromas cause little or no discomfort. On the shin, they are thought to arise from reaction to previous injuries such as shaving but trauma is less often related to vulva lesions. They tend to recur and should be managed conservatively.

Lipoma

Vulvar lipomas are uncommon and benign consisting of lobulated fat enclosed by a thin fibrous capsule. They can occur anywhere and in the anogenital area they usually involve the labia majora or buttock. They tend to be slow growing and are usually asymptomatic. They are more commonly seen in the third and fourth decades of life. Treatment of vulval lipomas should be conservative as surgery can cause scarring and disfigurement from removing subcutaneous fat which can extend deeply.

Hidradenatis suppurativa

Hidradenitis suppurativa (HS) is a chronic skin disorder characterised by skin abscesses, fistulas and scarring, generally affecting the anogenital and axillary areas. It is a common disease with an estimated prevalence of 1 per cent.[23] The aetiology is unknown although it appears on histological examination to be a disease of hair follicles rather than apocrine sweat glands. Recurrent and multiple boils and scarring makes this condition embarrassing and distressing. Treatment options are limited. First-line treatment includes topical antibiotics (e.g. metronidazole gel) or systemic antibiotics (e.g. low-dose minocycline). Second-line treatment with retinoids and immunosuppressive drugs may have limited response and should involve collaboration with dermatology.

Hidradenoma

Hidradenoma papilliferum (HP) is a rare, benign, cystic, papillary tumour. It is a sharply circumscribed nodule of ectopic breast tissue usually found on the labia majora or interlabial folds. It is often confused clinically with carcinoma of the vulva as it often ulcerates. Histologically, it is identical to an intraductal papilloma of the breast.

EBM

The supporting evidence for the management of common vulva disorders is limited mostly to uncontrolled observational studies or case series.

Vulval varicosities

Vulval varicosities are rare outwith pregnancy. They may present with pain, dyspareunia or general discomfort, especially when standing or later in day. Varicose swellings are most likely to involve the labia majora. An MRI scan of the pelvis may identify pelvic varicosities, local venous malformations of the vulva or vagina or arteriovenous malformations of the leg or ovarian vessels or other pelvic organs.[24] Isolated varicosities are managed conservatively in pregnancy but when symptomatic in non-pregnant women may be treated by incision and ligation or by sclerotherapy [D].

KEY POINTS

- Vulval itch is a very common complaint.
- The history required for vulva skin disorders differs from a standard gynaecological history to include information on other skin disorders and related factors.
- Examination requires good positioning of the patient with a good light source and a systematic approach to examining the whole ano-genital region.
- Skin biopsy is not always necessary unless you suspect malignant disease or the condition does not improve with first-line therapy.
- Advice on general care of vulva skin and avoiding irritants often benefits women with vulva skin disorders in addition to specific therapies.
- Lichen sclerosus is a lifelong condition but good symptom control and prevention of tissue destruction can be achieved with topical ultrapotent steroids.
- LS is associated with a 4 per cent risk of squamous cell cancer of the vulva and women should be aware of the signs or symptoms of malignant change.
- Surgery is rarely required for LS except to correct the effects of scarring such as apareunia or urinary retention.
- Lumps and bumps are common in the vulva area and can often be managed conservatively.

References

1. Crone AM, Stewart EJ, Wojnarowska F, Powell SM. Aetiological factors in vulvar dermatitis. *Journal of the European Academy of Dermatology & Venereology* 2000;14(3):181–6.
2. Utas S, Ferahbas A, Yildez. Patients with vulvar pruritus; patch test results. *Contact Dermatitis* 2008;58:296–8.
3. Simonart T *et al.* Vulvar lichen sclerosus: effect of maintenance treatment with a moisturizer on the course of the disease. *Menopause* 2008;15:74–7.
4. Cruickshank ME, Hay I. *The management of vulva skin disorders.* RCOG Green-top Guideline No 58, 2011.
5. Lynch PJ, Moyal-Barracco M, Scurry J, Stockdale C. 2011 ISSVD terminology and classification of vulvar dermatological disorders: an approach to clinical diagnosis. *JLGTD* 2012;16(4):339–44.
6. Cooper SM, Ali I, Baldo M, Wojnarowska F. The association of lichen sclerosus and erosive lichen planus of the vulva and autoimmune disease. *Arch Dermatol* 2008;1449(11):1432–5.
7. Carli P, Cattaneo A, de Magnis A, Biggeri A, Taddei G, Giannotti B. Squamous cell carcinoma arising in vulval lichen sclerosus: a longitudinal cohort study. *European Journal of Cancer Prevention* 1995;4:491–5.
8. Chi CC, Kirtschig G, Baldo M, Lewis F, Wojnarowska F. Systematic review and meta-analysis of randomized controlled trials on topical interventions for genital lichen sclerosus. *J Am Acad Dermatol* 2012;67:305–12.
9. Neill SM, Lewis FM, Tatnall FM, Cox NH. British Association of Dermatologists' guidelines for the management of lichen sclerosus 2010. *Br J Dermatol* 2010;163(4):672–82.
10. Hengge UR, Krause W, Hofmann H *et al.* Multicentre, phase II trial on the safety and efficacy of topical tacrolimus ointment for the treatment of lichen sclerosus. *British Journal of Dermatology* 2006;155(5):1021–1028.
11. Gurumurthy M, Cruickshank ME. The surgical management of complications of vulval lichen sclerosus. *European Journal of Obstetrics and Gynaecology and Reproductive Biology* 2012;162(1):79–82.
12. http://lichensclerosus.org/check-your-vulva/ (accessed 12/2/2014).
13. Helgesen AL, Gjersvik P, Jebsen P, Kirschner R, Tanbo T. Vaginal involvement in genital erosive lichen planus. *Acta Obstetricia et Gynecologica Scandinavica* 2010;89(7):966–70.
14. Simpson E, Littlewood S, Cooper S *et al.* Real life experience from UK multi-centre case-note audit of erosive vulval lichen planus. *British Journal of Dermatology* 2012;167(1):85–91.
15. Cheng S, Kirtchig G, Cooper S. Interventions for erosive lichen planus affecting mucosal sites. *Cochrane Library of Systematic Reviews* 2012;CD008092.
16. Personal communication Dr Ruth Murphy and Dr Rosalind Simpson, 2014.
17. Beikert FC, Le MT, Koeninger A, Technau K, Clad A. Recurrent vulvovaginal candidosis: focus on the vulva. *Mycoses* 2011;54(6):e807–10.
18. MacLean AB, Makwana M, Ellis PE, Cunnington F. Management of Paget's disease of the vulva. *Journal of Obstetrics & Gynaecology* 2004;24(2):124–8.
19. Mendivil AA, Abaid L, Epstein HD *et al.* Paget's disease of the vulva: a clinicopathologic institutional review. *International Journal of Clinical Oncology* 2012;17(6):569–74.
20. Gurumurthy M, Cairns M, Cruickshank ME. A case series of Zoon's vulvitis. *Journal of Lower Genital Tract Disease* 2010;14(1):56–8.
21. Wu H, Wang S, Wu L, Zheng S. A new procedure for treating sebaceous cyst. *Aesthetic Plastic Surgery* 2009;33(4):597–9.
22. http://www.nice.org.uk/nicemedia/live/12140/46577/46577.pdf

23. Nazary M, van der Zee HH, Prens EP, Folkerts G, Boer J. Pathogenesis and pharmacotherapy of hidradenitis suppurativa. *European Journal of Pharmacology* 2011;672(1–3):1–8.

24. Bell D, Kane PB, Liang S, Conway C, Tornos C. Vulvar varices: an uncommon entity in surgical pathology. *International Journal of Gynecological Pathology* 2007;26(1):99–101.

Chapter 105 Vulvodynia

Shuchi Dixit and David Nunns

INTRODUCTION

Vulvodynia has been defined by the ISSVD as vulval discomfort, most often described as a burning pain, occurring in the absence of relevant visible findings or a specific, clinically identifiable, neurological disorder.[1] Patients can be further classified by the anatomical site of the pain (e.g. generalised vulvodynia, hemivulvodynia, clitorodynia) and also by whether pain is provoked or unprovoked. Patients previously given a diagnosis of vestibulitis should now be diagnosed with vestibulodynia (localised provoked vulvodynia) (see Box 105.1). Some patients may have a combination of vulvodynia with another vulval problem e.g. herpes or thrush, and both conditions may require treatment.

Before a diagnosis of vulval pain syndrome can be made, infections and vulval dermatoses should be excluded.

PAIN PATHOPHYSIOLOGY

Clinical pain can either be inflammatory or neuropathic in origin. Inflammatory pain is associated with tissue damage or injury and clinically exhibits sensory hypersensitivity, which is characterised by hyperalgesia and allodynia. Hyperalgesia is the exaggerated response to noxious substances through a general increase in the responsiveness of tissues. Allodynia is

Box 105.1 ISSVD classification of vulval pain

Vulval pain related to a specific disorder
1. Infectious (e.g. candidiasis, herpes, etc.)
2. Inflammatory (e.g. lichen planus, lichen sclerosus, immunobullous disorders, etc.)
3. Neoplastic (e.g. Paget's disease, squamous cell carcinoma, etc.)
4. Neurologic (e.g. herpes neuralgia, spinal nerve compression, etc.)

Vulvodynia
1. Generalised
   i. Provoked (sexual, non-sexual or both)
   ii. Unprovoked
   iii. Mixed (provoked and unprovoked)
2. Localised (vestibulodynia – previously known as vulval vestibulitis, clitorodynia, hemivulvodynia, etc.)
   i. Provoked (sexual, non-sexual or both)
   ii. Unprovoked
   iii. Mixed (provoked and unprovoked

the production of pain by stimuli that do not usually cause pain, by a reduction in the sensory threshold of neurons. Hence, inflammatory pain seen with vestibulodynia is associated with pain on light touch and is usually localised. Neuropathic pain is usually caused by damage to either the central or peripheral nervous system and produces a diffuse burning, aching pain with intermittent flare-ups. Hyperalgesia and allodynia may not necessarily be present.

ASSESSMENT

History

An accurate pain history is essential to differentiate between the different subtypes. In addition to the nature of the pain, one should record any aggravating and relieving factors, with particular reference to sexual intercourse. Any past treatments should also be recorded to avoid duplication.

A psychosexual history is essential, as many women have significant dysfunction and may require a psychosexual referral [II].[2]

Examination

Identifying sites of vulval tenderness and discomfort can help in making a diagnosis. Clinical examination should also exclude other vulval conditions that can produce similar symptoms. Inflammatory vulval diseases such as lichen sclerosus and seborrhoeic dermatitis can cause vulval pain and soreness through excoriation, splitting and fissuring of the vulval skin, as well as itching. Some conditions may not be manifest at the time of examination, such as a tight posterior fourchette and the vulval fissuring.[3] Symptomatic dermographism is a rare cause of vulval pain, but this may be suggested by dermographism evident at other body sites.[4] Other less common causes of vulval pain are worth considering, including aphthous ulceration, erosive lichen planus and genital herpes simplex These conditions are less common but should be ruled out by adequate examination and investigation. Where diagnosis is unclear patients should be referred to a vulval service or clinic.

VESTIBULODYNIA (LOCALISED PROVOKED VULVODYNIA – FORMERLY VULVAL VESTIBULITIS)

Definition

Vestibulodynia is a cause of superficial dyspareunia and is characterised by vestibular tenderness on light touch.[5] This hyperaesthesia can be generalised throughout the vestibule or can be more focal, involving the opening of the ducts of the major vestibular glands or the posterior fourchette.[6]

Clinical features

Affected women are usually Caucasian, aged between 20 and 40 years, and present with a history of provoked pain such as superficial dyspareunia, tampon intolerance and pain during gynaecological examinations.[5,7] There is often a delay between the onset of symptoms and receiving a diagnosis, which varies from months to years. A 6-month period of time has been arbitrarily suggested from the onset of symptoms to making a diagnosis of vestibulodynia so as to exclude women recovering from acute vulval inflammation from other causes.[6]

As the condition is frequently chronic, a high level of psychological morbidity is common. Some patients are prone to stress and anxiety, which may play a role in developing symptoms [III].[2] Sexual dysfunction is common and frequently reported.[8] Reduced sexual arousal, more negative sexual feelings and less spontaneous interest in sex (not elicited by a partner) have all been described in vestibulodynia. These are all risk factors for significant psychosexual dysfunction such as vaginismus and anorgasmia, the management of which usually requires psychosexual input [III] (see Chapter xx).

Clinically, simply using a Q-tip applicator can identify vestibular tenderness. A defining feature of vestibulodynia is that the labial skin is non-tender. Vestibular erythema is a subjective finding that is often present on normal examination and is usually not helpful in making the diagnosis of vestibulodynia or in planning management.[9] The application of diluted acetic acid to the vulva does not assist in making a diagnosis [II].

Incidence

The incidence within gynaecology clinics in the UK remains unknown. However, the prevalence of vestibulodynia was 1.3 per cent of women attending a Central London GUM clinic.[10] Misdiagnosis is common.

Aetiology/risk factors

This remains unknown, but is likely to be multifactorial. It is often difficult to identify a cause, as symptoms usually develop insidiously. Recurrent attacks of vaginal candidiasis are frequently cited, but this may be due to initial misdiagnosis.

Prognosis

Up to 30 per cent of women with vestibulodynia may experience resolution of their symptoms without treatment and in 50 per cent of these, resolution can occur within 12 months [II].[6]

Management

The aims of management are to reduce vestibular tenderness and to identify the potential need for input from other disciplines, for example psychosexual counsellors.

General measures

Reassurance and an explanation of the condition are essential, and providing written information is helpful [II].[11] Strict vulval hygiene measures should be practised to reduce the chance of contact sensitivity [III].

Only one RCT addresses surgery, group therapy and biofeedback.[12] Good evidence for effective treatment is lacking. Many studies are methodologically flawed, for example low study numbers and short follow-up times.

Topical agents and vaginal dilators

No RCTs have compared topical agents. Local anaesthetic gel/ointment prior to sex and emollients are worthy of mention as first-line treatment [III]. Lidocaine gel together with the use of vaginal dilators can help desensitise the pelvic floor for patients who are fearful of sex and where secondary vaginismus may exist [II].[13]

Other topical agents include steroids and antifungal creams, which have been used with variable results, but no control arm existed in these studies.[14] Long-term empirical prescribing of topical treatments should be discouraged, as it places the woman at unnecessary risk of developing irritant dermatitis and contact allergy. Irritant dermatitis is common on the vulva and in essence is a chemical irritation to a topical treatment. It usually resolves when the irritant is removed.

Pain management and psychosexual counselling

A cognitive–behavioural assessment has been suggested to complement the physical treatments [Ib].[12] Over a series of sessions, a clinical psychologist can teach patients coping mechanisms and pain management strategies such as the pain-gate theory, and can address the patient's expectations of treatment, which might not necessarily be a cure for pain, but rather the ability to have penetrative sex. Fig. 105.1 outlines a connection between the psychological and psychosexual aspects of vulval pain connecting thoughts, emotions, behaviours and symptoms. Hence there is an important role that psychological therapies play in the overall management of vulval pain. For many women with vestibulodynia, sexual rehabilitation may be required and this can be structured over several sessions with a psychosexual counsellor, preferably with the woman's partner. It is important to stress that a referral for therapy does not mean that the pain is all in the mind.[21] Improving physical non-coital sexual contact, helping to overcome pelvic floor muscle hypertonia using sensate focus therapy, and addressing secondary psychosexual dysfunction such as low libido and anorgasmia will be of help to many.[8]

Surgery

The modified vestibulectomy is the procedure of choice, involving excision of a horseshoe-shaped area of the vestibule and inner labial fold followed by dissection of the posterior vaginal wall [II]. The vaginal tissue is then advanced to cover the skin defect. The complete response rate is around 60 per cent. Women who respond to lidocaine gel prior to sex have a more successful outcome.[15] The response rate can be further improved with post-operative psychosexual counselling, which is likely to help overcome the fear of sex after surgery [II].[13]

In an RCT, 78 women with vestibulodynia were randomised to one of three arms: (1) group cognitive–behavioural therapy (12 weeks' duration), (2) pelvic floor biofeedback therapy (12 weeks' duration), and (3) vestibulectomy.[12] At follow-up at 6 months, all patients reported significant improvements in pain scoring. Sexual functioning with surgery had the highest success rates; however, one concern was the high number of participants randomised to surgery who declined to be included in the study. The study did support both non-surgical treatments for vestibulodynia and suggested that patients prefer a behavioural approach to treatment than a surgical one.

Other treatments

Biofeedback therapy using surface electromyographic (sEMG) signals from the pelvic floor has been used successfully to help overcome pelvic floor muscle dysfunction in women with vestibulodynia [II].[16] Using portable home machines with a special vaginal skin sensor, 78 per cent of patients with apareunia had resumed penetrative sex and there was an objective improvement in the sEMG reading of the pelvic floor; however, many of these patients were also treated with amitriptyline. The system is not routinely available and experience in the UK is lacking. It is likely that patients may benefit from desensitising the vulval area using a variety of techniques; the optimal technique is not clear. Biofeedback or vaginal dilators may all work in a similar way.

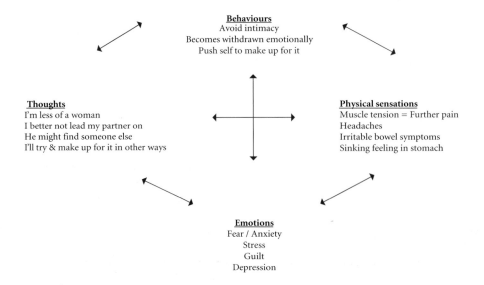

Behaviours
Avoid intimacy
Becomes withdrawn emotionally
Push self to make up for it

Thoughts
I'm less of a woman
I better not lead my partner on
He might find someone else
I'll try & make up for it in other ways

Physical sensations
Muscle tension = Further pain
Headaches
Irritable bowel symptoms
Sinking feeling in stomach

Emotions
Fear / Anxiety
Stress
Guilt
Depression

Fig. 105.1 Psychological and psychosexual therapy aspect of sexual pain

No evidence exists that dietary manipulations can improve outcome in vestibulodynia.

UNPROVOKED VULVODYNIA

Definition

Unprovoked vulvodynia is a cutaneous dysaesthesia causing non-localised vulval pain. Unlike with provoked pain, unprovoked vulvodynia gives more constant neuropathic-type pain in the vulva and occasionally the perianal area.[17]

Clinical features

The affected women are typically perimenopausal or post-menopausal and, like women with vestibulodynia, can present with a long history of multiple, inappropriate use of topical agents prior to a diagnosis.[18] Superficial dyspareunia is not consistently reported, as many women are less sexually active.[5] In addition, many experience rectal, perineal and urethral discomfort and there may be an overlap with other perineal pain syndromes.[17] Psychological morbidity is likely to be high as a consequence of chronic pain.

Clinical examination of the vulva is normal.

Incidence

The incidence is unknown, but, as with vestibulodynia, misdiagnosis is likely.

Aetiology/risk factors

These remain unknown.

Prognosis

The prognosis also remains unknown.

Management

The aims of treatment are pain relief and identification of the potential need for input from other disciplines.

General measures

Reassurance and an explanation of the condition are essential, and providing written information is helpful.[11] Strict vulval hygiene measures should be practised to reduce the chance of contact sensitivity.

No RCTs have been carried out to assess the management of this group of patients, and only case-controlled studies exist, which frequently contain small numbers of women.

Tricyclic antidepressants and neuroleptics

Amitriptyline (a tricyclic antidepressant) is of benefit and addresses the central and peripheral components of neuropathic pain seen in unprovoked vulvodynia [II].[16] A dose of 10 mg/day, increasing every week until the pain is controlled, has been suggested. The average dosage is 60 mg/day, although up to 150 mg/day can be used. Side effects may affect compliance. The duration of treatment is debatable, but 3–6 months has been suggested. Patients intolerant of the side effects can try dothiepin or nortriptyline. The neuroleptic gabapentin can be used as a second-line agent. In the only series to date of 17 patients with unprovoked vulvodynia, the complete response rate was 41 per cent for treatment with gabapentin with a follow-up period of 26 months [II].[19]

Surgery

Surgery is contraindicated in this group.

Other treatments

Acupuncture has shown limited promise in cases refractory to standard medical treatments. In one study comprising only 12 patients with unprovoked vulvodynia, two were completely cured [II].[20]

CONCLUSION

Women with vulvodynia form a heterogeneous group, with the clinical presentation reflecting physical, psychological and psychosexual factors. As with other chronic pain syndromes, a specific cause remains elusive and is probably multifactorial. A multidisciplinary approach to symptoms is likely to be of benefit to address the many complex issues surrounding vulval pain (Table 105.1). For some women who fail to respond to treatment, living and coping with pain become key issues in management. (Fig. 105.2.)

Table 105.1 The multidisciplinary approach to vulval pain syndromes

Health professional	Treatments offered
Clinician	Topical agents
	Tricyclic antidepressants/neuroleptics
	Modified vestibulectomy
Clinical psychologist	Cognitive–behavioural therapy
	Pain management
	Coping strategies
Psychosexual counsellors	Treatment of secondary sexual dysfunction
	Sensate focus therapy
	Increasing non-coital sexual activity
Physiotherapist	Biofeedback
	Pelvic floor muscle rehabilitation and desensitisation

The role of the general gynaecologist is assessment and then triage of the patient to the correct health professional depending on the needs of the patients. If the clinician is unsure of management or the patient does not respond to treatment then the patient should be referred to the local vulval service.

Algorithm for Managing Vulvodynia

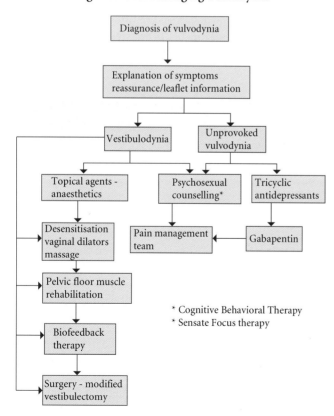

Fig. 105.2 Algorithm for managing Vulvodynia

KEY POINTS

- A good history and clinical examination are essential to distinguish between different vulvodynia subgroups.
- Surgery is only suitable for well-selected patients with vestibulodynia.
- Amitriptyline/gabapentin are treatments for unprovoked vulvodynia.
- A multidisciplinary approach can be helpful.
- Good evidence for effectiveness is lacking.
- It is important to escalate patients to senior colleagues for ongoing referral if 1) the patient has not responded to treatment, 2) the diagnosis is unclear, or 3) the symptoms are severe and there is a significant impact on function.

Key References

1. Haefner HK. Report of the International Society for the Study of Vulvovaginal Disease terminology and classification of vulvodynia. *J Low Genit Tract Dis* 2007;11(1):48–9.
2. Nunns D, Mandal D. Psychological and psychosexual aspects of vulval vestibulitis. *Genitourinary Med* 1997;73(6):541–4.
3. Harrington C. Presidential address. *In: Proceedings of the British Society for the Study of Vulval Disease Biennial Meeting*, 1999; Oxford, UK.
4. Lambiris A, Greaves MW. Urticaria: increasingly recognised but not adequately highlighted cause of dyspareunia and vulvodynia. *Acta Derm Venereol (Stockh)* 1996;77:160–1.
5. Friedrich EG. Vulvar vestibulitis syndrome. *J Reprod Med* 1987;32:110–14.
6. Peckham BM, Mak DG, Patterson JJ. Focal vulvitis: a characteristic syndrome and a cause of dyspareunia. *Am J Obstet Gynecol* 1986;154(4):855–64.
7. Marinnoff SC, Turner MLC. Vulvar vestibulitis syndrome: an overview. *Am J Obstet Gynecol* 1991;165:1228–33.
8. Schover LR, Youngs DD, Cannata RN. Psychosexual aspects of the evaluation and management of vulval vestibulitis. *Am J Obstet Gynecol* 1991;167(3):630–6.
9. Van Beurden W, van der Vange N, de Craen AJM *et al.* Normal findings in vulvar examination and vulvoscopy. *Br J Obstet Gynaecol* 1997;104:320–4.
10. Denbow ML, Byrne MA. Prevalence, causes and outcome of vulval pain in a genitourinary medicine clinic population. *Int J STI AIDS* 1998;9:88–91.
11. The Vulval Pain Society, PO Box 7804, Nottingham, NG3 5ZQ (send an s.a.e.).
12. Bergeron S, Binik YM, Khalife S, Pagidas K *et al.* A randomised comparison of group cognitive–behavioural therapy, surface electromyographic biofeedback and vestibulectomy in the treatment of dyspareunia resulting from vulvar vestibulitis. *Pain* 2001;91:297–306.

13. Abramov L, Wolman I, David MP. Vaginismus: an important factor in the evaluation and management of vulvar vestibulitis syndrome. *Gynaecol Obstet Inv* 1994;38:194–7.

14. Friedrich EG. Therapeutic studies on vulval vestibulitis. *J Reprod Med* 1988:33(6):515–18.

15. Kehoe S, Leusley D. An evaluation of modified vestibulectomy in the treatment of vulvar vestibulitis: preliminary results. *Acta Obstet Gynecol Scand* 1996;75:676–7.

16. Glazer HI. Treatment of vulval vestibulitis syndrome with electromyographic biofeedback of pelvic floor musculature. *J Reprod Med* 1995;40(4):283–90.

17. McKay M. Dysaesthetic vulvodynia. *J Reprod Med* 1993;38(1):9–13.

18. McKay M. Subsets of vulvodynia. *J Reprod Med* 1987;32:110–14.

19. Ben-David B, Friedman M. Gabapentin therapy for vulvodynia. *Anesth Analg* 1999;89:1459–60.

20. Powell J, Wojnarowska F. Acupuncture for vulvodynia. *J R Soc Med* 1999;92:579–81.

21. Woolf J. Too sore for sex: the mind–body interface. *IPM J* 2007;26:4–10.

Chapter 106 Pre-invasive disease

Nirmala Rai and Gabrielle Downey

MRCOG standards

The established standards relevant for this topic are:

Theoretical skills

- Understand the central role of human papillomavirus in the aetiology of cervical intraepithelial neoplasia.
- Understand the principles of organising population screening, the current NHS cervical screening programme and the implications of HPV positivity.
- Be confident about interpreting cervical cytology reports and counselling women accordingly.
- Be aware of the new changes to the cervical screening programme including HPV triage and 'test of cure'.
- Understand the principles and application of the national HPV vaccination programme.
- Be aware of the controversies in both screening and vaccination.

Practical skills

- Recognise pre-malignant conditions and cancer of cervix.
- Be able to counsel patients with abnormal cervical cytology/HPV tests.
- Understand indications and limitations of screening and investigative techniques of cytology, HPV testing and colposcopy.

INTRODUCTION

Worldwide, cervical cancer is the third most common cancer affecting women. Of the estimated 530,000 new cases in 2008, more than 85 per cent were in developing countries; in the same year 275,000 women died from it, about 88 per cent of whom were in the developing world. In developed nations, the figures for invasive cervical cancer are much lower. The disease has a relatively long natural history, and intervention and treatment in the pre-malignant phase is highly effective. The accessibility of the cervix and the availability of a simple test for the presence of pre-malignancy make it suitable for mass screening. Other malignancies and pre-malignancies of the lower genital tract are much less common and therefore most of this chapter focuses on the cervix. A causal relationship has been established beyond reasonable doubt between cervical cancer and infection with human papillomavirus (HPV). The association has been seen in virtually all cases worldwide, paving the way for tests based on viral detection to be integrally linked with screening.

CERVICAL INTRAEPITHELIAL NEOPLASIA, ITS PATHOGENESIS AND THE ROLE OF HPV INFECTION

Definitions

Pre-cancer of the cervix was first described at the end of the nineteenth century. Histologically areas were described where neoplastic cells replaced the entire thickness of the epithelium without breaching the basement membrane. This was referred to as carcinoma *in situ* (CIS). Retrospective studies found CIS lesions in women who subsequently went on to develop cervical cancer, and so the precursor nature of CIS came to be established. Subsequent prospective studies have confirmed these findings.[1,2] After exfoliative cytology was introduced, lesser degrees of change, not amounting to CIS, were recognised and termed 'dysplasia'. In order to rationalise the classification to encompass all degrees of change, the term cervical intraepithelial neoplasia (CIN) was introduced.[3] Pre-invasive changes were divided into grades 1, 2 and 3. Grades 1 and 2 corresponded to mild and moderate dysplasia respectively, and grade 3 combined severe dysplasia and CIS into one category. The definition implied a continuum of change from CIN-1 through to CIN-3 and invasive cancer. As knowledge of the natural history of pre-malignancy has grown, the concept of a continuum of change has been challenged. For practical purposes, there is now a two-stage grading, with CIN-1 becoming low-grade CIN (in which there is a significant chance of regression), and CIN-2 and CIN-3 being grouped together as high-grade CIN (Table 106.1). In North American and some European countries, this grouping has been formalised as the Bethesda Classification for cytological changes, consisting of low-grade squamous intraepithelial lesions (LSIL) and high-grade squamous intraepithelial lesions (HSIL).

Table 106.1 Glossary of terms

Term	Explanation
CIN	Cervical intraepithelial neoplasia, graded 1–3 depending on severity
VAIN	Vaginal intraepithelial neoplasia, graded 1–3 depending on severity
VIN	Vulval intraepithelial neoplasia, graded 1–3 depending on severity
AIS	Adenocarcinoma *in situ*, pre-invasive disease of glandular tissue
CIGN	Cervical intraepithelial glandular neoplasia, pre-invasive disease of glandular tissue graded low and high; high-grade CIGN = AIS
Pap smear	Cervical smear – cytological test described by Papanicolaou
ASCUS	Atypical squamous cells of uncertain significance – Bethesda system grade equating to borderline nuclear abnormalities
LSIL	Low-grade squamous intraepithelial lesion – Bethesda system grade equating to mild dyskaryosis/CIN-1
HSIL	High-grade squamous intraepithelial lesion – Bethesda system grade equating to moderate and severe dyskaryosis/CIN-2 and CIN-3
Dyskaryosis	A cytological term describing the nuclear abnormalities – not synonymous with dysplasia
Squamo-columnar junction (SCJ)	Where squamous and columnar tissue meet; this is not fixed, but is affected by metaplasia
Metaplasia	A physiological process whereby columnar epithelium is replaced by squamous tissue in response to the acid environment of the vagina
Transformation zone	That area on the cervix that has undergone metaplasia; it is bounded by the original SCJ and the present SCJ
Dysplasia	A histological term describing architectural abnormalities within tissue
LLETZ	Large loop excision of the transformation zone
LEEP	Loop electrosurgical excision procedure
DLE	Diathermy loop excision: taking a cone biopsy with an electrosurgical loop

Incidence

The UK has the second highest recorded incidence of CIN in the European Community. In 2010 in the UK there were 2900 new cases of invasive cervical cancer and 940 deaths, which equates to 8 women per day being diagnosed with cervical cancer and over 2 women per day dying of it.[4,5] The majority of deaths are in women aged over 50. There has been an increase in incidence rates of 60 per cent for women aged 25–34 years of age since 2002, which previously had seen a fall until then. This is attributed perhaps to an increase in HPV infection because of the increased proportion of women initiating sexual activity before the age of 16. Changes in smoking behaviour in women born after the 1970s are also proposed to be a factor contributing to the raised incidence. Another contributory factor is an increasing number of migrants from other countries without a screening programme being diagnosed with cervical disease after arrival in UK. There was an increase in incidence in 2009 across the UK which was attributed to the raised awareness brought on by the high-profile death of a young reality TV star; incidence has subsequently dropped below the rates for 2008. There has also been a statistically significant increase in the age-standardised incidence by 17 per cent for all ages in the UK.[4] Statistical modelling performed by the Imperial Cancer Research Fund (now a part of Cancer Research UK) has extrapolated that the current screening programme prevents around 3900–4500 deaths from cervical cancer per annum.[6,7]

It is difficult to estimate the total number of cases of CIN, as cancer registries only record cases of CIN-3, but there were around 24,070 cases of CIN-3 in England, Scotland and Wales registered in 2010 with the peak incidence being between 25 and 29 years of age.[8]

Aetiology

HPV infection is the essential prerequisite for the development of cervical malignancy. The most recent data on Dutch archived cervical cancer specimens, using sensitive methods of detecting HPV DNA, call into question whether HPV-negative cervical cancers actually exist: the estimated prevalence of HPV in cervical cancers is 99.7 per cent.[9] On the other hand, population-based studies have shown that genital HPV infection is extremely common with up to 80 per cent of sexually active women being HPV positive at some point during their lifetime. Using the incidence of genital warts as a marker the incidence appears to be rising five-fold in the female population and eight-fold in the male population, with approximately 15 per cent prevalence of the oncogenic HPV types 16 and 18.

While the likelihood of acquiring the infection is high, most infections are usually transient with 90 per cent of women clearing the infection within two years. Thus, the overwhelming majority of HPV infections will not lead to the development of cancer. Progression or regression depends on several factors that interfere with the host's ability to clear the virus.

LOWER GENITAL TRACT

The cell-mediated arm of the adaptive immune response is responsible for clearing HPV. If cell-mediated immunity is impaired, such as in transplant patients or in HIV-positive women, the virus will not be cleared and abnormalities may develop. How the virus results in cancer has now largely been defined. The virus lives in epithelial cells and is species specific. Genital infection with HPV can only be acquired through sexual contact. It is thought that the virus enters the epithelium through a breach in the skin integrity caused by microtrauma. The virus can remain and replicate within the cytoplasm (episomal) of the cell and is often cleared by the host immune system. Occasionally, the virus enters the cell's nucleus and this step towards oncogenesis is termed 'integration'. The cell no longer undergoes programmed cell death after 40–60 cycles but now becomes immortalised. The E6 and E7 oncoproteins are necessary for this, but vary in their ability to do so according to HPV type; E6 binds to the p53 cellular protein and E7 to the RB cellular protein, both of which are cell cycle regulators.[10,11] Interfering with the cell cycle allows DNA damage to accumulate, which may result in genetic instability and transformation of the cell into a malignant cell line. This process may be accelerated by cofactors.

Why persistent infection happens in what appears to be a healthy individual is largely unknown. Smoking is a recognised cofactor for the development of disease: local immunity within the cervix appears to be suppressed in women who smoke. Women who smoke and have pre-invasive disease of the lower genital tract should be advised to stop smoking and offered smoking cessation support. The major histocompatibility complex is responsible for presenting viral antigen to the host's immune system and there is limited evidence to suggest that women with particular human leukocyte antigen (HLA) types may have increased susceptibility to disease. The majority of HPV infections result in CIN-1 and 60 per cent of these will regress without the need for treatment, while approximately 10 per cent will progress to high-grade lesions. However, it should be noted that women with mild dyskaryosis have a 16–47 times increased incidence of invasive disease compared with the general female population.[12,13]

Cervical pre-cancer has a long natural history, which is one of the reasons why it is a suitable condition for screening. If a cancer is going to develop at all, it will take several years to do so, even from a CIN-3 lesion. It is unclear why some CIN-3 lesions become invasive, while others stay as intraepithelial disease, and it is not known how many CIN-3 lesions will become invasive, as prospective studies are unethical. However, the best prospective data suggest that at least 36 per cent of women with CIN-3 would develop invasive cancer if left untreated.[2]

Screening for cervical intraepithelial neoplasia

The test

The traditional Papanicolaou (Pap) smear test is used worldwide to screen for pre-cancerous cellular changes from the cervix. Although the test has been a significant factor in the reduction of the incidence of cervical cancer by the detection of pre-malignant cells the drive to improve the screening test has led to the development of liquid-based cytology. Traditionally, the cytology sample from the cervix was spread on a glass slide at the time of collection. Each slide would therefore have only a proportion of the cells collected from the cervix (around 20 per cent). In October 2003 liquid-based cytology (LBC) was introduced following a recommendation from NICE. LBC collects the whole sample from the sampling device in a liquid medium that is sent to a laboratory for processing. Cells are transferred from the transport liquid to a slide as a monolayer for examination. This technique reduces the proportion of inadequate smears and increases the detection of true dyskaryosis and improved recall rates. This also resulted in improved efficiency by laboratories as it improved the quality of the sample and reduced the workload per lab. It also reduced anxiety in women by reducing recall and giving quicker results. LBC is now the standard test used for the NHS cervical screening programme. There are two main types in use, Surepath™ and Thinprep®. The evaluation of the sentinel sites for the transport medium suggested that both mediums were equally efficient for HPV testing. An additional advantage of the new transport media is that they also allow screening for sexually transmitted infections if required.

HPV testing for triage of low-grade abnormal cytology and 'test of cure' following treatment was incorporated in January 2011 into the NHS cervical screening programme following the evaluation of the pilot studies conducted in six sentinel sites in England. It was concluded that the introduction of HPV testing for triage and 'test of cure' is not only feasible but also acceptable and cost effective and it was rolled out in England in 2012.[14]

More than 90 per cent of cervical cancers develop within the transformation zone, the upper limit of which is the squamo-columnar junction. It is therefore important that this area is adequately sampled by direct visualisation of the cervix. In order to quality assure the screening programme, all cytology samplers have a unique identification code.

Test performance

Cervical cytology is not a perfect test: there are false-positive results (i.e. no disease is actually present) and false-negative results (i.e. genuine disease is missed). False-positive rates vary from 7 to 27 per cent (high specificity) and false-negative rates from 20 to 50 per cent (low sensitivity). HPV testing has higher sensitivity for detecting CIN-2 or worse compared to cytology. Therefore HPV triage was introduced along with cytology with intent to improve outcomes and screening efficiency. About 98 per cent of the smears taken are adequate for diagnosis, and just under 10 per cent of adequate smears are 'not normal'. Most smear abnormalities are at the minor end of the spectrum.

According to the NHS cervical screening programme (2011–2012) (comparable with new British Society for Cervical

Cytology classifications), cervical smear abnormalities can be broken down as in Table 106.2.

In general, the proportion of normal smears increases in older women, but so does the proportion of abnormalities representing invasive cancer. Borderline changes and mild dyskaryosis are very common in young women; the proportion of moderate dyskaryosis is highest for women aged 20–29 years; and the proportion of severe dyskaryosis is highest in women aged 25–34 years.[13]

Table 106.2 Breakdown of cervical smear abnormalities

Type (*new BSCC classification in brackets*)	Per cent
Borderline nuclear abnormalities (*borderline change, squamous, and borderline change in endocervical cells*)	3.4
Mild dyskaryosis (*low-grade dyskaryosis*)	1.8
Moderate dyskaryosis (*high-grade dyskaryosis – moderate*)	0.5
Severe dyskaryosis (*high-grade dyskaryosis – severe*)	0.6
? Invasive or glandular abnormalities (*? invasive or ? glandular neoplasia endocervical non-cervical*)	0.0

The programme

By definition, a screening test is not diagnostic, but identifies a subgroup of the reference population at increased risk of the disease for which further tests should be carried out. Screening is always a trade-off between sensitivity and specificity. In this case, the reference population being screened comprises healthy, asymptomatic women.

No randomised trials have been undertaken to establish whether screening actually reduces mortality from cervical cancer. Evidence in support of screening has been extrapolated from reducing trends in incidence and mortality in those areas where screening has been introduced. This is most strikingly illustrated by considering data from Northern Europe: Iceland, Finland, Sweden and Denmark noted reductions in incidence and mortality soon after their screening programmes achieved target coverage of the population in the 1960s. Norway, on the other hand, with no organised programme in the 1960s, continued to show increasing incidence rates into the 1970s.[15]

A nationwide, organised (as opposed to opportunistic) cervical screening programme was introduced in England and Wales in 1988 with a national computerised call-and-recall system. The regions still have a degree of autonomy in planning their screening programme, but there is now a national coordinating network to ensure the adoption of common standards and working practices. The whole NHS cervical screening programme was rewritten in 2004 and a revised edition is available with new evidence (at present this is only available on the (BSCCP website).[16] This new programme differed from those that preceded it in that it incorporated all the available evidence and used this information to define a minimum standard and what was 'best practice'. There were significant changes to 1) the age to commence screening, 2) the screening interval, 3) actions to be taken following a mildly abnormal smear and 4) follow-up of both treated and untreated women. There were also guidelines dealing with immune-suppressed and HIV-positive women. In general, the principle of management was to keep 'low-risk' women in the community and 'high-risk' women in the colposcopy service. There were further changes introduced into the national screening programme i.e. HPV testing to triage low-grade (borderline and mild) abnormalities and test of cure following treatment which were rolled out from March 2012. There were regional variations within the UK in the commencement and cessation of screening which will be dealt with later in this chapter.

Main changes to the programme

The screening interval

The screening interval changed from 3- to 5-yearly to be defined as:

- 3-yearly to 49 years;
- 5-yearly thereafter to 64 years.

Evidence shows that a 3-yearly screening programme could prevent substantially more cancers than a 5-yearly programme in the younger woman with little extra cost.[17,18]

If maximum coverage for a 3-yearly programme is 91 per cent and the incremental gains become less and less thereafter with increasing screening frequency, therefore, in terms of cost–benefit, there is little justification for reducing the screening interval to less than 3 years in the younger age group.

The age to commence and stop screening

In England, Wales and Northern Ireland, screening begins at 25 years while it has been 20 years in Scotland. The incidence of cervical cancer in the under-25-year group is low and the incidence of transient infection and low-grade CIN is high. A recent review of the age to commence screening in England was undertaken as a result of media pressure following the death of a high-profile TV personality. The group concluded there was no new evidence to justify lowering the age of screening and good evidence to support the current policy of starting to screen at 25 years of age. Since 1 September 2013 Wales no longer invites women until they reach 25 and Scotland will change from 2015 onwards. Thus 25 will be the age to commence cervical screening throughout the UK. Cervical screening before 25 years of age may detect an abnormality that would resolve spontaneously, thus screening such young women could result in both physical and psychological morbidity with little evidence of benefit.

There are conflicting reports on the effect of large-loop excision of the transformation zone (LLETZ) on preterm

LOWER GENITAL TRACT

delivery. A systematic review and meta-analysis by Kyrigou *et al.*[19] reported an increase in preterm delivery following LLETZ. Since then more studies have been published which have suggested that the risk of preterm delivery may not be related to LLETZ but may be due to other confounding factors like smoking and socioeconomic status[20] and may be influenced by repeated LLETZ[21] or depth and volume of LLETZ.[22]

The reduction in mortality from cervical cancer in women over the age of 50 years is thought to be unrelated to the cervical screening process. Cervical screening is less effective in detecting CIN-3 in older women and the incidence of both CIN and cervical cancer over the age of 50 is low: 11/100,000 in well-screened women compared to 59/100,000 women in the population as a whole.[23] Women over the age of 50 who are diagnosed with cervical cancer usually have not fully participated in the cervical screening programme. The exit age of 65 years has been questioned, particularly on reducing the age of screening to 50 in women who have been well screened with a satisfactory negative history. The effectiveness of cervical screening in reducing invasive cancer varies with age, being greatest in younger age groups and least in women aged over 70 years. Age-specific declines in cervical cancer were confined to women aged 30 to 70 years with a nadir around ages 45–50 years.

HPV TRIAGE

Previous guidance recommended that women with 2 or 3 borderline dyskaryosis and 1 or 2 mild dyskaryosis cytology samples be referred for colposcopy. The reason was an underlying risk of high-grade lesions detected on biopsies in a significant number of women with low-grade smears. The risk of high-grade disease in low-grade dyskaryosis was reported to be as high as 40 per cent.[24] The difference in guidelines and in management was also influenced by availability of services and variable evidence regarding the risk of underlying high-grade disease.

The high-risk (HR) HPV-positive rate in borderline and mild dyskaryosis was 53.7 per cent and 83.9 per cent respectively in the sentinel site studies;[14] they also reported the positive predictive value of the HPV testing was 16.3 per cent and 6.1 per cent for CIN-2 or worse and CIN-3 or worse respectively. Studies have shown that HPV testing is acceptable to women. It also reduces anxiety in women because of the reduced number of repeat smears. Triage reduces requirement for repeat cytology and improves effective use of colposcopy services. However the overall referral rate to colposcopy is higher: hence it also increases pressure on the workforce because of increased colposcopy workload. Following the sentinel studies the operating framework for the NHS in England recommended implementation of HPV testing as triage for borderline and mild dyskaryosis for more patient-centred and cost-effective services.

Inclusion of HPV testing as a triage tool has introduced uniformity to the referral system of the screening programme. This has also reduced the time period of treatment and surveillance from a period of average 12 years to 9 months.[25] All smears reported as low-grade dyskaryosis (borderline/mild) are checked for HR-HPV DNA. This is called reflex HPV testing. HPV testing is done on the same sample that is taken for cytology. Women who are HR-HPV positive will be referred to colposcopy and women who are HPV negative will be returned to routine recall as women who are negative for HR-HPV are unlikely to develop cancer. If HPV testing is negative women are returned to routine recall as per national guidelines. Fig. 106.1 shows the HPV Triage protocol of the NHS cervical screening programme.

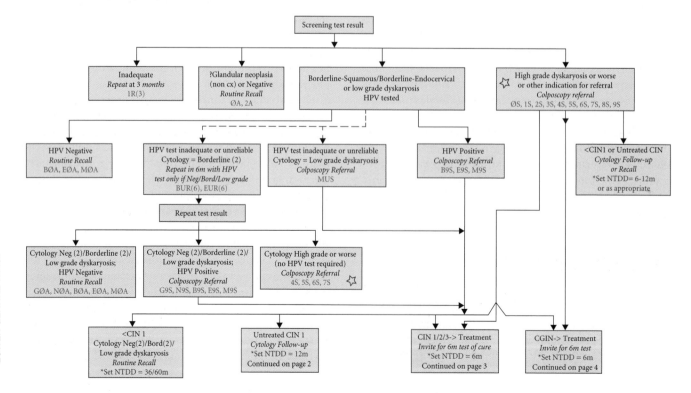

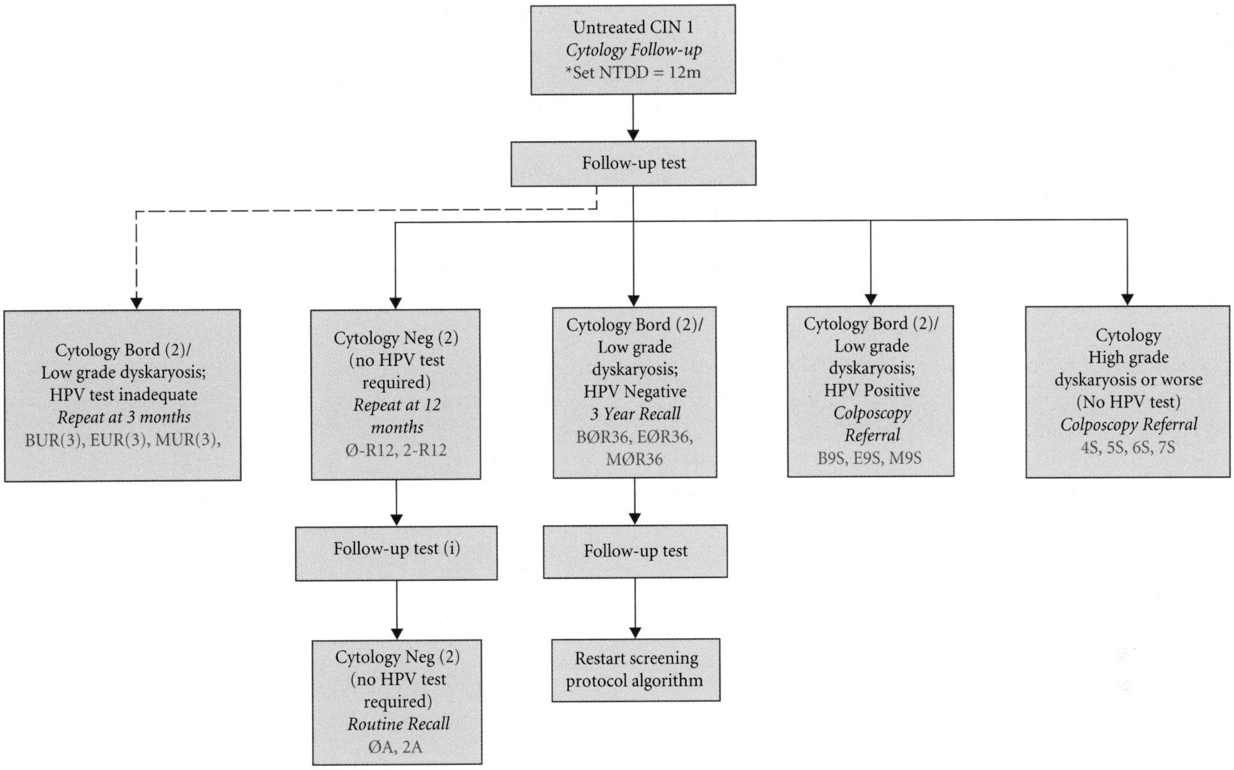

(i) The management of women with abnormal cytology at this second 12-month follow-up test will mirror that at the first 12-month repeat test.

Fig. 106.1 Flowchart for HPV-based triage (from reference 26, with permission)

The negative predictive value of the HR-HPV test is 93.8–99.7 per cent.[27] In a recent meta-analysis which evaluated the accuracy of hybrid capture assay (HC2) and other HR-HPV DNA assays for high grade CIN in ASCUS (atypical squamous cells of undetermined significance) triage (equivalent to borderline dyskaryosis), the pooled sensitivity was >90 per cent and significantly higher than that of repeat cytology; pooled specificity was >50 per cent and equivalent to cytology. The meta-analysis also found that other HPV DNA tests are comparable to HC2. The APTIMA mRNA test for five HPV types is not only equally sensitive but more specific too for detection of CIN-2$^+$ in comparison to HC2.[28]

On the other hand for LSIL (equivalent to mild dyskaryosis) though the pooled specificity for HPV triage in comparison to repeat cytology showed higher sensitivity, the specificity was significantly and substantially lower; similarly to ASCUS, testing with APTIMA viral mRNA is more specific without losing sensitivity.[28]

Referral to colposcopy

The referral system to colposcopy in England and Northern Ireland has changed significantly and is based on HPV reflex testing for triage. Women with low-grade dyskaryosis (borderline and mild) with HR-HPV positive and one moderate or severe dyskaryosis will be referred to colposcopy.

An economic model suggested that HPV triage is more cost effective compared to cytology.

Follow-up of treated and untreated women

Test of cure
The NHS Cervical Screening Programme follow-up protocols are shown in Fig. 106.2.

High-risk HPV testing is used to predict residual or recurrent disease more quickly and accurately. After treatment for either high-grade or low-grade disease women are tested for HR-HPV. Women with negative result have a very low risk of residual disease and can be followed up as per routine 3/5-year follow-up.[29] Pooled sensitivity in a meta-analysis showed HR-HPV to be more sensitive than cytology (93% vs 72%). The specificity in comparison to cytology was no better.[28]

There is no clear evidence suggesting that the diagnostic performance of cytology in combination with colposcopy for the detection of persistent disease after treatment for CIN is superior to cytology alone. However women treated for cervical glandular intraepithelial neoplasia (CGIN; see below) are at somewhat higher risk of developing recurrent disease than those with high-grade CIN.[30] In addition, recurrent CGIN is more difficult to detect by cytology. Smears should be taken for the same duration with the same frequency as after treatment

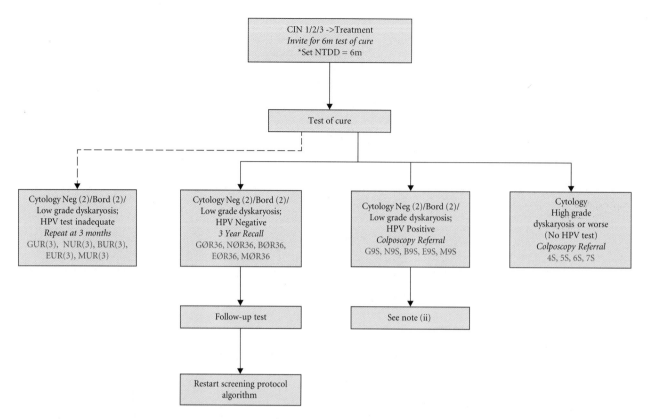

(ii) Women referred back to colposcopy (at TOC following treatment for CIN) due to borderline, low-grade dyskaryosis or negative cytology, who are HR-HPV positive, and who then have a satisfactory and negative colposcopy, can be recalled in 3 years.

of CIN-2/3 (minimum standard). Ideally, six-monthly smears would be taken for five years followed by annual smears for a further five years.

Management

Colposcopy

Further investigation of smear abnormalities is by colposcopy. A colposcope is a low-power binocular microscope that allows magnification from around ×4 to ×25. In the UK, colposcopy is a secondary investigation; in other countries that do not have organised cytological screening, it may be used as a primary tool.

It is important to recognise that the screening programme has the ability to generate considerable psychological morbidity.[31] Appropriate counselling at the time of or before colposcopy is important, and the vast majority of women can be reassured prior to the examination that they are extremely unlikely to have cancer. This is very important to emphasise.

The cervix is first examined at low magnification (×4–6). A saline-soaked cotton wool ball is then applied, which moistens the epithelium, allowing the underlying blood vessels to be examined under higher magnification (preferably ×16 or even ×25). A green filter may be used as it makes the capillaries stand out more clearly. The shapes of the capillaries are studied and the intercapillary distances estimated. Acetic acid (3 or 5%) is then applied to the cervix. Areas of CIN will appear as varying degrees of whiteness. This is termed 'acetowhiteness', in contrast to areas of hyperkeratosis or leukoplakia, which appear white before application of acetic acid. The exact reason why CIN tissue turns white with acetic acid is not fully understood. The cytoplasm becomes dehydrated so in areas of abnormality, where there is a high nuclear:cytoplasmic ratio in the cells, the nuclei become crowded and the light from the colposcope is reflected back. Such areas will therefore appear white. However, not all areas of high nuclear density are abnormal and so not all acetowhiteness necessarily correlates with CIN: areas of regenerating epithelium, subclinical papillomavirus infection and immature metaplasia may also appear acetowhite. One of the challenges facing the colposcopist is to decide which areas of acetowhiteness truly represent pre-malignancy and to avoid treating benign conditions. The classical vessel patterns of CIN are punctation and mosaicism. Bizarre-shaped vessels suggest cancer.

Another test used in colposcopy involves the application of Lugol's iodine solution to the cervix. Normal squamous epithelium contains glycogen and stains dark brown when Lugol's iodine is applied. Conversely, pre-malignant and malignant squamous tissue contains little or no glycogen and does not stain with iodine. This is Schiller's test: areas that are non-staining with iodine are referred to as Schiller-positive and those that take up iodine as Schiller-negative. The test may be used following acetic acid colposcopy.

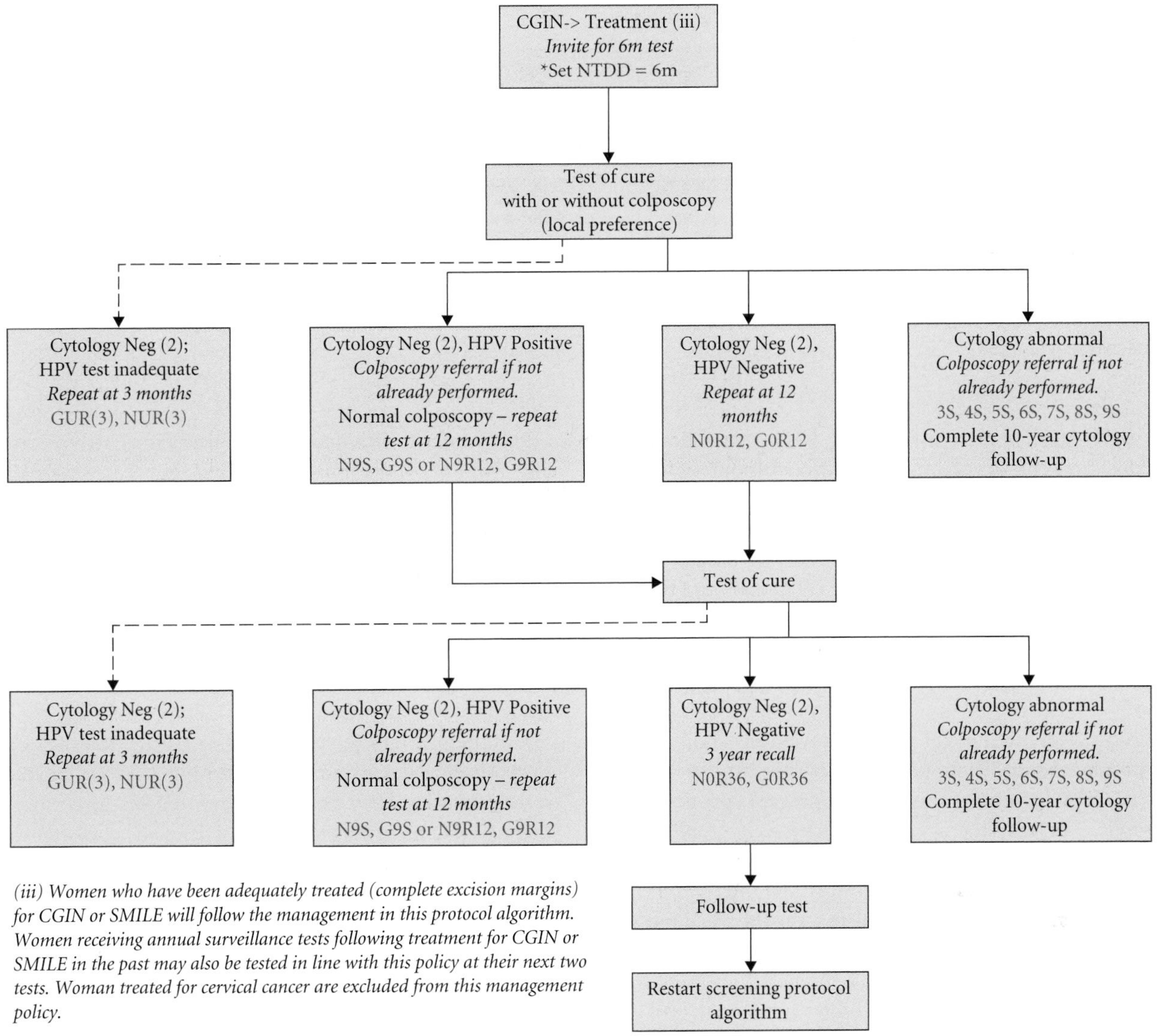

Fig. 106.2 Follow-up protocols based on HPV test of cure (from reference 26 with permission)

Dynamic Spectral Imaging System (DySIS) and Niris are adjunctive colposcopic imaging systems that are newly available for examination of the cervix. DySIS uses photonics and computer-assisted methods to map and provide quantitative assessment of acetowhite areas. It is an objective assessment and identifies abnormal lesions to guide biopsy. It shows higher sensitivity to identify high grade lesions and NICE guidance recommends that DySIS should be considered when new colposcopic equipment is bought by the NHS as it is cost effective and works well. Niris uses near-infrared light to scan epithelial tissue and the rebound scattered optical light is analysed to provide an image data in real time. NICE does not recommend Niris as it is not cost effective.[32]

Treatment

High-grade lesions (CIN-2/3) should be treated, but there is some debate about whether and when CIN-1 should be treated, as a large proportion (60 per cent) will resolve spontaneously. If it is decided that treatment is needed, there are several options. Abnormal tissue can be removed (excisional techniques) or it can be destroyed (ablative techniques) (Table 106.3). Removing the entire transformation zone has the advantage of allowing a large specimen to be examined: the pathologist can comment on the most severe abnormality and can assess whether all the abnormal tissue has been removed. Destroying the transformation zone does not allow this, so it is mandatory to establish the diagnosis by taking a small biopsy before treatment. However, punch biopsy has been shown to be an inaccurate investigation when compared with subsequent loop excision from the same cervix.[33]

Randomised trial data on the different methods of treating CIN do not point to one overwhelmingly superior technique.

Cryotherapy is cheap and easy to use, with low morbidity. It should be used as a double freeze–thaw–freeze

Table 106.3 Treatment modalities for cervical intraepithelial neoplasia

Excisional techniques	Ablative techniques
LLETZ – removal of the transformation zone using an electrodiathermy loop; requires local, regional or general anaesthesia	Radical electrodiathermy – burning the transformation zone; usually requires regional or general anaesthesia
Laser cone – removal of the transformation zone using the laser; requires local, regional or general anaesthesia	Cold coagulation – destroying the transformation zone by applying a probe heated to 100–120°C; usually requires local anaesthesia
Knife cone biopsy – taking a cone with a knife; usually requires regional or general anaesthesia	Cryocautery – freezing the tissue; does not require any anaesthesia
Hysterectomy – may be suitable if the woman has other gynaecological problems	Laser – vaporising the tissue; requires local, regional or general anaesthesia

technique. Success rates for treating CIN-3 vary between 77 and 93 per cent. Cryotherapy is a reasonable option for the treatment of low-grade disease, but not of high-grade disease. It may be suitable in resource-poor situations. All of the other ablative and excisional methods achieve cure (or success) rates of 90–98 per cent.[34] Women who are treated should be followed as per test-of-cure protocol.

Current treatments rely on the destruction or excision of affected tissue. However, with expanding knowledge about the role of HPV and the body's immune response to it, new immunological methods of disease prevention and therapy have been proposed. These aim to address the cause of the disease (i.e. HPV infection) and to either prevent (prophylactic vaccination) or treat (therapeutic vaccination) it. Prophylactic vaccination targets the viral capsid and aims to prevent infection or the early spread of infection through the production of neutralising antibody (see section on the vaccination programme and the potential for prevention). Therapeutic vaccines aim to boost the host's cell-mediated immune arm to attack established infection and have not shown efficacy to date.

Screening for HPV infection

As HPV infection is strongly implicated in the genesis of CIN and cervical cancer, it is logical to ask whether viral detection could improve the screening process. Two methods of detecting HPV that have been commonly used for population screening are the PCR and the hybrid capture system. Data from studies using earlier methodology can be disregarded. Applications of HPV testing can be at a primary or secondary level. Most published data refer to HPV testing as an adjunct to cytology and test the hypothesis that HPV detection improves the accuracy of cytology alone.[35,36] Qualitative identification of HPV in women presenting with a high-grade smear is pointless, as the vast majority will be HR-HPV-positive anyway. It is becoming apparent that the same is true for women who have mild dyskaryosis (or LSIL). However, in women with a borderline smear, it may be more discriminatory. This is particularly so in situations in which the background prevalence of infection is lower (such as in women over 30 or 35 years of age). Testing with mRNA assays in research trials has also been used in search of a better test. The APTIMA[37] and Pretect

HPV-Proofer[38] mRNA testing has been shown to be more specific without compromising sensitivity but these markers' current ranges are lower than the full range of HR-HPV testing. Quantitative HPV estimation has been suggested as being more discriminatory than qualitative estimation. Methods of quantification vary and have limited reproducibility. Furthermore, data suggest that viral load varies in the natural history of disease and may be of limited predictive value.[39]

Increasing knowledge of HPV and improvement in HPV-related assays have prompted consideration of using the HPV test as the primary screening method instead of the adjunct to cytology as it used now. In December 2012 a pilot study of screening using HPV as the primary tool was announced for England. The screening algorithm is detailed below. It included all women aged 25–64 on routine call/recall and early recall. The recall was 3 years for age 25–49 years and 5 years for women >/= 50 years. The routine recall was extended to 6 years for all age groups in the second year of the pilot. Fig. 106.4 shows the NHS HPV primary screening algorithm.

New data are available from a population-based cohort study using HPV testing as the primary test for cervical screening. Participation was higher in all age groups and detection rates were reported to be three times higher than cytology. The overall rate of referral to immediate colposcopy was similar to cytology, but increased by 4.6 per cent when considered together with the 1-year repeat that was done for women who were cytology negative in the first round. The 1-year repeat also contributed to 23 per cent of the CIN-2+ cases, underlying the importance of the need for high compliance with the screening algorithm. A higher specificity for CIN-2+ was reported with cut-offs of greater than 1.00 Relative Light Units/Positive Controls ratio (RLU/PC) for HC2 positivity. The benefits are the earlier detection of CIN and reduced need for repeat testing. An important concern to consider is the response of women to HPV testing and a perceived association by the public of HPV positivity with sexually transmitted infection.

Whilst HPV testing for primary screening may improve cost effectiveness and effectiveness of the colposcopy service in general one must bear in mind whether it would lead to unnecessary colposcopy and possible overdiagnosis and psychological stress. HPV screening is not recommended in women under the age of 30 due to high clearance of infection. Over 35 years HR-HPV testing mostly detects high-grade

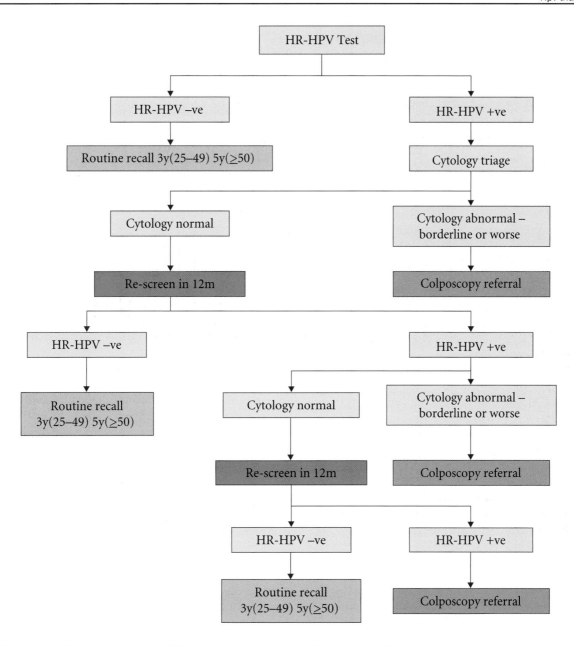

Fig. 106.3 NHS cervical screening programme: HPV primary screening algorithm (from reference 40 with permission)

non-regressive lesions and makes it beneficial. HPV testing between 30 and 35 is debatable but evidence suggests detection of more high-grade non-regressive lesions compared to cytology and hence HPV testing is being considered as beneficial.[41] A systematic review of the surveys undertaken to find out if women were ready for the new screening protocol reported women to have concerns about HPV diagnosis and associated problems of disclosure of STIs and its impact on relationships. However despite the negative concerns repeat HPV testing was a preferable alternative to repeat cytology. It also highlighted the fact that much more needs to be done to educate women regarding HPV and improved information had a more positive impact.[42] There also may be an interpretation bias of cytology as the cytologists would be aware of HR-HPV-positive results. There also may be a reluctance on the part of the clinicians to discharge patients

to community and may lead to over-interpretation of mildly abnormal colposcopies resulting in more negative biopsies being taken.

Other tests like HPV genotyping, viral load analysis, p16-INK4A staining, E6/E7 expression analysis and promotor methylation analysis of tumour supression genes have been proposed as triage tools but so far cytology remains the best available triage tool.[43-46] A promising alternative to cytology is p16-INK4A staining but for further confirmation larger studies are required.[47]

Results are awaited from the various trials and pilot studies but it seems likely that cervical screening in future may be more HPV based than cytology. Education of women and clinicians, training, quality assurance, programme management and audits to maintain standards will all be crucial in maintaining the success of the cervical programme.

GLANDULAR PRE-INVASIVE DISEASE

Adenocarcinoma *in situ* (AIS), or high-grade cervical intraepithelial glandular neoplasia (CIGN) of the cervix, is a rare condition. It presents a particular challenge to the colposcopist, who may only see a few cases per year. Cytology screening for this condition is unsatisfactory, and the disease has no reliable colposcopic features. Diagnosis is often made by chance during the treatment of squamous pre-invasive disease, which commonly (30 per cent) coexists with AIS. Although the entire endocervical canal can be the site of disease, most lesions lie within 1 cm of the squamo-columnar junction. Skip lesions are rare, making fertility-sparing surgery a possibility, provided that endocervical margins are clear of disease. Recurrent disease occurs in 14 per cent of cases when cone margins are free of disease and rises to more than 50 per cent if the margins are involved. The method of conisation is immaterial provided that a large enough specimen is taken and that the pathologist can evaluate the endocervical and lateral margins. There are no guidelines on the optimal follow-up of conservatively managed women; however, most would recommend that regular endocervical cytology be performed in addition to conventional cytology and colposcopy.[48]

KEY POINTS

- Virtually all cervical cancer is related to HPV infection [B].
- Cervical sampling now utilises liquid-based cytology.
- The treatment methods (other than cryotherapy) to eradicate CIN are all equally effective [A].
- HPV is an extremely common infection that rarely causes cancer [C].
- Organised cervical cytology with HPV testing programmes has been shown to reduce the incidence of invasive cancer [C].
- HR-HPV testing detects 30% more CIN-2+ and 22% more CIN-3+ in women over 30 years with 4–6% lower specifity.
- Negative HR-HPV test offers 50% better protection against CIN-3+ in comparison to a negative cytology.
- The screening of teenagers cannot be justified [E].
- Screening for HPV infection is not yet routinely recommended.
- Neither cytology nor colposcopy is a reliable method for detecting glandular disease [D].

THE VACCINATION PROGRAMME AND THE POTENTIAL FOR PREVENTION

Most, if not all, would now accept the central role played by oncogenic human papillomaviruses in the development of CIN and cervical cancer. Furthermore, there is also some understanding of the role played by the host's immune system in preventing and eradicating infection. It was therefore inevitable that attempts would be made to exploit the virus's immunogenicity and develop vaccines to prevent infection.

There are now two commercially available vaccines, one a quadrivalent vaccine (Gardasil™) directed against HPV-6, -11, -16 and -18; the second is a bivalent vaccine (Cervarix™) directed against HPV-16 and -18. The design of both vaccines uses the ability of viral capsid proteins to self-assemble into virus-like particles (VLPs). The VLPs present the same antigenic signature to the host's immune system as a 'real' virus, but as they do not contain any internal DNA they are biologically non-infective and non-transforming.

Several large randomised studies have now been completed and published and they have shown that both types of vaccine effectively increase specific IgG, reduce or eliminate infection with type-specific virus and effectively eliminate pre-invasive disease related to the vaccinated subtypes.[49,50] As we believe that up to 70 per cent of cervical cancers are the result of infections caused by either HPV-16 or -18, there is an expectation that a vaccination programme, if systematically applied, will result in a significant reduction in the burden of invasive and pre-invasive disease.

There are, however, some unanswered questions. The duration of the effect is unknown; although it would appear that it is at least 5 years.[51] Recent modelling of long-term antibody persistence predicted that anti-HPV-16 and anti-HPV-18 will remain detectable for at least 20 years.[52] An immunological-based study reported anti-HPV-16 antibodies to be persistent above those induced from natural infection for at least 12 years or potentially even for a lifetime.[53] These studies suggest that a booster dose may be not required. However, there is no guidance as yet as to when and how often, if any, booster vaccinations may be required. Although there is some evidence that vaccinating against one subtype may provide cross-resistance with other subtypes, we must still accept that up to 30 per cent of oncogenic subtypes remain potential threats to carcinogenesis and thus it is strongly recommended that despite the introduction of a vaccination programme, women should still be enrolled into the cervical screening programme.[54] Whether the natural spectrum of HPVs will be altered by widespread introduction of the vaccines is also unknown. There does not appear to be any evidence as yet of an increasing prevalence of non-16/18 HPV, although this effect will probably take decades to become noticeable.

The vaccines have not been shown to confer any significant benefit to those who have already been exposed to HPV and the current focus is schoolgirls aged 12 to 13 years with retrograde catch-up of older groups. The vaccination programme commenced in 2008 and is organised through schools. The NHS initially opted for the bivalent vaccine (Cervarix) and the quadrivalent vaccine (Gardasil) was available only on a private basis. The quadrivalent vaccine offers the advantage of additional protection against vulvovaginal warts. The quadrivalent vaccine, as well as protection against 16 and 18, also offers protection against HPV-6 and -11 that are responsible for causing 90 per cent of vulvovaginal warts. In

November 2011, the Department of Health (DH) announced that the UK HPV immunisation programme would switch to Gardasil. Since September 2012 the NHS has adopted Gardasil in line with DH recommendations. However, there is no evidence to suggest vaccinating boys alters CIN or HPV infection rates.

Prevention of HPV infection is a desirable goal and now, for the first time, there is clear evidence that at least some cervical cancer can be prevented. Further developments can be expected in this field and trials are underway to explore the therapeutic benefits of the vaccine. Further developments could develop, particularly in the immunological interventions. This may provide benefit to women already exposed and at risk of developing persistent disease.

VAGINAL INTRAEPITHELIAL NEOPLASIA

Pre-invasive disease of the vagina is extremely uncommon (about 150 times less common than CIN). In 70 per cent of cases of vaginal intraepithelial neoplasia (VAIN), there will be associated CIN. The average age of the woman with VAIN tends to be higher than for CIN. The major predisposing factor is the same, namely oncogenic HPV, but the reason for the lower incidence is the relative stability of the epithelium compared with the metaplastic cervical epithelium. Women exposed to diethylstilboestrol *in utero* have a higher incidence of VAIN and clear cell carcinoma of the vagina as here the areas of metaplastic transformation extend on to the vagina. Around 25 per cent of women with VAIN will have had a hysterectomy previously, for either CIN or a benign condition. Like CIN, VAIN is graded 1–3, but in common with vulval intraepithelial neoplasia (VIN), the invasive potential is less than for CIN. Treatment of VAIN-3 is by surgical excision; it is usually best removed vaginally. Small areas of VAIN can be removed with local excision or laser ablation. Prior to destructive treatment it is essential that invasion has been ruled out and it is best suited in patients where the entire lesion is visible. Medical treatment with 5-fluorouracil and imiquimod has also been described as an effective treatment.[55] Treatment of multiple lesions or involvement of the upper vaginal wall or following hysterectomy (in the vault involving suture line or dimples) may be difficult and a multimodal approach may be necessary and may even necessitate a vaginectomy which may be best performed by a combined abdomino-vaginal approach and an experienced surgeon. Chemosurgery using 5-fluorouracil prior to diathermy ablation is an experimental treatment that has shown some promising results. Radiotherapy (brachytherapy) is an alternative treatment for women who may not be suitable for surgery. Lower grades of disease can be observed. For women who have had a hysterectomy in which VAIN is seen at the vaginal vault, there may still be disease buried above the vault in the cuff that was closed over at hysterectomy. In view of this, if high-grade VAIN is detected at the vault of the vagina, it should be treated by excision rather than destruction.

VULVAL INTRAEPITHELIAL NEOPLASIA

Pre-malignant disease of the vulva is much less common than its cervical counterpart. HPV infection is recognised as a major factor in the aetiology of some, though not all, vulval intraepithelial neoplasia. The HPV types most commonly associated with VIN are HPV-16 and -33. HPV-associated VIN is increasing in incidence, particularly in younger women.[56] This increase may be explained by a number of factors, such as increased awareness amongst medical practitioners leading to improved detection, increased smoking by younger women, or changing sexual attitudes and increased exposure to HPV. These women should be examined for other intraepithelial neoplasia of the anogenital tract.

The pre-malignant potential of VIN has been estimated to range from 4 per cent for treated cases to 80 per cent for untreated cases.[57,58] Most published series estimate a risk of 10 per cent or less.

VIN affects mainly the labia minora and the perineum. It can take a variety of forms and can be difficult to diagnose. Up to 60 per cent of affected women may complain of itching, soreness and burning, but many are asymptomatic and the abnormality can be a chance finding on examination.[59] The lesions may extend to the perianal and anal mucosa. Diagnosis is made by examining the vulva with a good light source, such as the colposcope at low magnification, and by taking representative biopsies. Like CIN, VIN is graded 1–3 in increasing severity of abnormal cell maturation and stratification. However, there are some striking differences between VIN and CIN (Table 106.4).

Current treatments for VIN are suboptimal in terms of their poor clinical response rates, high relapse rates and associated physical and psychological morbidities. The high recurrence rates following many therapies may reflect that they fail to remove the reservoir of HPV present in the vulval skin. Low-grade VIN should be observed. VIN-3 lesions can be treated by local excision or laser vaporisation. Recurrences of 39 and 70 per cent have been described after surgical excision and laser ablation, respectively.[60,61]

A topical immunomodulator called imiquimod may be of use in the management of women with VIN, although it remains experimental at present. Cidofovir is also shown to have a clinical and histological response in the treatment of VIN and promises benefit.[62] A randomised multicentre clinical trial (RT3 VIN) examines cidofovir and imiquimod in the treatment of VIN.[63]

Table 106.4 Comparison of characteristics of vulval intraepithelial neoplasia grade 3 (VIN-3) and cervical intraepithelial neoplasia grade 3 (CIN-3)

	VIN-3	CIN-3
Proportion of cases of disease adjacent to malignancy	25%	90%
Invasive potential	Low (<10%)	Significant (40%)
Time to progress to invasion	20-30 years	10-15 years
Spontaneous regression	Up to 40%	Low

Non-HPV intraepithelial neoplasia is termed 'differentiated VIN' and oncogenesis involves alternative pathways to the HPV model. There appears to be an association with some inflammatory vulval epithelial disorders, such as lichen sclerosus, but the condition is poorly understood.

KEY POINTS

- VIN is uncommon and there is little evidence base on the subject.
- VIN in younger women is strongly associated with HPV [C].
- The most common presenting symptom is pruritus [D].
- Lesions may be multifocal and have a variety of appearances.
- Multicentric disease should be considered when VIN is diagnosed.
- Conservative surgery is currently the basis of treatment [E].
- Long-term follow-up is essential as recurrence is common [D].

MULTICENTRIC INTRAEPITHELIAL NEOPLASIA

There is a small group of women in whom intraepithelial neoplastic changes can be detected at more than one site in the lower genital tract. The sites involved are the cervix, vagina, vulva, perineum, anal canal and natal cleft. Although the number of women affected by multicentric intraepithelial neoplasia (MIN) is small, the number appears to be increasing, which may be a true reflection of more disease or it may be a result of increased awareness and detection. The aetiology of MIN is a combination of HPV infection and host immunosuppression of varying degrees. Patients with compromised cell-mediated immunity, such as women who have had organ transplantation or who carry HIV, often have recognisable HPV-associated changes in numerous sites in the lower genital tract. Conversely, women with humoral immunodeficiency do not have an increased risk of HPV-associated lesions.

MIN may be detected in a woman who has repeated abnormal smears despite treatment for CIN, or in a woman being assessed for VIN. Genito-urinary physicians who perform colposcopy may also encounter MIN in HIV-positive women under their care.

At the time of writing, there are no national guidelines for the management of women with MIN. Such cases are often complex and become chronic, with women sometimes having repeated surgery over several years. It is therefore important to be aware that these women may suffer adverse psychological sequelae as a result of their condition. As their numbers are small, women with MIN should be managed in large centres to concentrate experience and expertise. Investigations should be individualised, but may include multiple colposcopically directed biopsies, HPV typing, HIV testing and tests of T-cell function. Management aims to exclude invasive cancer and control symptoms while preserving anatomical and functional integrity where possible. The treatments of lesions of the vagina and vulva are described above. Lesions of the perineum and anal canal may require an initial colostomy prior to skin grafting. Such cases require a multidisciplinary team comprising a gynaecologist, colorectal surgeon, plastic surgeon, stoma nurse and possibly a psychologist.

New immunomodulating therapies currently under investigation, such as therapeutic vaccination and imiquimod, hold out some hope for women affected with MIN. Research to date suggests that they are suitable for around 30 per cent of cases and thus upholds the theory that MIN has varied causes.

KEY POINTS

- MIN is a rare condition and there is no evidence base.
- There is an association with conditions in which cell-mediated immunity is impaired [D].
- It is often a chronic, relapsing condition [D].
- The key aim of management is to do the least required to exclude invasion and control symptoms [E].

SUMMARY

Lower genital tract pre-malignancy is an important area of gynaecology. Most of the pre-cancers in this area have an association with HPV, but HPV infection is extremely common and causes no problems in the majority of individuals affected. Organised national screening seems to have been effective in reducing the incidence of, and mortality from, cervical cancer, but there has been a cost to pay in terms of over-investigation and treatment of women who have very minor changes that are unlikely ever to progress to cancer. Pre-cancers of the vagina, vulva and perineum are much less common, but require specialised skills for accurate diagnosis and appropriate management. Current treatment modalities for the pre-cancers involve ablation or excision. As our knowledge of the aetiology of lower genital tract pre-malignancy expands, it may be possible to target the underlying cause more accurately through the use of therapeutic and prophylactic vaccinations.

Published Guidelines

NHSCSP. Guideline No. 20. Sheffield: NHSCP, 2004.

NHSCSP. *Achievable standards and benchmarks for reporting and criteria for evaluating cervical cytopathology.* NHSCSP publication No. 1. Sheffield: NHSCP, May 2000.

NHSCSP. External quality assessment scheme for gynaecological cytopathology: protocol and standard operating procedures. NHSCSP publication No. 15. Sheffield: NHSCP, 2009.

All guidelines from www.cancerscreening.nhs.uk/cervicalpublications.

Key References

1. Koss LG, Stewart FW, Foote FW *et al.* Some histological aspects of the behaviour of epidermoid carcinoma *in situ* and related lesions of the uterine cervix. *Cancer* 1963;16:1160.
2. McIndoe WA, McLean MR, Jones RW, Mullins PR. The invasive potential of carcinoma *in situ* of the cervix. *Obstet Gynecol* 1984;64:451–8.
3. Richart RM. Natural history of cervical intraepithelial neoplasia. *Clin Obstet Gynecol* 1968;10:748.
4. Cancer Research UK. Cancer incidence statistics 2010. London: Cancer Research UK. Available from: http//info.cancerresearchuk.org/images/excels/cs_inc_t8.2.xls.
5. Cancer Research UK. Cancer incidence statistics 2010. Available from: http//info.cancerresearchuk.org/images/excels/cs_mort_6.6.2.xls.
6. Peto J, Gilham C, Fletcher O *et al.* The cervical cancer epidemic that screening has prevented in the UK. *Lancet* 2004;364:249–56.
7. Sasieni PD, Cuzick J, Lynch-Farmery E. Estimating the efficacy of screening by auditing smear histories of women with and without cervical cancer. The National Coordinating Network for Cervical Screening. *Br J Cancer* 1996;73:1001–5.
8. United Kingdom cancer information system (UKCIS) 2014.
9. Walboomers JMM. Human papillomavirus is a necessary cause of invasive cervical cancer worldwide. *J Pathol* 1999;189:12–19.
10. Werness BA, Levine AJ, Howley PM. Association of human papillomavirus types 16 and 18 E6 proteins with p53. *Science* 1990;248:76–9.
11. White E. p53 guardian of Rb. *Nature* 1994;371:21–22.
12. Robertson JH, Woodend BE, Crozier EH, Hutchinson J. Risk of cervical cancer associated with mild dyskaryosis. *BMJ* 1988;297:18–21.
13. Soutter WP. The management of a mildly dyskaryotic smear: immediate referral to colposcopy is safer. *BMJ* 1994;309:591–2.
14. Kelly RS, Patnick J, Kitchener HC, Moss SM on behalf of the NHSCSP HPV Special Interest Group. HPV testing as a triage for borderline or mild dyskaryosis on cervical cytology: results from the Sentinel Sites study. *British Journal of Cancer* 2011;105:983–8.
15. Laara E, Day NE, Hakama M. Trends in mortality from cervical cancer in the Nordic countries: association with organised screening programmes. *Lancet* 1987;I:1247–9.
16. National Health Service Cervical Screening Programme. Guideline No. 20. Sheffield: NHSCP, 2004.
17. Herbert A, Stein K, Bryant TN *et al.* Relation between the incidence of invasive cervical cancer and the screening interval: is a five year interval too long? *J Med Screen* 1996;3:140–5.
18. Sasieni P, Adams J. Effect of screening on cervical cancer mortality in England and Wales: analysis of trends with an age cohort model. *BMJ* 1999;318:1244–5.
19. Kyrgiou M, Koliopoulos G, Martin-Hirsch P, Arbyn M, Prendiville W, Paraskevaidis E. Obstetric outcomes after conservative treatment for intraepithelial or early invasive cervical lesions: systematic review and meta-analysis. *Lancet* 2006;367(9509):489–98.
20. Cruickshank ME, Flannelly G, Campbell DM, Kitchener HC. Fertility and pregnancy outcome following large loop excision of the cervical transformation zone. *Br J Obstet Gynaecol* 1995;102(6):467–70.
21. Castanon A, Brocklehurst P, Evans H *et al.*; PaCT Study Group. Risk of preterm birth after treatment for cervical intraepithelial neoplasia among women attending colposcopy in England: retrospective-prospective cohort study. *BMJ* 2012;345:e5174.
22. Khalid S, Dimitriou E, Conroy R *et al.* The thickness and volume of LLETZ specimens can predict the relative risk of pregnancy-related morbidity. *BJOG* 2012;119(6):685–91.
23. Van Wijngaarden WJ, Duncan ID. Rationale for stopping cervical screening in women over 50. *BMJ* 1993;306:967.
24. Bolger BS, Lewis BV. A prospective study of colposcopy in women with mild dyskaryosis or koilocytosis. *Br J Obstet Gynaecol* 1988;95(11):1117–19.
25. NHSCSP. *HPV Triage and Test of Cure Implementation.* NHSCSP Good practice guide no.3, 2011.
26. Moss S, Gray A, Legood R, Vessey M, Patnick J, Kitchener H. Liquid Based Cytology/Human Papillomavirus Cervical Pilot Studies Group. Effect of testing for human papillomavirus as a triage during screening for cervical cancer: observational before-and-after study. *BMJ* 200614;332(7533):83–5.
27. Arbyn M, Ronco G, Anttila A, Meijer CJ, Poljak M, Ogilvie G, Koliopoulos G, Naucler P, Sankaranarayanan R, Peto J. Evidence regarding human papillomavirus testing in secondary prevention of cervical cancer. *Vaccine.* 2012 Nov 20;30 Suppl 5:F88–99.

28. Arbyn M, Ronco G, Anttila A *et al.* Evidence regarding human papillomavirus testing in secondary prevention of cervical cancer. *Vaccine* 2012;30 Suppl 5:F88–99.

29. Kitchener HC, Walker PG, Nelson L *et al.* HPV testing as an adjunct to cytology in the follow-up of women treated for cervical intraepithelial neoplasia. *BJOG* 2008;115(8):1001–7.

30. Teshima S, Shimosato Y, Kishi K *et al.* Early stage adenocarcinoma of the uterine cervix. Histopathalogic analysis with consideration of histogenesis. *Cancer* 1985;56:167–72.

31. Marteau TM, Walker P, Giles J, Smail M. Anxieties in women undergoing colposcopy. *Br J Obstet Gynaecol* 1990;97:859–61.

32. NICE. Adjunctive colposcopy technologies for examination of the uterine cervix - DySIS and the Niris Imaging System (DG4). NICE, 2012.

33. Buxton EJ, Luesley DM, Shafi MI, Rollason T. Colposcopically directed punch biopsy: a potentially misleading investigation. *Br J Obstet Gynaecol* 1991;98:1273–6.

34. Martin-Hirsch PL, Paraskevaidis E, Kitchener H. Surgery for cervical intraepithelial neoplasia. *Cochrane Database Syst Rev* 2001;(4):CD001318.

35. Bavin PJ, Giles JA, Deery A *et al.* Use of semi-quantitative PCR for human papillomavirus DNA type 16 to identify women with high-grade cervical disease in a population presenting with a mildly dyskaryotic smear report. *BrxJ Cancer* 1993;67:602–5.

36. Cuzick J, Terry G, Ho L *et al.* Type-specific human papillomavirus DNA in abnormal smears as a predictor of high-grade cervical intraepithelial neoplasia. *Br J Cancer* 1994;69:167–71.

37. Arbyn M1, Roelens J, Cuschieri K *et al.* The APTIMA HPV assay versus the Hybrid Capture 2 test in triage of women with ASC-US or LSIL cervical cytology: a meta-analysis of the diagnostic accuracy. *Int J Cancer* 2013;132(1):101–8.

38. Ratnam S, Coutlee F, Fontaine D *et al.* Clinical performance of the PreTect HPV-Proofer E6/E7 mRNA assay in comparison with that of the hybrid capture 2 test for identification of women at risk of cervical cancer. *J Clin Microbiol* 2010;48(8):2779–85.

39. Woodman CB, Collins S, Winter H *et al.* Natural history of cervical human papillomavirus infection in young women: a longitudinal cohort study. *Lancet* 2001;357:1831–6.

40. Cuzick J, Arbyn M, Sankaranarayanan R *et al.* Overview of human papillomavirus-based and other novel options for cervical cancer screening in developed and developing countries. *Vaccine* 2008;26Suppl 10:K29–41.

41. Cuzick J, Mayrand MH, Ronco G, Snijders P, Wardle J. Chapter 10: New dimensions in cervical cancer screening. *Vaccine.* 2006 Aug 31;24 Suppl 3:S3/90–7.

42. Hendry M, Pasterfield D, Lewis R *et al.* Are women ready for the new cervical screening protocol in England? A systematic review and qualitative synthesis of views

43. Cuzick J, Mayrand MH, Ronco G, Snijders P, Wardle J. Chapter 10: New dimensions in cervical cancer screening. *Vaccine* 2006;24 Suppl 3:S3/90–7.

44. Wentzensen N, von Knebel Doeberitz M. Biomarkers in cervical cancer screening. *Dis Markers* 2007;23(4):315–30.

45. von Knebel-Doeberitz M, Syrjänen KJ. Molecular markers: how to apply in practice. *Gynecologic Oncology* 2006;103:18–20.

46. Petry KU, Schmidt D, Scherbring S *et al.* Triaging Pap cytology negative, HPV positive cervical cancer screening results with p16/Ki-67 Dual-stained cytology. *Gynecol Oncol* 2011;121(3):505–9.

47. Carozzi F, Confortini M, Dalla Palma P *et al.* Use of p16-INK4A overexpression to increase the specificity of human papillomavirus testing: a nested substudy of the NTCC randomised controlled trial. *Lancet Oncol.* 2008;9(10):937–45.

48. Etherington IJ, Luesley DM. Adenocarcinoma *in situ* of the cervix – controversies in diagnosis and treatment. *J Lower Genital Tract Dis* 2001;5:94–8.

49. Paavonen J, Jenkins D, Bosch FX *et al.* Efficacy of a prophylactic adjuvanted bivalent L1 virus-like-particle vaccine against infection with human papillomavirus types 16 and 18 in young women: an interim analysis of a phase III double-blind, randomised controlled trial. *Lancet* 2007;369:2161–70.

50. Joura EA, Leodolter S, Hernandez-Avila M *et al.* Efficacy of a quadrivalent prophylactic human papillomavirus (types 6, 11, 16, and 18) L1 virus-like-particle vaccine against high-grade vulval and vaginal lesions: a combined analysis of three randomised clinical trials. *Lancet* 2007;369:1693–702.

51. Harper DM, Franco EL, Wheeler CM *et al.* Sustained efficacy up to 4.5 years of a bivalent L1 virus-like particle vaccine against human papillomavirus types 16 and 18: follow-up from a randomised control trial. *Lancet* 2006;367:1247–55.

52. David M-P, Hardt K, Tibaldi F *et al.* Modelling of long-term persistence of anti-HPV-16 and anti-HPV-18 antibodies induced by an AS04-adjuvanted cervical cancer vaccine. Abstract presented at EUROGIN, Nice, France, November 2008.

53. Fraser C, Tomassini JE, Xi L *et al.* Modelling the long-term antibody response of a human papillomavirus (HPV) virus-like particle (VLP) type 16 prophylactic vaccine. *Vaccine* 2007;25(21):4324–33.

54. Jenkins D. A review of cross-protection against oncogenic HPV by an HPV-16/18 AS04-adjuvanted cervical cancer vaccine: importance of virological and clinical endpoints and implications for mass vaccination in cervical cancer prevention. *Gynecol Oncol* 2008;110 (Suppl. 1):S18–25.

55. Gurumurthy M, Cruickshank ME. Management of vaginal intraepithelial neoplasia. *J Low Genit Tract Dis* 2012;16(3):306–12.

56. Jones RW, Baranyai J, Stables S. Trends in squamous cell carcinoma of the vulva: the influence of vulvar intraepithelial neoplasia. *Obstet Gynecol* 1997;90:448–52.

57. Iversen T, Tretli S. Intraepithelial and invasive squamous cell neoplasia of the vulva: trends in incidence, recurrence and survival in Norway. *Obstet Gynecol* 1994;6:969–972.

58. Jones RW, Rowan DM. Vulvar intraepithelial neoplasia 3: a clinical study of the outcome in 113 cases with relation to the later development of invasive vulvar cancer. *Obstet Gynecol* 1994;5:741–5.

59. Campion MJ, Singer A. Vulvar intraepithelial neoplasia: clinical review. *Genitourinary Med* 1987;63:147–52.

60. DiSaia PJ, Rich WM. Surgical approach to multifocal carcinoma *in situ* of the vulva. *Am J Obstet Gynecol* 1981;140:136–45.

61. Townsend DE, Levine RU, Richart RM *et al.* Management of vulvar intraepithelial neoplasia by carbon dioxide laser. *Obstet Gynecol* 1982;60:49–52.

62. Tristram A, Fiander A. Clinical responses to Cidofovir applied topically to women with high-grade vulval intraepithelial neoplasia. *Gynecol Oncol* 2005;99(3):652–5.

63. Tristram A, Hurt CN, Madden T, Powell N, Man S, Hibbitts S, Dutton P, Jones S, Nordin AJ, Naik R, Fiander A, Griffiths G. Activity, safety, and feasibility of cidofovir and imiguimod for treatment of vulval intraepithelial neoplasia (RPVIN): a multicentre. open-label, randomised. phase 2 trial. *Lancet Oncol.* 2014;15:1361-8. doi: 10.1016/S1470-2045(14)70456-5.

SECTION ELEVEN

Gynaecological Oncology

Chapter 107 Endometrial cancer

Mahalakshmi Gurumurthy and Margaret Cruickshank

MRCOG standards

Theoretical skills

- Be able to describe pelvic anatomy.
- Understand the epidemiology and aetiology of malignant conditions of the uterus.
- Be able to manage pre-malignant conditions of the endometrium (including referral as appropriate).
- Be able to describe the diagnostic and imaging techniques in the diagnosis of endometrial cancer.
- Be able to describe the role of hysteroscopy and endometrial biopsy in the diagnosis of endometrial cancer.
- Be able to council and plan the initial management of endometrial cancer.
- Be able to describe the FIGO classification for endometrial cancer.
- Be aware of genetic abnormalities in relation to development of endometrial cancer.
- Be able to describe the indications, techniques, complications, and outcomes of oncological surgery, radiotherapy and chemotherapy.
- Understand the principles of symptom relief, palliative and terminal care.

Practical skills

- Be confident to perform outpatient endometrial biopsy.
- Be able to provide counselling to patients with endometrial cancer.

INTRODUCTION

Endometrial cancer usually arises in post-menopausal women. The incidence continues to increase in many developed countries and it is now the most common gynaecological cancer in the UK with more than 8000 cases in 2010.[1] Seventy-five per cent of women present with stage I disease and for most of them the management is surgical and the prognosis is very good.

INCIDENCE

Endometrial cancer is the fourth most common cancer in women in the UK. In 2010, there were 8288 new cases or 26 per 100,000 women per year (European age-standardised). This compares with 6531 new cases (17 per 100,000 women per year) in 2005 and 4850 new cases in 1997 (Office of National Statistics), demonstrating an upward trend in the incidence. This increase is most marked in the age group 60–79 years, while the rate in women aged less than 50 years has remained stable. Endometrial cancer is rare in women before the age of 40, at less than 2 per 100,000 women. The incidence increases between the ages of 40 and 55, thereafter reaching a plateau. The incidence of endometrial cancer is four-fold higher in developed countries and is significantly higher in Wales compared to the other constituent countries of the UK.[1]

Survival has been improving and the five-year age-standardised relative survival is 77 per cent (CRC Cancer Statistics for England and Wales, 2000–2001) compared with 61 per cent for women diagnosed in 1971–75. However the survival figures remained the same between the two time periods (2005–2009 and 2000–2001). For stage I disease, there is an overall five-year survival of 85 per cent, but this falls to 25 per cent for stage IV disease.

AETIOLOGY

Women with relatively high levels of circulating oestrogens or prolonged oestrogenic influence are a recognised high-risk group for type 1 endometrial cancer. Type 1 tumours are more common and have a more favourable prognosis compared to type 2 tumours. Type 2 tumours include serous and clear-cell carcinomas which develop in association with endometrial atrophy. They are usually seen in the older patient. Type 1 tumours develop in a background of thickened endometrium and are well, moderately or poorly differentiated endometrioid tumours. They are seen in the following situations:

- obesity, due to the peripheral conversion of androgens in adipose tissue;
- tamoxifen therapy;
- oestrogen therapy unopposed by progestogens;

- polycystic ovarian syndrome (PCOS);
- early menarche and late menopause.

In contrast, type 2 endometrial cancers, which are more aggressive, have differing aetiology and pathogenesis. They are more common in post-menopausal women with a background of atrophic endometrium.

Endometrial hyperplasia (simple and complex types with or without atypia) results from protracted oestrogen stimulation. Those cases without atypia are benign, but when cellular atypia is present this is considered to be pre-malignant. The malignant progression ranges from 1 per cent for a simple hyperplasia to 25–82 per cent for complex atypical hyperplasia.

OBESITY

The rising incidence is associated with the obesity epidemic at a time when the use of HRT has fallen. This suggests that obesity is responsible for the rising incidence and everyday clinical experience confirms the increasing proportion of morbidly obese women amongst women with endometrial cancer. A recent epidemiological study has indicated that the malignancy most strongly associated with obesity is endometrial cancer.[2]

OESTROGEN REPLACEMENT

The use of unopposed oestrogen replacement therapy (ERT) is clearly linked to endometrial cancer and more than doubles the risk (RR 2.3 for users compared with non-users, 95% CI 2.1–2.5) [A].[3] This meta-analysis of 30 studies found significant heterogeneity between the studies analysed, which was mostly due to differences in the dose and duration of oestrogen. Higher doses of oestrogen and duration of use of ten or more years have a relative risk of 9.5 (95% CI 7.4–12.3). The risk does reduce after stopping ERT and interrupted use does not lower the risk compared with daily use. This analysis clearly showed that there is a substantial risk from unopposed ERT and this should only be used for hysterectomised women.

The highest risk of HRT is for atypical endometrial hyperplasia, but there is also an effect on advanced cancer and mortality. The concurrent use of a progesterone reduces the relative risk to that of a non-ERT-user (RR 0.8, 95% CI 0.6–1.2), but the direction of this effect does vary between case–control and cohort studies. Unopposed ERT increases the rate of irregular bleeding and non-adherence to treatment [A].[4] The addition of progesterone, whether cyclical or sequential, prevents the development of endometrial hyperplasia and improves compliance. Irregular bleeding is more likely with a continuous than with a sequential preparation (OR 2.3, 95% CI 2.1–2.5), but with longer duration of therapy, continuous is more protective than sequential in preventing endometrial hyperplasia. The UK Million Women study,[5] a prospective cohort study of 716,738 post-menopausal women, confirmed an increased risk in the order of 50 per cent among current users of ERT and 80 per cent in those using tibolone preparations. There was a reduced risk for ever vs never users of continuous combined therapy (RR 0.71, 95% CI 0.56–0.90, p = 0.005), but no significant difference in risk with combined cyclical preparations (RR 1.05, 95% CI 0.91–1.22, p = 0.5). BMI significantly affected these risks with the adverse effects of tibolone and ERT greatest in non-obese women, and the benefits of combined HRT greatest in obese women. The counteraction of progesterone on oestrogens on the endometrium is greater the more days every month that they are added to oestrogen and the higher the women's BMI [C].

GENETIC PREDISPOSITION

Endometrial cancer in women under the age of 45 may be associated with Lynch type II familial cancer syndrome, which is known as hereditary non-polyposis colorectal cancer (HNPCC). There does not appear to be a site-specific inherited form of endometrial cancer, but it is associated with a genetic predisposition as a component of the HNPCC syndrome. Families affected with this syndrome have a predisposition to bowel cancer and also to ovarian tumours. The other tumours associated with this syndrome are of small bowel, pancreas, skin and brain. A retrospective cohort study in Australia found that around one quarter of women with Lynch-associated colon cancer over the age of 70 developed endometrial cancer.[6]

PATHOLOGY

The uterine corpus lies above the level of the internal cervical os and is composed of the fundus above the tubal ostiae and the body below. The blood supply is the uterine artery, a branch of the anterior division of the internal iliac artery. There is collateral blood supply via the tubal artery from the ovarian artery, a direct branch from the aorta. Correspondingly lymphatic drainage from the fundus of the uterus drains to the para-aortic nodes at the level of the renal veins. The lymphatic drainage from the body of the uterus passes with the uterine artery to the internal, external and common iliac nodes and obturator fossa nodes.

The FIGO Committee on Gynaecologic Oncology recommends that endometrial cancer is surgically staged.[7] This includes histological verification of the tumour type, grading and the extent of tumour. The degree of tumour differentiation has an important impact on the natural history of the disease and on treatment selection. Ninety-five per cent of uterine cancers are adenocarcinomas arising from the endometrium. They are graded with regard to the degree of cell differentiation (Table 107.1).

Table 107.1 Grading of tumour differentiation

G1	5% or less of a non-squamous or non-morular solid growth pattern
G2	6–50% of a non-squamous or non-morular solid growth pattern
G3	50% or more of a non-squamous or non-morular solid growth pattern

Notable nuclear atypia that is inappropriate for the architectural grade raises it to the next tumour grade. Nuclear grading takes precedence in serous and clear-cell adenocarcinomas. Histopathological reporting should include:

- depth of myometrial invasion;
- tumour grade;
- histological subtype;
- presence or absence of hyperplasia in adjacent non-neoplastic endometrium;
- lymphovascular space invasion;
- lymph node involvement;
- involvement of cervix or adnexae;
- the status of peritoneal washings taken at surgery.

There are clearly recognised risk factors for lymph node involvement, distant metastasis and poor survival. These are tumour grade, non-endometrial tumour, deep myometrial invasion and lympho-vascular invasion. Papillary serous adenocarcinomas and clear-cell carcinomas are high-risk subtypes and they are associated with about 50 per cent of all relapses. Their five-year survival rates are 27 and 42 per cent, respectively. Mucinous, squamous and undifferentiated tumours are rare.

Histopathology by WHO/International Society of Gynaecological Pathology classification

WHO classification of endometrial carcinomas (2003):

- Adenocarcinoma
- Endometrioid
- Variant with squamous differentiation
- Villoglandular variant
- Secretory variant
- Ciliated cell variant
- Mucinous
- Serous
- Clear cell
- Mixed cell carcinoma
- Squamous cell carcinomas
- Transitional carcinomas
- Small cell carcinoma
- Undifferentiated carcinoma
- Carcinosarcoma

PRESENTATION AND DIAGNOSIS

Endometrial cancer usually presents with vaginal bleeding in post-menopausal women. Post-menopausal bleeding (PMB) is defined as bleeding from the genital tract one or more years after a woman's last period. Women who continue to menstruate after the age of 55 also merit investigation. Up to 10 per cent of women with PMB will have an endometrial carcinoma. The likelihood of an underlying cancer increases with age at presentation.

INVESTIGATION OF POST-MENOPAUSAL BLEEDING

Most women with PMB can be investigated effectively and safely as outpatients.

Transvaginal ultrasound scanning is an accurate method of excluding endometrial cancer [B]. Women can be assessed quickly and triaged for endometrial biopsy on the basis of their scan findings. TVS limits the need for endometrial biopsy to women with an endometrial thickness of ≤5 mm, an irregular endometrial outline or fluid within the uterine cavity. The majority of women have a thin, regular endometrium and can be reassured at a first visit without further investigation. A meta-analysis[8] summarised accuracy data using likelihood ratios for various cut-off levels of abnormal endometrial thickness (measuring the thickness of both layers). The most common cut-offs were 4 mm (nine studies) and 5 mm (21 studies). Using the pooled estimates from four studies which used the best-quality criteria, a thickness of >5 mm raised the probability of carcinoma from 14.0 per cent (95% CI 13.3–14.7) to 31.3 per cent (95% CI 26.1–36.3) and a thickness <5 mm reduced the risk to 2.5 per cent (95% CI 0.9–6.4) [A]. This reduces the need for further intervention, service costs and patient anxiety, and provides rapid reassurance for those women with a normal result.

There are a number of devices for taking outpatient endometrial biopsies which have been compared in prospective studies. Samples taken by Pipelle are comparable with the Vabra and Novak aspirators in terms of specimen adequacy and diagnostic accuracy. In addition, this method produces less patient discomfort. Dilatation and curettage (D&C) is no longer recommended for the investigation of PMB.[9] However, hysteroscopy with biopsy is preferable as the first line of investigation in women taking tamoxifen who experience post-menopausal bleeding.[9] Hysteroscopy is often used to investigate PMB, as it allows direct inspection of the endometrium. It can detect 95 per cent of intrauterine abnormalities and is a sensitive means of identifying polyps and sub-mucous fibroids [B]. It can be used in the outpatient setting, and outpatient hysteroscopy is highly acceptable to women [B], although general anaesthesia may sometimes be necessary.

Dedicated PMB clinic

A dedicated clinic allows rapid assessment and reassurance for women with PMB using a one-stop clinic approach. Most clinics provide TV scanning by appropriately trained staff. Women with a history that meets the criteria of PMB can be fast-tracked to this service, with written information provided in primary care prior to their visit. The diagnosis of cancer can be excluded for most women at their first visit. Endometrial biopsy and outpatient hysteroscopy should be provided for those women with an abnormal scan result at their first assessment. The majority of consultant gynaecologists in a Scottish audit supported such outpatient investigation [C].

EBM: Diagnosis of endometrial cancer

- A meta-analysis of 35 studies found TVS scanning to be an accurate means of excluding endometrial cancer.
- Initial assessment of PMB should be provided as an outpatient service and TVS used to assess the endometrium.
- Seven prospective studies have evaluated TVS in women with PMB, comparing it against D&C or outpatient endometrial biopsy.
- The cost effectiveness and clinical effectiveness of outpatient investigation of PMB have not been evaluated.

WOMEN ON TAMOXIFEN

Tamoxifen is a non-steroidal oestrogen antagonist, which is used widely as adjuvant treatment for post-menopausal women who have breast carcinoma. The absolute improvement in recurrence is greatest during the first five years of treatment [A].[9] Tamoxifen has been shown to decrease the overall progression of the disease and to prevent disease in the contralateral breast. Long-term tamoxifen use is controversial due to its oestrogenic effects on the endometrium. Although it acts as an anti-oestrogen on breast cancer cells, it has a mild oestrogenic effect on the endometrium, bone and cardiovascular system.

Long-term use is associated with proliferative endometrium, and a spectrum of benign and malignant changes of the endometrium has been reported, including hyperplasia, polyps and carcinoma. The incidence of endometrial carcinoma in post-menopausal women taking tamoxifen is significantly higher than in women not on tamoxifen [A].[10]

However, the absolute decrease in contralateral breast cancer is twice as large as the absolute increase in endometrial cancer, and overall the benefits of tamoxifen are greater than the risks.

Post-menopausal women who have a uterus and are taking tamoxifen should be advised of these effects.

Abnormal bleeding needs to be investigated fully and promptly. A Pipelle biopsy is appropriate as the first line of investigation, but a negative result is not conclusive. Women with a negative result still require hysteroscopy. TVS can be useful in triaging the urgency of further investigation. The fact that the ultrasonic appearances can be misleading needs to be considered. Tamoxifen has a sono-translucent effect on both the endometrial stroma and the myometrium. This can give rise to false-positive reports in cases of cystic atrophy, which appears as thickened cystic endometrium on scan. Histology confirms this to be multiple cystic spaces lined by atrophic epithelium within a dense fibrous stroma. Hysteroscopy may be the investigation of choice in this situation as it allows direct inspection of the endometrium, and full-thickness biopsies can be taken at the same procedure.[7]

There is no evidence that asymptomatic women on tamoxifen should be screened for endometrial changes [C]. Asymptomatic women taking tamoxifen have a greater endometrial thickness on TVS scan. Comparatively, those who present with bleeding have a significantly thicker endometrium and are more likely to have endometrial pathology [B][11] and women with endometrial pathology are also more likely to present with symptoms. Outpatient hysteroscopy, although a good screening tool, is not as useful when biopsies are necessary. A randomised, cross-over study comparing TVS with outpatient hysteroscopy found the former together with sonohysterogram more sensitive, specific and acceptable to women.[12] There is no clinical or cost-effectiveness evidence to support the endometrial screening of asymptomatic women on tamoxifen [B], and the benefit in terms of breast cancer mortality far outweighs the risk to the endometrium. The evidence, however, is less clear for healthy women taking tamoxifen to reduce their risk of breast cancer. The International Breast Cancer Intervention Study 1 (IBIS 1)[13] reported on the risk:benefit ratio of tamoxifen as preventative treatment in women at increased risk of breast cancer. This trial randomised 7145 women aged 35–70 years to five years of tamoxifen or placebo. There was a non-significant increase in endometrial cancers in the tamoxifen group. Although there was a 32 per cent risk reduction in breast cancer, the risk:benefit ratio was not clear due to increased deaths from other causes, including thromboembolic disease. An earlier American trial, the Breast Cancer Prevention Trial (BCPT-P-1), was stopped early when a 45 per cent decrease in new breast cancers was reported in the tamoxifen arm. There was also an increase in endometrial cancers. Newer selective oestrogen receptor modulators (SERMs) have a similar profile to tamoxifen without the uterotrophic effects. The IBIS 2 trial is looking into the effects of anastrazole (aromatase inhibitor) on breast cancer prevention in post-menopausal women. It will be interesting to await the results of the effects of anastrazole on breast and endometrium.

EBM: Tamoxifen and the endometrium

- A systematic review of 55 RCTs of adjuvant tamoxifen vs no tamoxifen before recurrence and with at least five years of follow-up data shows that tamoxifen substantially improves the ten-year survival of women with oestrogen-receptor-positive breast cancer. It also found that the incidence of endometrial cancer increases by a factor of 2 at one to two years and by a factor of 4 after five years of tamoxifen treatment.
- There is no evidence to support the screening of asymptomatic women on tamoxifen for endometrial abnormalities.

STAGING

The staging of endometrial cancer is surgico-pathological. Tumour grade and the depth of myometrial involvement are the main determinants of extrauterine spread. These two pathological criteria along with extensive lympho-vascular space invasion are often used to determine the risk of recurrence and to select women for postoperative radiotherapy. Metastatic spread occurs characteristically to the pelvic nodes initially and in 4 per cent of cases could have isolated para-aortic lymph node involvement. Distant metastasis is uncommon at presentation. The most common sites of distant spread are the vagina and lungs, but the inguinal and supraclavicular lymph nodes, liver and brain may also be involved. (See Table 107.2.)

Radiological imaging

Pre-operative evaluation and planning for treatment require clinical staging. The risk of pelvic and para-aortic lymph node involvement depends on the stage, grade and myometrial invasion. Twelve per cent of women with stage I disease will have lymph node metastasis. With grade 3 disease, this rises to 18 per cent, and when there is deep myometrial involvement, to 22 per cent. Without proper assessment and a treatment plan based on the risk of nodal disease, the prognosis is poorer [C].[14]

Endometrial biopsy will already have confirmed the diagnosis and given information on the tumour grade. Myometrial invasion can be assessed by TVS or MRI. TVS can assess the depth of myometrial invasion and can be used to triage women for appropriate management at a cancer centre or cancer unit. Although TVS is quicker and relatively cheap, it is less accurate than MRI. MRI appears to be the optimum method of evaluating the soft-tissue structures of the pelvis, including myometrial invasion and the status of the pelvic lymph nodes with acceptable accuracy and specificity, although micrometastasis will not be detected, reducing the overall sensitivity. CT scanning is less useful in imaging these

Table 107.2 FIGO tumour classification 2009

Stage I[a]	Tumour confined to the corpus uteri
IA[a]	No or less than half myometrial invasion
IB[a]	Invasion equal to or more than half of the myometrium
Stage II[a]	Tumour invades cervical stroma, but does not extend beyond the uterus[b]
Stage III[a]	Local and/or regional spread of the tumour
IIIA[a]	Tumour invades serosa of the uterus and/or adnexae[c]
IIIB[a]	Vaginal and/or parametrial involvement[c]
IIIC[a]	Metastasis to pelvic and/or para-aortic lymph nodes
IIIC1	Positive pelvic nodes
IIIC2	Positive para-aortic lymph nodes with or without positive pelvic nodes
Stage IV[a]	Tumour invades bladder and/or bowel mucosa and/or distant metastasis
IVA[a]	Invasion of bladder and/or bowel mucosa
IVB[a]	Distant metastasis, including intra-abdominal and/or inguinal lymph nodes

[a] G1, G2 or G3.

[b] Endocervical glandular involvement only should be considered as stage I and no longer as stage II.

[c] Positive cytology has to be reported separately without changing the stage.

soft tissues. The results are similar in predicting nodal disease, but less accurate at assessing the depth of myometrial invasion [B] and cervical involvement, but may be useful for women with high-risk histology to detect extra-pelvic disease. A chest X-ray should also be performed for staging, as the lungs are a common metastatic site.

Endometrial cancer imaging

MRI is the imaging method of choice for pre-treatment staging to assess myometrial invasion, cervical involvement and lymph node status.

MANAGEMENT

Women with disease localised to the corpus are usually curable by surgery. There are variations in the definition of intermediate and high risk, but the high-risk group generally includes deep myometrial invasion and grade 3 tumours including the type 2 tumours. High-risk features are associated with a poorer prognosis because of the increased risk of nodal disease and recurrence.

Women with endometrial cancer are often elderly with other medical problems, and pre-operative assessment for fitness for an anaesthetic and surgery is essential. Survival rates are reduced by 20 per cent when primary surgery is not feasible.

Early-stage disease

Most women present with early-stage disease and primary surgery is fundamental to achieving a cure. As laparoscopic surgery has become a common surgical practice, the treatment of choice should be total laparoscopic hysterectomy and bilateral salpingo-oopherectomy (TLH/BSO) if possible. It is not necessary to remove a vaginal cuff or parametrial tissue for early-stage disease [C]. Recurrence at the vaginal vault is related to recognised risk factors and particularly cervical stromal involvement – factors that reflect lymphatic vessel involvement. Endocervical glandular involvement only is now considered as stage I disease. Additional staging for type 2 tumours and high-grade type 1 tumours should be done which includes omental biopsy and peritoneal washings. Para-aortic lymph node dissection for stage I high-grade tumours is still contentious and not practised routinely.

Stage II disease could be treated the same as stage I disease by TLH/BSO or total abdominal hysterectomy (TAH)/BSO. Sometimes when there is obvious cervical stromal involvement on imaging, the treatment options are modified radical hysterectomy (Piver II) or radical hysterectomy with pelvic lymphadenectomy (Piver III) or TAH/BSO with lymphadenectomy followed by post-operative radiotherapy. However, lymphadenectomy and radiotherapy do carry the additional morbidity of lymphoedema which can develop years after treatment.

The choice of treatment depends on the tumour site, size and the fitness of the patient when considering the feasibility of extirpative surgery. The LAP-2 trial comparing laparoscopy versus laparotomy for surgical management of women with stage I–IIA uterine cancer (FIGO 2003 staging) found laparoscopic surgical management to be superior for short-term safety and length of stay. Laparoscopy was associated with similar overall and disease-free survival compared to laparotomy.[15] This has been highlighted in the Cochrane review supporting laparoscopy in the initial surgical management of women with endometrial cancer.[16]

Role of lymphadenectomy

The role of pelvic lymphadenectomy has been advocated to improve surgical staging, but there is no clear evidence that it improves survival or that it rationalises the use of radiotherapy by excluding extrauterine disease. A recently reported RCT (MRC ASTEC trial) on the management of endometrial cancer[17] has shown that lymphadenectomy did not improve recurrence-free, disease-free or overall survival. The hazard ratio (adjusted for baseline characteristics and pathology) was 1.04 (0.74–1.45; p = 0.83) and for recurrence-free survival was 1.25 (0.93–1.66; p = 0.14). The rate of reported post-surgical morbidity in ASTEC was low, but there were more cases of ileus, deep venous thrombosis (DVT), lymphocyst and major wound dehiscence reported in the women who had been randomised to lymphadenectomy.

Another large RCT of lymphadenectomy in endometrial cancer was reported just prior to ASTEC. In this Italian trial,[18] there was again no evidence of a survival benefit despite improved surgical staging in the lymphadenectomy arm (13.3 vs 3.2 per cent). These trials indicate that routine lymphadenectomy is not beneficial in early-stage endometrial cancer.

Who should perform surgery?

Endometrial cancer categorised as low risk following full pre-operative assessment can be safely treated by TLH/BSO or TAH/BSO by a general gynaecologist with a cancer lead status. Women with high-risk disease with a risk of cervical or pelvic node involvement or type 2 tumours should be referred to a specialist gynaecological oncologist.

Role of radiotherapy

There have been no RCTs comparing surgery and primary radiotherapy. Women with intermediate- or high-risk early-stage disease considered to be at increased risk of recurrence are often given post-operative adjuvant radiotherapy.

Moderate and high risk patients include:

- 1b, G3;
- type 2 (serous papillary, clear cell) with any myometrial invasion;
- grade 3, ≥60 years with any myometrial invasion;
- >50% myometrial invasion, grade 1/2, ≥60 years;
- stage II (any grade).

The main role for radiotherapy is as adjuvant treatment following surgery to reduce the risk of pelvic relapse. Radiotherapy cure can be achieved in women with early-stage disease who are entirely unfit for surgery, but this is suboptimal treatment with risks of intrauterine failure.

Vault brachytherapy is used to prevent vault recurrence, and external-beam therapy to the pelvis is used to treat the parametrium and pelvic sidewalls. It should be remembered that there is no evidence to show that radiotherapy improves survival in an unselected patient population. A meta-analysis of over 2000 patients in RCTs on the management of endometrial cancer (MRC ASTEC/EN.5, PORTEC 1 and GOG 99)[19] has shown no benefit from external-beam radiotherapy for early-stage endometrial cancer at intermediate and high risk in terms of disease-specific, recurrence-free or overall survival. Although there is a small reduction in isolated local pelvic recurrence, this does not confer any advantage to overall or recurrence-free survival. A meta-analysis of five randomised trials from Johnson and Cornes (2007) found a statistically significant survival advantage for patients receiving external-beam radiotherapy following hysterectomy for high-risk tumours (Ic grade 3; FIGO 2003 staging[20]). The isolated local recurrence rate without external-beam radiotherapy is small and can be reduced with local brachytherapy which is associated with less toxicity.

The recently reported post-operative radiation therapy in endometrial carcinoma (PORTEC)-2 trial has shown that brachytherapy is as effective as external-beam radiation in high–intermediate-risk patients with fewer radiation effects and should be the treatment of choice for these women.[21]

Currently, women are selected with care for post-operative radiotherapy because of the impact of the treatment regime and the associated complications related to quality of life. The incidence of bowel complications is 3 per cent and can be higher after pelvic lymphadenectomy. The PORTEC trial[22] reported treatment-related complications in 25 per cent of radiotherapy patients, although a fifth of these were grade 1. Most of the complications were associated with the gastro-intestinal tract. The symptoms resolved after some years in 50 per cent of women. Grade 1–2 genito-urinary symptoms occur in 8 per cent of women treated by surgery and radiotherapy, compared with 4 per cent of women treated by surgery alone. Two per cent of women discontinued radiotherapy due to acute related symptoms. In addition, patients with acute morbidity have an increased risk of late radiotherapy complications, including rectal bleeding, fistulae or radiation damage to the small or large bowel.

The prognosis for most women with endometrial cancer is good, and therefore any impact of radiotherapy on survival will come from salvaging the small number of patients who develop a pelvic recurrence.

Progesterone therapy

Progesterone therapy for women who have had surgery for early-stage endometrial cancer is not recommended, as overall survival is not improved [A].[23] Although deaths from endometrial cancer (OR 0.88, 95% CI 0.71–1.01) and the rate of disease relapse are reduced (OR 0.81, 95% CI 0.65–1.01), non-endometrial cancer-related deaths are more common (OR 1.33, 95% CI 1.02–1.73) [C]. However, progesterone therapy (either as a Mirena coil or high-dose medroxyprogesterone acetate) as a primary treatment of complex atypical hyperplasia and grade 1 stage IA endometrial cancer for women who wish to retain fertility or in inoperable cases has been used.

Hormone replacement therapy

Traditionally, ERT has not been advocated in the first two years following surgery for endometrial cancer because of the concern of activating any residual disease. However it is advisable to avoid ERT in women with endometrial stromal sarcoma, which are highly oestrogen-dependent tumours. There is, however, no evidence to support this, and the benefits of ERT may outweigh any theoretical risks [C]. In women aged 45 years or less, treated for early-stage disease, ovarian preservation has no effect on cancer-specific survival (HR 0.58, 95% CI 0.14–2.44) or overall survival (HR 0.65, 95% CI 0.34–1.35).[24]

Advanced-stage disease

At presentation, only 13 per cent of women have stage III and 3 per cent stage IV disease. In general, women with stage III disease have been treated with surgery and radiation or radiotherapy alone. Treatment with chemotherapy is increasing and is discussed below. Laparotomy will allow staging and tumour-reductive surgery including hysterectomy if possible. However, side-wall extension will prevent tumour resection. Radiotherapy is used when surgery is inappropriate or incomplete. This may be a combination of intracavitary and external-beam radiation, and cure rates of 30 and 20 per cent for stage III and IV disease, respectively, have been reported. If the woman is not fit for either surgery or irradiation, progesterone therapy is appropriate [C]. If radiotherapy achieves significant tumour shrinkage, 'adjuvant' surgery should be considered.

With stage IV disease, the tumour site and the resultant symptoms will dictate management. Chemotherapy is usually offered first. Bulky pelvic disease or heavy vaginal bleeding may be controlled by radiation, either intracavitary or external beam, or in combination. Local radiation can palliate symptomatic metastasis (e.g. to the lung, brain or bone).

Role of chemotherapy

There is no evidence that chemotherapy has an adjuvant role in primary treatment of low-risk disease. There is emerging evidence from phase 2 and 3 trials to support the selection of intermediate or high-risk women or those with advanced disease for adjuvant chemotherapy. The diagnosis of advanced endometrial cancer confers a relatively poor prognosis. Traditionally, treatment for women with stage III endometrial cancer has relied on radiotherapy, while women with stage IV disease have been treated with palliative chemotherapy. There has been a gradual shift towards incorporating chemotherapy into the treatment of women with stage III and IV endometrial cancer. There has been a series of Gynecologic Oncology Group (GOG) phase 1–3 studies to investigate the effectiveness of different combinations of chemotherapeutic agents for systemic control of disease with or without radiotherapy for enhanced loco-regional control. Acute and chronic toxicities are higher in women treated with chemotherapy rather than radiotherapy alone, but with improved response rates. The most effective agents for endometrial cancer appear to be carboplatin and paclitaxel. Two prospective randomised trials have demonstrated a superior response rate to doxorubicin and cisplatin as compared with doxorubicin alone; however, survival rates for the two regimens were similar. More recently, paclitaxel has been included in triplet regimens. When combined with a platinum agent, response rates of greater than 40 per cent have been reported. A doublet regime of doxorubicin and paclitaxel has been investigated by the GOG (GOG 163) as an alternative to doxorubicin and cisplatin for women with advanced or recurrent disease. Both regimes had similar response and survival, but there was no difference in progression-free or overall survival. The most recent GOG trial compared doxorubicin and cisplatin to doxorubicin, cisplatin and paclitaxel. The triplet regimen had a statistically significant improved response rate, progression-free and overall survival, but at the cost of higher toxicity. The GOG is currently conducting a trial (GOG 209) comparing paclitaxel and carboplatin to doxorubicin, cisplatin and paclitaxel in women with advanced or recurrent disease because, if equivalent, paclitaxel and carboplatin are less toxic.

PORTEC-3,[25] a randomised phase 3 trial comparing concurrent chemoradiation plus adjuvant chemotherapy with pelvic radiation alone, in high-risk and advanced-stage endometrial cancer, opened in 2008 and aims to recruit 500 women over five years. For clear-cell endometrial cancer, a review by the Society of Gynecologic Oncology[26] recommends comprehensive surgical staging and platinum-based adjuvant chemotherapy with taxol and/or doxorubicin. Radiotherapy has not been shown to be clearly beneficial for clear-cell endometrial cancer.

EBM: Treatment of endometrial cancer

- Two surgical RCTs relating to early-stage endometrial carcinoma with intermediate- or high-risk features show that pelvic lymphadenectomy does not increase survival and is not recommended as a routine in addition to TLH/BSO.
- Two meta-analyses show that laparoscopic surgery is as clinically effective as abdominal hysterectomy and is associated with lower post-operative morbidity, although operating time is longer.
- A meta-analysis has shown adjuvant radiotherapy reduces the rate of pelvic recurrence, but without any improvement in overall survival and a 50 per cent increase in moderate and severe complications and late radiotherapy sequelae.
- A meta-analysis of six RCTs and a large RCT have both shown no reduction in death rates for endometrial cancer with progesterone therapy.
- The use of combined chemotherapy appears beneficial in women with high-risk histological tumours, but with increased toxicity.

PROGNOSIS

Survival is related to stage at presentation and grade of tumour (Table 107.3). There is a wide variation in rates of recurrence with early-stage disease, from 10 per cent in low-risk women (stage Ia G1 disease) to almost 50 per cent in high-risk women (stage Ic G3 disease). The latest revision of FIGO staging reflects more clearly clinically relevant factors. When the only evidence of extrauterine spread is positive peritoneal washings, the influence on outcome is unclear, and there is no evidence that adjuvant therapy is of value unless extrauterine disease is present [C].[27,28]

Table 107.3 Five-year survival rates for endometrial adenocarcinoma by stage

Stage	Five-year survival (%)
Stage I	80
Stage II	65
Stage III	30
Stage IV	10

PALLIATIVE CARE

Palliation for women with endometrial cancer should be approached with a multidisciplinary team and in a holistic way. This should be discussed with women who have advanced-stage disease with a poor ECOG performance status or widespread recurrence. (Eastern Cooperative Oncology Group is used to assess functional status of a patient. It is graded from 0-5 with 0 being the ideal performance status and 5 corresponds to death). Palliative care could be offered in the secondary care, respite or community setting. The multidisciplinary team comprises the gynaecological oncologist, cancer nurse specialist, medical and clinical oncologists, palliative care team, GP and the community team. Vaginal bleeding can be controlled initially with high-dose progestogens but if heavy or uncontrolled, radiotherapy may be used with palliative intent. Various other symptoms include nausea, constipation, poor appetite and pain. A decision for a palliative approach should be discussed with the woman and her family by the oncological team. Access to the cancer nurse specialist and the community team should be offered to the woman.

Recurrent disease

Women with recurrence limited to the pelvis who have not previously received radiotherapy may be salvaged by radiotherapy, with a five-year survival of about 25–50 per cent. For women with localised vaginal vault recurrence following external beam radiotherapy and who have an acceptable ECOG performance status; the decision for pelvic exenteration should be considered after in depth discussion by the Multidisciplinary team. Para-aortic lymph nodes may be palliated by radiotherapy and, as with localised pelvic recurrence, this can be curative when there has been no previous irradiation. The prognosis for distant metastatic endometrial cancer is poor and management concentrates on symptom control.

KEY POINTS

- Investigation of PMB should be provided as a rapid-access outpatient service.
- Understand the two types of endometrial cancer (type 1 and type 2) and their differing management.
- The benefits of tamoxifen in breast cancer treatment outweigh the increased risk of endometrial cancer. Any abnormal vaginal bleeding while on tamoxifen requires full investigation.
- Surgery with total laparosocpic hysterectomy and bilateral salpingo-oopherectomy offers good prognosis in early-stage disease, but routine systematic pelvic lymphadenectomy is not recommended as it does not improve survival.
- Endometrial carcinoma is radiosensitive, but the benefits of loco-regional control from external-beam radiotherapy do not improve survival and it is not recommended for early-stage intermediate-risk endometrial cancer (<Ib, G3).
- Adjuvant radiotherapy should be restricted to early-stage high-risk disease and advanced disease.
- Combined chemotherapy has an increased role in the treatment of high-risk endometrial cancer.
- Progesterones will produce a clinical response in about 20 per cent of women with recurrent disease [C] and appear to be more effective in women with a long disease-free interval prior to recurrence. Standard agents are megoestrol and medroxyprogesterone. Chemotherapy may have a limited palliative role for women with advanced or recurrent disease not amenable to radiation.

SUMMARY

Endometrial cancer usually presents with PMB at an early stage. Staging is surgical/pathological, and pre-operative imaging should include a chest X-ray and imaging for depth of myometrial penetration. Early-stage disease should be managed by TLH and BSO, with peritoneal washings which are reported separately, but without changing the stage. Pelvic lymphadenectomy is not recommended. While post-operative radiotherapy reduces the rate of local recurrence, it does not improve overall survival and it is associated with increased toxicity. Brachytherapy is the adjuvant treatment of choice for high–intermediate-risk disease with external-beam radiation being restricted to high-risk early disease.

Published Guidelines

SIGN. *Investigation of post-menopausal bleeding.* SIGN Guideline Publication 61. ISBN 1899893 13 X. September 2002.

Royal College of Pathologists. *Minimum dataset for the histopathological reporting of atypical hyperplasia and adenocarcinoma in endometrial biopsy and curettage hysterectomy specimens.* Royal College of Pathologists, 2001. Available from: www.rcpath.org/resources/pdf/datasetreendometrialcancer.pdf.

RCOG. Recommendations arising from the 37th Study Group: *Hormones and Cancer.* RCOG Study Group Recommendations. London: RCOG Press, 1999. Available from: ‹www.rcog.org.uk/study/hormones›.

Key References

1. CRUK website. *UK Uterus (Womb) Cancer incidence statistics.* Last accessed December 2013. Available from: http://info.cancerresearchuk.org/cancerstats/ incidence/common cancers/ and http://infor.cancerresearchuk.org/cancer stats/types/uterus/incidence/.

2. Renehan A, Tyson M, Egger M *et al.* Body mass index and incidence of cancer: a systematic review and meta-analysis of prospective observational studies. *Lancet* 2008;371:569–78.

3. Grady D, Gebretsadik T, Kerlikowske K *et al.* Hormone replacement therapy and endometrial cancer risk: A meta-analysis. *Obstet Gynecol* 1995;85:304–13.

4. Lethaby A, Farquhaar C, Sarkis A *et al.* Hormone replacement therapy in post-menopausal women: Endometrial hyperplasia and irregular bleeding. *Cochrane Database Syst Rev* 2000;2:CD000402.

5. Beral V, Bull D, Reeves G. Endometrial cancer and hormone replacement therapy in the Million Women Study. *Lancet* 2005;365:1543–51.

6. Obermair A, Youlden D, Young J *et al.* Risk of endometrial cancer for women diagnosed with HNPCC-related colorectal carcinoma. *Int J Can* 2010;127: 2678–84.

7. FIGO Committee on Gynecologic Oncology. Revised FIGO staging for carcinoma of the vulva, cervix and endometrium. *Int J Gynaecol Obstet* 2009;105:103–4.

8. Chien PFW, Voit D, Clark TJ *et al.* Ultrasonographic endometrial thickness for diagnosing endometrial pathology in women with post-menopausal bleeding: A meta-analysis. *Acta Obstet Gynecol Scand* 2002;81:799–816.

9. SIGN. *Investigation of post-menopausal bleeding.* SIGN Guideline Publication 61. ISBN 1899893 13 X. September 2002.

10. Early Breast Cancer Trialists' Collaborative Group. Tamoxifen for early breast cancer. *Lancet* 1998;351:1451–67.

11. Marconi D, Exacoustos C, Cangi B *et al.* Transvaginal sonographic and hysteroscopic findings in post-menopausal women receiving tamoxifen. *J Am Assoc Gynecol Laparosc* 1997;4:331–9.

12. Timmerman D, Deprest J, Bourne T *et al.* A randomised trial on the use of ultrasonography or office hysteroscopy for endometrial assessment in post-menopausal patients with breast cancer who were treated with tamoxifen. *Am J Obstet Gynecol* 1998;179:62–70.

13. IBIS investigators. First results from the International Breast Cancer Intervention Study (IBIS-1): A randomised prevention trial. *Lancet* 2002;360:817–24.

14. Creasman WT, Morrow CP, Bundy BN *et al.* Surgical pathologic spread patterns of endometrial cancer: a Gynecologic Oncology Group study. *Cancer* 1987;60:2035–41.

15. Walker JL, Piedmonte MR, Spirtos NM *et al.* Recurrence and survival after random assignment to laparoscopy versus laparotomy for comprehensive surgical staging of uterine cancer: Gynecologic Oncology Group LAP2 Study. *Journal of Clinical Oncology* 2012;30:695-700.

16. Galaal K, Bryant A, Fisher AD *et al.* Laparoscopy versus laparotomy for the management of early-stage endometrial cancer. *Cochrane Database of Systematic Reviews* 2012;9:CD006655.

17. ASTEC Study Group. Efficacy of systematic pelvic lymphadenectomy in endometrial cancer (MRC ASTEC trial): A randomised study. *Lancet* 2009;373:125–36.

18. Panici PB, Basile S, Maneschi F *et al.* Systematic pelvic lymphadenectomy vs no lymphadenectomy in early-stage endometrial carcinoma: randomised clinical trial. *J Natl Cancer Inst* 2008;100:1707–16.

19. ASTEC/EN.5 Study Group. Adjuvant external-beam radiotherapy in the treatment of endometrial cancer (MRC ASTEC abd NCIC CTG EN.5 randomised trials): Pooled trial results, systematic review and meta-analysis. *Lancet* 2009;373:97–9.

20. Johnson N, Cornes P. (2007) Survival and recurrent disease after postoperative radiotherapy for early endometrial cancer: systematic review and meta-analysis. *Br J Obstet Gynaecol,* 114:1313-20.

21. Nout RA, Smit VTHBM, Putter H for the PORTEC Study Group. Vaginal brachytherapy versus pelvic external-beam radiotherapy for patients with endometrial cancer of high–intermediate risk (PORTEC-2): an open-label, non-inferiority, randomised trial. *Lancet* 2010;375:816–23.

22. Creutzberg CL, van Putten WLJ, Koper PC *et al.* Surgery and postoperative radiotherapy versus surgery alone for patients with stage I endometrial carcinoma: Multicentre randomized trial. *Lancet* 2000;355:1404–11.

23. Martin-Hirsch PL, Lilford RJ, Jarvis GJ. Adjuvant progesterone therapy for the treatment of endometrial cancer: Review and meta-analysis of published randomised controlled trials. *Eur J Obstet Gynecol Reprod Biol* 1996;65:2201–7.

24. Wright JD, Buck AM, Shah M *et al.* Safety of ovarian preservation in premenopausal women with endometrial cancer. *J Clin Oncol* 2009;27:1214–19.

25. PORTEC-3. Available from: www.clinicalresearch.nl/portec3/.

26. Olawaiye AB, Boruta DM. Management of women with clear-cell endometrial cancer: a Society of Gynecologic Oncology (SGO) review. *Gynecol Oncol* 2009;113:277–83.

27. Kadar N, Homesley HD, Malfetano JH. Positive peritoneal cytology is an adverse factor in endometrial carcinoma only if there is other evidence of extrauterine disease. *Gynecol Oncol* 1992;46:145–9.

28. Benedetti Panici P, Basile S, Maneschi F *et al.* Systematic pelvic lymphadenectomy vs no lymphadenectomy in early-stage endometrial carcinoma: Randomised clinical trial. *J Natl Cancer Inst* 2008;100:1707–16.

Chapter 108 Cervical cancer

Pierre L Martin-Hirsch

MRCOG standards

The established standards relevant for this topic are:

Theoretical skills
- Revise the anatomy of the cervix, blood supply and lymphatics.
- Understand the epidemiology and pathology of disease.
- Know the optimum pre-treatment assessment.
- Know how to manage surgically and non-surgically.

Practical skills
- Be able to recognise suspicious cervical lesions.
- Be able to take appropriate diagnostic biopsies.
- Be able to counsel patients with regard to diagnosis, management options and prognosis.

EPIDEMIOLOGY

Cervical cancer is the most common form of cancer in women in developing countries and the third most common form of cancer in women in the world as a whole. Three quarters of affected women live in developing countries and it is estimated that up to 450,000 new cases of invasive cancer of the cervix occur per year in these countries, leading to 275,000 deaths. Cervical cancer accounts for 6 per cent of all malignancies in women.

There were an estimated 11,818 new cases of invasive cancer of the cervix and 3939 deaths in the United States in 2010. In the United Kingdom in 2010, there were 2851 registrations and 972 deaths. Although cervical screening has been carried out in the UK since the 1960s, the benefits of screening are only now becoming apparent, following the reorganisation of the service in 1988. The incidence of cervical cancer has fallen in the UK by 44 per cent since 1975, and mortality from 7.1 per 100,000 in 1988 to 2.4 per 100,000 in 2011.

This decrease is almost certainly due to the widespread coverage of screening, which rose from less than 35 per cent in 1988 to 85 per cent in 1998 through the introduction of an effective call–recall system for cervical screening. The reduction in deaths is due to a reduction in both incidence and the proportion of advanced disease with around a third of cancers being diagnosed as stage I. The incidence rate for cervical cancer peaks at 17 per 100,000 women at the age range of 30–40 years, declines in incidence for older age groups but peaks again in the early 80s age band.

Epidemiological studies convincingly demonstrate that the major risk factor, indeed a necessary event, for the development of pre-invasive and invasive carcinoma of the cervix is human papillomavirus infection, which far outweighs other known risk factors such as high parity, increasing number of sexual partners, young age at first intercourse, low socioeconomic status and positive smoking history. In an international study consisting of 1000 specimens collected from patients with invasive cervical cancer in 32 hospitals in 22 countries, HPV DNA was present in 99.7 per cent of cervical cancers.[1] HPV-16 was the predominant type in all countries except Indonesia, where HPV-18 was more common.[1] The advent of prophylactic vaccines directed against types 16/18 HPV could reduce the incidence of cervical cancer by at least 70 per cent in a high-coverage population.[2]

PATHOLOGY

Squamous cell and adenosquamous carcinomas comprise approximately 85 per cent and adenocarcinoma approximately 15 per cent of cervical cancers. Squamous carcinomas are large-cell keratinising, large-cell non-keratinising and small-cell types. The rare but dangerous small-cell neuroendocrine type typically behaves like similar disease arising from the bronchus. Adenocarcinomas can be pure or mixed with squamous cell carcinomas – the adenosquamous carcinoma. About 80 per cent of cervical adenocarcinomas are made up of cells of the endocervical type with mucin production. The remaining tumours are populated by endometrioid, clear cell, intestinal or a mixture of more than one type of cell.

KEY POINTS

- Cervical cancer is the most common form of cancer in women in developing countries.
- The incidence of and deaths from cervical cancer are decreasing in the UK due to cervical screening.
- HPV DNA is present in virtually 100 per cent of cervical cancers.
- Squamous cell and adenosquamous carcinomas comprise approximately 85 per cent and adenocarcinomas approximately 15 per cent of cervical cancers.

CLINICAL MANAGEMENT

The goals of the management of cervical cancer are to stage the disease and to treat both the primary lesion and other sites of spread. Cervical cancers spread by direct spread into the cervical stroma, parametrium and beyond, and by lymphatic metastasis into parametrial, pelvic sidewall and para-aortic nodes. Blood-borne spread is unusual. Among the major factors that influence prognosis are:

- stage;
- volume;
- grade of tumour;
- histological type;
- lymphatic spread;
- vascular invasion.

In a large surgico-pathological staging study of patients with clinical disease confined to the cervix, the factors that predicted lymph node metastases and a decrease in disease-free survival were capillary–lymphatic space involvement by tumour, increasing tumour size and increasing depth of stromal invasion.[3,4] A similar study of 626 patients with locally advanced disease demonstrated that para-aortic and pelvic lymph node status, tumour size, clinical stage, patient age and performance status were all significant prognostic factors for a reduction in progression-free interval and survival.[5] The incidence of para-aortic and pelvic lymph node disease according to stage is illustrated in Table 108.1.

Staging

Women should be fully staged using the FIGO system (Table 108.2). FIGO staging is based largely on clinical assessment, chest X-ray and cystoscopy. Radiological staging, particularly by MRI, which permits more accurate determination of disease extent,[12] also permits assessment of lymph node status. Routine use of imaging enhances the selection of women in whom surgery alone is likely to be curative. MRI has become so accurate at staging disease that examination under anaesthetic combined with cystoscopy is often not required. In a limited number of pilot studies, positron emission tomography has demonstrated enhanced accuracy at diagnosing involved lymph nodes and local invasion, but more robust

Table 108.1 Incidence of nodal disease in cervical cancer according to stages[6-11]

Stage	No.	Positive pelvic lymph nodes (%)	Positive para-aortic lymph nodes (%)
IA1 (<1 mm)	23	0	0
IA1 (1–3 mm)	156	0.6	0
IA2 (3–5 mm)	84	4.8	<1
IB	1926	15.9	2.2
IIA	110	24.5	11
IIB	324	31.4	19
III	125	44.8	30
IVA	23	55	40

studies are required. If performed prior to pelvic exenteration a whole-body PET or PET/CT scan may improve selection of patients and therefore improve survival and reduce morbidity. If performed prior to radiotherapy a whole-body PET or PET/CT scan may change planned radiotherapy fields.

Treatment

Specialised gynaecological oncology teams should determine the management of women with cervical cancer. Decisions about how best to treat early disease in young women in particular require considerable experience. Both surgery and radiotherapy are effective in early-stage disease, whereas locally advanced disease relies on treatment by radiation or chemoradiation. Surgery does provide the advantage of conservation of ovarian function.

Factors that influence the mode of treatment include stage, age and health status. Radiation can be used for all stages, whereas surgery should only be considered an option for early-disease, stage I and stage IIA. A large randomised trial reported identical five-year overall and disease-free survival rates when comparing radiation therapy with radical hysterectomy, but women who had surgery and adjuvant radiotherapy suffered significantly higher morbidity than those who had either surgery or radiotherapy alone [B].[13]

There are clear advantages to surgery in women at low operative risk. Surgery permits conservation of ovarian function in pre-menopausal women and also reduces the risk of chronic bladder, bowel and sexual dysfunction associated with radiotherapy. Complications in the hands of skilled surgeons are uncommon. Surgery also permits the assessment of risk factors, such as lymph node status, that will ultimately influence prognosis. Complications of surgery include fistulae (≤1 per cent), lymphocyst, primary haemorrhage and bladder injury. Chronic bowel and bladder problems that require medical or surgical intervention occur in up to 8–13 per cent of women[13] due to parasympathetic denervation secondary to surgical clamping at the lateral excision margins.

Table 108.2 FIGO staging

Stage I	Stage I	Carcinoma strictly confined to the cervix; extension to the uterine corpus does not affect the stage
	Stage IA	Invasive cancer identified only microscopically. All gross lesions, even with superficial invasion, are stage IB cancers. Invasion is limited to measured stromal invasion with a maximum depth of 5 mm and no wider than 7 mm
	Stage IA1	Measured invasion of the stroma no greater than 3 mm in depth and no wider than 7 mm diameter
	Stage IA2	Measured invasion of stroma greater than 3 mm, but no greater than 5 mm in depth and no wider than 7 mm in diameter
	Stage IB	Clinical lesions confined to the cervix or preclinical lesions greater than stage IA
	Stage IB1	Clinical lesions no greater than 4 cm in size
	Stage IB2	Clinical lesions greater than 4 cm in size
Stage II	Stage II	Carcinoma that extends beyond the cervix, but has not extended on to the pelvic wall. The carcinoma involves the vagina, but not as far as the lower third
	Stage IIA1	No obvious parametrial involvement. Involvement of up to the upper two thirds of the vagina, <4 cm
	Stage IIA2	No obvious parametrial involvement. Involvement of up to the upper two thirds of the vagina, >4 cm
	Stage IIB	Obvious parametrial involvement, but not on to the pelvic sidewall
Stage III	Stage III	Carcinoma that has extended on to the pelvic sidewall. On rectal examination, there is no cancer-free space between the tumour and the pelvic sidewall. The tumour involves the lower third of the vagina. All cases with a hydronephrosis or non-functioning kidney should be included, unless they are known to be due to other causes
	Stage IIIA	No extension on to the pelvic sidewall, but involvement of the lower third of the vagina
	Stage IIIB	Extension on to the pelvic sidewall or hydronephrosis or non-functioning kidney
Stage IV	Stage IV	Carcinoma that has extended beyond the true pelvis or has clinically involved the mucosa of the bladder and/or rectum
	Stage IVA	Spread of the tumour on to adjacent pelvic organs
	Stage IVB	Spread to distant organs

Stage IA disease

Micro-invasive disease is one in which neoplastic cells invade from the epithelium to a maximum depth of 5 mm and a maximum horizontal spread of 7 mm. Any invasion beyond these dimensions upstages the disease to stage IB. The identification of early disease allows the selection of a group of women who are not at risk of lymph node disease and can be treated with less aggressive and, importantly, fertility-sparing therapy.

Micro-invasive disease comprises 20 per cent of invasive cancers. Stage IA1 disease (invasion ≤3 mm) is rarely associated with lymph node metastases (see Table 108.1). This disease should be formally diagnosed by cone biopsy or diathermy excision. Knife cone biopsy does not cause any thermal damage, and the extent of disease may be more accurately assessed than on a loop excision specimen. If the disease and any associated intraepithelial neoplasia are removed with clear margins, no further treatment is necessary. If disease is present at the margins, further excision or hysterectomy is required. A simple abdominal total hysterectomy is sufficient, as there is no risk of parametrial involvement. Because invasive disease of ≤3 mm invasion is associated with a very low risk of lymph node disease (see Table 108.1), lymphadenectomy is not indicated. Lymphadenectomy should, however, be considered for stage IA2 (invasion 3–5 mm) disease as the

rate of node involvement reaches 5 per cent, particularly if the tumour is poorly differentiated.

Stage IB–IIA

Stage IB is divided into IB1 (≤4 cm diameter) and IB2 (>4 cm diameter); stage IIA means upper vaginal, but not parametrial involvement.

Surgical therapy for stage IB and IIA tumours ≤4 cm across usually involves radical hysterectomy and pelvic lymphadenectomy. Radical hysterectomy involves removing the tumour with adequate disease-free margins, by means of excising the parametrial tissue around the cervix and upper vagina, with removal of part or all of the cardinal and uterosacral ligaments, depending on the extent of the dissection. More radical dissections are associated with a higher incidence of peri-operative morbidity and chronic bladder and bowel dysfunction with no survival advantage [B].[15]

The lymph node dissection should include obturator, internal, external and common iliac nodes. The presence of suspicious lymph nodes on pre-operative MR scan in early-stage disease should dictate chemoradiation as a sole treatment modality. If there is any doubt of the nature of enlarged nodes laparoscopic biopsy or PET imaging should be considered before the treatment plan is finally decided

GYNAECOLOGICAL ONCOLOGY

Lymphadenectomy may result in lymphocyst formation. Lymphoedema following pelvic lymphadenectomy can occur, although its incidence increases if adjuvant radiotherapy is given.

In cases in which positive nodes are encountered, there are differing views. Some would advocate abandoning surgery in favour of radical chemoradiation. Others would argue that, if possible, radical surgery should be completed to achieve an adjuvant setting for radiotherapy. If suspicious nodes are identified and confirmed to be diseased at frozen section, it is probably best to remove resectable nodes and treat with chemoradiation, including brachytherapy, which requires the uterus to be *in situ*. Radical surgery followed by radical radiotherapy is associated with increased morbidity.

Adjuvant radiotherapy is normally recommended for women with resected positive pelvic nodes to reduce the risk of recurrence. Patients with 'close' vaginal margins (≤ 0.5 cm) may also benefit from pelvic irradiation.[15]

Indirect evidence from non-randomised studies suggests that radiotherapy can improve pelvic control, but there is no firm evidence of increased survival [C].[17,18] Careful preoperative radiological imaging reduces the risk of encountering unexpected lymphadenopathy or unexpectedly large tumours.

Because bulky IB tumours have a higher risk of positive nodes and close surgical margins, these are now regarded by many as being better treated with chemoradiation as opposed to surgery or radiotherapy alone. Some women with small-volume stage IB disease who wish to conserve their fertility might be suitable for trachelectomy (radical excision of the cervix) combined with either laparoscopic or open lymphadenectomy. The most common approach is a vaginal trachelectomy; however, more recently some surgeons are favouring an abdominal approach facilitating greater excision of the parametrium with this technique. Meta-analyses and large UK case series based on the vaginal approach have demonstrated recurrence rates of around 4 per cent, and a 70 per cent term delivery rate.[19,20] Some surgeons recommend the insertion of an abdominal isthmic cervical cerclage to reduce the risk of late miscarriage. Indeed, in selected cases of IB1 disease that are just greater than 7 mm in horizontal spread, a large-cone biopsy may be adequate for central control, even though it may need to be combined with lymphadenectomy.

Stage IIB and above

It is not feasible to perform surgery with curative intent in these advanced stages of disease. Radical radiotherapy and chemoradiation are the only modalities of treatment that offer the potential for cure. One randomised trial has suggested that pre-operative chemotherapy to shrink disease followed by radical surgery may be superior to radical radiotherapy, but this has not been confirmed.[21] It is inevitable that pre-operative chemotherapy followed by surgery will still require some women to undergo adjuvant or non-adjuvant radiotherapy that is more likely to result in unacceptable toxicity.

Radical radiotherapy

Radical radiotherapy is indicated for women unfit for surgery, or with bulky stage IB2 disease and more advanced disease. The goals of such treatment are to treat primary disease and to control metastatic pelvic lymph nodes. The radical dose is delivered by external-beam (teletherapy) and intracavitary treatment (brachytherapy). The standard technique now is of remote after-loading (e.g. using the Selectron). Intracavitary treatment is designed to give high doses locally to the primary site. Teletherapy is designed to treat any pelvic spread. The challenge in administering radiotherapy is in achieving an optimal dose throughout the primary tumour and pelvic sidewall without causing high morbidity. The peripheral field of treatment of intracavitary radiotherapy delivers an insufficient dose to treat the pelvic sidewalls. The dose-limiting normal tissues within the pelvis are the rectum posteriorly, the bladder anteriorly and any loops of small bowel within the pelvic radiation fields.

Prescribing rules have been devised for determining the precise dose of radiotherapy within the pelvis, and improved planning by CT has enabled more accurate targeting of external-beam radiation in particular. An example is the Manchester system. This uses a number of predetermined source sizes and radioactive loadings such that a constant dose rate is delivered to a point A. Point A is defined as a point 2 cm lateral to the central axis of the uterus and 2 cm from the lateral fornix. A second point (B) lying in the same plane 3 cm lateral to point A is used to determine the dose to parametrial tissues. Following the insertion of the sources for each patient, a dose distribution is calculated. The total dose is a product of the dose rate and treatment time. The usual doses delivered are 70–80 Gy to point A and 60 Gy to point B, limiting the bladder and rectal dose to 60 Gy. To achieve this, it is necessary to have adequate packing to keep the bladder and bowel away from the intracavitary source. External-beam radiation is usually given two to three weeks after intracavitary treatment to allow for involution of the primary disease. External-beam radiotherapy is fractionated over 20–30 days' treatment, as this technique allows a cancericidal effect while enabling normal tissue recovery between fractions.

Routine extended field radiotherapy designed to include para-aortic nodes has not been proven to improve survival compared with pelvic radiotherapy alone, and it is associated with significantly more gastrointestinal complications [B].[22] While there does not appear to be significant benefit from extended field irradiation for all cases, para-aortic node irradiation is appropriate in cases of proven para-aortic node involvement as indicated by diagnostic imaging or surgical staging.

Chemoradiation

Five randomised trials from the US[23–27] have shown an overall survival advantage for cisplatin-based therapy given concurrently with radiation therapy [B]. The patient populations in these studies included women with FIGO stages IB2–IVA cervical cancer treated with primary radiation therapy and women with FIGO stages I–IIA disease found to have poor prognostic factors (metastatic disease in pelvic lymph nodes, parametrial disease or positive surgical margins) at the time of primary surgery. Although the trials vary somewhat in terms of stage of disease, dose of radiation and schedule of cisplatin and radiation, they all demonstrate significant survival benefit for this combined approach, the risk of death from cervical cancer being decreased by 30 per cent. These trials reported higher rates of short- and medium-term complications with chemoradiation, and although longer follow-up is required to examine the true morbidity of this treatment regimen, there is now international acceptance that chemoradiation is superior to radiation alone.

Recurrent cervical cancer

Treatment for recurrent cervical cancer depends on the mode of primary therapy and the site of recurrence. Women who have had initial treatment by surgery should be considered for radiotherapy, and those who have had radiotherapy should be considered for exenterative surgery, provided the recurrence is central and there is no evidence of distant recurrence. These women require very careful pre-operative assessment and counselling in order to understand the consequences of defunctioning surgery. Exenterative surgery in carefully selected cases can result in five-year survival of 50 per cent [D]. Positive nodes at the time of attempted salvage surgery and positive resection margins are associated with a poor prognosis. Anterior exenteration requires excision of the bladder and most of the vagina *en bloc* with the recurrence, and posterior exenteration requires excision of the sigmoid rectum with formation of a colostomy. Sometimes a combination of the two is required. This type of surgery should only be undertaken by teams of highly skilled pelvic surgeons. Relapse within two years of primary treatment, the presence of hydronephrosis and symptoms of pain are all associated with poorer outcomes in terms of exenterative surgery.

Palliation of progressive cervical disease

Chemotherapy is palliative and should be reserved for patients who are not considered curable by the other two treatment modalities. Urinary tract symptoms are particularly common in advanced cervical disease. Ureteric obstruction with subsequent pain, infection and ultimately impaired renal function are common features. Mechanical diversion by nephrostomy or ureteric stenting is only usually justified as part of treatment with curative intent. Fistulae can occur in late-stage disease and can cause intolerable symptoms. If there is a prospect of surviving more than 8 weeks, palliative surgery should be offered in order to divert faeces or urine.

In progressive late-stage disease, there is usually ureteric obstruction, which heralds a terminal phase. Pain can be particularly distressing due to infiltration of the lumbosacral nerve plexuses. Meticulous attention to pain control and psychological and emotional support are essential.

KEY POINTS

- Early micro-invasive disease can be treated by cone biopsy or excisional treatment alone [C].
- Surgery and radiotherapy for stage IB/IIA disease have similar five-year overall and disease-free survival rates, but women who have had surgery and adjuvant radiotherapy combined have significantly higher morbidity than those who have had either surgery or radiotherapy alone [B].
- Pre-operative imaging with MRI scans reduces the number of women undergoing both modalities of treatment [C].
- Chemoradiation increases survival over radiotherapy alone for advanced disease, but toxicity is increased [B].

References

1. Walboomers JM, Jacobs MV, Manos MM *et al.* Human papillomavirus is a necessary cause of invasive cervical cancer worldwide. *J Pathol* 1999;189:12–19.
2. Cuzick J, Castanon A, Sasieni P. Predicted impact of vaccination against human papillomavirus 16/18 on cancer incidence and cervical abnormalities in women aged 20–29 in the UK. *Br J Cancer* 2010;102:933–9.
3. Delgado G, Bundy BN, Fowler WC *et al.* A prospective surgical pathological study of stage I squamous carcinoma of the cervix: a Gynecologic Oncology Group study. *Gynecol Oncol* 1989;35:314–20.
4. Zaino RJ, Ward S, Delgado G *et al.* Histopathologic predictors of the behavior of surgically treated stage IB squamous cell carcinoma of the cervix. A Gynecologic Oncology Group study. *Cancer* 1992;69:1750–8.
5. Stehman FB, Bundy BN, DiSaia PJ *et al.* Carcinoma of the cervix treated with radiation therapy. I. A multivariate analysis of prognostic variables in the Gynecologic Oncology Group. *Cancer* 1991;67:2776–85.
6. Boyce, Fruchter R, Nicastri AD *et al.* Prognostic factors in stage I carcinoma of the cervix. *Gynecol Oncol* 1981;12:154–65.
7. Inoue T, Okumura M. Prognostic significance of parametrial extension in patients with cervical carcinoma stages IB, IIA, and IIB. A study of 628 cases treated by radical hysterectomy and lymphadenectomy with or without postoperative irradiation. *Cancer* 1984;54:1714–19.
8. Lohe KJ. Early squamous cell carcinoma of the uterine cervix. *Gynecol Oncol* 1978;6:10–30.
9. van Nagell J, Donaldson ES, Wood EG, Parker JC. The significance of vascular invasion and lymphocytic infiltration in invasive cervical cancer. *Cancer* 1978;41:228–34.
10. Tinga DJ, Timmer PR, Bouma J, Aalders JG. Prognostic significance of single versus multiple lymph node

metastases in cervical carcinoma stage IB. *Gynecol Oncol* 1990;39:175–80.

11. Nahhas WA, Sharkey FE, Whitney CW *et al.* The prognostic significance of vascular channel involvement and deep stromal penetration in early cervical carcinoma. *Am J Clin Oncol* 1983;6:259–64.

12. Scheidler J, Hricak H, Yu KK *et al.* Radiological evaluation of lymph node metastases in patients with cervical cancer. A meta-analysis. *J Am Med Assoc* 1997;278:1096–101.

13. Landoni F, Maneo A, Colombo A *et al.* Randomised study of radical surgery versus radiotherapy for stage IB–IIA cervical cancer. *Lancet* 1997;350:535–40.

14. Fujikawa K, Miyamoto T, Ihara Y *et al.* High incidence of severe urologic complications following radiotherapy for cervical cancer in Japanese women. *Gynecol Oncol* 2001; 80: 21–3.

15. Landoni F, Maneo A, Cormio G *et al.* Class II versus class III radical hysterectomy in stage IB–IIA cervical cancer: a prospective randomized study. *Gynecol Oncol* 2001;80:3–12.

16. Estape RE, Angioli R, Madrigal M *et al.* Close vaginal margins as a prognostic factor after radical hysterectomy. *Gynecol Oncol* 1998;68:229–32.

17. Soisson AP, Soper JT, Clarke Pearson DL *et al.* Adjuvant radiotherapy following radical hysterectomy for patients with stage IB and IIA cervical cancer. *Gynecol Oncol* 1990; 37: 390–5.

18. Kinney WK, Alvarez RD, Reid GC *et al.* Value of adjuvant whole-pelvis irradiation after Wertheim hysterectomy for early-stage squamous carcinoma of the cervix with pelvic nodal metastasis: a matched-control study. *Gynecol Oncol* 1989;34:258–62.

19. Plante M, Renaud MC, Hoskins IA, Roy M. Vaginal radical trachelectomy: a valuable fertility-preserving option in the management of early-stage cervical cancer. A series of 50 pregnancies and review of the literature. *Gynecol Oncol* 2005;98:3–10.

20. Shepherd JH, Spencer C, Herod J, Ind TE. Radical vaginal trachelectomy as a fertility-sparing procedure in women with early-stage cervical cancer: cumulative pregnancy rate in a series of 123 women. *BJOG* 2006;113:719–24.

21. Sardi JE, Giaroli A, di Paola G *et al.* Long-term follow-up of the first randomized trial using neoadjuvant chemotherapy in stage IB squamous carcinoma of the cervix: the final results. *Gynecol Oncol* 1997;67:61–9.

22. Haie C, Pejovic MH, Gerbaulet A *et al.* Is prophylactic para-aortic irradiation worthwhile in the treatment of advanced cervical carcinoma? Results of a control-led clinical trial of the EORTC radiotherapy group. *Radiother Oncol* 1988;11:101–12.

23. Whitney CW, Sause W, Bundy BN *et al.* Randomized comparison of fluorouracil plus cisplatin versus hydroxyurea as an adjunct to radiation therapy in stage IIB–IVA carcinoma of the cervix with negative para-aortic lymph nodes: a Gynecologic Oncology Group and Southwest Oncology Group study. *J Clin Oncol* 1999;17:1339–48.

24. Morris M, Eifel PJ, Lu J *et al.* Pelvic radiation with concurrent chemotherapy compared with pelvic and para-aortic radiation for high-risk cervical cancer. *N Engl J Med* 1999;340:1137–43.

25. Rose PG, Bundy BN, Watkins EB *et al.* Concurrent cisplatin-based radiotherapy and chemotherapy for locally advanced cervical cancer. *N Engl J Med* 1999;340:1144–53.

26. Keys HM, Bundy BN, Stehman FB *et al.* Cisplatin, radiation, and adjuvant hysterectomy compared with radiation and adjuvant hysterectomy for bulky stage IB cervical carcinoma. *N Engl J Med* 1999;340:1154–61.

27. Peters WA 3rd, Liu PY, Barrett RJ 2nd *et al.* Concurrent chemotherapy and pelvic radiation therapy compared with pelvic radiation therapy alone as adjuvant therapy after radical surgery in high-risk early-stage cancer of the cervix. *J Clin Oncol* 2000;18:1606–13.

Chapter 109 Benign and malignant ovarian masses

Sudha Sundar

MRCOG standards

- To understand and demonstrate appropriate knowledge in relation to: epidemiology, aetiology, genetic associations, diagnosis, prevention, screening, management, staging, prognosis, complications and anatomical considerations of pre-malignant and malignant conditions of the ovary.
- To understand and demonstrate appropriate knowledge in relation to: indications, techniques, complications and outcomes of oncological surgery, radiotherapy and chemotherapy for ovarian cancer.

INTRODUCTION

By the age of 65, 4 per cent of women will have been admitted to hospital with an ovarian cyst, making this the fourth most common gynaecological cause for hospital admission in England. Ovarian masses are common in pre-menopausal women and up to 10 per cent of women will undergo surgery during their lifetime for the presence of an ovarian mass.[1] Among pre-menopausal patients, more than 90 per cent of surgically managed cases are benign, as opposed to just 60 per cent in the post-menopausal population. Although differentiating malignant from benign disease is critical in optimising management for the individual, non-invasive diagnosis continues to be elusive. Women with complex masses considered benign can undergo laparoscopic or conservative management, whereas women with malignancy who undergo thorough surgery by gynaecological oncologist have the best outcomes.[2,3]

Ovarian cancer is the fifth most common cancer among women in the UK (2010), accounting for 4 per cent of all new cases of cancer in females. In 2010 there were 7011 new cases of ovarian cancer in the UK. The crude incidence rate shows that there are 22 new ovarian cancer cases for every 100,000 females in the UK.[4] Ovarian cancer is the fourth most common cause of cancer death among females in the UK, accounting for 6 per cent of all female deaths from cancer with 4272 deaths in 2011.[5]

The lifetime risk of developing ovarian cancer is 1 in 54.[6] Eighty per cent of patients will present at advanced stage and all-stage 5-year survival rate is about 40 per cent. Ovarian cancer is predominantly a disease of older, post-menopausal women; however 1000 women under 50 will be diagnosed annually.[6] Ovarian cancer survival is stage dependent (5-year relative survival 92% Stage I vs 5% Stage IV).[7] Five-year survival from ovarian cancer has increased significantly over the last decade. This may be as a result of improved chemotherapy regimens, treatment by dedicated multidisciplinary teams and radical surgery performed by gynaecological oncologists.

HISTOPATHOLOGY AND CLASSIFICATION OF OVARIAN MASSES

An ovarian mass may be neoplastic or physiological, and most adnexal masses are benign. The current edition of *International Classification of Tumours*, published by the WHO,[7] provides a classification of ovarian tumours that has been universally accepted.[8] Epithelial tumours are derived from the surface epithelium of the ovary and are further classified as benign, borderline or malignant, according to cell type and behaviour (Figs. 109.1 and 109.2).

Epithelial tumours account for 60–65 per cent of all ovarian tumours and approximately 90 per cent of those that are malignant. Sex-cord stromal tumours are, as their name suggests, derived from the sex cords and stroma of the ovary and account for approximately 8 per cent of all ovarian tumours. Germ-cell tumours, derived from the germ cells, account for 30 per cent of ovarian tumours, largely in the form of mature cystic teratomas (dermoid cysts). Although germ-cell tumours account for only 1–3 per cent of all ovarian malignancies, they represent more than 60 per cent of ovarian cancers in children and adolescents.

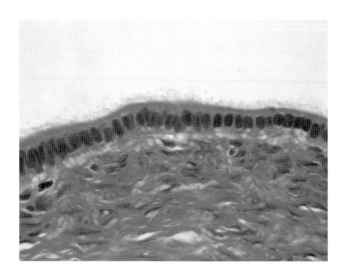

Fig. 109.1 Haematoxylin and eosin staining of a section of tumour demonstrating the typical epithelium of a benign serous cystadenoma – note single layer and bland appearance

Note: the term **ovarian cancer** is used in this chapter to include not only epithelial ovarian malignancies, but also malignant sex-cord stromal and germ-cell neoplasms.

Epithelial ovarian tumours

The ovary first appears in fetal life as an aggregation of cells covered with primitive coelomic epithelium. Subsequently, germ cells migrate from the yolk sac into the gonadal area. The coelomic epithelium that covers the ovary also gives rise to a variety of epithelia of Müllerian origin, which line the genital tract structures, including the Fallopian tubes, the uterus and the cervix, and are similar to those found in epithelial tumours of the ovary. Well-differentiated serous carcinoma resembles epithelium of the Fallopian tube, whereas the cell type in endometrioid tumours has a similar appearance to the cells found in endometrial glands. The WHO classification of epithelial ovarian tumours is based on this similarity in cell type (Table 109.1).

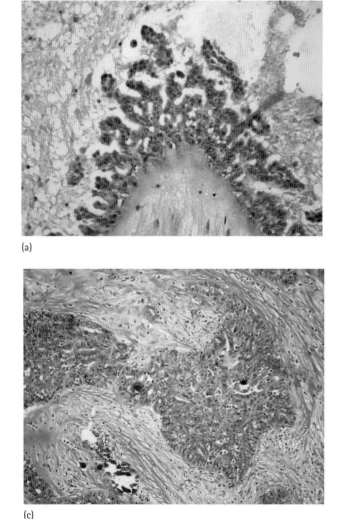

(a)

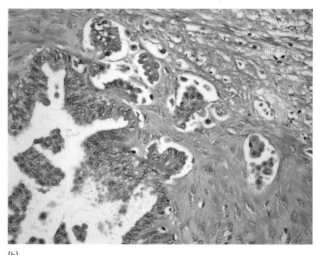

(b)

(c)

Fig. 109.2 Haematoxylin and eosin sections from borderline, micro-invasive and malignant ovarian tumours demonstrating increasing architectural complexity and nuclear pleomorphism. (a) Borderline serous ovarian tumour. (b) Borderline serous ovarian tumour with micro-invasion. (c) Invasive serous cystadenocarcinoma

Table 109.1 WHO clasification of tumours of the ovary[a,b]

Epithellial tumours	
Serous Tumours	
Benign	
Serous cystadenoma	8441/0
Serous adenofibroma	9014/0
Serous surface papilloma	8461/0
Borderline	
Serous borderline tumour/Atypical proliferative serous tumour	8442/1
Serous borderline tumour - micropapillary variant / Non-invasive low-grade serous carcinoma	8460/2*
Malignant	
Low-grade serous carcinoma	8460/3
High-grade serous carcinoma	8461/3
Mucinous tumours	
Benign	
Mucinous cystadenoma	8470/0
Mucinous adenofibroma	9015/0
Borderline	
Mucinous borderline tumour/Atypical proliferative mucinous tumour	8472/1
Malignant	
Mucinous carcinoma	8480/3
Endometrioid tumours	
Benign	
Endometriotic cyst	
Endometrioid cystadenoma	8380/0
Endometrioid adenofibroma	8381/1
Borderline	
Endometrioid borderline tumour/Atypical proliferative endometrioid tumour	8380/1
Malignant	
Endometrioid carcinoma	8380/3
Clear cell tumours	
Benign	
Clear cell cystadenoma	8443/0
Clear cell adenofibroma	8313/0
Borderline	
Clear cell borderline tumour/Atypical proliferative clear cell tumour	8313/1
Malignant	
Clear cell carcinoma	8310/3

Brenner tumours	
Benign	
Brenner tumour	9000/0
Borderline	
Borderline Brenner tumour/Atypical proliferative Brenner tumour	9000/1
Malignant	
Malignant Brenner tumour	9000/3
Seromucinous tumours	
Benign	
Seromucinous cystadenoma	8474/0*
Seromucinous adenofibroma	9014/0*
Borderline	
Seromucinous borderline tumour/Atypical proliferative seromucinous tumour	8474/1*
Malignant	
Seromucinous carcinoma	8474/3*
Undifferentiated carcinoma	8020/3
Mesenchymal tumours	
Low-grade endometrioid stromal sarcoma	8931/3
High-grade endometrioid stromal sarcoma	8930/3
Mixed epithelial and mesenchymal tumours	
Adenosarcoma	8933/3
Carcinosarcoma	8980/3
Sex cord-stromal tumours	
Pure stromal tumours	
Fibroma	8810/0
Cellular fibroma	8810/1
Thecoma	8600/0
Luteinized thecoma associated with sclerosing peritonitis	8601/0
Fibrosarcoma	8810/3
Sclerosing stromal tumour	8602/0
Signet-ring stromal tumour	8590/0
Microcystic stromal tumour	8590/0
Leydig cell tumour	8650/0
Steriod cell tumour	8760/0
Steriod cell tumour, malignant	8760/3
Pure sex cord tumours	
Adult granulosa cell tumour	8620/3
Juvenile granulosa cell tumour	8622/1
Sertoli cell tumour	8640/1
Sex cord tumour with annular tubules	8623/1

Table 109.1 WHO clasification of tumours of the ovary[a,b] (*continued*)

Mixed sex cord-stromal tumours	
Sertoli-Leydig cell tumours	
well differentiated	8631/0
Moderately differentiated	8631/1
With heterologous elements	8634/1
Poorly differentiated	8631/3
With heterologous elements	8634/3
Retiform	8633/1
With heterologous elements	8634/1
Sex cord-stromal tumours, NOS	8590/1
Germ cell tumours	
Dysgerminoma	9060/3
Yolk sac tumour	9071/3
Embryonal carcinoma	9070/3
Non-gestational choriocarcinoma	9100/3
Mature teratoma	9080/0
Immature teratoma	9080/3
Mixed germ cell tumour	9085/3
Monodermal teratoma and somatic-type tumours arising from a dermoid cyst	
Struma ovarii, benign	9090/0
Struma ovarii, malignant	9090/3
Carcinoid	8240/3
Strumal carcinoid	9091/1
Mucinous carcinoid	8243/3
Neuroectodermal-type tumors	
Sebaceous tumours	
Sebaceous adenoma	8410/0
Sebaceous carcinoma	8410/3
Other rare monodermal teratomas	
Carcinomas	
Squamous cell carcinoma	8070/3
Others	
Germ cell-sex cord-stromal tumours	
Gonadoblastoma, including gonadoblastoma with malignant germ cell tumour	9073/1
Mixed germ cell-sex cord-stromal tumour, unclassified	8594/1*

Miscellaneous tumours	
Tumours of rete ovarii	
Adenoma of rete ovarii	9110/0
Adenocarcinoma of rete ovarii	9110/3
Wolffian tumour	9110/1
Small cell carcinoma, hypercalcaemic type	8044/3*
Small cell carcinoma, pulmonary type	8041/3
Wilms tumour	8960/3
Paraganglioma	8693/1
Solid pseudopapillary neoplasm	8452/1
Mesothelial tumours	
Adenomatoid tumour	9054/0
Mesothelioma	9050/3
Soft tissue tumours	
Myxoma	8840/0
Others	
Tumour-like lesions	
Follicle cyst	
Corpus luteum cyst	
Large solitary luteinized follicle cyst	
Hyperreactio luteinalis	
Pregnancy luteoma	
Stromal hyperplasia	
Stromal hyperthecosis	
Fibromatosis	
Massive oedema	
Leydig cell hyperplasia	
Others	
Lymphoid and myeloid tumours	
Lymphomas	
Plasmacytoma	9734/3
Myeloid neoplasms	
Secondary tumours	

[a]The Morphology codes are from the International Classification of Diseases for Oncology (ICD-O) {575A}. Behaviour is coded /0 for benign tumours, /1 for unspecified, borderline or uncertain behaviour, /2 for carcinoma *in situ* and grade III intraepithelial neoplasia and /3 for malignant tumours;[b] The classification is modified from the previous WHO classification of tumours {1906A}, taking into account changes in our understanding of these lesions; *These new codes were approved by the IARC/WHO Committee for ICD-O in 2013.

Approximately 90 per cent of ovarian cancers are carcinomas (malignant epithelial tumours) and, based on histopathology, immunohistochemistry and molecular genetic analysis, at least five main types are currently distinguished: high-grade serous carcinoma (HGSC, 70 per cent); endometrioid carcinoma (EC, 10 per cent); clear-cell carcinoma (CCC, 10 per cent); mucinous carcinoma (MC, 3 per cent); and low-grade serous carcinoma (LGSC, <5 per cent).

It is now understood that primary mucinous cancers of the ovary are rare, and the majority of mucinous cancers that were attributed to ovarian origin are in fact metastases from the intestinal tract. Bilaterality of epithelial ovarian malignancies is common. Although endocrine function is most commonly a feature of sex-cord stromal tumours, it may also occur in association with epithelial ovarian tumours. Paraneoplastic syndromes are a rare feature of these tumours.

Sex-cord stromal tumours

These tumours are composed of granulosa cells, theca cells, Sertoli cells, Leydig cells, fibroblasts or the precursors of these cells in varying proportions. The classification of these tumours (based on the WHO classification) is shown in Table 109.1. They may be associated with an oestrogenic, androgenic or (more rarely) progestogenic effect, but functional activity does not correlate with the appearance of the cell. Many of these tumours are benign and most of the clinically malignant forms are granulosa cell tumours. Fibromas are well known for their association with ascites and right hydrothorax (Meigs syndrome).

Germ-cell tumours

Approximately 30 per cent of benign and malignant ovarian tumours are of germ-cell origin (Table 109.1). However, as only a small proportion are malignant, they account for less than 5 per cent of all ovarian cancers. Nonetheless, they are the commonest ovarian malignancy in the first two decades of life.

Dysgerminoma is the commonest germ-cell malignancy, and 75 per cent of cases present with stage I disease. In contrast with other malignant germ-cell tumours, 10–15 per cent are bilateral, with contralateral involvement usually being microscopic. Five to 10 per cent occur in phenotypic females with abnormal gonads (androgen insensitivity syndrome or gonadal dysgenesis).

Teratomas are tumours that are composed of tissue derived from two or three embryonic layers. The mature cystic teratoma is the commonest ovarian germ-cell tumour and is usually benign. Most are unilateral, but 15–20 per cent are bilateral. They are the commonest ovarian tumours leading to torsion. Hair and teeth may be present in the cysts, the latter resulting in the classical appearance on plain abdominal X-ray. Malignant transformation is reported in up to 2 per cent, squamous carcinoma being the commonest malignancy to develop. A diagnosis of struma ovarii is made when these tumours are predominantly composed of thyroid tissue. Primary ovarian carcinoid tumours are also variants of monodermal teratomas and usually have a favourable prognosis. However, secondary carcinoids (not associated with a monodermal teratoma) are usually metastatic from the gastrointestinal tract and have a poor prognosis.

Immature teratoma is the second commonest germ-cell malignancy and accounts for approximately 20 per cent of ovarian malignancies in females under 20 years of age. Virtually all immature teratomas are unilateral and they are currently classified according to a grading system that is based on the degree of differentiation and the quantity of immature tissue.

Embryonic markers

Most patients with ovarian yolk sac tumours have elevated levels of alpha-fetoprotein (AFP), but normal levels do not exclude this diagnosis. Embryonal carcinomas are extremely rare. They usually secrete beta-human chorionic gonadotrophin (b-hCG) and may secrete AFP. Ovarian choriocarcinoma secretes b-hCG and polyembryoma secretes b-hCG and AFP. These are also very rare tumours. The commoner immature teratoma and pure dysgerminoma do not secrete these tumour markers.

Gonadoblastoma

This rare tumour consists of admixed germ-cell and sex-cord stromal elements. This is usually a tumour of the second decade of life and rarely occurs in normal ovaries. Eighty per cent occur in phenotypic females who are virilised, and 20 per cent in phenotypic males with developmental abnormalities of the external genitalia. The most common karyotypes are 46XY and 45XO/46XY (mosaic).

Secondary ovarian malignancies

Up to 10 per cent of ovarian masses are metastases from some other organ and in many cases the ovarian metastases are detected before the primary tumour. The most common metastatic cancers are those arising from the colon, stomach, breast and, of course, the female genital tract. Bilaterally enlarged ovaries that contain signet-ring cells on microscopic assessment have been named after Krukenberg, who described these ovarian tumours in patients with metastatic gastric or (less commonly) colonic cancer.

Primary peritoneal carcinoma

Primary peritoneal carcinoma is a highly malignant tumour arising from the peritoneum and resulting in signs and symptoms very similar to those of primary epithelial ovarian cancer. Rare benign and borderline variants have been described. Thus a patient who has previously had both ovaries removed may develop a condition that clinically simulates ovarian cancer. Primary peritoneal cancer and primary Fallopian tube cancer are rare malignancies but share many similarities with ovarian cancer. Clinically, these three cancers are managed in a similar manner.

Primary Fallopian tube cancer

This rare cancer accounts for approximately 0.3 per cent of all female genital tract cancers. The classical presenting triad consists of:

- a prominent watery discharge (hydrops tubae profluens);
- pelvic pain;
- a pelvic mass.

It is similar to primary epithelial ovarian cancer in histological appearance and clinical behaviour. Management is therefore essentially the same.

Rare ovarian tumours

Rare ovarian tumours include primary small-cell carcinoma and various types of sarcoma, all having a poor prognosis. Lymphoma or extramedullary leukaemia may also manifest initially as an ovarian tumour.

Molecular classification of ovarian cancer

Currently, on the basis of molecular characteristics, ovarian cancer can be divided into two types – type 1 which comprises clear-cell, mucinous, endometrioid and low-grade serous cancer histology, and type 2 which comprises high-grade serous cancers. Type 1 cancers tend to be slow growing, indolent and more likely to be detected earlier by ultrasound whereas type 2 cancers are typically fast growing. Paradoxically type 1 cancers can prove harder to treat as most respond less well to chemotherapy. Improved understanding of ovarian cancer biology has led to a fundamental rethink of the origin of ovarian cancer.

The theory of 'incessant ovulation' causing ovarian cancer on the epithelial surface of the capsule has now been replaced after greater insight into genetic drivers of this disease. It is now believed that many serous ovarian cancer arises in the fimbrial end of the fallopian tube and disseminates within the peritoneal cavity. It is likely that high-grade serous cancer, Fallopian tube cancer and primary peritoneal cancer are different phenotypes of the same biological disease entity.[9]

With advancements in gene-sequencing technology, landmark studies have revealed that *p53* is mutated in almost all serous ovarian cancer, whereas other histology types have specific molecular alterations (e.g. ARID1A in clear-cell cancers).[10] A greater understanding of these will lead to improved treatments in the next decade.

Germline *BRCA* mutations have been detected in almost 17 per cent of all high-grade serous cancer, and there is a

sound case for *BRCA* testing in every patient with high-grade serous cancer.[11] Whilst this approach carries implications in terms of resource and the impact on extended family members, patients with BRCA mutations in ovarian cancer may also benefit from a newer class of drugs – poly ADP ribose polymerase inhibitors.

KEY POINTS

- The mature cystic teratoma is the commonest ovarian germ-cell tumour, is benign and the commonest ovarian tumour leading to torsion.
- 90 per cent of malignant ovarian tumours are epithelial, but germ-cell tumours account for 60 per cent of ovarian cancers in adolescents and children.
- High-grade serous ovarian cancers probably arise from the fimbrial end of the Fallopian tube.
- 17 per cent of patients with high-grade serous ovarian cancer have germline mutations of the *BRCA* gene.
- Bilaterality of epithelial ovarian malignancies is common.
- Up to 10 per cent of ovarian masses are secondary to metastases from some other organ.

EPIDEMIOLOGY, INCIDENCE AND AETIOLOGY OF EPITHELIAL OVARIAN CANCER

In 2008, it was estimated that 225,500 women were diagnosed with ovarian cancer and 140,200 women died from this disease worldwide. Thus ovarian cancer is the eighth most common type of cancer and the seventh most common cause of cancer-related death among women. Like many other types of cancer, there is substantial geographical variation in ovarian cancer incidence and mortality, with a higher incidence in economically developed regions of the world.[12] In England and Wales, ovarian cancer is the second most common gynaecological malignancy to uterine cancer but ovarian cancer accounts for more deaths in these countries than the other gynaecological malignancies together.

The incidence and mortality rates are influenced by country of origin and race. In general, epithelial ovarian cancer is most common and most lethal in industrialised countries (excepting Japan) and has the lowest rates in the non-industrialised world. In contrast, germ-cell tumours represent up to 15 per cent of ovarian cancers in black and oriental populations, in whom epithelial ovarian cancers are less common.

Most epithelial ovarian cancers occur in post-menopausal women, with less than 1 per cent affecting females under the age of 21 years. In this age group, more than 60 per cent of ovarian malignancies are of germ-cell origin.

Precursor lesions to epithelial ovarian cancer

Patients with *BRCA* mutation (breast–ovarian cancer syndrome) undergoing risk-reducing salpingo-oophorectomy were found to have high-grade serous tubal intraepithelial carcinoma (STIC) not in the ovary but in the Fallopian tube and, particularly, in the fimbria. Although not considered invasive lesions, STICS have been known to metastasise; it is likely that these lesions are the earliest phase of epithelial ovarian cancer. In addition, precursor tubal lesions termed '*p53* signatures' have been found in one third of all women and are believed to represent the initial events of serous carcinogenesis: DNA damage of secretory cells and *p53* mutations.[13]

Opportunistic postpartum salpingectomy is now being evaluated in British Columbia as a prevention strategy for epithelial ovarian cancer. Long-term incidence and mortality data are eagerly awaited.[14]

Aetiology

Environmental factors

The causes of ovarian cancer and environmental factors contributing to these are not clearly defined. In general, combined oral contraception and factors that limit the number of ovulations are associated with a reduced risk of ovarian cancer.

Genetic factors contributing to ovarian cancer

The concept that there is a familial predisposition to ovarian cancer was initially suggested by epidemiological studies that have consistently documented an increased relative risk for ovarian cancer associated with a family history of the disease.

There is a growing recognition that hereditary ovarian cancers are likely to represent about 20 per cent of all ovarian cancers. In 1994, following intense linkage analysis, a large gene was cloned and sequenced and confirmed to be the *BRCA1* – BReast CAncer 1 – gene. Confirmatory studies have identified more than 100 mutations. It has been estimated that germline mutations in *BRCA1* are responsible for approximately 5 per cent of ovarian cancers in women less than 40 years of age.

Although the estimated risk of developing either ovarian or breast cancer by the age of 70 is 82 per cent, most carriers do not develop both diseases, and thus the penetrance for development of ovarian cancer is lower and estimated at 42 per cent. Mutations in the *BRCA2* gene also increase the risk of ovarian cancer in carriers, the site of mutation possibly correlating with risk, as in the case of *BRCA1*.

HNPCC has been classified into two syndromes termed Lynch I and II. The latter has an association with cancers at other sites, including the ovary and endometrium. The genes responsible for HNPCC have now been identified. The lifetime risk of ovarian cancer among gene carriers has not been precisely documented but may be as high as seven times that of non-carriers.

Other gene mutations that confer an increased risk of ovarian carcinoma, include RAD51C and RAD51D, however testing for these is not in routine practice. Narod and colleagues have reported in a case–control study that women from families with hereditary ovarian cancer syndromes reduce their risk of developing ovarian cancer by ever use of the combined oral contraceptive pill.[15] Risk-reducing salpingo-oophorectomy (RRSO) has been widely adopted as a key component of breast and gynaecological cancer risk-reduction for women with *BRCA1* and *BRCA2* mutations once they have completed their families.[16]

SCREENING FOR OVARIAN CANCER

The possibility of pre-symptomatic genetic testing raises a number of medical, psychological, ethical, legal and social issues. Due to the limitations of genetic testing at the present time, it is imperative that it is offered only to high-risk individuals in cases for which the result of the test will affect medical management. In this context it must be remembered that a woman with a single affected relative has a lifetime risk of developing ovarian cancer of only 3–4 per cent (see Published guidelines).

Women who are at high risk for developing ovarian cancer (i.e. 10 per cent or more lifetime risk based on family history) may be offered ovarian screening. A large study, UK Familial Ovarian Cancer Screening Study (UKFOCSS), is due to report results soon, after a surveillance strategy of CA125 and ultrasound in *BRCA* carriers to detect ovarian cancer early.

However, data regarding the efficacy or potential morbidity of ovarian screening in the asymptomatic general population are lacking. Screening this population is contraindicated until such time as studies show that it is justified (see Published guidelines).

It is also unclear if ongoing surveillance should be offered for women who are deemed to be at 10 per cent or more risk of developing ovarian cancer, but if provided then it should be done in the context of familial screening clinics, usually run jointly by a clinical geneticist and a gynaecological oncologist. However initial assessment should be available to consider management choices and to highlight current uncertainties surrounding surveillance for high-risk women. Women who attend general gynaecological clinics with concerns about their familial risk of ovarian cancer should be referred to such services. They will be asked to complete a questionnaire which enables their risk to be calculated objectively and then rational choices can be made regarding whether to offer screening.

Two large trials on screening and testing asymptomatic populations for ovarian cancer have been conducted. In the

PLCO (prostate, lung, colon and ovarian cancer screening) trial conducted in the US, women between 55 and 74 were tested with Ca125 and ultrasound.[17] This trial found no benefit in terms of cases or stage of ovarian cancer detected. The UK Collaborative Trial of Ovarian Cancer Screening (UKCTOCS) is a large trial evaluating an algorithm (risk of ovarian cancer algorithm) which is based on changing levels of CA125 and a rigorous ultrasound protocol. Preliminary results from this trial suggest that screening strategies using ultrasound and CA125 levels are feasible but further results are awaited on the impact on mortality of such strategies.[18] It has completed recruitment and results are expected in 2015.[18] Currently, there is no evidence to support screening for ovarian cancer in asymptomatic women.

Symptoms of ovarian cancer

In 2011 NICE, the UK body which advises on standards of clinical care, issued guidance on the recognition and initial management of ovarian cancer.[19] NICE recommended that symptoms considered 'suspicious' should trigger diagnostic testing in the primary care setting and referral to rapid-access clinics based in secondary care within 2 weeks (2-week-wait clinics). NICE guidance aimed to improve cancer mortality by permitting primary care access to rapid diagnostic testing previously only accessible via secondary care, thereby aiding earlier diagnosis in ovarian cancer, and earlier interventions. The objectives underpinning this guidance were to diagnose the disease at an earlier stage and thus improve mortality. NICE recommended a diagnostic pathway involving sequential testing of serum CA125 followed by an abdomino-pelvic ultrasound if the serum CA125 was $\geq$35 IU/L in women presenting to primary care with symptoms on a persistent or frequent basis of: persistent abdominal distension/'bloating', feeling full and/or loss of appetite, pelvic/abdominal pain, increased urinary urgency and/or frequency, unexplained weight loss, fatigue, or changes in bowel habit. No age limits were issued at the time of guidance; however it was emphasised that the high-risk group were those aged over 50 years. Of note, both diagnostic tests were recommended to be performed in the primary care setting. No guidance on what constituted an abnormal ultrasound was issued.

NICE recommendations were based on evidence from case–control studies. Since guidance was issued, two well-conducted prospective studies have been published demonstrating that symptom-triggered diagnostic testing with CA125 and ultrasound for ovarian cancer does not result in a stage shift in ovarian cancer but may result in lesser volume stage 3 disease being detected.[20,21] At present, the impact on mortality with a strategy of symptom-triggered diagnostic testing is not known. The ROCkeTS trial aims to identify the best tests and diagnostic pathways in pre and postmenopausal women with symptoms in primary and secondary care and wil report in 2018, www.birmingham.ac.uk/ROCKETS.

KEY POINTS

Aetiology of ovarian cancer

- Postpartum salpingectomy is a potential prevention strategy for epithelial ovarian cancer.
- Pregnancy, breastfeeding, tubal ligation, hysterectomy and the combined oral contraceptive pill protect against the development of epithelial ovarian cancer.
- Hereditary ovarian cancers are unlikely to represent more than 20 per cent of all ovarian cancers.
- Bilateral salpingo-oophorectomy is protective in *BRCA* mutation carriers [I].
- HNPCC has an association with cancer of the ovary and endometrium.

MANAGEMENT OF THE ADNEXAL MASS

An adnexal mass may present either as a result of symptoms, which may be severe in the case of a cyst accident, or as an incidental finding when performing a pelvic examination or radiological investigation. Cyst accidents include torsion, haemorrhage and rupture. Pelvic pain radiating down the inner aspect of the leg is a common presenting symptom, and torsion classically presents as severe pain associated with vomiting. Although rupture of a small cyst may be asymptomatic with few associated signs, the abdomen of a patient experiencing a cyst accident is usually tender, with guarding and rigidity. Rupture of a large cyst may produce signs of peritonitis, particularly if the cyst contents are irritant (e.g. endometriotic cyst or dermoid cyst), and the patient may be shocked in cases of extensive rupture or continuing haemorrhage.

Investigation

A complete history and examination are essential, as the diagnosis is usually based on clinical findings. The history should include information about the duration and growth of the mass. Symptoms, past history or family history increasing the likelihood of malignancy should be sought. The duration of use of combined oral contraception should be noted. General, abdominal, vaginal and rectal examinations are mandatory.

Full blood count, group and save, serum amylase, urea, electrolytes and liver function tests should be performed. Tumour markers should be measured if the mass is complex; if this information is not available, serum may be stored until histopathology has been reported. Pregnancy must be excluded and urinalysis performed. A midstream specimen of urine should be sent for culture and sensitivity. Other investigations may be indicated by the patient's condition, for example cross-match and coagulation screen in cases of haemorrhage.

A pelvic ultrasound, preferably transvaginal, will reveal the dimensions and morphology of the mass and is the single most important investigation in predicting whether an ovarian mass is benign or malignant. Most ovarian masses are cystic, but the presence of solid areas makes a tumour most likely and a malignancy possible. However, some benign tumours are solid, for example thecoma, fibroma and Brenner tumours. Thickened walls and septae are other features of malignancy. The results of colour Doppler imaging have been disappointing, and this technique has not proven superior to morphological assessment.

Diagnosis of adnexal mass

The triage of an adnexal mass into possibly benign or malignant categories can be challenging and a number of tests have been investigated in the literature.

It is important here to distinguish between post-menopausal women and pre-menopausal women, in whom the risk of ovarian cancer is low, benign adnexal cysts are very common and CA125 can be elevated frequently. A number of non-specific conditions, including menstruation, endometrioisis and peritoneal irritation secondary to haemorrhage, can contribute to a raised CA125 level. RCOG guidelines on managing pre-menopausal women with ovarian cyst recommend that patients be referred to a gynaecological oncologist if CA125 >200.[1] Alternatively, International Ovarian Tumour Analysis (IOTA) is a consortium of experts in ultrasound who have established ultrasound models hat can differentiate benign and malignant ovarian tumours.[1] (see Published guidelines).

In post-menopausal women, RCOG recommends use of the Risk of Malignancy Index (see below). However, normal levels of CA125 are found in 50 per cent of stage I ovarian cancers. Equally CA125 levels are also raised in benign conditions such as hepatorenal disease, diverticulitis, chest complaints and benign cysts. Human epididymis protein 4 (He4) is a new marker, not in routine practice in the UK, which may be of benefit.[22]

Jacobs and colleagues included ultrasound findings and menopausal status with CA125 in an algorithm termed the 'Risk of Malignancy Index' (RMI) and reported 87 per cent sensitivity, 89 per cent specificity and 75 per cent positive predictive value (given an RMI cut-off value of 200).[8] The RMI is the product of the serum CA125 level (in units per millilitre), the ultrasound score (0, 1 or 3) and the menopausal status (1 if pre-menopausal, 3 if post-menopausal: see Table 109.2). The ultrasound score is calculated by giving one point for each of the following findings:

- multilocular cyst;
- solid areas;

Table 109.2 An example of a protocol for triaging women using the risk of malignancy index (RMI)

RMI	Women (%)	Risk of cancer (%)
Low <25	40	<3
Moderate 25–250	30	20
High >250	30	75

- bilateral lesions;
- metastases;
- ascites.

The RMI provides a means of triaging women for referral to a gynaecological oncologist. The cut-off for referral to a cancer centre varies according to local practice.

ORGANISATION OF CARE IN THE UK

The use of the RMI has been endorsed by both RCOG and NICE guidelines (see Published guidelines). Since the introduction of Improving Outcomes Guidance in the United Kingdom in 1999[23], gynaecological cancer care is delivered in a hub-and-spoke model. With respect to ovarian cancer, cancer units triage patients with adnexal masses. In general, women are referred for management in the cancer centre for surgery by a gynaecological oncologist when the RMI is over 250. All women with RMI >250 should be discussed at the cancer centre multidisciplinary team meeting.

The appropriate location for the management should reflect the new structure of cancer care in the UK.[3,4] As the risk of malignancy increases, the appropriate location for management changes, so that while a general gynaecologist might manage women with a low risk of malignancy, those at intermediate risk should be managed in a cancer unit and those at high risk in a cancer centre. It is recommended that ovarian cysts in post-menopausal women should be assessed using CA125 and transvaginal grey-scale sonography. There is no routine role yet for 3D or Doppler ultrasound, MRI, CT or PET. The best prognosis for women with ovarian cancer is offered if a laparotomy and full staging procedure is carried out by a trained gynaecological oncologist.

RCOG guidance states that women should be managed as below.

Low risk: Less than 3% risk of cancer:

- Management in a gynaecology unit.
- Simple cysts less than 5 cm in diameter with a serum CA125 level of less than 30 may be managed conservatively.
- Conservative management should entail repeat ultrasound scans and serum CA125 measurement every four months for one year.
- If the cyst does not fit the above criteria or if the woman requests surgery then laparoscopic oophorectomy is acceptable.

Moderate risk: approximately 20% risk of cancer:

- Management in a cancer unit.
- Laparoscopic oophorectomy is acceptable in selected cases.
- If a malignancy is discovered then a full staging procedure should be undertaken in a cancer centre.

High risk: greater than 75% risk of cancer:

- Management in a cancer centre.
- Full staging procedure as described above.

Conservative and surgical management

Management depends on the presentation (cyst accident or asymptomatic finding) and the risk of malignancy. Surgical intervention is usually required when an ovarian cyst presents with acute symptoms, although a conservative approach may be taken in mild cases where the findings indicate a low risk of malignancy. Most functional cysts can be managed conservatively and disappear spontaneously within two cycles if managed with combined oral contraceptives or observation alone.[9] Patients with peritonitis or hypovolaemic shock require prompt resuscitation. RCOG recommends conservative management in post-menopausal women with simple unilateral cysts <5 cm and CA125 <30. These cysts can be kept under surveillance with regular transvaginal ultrasound scans and CA125 levels and women discharged from follow-up if the cyst resolves or remains unchanged at the end of one-year follow-up.

The benefits of laparoscopic surgery are widely reported, and large studies have been published demonstrating the safety and efficacy of this approach (see Published guidelines). However, specialised and skilled gynaecologists performed the surgery in these series, and the unfortunate consequences of laparoscopic management of undiagnosed ovarian cancers have been reported. If an adequate pre-operative assessment indicates that the risk of malignancy is low, a laparoscopic approach should be considered. However, laparoscopic aspiration of cysts should not be performed to make a diagnosis of cancer, as the negative predictive value of cyst fluid cytology is low in most departments and aspiration adversely affects the prognosis of a stage I malignancy. Furthermore, therapeutic aspiration of ovarian cysts is usually ineffective, as most recur. It is recommended that an RMI should be used to select women for laparoscopic surgery, to be undertaken by a suitably qualified surgeon. It is recommended that laparoscopic management of ovarian cysts in postmenopausal women should involve oophorectomy (usually bilateral) rather than cystectomy. In a post-menopausal woman the appropriate laparoscopic treatment for an ovarian cyst, which is not suitable for conservative management, is oophorectomy, with removal of the ovary intact in a bag without cyst rupture into the peritoneal cavity.

Patients at intermediate risk of malignancy may also be considered for laparoscopic assessment when the operator is skilled, there is a safe method of retrieval of the mass and there are facilities for prompt frozen section analysis. In this situation, access to immediate surgical staging must be available. All patients with obvious malignancy should be referred to a gynaecological oncologist for further management. The role of laparoscopy in the management of ovarian cancer is not proven and is not in routine practice in the UK.

At laparoscopy, a careful assessment is performed and washings taken. If the findings are suspicious for malignancy, a biopsy is taken if metastases or surface excrescences are identified. An appropriate procedure is then rescheduled following the results of histopathology (see below). If there are no suspicious findings, the surgeon may proceed to cystectomy or oophorectomy as indicated.

> ### KEY POINTS
>
> - At the present time, there is no role for ovarian screening in the asymptomatic population.
> - All women presenting with vague pelvi-abdominal symptoms warrant a complete history and examination, including vaginal.
> - The RMI is used to stratify the risk of ovarian cancer for women with an ovarian cyst and to identify cases for referral to a gynaecological oncologist.

CLINICAL MANAGEMENT OF OVARIAN CANCER

Clinical presentation and diagnosis

Primary ovarian cancer is most common in women in the seventh decade of life. Hereditary cancers usually present in younger women, occurring approximately 10 years earlier. Most women with Ovarian cancer have non specific symptoms. A complete history and examination are essential to make the diagnosis, to identify patients with secondary ovarian malignancy and to assess fitness for surgical and non-surgical management.

Symptoms

When the tumour is confined to the ovary, the patient may present with pressure symptoms (urinary frequency, constipation, pelvic pain/pressure, dyspareunia) and, rarely, symptoms of a cyst accident. In advanced-stage disease, symptoms are usually due to metastases affecting the bowel and mesentery, and ascites. Resulting symptoms (bloating, constipation, early satiety, loss of appetite) may be misinterpreted as irritable bowel syndrome. Symptoms due to pressure effects in the pelvis may also occur. Abnormal vaginal bleeding (in pre-menopausal and post-menopausal women) is a less common presenting feature. Unfortunately, given that symptoms in ovarian cancer are so vague, delays in presentation to the GP and subsequent delay in diagnosis are common and well known.

Clinical signs

Assessment should include examination of supraclavicular, axillary and inguinal nodes, breast examination, chest examination (pleural effusion) and abdominal examination, including assessment of liver size. In women presenting with the above symptoms, a pelvic examination (including per-rectal examination) is mandatory. The presence of a solid, irregular mass is highly suspicious, particularly when associated with an upper abdominal mass (omental cake).

Investigations

Investigations are performed to assess the likelihood of malignant disease, to assess fitness for anaesthesia and surgery, and to plan the extent of surgery. Ultrasonography (see above) should include assessment not just of the pelvis but also of the kidneys and liver. Liver parenchymal metastases increase the likelihood of a non-ovarian primary, and significant hydronephrosis should be identified pre-operatively. Chest imaging is essential. CA125 (see above) and carcinoembryonic antigen (CEA) levels should be measured, the latter to identify primary gastrointestinal malignancy. In young women <40 years, AFP and b-hCG levels should also be measured, as germ-cell tumours are the commonest gynaecological malignancy in the first two decades of life. Full blood count, urea, creatinine, electrolytes and liver function tests (including total protein and albumin) should also be done.

CT scan of the abdomen and pelvis can be very helpful in delineating the extent of upper abdominal disease and can guide choice between primary surgery or chemotherapy. MRI of the pelvis may also assist surgical planning in patients with a fixed pelvic mass to determine adherence to large bowel or the pelvic sidewalls. A chest X-ray must be performed to assess the possibility of Stage IV disease (see Table 109.3). In patients with abnormal vaginal bleeding, full assessment of the cervix and uterus, including outpatient endometrial biopsy, should be considered as an ovarian mass may be the site of secondary spread from a primary cervical or endometrial carcinoma. Endoscopy of the upper or lower gastrointestinal tract is indicated in women whose symptoms, tumour marker profile or CT suggest a primary gastrointestinal malignancy.

Staging of primary ovarian cancer

Ovarian cancers are staged according to FIGO recommendations (Table 109.4). Staging is based on findings at laparotomy, but pre-operative assessment is required to assess extraperitoneal spread. Accurate staging is of paramount importance, as it determines not only prognosis but also to a large extent the requirement for adjuvant treatment. FIGO reports the five-year survival of patients with stage I disease as 70 per cent. This is in contrast to survival rates of more than 90 per cent reported in studies on patients with properly staged disease, and suggests that a significant proportion of women are not undergoing careful surgical staging. Gynaecological Cancer Intergroup (GCIG) recommendations to FIGO staging suggest that in early-stage disease, grading and in advanced disease, the amount of residual disease must be reported.

FIGO staging (Table 109.4)

Staging for ovarian cancer was revised at the end of 2013.[24] The new classification allows for surgical rupture of cyst to be clearly distinguished from pre-operative rupture and also quantifies the extent of lymph node metastasis.

Technique for surgical staging

A midline incision extending above the umbilicus is essential to allow adequate access for thorough surgical staging and should be performed whenever an ovarian malignancy is anticipated. A systematic exploration of all peritoneal surfaces and viscera is performed. The staging laparotomy involves the following steps:

- sending ascites or peritoneal washings for cytological assessment;
- performing a total abdominal hysterectomy and bilateral salpingo-ophorectomy (TAH/BSO);
- omentectomy;
- peritoneal biopsies of all suspicious areas;
- assessment of pelvic and para-aortic lymph nodes;
- careful assessment of upper abdomen including diaphragm, liver, spleen, lesser sac, Morrison's pouch

The rationale for TAH/BSO is the high incidence of bilateral tumours (metastatic or primary) and metastases to the uterus. Furthermore, the endometrium may be the site of a coincidental primary carcinoma, particularly in the case of endometrioid carcinoma of the ovary. The omentum is removed, as it is the major site of abdominal metastases. An infra-colic omentectomy is most universally performed, but a supracolic procedure may be preferable and, indeed, is often essential to achieve adequate cytoreduction of gross omental disease. Washings may be positive in apparent stage Ia disease, substantially altering decision making with regard to adjuvant treatment.

Table 109.3 illustrates the rate of occult metastases when adequate surgical staging is performed by combining results from 13 published series involving a total of over 1000 cases.

Appendicectomy has not yet been universally accepted as part of the standard procedure but is currently under consideration. However, the appendix is commonly the site of metastases in advanced-stage disease and is reported to be a site of occult disease in a significant proportion of apparent stage I disease as

Table 109.3 Metastases in apparent early-stage epithelial ovarian carcinoma, presented as percentages. Adapted with permission from: Moore DH. Primary surgical management of early epithelial ovarian carcinoma. *In*: Rubin CR, Sutton GP (eds). *Ovarian Cancer*. 2nd edn. Philadelphia: Lippincott Williams and Wilkins, 2001, 201–18.

Percentage of cases with occult metastases	
Diaphragm	7.6
Omentum	7.1
Cytology	18.8
Peritoneum	9.8
Pelvic lymph nodes	8.9
Para-aortic lymph nodes	12.3

Table 109.4 International Federation of Gynecology and Obstetrics (FIGO) 2013 staging

Stage I	Tumour is confined to the ovary/ovaries or Fallopian tube(s)
IA	Only one ovary or Fallopian tube is affected by the tumour, the ovary capsule is intact
	No tumour is detected on the surface of the ovary or Fallopian tube
	Malignant cells are not detected in ascites or peritoneal washings
IB	Both ovaries or Fallopian tubes are affected by the tumour, the ovary capsule is intact
	No tumour is detected on the surface of the ovaries or Fallopian tube
	Malignant cells are not detected in ascites or peritoneal washings
IC	The tumour is limited to one or both ovaries or Fallopian tubes, with any of the following: Surgical spill The ovary capsule is ruptured before surgery The tumour is detected on the ovary or fallopian tube surface Malignant cells are detected in the ascites or peritoneal washings
Stage II	Tumour involves one or both ovaries or Fallopian tubes with pelvic extension (below pelvic brim) or primary peritoneal cancer
IIA	The tumour has extended and/or implanted into the uterus and/or the fallopian tubes and/or ovaries
IIB	The tumour has extended to another organ in the pelvis
Stage III	The tumour involves one or both ovaries or Fallopian tubes, or primary peritoneal cancer, with confirmed (cytologically or histologically) spread to the peritoneal surfaces involving both pelvic and abdominal peritoneum and/or metastasis to the retroperitoneal lymph nodes
IIIA1	Positive retroperitoneal lymph nodes only (cytologically or histologically proven) Metastasis up to 10 mm in greatest dimension Metastasis more than 10 mm in greatest dimension
IIIA2	Microscopic extrapelvic peritoneal involvement with or without positive retroperitoneal lymph nodes
IIIB	Microscopic peritoneal metastasis beyond the pelvis 2 cm in greatest dimension, with or without metastasis to the retroperitoneal lymph nodes
IIIC	Microscopic peritoneal metastasis beyond the pelvis 2 cm in greatest dimension, with or without metastasis to the retroperitoneal lymph nodes (includes extension of tumour to capsule of liver and spleen without parenchymal involvement of either organ)
Stage IV	Distant metastasis beyond the peritoneal cavity (including parenchymal liver/splenic metastases and extra-abdominal metastases
IVA	Pleural effusion with positive cytology
IVB	Parenchymal metastases and metastases to extra-abdominal organs (including inguinal lymph nodes and lymph nodes outside of the abdominal cavity)

well. Furthermore, the ovary may be a site of secondary disease in the rare case of an appendiceal primary and may be associated with pseudomyxoma peritoneii. It should be removed if it appears abnormal at laparotomy.

SURGICAL AND NON-SURGICAL MANAGEMENT OF OVARIAN CANCER

The management of ovarian cancer is discussed below in seven consecutive sections.

Primary surgery: early epithelial ovarian cancer

In cases of early-stage disease, the surgical objective is to identify occult metastases through meticulous systematic exploration. The commonest pattern of metastatic spread of epithelial ovarian cancer is transcoelomic. The cells disseminate and implant along the peritoneal surfaces following the circulatory path of peritoneal fluid. Lymphatic dissemination to pelvic and para-aortic nodes is also common and may occur in apparent early-stage disease. Haematogenous spread is uncommon at the time of diagnosis, but the liver and lung are the preferred sites. The importance of adequate surgical staging in apparent early disease cannot be overemphasised.

The standard surgical procedure for early-stage disease has already been described. However, when operating on a young patient for whom fertility is important, it is advisable to perform an adequate staging procedure while minimising the risk to future fertility. Although frozen section may be useful if it produces a definitive diagnosis of malignancy, the heterogeneity and size of ovarian malignancies result in under-diagnosis in a considerable proportion of cases. Delaying a sterilising procedure until the final histopathology is available allows a decision regarding further surgical management to be made in consultation with the patient. An initial procedure in such a case would involve complete surgical staging as described, but the uterus and contralateral ovary would be left *in situ* following careful inspection. A decision regarding completion of surgery and adjuvant treatment should then be made in consultation with the patient and based on the advice of the cancer centre's multidisciplinary team.

Laparotomy is currently the gold-standard surgical procedure for the diagnosis and staging of early ovarian cancer. The role of laparoscopy is undefined and it should only be used as part of well-designed prospective clinical trials.

Primary surgery: advanced epithelial ovarian cancer

In contrast with early ovarian cancer, the surgical emphasis in advanced disease is on tumour cytoreduction. Cytoreductive surgery typically involves performing a TAH/BSO, complete omentectomy and resection of any metastases.

Complete cytoreduction i.e. removal of all visible cancer deposits is the goal of surgery in ovarian cancer. If this is not possible, the surgeon aims to reduce the tumour load to achieve 'optimal' status (no residual disease >1 cm).

Resectability of disease depends not only on the skill of the surgeon, but also on the site of disease. Optimal cytoreduction is unlikely if there is extensive disease in the liver parenchyma, porta hepatis or root of the small bowel mesentery.

Retrospective data suggest that this type of surgery is feasible in 70–90 per cent of cases when performed by a gynaecological oncologist.

Ultra-radical surgery in ovarian cancer

Recently, centres of excellence from the United States and Europe have published single institutional case series that demonstrate a marked improvement in progression-free and overall survival by the utilisation of complex surgical procedures (radical and ultra-radical surgery) that result in complete removal of all cancer deposits in addition to standard surgery to remove the uterus and ovaries.[25-28] A Cochrane review of studies comparing standard vs radical/ultra-radical surgery showed that the utilisation of extensive surgery to remove all cancer deposits in addition to conventional

surgery can significantly improve survival in women with carcinomatosis (adjusted HR = 0.64, 95% CI 0.41–0.98).[29] NICE recommends that complete cytoreduction be the aim of surgery in ovarian cancer. Currently, there is no RCT evidence evaluating supra-radical surgery and other key factors including the quality of life in these women are not known. Verleye *et al.* have published a series of quality standards to be maintained in patients undergoing surgery in ovarian cancer.[30]

Major morbidity from such procedures is approximately 1–3 per cent and operative mortality 1 per cent. Although prognosis depends on the extent of residual disease following surgery, it is also determined by the patient's age, the volume of ascites and performance status (independent prognostic variables). In planning management, these factors must be taken into consideration.

A prospective multicentre observational study of outcomes, including patient reported outcomes (Quality of life) is now underway, www.birmingham.ac.uk/SOCQER. It is also possible that the biology of the disease determines resectability and prognosis. The only prospective randomised trial of cytoreductive surgery [Ib][11] has demonstrated a survival advantage for patients randomised to a second resection of disease as an interval procedure.[31]

TIMING OF SURGERY – PRIMARY SURGERY VERSUS INTERVAL DEBULKING SURGERY AFTER NEOADJUVANT CHEMOTHERAPY

It has been known for some time that patients who have no residual disease after surgery and those who respond to platinum – 'platinum sensitive' patients – have the best survival after ovarian cancer. Two important trials have investigated the role of timing of surgery with relation to chemotherapy – EORTC and CHORUS. These multicentre RCTs investigated whether primary surgery followed by chemotherapy or surgery after neoadjuvant chemotherapy (chemotherapy where three or four cycles are given pre-surgery) would lead to more complete cytoreductive surgery and survival. Both trials have now reported and are consistent in their findings that in patients with large tumour burden and poor performance status, both approaches – primary surgery or interval debulking surgery after neoadjuvant chemotherapy had similar survival outcomes. Interval debulking surgery was associated with lesser morbidity and a reduced number of major resections.[32]

It is therefore clear that women who have complete interval cytoreduction have outcomes equivalent to those of patients who have optimal surgery performed as a primary procedure. Therefore, in cases in which initial surgery has involved biopsy only, with no attempt at cytoreduction of advanced disease, it is reasonable to consider definitive surgery after three cycles of chemotherapy, with three further cycles being given following surgery.

GYNAECOLOGICAL ONCOLOGY

KEY POINTS

- The importance of adequate surgical staging in apparent early-stage ovarian cancer cannot be overemphasised.
- Primary cytoreductive surgery followed by chemotherapy has similar survival outcomes to interval debulking surgery in patients with advanced ovarian carcinoma, in patients with poor performance status and large tumour burden.

CHEMOTHERAPY

In general, it is agreed that patients with (adequately staged) low-grade stage IA and IB disease have a very good prognosis and do not require adjuvant treatment [Ia].

However, patients with early-stage disease and poor prognostic factors *may* benefit from adjuvant treatment, as they have a substantial risk of micrometastases. Two large randomised trials addressing this issue (ICON-1 and ACTION – over 900 patients studied) demonstrate a statistically significant improvement in recurrence-free survival and overall survival in women receiving adjuvant chemotherapy if they had not been completely staged at surgery. A multivariate analysis of studies of prognostic variables involving 1545 patients found that degree of differentiation and cyst rupture were independent poor prognosticators. This topic has been reviewed by Winter-Roach *et al.*[33]

Currently, for patients with high-risk early-stage disease and for advanced-stage ovarian cancer, the recommended standard treatment is combination chemotherapy with carboplatin and paclitaxel, or carboplatin alone, for six cycles. The latter is usually preferred in less fit patients.

Pelvic radiation alone is not as effective as adjuvant treatment but may be occasionally used to palliate isolated pelvic recurrence, for example a bleeding mass at the vaginal vault.

ICON-7 is a multicentre RCT that evaluated the addition of an antiangiogenic agent, bevazicumab, to carboplatin/taxol chemotherapy. This trial demonstrated that in stage IV cancer and in those with residual disease after surgery, bevazicumab concurrent with chemotherapy and maintenance up to 12 months showed significant improvement in survival over standard chemotherapy.[34] The drug is also commonly used in recurrent cancer, in the first relapse setting. Intraperitoneal chemotherapy also shows great promise after a number of trials demonstrated that administering chemotherapy intraperitoneally confers significant improvement in survival after the patient has been completely cytoreduced. However, critics of intraperitoneal chemotherapy point to the high toxicity rates associated with this form of treatment. At the present time, the role of intraperitoneal chemotherapy is unclear. The PETROC trial should finally address this question comprehensively and is ongoing.

Although 70 per cent of patients receiving adjuvant chemotherapy will respond initially to platinum-based chemotherapy at least half will relapse within 18 months. Treatment at relapse is palliative in intent. With the increasing use of supportive factors such as granulocyte colony-stimulating factor (G-CSF) in chemotherapy, patients receive more cycles of chemotherapy and more lines of chemotherapy than previously and survival for five to six years is achievable in a minority. Carboplatin and taxol are first choice for relapse six or more months (platinum-sensitive or partially sensitive disease) after completing previous chemotherapy. Second-line chemotherapy (combinations different to carboplatin with or without taxol) is indicated in cases of recurrent or progressive platinum-resistant or refractory disease. Response rates are much lower than for primary treatment for second-line therapy (15–35 per cent vs 80 per cent), although better response rates are found in women with longer disease-free intervals before recurrence. In patients with platinum-sensitive disease (i.e. women with a progression-free interval of at least 12 months since platinum-based therapy), re-treatment with platinum or paclitaxel is appropriate. In platinum-resistant cases, an agent without cross-resistance is required. These include alkylating agents (liposomal doxorubicin), gemcitabine, anthracyclines, topoisomerase inhibitors (etoposide, topotecan) and others (tamoxifen). There is some evidence from observational studies that tamoxifen may produce a response in a modest proportion of women with relapsed ovarian cancer. Single-agent regimens are often adopted due to ease of administration and low toxicity.

The OVO5 trial clarifies that monitoring patients who have been treated for ovarian cancer with serial CA125 and administering chemotherapy on the basis of rising CA125 levels in asymptomatic patients does not improve survival in comparison to re-treatment with chemotherapy when the patient becomes symptomatic of recurrence.[35]

This means it is reasonable to manage patients with symptom-based follow-up rather than serial measurements of CA125.

KEY POINTS

- Additional therapy may be considered for patients who have early-stage disease associated with high-risk factors.
- Standard adjuvant therapy for ovarian cancer involves intravenous chemotherapy.
- Response rates to second-line chemotherapy are much lower than for primary treatment.
- Patients with low-grade stage IA and IB disease do not require adjuvant treatment [Ia].
- In stage I invasive epithelial ovarian carcinoma, degree of differentiation, capsular penetrance, surface excrescences, malignant ascites and cyst rupture are independent poor prognosticators [Ia].
- Platinum-based therapy is better than non-platinum therapy [Ia] and combination therapy improves survival compared with platinum alone [Ia].
- The addition of bevazicumab to chemotherapy marginally improves survival in a subset of patients with stage IV or incompletely resected disease but is associated with more morbidity.

SECONDARY CYTOREDUCTIVE SURGERY

As complete cytoreductive surgery is associated with improved outcomes in patients with advanced ovarian cancer, it has been suggested that there is a role for debulking in patients with persistent or recurrent disease. This group of patients is highly heterogeneous, but may be broadly categorised as follows:

- patients with persistent disease following completion of primary treatment;
- patients with recurrent disease after completion of primary treatment.

Patients with persistent or recurrent disease following completion of primary treatment

Patients whose disease progresses during chemotherapy, those with persistent disease at the completion of chemotherapy and those who develop recurrence early have a limited median survival. Treatment should therefore be directed at optimising quality of life. As a result, cytoreductive surgery is rarely indicated in these groups. However, patients who have had complete clinical responses to primary treatment and who develop localised recurrences, with no ascites after a disease-free interval of six months or more, may benefit from cytoreductive surgery. Best prognostic indicators suggest reserving this approach for single-site recurrence with good performance status, no ascites and where optimal debulking had previously been achieved. A large multicentre trial is now underway (DESKTOPIII) to address the issue of whether secondary surgery or chemotherapy is better for survival in this setting.

PALLIATIVE SURGERY

The most common indication for palliative surgery is bowel obstruction, which is a common feature of recurrent disease but may also be the presenting feature in undiagnosed patients. Most patients have small-bowel obstruction, approximately one third have large-bowel obstruction and a minority have both. However, in many cases of small-bowel obstruction due to ovarian cancer, the site of obstruction is not single and on occasions the entire small bowel is rendered dysfunctional due to extensive peritoneal and mesenteric involvement (carcinomatous ileus). As these latter cases are not amenable to surgery, careful case selection is the essence of good management. Surgery may involve bowel resection, but most commonly intestinal bypass and/or stoma formation is required.

The median survival for patients undergoing palliative surgery for bowel obstruction is 3–12 months. Those who are young, with a good nutritional status (normal albumin levels) and who do not have rapidly accumulating ascites have the best prognosis. Reported morbidity and mortality rates are 30 per cent and 10 per cent respectively.

TARGETED THERAPIES IN OVARIAN CANCER

Given current survival rates there is great scope to improve survival from ovarian cancer with targeted therapies. Current large trials investigate PARP inhibitors for patients with *BRCA* mutations. Recent drugs that have shown positive improvements in progression-free and overall survival in the recurrence setting are bevazucimab, an antiangiogenic agent, and cediranib, a multiple tyrosine kinase inhibitor. Several targeted agents are in early-phase trials and in the pipeline. However scheduling of these agents with conventional chemotherapy and choice of which agent to use to obtain optimal benefit for the patient are questions that have not been answered. Funding of these agents remains under purview of NICE reviews.

MANAGEMENT OF RARER TUMOUR TYPES

Borderline ovarian tumours

Approximately 15 per cent of epithelial ovarian tumours are borderline (tumours of low malignant potential). They affect younger women than primary epithelial ovarian cancers and may present in pregnancy. They are usually of low stage and have a very good prognosis. Surgical resection is the primary modality of treatment, as there are no prospective data suggesting that adjuvant treatment prolongs survival. Pre-menopausal women who wish to preserve fertility may be treated by conservative surgery (recurrence rate is about 7 per cent in women managed by conservative surgery). Nonetheless, it should be emphasised that a small subgroup of these patients has rapidly progressive disease and a poor prognosis. Long-term follow-up is advised, as late recurrences do occur. Higher stage, incomplete staging, residual tumour after surgery and cystectomy rather than oophorectomy are independent prognostic factors for disease recurrence.[36]

Germ-cell tumours of the ovary

Adequate surgical staging, removal of primary tumour and adjuvant chemotherapy is current standard therapy for germ-cell tumours of the ovary. As these malignancies usually occur in young women, conservation of the contralateral ovary and uterus is appropriate. However, the importance of a complete and thorough staging procedure cannot be underestimated – patients with stage IA dysgerminoma and stage I, grade 1 immature teratoma require no further therapy if comprehensively staged. All other patients should be treated with three or more cycles of combination chemotherapy (bleomycin, etoposide and cisplatin). Most patients with these tumours are cured of disease and most survivors can anticipate normal menstrual and reproductive function. Tumour markers are often useful in monitoring disease and planning management. In the UK, the care of women with germ-cell tumours is centralised, with three key centres at Charing Cross, Dundee and Sheffield coordinating care. This is likely to improve outcomes and facilitate research in this poorly studied field.

Sex-cord stromal tumours

Although they are reported to be most common among post-menopausal women, these tumours often affect children and young adults. They are the most hormonally active of all ovarian tumours and there is an association with endometrial hyperplasia and well-differentiated adenocarcinoma of the endometrium. Surgery is the cornerstone of management, but early-stage disease may be managed by unilateral oophorectomy and endometrial biopsy when fertility sparing is important. Late recurrence is the hallmark of these tumours.

Pseudomyxoma peritoneii

This condition involves the accumulation of gelatinous material in the peritoneal cavity. It occurs in association with mucinous tumours of the appendix and/or ovary. It is extremely rare and has a very poor prognosis. Cases should be referred for specialist opinion as early as possible. There are two centres in the UK, at the Christie Hospital in Manchester and in Basingstoke. A histopathological diagnosis of pseudomyxoma ovarii would warrant such a referral.

QUALITY OF LIFE

Most patients with ovarian cancer present late and die of the disease. Cure is the ultimate goal of patient and oncologist, but is not achieved for the majority. Therefore a careful balance must be struck between the pursuit of that goal and optimisation of the quality of the period of life remaining. Specific treatments and their potential impact on disease must be weighed against the morbidity of each therapy. The optimum balance between these opposing aims will be different for each patient. The informed patient's voice is critical to finding the best compromise for her and should be heard. Management decisions should be made with the balance of probabilities and the patient's desires clearly in focus.

CONCLUSION

The management of ovarian cancer represents a major challenge and requires close multidisciplinary team working amongst medical, clinical and surgical oncologists, radiologists, pathologists, clinical nurse specialists and specialists in palliative care. The centralisation of gynaecological cancer services has improved compliance with management guidelines, provided specialist training and treatment, facilitated research and consequently improved patient care and outcomes which are particularly pertinent to the care of women with ovarian cancer.

Published Guidelines

RCOG guideline no 34. *Management of ovarian cysts in post-menopausal women.* http://www.rcog.org.uk/files/rcog-corp/GTG34OvarianCysts.pdf

RCOG guideline no 62. *Management of ovarian cysts in pre-menopausal women.* http://www.rcog.org.uk/files/rcog-corp/GTG62_021211_OvarianMasses.pdf

NICE guidance (CG122). *Recognition and initial management of ovarian cancer.* http://www.nice.org.uk/cg122.

NICE Interventional Procedures guidance. *Ultra-radical (extensive) surgery for advanced ovarian cancer.* https://www.nice.org.uk/guidance/ipg470.

References

1. RCOG/BSGE. Green-top guideline No: 62. *Management of suspected ovarian masses in pre-menopausal women.* London: RCOG, November 2011.
2. Vernooij F, Heintz AP, Witteveen PO, van der Heiden-van der Loo M, Coebergh JW, van der Graaf Y. Specialized care and survival of ovarian cancer patients in The Netherlands: nationwide cohort study. *J Natl Cancer Inst* 2008;100(6):399–406.
3. Vernooij F, Heintz P, Witteveen E, van der Graaf Y. The outcomes of ovarian cancer treatment are better when provided by gynecologic oncologists and in specialized hospitals: a systematic review. *Gynecol Oncol* 2007;105(3):801–12.
4. CRUK. http://www.cancerresearchuk.org/cancer-info/cancerstats/types/ovary/incidence/uk-ovarian-cancer-incidence-statistics, 2014.
5. CRUK. http://www.cancerresearchuk.org/cancer-info/cancerstats/types/ovary/mortality/, 2014.
6. CRUK. http://www.cancerresearchuk.org/cancer-info/cancerstats/types/ovary/incidence/uk-ovarian-cancer-incidence-statistics, 2013.
7. IARC WHO Classification of Tumours of Female Reproductive Organs. Fourth Edition, 2014.
8. CRUK. http://www.cancerresearchuk.org/cancer-info/cancerstats/types/ovary/survival/ovarian-cancer-survival-statistics, 2013.

9. Vaughan S, Coward JI, Bast RC, Jr et al. Rethinking ovarian cancer: recommendations for improving outcomes. *Nat Rev Cancer* 2011;11(10):719–25.

10. Network CGAR. Integrated genomic analyses of ovarian carcinoma. *Nature* 2011;474(7353):609–15.

11. Alsop K, Fereday S, Meldrum C et al. BRCA mutation frequency and patterns of treatment response in BRCA mutation-positive women with ovarian cancer: a report from the Australian Ovarian Cancer Study Group. *J Clin Oncol* 2012;30(21):2654–63.

12. Lowe KA, Chia VM, Taylor A et al. An international assessment of ovarian cancer incidence and mortality. *Gynecol Oncol* 2013;130(1):107–14.

13. Lee Y, Miron A, Drapkin R et al. A candidate precursor to serous carcinoma that originates in the distal fallopian tube. *J Pathol* 2007;211(1):26–35.

14. McAlpine JN, Hanley GE, Woo MM et al. Opportunistic salpingectomy: uptake, risks, and complications of a regional initiative for ovarian cancer prevention. *Am J Obstet Gynecol* 2014; 210(5):471.e1–11

15. Narod SA, Sun P, Risch HA. Ovarian cancer, oral contraceptives, and BRCA mutations. *N Engl J Med* 2001;345(23):1706–7.

16. Manchanda R, Burnell M, Abdelraheim A et al. Factors influencing uptake and timing of risk-reducing salpingo-oophorectomy in women at risk of familial ovarian cancer: a competing risk time to event analysis. *BJOG* 2012;119(5):527–536.

17. Buys SS, Partridge E, Black A et al. Effect of screening on ovarian cancer mortality: the Prostate, Lung, Colorectal and Ovarian (PLCO) Cancer Screening Randomized Controlled Trial. *JAMA* 2011;305(22):2295–303.

18. Menon U, Gentry-Maharaj A, Hallett R et al. Sensitivity and specificity of multimodal and ultrasound screening for ovarian cancer, and stage distribution of detected cancers: results of the prevalence screen of the UK Collaborative Trial of Ovarian Cancer Screening (UKCTOCS). *Lancet Oncol* 2009;10(4):327–40.

19. NICE. *The recognition and initial management of ovarian cancer* (CG122). NICE, April 2011.

20. Gilbert L, Basso O, Sampalis J et al. Assessment of symptomatic women for early diagnosis of ovarian cancer: results from the prospective DOvE pilot project. *Lancet Oncol* 2012;13(3):285–91.

21. Andersen MR, Lowe KA, Goff BA. Value of symptom-triggered diagnostic evaluation for ovarian cancer. *Obstet Gynecol* 2014;123(1):73–9.

22. Wu L, Dai ZY, Qian YH, Shi Y, Liu FJ, Yang C. Diagnostic value of serum human epididymis protein 4 (HE4) in ovarian carcinoma: a systematic review and meta-analysis. *Int J Gynecol Cancer* 2012;22(7):1106–12.

23. NHS Executive, Department of Health. *Guidance on Commissioning Cancer Services. Improving Outcomes in Gynaecological Cancers.* 1999. http://webarchive.nationalarchives.gov.uk/20130107105354/http://www.dh.gov. uk/prod_consum_dh/groups/dh_digitalassets/@dh/en/documents/digitalasset/dh_4083846.pdf

24. Prat J. Staging classification for cancer of the ovary, fallopian tube, and peritoneum. *Int J Gynaecol Obstet* 2014;124(1):1–5.

25. Aletti GD, Podratz KC, Moriarty JP, Cliby WA, Long KH. Aggressive and complex surgery for advanced ovarian cancer: an economic analysis. *Gynecol Oncol* 2009;112(1):16–21.

26. Chi DS, Eisenhauer EL, Zivanovic O et al. Improved progression-free and overall survival in advanced ovarian cancer as a result of a change in surgical paradigm. *Gynecol Oncol* 2009;114(1):26–31.

27. Eisenhauer EL, Abu-Rustum NR, Sonoda Y, Aghajanian C, Barakat RR, Chi DS. The effect of maximal surgical cytoreduction on sensitivity to platinum-taxane chemotherapy and subsequent survival in patients with advanced ovarian cancer. *Gynecol Oncol* 2008;108(2):276–81.

28. Eisenhauer EL, Abu-Rustum NR, Sonoda Y et al. The addition of extensive upper abdominal surgery to achieve optimal cytoreduction improves survival in patients with stages IIIC-IV epithelial ovarian cancer. *Gynecol Oncol* 2006;103(3):1083–90.

29. Ang C, Chan KK, Bryant A, Naik R, Dickinson HO. Ultra-radical (extensive) surgery versus standard surgery for the primary cytoreduction of advanced epithelial ovarian cancer. *Cochrane Database Syst Rev* 2011;4:CD007697.

30. Verleye L, Ottevanger PB, van der Graaf W, Reed NS, Vergote I. EORTC-GCG process quality indicators for ovarian cancer surgery. *Eur J Cancer* 2009;45(4):517–526.

31. van der Burg ME, van Lent M, Buyse M et al. The effect of debulking surgery after induction chemotherapy on the prognosis in advanced epithelial ovarian cancer. Gynecological Cancer Cooperative Group of the European Organization for Research and Treatment of Cancer. *N Engl J Med* 1995;332(10):629–34.

32. Vergote I, Trope CG, Amant F et al. Neoadjuvant chemotherapy or primary surgery in stage IIIC or IV ovarian cancer. *N Engl J Med* 2010;363(10):943–53.

33. Winter-Roach B, Hooper L, Kitchener H. Systematic review of adjuvant therapy for early stage (epithelial) ovarian cancer. *Int J Gynecol Cancer* 2003;13(4):395–404.

34. Perren TJ, Swart AM, Pfisterer J et al. A phase 3 trial of bevacizumab in ovarian cancer. *N Engl J Med* 2011;365(26):2484–96.

35. Rustin GJ, van der Burg ME, Griffin CL et al. Early versus delayed treatment of relapsed ovarian cancer (MRC OV05/EORTC 55955): a randomised trial. *Lancet* 2010;376(9747):1155–63.

36. du Bois A, Ewald-Riegler N, de Gregorio N et al. Borderline tumours of the ovary: A cohort study of the Arbeitsgemeinschaft Gynakologische Onkologie (AGO) Study Group. *Eur J Cancer* 2013;49(8):1905–14.

Chapter 110 Vulval and vaginal cancer

John Tidy

INTRODUCTION

Vulval and vaginal cancers are rare, accounting for about 1000 new cases per year in the UK. It is important to recognise the symptoms and signs associated with these cancers to make an early diagnosis. As in all cancers, appropriate treatment at an early stage in the disease will lead to a better outcome for the patient, as reported by a population-based study of a series of 411 women in the West Midlands [D].[1] Most of the evidence for the management of these cancers is derived from case-controlled series, and the rarity of these tumours is a major obstacle in undertaking randomised trials.

VULVAL CANCER

Vulval cancer is a disease primarily of the older age group, with the majority of cases presenting between the ages of 60 and 75. An increasing proportion of young women do present with this disease and therefore this diagnosis must always be borne in mind.

Approximately 800 new cases of vulval cancer are diagnosed in the UK each year. The incidence has remained steady over the past three to four decades despite the increasing recognition of patients with vulval intraepithelial neoplasia (VIN). The majority (90–95 per cent) of vulval carcinomas are of squamous origin, although adenocarcinomas can arise from the Bartholin's gland and also in conjunction with Paget's disease of the vulva. Melanoma of the vulva is the second most common malignancy arising in the vulva, accounting for 4–9 per cent of cases. Basal cell and verrucous carcinomas also occur in the vulva.

Aetiology

Pathology

Certain pre-existing vulval dermatoses are known to be associated with the development of vulval carcinoma. VIN is often found in association with vulval cancer and VIN-3 is regarded as a pre-invasive condition. The risk of this condition progressing to invasive cancer is highly variable, according to the literature. In women who have previously been treated for VIN, the risk is estimated at between 7 and 8 per cent,[2] whereas in one study in which women remained untreated, the progression rate of VIN to invasive cancer was 80 per cent at 10 years [D].[3] Lichen sclerosus is a common vulval inflammatory dermatosis affecting older women and is generally thought to carry an increased chance of malignant progression, although the exact risk is unknown because the ascertainment of LS is inexact. Recently it has been postulated that women with LS who develop differentiated VIN are at greatest risk of progressing to invasive cancer.[4] Differentiated VIN is more frequently associated with invasive cancers compared with undifferentiated VIN and other dermatoses. In the past this condition may have gone unrecognised and so unreported. Extramammary Paget's disease of the vulva is a rare form of VIN and is occasionally associated with cancer of the apocrine gland.

Molecular biology

Approximately 30 per cent of all vulval cancers are associated with human papillomavirus and about 80–90 per cent of these vulval cancers develop in women under the age of 50.

Variations in the cell-cycle regulatory protein p53 are reported in approximately 30 per cent of cancers and for the remainder there currently appears to be no aetiological or molecular biological event. Recent studies have shown similar molecular changes, including alterations in p53 expression, to be present in both vulval cancer and the surrounding LS.

Smoking may be an important cofactor in the development of HPV-related VIN and is linked to a lower survival rate for women with vulval cancer.

> ## KEY POINTS
>
> ### Vulval cancer: epidemiology and pathology
> 1. Vulval cancer is uncommon and most evidence arises from observational studies and case series.
> 2. Population-based observational studies confirm better outcomes with early detection.
> 3. There appear to be different aetiologies; one linked to infection with oncogenic HPV and another linked to pre-existing vulval maturation disorders.
> 4. The reported malignant potential of VIN varies between 5 and 80 per cent. This probably reflects the variations in the observational studies rather than a widely varying biological effect.

Diagnosis

Women with vulval cancer usually present with symptoms, although an asymptomatic mass may be an unusual presentation. The associated symptoms are usually vulval soreness and itching and there may be a mass that is painful and bleeds. Investigation of post-menopausal bleeding should always include examination of the vulva. The most common site of involvement is the labium majus (about 50 per cent of cases). The labium minus accounts for 15–20 per cent of cases. The clitoris and Bartholin's glands are less frequently involved. In the majority of cases, a vulval cancer is obvious to the alert clinician, but very early cancers may be clinically indistinguishable from florid warty VIN.

Investigations

When women present with vulval symptoms, a full clinical examination should be performed, paying particular attention to palpation of the groins for lymphadenopathy. A full-thickness biopsy should be taken from the tumour and should include the interface between the apparent normal surrounding tissue and the cancer. This allows for the most accurate histological interpretation and for the depth of invasion to be assessed, which is important in determining the future management. The cervix should be visualised to exclude a cervical cancer, which may occasionally coexist. Assessment of the inguinal glands is not absolutely reliable with any imaging technique at present, but should there be a clinical suspicion of inguinal lymph node enlargement, a

CT or MRI assessment of the pelvis should be undertaken to exclude obvious pelvic lymphadenopathy.

Treatment

There is increasing emphasis placed on the individualisation of treatment for women with vulval cancer. In deciding the optimum treatment, it is best to consider early and advanced vulval cancers separately and to manage the primary lesion and the regional lymph glands on individual merit. Because of the rarity of vulval cancer, and the need for careful assessment to optimise both vulval preservation and care, these women should be managed by specialised gynaecological oncologists in cancer centres. In addition to imaging, the pathological assessment of these tumours is extremely important in forming decisions about adjuvant treatment. All cases must be discussed at the local specialist gynaecological oncology MDT meeting.

Early stage vulval cancer

Primary lesion
Treatment of the primary lesion is in part determined by the risk of local vulval recurrence and the risk of groin node involvement at the time of diagnosis. A retrospective surgical–pathological study of 135 cases found that if a pathological disease-free margin of 8 mm can be achieved, the risk of local recurrence is zero [D].[5] Therefore the primary lesion should be excised with a 1-cm disease-free margin including the deep margin. The 1-cm margin will allow for tissue shrinkage due to fixation of the specimen. In most early cancers this can be achieved by a wide radical local excision and will allow for the preservation of non-involved structures. If the primary lesion is associated with a vulval maturation disorder or VIN, this may be removed as well. However, if the VIN is very widespread, this could necessitate a very large excision requiring myocutaneous flaps. Under these circumstances it may not be considered essential to remove all VIN as part of the primary surgical procedure to remove a carcinoma. Re-excision of the vulval lesion to achieve at least 1 cm of disease-free margin has been the standard of care but recent data have shown a low rate of residual disease but high rate of surgical complications. Careful observation and re-excision of any new disease may be a suitable alternative approach.[6]

Regional lymph nodes
Depth of invasion is the best predictor of risk of nodal metastasis in vulval cancer. The most recent staging criteria for vulval cancer (Table 110.1) have recognised the concept of micro-invasive or superficially invasive vulval cancer (Stage IA), as the risk of nodal involvement in tumours with depth of invasion up to 1 mm is virtually zero [D].[7] These tumours may therefore be treated by wide local excision alone.

Lateral vulval tumours
The management of regional lymph nodes can be modified for patients presenting with lateral vulval tumours. Although there is extensive lymphatic crossover in the midline of the

Table 110.1 Staging of vulval cancer. FIGO classification 2009

Stage I	Tumour confined to the vulva
IA	Lesion ≤2 cm in size, confined to vulva or perineum and with stromal invasion ≤1 mm invasion*, no nodal metastasis
IB	Lesion >2 cm in size or with stromal invasion >1 mm invasion*, confined to vulva or perineum, with negative nodes
Stage II	Tumour of any size with extension to adjacent perineal stuctures (one third lower urethra, one third lower vagina, anus) with negative nodes
Stage III	Tumour of any size with extension to adjacent perineal stuctures (one third lower urethra, one third lower vagina, anus) with positive inguino-femoral lymph nodes
IIIA	(i) With lymph node metastasis (≥5 mm), or (ii) 1-2 lymph node metastases (<5 mm)
IIIB	(i) With 2 or more lymph node metastases (≥5 mm), or (ii) 3 or more lymph node metastases (<5 mm)
IIIC	With positive nodes with extracapsular spread
Stage IV	Tumour invades other regional (two thirds upper urethra, two thirds vagina) or distant structures
IVA	Tumour invades any of the following: (i) upper urethra and/or vaginal mucosa, bladder mucosa, rectal mucosa or fixed to pelvis bone, or (ii) fixed or ulcerated inguino-femoral lymph nodes
IVB	Any distant metastasis including pelvic lymph nodes

* The depth of invasion is defined as the measurement of the tumour from the epithelial–stromal junction of the adjacent most superficial dermal papilla to the deepest point of the invasion.

vulva, lateral tumours (i.e. those with the medial border at least 2 cm lateral to a line drawn between the clitoris and the anus) require only an ipsilateral inguinal node dissection. If the ipsilateral nodes are negative, the contralateral nodes are rarely involved [D].[8] However, should these nodes be positive, a contralateral node dissection should be undertaken. In a prospective trial, the outcome for 26 women who underwent ipsilateral lateral groin node dissection alone was similar when compared with historical controls [C].[9]

Inguinal node dissection

Surgical dissection of inguinal nodes is considered mandatory in early-stage vulval cancer when depth of invasion is greater than 1 mm. A randomised trial comparing inguinal node dissection with radiotherapy to the groin in women with clinically normal inguinal nodes found a survival advantage in favour of the surgical arm; however, this trial has been criticised because an inadequate dose of radiotherapy was given to the inguinal nodes.[10] A subsequent systematic review, of only three eligible studies, suggested that surgery is superior to radiotherapy [A].[11]

Attempts have been made to reduce the morbidity associated with this procedure. Unfortunately, superficial inguinal node dissection, which removes only the lymph nodes above the cribriform fascia, is associated with a higher rate of inguinal recurrence compared with inguino-femoral node dissection, which removes tissue below the cribriform fascia (this is the layer deep to the fascia lata) and medial to the femoral vein. In a prospective clinical trial, 155 women underwent a superficial inguinal node dissection and although the overall survival rate was the same compared with a series of historical controls, the rate of inguinal node recurrence was significantly higher.[9] It is therefore recommended that a full dissection should still be performed in cases of early vulval cancer [C]. The routine removal of pelvic lymph nodes in early stage vulval cancer is not recommended. Recent data have suggested that by sparing the long saphenous vein, the short-term and long-term morbidity associated with lymphoedema may be reduced [D].

Another approach to reduce morbidity is the identification and removal of the sentinel node. The idea depends on the sentinel node (i.e. the first node to drain the vulval tumour) being identified and, if histologically normal, the remainder of the inguinal lymph node dissection could be omitted. The most reliable technique is probably a hybrid of pre-operative intralesional injection of radiolabelled technetium combined with intralesion injection of blue dye at the time of surgery and scanning of the nodal tissue for a radioactive signal. In the collected series to date, the sentinel node – the anatomical location of which is highly variable – has been identified in almost 100 per cent of cases and there have been only a very few cases reported in which the sentinel node was normal but other nodes were positive for tumour [C].[12] In the GROINSS-V study a sentinel node procedure was performed in 623 groins of 403 women with squamous cancer of the vulva. Out of 259 women with unifocal disease and negative sentinel node, six developed groin recurrence (2.3 per cent). Women who had a positive sentinel node and underwent a full groin excision experienced significantly more morbidity. The current study, GROINSS-VII, is evaluating a protocol in which women with negative nodes have no further groin surgery and those with a positive sentinel node are offered radiation therapy without full groin dissection.[13]

Advanced vulval cancer

Women in whom the cancer has spread beyond the vulva will benefit from a multimodality approach to their management. Neoadjuvant chemotherapy and radiotherapy can be used to shrink the tumour and so permit surgery, which may preserve urethral and anal sphincter function. Reconstructive surgery can potentially reduce physical morbidity by filling large tissue defects and may reduce psychological morbidity as well.

Surgery to the primary lesion

The size and location of the tumour will influence the surgical approach to the primary lesion. The surgical goal is to remove the tumour with at least a 1 cm disease-free margin. In the majority of cases a triple-incision technique can be employed.

Several clinical series have shown that the incidence of skin bridge recurrence between the primary lesion and the inguinal node dissection is low, even if there is evidence of lymphatic channel involvement [D].[14] However, if there is evidence of tumour within the skin bridge between the primary tumour and the inguinal nodes at the time of surgery, a radical vulvectomy with en-bloc inguinal node dissection (butterfly incision) should be considered. If extensive areas of vulval tissue need to be removed, reconstructive surgery with the use of skin grafts or myocutaneous flaps may be essential to achieve healing.

Management of inguinal nodes

In cases in which there is clinical suspicion of inguinal node involvement, an inguinal node dissection should be undertaken. As stated above, if there is concern about lymphatic permeation, an en-bloc dissection should be considered. In cases in which the nodes are fixed or ulcerated, biopsy of these or fine-needle aspiration should be considered, followed by radiotherapy to the inguinal and pelvic lymph nodes. Surgical removal of large inguinal or pelvic nodes should be attempted if feasible, since standard radiotherapy doses to the inguinal nodes may be inadequate to bring about a complete regression.

KEY POINTS

Surgical management of vulval cancer

- Vulval cancer should be managed in cancer centres.
- Vulval tumours should be excised with a minimum margin of 10 mm of normal epithelium.
- This will vary from a wide local excision to radical vulvectomy, depending on the size of the tumour and the nature of adjacent epithelium.
- Lymphadenectomy is required for all but superficially invasive squamous tumours.
- Routine lymphadenectomy is not required for basal-cell and verrucous carcinomas and melanomas.
- Lateral tumours initially require only ipsilateral lymphadenectomy.
- Formal inguino-femoral lymphadenectomy remains the procedure of choice.
- A triple-incision technique will suffice unless there is evidence of skin bridge involvement at the outset, when an en-bloc approach should be used.
- Pelvic lymphadenectomy is not routinely used in the treatment of vulval cancer.
- Advanced disease requires a multimodality approach.

The management of other vulval cancers

Basal-cell carcinomas and verrucous carcinomas of the vulva are usually only superficially invasive to a depth of 1 mm and are rarely associated with lymph node metastases.

These tumours can be adequately managed by means of a wide local excision. Basal-cell carcinomas can be treated with radiotherapy if surgery would compromise the sphincter function, but this is rarely necessary.

Melanomas of the vulva should be managed by wide local excision. Inguinal node dissection does not influence outcome in these cases, and management should be determined as for the criteria for other sites of cutaneous melanoma. Close liaison with the melanoma MDT is recommended.

Cancer can develop within the Bartholin's gland and may be either squamous or adenocarcinoma. Its management is the same as for squamous vulval cancer.

Neoadjuvant therapy

Radiotherapy may be given pre-operatively to the primary lesion to allow for tumour shrinkage. This is particularly useful if primary surgery would necessitate removal of the urethral or anal sphincters. A total maximum dose of 55 Gy may be given with concurrent 5-fluorouracil (5-FU). Subsequent tumour shrinkage may then enable the preservation of sphincters.

Radical chemoradiotherapy with curative intent

Radical radiotherapy with chemotherapy may be used as an alternative to surgery in the management of advanced squamous vulval carcinomas. There are no published data comparing surgery with chemoradiotherapy in the primary treatment of vulval cancer. Radical radiotherapy alone in the UK has usually been confined to patients who decline surgery or in whom medical morbidity prevents surgery. The recommended dose of radiotherapy is 65 Gy with concurrent 5-FU and cisplatin. In a study of 14 women who were not candidates for standard surgery (nine stage III and five stage IV), nine (64 per cent) had a complete response to radiation (50–65 Gy) in combination with cisplatin (50 mg/m^2) and 5-FU (100 mg/m^2 per 24 to 96 hours).[15]

Adjuvant radiotherapy

Surgical margins

Post-operative radiotherapy should be considered in patients with close or positive surgical margins. There is no minimum disease-free margin at which radiotherapy should be considered. However, patients with <4.8 mm of disease-free margin have a 57 per cent chance of disease recurrence.[5] Where possible, consideration should be given to re-excision of the vulva to improve the disease-free margin rather than radiotherapy [E].

Inguinal nodes

Post-operative radiotherapy should be considered in patients who have nodal involvement with metastatic disease. Several case series have found that prognosis is only affected when two or more nodes are involved [D]. The presence of extracapsular spread in any lymph node is an adverse factor and warrants adjuvant treatment [D]. Adjuvant radiotherapy should be confined to the affected side and should include pelvic nodes as well. In a randomised trial comparing adjuvant pelvic radiotherapy with pelvic lymphadenectomy, in 114 women with positive inguinal nodes, there was a significant survival advantage (68 per cent vs 54 per cent at 2 years) in favour of radiotherapy [B].[16] A total dose of radiotherapy between 45 and 50 Gy without 5-FU is recommended.

KEY POINTS

Non-surgical management of vulval cancer

- Vulval tumours can be treated by primary radical radiotherapy if surgery is declined or not possible.
- Adjuvant radiotherapy is recommended when surgical margins are inadequate (<8 mm) if re-excision might compromise function.
- Radiotherapy to the groin and pelvic node sites is recommended if more than one node is involved or there is evidence of any extracapsular spread.
- Radiotherapy may be used prior to surgery to attempt to reduce the morbidity and functional loss associated with surgery in large lesions.
- Radiotherapy with concurrent chemotherapy may improve outcome, but as yet there are no data in support of this approach.

Treatment-related morbidity

A more conservative approach to the management of vulval cancer and individualisation of care have led to a reduction in treatment-related morbidity. However, there still remains a significant rate of wound infection and wound breakdown. Lymphoedema of the legs is a major cause of long-term morbidity and there are also high levels of psychological and psychosexual morbidity associated with the disfiguring nature of the surgery employed.

Morbidity associated with recurrent disease

Recurrent disease affecting the vulva itself should be managed by further surgical excision and, if necessary, radiotherapy. Recurrence involving the inguinal nodes or pelvic nodes should be treated with radiotherapy. However, this can usually only be palliative, and most patients with groin recurrence die of the disease.

Follow-up of treated patients

Patients should be followed up on a 3-monthly basis for the first 2 years following treatment, as this allows for the detection of early recurrence and the management of treatment-related morbidity. Once they have completed 2 years of follow-up, they may be seen 6-monthly for the following 3 years.

VAGINAL CANCER

Vaginal cancers are rare gynaecological tumours accounting for only 1–2 per cent of all gynaecological cancers. The majority of vaginal cancers are squamous in origin (about 85 per cent), but adenocarcinoma can also develop in young women between the ages of 17 and 21 and is associated with a higher incidence of metastatic disease to the lymph nodes and lungs. Melanomas and sarcomas are rare causes of vaginal cancer. Clear-cell adenocarcinomas of the vagina are linked to women with a history of in-utero exposure to diethylstilboestrol (DES). An increased incidence of this tumour was first reported in the mid-1970s, but there has been a steady decline in its incidence over recent years with the withdrawal of DES from clinical practice.

Aetiology

Little is known about the aetiology of vaginal cancer, but it is presumed to share similarities with vulval and cervical cancer. Vaginal intraepthelial neoplasia (VAIN) grade 3 is a recognised pre-cancerous condition affecting the vagina and it is frequently seen in combination with cervical intraepithelial neoplasia (CIN). It may occur in one of two ways: as a lateral extension of the CIN out onto the vaginal fornices at the time of treatment for CIN, or in women who have previously undergone hysterectomy for CIN, which was incompletely excised by this procedure. In these latter cases, the VAIN is often found within the surgical margin of the vaginal vault. The percentage of women who present with this condition and who subsequently develop vaginal cancer is unknown, but there is a significant risk of invasive disease. Factors that influence the outcome of vaginal cancer are the size of the tumour and the age of the patient.

Diagnosis

The diagnosis of vaginal cancer may be suspected at the time of colposcopic examination of the vagina. An adequate biopsy, which includes the entire thickness of vaginal epithelium, should be obtained for histological confirmation. This is important, as the depth of invasion of the tumour into the vaginal mucosa and muscle is significant in the staging of the disease (Table 110.2). A diagnosis of cancer of the vagina can only be made with certainty in the presence of a normal cervix or following hysterectomy, as described above.

Investigations

The cervix should be carefully examined if still *in situ* to exclude cervical involvement. An MRI of the pelvis will help to determine the extent of any spread from the vagina and also the status of the regional pelvic nodes.

Table 110.2 Staging of vaginal cancer. FIGO classification 2006

I	Tumour confined to vagina
II	Tumour invades paravaginal tissues but not to pelvic sidewall
III	Tumour extends to pelvic sidewall
IVA	Tumour invades mucosa of bladder or rectum and/or extends beyond the true pelvis
IVB	All cases with distant metastases

Treatment

In planning definitive treatment, consideration should be given not only to the stage of disease at presentation, but also to the size and location of the tumour. Surgery in combination with pelvic radiotherapy, when appropriate, can be effective in the management of stage I and II disease, with survival rates of 68 per cent and 48 per cent respectively [D].[17]

Stage I vaginal cancer

Tumours <0.5 cm deep

Early vaginal cancer may be managed either by surgery or by intracavity radiotherapy. Surgery should include wide local excision or total vaginectomy with reconstruction of the vagina where possible. Intracavity treatment with 60–70 Gy to the tumour should be given and in cases where the tumour lies within the lower third of the vagina, external-beam radiotherapy to the pelvic and inguinal lymph nodes should be considered.

Tumours >0.5 cm deep

Surgery for this condition should include wide vaginectomy, pelvic lymphadenectomy and reconstruction of the vagina where possible. For lesions in the lower third of the vagina, inguinal lymphadenectomy should be performed as well. Radiotherapy for this condition should be a combination of brachytherapy to the tumour and external-beam radiotherapy to the pelvic and inguinal nodes if the tumour is present in the lower third of the vagina.

Although surgery or radiotherapy can be used in the primary management of stage I disease, the usual practice in the UK has been to offer radiotherapy, which has the advantage of vaginal preservation.

Stage II vaginal cancer

Radical surgery can be considered for this condition and should include radical vaginectomy with lymph node dissection or possibly pelvic exenteration. Radiotherapy may also be used, with a combination of brachytherapy to the tumour and external-beam radiotherapy to the pelvic and inguinal lymph nodes.

Stage III and IV vaginal cancer

These cases should be managed by a combination of brachytherapy to the primary tumour and external-beam radiotherapy to the pelvis and inguinal lymph nodes.

Morbidity

Treatment-related morbidity can be significant. Sexual dysfunction due to vaginal atrophy and damage to the bladder and rectum are not infrequent. Recurrent vaginal cancer can be treated with radical pelvic radiotherapy if recurring after surgery. If disease recurs after radiotherapy, palliative surgery may be possible in selected cases.

Follow-up

Patients should be followed up on a 3-monthly basis for the first 2 years following treatment, as this allows for the detection of early recurrence and the management of treatment-related morbidity. Once they have completed 2 years of follow-up, they may be seen 6-monthly for the following 3 years.

KEY POINTS

Vaginal cancer
- There is limited published evidence concerning the treatment of vaginal cancers.
- Case series support the use of surgery in selected cases, with cure rates similar to those of primary radiotherapy in early-stage disease.
- A combination of brachytherapy and external beam radiation has the advantage of vaginal preservation.

SUMMARY

Vulval and vaginal cancers are rare and affect an older age range. Individualisation of care has led to a reduction in morbidity without affecting cure rates. Multimodality treatment is often required in advanced cases. All vulval and vaginal cancers should be managed at a cancer centre.

Published Guidelines

RCOG. *Management of Vulval Cancer*. London: RCOG, 2006.

Key References

1. Rhodes CA, Cummins C, Shafi MI. The management of squamous cell vulval cancer: a population based retrospective study of 411 cases. *BJOG* 1998; 105:200–5.
2. Herod JJ, Shafi MI, Rollason TP, Jordan JA, Luesley DM. Vulvar intraepithelial neoplasia: long-term follow-up of treated and untreated women. *BJOG* 1996;103:446–52.
3. Jones RW, Baranyai J, Stables S. Trends in squamous cell carcinoma of the vulva: the influence of vulvar intraepithelial neoplasia. *Obstet Gynecol* 1997;90:448–52.
4. Eva LJ, Ganesan R, Chan KK, Honest H, Luesley DM. Differentiated-type vulval intraepithelial neoplasia has

GYNAECOLOGICAL ONCOLOGY

a high-risk association with vulval squamous cell carcinoma. *Int J Gynecol Cancer* 2009;19:741–4.

5. Heaps JM, Yao SF, Montz FJ, Hacker NF, Berek JS. Surgical–pathological variables predictive of local recurrence in squamous cell carcinoma of the vulva. *Gynecol Oncol* 1990;38:309–14.

6. Ioffe YJ, Erickson BK, Foster KE *et al.* Low yield of residual vulvar carcinoma and dysplasia upon re-excision for close or positive margins. *Gynecol Oncol* 2013;129:528–32.

7. Sedlis A, Homesley H, Bundy BN *et al.* Positive groin lymph nodes in superficial squamous cell vulvar cancer: a Gynecologic Oncology Group study. *Am J Obstet Gynecol* 1987;156:1159–64.

8. Homesley HD, Bundy BN, Sedlis A *et al.* Assessment of current International Federation of Gynecology and Obstetrics staging of vulvar carcinoma relative to prognostic factors for survival (a Gynecologic Oncology Group study). *Am J Obstet Gynecol* 1991;164:997–1004.

9. Stehman FB, Bundy BN, Dvoretsky PM *et al.* Early stage I carcinoma of the vulva treated with ipsilateral superficial inguinal lymphadenectomy and modified radical hemivulvectomy: a prospective study of the Gynecologic Oncology Group. *Obstet Gynecol* 1992;79:490–7.

10. Stehman FB, Bundy BN, Thomas G. Groin dissection versus groin radiation in carcinoma of the vulva: a Gynecologic Oncology Group study. *Int J Rad Oncol Biol Phys* 1992;24:389–96.

11. van der Velden J, Ansink A. Primary groin irradiation vs primary surgery for early vulvar cancer (Cochrane Review). *In: The Cochrane Library*, Issue 3. Oxford: Update Software, 2001.

12. Ayhan A, Celik H, Dursun P. Lymphatic mapping and sentinel node biopsy in gynaecological cancers: a critical review of the literature. *W J Surgical Oncol* 2008;6:53–65.

13. Van der Zee AGJ, Oonk MW, De Hulla JA *et al.* Sentinel node dissection is safe in the treatment of early-stage vulval cancer. *J Clin Oncol* 2008;26:884-9.

14. Hacker NF, Leuchter RS, Berek JS, Castaldo TW, Lagasse LD. Radical vulvectomy and bilateral inguinal lymphadenectomy through separate groin incisions. *Obstet Gynecol* 1981;58:574–9.

15. Cunningham MJ, Goyer RP, Gibbons SK, Kredentser DC, Malfetano JH, Keys H. Primary radiation, cisplatin, and 5-fluorouracil for advanced aquamous carcinoma of the vulva. *Gynecol Oncol* 1997;66:258–61.

16. Homesley HD, Bundy BN, Sedlis A, Adcock L. Radiation therapy versus pelvic node resection for carcinoma of the vulva with positive groin nodes. *Obstet Gynecol* 1986;68:733–9.

17. Tjalma WAA, Monaghan JM, Lopes AB, Naik R, Nordin AJ, Weyler JJ. The role of surgery in invasive squamous carcinoma of the vagina. *Gynecol Oncol* 2001;81:360–5.

Chapter 111 Gestational trophoblastic disease

Fieke E M Froeling and Michael J Seckl

MRCOG standards

Theoretical skills

- Understand the pathogenesis.
- Have good knowledge of gynaecological diagnosis and management.
- Have an appreciation of the needs for monitoring and/or medical intervention.

Practical skills

- Be able to counsel a woman with gestational trophoblastic disease.
- Be able to recognise the clinical features of gestational trophoblastic disease.
- Be able to perform evacuation of molar pregnancy under supervision.

INTRODUCTION

Gestational trophoblastic disease (GTD) is an uncommon complication of pregnancy. An average consultant obstetrician may deal with only one new case every second year. The term gestational trophoblastic disease describes a group of inter-related diseases, including the pre-malignant disorders of partial and complete hydatidiform mole (PHM and CHM) and the malignant diseases of invasive mole, choriocarcinoma and the rare placental site trophoblastic tumour/epithelioid trophoblastic tumour (PSTT/ETT). The malignant diseases are also collectively named gestational trophoblastic neoplasia (GTN). Although persistent GTD most commonly follows a molar pregnancy, it can be seen after any type of gestation, including term pregnancy, abortion and ectopic pregnancy. Gestational trophoblastic tumours produce hCG which is important in the diagnosis, management and follow-up of these patients, providing an example of an 'ideal' tumour marker. The first complete responses to methotrexate chemotherapy were described in the 1950s, and presently almost 100 per cent of patients are cured.

EPIDEMIOLOGY

The incidence and aetiological factors of GTD have been difficult to assess. As GTD follows all kinds of pregnancies, the denominator for the incidence should ideally include all livebirths, stillbirths, abortions and ectopic pregnancies. The accepted convention, however, has been to report incidence data according to the livebirth rate. Furthermore, reports from different countries often use different denominators, and figures for hospital-based populations are likely to overestimate the incidence compared with community-based figures, particularly in developing countries. Under-reporting may also occur, especially, but not uniquely, in communities where medical attention is suboptimal.

In the UK, all patients are nationally registered with central pathology review and the incidence is estimated at 3 per 1000 pregnancies for PHM and 1–3 per 1000 pregnancies for CHM. The incidence is approximately twice as high in some Asian countries and also in native Americans, which can be a reflection of discrepancies between hospital- and population-based data, availability of central pathology review or true differences because of dietary and genetic influences.[1] Maternal age appears to be the most consistent risk factor associated with molar gestation. Age-specific incidence reports usually reveal a 'J curve', with extremes of reproductive life associated with an increased incidence. Pregnancies below the age of 15 years have a moderately increased risk, whereas those occurring over the age of 50 years are associated with a substantially increased risk. This increased incidence in the youngest and oldest age groups seems to be a consistent finding in all regions and races. Women who have had a previous mole have an increased risk of further molar pregnancies. Following one mole, the risk of a further complete or partial mole is 1–2 per cent. After two molar pregnancies the risk of a third mole increases substantially to 15–20 per cent and is not decreased by changing partner. Occasionally, family clusters have been seen, implicating an underlying genetic disorder in such cases. Nutritional factors also appear to be risk factors for molar pregnancy in some populations, with a low dietary intake of carotene and animal fat reported to be associated with an increased incidence of CHM.[1]

The incidence of choriocarcinoma and PSTT is less clear. Following a term delivery, choriocarcinoma develops in approximately 1 in 50,000 women. However, CHM precedes choriocarcinoma in 29–83 per cent of cases and therefore the overall incidence of choriocarcinoma is probably much higher. Rarely, PHMs can give rise to choriocarcinoma or PSTT. PSTT is the rarest form of GTD, representing 0.2 per cent of all registered cases of GTD in the UK.[2]

PATHOLOGY AND GENETICS

All forms of GTD arise from components of the placenta, either the villous trophoblast (hydatidiform moles and choriocarcinoma) or the interstitial trophoblast (PSTT). Most complete and partial moles have distinct morphological characteristics (Table 111.1) but suspected cases should be reviewed by specialist histopathologists. Complete hydatidiform moles are usually diploid and androgenic in origin, the most common type being 46XX from duplication of the haploid genome of a single sperm (~ 80%). In approximately 20 per cent, a molar pregnancy develops from dispermic fertilisation. In either scenario, the maternal chromosomes are lost before or after fertilisation (Fig. 111.1A, B). Some patients with recurrent CHM can have a biparental karyotype due to familial recurrent hydatidiform mole (FRHM), an autosomal recessive disease (Fig. 111.1C). Mutations in two genes, *NLRP7* and, more rarely, *KHDC3L*, have been associated with this condition.[3] PHMs are generally triploid, most often from dispermic fertilisation of normal ova (Fig. 111.1D). When a fetus is present it often has the features of triploidy, including growth retardation and multiple congenital malformations, and is never viable.

In current-day practice, the earlier evacuation of suspected molar pregnancies has meant that there is more likelihood of misdiagnosis by the pathologists as classical features may be less well developed. Complete moles are now often characterised by subtle morphological abnormalities that may result in their misclassification as partial moles or non-molar abortions, especially when associated with chromosomal abnormalities. Abortions due to trisomy, monosomy, maternally derived triploidy and translocations often develop some degree of hydropic change which can cause diagnostic confusion with molar pregnancies. CHM can be excluded with the help of additional techniques such as immunostaining with p57^{KIP2}, an imprinted marker expressed only by the maternal genome and therefore negative in CHM but positive in non-molar pregnancies or PHM. Ploidy analysis by in-situ hybridisation or flow cytometry (triploid in PHM) or molecular genotyping can help to distinguish PHM from CHM and non-molar hydropic abortions.[4] The clinical entity of invasive mole occurs when a complete or, less commonly, a partial mole invades deeply into the myometrium. Unfortunately, there are no pathological or molecular features that reliably predict which patients will develop persistent GTD (malignant change in a CHM or PHM) and therefore all patients with an evacuated molar pregnancy will need surveillance with hCG.

Gestational choriocarcinoma is the malignant form of GTD and may originate from a previous hydatidiform mole

Table 111.1 Pathological features of complete and partial hydatidiform mole

		CHM	PHM
Macroscopic		Characteristic grape-like structures	Can resemble an hydropic abortion with avascular and oedematous villi*
			May have recognisable fetal tissues
Microscopic		Diffusely hydropic villi	Patchy villous hydropic change
		Diffuse trophoblast hyperplasia	Patchy trophoblast hyperplasia
		Stromal hypercellularity	Scattered, abnormally formed villi with trophoblastic pseudo-inclusions
		Stromal karyorrhectic debris	
		Collapsed villous blood vessels	
		Usually appropriately diagnosed from uterine products	Often misdiagnosed as hydropic abortion or CHM
Karyotype		46XX (androgenic monospermic, majority)	69XXY
		46XY (androgenic dispermic, around 20%)	
		46XX (biparental, rare cases of familial recurrent HM, <1%)	

*Usually spontaneous abortion, in which the embryo either never developed or ceased development very early in gestation. Macroscopically, the hydrophobic changes can resemble molar pregnancies, in particular PHM

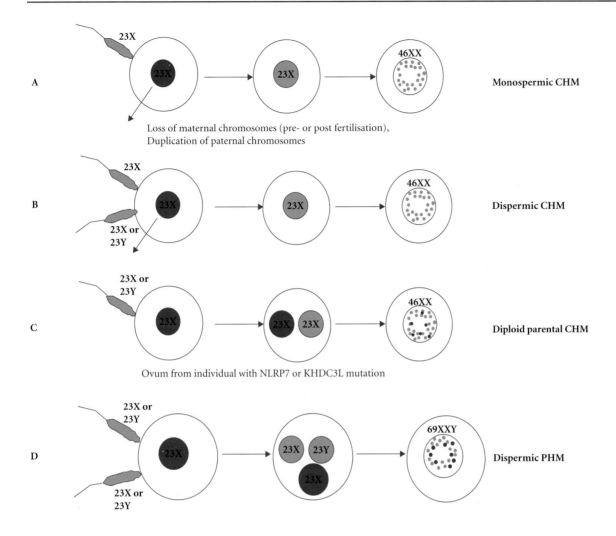

Fig. 111.1 The origins of molar pregnancies

or from a normal conception. The definitive histopathological diagnosis of choriocarcinoma requires the demonstration of a dimorphic population of both cytotrophoblast and syncytiotrophoblast without the presence of formed chorionic villi, plus evidence of myometrial invasion. However, because of the availability of a sensitive tumour marker, the majority of patients are treated without the benefit of a histological diagnosis. Gestational choriocarcinoma metastasises widely, particularly to the lungs, pelvic organs and brain.

PSTT and the newly recognised variant ETT may develop after any type of pregnancy and originate from intermediate trophoblastic tissue. They produce less hCG, grow more slowly, infiltrating and pushing apart the myometrial cells, and metastasise later in their disease course with a slightly increased propensity for involving the lymphatics.[1] After the placenta is lost from the uterus, small nodules of placental tissue can remain in the myometrium. These usually resorb over time but in some, they persist as placental site nodules (PSNs). We have recently realised that these may develop

atypical features (atypical placental site nodules: APSNs) that include increased mitoses and can progress to PSTT/ETT.[5]

CLINICAL FEATURES

The majority of patients with PHM or CHM are diagnosed prior to 16 weeks of gestation and most patients present with vaginal bleeding in the first trimester. The clinical presentation of CHM has changed considerably over the past few decades. Excessive uterine size, anaemia, hyperemesis, pre-eclampsia, theca lutein cysts, hyperthyroidism and metastatic disease are seen far less often, except in countries with less well-developed healthcare systems. Invasive mole can produce heavy bleeding, lower abdominal pain or intraperitoneal haemorrhage. Occasionally, the bladder or rectum is infiltrated, producing haematuria or rectal bleeding. Invasive moles may regress spontaneously or they may embolise, particularly to the lungs, but they do not usually exhibit the progression of true malignancy.

The clinical features of a PHM are usually less severe than those of a CHM and this condition is frequently diagnosed on histological review of curettings from what appeared clinically to be a miscarriage. Even in earlier studies, increased uterine size, theca lutein cysts and pre-eclampsia were seen in only a small percentage of cases.[6,7]

DIAGNOSTIC INVESTIGATIONS

The classic 'snowstorm' sonographic pattern of CHM seen in the second trimester, with associated theca lutein ovarian cysts, is rarely seen due to earlier presentation with bleeding. Ultrasound in the first trimester will show no clear evidence of a normal pregnancy and so prompt early evacuation. The sonographic features are not diagnostic of CHM or PHM and histological analysis by a specialist histopathologist is essential in making the correct diagnosis.[8] In locally invasive moles, increased areas of echogenicity are seen within the myometrium.

Trophoblastic disease is virtually unique in that it produces a specific marker in the form of hCG, which can be measured in urine and/or blood and correlates precisely with the amount of disease present. This is a large placental glycoprotein composed of two peptide subunits and is produced naturally during pregnancy. The alpha subunit is similar to those of other pituitary glycoprotein hormones, but the beta subunit is specific to hCG alone. Higher than normal levels of hCG (particularly when >200,000 IU/L) are suggestive of molar pregnancy but, in particular, in PHM the levels are only infrequently above the range for a normal pregnancy. As a diagnostic marker for molar pregnancy, hCG measurement is therefore of limited value.

Assays to detect hCG use antibodies that detect the beta subunit. However, beta hCG can exist in a number of forms/fragments including nicked hCG, beta-core, C-terminal segment, hyperglycosylated hCG and free beta subunit. When it is measured in trophoblastic disease it is therefore important that the assay being used detects all main forms of hCG.[1]

EVACUATION OF MOLAR PREGNANCY

Suction curettage is the method of choice for evacuation of molar pregnancies and because of the lack of fetal parts in CHM, a suction catheter of up to 12 mm is usually sufficient. Sharp curettage is now not generally recommended because of the possibility of uterine perforation and of increasing the risk of Asherman's syndrome (uterine synechiae). Ultrasound during the procedure can help to guide the procedure and ensure complete uterine evacuation. Following suction curettage of a PHM, patients should have anti-RhD prophylaxis.

Medical termination should be avoided where possible. There is a theoretical concern about the routine use of potent oxytocic agents because of the possibility of forcing trophoblastic tissue into the venous spaces of the placental bed and disseminating disease to the lungs. It is recommended that, when necessary, ergometrine which produces sustained rather than rhythmic contractions is only commenced once evacuation is complete. Ergometrine is preferred to syntocinon due to its persistent uterotonic effect. If there is significant haemorrhage prior to or during evacuation and some degree of control is needed, such agents may be used according to clinical judgement. It is also suggested that prostaglandin analogues should be reserved for cases for which oxytocic therapy is ineffective. Since evacuation of a large mole is a rare event, advice and help from an experienced colleague should be sought where appropriate. In partial molar pregnancies where the size of fetal parts deters the use of suction curettage, medical termination can be used. Data from the management of molar pregnancies with mifepristone are incomplete; evacuation of complete mole with this agent may be best avoided, as it increases the sensitivity of the uterus to prostaglandins.

The difficulty in making the diagnosis before evacuation mandates the histological assessment of material obtained from incomplete miscarriages. Also, since persistent trophoblastic disease may develop after any pregnancy, all products of conception obtained after evacuation performed for persisting symptoms should be histologically examined.[9]

> ### EBM
> Though there is much published on evacuation of molar pregnancy, the above text reflects mainly UK expert opinion and practice [C].

Twin molar pregnancy

Twin pregnancies comprising a normal fetus and a hydatidiform mole are estimated to occur in between 1:20,000 and 1:100,000 pregnancies. A successful pregnancy outcome occurs in around 40 per cent of cases, with no obvious increase in the risk of malignant change.[10] Based on these results, it appears reasonably safe to allow patients with twin pregnancies in which one of the conceptions is a CHM or PHM to continue to term, provided there are no other complications.

Ectopic molar pregnancy

As with normal pregnancy, hydatidiform mole may occur in ectopic sites, most often in the Fallopian tube. Tubal ectopic moles are rare and overdiagnosed, but strict follow-up of confirmed cases is essential, as these are more likely to require chemotherapy for persistent disease [E].[11]

REGISTRATION

In the UK, a trophoblastic registration scheme has been in operation since it was initiated by RCOG in 1973. Three centres – in London (Charing Cross Hospital), Sheffield (Weston Park Hospital) and Dundee (Ninewells Hospital) – coordinate the registration and monitoring of all patients. However, only Charing Cross and Weston Park have the specialist facilities to offer appropriate chemotherapy. Patients with CHM or PHM, twin pregnancy with complete or partial hydatidiform mole, limited macroscopic or microscopic molar change judged to require follow-up, choriocarcinoma, PSTT or APSNs should all be registered. Recently the service has expanded to include patients with APSNs as a small proportion of patients with this pathological abnormality may go on to develop PSTT/ETT.

Persistent trophoblastic disease (gestational trophoblastic neoplasia)

After any molar pregnancy, the onset of malignant change or persistent GTD is nearly always indicated by a persistently elevated hCG or continuing clinical symptoms, particularly vaginal bleeding. In the UK, this occurs after 15 per cent of CHM and 0.5–1 per cent of PHM.[1] Excessive uterine size, markedly elevated hCG levels and prominent theca lutein cysts may predict persistent trophoblastic disease. The UK surveillance scheme involves periodic assays of urine and/or serum hCG being performed for six months or longer, depending on when the hCG level reaches normal. This has ensured that the great majority of patients requiring chemotherapy for persistent disease are recognised early.

We have been able to adopt a conservative approach using stringent criteria for the initiation of chemotherapy (Box 111.1). Based on recent data, which showed that continued observation six months after evacuation was safe and effective, the previous UK and FIGO recommendation to start chemotherapy if the hCG was still elevated but falling six months after evacuation has been omitted (as long as the hCG continues to fall).[5,12]

Box 111.1 Indications for chemotherapy

Indications for chemotherapy

Plateaued or rising hCG levels that are plateaued over three consecutive or rising over two consecutive samples after evacuation

Heavy vaginal bleeding or evidence of gastrointestinal or intraperitoneal haemorrhage

Histological evidence of choriocarcinoma

Evidence of metastases in the brain, liver, gastrointestinal tract or radiological opacities of >2 cm on chest radiograph

Pulmonary, vulval or vaginal metastases unless hCG falling

Serum hCG of ≥20,000 IU/L more than four weeks after evacuation (risk of uterine perforation)

The role of repeat curettage for patients with stage I disease (Table 111.2) in reducing the need for chemotherapy remains controversial. Current data suggest that it should only be considered in patients where the hCG is still <5,000 IU/L and the abnormalities on ultrasound are confined to the uterine cavity. In all other cases the chances of avoiding chemotherapy seem to be very low. Indeed, given that cure rates of almost 100 per cent are obtained with chemotherapy, versus the risks involved with suction curettage, chemotherapy is the treatment of choice.[1]

EBM

The indications for when to use chemotherapy vary internationally. The above guidance relies on retrospective, uncontrolled but substantial data from UK studies [C].

CHOICE OF CHEMOTHERAPY

Once the decision has been made to initiate chemotherapy, the regimen is chosen by assessing the patient's prognostic risk.[13] This involves using a number of factors from the history, examination and investigations to allow the patient to be assigned to a risk group, which in turn facilitates the selection of the least toxic, most effective treatment for that individual (Table 111.3). The most important prognostic variables include the duration of the disease (risk of drug resistance of GTN varies inversely with time), the serum hCG concentration (correlation with viable tumour volume) and the presence of liver and/or brain metastases. Patients will need a Doppler pelvic ultrasound and, as pulmonary metastases are most common, a chest X-ray (CXR). Since possible pulmonary micrometastases do not influence the outcome, CT of the chest is not needed if the CXR is normal. However, if pulmonary lesions are seen, a CT of the body and MRI of the brain are indicated to exclude more widespread disease.

In 2000, an international committee recommended a combined FIGO anatomical staging and prognostic scoring system, which was accepted in 2002. All centres managing GTN should now use this scoring system to allow comparison of data.[13] The majority of patients have a FIGO score of 0–6 and have disease at low risk of becoming resistant to single-agent chemotherapy with methotrexate or actinomycin D; those with a FIGO score greater than 6 are at high risk of drug resistance and should therefore be treated with combination-agent chemotherapy. Several treatment regimens have been developed for both low- and high-risk GTN. The most commonly used first-line treatment for low-risk disease is methotrexate with folinic acid rescue (MTX/FA). For high-risk disease, Charing Cross Hospital developed a treatment regimen consisting of EMA (etoposide, methotrexate, actinomycin D) alternated weekly with CO (cyclophosphamide and vincristine); this has been adopted worldwide and

Table 111.2 FIGO scoring system 2000 for gestational trophoblastic neoplasia (here, with some adaptations)

FIGO 2000 scoring system				
Prognostic factor score	0	1	2	4
Age (years)	<40	≥ 40	-	-
Antecedent pregnancy (AP)	Mole	Abortion	Term	-
Interval (months) from end of AP to chemotherapy	<4	4–6	7–12	>12
Serum hCG (IU/l)	$<10^3$	10^3–10^4	10^4–10^5	$>10^5$
Largest tumour mass	-	3–5 cm	>5 cm	-
Number of metastases	0	1–4	5–8	>8
Site of metastases	Lung	Spleen and kidney	GI tract	Brain and liver
Prior chemotherapy	-	-	Single drug	≥ 2 drugs

The total score is calculated by adding the individual scores for each prognostic factor. Low risk, 0–6; high risk, ≥ 7.

FIGO staging system, to be used for PSTT		
I	Disease confined to the uterus	
II	Disease extending into the pelvis	
III	Disease spread to lungs and/or vagina	
IV	All other metastatic sites including liver, kidney, spleen and brain	

Table 111.3 Treatment regimens for low-risk and high-risk disease

Treatment for low-risk patients	
Methotrexate (MTX)	50 mg intramuscular, repeated every 48 hours for total of 4 doses
Folinic acid	15 mg orally 30 hours after each MTX injection
Cycles repeated every 2 weeks	
Treatment for high-risk patients	
EMA Day 1	
Etoposide	100 mg/m^2 IV over 30 minutes
Actinomycin D	0.5 mg IV bolus
Methotrexate	300 mg/m^2 over 12 hours
EMA Day 2	
Etoposide	100 mg/m^2 IV over 30 minutes
Actinomycin D	0.5 mg IV bolus
Folinic acid	15 mg IV or orally every 12 hours for 4 doses (starting 24 hours after commencing the MTX infusion)
CO Day 8	
Vincristine	1 mg/m^2 IV bolus
Cyclophosphamide	600 mg/m^2 IV over 30 minutes
EMA alternates with CO every week	

is most commonly used within the UK as first-line treatment for high-risk disease (Table 111.3). Overall, the cure rate approaches 100 per cent and both the low- and high-risk treatments have no significant effect on subsequent fertility.[5,14]

POSTPARTUM CHORIOCARCINOMA

This is a very rare and serious complication with a reported UK incidence of 1 in 50,000 livebirths. Most cases present with abnormal vaginal bleeding following delivery, and diagnosis may be delayed, with many patients presenting with metastatic disease. Any woman of child-bearing age with metastatic disease should have her hCG level measured. If this is elevated the patient should be urgently discussed with the national specialist GTD centre as biopsy to confirm the diagnosis may promote life-threatening haemorrhage and may not be necessary. Instead, prompt recognition and early transfer to the specialist national centres is likely to maximise chances of cure with chemotherapy.

THE ROLE OF SURGERY

Older patients with stage I disease who are fit and have completed their family may request a hysterectomy. They should however be advised that although hysterectomy eliminates the complications of local invasion, it does not prevent metastatic disease or the possible need for chemotherapy and that therefore monitoring of hCG concentrations should still be done. As GTD is highly chemosensitive, the need for surgical intervention once the diagnosis has been established is small. At present, there are essentially two indications for hysterectomy, namely to control severe uterine haemorrhage and to eliminate disease that is confined to the uterus and

Box 111.2 Indications for hysterectomy

Indications for hysterectomy in the management of gestational trophoblastic disease

Choice (older patient, localised disease, family complete)

Excessive uterine bleeding (before, during or after treatment) that cannot be controlled by embolisation

Chemoresistant (localised) uterine tumour

Placental site trophoblastic tumour/epitheliod trophoblastic tumour

resistant to chemotherapy (Box 111.2). In order to minimise the risk of causing trophoblastic emboli, the vessels draining the uterus should be ligated at an early stage and the uterine tissues should be handled as gently as possible. Conservative uterine surgery, whereby local excision of a bleeding invasive trophoblastic tumour is performed, may be reasonable in young women, as their disease may then be cured medically, thus preserving their fertility.

A rare problem is that of vaginal bleeding after completion of successful chemotherapy due to a post-molar arterio-venous malformation. Selective embolisation or ligation may preserve fertility, but sometimes hysterectomy is necessary.

Surgery also has an important role, in selected patients, for the removal of chemotherapy-resistant metastases. Thoracotomy – for which the indications are previous multi-agent chemotherapy, a solitary lung lesion confined to one lung and no other sites of active disease – may achieve remission in over two thirds of patients. Stereotactic radiosurgery (and less frequently resection) is now recommended in the UK for the treatment of accessible deposits before starting chemotherapy because of the risk of precipitating haemorrhage.

PSTT/ETT

Surgery provides the cornerstone of management for the rare placental site trophoblastic tumours. These tumours have a slow growth rate and can present many years after term delivery, non-molar miscarriage or complete mole. The usual presentation is with local disease leading to vaginal bleeding or amenorrhoea, but they may also metastasise, particularly to the lung. Surgery alone is the treatment of choice for localised disease; combination chemotherapy is needed for metastatic PSTT. In contrast to choriocarcinoma, once the hCG has normalised residual masses are removed surgically, including the uterus as this can potentially harbour microscopic disease.[2]

ROUTINE FOLLOW-UP

Patterns of clinical and hCG surveillance for further molar problems vary across the world, determined by local factors and also by knowledge of the difference in risk of sequelae between complete and partial moles. The clinical course of partial mole is almost invariably 'benign'. Persistent trophoblastic disease after partial mole is much less common than after complete mole and almost all cases are low risk. However, it has been confirmed that partial mole can transform into choriocarcinoma or PSTT.[15]

All patients with confirmed PHM as well as CHM should undergo hCG follow-up. In the UK, patients who have received chemotherapy for persistent trophoblastic disease will continue with weekly serum hCG for six weeks post-chemotherapy, then in serum and urine two weekly until six months, before switching to just urine assessments monthly with decreasing frequency until eventually they send samples just six monthly. Follow-up is currently for life until there are sufficient data to know when it is safe to stop monitoring. As a few patients have relapsed following subsequent pregnancies years later, an hCG sample is requested six and ten weeks at the end of each new pregnancy.[1] However, the risk of molar problems is greatest in the first 12 months following chemotherapy with an overall relapse rate of about 3 per cent. To enable efficient hCG follow-up, patients are therefore advised to delay a further pregnancy beyond this period. Some patients either ignore this advice or accidentally become pregnant during this time; fortunately, in the vast majority of cases, the outcome is good.[1] Current advice is therefore to avoid early pregnancy but, when it does occur, to allow the pregnancy to continue with careful clinical, ultrasound and hCG monitoring.

CONTRACEPTION

Early studies from Charing Cross Hospital suggested that women who used oral contraceptives before the hCG had normalised after evacuation of a molar pregnancy had a slower rate of hCG decrease and increased risk of developing persistent trophoblastic disease.[16] However, at least two other studies in the US and elsewhere have noted no increased risk with oral contraceptive use. Moreover, a recent study in UK women using more modern low-dose contraceptive pills also failed to show any evidence of increased risk of malignant sequelae after molar pregnancy. Consequently, it seems sensible to allow women to use the oral contraceptive to prevent a further pregnancy following molar evacuation. There is agreement that intrauterine contraceptive devices should be avoided until hCG levels are normal, because of the risk of uterine perforation and bleeding.

AUDITABLE OUTCOMES

These auditable outcomes are recommended by RCOG:

1 The proportion of women with GTD registered with the relevant screening centre;
2 The proportion of women with a histological diagnosis of molar pregnancy who have an ultrasound diagnosis of molar pregnancy prior to uterine evacuation;
3 The proportion of women who undergo medical management for evacuation of products of conception with an ultrasound diagnosis of molar pregnancy.

KEY POINTS

The following RCOG recommendations[9] are based on limited but robust evidence that relies on expert opinion and has the endorsement of respected authorities.
1. Registration of any molar pregnancy is essential.
2. Ultrasound has limited value in detecting partial molar pregnancies.

---

3. In twin pregnancies with a viable fetus and a molar pregnancy, the pregnancy can be allowed to proceed after appropriate counselling.
4. Surgical evacuation of molar pregnancies is advisable.
5. Routine repeat evacuation after the diagnosis of a molar pregnancy is not warranted.
6. The combined oral contraceptive pill and hormone replacement therapy are safe to use after hCG levels have reverted to normal.
7. Women should be advised not to conceive until the hCG level has been normal for six months or follow-up has been completed (whichever is sooner).

Published Guidelines

Seckl MJ, Sebire NJ, Fisher RA *et al.* Gestational trophoblastic disease: ESMO Clinical Practice Guidelines for diagnosis, treatment and follow-up. *Ann Oncol* 2013;24 Suppl 6:vi39–vi50.
RCOG. *The management of gestational trophoblastic disease.* Green-top Guideline No. 38. London: RCOG, 2010.
Hancock BW, Berkowitz R, Seckl M, Cole L. *Gestational Trophoblastic Diseases.* 3rd edn. Sheffield: International Society for the Study of Trophoblastic Disease, 2009. Available from: www.isstd.org

Key References

1. Seckl MJ, Sebire NJ, Berkowitz RS. Gestational trophoblastic disease. *Lancet* 2010;376(9742):717–29.
2. Schmid P, Nagai Y, Agarwal R *et al.* Prognostic markers and long-term outcome of placental-site trophoblastic tumours: a retrospective observational study. *Lancet* 2009;374(9683):48–55.
3. Murdoch S, Djuric U, Mazhar B *et al.* Mutations in NALP7 cause recurrent hydatidiform moles and reproductive wastage in humans. *Nat Genet* 2006;38(3):300–2.
4. Paradinas FJ. The diagnosis and prognosis of molar pregnancy. The experience of the National Referral Centre in London. *Int J Gynaecol Obstet* 1998;60:S57–64.
5. Seckl MJ, Sebire NJ, Fisher RA *et al.* Gestational trophoblastic disease: ESMO Clinical Practice Guidelines for diagnosis, treatment and follow-up. *Ann Oncol* 2013;24 Suppl 6:vi39–vi50.
6. Hou JL, Wan XR, Xiang Y, Qi QW, Yang XY. Changes of clinical features in hydatidiform mole: analysis of 113 cases. *Journal of Reproductive Medicine* 2008;53(8):629–33.
7. Berkowitz RS, Goldstein DP, Bernstein MR. Natural history of partial molar pregnancy. *Obstetrics and Gynecology* 1985;66(5):677–81.
8. Fowler DJ, Lindsay I, Seckl MJ, Sebire NJ. Histomorphometric features of hydatidiform moles in early pregnancy: relationship to detectability by

ultrasound examination. *Ultrasound Obstet Gynecol* 2007;29(1):76–80.

9. RCOG. *The management of gestational trophoblastic disease.* London: RCOG, 2010 [updated February 2010]. Available from: http://www.rcog.org.uk/files/rcog-corp/GT38ManagementGestational0210.pdf.

10. Sebire NJ, Foskett M, Paradinas FJ *et al.* Outcome of twin pregnancies with complete hydatidiform mole and healthy co-twin. *Lancet* 2002;359:2165–6.

11. Hassadia A, Kew FM, Tidy JA, Wells M, Hancock BW. Ectopic gestational trophoblastic disease: a case series review. *Journal of Reproductive Medicine* 2012;57(7–8):297–300.

12. Agarwal R, Teoh S, Short D, Harvey R, Savage PM, Seckl MJ. Chemotherapy and human chorionic gonadotropin concentrations 6 months after uterine evacuation of molar pregnancy: a retrospective cohort study. *Lancet* 2012;379(9811):130–5.

13. FIGO staging for gestational trophoblastic neoplasia 2000. FIGO Oncology Committee. *Int J Gynaecol Obstet* 2002;77(3):285–7.

14. Woolas RP, Bower M, Newlands ES, Seckl MJ, Short D, Holden L. Influence of chemotherapy for gestational trophoblastic disease on subsequent pregnancy outcome. *British Journal of Obstetrics and Gynaecology* 1998;105:1032–5.

15. Seckl MJ, Fisher RA, Salerno GA *et al.* Choriocarcinoma and partial hydatidiform moles. *Lancet* 2000;356:36–9.

16. Stone M, Dent J, Kardana A, Bagshawe KD. Relationship of oral contraceptive to development of trophoblastic tumour after evacuation of hydatidiform mole. *Brit J Obstet Gynaecol* 1976;86:913–6.

Chapter 112 Rare tumours

Nicholas Reed

MRCOG Standards

Theoretical skills

- To understand the epidemiology, aetiology, pathology, clinical characteristics and prognostic features of rare gynaecological cancers.
- To understand the most appropriate way to manage these rare and uncommon tumours.
- Specific mention is made of referral pathways and processes for ensuring that optimal care is offered to patients with these rare tumours.

Practical skills

- To be able to manage in broad terms a rare tumour and know the pathway for referrals to specialist multidisciplinary teams.
- To recognise that in some circumstances, fertility-sparing surgery may be offered.
- To be able to share follow-up care with regional teams.

KEY POINTS

- These are by definition rare cancers and many fall into the category of ultra-rare or orphan tumours. Orphan disease status has been defined as fewer than 500 cases per million population whilst ultra-orphan is described as fewer than 4 cases per million population.
- All of these tumours should be managed by multidisciplinary teams composed of experts who have a recognised interest in the field.
- Consideration should be given to supra-regionalisation of care especially in smaller countries.
- Histopathological review is essential as there is a high rate of reclassification with central review.
- Registries of rare tumours should be set up to help document the true incidence, along with the development of tumour banks.
- Careful consideration should be given to fertility-preserving surgery in younger women where clinically appropriate.
- National and international guidelines are needed to improve quality of care.

DEFINITION, INCIDENCE AND PREVALENCE

This chapter focuses on rare gynaecological cancers which represent an extraordinarily high number of the gynaecological cancers. Over a third of gynaecological cancers fall into the rare or uncommon group, which is the highest for any of the common solid cancers.[1] There are a number of definitions of the term 'rare' but incidences range from around 30 to 100 cases per million population. The latter number, used by NICE, described an incidence up to 7000 cases per annum but this is likely to include many cancers considered to be of 'intermediate commonness'.[2] There is no universally agreed standard definition. Most of these tumours by definition will have an incidence of less than 2000 cases per annum in the UK (less than 50 per million population) so while the incidence of these tumours is by definition low, the relative prevalence may be higher as some of them are slow growing and be associated with late relapses, for example many sex cord and stromal tumours and low-grade uterine sarcomas.

This therefore means that there is obviously less experience and less evidence base on which to support management. In view of their rarity, it is thus necessary to state that there is usually no established standard of care for these tumours but the points below will offer guidance for their management. There are well-established guidelines which include the rarer tumours, specifically by ESMO (European Society of Medical Oncology) which covers non-epithelial cancers,[3] and by the NCCN (National Comprehensive Cancer Network)[4] and in a recently published textbook on rare gynaecological cancers.[5]

However to complicate matters further, the classifications of some of the commoner gynaecological cancers are now being subdivided, for example ovarian epithelial cancers are now subdivided into five types, namely high-grade and low-grade serous, endometrioid, clear cell and mucinous. Whilst high-grade serous account for over 70 per cent, the remaining four types of these would fall within the definition of rare cancers as they account for less than 25 per cent of ovarian

Table 112.1 EOC [epithelial ovarian cancer] histotype and molecular pathway

Ovarian cancer	Pathway
High-grade serous	P53, PI3K, mTOR
Low-grade serous	KRAS
Endometrioid	KRAS, B-catenin, MSI
Mucinous	KRAS (50%), BRAF (20%)
Clear cell	ARID1A (50%) PIK3

epithelial cancers. This is not simply due to histotyping on morphological grounds but takes account of the aetiology and different molecular pathways that are recognised to cause tumour development (see Table 112.1). Furthermore the recognition of the different pathways has led to new therapeutic approaches that target these pathways, commonly known as personalised or stratified medicine. This approach will be applied to many other tumours in the course of the next few years as our knowledge of molecular pathways increases.[6-8] This is excellently reviewed in a recent review paper by Merritt and Cramer, with the only danger being the built-in obsolescence of these kinds of papers due to rapidly evolving technology.

However there are many other uncommon gynaecological cancers including carcinosarcomas, small cell tumours, sex cord and stromal tumours, germ cell tumours and the miscellaneous sarcomas of the genital tract (Table 112.2). The incidence of many of these will be less than 10 per million population, sometimes significantly lower, so they may be considered 'ultra-rare', although some of these tumours have a relatively higher prevalence due to their slow natural pattern of relapse.

A topical debate is whether it is better to classify these tumours by site of origin, by histological type or increasingly by the molecular pathways that are involved and this latter is gradually taking precedence and probably will be important in terms of defining future treatment strategies. For example, are small cell cancers of the ovary and cervix the same? Probably not especially as there are at least two types of small cell ovarian cancer! Translational medicine is emerging as the basis of the new classification systems that unite them. Similarly mucinous tumours may occur in a variety of gynaecological organs but to date there is no common identified pathway, and there is even greater debate as to whether so-called primary ovarian mucinous carcinomas do really arise in the ovary but from the GI tract. Hence the classification systems do to some extent mix and match using organ site morphology and molecular pathways.

The list above is not exhaustive but is meant to illustrate that some rarer variants apply across the board such as mucinous, clear cell and small cell, but others are specific to the organ such as granulosa cell tumours and sex-cord/stromal tumours of the ovary and the smooth muscle and stromal tumours of uterus.

EPIDEMIOLOGY

Because of their relative rarity it is often not possible to comment on the epidemiology. No particular patterns have been established and relatively few of these tumours have as yet been identified to be hereditary. The molecular pathways have often yet to be identified. One example recently established a FOXL2 pathway in adult granulosa cell tumours.[9] The previously referred-to papers also discuss pathways in rarer ovarian cancer subtypes.[6-8]

Table 112.2 Examples of rare and uncommon cancers of gynaecological organs, comparing anatomical site of origin with histological type

Ovary	Cervix	Corpus	Vagina and vulva
Small cell cancers of pulmonary type, SCCOPT	Small cell cancers	Small cell cancers	Small cell cancers
Small cell cancers of hypercalcaemic type, SCCOHT			
Sarcomas	Sarcomas	Carcinosarcomas	Sarcomas
Germ cell tumours		Stromal sarcomas	
Sex cord and stromal tumours			Smooth muscle tumours incl. LMS and STUMP
Low-grade serous		Serous tumours	
Mucinous	Mucinous	Mucinous	
Endometrioid			
Clear cell	Clear cell	Clear cell	
Carcinoid tumours	Adeno-carcinomas	Adenosarcomas	Adenoid-cystic

STUMP, smooth muscle tumour of unknown malignant potential
LMS, leiomyosarcoma

PRESENTATION

Because of the diverse nature of these tumours it is not possible to discuss this in detail. Ovarian rare cancers may present with bloating in the same way as common epithelial cancers, but post-menopausal bleeding may be less likely in the rarer uterine tumours as they do not often develop in the endometrial layer. There may be very varied ways in which these tumours are diagnosed. There are a few more obvious patterns. For example in younger women with ovarian tumours, there should be a greater suspicion of germ cell tumours or sex cord and stromal tumours, whilst the finding of hypercalcaemia or syndrome of inappropriate anti-diuretic hormone (SIADH) secretion may suggest a small cell tumour of the ovary. Post-menopausal bleeding associated with endometrial hyperplasia and a solid adnexal mass may raise suspicion of a functioning sex cord tumour. Menorrhagia in the peri-menopausal women is common, as are fibroids. It remains challenging to identify the occasional patient who has an occult uterine sarcoma and it is hoped that new imaging techniques may help to identify these in the future.

MANAGEMENT

Evidence based medicine

For the vast majority of these tumours, there are no randomised clinical trials pertinent to the management of rare gynaecological cancers. Most of the evidence is based on small phase-2 studies, institutional series reports and case reports. Recently published guidelines from the GCIG have been published at the end of 2014. They are principally based on evidence grades C, D and E. The promotion of clinical trials and studies is to be encouraged and supported through international collaboration.

These patients should be investigated and assessed in the standard manner and staging and histological diagnosis are the key points in the management of these tumours. They should all be presented and discussed at the MDT meeting. Discussion should take place with radiologists to select the most appropriate imaging. This may include ultrasound, CT, MRI and PET-CT. MRI is tending to emerge as the better imaging technique for scanning pelvic masses but CT or PET-CT are more useful in searching for distant metastases. Tumour markers again may be useful depending on the tumour type, and in germ cell tumours they may be diagnostic whilst in sex cord and stromal tumours, they may be valuable in diagnosis and serial monitoring and follow-up. In the younger woman with an ovarian mass, it is necessary to check for elevated AFP and beta-hCG to exclude a germ cell tumour, and in sex cord/stromal tumours beta inhibin and AMH may be useful for diagnosis and serial monitoring; in the post-menopausal woman FSH, LH and oestradiol levels can be measured. These tumour markers also have an important role in follow-up.

When surgery is considered, discussions will take place regarding whether this should be done locally or centrally in the gynaecological oncology centre, and whether surgery is 'radical' or fertility sparing.[10,11] If there are any unusual or suspicious features then it would be a wise counsel to recommend that these patients are referred to the specialist gynaecological oncology team so that appropriate surgical staging can be carried out if clinically indicated. Even in the emergency situation, it should be rare that a decision cannot wait 12–24 hours to discuss with a specialist team especially when fertility-sparing surgery is an option.

For post-menopausal women with ovarian and uterine suspected tumours, the standard of care will usually include total hysterectomy, bilateral salpingo-oophorectomy and consideration of omentectomy and nodal dissection. However, many of these tumours do occur in younger women and this requires careful consideration and discussion of fertility preserving procedures. This may require a two-step procedure. Curative treatment should always be offered to younger women, and particularly for suspected germ cell tumours fertility-sparing surgery should be at the forefront of the mind when planning the procedure as chemotherapy is highly effective and fertility can usually be preserved in spite of additional treatments. This again should be carefully discussed and documented at the MDT which will take into account the tumour markers, imaging and other factors. This will include taking into account the patient's wishes where possible. For some conditions, supra-regional services may be considered; good examples of these include management of trophoblastic cancers, and this could be extended to other rare tumour types.

Post-operative management

Pathology

Specialist pathology review is essential by a histopathologist with a recognised subspeciality interest in gynaecological pathology. These rare tumours are often quite difficult to interpret and the differential diagnosis may be quite wide. Even with specialist immunocytochemistry there may be some degree of uncertainty about the final diagnosis. Within the UK, the British Association for Gynaecological Pathologists and their network may be valuable in arranging cross-referral for second opinions.

If the specimen indicates that this is a tumour associated with secretion of tumour markers then post-operatively this should be checked, but a strong case can be made for storing serum on all younger patients pre-operatively so that analysis of the markers can be taken if the germ cell or sex cord tumour is identified. The GCIG published their rare tumour guidelines in late 2014 in a supplement to the *International Journal of Gynaecological Cancer*.[13,14]

Adjuvant treatments

Full and thorough staging is essential to allow decisions on the need for any adjuvant therapy or surveillance programme. All cases should be discussed at the MDT. For many cases which are stage I, a watch-and-see policy with surveillance may be advised. This will include frequent measurement of tumour markers and scans as determined by appropriate protocols. Again due to the diversity of these tumours it is not possible to cover all of these. However a number of these tumours may be associated with a greater risk of late relapse, sometimes well beyond 10 years, for example sex cord and stromal tumours, uterine STUMPs, low-grade leiomyosarcomas and endometrial stromal sarcomas. Thus these are patients who need longer-term follow-up, beyond the standard five years and arguably lifelong. Locally available protocols should identify how frequently clinical examination and imaging should be done. However because of their risk of late relapse, follow-up beyond the normal five years will be advised for selected rare subtypes.

For more advanced cancers additional treatment will be required. The type of chemotherapy for germ cell tumours is well established and usually involves treatment with the BEP (bleomycin, etoposide, cisplatin) regime or variants of this, usually between two and four cycles depending on the prognostic factors.[3,12] For advanced sex cord and stromal tumours again regimes such as BEP or EP or carboplatin/paclitaxel will tend to be used. Some more slowly growing tumours with strong expression of oestrogen or progestogen receptor positivity may be treated with hormonal therapy. This will include low-grade endometrial stromal sarcomas (LGESS), low-grade leiomyosarcomas (LMS) and some sex cord tumours. At the opposite end of the spectrum are high-grade undifferentiated sarcomas (HGUS) and highly mitotic leiomyosarcomas; they are particularly challenging to treat with few patients surviving beyond 24 months. Although adjuvant chemotherapy often with a doxorubicin- or doxorubicin and ifosfamide-based regime is offered, the prognosis is usually very poor. Several new studies are investigating the use of adjuvant treatments including chemotherapy for LMS (GOG Trial 277) and molecular targeting in HGUS.

For uterine and ovarian carcinosarcomas, adjuvant treatment with carboplatin and paclitaxel is frequently advised and radiotherapy is usually not given unless there is residual disease. The only two randomised trials (GOG 150 and EORTC 55874) failed to show any overall survival benefit for radiation in this group.[15,16] For LMS there is at present no documented evidence to support the use of adjuvant radiation or chemotherapy outwith the clinical trial setting, but the current GOG study (protocol 277) is investigating adjuvant chemotherapy. Ovarian carcinosarcomas tend to be treated like epithelial ovarian cancers although probably carry a worse prognosis.

The small cell cancers of ovary, cervix and uterus are very rare and there is no commonly accepted regime. Schedules such as platinum and etoposide or carboplatin and paclitaxel are commonly used. Much lively debate centres around the role of adjuvant radiotherapy in small cell ovarian cancer. It is probably necessary to use multiple modality therapy in these patients and even then only about one third will be long-term survivors. For the ultra-rare gynaecological cancers, there are usually no guidelines so these must be discussed at MDT.

Arguments can be made for supra-regional specialisation as is seen with gestational trophoblastic tumours (GTTs) and shared-care follow-up with local services.

Follow-up

It is important that all these patients are followed up but there are issues as to how to follow them up, who should follow them up, where they should be followed up and for how long. It is the author's belief that these uncommon and rare tumours should be followed up by the specialist MDTs in the gynaecological cancer centres, whether it be the gynaecological, surgical, clinical or medical oncologist. Access to specialist opinion is the key factor. There should be local champions or enthusiasts who take on the mantle to oversee their care and write the local guidelines which should fit in with best available evidence and any national guidelines. Where there are issues of remoteness of the cancer centre from the patient's home it may be possible to offer some form of shared care. Nevertheless management by an experienced team is important. Patients will generally be seen at intervals of around three to four months in the first and second year and then switch to six-monthly visits thereafter but certain subgroups will be seen more frequently, for example stage I germ cell tumours on surveillance will be seen much more frequently in the first two years with monitoring of tumour markers and imaging as per locally agreed protocols to detect early recurrence which can be salvaged. This differs from epithelial ovarian cancers where intervention due to rising markers does not influence survival, but in some of these rarer cancers, rising markers and imaging may lead to interventions that can improve outcome. Imaging protocols will need to be developed where unexpected malignancy has been identified after surgery, often for uterine sarcomas and some germ cell and sex cord ovarian tumours; immediate post-operative CT scan should be carried out for 'baseline purposes' and again depending on the tumour type it may be necessary to image at six and 12 months and annually or bi-annually for up to five years. HRT is also controversial, especially in tumours that may show high levels of expression of oestrogen and/or progestogen. The cautious approach is to withhold its use but consider using it in carefully selected cases where symptoms affect quality of life and the patient is fully informed of the potential risk.

KEY POINTS

- These tumours are by definition uncommon although some of the larger cancer centres will see relatively more as they often act as referral centres. Because of their complexity they must be managed by MDTs and within the cancer centres it may be desirable for a small number of individuals to take on the responsibility of looking after these tumours so that they can individually develop greater expertise and competence.
- In younger women fertility-sparing surgery should always be considered as an option and discussed before rushing in to

- do a pelvic clearance and careful discussion at the tumour board should always be carried out.
- Setting up of registries and databases is important to record the numbers of patients being treated and this is also useful for access to histological material, serum, biomarkers and material for translational research which will be important in managing these patients in the future.
- National or international guidelines are being introduced to try to harmonise the treatment but this will not always be simple or straightforward. The GCIG is trying to facilitate clinical trials in these rare tumours but again there are huge issues regarding confidentiality and security of international data and tissue transfer and additionally motivation to go through the huge effort of submitting protocols through national ethics committees when only one or two patients may be seen a year. Suitably motivated centres will do this. An argument could be made for having supra-regional centres to deal with some of these rarer tumours within each nation together with a more enlightened approach to dealing with ethical issues for trials in rare conditions.

CONCLUSIONS

Gynaecological cancers include a high proportion of rare and uncommon diseases. These cause major clinical challenges, particularly in younger patients where issues of fertility-sparing surgical approaches must always be considered. Patients must be discussed at multidisciplinary teams. Specialist imaging and histopathology opinions are essential to the basic MDT who will carry out the surgery and adjuvant chemotherapy or radiotherapy. Localised databases are important to learn more about these tumours and, for the future, the identification of molecular pathways is likely to bring about improvements in diagnosis and treatment.

References

1. Gatta G, van der Zwan J, Casali P G *et al*. The RARECARE working group. Rare neuroendocrine tumours: Results of the surveillance of rare cancers in Europe project. *European Journal of Cancer* 2011;47:2493–511.
2. NICE. *Guide to the Methods of Technology Appraisal.* Section 6.2.10. NICE, 2013. http://www.nice.org.uk/media/ D45/1E/GuideToMethodsTechnologyAppraisal2013.pdf.
3. http://www.esmo.org/Guidelines-Practice/Clinical-Practice-Guidelines.
4. http://www.nccn.org/professionals/physician_gls/f_guidelines.asp
5. Reed NS, Siddiqui N, Green JA, Gershenson D, Connor R. *A Guide to Rare and Uncommon Gynaecological Cancers.* Springer Verlag, 2011.
6. Kurman R. Pathogenesis of ovarian cancer. lessons from morphology and molecular biology and their clinical implications. *Int J Gynecol Pathol* 2008;27(2):151–60.
7. Le-Ming S. Special Issue: Genes and Pathways in the Pathogenesis of Ovarian Cancer. *International Journal of Molecular Sciences* 2013.
8. Merrit M, Cramer DA. Molecular pathogenesis of endometrial and ovarian cancer. *Cancer Biomark* 2010;9(0): doi:10.3233/CBM-2011-0167.
9. Rosario R. *et al*. Adult granulosa cell tumours (GCT): Clinico-pathological outcomes including FOXL2 mutational status and expression. *Gynecol Oncol* 2013. http://dx.doi.org/10.1016/j.ygyno.2013.08.031
10. Denschlag D, Reed NS, Rodolakis A. Fertility-sparing approaches in gynecologic cancers: a review of ESGO task force activities. *Curr Oncol Rep* 2012;14(6):535–8.
11. Morice P, Denschlag D, Rodolakis A *et al*. Recommendations of the Fertility Task Force of the European Society of Gynecologic Oncology about the conservative management of ovarian malignant tumors. *Int J Gynecol Cancer* 2011;21(5):951–63.
12. Reed N, Millan D, Verheijen R, Castiglione M. ESMO Guidelines Working Group. Non-epithelial ovarian cancer: ESMO Clinical Practice Guidelines for diagnosis, treatment and follow-up. *Ann Oncol* 2010;21Suppl 5:v31–6.
13. GCIG. http://www.gcig.igcs.org.
14. GCIG. Rare tumour guidelines.*International Journal of Gynaecological Cancer* 2014;24(3) S1–S122.
15. Wolfson AH, Brady MF, Rocereto TF *et al*. A Gynecologic Oncology Group randomized trial of whole abdominal irradiation (WAI) vs. cisplatin-ifosfamide and mesna (CIM) as post surgical therapy in stage I–IV carcinosarcoma (CS) of the uterus. *Gynecol Oncol* 2007;107(2):177–85.
16. Reed N.S, Mangioni C, Malmstrom H *et al*. First results of a randomised trial comparing radiotherapy versus observation postoperatively in patients with uterine sarcomas: an EORTC-GCG study. *Eur J Cancer* 2008;44(6):808–18.

Index

Note: Page numbers ending in "f" refer to figures. Page numbers ending in "t" refer to tables.